F U N D A M E N T A L
Neuroscience
for Basic and Clinical Applications

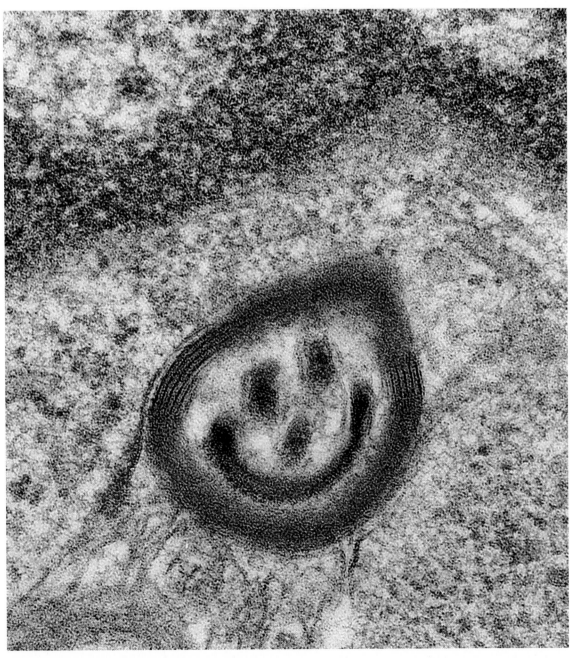

As seen in this unretouched photograph of a small myelinated axon, mitochondria may assume a variety of sizes, shapes, and orientations.

EDITED BY **Duane E. Haines, Ph.D.**

*Professor and Chairman of the Department of Anatomy
and Professor of Neurosurgery and Professor of Neurology
at The University of Mississippi Medical Center,
Jackson, Mississippi*

Contributors

M. D. ARD. Ph.D.
J. R. BLOEDEL, M.D., Ph.D.
N. F. CAPRA, Ph.D.
R. B. CHRONISTER, Ph.D.
J. J. CORBETT, M.D.
J. D. DICKMAN, Ph.D.
T. M. DWYER, M.D.
O. B. EVANS, M.D., Ph.D.
J. D. FRATKIN, M.D.
S. G. P. HARDY, Ph.D.
J. A. LANCON, M.D.
J. C. LYNCH, Ph.D.
T. P. MA, Ph.D.
P. J. MAY, Ph.D.
G. A. MIHAILOFF, Ph.D.
J. P. NAFTEL, Ph.D.
A. D. PARENT, M.D.
F. A. RAILA, M.D.
R. W. ROCKHOLD, Ph.D.
M. E. SANTIAGO, M.D.
K. M. SIMPSON, Ph.D.
A. C. TERRELL, M.S., R.T. (R.) (M.R.)
S. WARREN, Ph.D.
R. P. YEZIERSKI, Ph.D.

Illustrators

M. P. SCHENK, B.S., M.S.M.I, CMI, FAMI; W. K. CUNNINGHAM, B.A., M.S.M.I.; AND M. E. KIRKMAN, B.A., M.S.M.I.

Photographer

G. W. ARMSTRONG, R.B.P.

Computer Graphics

W. A. BUHNER II, B.S.

Typist

L. K. BOYD

FUNDAMENTAL
Neuroscience
for Basic and Clinical Applications

THIRD EDITION

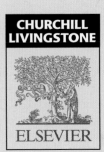

CHURCHILL
LIVINGSTONE

ELSEVIER

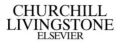

CHURCHILL
LIVINGSTONE
ELSEVIER

1600 John F. Kennedy Blvd.
Ste 1800
Philadelphia, Pa 19130-2899

FUNDAMENTAL NEUROSCIENCE FOR BASIC AND CLINICAL
APPPLICATIONS

ISBN-9780443067518
ISBN-0443067511

Notice

Library of Congress Cataloging-in-Publication Data

Fundamental Neuroscience for Basic and Clinical Applications/edited by Duane E. Haines. — 3rd ed.
   p. ; cm.
      Includes bibliographical references and index.
      ISBN 0-443-06751-1
   1. Neurosciences.
   [DNLM: 1. Nervous System—anatomy & histology. 2. Nervous System Physiology. 3. Neurons.
   WL 101 F981 2006] I. Haines, Duane E.
   QP355.2.F86 2006
   612.8—dc22   2005049667

Previous editions copyrighted 2002 and 1997; Spanish edition 2003.

Acquisitions Editor: Inta Ozols
Developmental Editor: Katie Miller
Publishing Services Manager: Tina Rebane
Project Manager: Mary Anne Folcher
Design Direction: Karen O'Keefe Owens

Printed in China

Last digit is the print number: 9 8 7 6 5 4 3 2 1

Contributors

MARCH D. ARD, PH.D.
Associate Professor, Department of Anatomy, The University of Mississippi Medical Center, Jackson, Mississippi
The Cell Biology of Neurons and Glia; The Ventricles, Chroid Plexus, and Cerebrospinal Fluid

JAMES R. BLOEDEL, M.D., PH.D.
Vice Provost for Research Administration, Departments of Health and Human Performance and Biomedical Sciences, Iowa State University, Ames, Iowa
The Cerebellum

NORMAN F. CAPRA, PH.D.
Associate Professor, Department of Oral and Craniofacial Biological Sciences, The University of Maryland School of Dentistry, Baltimore, Maryland
The Somatosensory System I: Tactile Discrimination and Position Sense; The Somatosensory System II: Touch, Thermal Sense, and Pain

ROBERT B. CHRONISTER, PH.D.
Associate Professor, Department of Anatomy, University of South Alabama College of Medicine, Mobile, Alabama
The Hypothalamus; The Limbic System

JAMES J. CORBETT, M.D.
Chairman and Professor, Department of Neurology, The University of Mississippi Medical Center, Jackson, Mississippi
The Ventricles, Choroid Plexus, and Cerebrospinal Fluid; The Visual System; Visual Motor Systems; The Neurological Examination

J. DAVID DICKMAN, PH.D.
Associate Professor, Department or Anatomy and Neurobiology, Washington University, St. Louis, Missouri
The Vestibular System

TERRY M. DWYER, M.D., PH.D.
Professor, Department of Physiology and Biophysics, The University of Mississippi Medical Center, Jackson, Mississippi
The Electrochemical Basis of Nerve Function

OWEN B. EVANS, M.D.
Chairman and Professor, Department of Pediatrics, The University of Mississippi Medical Center, Jackson, Mississippi
Development of the Nervous System

JONATHAN D. FRATKIN, M.D.
Associate Professor, Department of Pathology, The University of Mississippi Medical Center, Jackson, Mississippi
The Cell Biology of Neurons and Glia

DUANE E. HAINES, PH.D.
Chairman and Professor, Department of Anatomy, The University of Mississippi Medical Center, Jackson, Mississippi
Orientation to Structure and Imaging of the Central Nervous System; The Ventricles, Choroid Plexus, and Cerebrospinal Fluid; The Meninges; A Survey of the Cerebrovascular System; The Spinal Cord; An Overview of the Brainstem; The Medulla Oblongata; The Pons and Cerebellum; The Midbrain; A Synopsis of Cranial Nerves of the Brainstem; The Diencephalon; The Telenecephalon; Motor System I: Peripheral Sensory, Brainstem, and Spinal Influence on Anterior Horn Neurons; Motor System II: Corticofugal Systems and the Control of Movement; The Cerebellum

S. G. PATRICK HARDY, PH.D.
Consultant, Department of Anatomy, The University of Mississippi Medical Center, Jackson, Mississippi
Viscerosensory Pathways; Visceral Motor Pathways; The Hypothalamus; The Limbic System

CRAIG K. HENKEL, PH.D.
Professor, Department of Neurobiology and Anatomy, Bowman Gray School of Medicine of Wake Forest University, Winston-Salem, North Carolina
The Auditory System

JOHN A. LANCON, M.D.
Associate Professor, Department of Neurosurgery, The University of Mississippi Medical Center, Jackson, Mississippi
The Ventricles, Choroid Plexus, and Cerebrospinal Fluid; A Survey of the Cerebrovascular System

JAMES C. LYNCH, PH.D.
Professor, Department of Anatomy, The University of Mississippi Medical Center, Jackson, Mississippi
The Visual System; The Cerebral Cortex

TERENCE P. MA, PH.D.
Associate Professor, Touro University–Nevada, School of Osteopathic Medicine, Henderson, Nevada
The Basal Nuclei

PAUL J. MAY, PH.D.
Professor, Department of Anatomy, The University of Mississippi Medical Center, Jackson, Mississippi
The Midbrain; Visual Motor System

GREGORY A. MIHAILOFF, PH.D.
Professor, Division of Basic Sciences – Anatomy, Arizona College of Osteopathic Medicine, Glendale, Arizona
The Spinal Cord; An Overview of the Brainstem; The Medulla Oblongata; The Pons and Cerebellum; The Midbrain; A Synopsis of Cranial Nerves of the Brainstem; The Diencephalon; The Telencephalon; Motor System I: Peripheral Sensory, Brainstem, and Spinal Influence on Anterior Horn Neurons; Motor System II: Corticofugal Systems and the Control of Movement; The Cerebellum

JOHN P. NAFTEL, PH.D.

Professor, Department of Anatomy, The University of Mississippi Medical Center, Jackson, Mississippi
The Cell Biology of Neurons and Glia; Viscerosensory Pathways; Visceral Motor Pathways

ANDREW D. PARENT, M.D.

Chairman and Professor, Department of Neurosurgery, The University of Mississippi Medical Center, Jackson, Mississippi
The Hypothalamus

FRANK A. RAILA, M.D.

Professor Emeritus, Department of Radiology, The University of Mississippi Medical Center, Jackson, Mississippi
Orientation to Structure and Imaging of the Central Nervous System

ROBIN W. ROCKHOLD, PH.D.

Professor, Department of Pharmacology and Toxicology, The University of Mississippi Medical Center, Jackson, Mississippi
The Chemical Basis for Neuronal Communication

MARIA E. SANTIAGO, M.D.

Department of Neurology, G V Sonny Montgomery VA Medical Center, Jackson, Mississippi
The Neurological Examination

KIMBERLY L. SIMPSON, PH.D.

Assistant Professor, Department of Anatomy, The University of Mississippi Medical Center, Jackson, Mississippi
Olfaction and Taste

ALLEN C. TERRELL, M.S., R.T. (R) (MR)

Director, Imaging Services, Riverpark Imaging Center, Vidalia, Lousiana
Orientation to Structure and Imaging of the Central Nervous System

SUSAN WARREN, PH.D.

Associate Professor, Department of Anatomy, The University of Mississippi Medical Center, Jackson, Mississippi
The Somatosensory System I: Tactile Discrimination and Position Sense; The Somatosensory System II: Touch, Thermal Sense, and Pain

ROBERT P. YEZIERSKI, PH.D.

Director, Center for Pain Research, University of Florida, College of Dentistry, Gainesville, Florida
The Spinal Cord; Somatosensory System I: Tactile Discrimination and Position Sense; The Somatosensory System II: Touch, Thermal Sense, and Pain

Preface

The title of the Third Edition of this book has been changed to *Fundamental Neuroscience for Basic and Clinical Applications.* This recognizes two important points that most educators have at the forefront of their thinking. First, the methods used to teach neuroscience have evolved in recent years. Rather than teach anatomy or connections within the nervous system for their own intrinsic value, the trend now is to truly integrate basic science and clinical information. In many situations, the clinical case acts as a springboard to introduce or understand basic science concepts. Clinical information helps to build an understanding of basic neuroscience. Second, accrediting and licensing bodies that govern the various branches of medicine, dentistry, and allied health, as broadly defined, have given clear hints that the integration of basic science and clinical information is a highly desirable educational goal.

The modification of the title of this book not only recognizes these points, but, more importantly, reflects the significant changes and additions (both great and small) that have been made in this new edition of *Fundamentals of Neuroscience.* The main goal has been to introduce additional relevant clinical information, to integrate clinical and basic science information in a more effective manner, and to introduce new anatomical information *only* if it enhances the understanding of clinical concepts. The emphasis is clearly shifted to an even more clinically oriented approach.

While it is not possible to describe each individual change and addition, some of the more significant and comprehensive modifications are mentioned here.

First, a Synopsis of Clinical Points appears at the end of each chapter. This table summarizes the main clinical issues discussed in the chapter, and each point is keyed to the page(s) in the chapter(s) where the fact or concept is discussed in more detail. This provides a format to review the main clinical points, and makes it easy to review the clinical points in their full context if needed.

Second, numerous new MRI, angiograms, and CT are introduced throughout the book. These are used primarily to illustrate clinical examples but also to show important anatomical points as they are seen in the types of images commonly used in the clinical setting. Complementing these images are new line drawings that also illustrate clinical information, such as the locations of aneurysms,

herniation syndromes, segments of cerebral arteries, and the course of the vertebral arteries.

Third, several of the pathways routinely evaluated during a neurological examination are shown in MRI orientation. This innovation shows the reader the locations and relationships of these pathways as they appear in a clinical orientation. Complementing these pathway illustrations are representative levels of the brainstem in MRI on which nuclei and pathways are superimposed at each respective level. This novel approach serves to emphasize the point that while students may learn the structures of the brain in an *anatomical orientation*, when they observe MRI or CT of the neurologically compromised patient in the clinical setting the brain will be viewed in a *clinical orientation.*

Fourth, new and relevant developmental points have been introduced including, but not limited to, lobar holoprosencephaly, heterotopia, megacolon, and pituitary development.

Fifth, a variety of basic concepts are discussed, such as afferent versus efferent, sign versus symptom, and examination versus evaluation—all of which are essential to honing clinical and diagnostic skills.

Sixth, the basic histologic characteristics of primary central nervous system tumors are introduced. These include synoptic text and illustrations of gliomas, meningiomas, and tumors of the choroid plexus. Although treated briefly, they serve as an introduction to later academic experiences.

Seventh, examples of cranial nerves in MRI have been added to several chapters. This serves to emphasize the fact that the subarachnoid space contains, in addition to cerebrospinal fluid, enormously important structures such as roots of cranial nerves and blood vessels.

This Edition continues to follow the official international list of anatomical terms for neuroanatomy (Terminologia Anatomica, Thieme, 1998). We have made a concerted effort to include the most current and most correct terminology; if some terms have eluded us these will be corrected in future printings.

The editor and contributors want to improve this edition when and where we can. We welcome comments, corrections, and suggestion from students, colleagues, and any other users of this book.

Acknowledgments

As was the case for previous Editions of *Fundamental Neuroscience for Basic and Clinical Applications*, this new Edition reflects the efforts of the various contributors and the valuable input that we have received from our students and colleagues. We especially thank students, here at the University of Mississippi Medical Center (UMMC) and many other Medical Centers and Schools, for their probing interest which has allowed us to better address their present and future educational needs.

A special thanks is extended to many colleagues who have provided valuable input to this, and earlier, Editions including, Drs. V. K. Arand, D. E. Angelaki, M. Behari, R. H. Baisden, A. J. (Tony) Castro, S. C. Crawford, J. L. Culberson, E. Dietrichs, J. T. Ericksen, W. C. Hall, R. Hoffman, J. S. King, W. M. King, G. R. Leichnetz, G. F. Martin, I. J. Miller, E. Mugnaini, R. S. Nowakowski, R. Nieuwenhuys, D. F. Peeler, A. Peters, J. D. Porter, J. A. Rafols, W. A. Roy, L. F. Schweitzer, D. L. Tolbert, and M. L. Woodruff. The photographs of Golgi-stained material in Chapters 26 and 27 are from the Clement A. Fox Collection at Wayne State University and through the courtesy of Dr. Rafols. The photograph of the unipolar brush cell in Chapter 27 was generously provided by Dr. Enrico Mugnaini, Northwestern University Institute for Neuroscience, and Dr. Madhuri Behari, All India Institute of Medical Sciences, who generously supplied the MRI image of a Wilson patient in Chapter 26. Dr. Richard Miller, UMMC, kindly provided the images of congenital megacolon in Chapters 5 and 29. The photograph on the half-title page was provided by Drs. Ross Kosinski and Greg Mihailoff.

A number of individuals at UMMC have gone out of their way to provide special help with this new Edition; this has included giving general advice and suggestions, proofreading of clinical information, suggesting of cases, interpretating of images, providing unusually good CT and MRI, and responding in a timely manner for requests for specific types of images. The individuals so involved are Mr. J. Barnes (Senior MRI Technologist – Pathology), Dr. O. B. Evans (Pediatrics), Dr. J. Fratkin (Pathology), Dr. R. Halpert (Radiology), Mr. W. (Eddie) Herrington (Chief CT/MRI Technologist), Dr. J. Lancon (Neurosurgery), and Dr. S. Subramony (Neurology). We are also greatly indebted to our colleagues in the Department of Neurosurgery (Drs. Parent, Badar, Harkey, Hoekema, Lancon, Esposito, Mandybur, and Ross) and in the Department of Neurology (Drs. Corbett, Herndon, Subramony, Santiago, Uschmann, and Zubkov) who have given valuable suggestions and insights or information for this new Edition. The Editor is also very grateful for their collective patience with his repeated queries.

Three of the original contributors are not participating in this Edition: Drs. Paul Brown, James Hutchins, and Robert Sweazey. The neurophysiology chapter has been completely rewritten by a new author with many new illustrations. The chapters by Hutchins and by Sweazey have new first authors, but recognizing that these chapters are revised and not totally rewritten, their names appear as co-authors of these chapters for this Edition. The Editor expresses his sincere appreciation to these three individuals for their contributions to previous Editions of this book.

All of the artwork and photography (but not including specifically acknowledged photographs) was done in the Department of Biomedical Illustration Services at UMMC. The authors are indebted to Mr. Michael P. Schenk (Director of the Department) and his colleagues, Mr. W. K. Cunningham, Mr. G. W. Armstrong, and Mr. W. A. Buhner II, for their exemplary efforts. Mr. Schenk modified some existing artwork and produced many new pieces, labeled all MRI/CT, and collaborated with Mr. Cunningham in the generation of new artwork, including that combining pathways with MRI. All photography was done by Mr. Armstrong. He produced many new images, especially of clinical examples, for this new Edition. Mr. Buhner scanned 2x2 slides and generated outstanding photographs of a variety of clinical examples that could be retrieved only through this approach. The Editor is enormously appreciative of their patience and cooperation in getting the best-quality artwork and photographs for this book.

Ms. Lisa Boyd did an outstanding job of typing all new and modified text, inserting numerous changes, and checking everything over and over to make sure nothing was missed. Her efforts and very good-natured cooperation were essential to the development of this third Edition. The Editor is greatly appreciative and each contributor, even though many are not aware, also relied on Lisa to get their final draft done.

Production of this finely done and visually appealing book would not have been accomplished without Churchill Livingstone, Elsevier. I am very grateful to Ms. Inta Ozols, my Editor, for her cooperation and for smoothing out many little rough spots in the road, Ms. Madelene Hyde (Marketing) for insights and suggestions, Ms. Mary Anne Folcher (Senior Project Manager), and Mr. Andy Chapman and Ms. Karen O'Keefe Owens (Designers). I am especially indebted to Ms. Katie Miller (Associate Developmental Editor) who received the manuscript, carefully reviewed every page, and saw it into the production process. Last, but certainly not least, the Editor expresses a special thanks to his wife, Gretchen (now Grandma Gretchen); she was an important element in getting everything done.

Contents

SECTION 2
Regional Neurobiology

SECTION 3
Systems Neurobiology

Section 1

Essential Concepts

Chapters 1–5

Chapter 1

Orientation to the Structure and Imaging of the Central Nervous System

D. E. Haines, F. A. Raila, and A. C. Terrell

Our nervous system makes us what we are. Personality, outlook, intellect, coordination (or lack thereof), and the *many* other characteristics that are unique to each of us are the result of complex interactions within our nervous system. Information is received from the environment by sensory receptors and transmitted into the brain or spinal cord. Once inside the brain or spinal cord, this sensory information is processed and integrated, and an appropriate response is initiated.

The nervous system can be viewed as a scale of structural complexity. Microscopically, the individual structural and functional unit of the nervous system is the *neuron*, or nerve cell. Interspersed among the neurons of the central nervous system are supportive elements called *glial cells*. At the macroscopic end of the scale are the large divisions (or parts) of the nervous system that can be handled and studied without magnification. These two extremes are not independent but form a continuum; functionally related neurons aggregate to form small structures, which combine to form larger structures, and so on. Communication takes place at many different levels, the end result being a wide range of productive or life-sustaining nervous activities.

Overview

Central, Peripheral, and Visceromotor Nervous Systems

The human nervous system is divided into the *central nervous system* (CNS) and the *peripheral nervous system* (PNS) (Fig. 1-1A). The CNS consists of the brain and spinal cord. Because of their locations in the skull and vertebral column, these structures are the most protected in the body. The PNS is made up of nerves that connect the brain and spinal cord with peripheral structures. These nerves innervate muscle (skeletal, cardiac, smooth) and glandular epithelium and contain a variety of sensory fibers. These sensory fibers enter the spinal cord via the posterior (dorsal) root, and motor fibers exit through the anterior (ventral) root. The *spinal nerve* is formed by the joining of posterior (sensory) and anterior (motor) roots and is, consequently, a *mixed nerve* (Fig. 1-1B). In the case of *mixed cranial nerves*, the sensory and motor fibers are combined into a single root.

The *visceromotor nervous system* (also called *visceral motor*) is a functional division of the nervous system that has parts in both the CNS and the PNS (Fig. 1-1). It is made up of neurons that innervate *smooth muscle, cardiac muscle, or glandular epithelium or combinations of these tissues*. These individual *visceral tissues*, when combined, make up *visceral organs* such as the stomach. The visceromotor nervous system is also called the *autonomic* or *vegetative nervous system* because it regulates motor responses outside the realm of conscious control.

Neurons

At the histologic level, the nervous system is composed of *neurons* and *glial cells*. As the basic structural and functional units of the nervous system, neurons are specialized to receive information, transmit electrical impulses, and influence other neurons or effector tissues. In many areas of the nervous system, neurons are structurally modified to serve particular functions. At this point, however, we shall consider the neuron only as a general concept.

A *neuron* consists of a *cell body (perikaryon or soma)* and the processes that emanate from the cell body (Fig. 1-2). Collectively, neuronal cell bodies constitute the *gray matter* of the CNS. Named and usually function-specific clusters of cell bodies in the CNS are called *nuclei* (singular, *nucleus*). Typically, *dendrites* are those processes that ramify in the vicinity of the cell body, whereas a single, longer process called the *axon* carries impulses to a more remote destination. The *white matter* of the CNS consists of bundles of axons that are wrapped in a sheath of insulating lipoprotein called *myelin*.

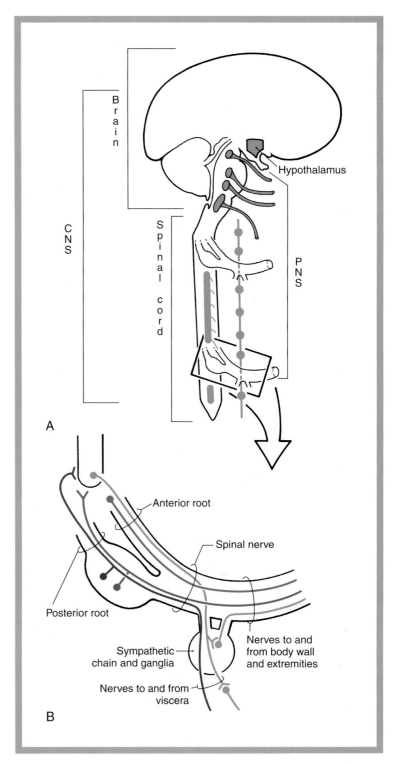

Figure 1-1. (A) General relationships of central (CNS), peripheral (PNS), and visceromotor nervous systems. Visceromotor regions of CNS and PNS are shown in *red*. **(B)** Enlargement of the *boxed area* in **A** shows the relationships of efferent (outgoing, motor) and afferent (incoming, sensory) fibers to spinal nerves and roots. Motor fibers are general visceral efferent (visceromotor; *red*) and general somatic efferent *(green)*; sensory fibers are general somatic afferent *(blue)* and general visceral efferent *(grey)*.

In general there is a direct relationship between (1) the diameter of the axon, (2) the thickness of the myelin sheath, (3) the distance between the nodes of the myelin sheath (nodes of Ranvier), and (4) the conduction velocity of the nerve fiber. Axons with a large diameter have thick myelin sheaths with longer internodal distances and therefore exhibit faster conduction velocities. Likewise, axons with a thin diameter that have thin myelin sheaths with shorter internodal distances have slower conduction velocities. The axon terminates at specialized structures called *synapses* or, in the case of those neurons that

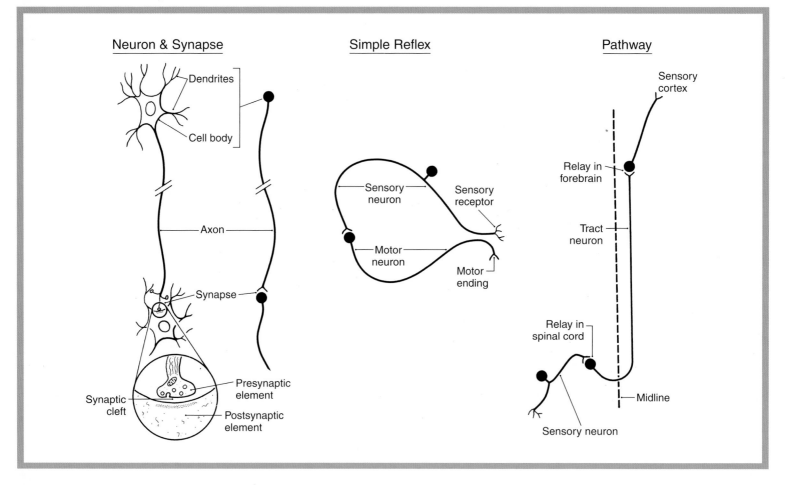

Figure 1-2. A representative neuron and synapse, a simple (monosynaptic) reflex, and a pathway.

innervate muscles, as *motor end plates (neuromuscular junctions),* which function much like synapses.

The generalized synapse shown in Figure 1-2 is the most common type seen in the CNS and is sometimes called an *electrochemical synapse.* It consists of a *presynaptic element,* which is usually part of an axon; a gap called the *synaptic cleft;* and the *postsynaptic region* of the innervated neuron or effector structure. Communication across this synapse is accomplished as follows. An electrical impulse (the *action potential*) causes the release of a neuroactive substance (a *neurotransmitter, neuromodulator,* or *neuromediator*) from the presynaptic element into the synaptic cleft. This substance is stored in *synaptic vesicles* in the presynaptic element and is released into the synaptic space by the fusion of these vesicles with the cell membrane (Fig. 1-2).

The neurotransmitter diffuses rapidly across the synaptic space and binds to receptor sites on the postsynaptic membrane. Based on the action of the neurotransmitter at receptor sites, the postsynaptic neuron may be excited (lead to generation of an action potential) or inhibited (prevent generation of an action potential). Neurotransmitter residues in the synaptic cleft are rapidly inactivated by other chemicals found in this space. In this brief example, we see that (1) the neuron is structurally specialized to receive and propagate electrical signals, (2) this propagation is accomplished by a combination of electrical and chemical events, and (3) the transmission of signals across the synapse is in one direction (unidirectional), that is, from the presynaptic neuron to the postsynaptic neuron. There are a number of neurologic disorders that represent a failure of neurotransmitter action at the synapse or at the receptors on the postsynaptic membrane.

Figure 1-2 shows the convention that is used for illustrating neurons as elements of reflex arcs and pathways in this book.

The dendrites and cell body (the "receiving" parts of the neuron) are represented by a large dot, and the axon (the "sending" part of the neuron) is represented by a line, which terminates in a fork or "Y" at the synapse.

Reflexes and Pathways

The function of the nervous system is based on the interactions of neurons with one another. Figure 1-2 illustrates one of the simplest types of neuronal circuits, a reflex arc composed of only two neurons. This is called a *monosynaptic reflex arc,* because only one synapse is involved. In this example, the peripheral end of a sensory fiber responds to a particular type of input. The resulting action potential is conducted by the sensory fiber into the spinal cord, where it influences a motor neuron. The axon of the motor neuron conducts a signal from the spinal cord to the appropriate skeletal muscle, which responds by contracting. This is an example of a *muscle stretch reflex* (or tendon reflex), which is actually one of the more commonly tested reflexes in clinical medicine. *Reflexes are involuntary responses to a particular bit of sensory input.* For example, the physician taps on the patellar tendon and the leg jerks; the patient does not think about it—the motor response just happens. The lack of a reflex *(areflexia),* an obviously weakened reflex *(hyporeflexia),* or an excessively active reflex *(hyperreflexia)* is usually indicative of a neurologic disorder.

By building on these summaries of the *neuron* and of the *basic reflex arc,* we shall briefly consider what neuronal elements constitute a *pathway.* If the patient bumps his or her knee and not only hits the patellar tendon but also damages the skin over the tendon, two things happen (Fig. 1-2). First, impulses from receptors in the tendon travel through a reflex arc that causes the leg to jerk *(knee jerk,* or *patellar reflex).* The synapse for this reflex arc is located in the lumbosacral spinal cord. Second, impulses from pain receptors in the damaged skin are transmitted in the lumbosacral cord to a second set of neurons that convey them via ascending axons to the forebrain. As can be seen in Figure 1-2, these axons cross the midline of the spinal cord and form an ascending tract on the contralateral side. In the forebrain, these signals are passed to a third group of neurons that distribute them to a region of the cerebral cortex specialized to interpret them as pain from the knee.

This three-neuron chain constitutes a *pathway*, a series of neurons designed to carry a specific type of information from one site to another (Fig. 1-2). Some pathways carry information to a level of conscious perception (we not only recognize pain but know that it is coming from the knee), and others convey information that does not reach the conscious level. It is common to refer to all the neurons comprising a pathway, and conducting a specific type of information, as a *system*. For example, the *anterolateral system* conducts pain and thermal information, the *posterior column–medial lemniscus system* conducts vibratory and position sense, and the *corticospinal system* conducts information from the cerebral cortex to the spinal cord. We will see many examples of pathways and systems in later chapters.

Regions of the Central Nervous System

Spinal Cord
The spinal cord is located inside the vertebral canal and is rostrally continuous with the medulla oblongata of the brain (Fig. 1-3). An essential link between the PNS and the brain, it conveys sensory information originating from the body wall, extremities, and gut and distributes motor impulses to these areas. Impulses enter and leave the spinal cord through the 31 pairs of spinal nerves (Fig. 1-1; see also Fig. 9-2). The spinal cord contains sensory fibers and motor neurons involved in reflex activity and ascending and descending pathways (many are called *tracts*) that link spinal centers with other parts of the CNS. Ascending pathways convey sensory information to higher centers, whereas descending pathways influence the activity of neurons in the spinal cord gray matter.

Medulla Oblongata
At the level of the foramen magnum, the spinal cord is continuous with the most caudal part of the brain, the *medulla oblongata*, commonly called the *medulla* (Fig. 1-3). The medulla consists of (1) neurons that perform functions associated with the medulla and (2) ascending and descending tracts that pass through the medulla on their way from or to the spinal cord. In general, fibers that descend through the medulla are involved in motor functions, whereas fibers that ascend through it carry sensory information. Some of the neuronal cell bodies of the medulla are organized into nuclei associated with specific cranial nerves. The medulla contains the nuclei for the glossopharyngeal (cranial nerve IX), vagus (X), and hypoglossal (XII) nerves, as well as portions of the nuclei for the trigeminal (V), vestibulocochlear (VIII), and spinal accessory (XI) nerves. It also contains important relay centers and nuclei that are essential to the regulation of respiration, heart rate, and various visceral functions.

Pons and Cerebellum
Embryologically, the pons and cerebellum originate from the same segment of the developing neural tube. However, in the adult the *pons* forms part of the *brainstem* (the other parts being the *midbrain* and *medulla*) and the cerebellum is a *suprasegmental* structure because it is located posterior (dorsal) to the brainstem (Fig. 1-3).

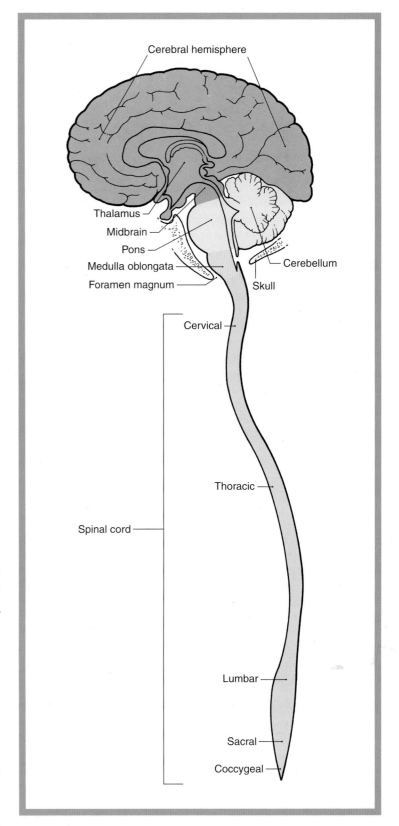

Figure 1-3. The basic divisions of the central nervous system.

Like the medulla, the pons contains many neuronal cell bodies, some of which are organized into cranial nerve nuclei, and it is traversed by ascending and descending tracts. The pons contains the nuclei of the abducens (VI) and facial (VII) nerves and portions of the nuclei for the trigeminal (V) and vestibulocochlear (VIII) nerves. The anterior (ventral) part of the pons contains large populations of neurons *(pontine nuclei)* that form a relay station between the cerebral cortex and cerebellum and descending motor fibers that travel to all spinal levels.

The cerebellum is connected with diverse regions of the CNS. Functionally, the cerebellum is considered part of the motor system. It serves to coordinate the activity of individual muscle groups to produce smooth, purposeful, synergistic movements.

Midbrain

Rostrally, the pons is continuous with the midbrain (Fig. 1-3). This latter part of the brain is, quite literally, the link between the brainstem and the forebrain. Ascending or descending pathways to or from the forebrain must traverse the midbrain. The nuclei for the oculomotor (III) and trochlear (IV) cranial nerves, as well as part of the trigeminal (V) complex, are found in the midbrain. Other midbrain centers are concerned with visual and auditory reflex pathways, motor function, the transmission of pain, and visceral functions.

Thalamus

The forebrain consists of the *cerebral hemispheres* and the large groups of neurons that compose the *basal nuclei* and the *thalamus* (Fig. 1-3). We shall see later that what is commonly called the thalamus actually consists of several regions—for example, the hypothalamus, subthalamus, epithalamus, and dorsal thalamus. The thalamus is also commonly called the *diencephalon*, a term that reflects its embryologic origin.

The thalamus is rostral to the midbrain and almost completely surrounded by elements of the cerebral hemisphere. Individual parts of the thalamus can be seen in detail only when the brain is cut in coronal or axial planes.

With the exception of olfaction, all sensory information that eventually reaches the cerebral cortex must pass through the thalamus. One function of the thalamus, therefore, is to receive sensory information of many sorts (such as temperature, pain, and vision) and to distribute it to the specific regions in the cerebral cortex that are specialized to decode it. Other areas of the thalamus receive input from pathways conveying information on, for example, position sense or the tension in a tendon or muscle. This input is relayed to areas of the cerebral cortex that function to generate smooth, purposeful movements.

Although quite small, the hypothalamus is extremely important. It functions in sexual behavior, feeding, hormonal output of the pituitary gland, body temperature regulation, and a wide range of visceromotor functions. Through descending connections, the hypothalamus influences visceral centers in the brainstem and spinal cord.

Cerebral Hemispheres

The largest and most obvious parts of the human brain are the two cerebral hemispheres. Each hemisphere is composed of three major subdivisions. First, the *cerebral cortex* is a layer of neuronal cell bodies about 0.5 cm thick that covers the entire surface of the hemisphere. This layer of cells is thrown into elevations called *gyri* (singular, *gyrus*) separated by creases called *sulci* (singular, *sulcus*).

The second major part of the hemisphere is the *subcortical white matter*, which is made up of myelinated axons that carry information to or from the cerebral cortex. The largest and most organized part of the white matter is the *internal capsule*. This bundle contains fibers passing to and from the cerebral cortex such as *corticospinal* and *thalamocortical* fibers.

The third major component of the hemisphere is a prominent group of neuronal cell bodies collectively called the *basal nuclei* (also called the *basal ganglia*). These prominent forebrain centers are involved in motor function. Parkinson disease, a neurologic disorder associated with the basal nuclei, is characterized by a profound impairment of movement.

The gyri and sulci that make up the cerebral cortex are named, and many are associated with particular functions. Some gyri receive sensory input, such as vision or general sensation, whereas others give rise to fibers that project to the spinal cord where they influence spinal neurons (including those motor neurons in the anterior horn) and to motor nuclei of cranial nerves. The cerebral cortex also has association areas that are essential for analysis and cognitive thought.

Functional Systems and Regions

A *functional system* is a set of neurons linked together to convey a particular block of information or accomplish a particular task. In this respect, *systems* and *pathways*, in some cases, may be quite similar, and occasionally their meanings may overlap.

Anatomic parts of the CNS, such as the medulla and pons, are commonly called *regions*. The study of their structure and function, called *regional neurobiology*, is the focus of the second section of this book. *Systems* and *pathways*, however, generally traverse more than one region. The system of neurons and axons that allows you to feel the edge of this page, for example, crosses every region of the nervous system between your fingers and the somatosensory cortex of the cerebral hemisphere. The study of functional systems, called *systems neurobiology*, is the focus of the third section of this text. It is important to remember that the *functional characteristics of regions coexist with those of systems*.

Let us consider an example of how the interrelation of systems and regions can be important clinically. The signals that influence movements of the hand originate in the cerebral cortex. Neurons in the hand area of the *motor cortex* send their axons to cervical levels of the spinal cord, where they influence spinal motor neurons that innervate the muscles of the forearm. These are called *corticospinal fibers*, because their cell bodies are in the cerebral cortex (*cortico-*) and their axons end in the spinal cord (*-spinal*). These fibers pass through the subcortical white matter, the entire brainstem, and upper levels of the cervical spinal cord. En route they pass near nuclei and fiber tracts that are specific to that particular region (Fig. 1-4). In the midbrain, for example, they pass near fibers of the oculomotor nerve, which originate in the midbrain and control certain extraocular muscles. In the medulla, they pass near fibers that originate in the medulla and innervate the musculature of the tongue. An injury to the midbrain, therefore, could cause motor problems in the hand (*systems damage*) combined with partial paralysis of eye movement (*regional damage*). In similar fashion, an injury to the medulla could cause the same hand problem but now in association with partial paralysis of the tongue rather than with eye movements. As we study the nervous system, we shall see that *successful diagnosis of patients with neurologic disorders will depend on, among other things, a good understanding of both regional and systems neurobiology*.

Localizing Signs and Localization

The example (Fig. 1-4) of corticospinal fibers that innervate spinal motor neurons serving the hand coupled with neuron cell bodies in the midbrain that innervate eye muscles via the oculomotor nerve also illustrates the concept of *localizing signs*. Brain injury that results in a weakness or paralysis of the upper extremity generally localizes the lesion only to one cerebral hemisphere or perhaps to one side of the brainstem. The clinical examination does not tell us which region of the brain is injured (internal capsule, midbrain, pons, or medulla) or, for that matter, even whether the lesion is in the upper portions of the cervical spinal cord. However, if the paralysis of the upper extremity is coupled with a partial paralysis of eye movement, the lesion can be *specifically localized to the midbrain*. In this example, the lesion in the midbrain damages the fibers of the oculomotor nerve that are specific to this level, while the corticospinal fibers

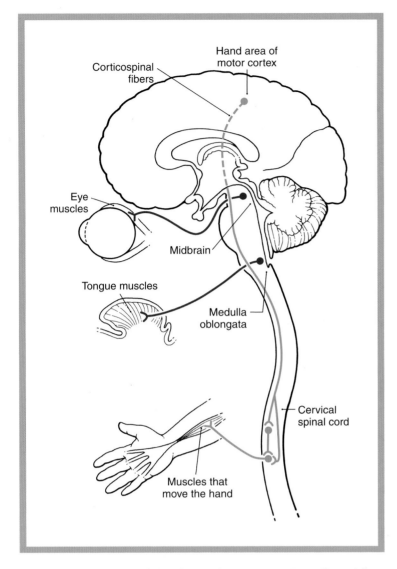

Figure 1-4. An example of the relation of systems to regions. Fibers of the motor system that control band movement descend from the motor cortex to the cervical spinal cord. In the cord these fibers influence motor neurons that control hand and forearm muscles. Injury at any point along the way can damage fibers of the system and structures specific to the region. For example, injury to the midbrain could damage both fibers to the hand and fibers to the eye muscles whereas injury to the medulla could damage both fibers to the hand and fibers to the tongue musculature.

are injured as they traverse the midbrain (Fig. 1-4). In general, cranial nerve signs are more helpful than long-tract signs in localizing the lesion; that is, they are better *localizing signs*. Many examples of localizing signs are seen in later chapters.

Another general concept of *localization* states that certain combinations of neurologic deficits may indicate involvement of one of three general locations of the CNS. First, deficits (motor or sensory) located on the same side of the head and body frequently signify lesions in the cerebral hemisphere. Second, deficits on one side of the head and on the opposite side of the body generally indicate a lesion in the brainstem. Such deficits are called *crossed* (or *alternating*) *deficits*. Third, deficits of the body only usually suggest a lesion in the spinal cord. Although there are exceptions to these general rules, we shall see that they hold true in many clinical situations.

The Concept of Afferent and Efferent

The terms *afferent* and *efferent* are used to describe a variety of structures in the human body, such as nerve fibers, small vessels, or lymphatics. Afferent refers to conduction (of an impulse

on a nerve, or fluid in a vessel) toward a structure; this is an incoming bit of information. Efferent refers to conduction (impulse or fluid) away from a structure; this is an outgoing bit of information.

In this respect, the posterior root of the spinal nerve is *afferent* since it conducts impulses toward the spinal cord and, at the same time it is a *sensory* root, while the anterior root is *efferent* since it conducts impulses away from the spinal cord and, at the same time it is a *motor* root (Figs. 1-1 and 1-2). This has given rise to the widely held, but incorrect, view that afferent nerve fibers are always sensory and efferent nerve fibers are always motor. While this may be true for the restricted examples of spinal and cranial nerves, the terms *afferent* and *efferent* can also be used to designate bundles of fibers (axons) traveling toward, or away from, a specific nucleus.

Whether a bundle of axons is afferent or efferent, in relation to a specific nucleus, depends on *what reference point is selected to define the bundle and its relationships*. For example, the neuron cell body in nucleus A in Figure 1-5 gives rise to an axon that is an *efferent of nucleus A* (conducting away from) but at the same time this axon is an *afferent of nucleus B* (coming toward). If nucleus B is chosen as the reference point, it would be described as receiving afferent input from nucleus A and sending efferent impulses to nucleus C (Fig. 1-5). The use of these terms is commonplace when describing connections within the nervous system (systems neurobiology). With reference to an example described in the previous section, corticospinal fibers are efferents of the cerebral cortex and, at the same time, afferents to the spinal cord.

Posterior (Dorsal), Anterior (Ventral), and Other Directions in the Central Nervous System

By convention, directions in the human CNS—such as *posterior* (*dorsal*) and *anterior* (*ventral*), *medial* (toward or at the midline) and *lateral* (away from the midline), *rostral* (or *rostrad*, a direction toward the nose) and *caudal* (or *caudad*, a direction toward the tail)—are absolute with respect to the central axis

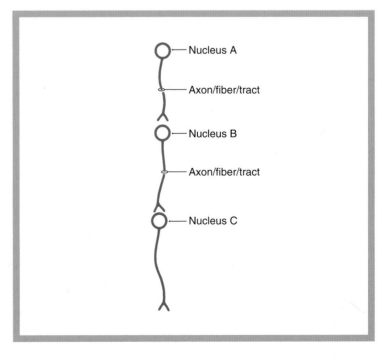

Figure 1-5. Diagrammatic representation of the use of the terms *afferent* and *efferent* when describing information conducted toward, or away from, a particular reference point.

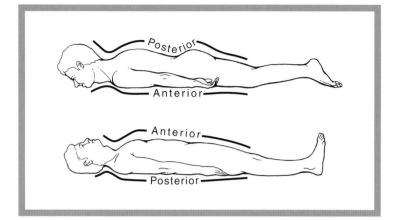

Figure 1-6. The anatomic directions of the body are absolute with respect to the axes of the body, not with respect to the position of the body in space.

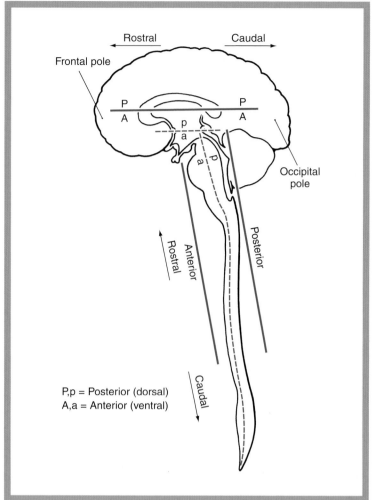

P,p = Posterior (dorsal)
A,a = Anterior (ventral)

Figure 1-7. The central axis and anatomic directions of the central nervous system (CNS). The *dashed line* shows the long (rostrocaudal) axis of the CNS. The long axis of the spinal cord and brainstem forms a sharp angle with the long axis of the forebrain. Posterior (dorsal) and anterior (ventral) orientations are also shown.

of the brain and spinal cord. In similar manner, the anatomic orientation of the body in space is related to its central axis. For example, if the patient is lying on his or her stomach, the posterior surface of the trunk is up and its anterior surface is down (Fig. 1-6). If the patient rolls over, the back remains the posterior surface of the patient's body even though it now faces down.

As shown in Figure 1-7, the spinal cord and the brainstem (medulla, pons, and midbrain) form a nearly straight line that is roughly parallel with the superoinferior axis of the body. Therefore, anatomic directions in these regions of the CNS coincide roughly with those of the body as a whole. The pons is rostral to the medulla, for instance, and the cerebellum is posterior (dorsal) to the pons.

The situation is different in the forebrain because during embryonic development the forebrain rotates (at the cephalic flexure) relative to the midbrain until its rostrocaudal axis corresponds to a line drawn from the forehead to the occiput (from the frontal to the occipital poles of the cerebral hemispheres). This rotation creates a sharp angle in the long axis of the CNS at the midbrain-thalamus junction. Consequently, the long axis of the CNS bends at the midbrain-thalamus junction, and the directions posterior and anterior follow accordingly (Fig. 1-7).

In the cerebral hemisphere (forebrain), *posterior (dorsal)* is toward the top of the brain, *anterior (ventral)* is toward the base of the brain, *rostral* is toward the frontal pole, and *caudal* is toward the occipital pole. Anatomic directions in the forebrain relate to its long axis; therefore, the posterior side of the forebrain structures faces the vertex of the head and the anterior aspect of the forebrain faces the base of the skull (Fig. 1-7). *Posterior* and *dorsal* and *anterior* and *ventral* are considered synonymous and *are commonly and frequently used interchangeably.*

It is also important to understand that these directional terms are extremely valuable when describing the relative position of a structure within the brain or spinal cord or describing the relative positions of two structures to each other. For example, the midbrain is *rostral to the pons but caudal to the thalamus* (Fig. 1-3). The midbrain is selected as the reference point and adjacent structures described in relation to it. Also, directional terms, such as *posterior* and *lateral,* can be combined to describe a structure that occupies an intermediate position. For example, the nuclei in the spinal cord transmitting sensory information can be described as *posterolateral* to the central canal. There are innumerable examples of directional terms being used in this manner in human neurobiology.

Symptom or Sign?

These terms are used literally everyday in countless physician's offices or in hospital settings and serve to form an essential and important part of the physician-patient relationship — that is, the communication of information that will result in proper and successful medical treatment. It is useful to establish what constitutes a *symptom* versus a *sign* at this early point. These concepts and definitions will be frequently revisited throughout subsequent chapters, especially those in which clinical information is emphasized.

Symptom

A *symptom* is a departure from any normal state of structure or function that is *experienced by the patient.* In other words, something is wrong and the patient knows it. Symptoms may develop slowly, almost imperceptively, as in a slow-growing tumor or as part of the aging process, or appear suddenly, as in hemorrhage or trauma. A symptom, such as pain, may be clear to the patient (a symptom) but difficult for the attending physician to evaluate. A symptom is a *subjective indicator* of a presumably abnormal process.

Sign.   A *sign* is a departure from any normal state of structure or function that is *discovered, observed, and evaluated by a health care professional upon examining the patient.* In this situation,

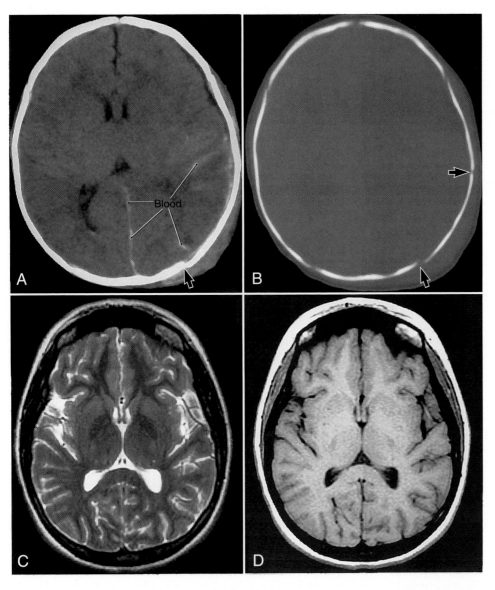

Figure 1-8. CT scans (**A**, **B**) of a 2-month-old infant who was a victim of the shaken baby syndrome and MR images of a normal 20-year-old woman (**C**, **D**). On the CT study, note that brain detail is less than on the MR images but that the presence of blood (**A**, in the interhemispheric fissure between the hemisphere and in the brain substance) is obvious. In the same patient, the bone window (**B**) clearly illustrates the outline of the skull but also clearly shows skull fractures (*arrows* in **A** and **B**). In this infant, the ventricles on the left are largely compressed and the gyri have largely disappeared owing to pressure from bleeding into the hemisphere. The pressure results in the effacement of the sulci and gyri on the left side. In the T2-weighted image (**C**), cerebrospinal fluid is white, internal brain structures are seen in excellent detail, and vessels are obvious. In the T1-weighted image (**D**), cerebrospinal fluid is dark and internal structures of the brain are somewhat less obvious.

the clinical problem (be it great or small) is seen and can be evaluated by the physician. It is possible that a patient may have signs of a disease process, seen during the examination, that he or she is unaware of; the patient has *signs but no symptoms*. A sign is an *objective indicator* of a presumably abnormal process.

Clinical Images of the Brain and Skull

Modern technology has given us the tools to view the living brain and skull in some detail. In addition, arteries and veins of the brain and of the meninges can be visualized by mapping the movement of blood through these vascular structures. The resultant images are powerful tools to use in the diagnosis of the neurologically impaired patient.

The most routinely used methods to image the brain and skull are computed tomography (CT) and magnetic resonance imaging (MRI) (Fig. 1-8). As we shall see, CT is especially useful in visualizing the skull and the brain in the early stages of subarachnoid hemorrhage. On the other hand, MRI, using T1-weighted or T2-weighted techniques, shows brain anatomy in elegant detail, cisternal relationships, cranial nerves, and a wide variety of clinical abnormalities.

Magnetic resonance angiography (MRA) visualizes arteries and veins by measuring the velocity of flow in these structures (Fig. 1-9). The resultant images show detail of vascular structures that, in some situations, may be superior to that seen on angiograms. Arterial structures may be selectively imaged, or

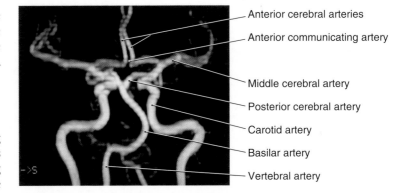

Figure 1-9. MR angiography of the internal carotid artery and the vertebrobasilar systems.

combinations of arterial and venous structures or only venous structures can be visualized. Some clinicians refer to these images of venous structures as MRVs (magnetic resonance venograms).

Computed Tomography

CT is an x-ray imaging technique that measures the effects that tissue density and the various types of atoms in the tissue have on x-rays passing through that tissue (Table 1-1; see also Fig. 1-8A, B). Changes in the emerging x-ray beam are measured by detectors.

Table 1-1. Appearance of Tissues Imaged by CT and MRI

Modality	Tissue						
	Bone	*CSF*	*Gray Matter*	*White Matter*	*Fat*	*Air*	*Muscle*
CT*	↑↑↑	↓↓	↓	↓↓	↓	↓↓↓	↑↑
MRI/T1†	↓↓↓	↓↓↓	↓↓	↓	↑↑	↓↓↓	↓↓
MRI/T2†	↓↓↓	↑↑↑	↓↓	↓↓↓	↑	↓↓↓	↓↓–↓↓↓

*Measures tissue density.
†Measures tissue signal.
↑↑↑–↑ represents very white to light gray:

↓–↓↓↓ represents light gray to very black:

CSF, cerebrospinal fluid; CT, computed tomography; MRI, magnetic resonance imaging.

The higher the atomic number, the greater the ability of the atom to attenuate, or stop, x-rays. These attenuation transmission intensities emerging from the tissue are transformed by a computer into numbers that represent values found in all the points located in the volume of the tissue slice. These values are expressed in Hounsfield units (HUs). HU values, also known as CT numbers, are used in an arbitrary scale in which bone is specified as +1000 (and is very white; Fig. 1-8A, B), water as zero, and air as −1000 (and is very black). Approximate numbers are +100 for blood, +30 for brain, and +5 for cerebrospinal fluid (CSF). Using this scale, the HU values, or CT numbers, represent specific shades of gray for each of the various points located in the slice (Tables 1-1 and 1-2; see also Fig. 1-8A, B). The resultant image is seen on a computer monitor, or it can be transferred to x-ray film.

Present-generation CT scanners, known as helical (spiral) scanners, image a continuous spiral slice through a preselected body region very quickly. Computer software converts this information into contiguous slices of a chosen thickness. This technique eliminates movement artifacts and enables reconstruction of soft tissues, bone, or contrast medium–enhanced vessels into three-dimensional images that can be manipulated in any plane.

CT is a fast and accurate method of detecting recent subarachnoid hemorrhage (Table 1-2; see also Fig. 1-8A). An acute subarachnoid hemorrhage in a noncontrast CT scan appears hyperdense (white) in contrast to the subarachnoid spaces and cisterns, which normally are hypodense (dark).

Enhanced CT is a technique using an iodinated contrast material injected intravenously followed by CT examination. Iodine has a large atomic number and attenuates x-rays. As a result, vasculature is visualized as hyperdense (white) structures. This contrast material may also enhance neoplasms or areas of inflammation, because the contrast agent leaks from the vessels into the cellular spaces owing to a breakdown of the blood-brain barrier. Imaged in this way, the tumor, inflamed meninges, or brain parenchyma will show varying degrees of enhancement or hyperdensity (varying degrees of whiteness).

Table 1-2. Differences in CT Density and MRI Signals in Representative Clinical Examples

Clinical Problem	CT*	MRI	
		T1†	*T2†*
Acute SAH	↑↑↑	0	0
Subacute SAH	↑↑	0–↑	0
Tumor	0	0	↑–↑↑
Enhanced tumor	↑↑↑	↑↑↑	↑↑↑
Acute infarct	0	0–↑	↑–↑↑
Subacute infarct	0–↑	0–↓↓	↑↑–↑↑↑
Acute ischemia	0	0–↓	↑–↑↑
Subacute ischemia	0–↑	0–↓↓	↑↑–↑↑↑
Edema	0–↑	0–↓	↑–↑↑

*Measures tissue density.
†Measures tissue signal.
↑↑↑–↑ represents very white to light gray:

↓–↓↓↓ represents light gray to very black:

0 represents no change from normal.
CT, computer tomography; MRI, magnetic resonance imaging; SAH, subarachnoid hemorrhage.

Magnetic Resonance Imaging (Tables 1-1 and 1-2; see also Fig. 1-8C, D)

Protons (hydrogen) constitute a large proportion of body tissue. These atoms have a nucleus and a shell of electrons and a north and a south pole, and they spin around an angulated axis like small planets. As the electrons move with the spinning atom, they induce an electrical current that creates a magnetic field. These atoms function somewhat like little spinning bar magnets. They are aligned randomly because of the changing magnetic effects on each other. When these protons are exposed to a powerful magnet, they stop pointing randomly and align themselves in parallel with the external magnetic field but at different energy levels. The stronger the external magnetic field, the faster the frequency of the spin at that angle. When undergoing an MRI examination, the patient becomes a magnet, with all the protons aligning along the external magnetic field and spinning at an angle with a certain frequency.

A radio wave is an electromagnetic wave. When sent as a short burst into the magnet containing the patient, it is known as a radiofrequency (RF) pulse. This RF pulse can vary in frequency strength. Only when the frequency strength of the RF pulse matches the frequency strength of the angulated spinning proton will the proton absorb energy from the radio wave. This phenomenon is called *resonance* and is the "resonance" in "magnetic resonance imaging." This results in a twofold effect:

it cancels out the magnetic effects of certain protons, and it raises the energy levels and magnetic effects of another group of protons. When the radio wave is turned off, the canceled-out protons gradually return to their original state and strength of magnetization, which is called *relaxation* and is described by a time constant known as T1 (Fig. 1-8D). The protons that aligned themselves at a higher energy level and magnetization also start to lose their energy (relaxation), and this time constant is known as T2 (Fig. 1-8C). The T1 relaxation time is longer than the T2 relaxation time. The "de-excited" or relaxed protons release their energy as an "echo" of radio waves. A receiver coil (antenna) absorbs this information, and a computer determines the characteristics of the emitted radio waves from all the specific points in that section of the body. The MR image is then constructed and transferred to a computer monitor or x-ray film. T1-weighted or T2-weighted images can be obtained by using varying times to receive the echoes (TE).

Conventional *spin-echo* sequences generate images that may be T1 weighted or T2 weighted according to the time interval in milliseconds between each exciting radio wave. This is called *repetition time* (TR). The time interval, in milliseconds, required to collect these radio waves from the relaxing protons is called *echo time* (TE). With spin-echo pulse sequences, the shorter the TR and TE, the more the image is considered T1 weighted. The longer the TR and TE, the more the image is considered T2 weighted.

The contrast material used for enhancing tumors and blood vessels is the paramagnetic rare earth gadolinium. It is chelated

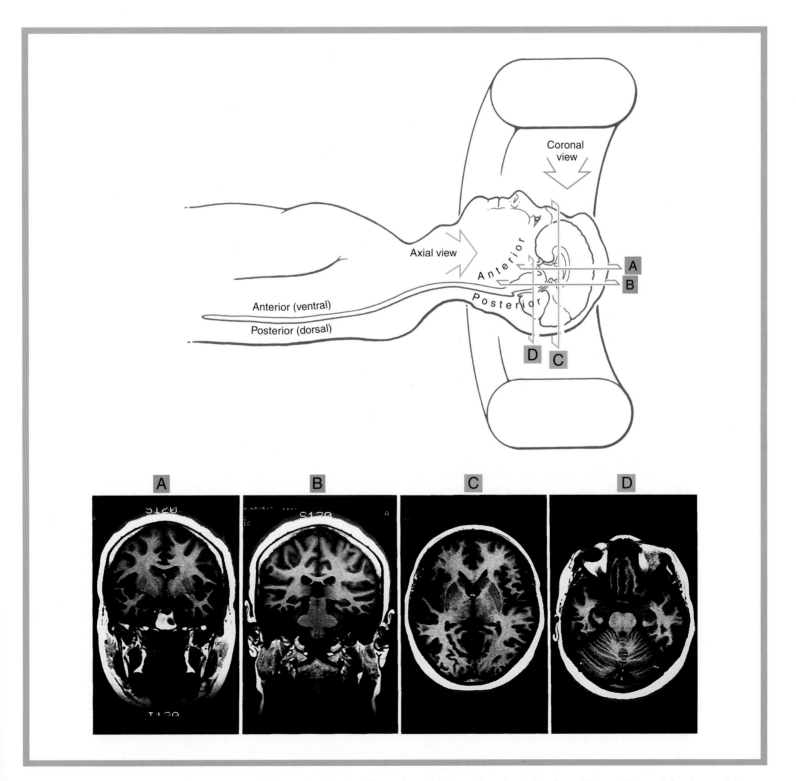

Figure 1-10. The relation of imaging planes to the brain. The diagram shows the usual orientation of a patient in an MRI machine and the planes of the four scans (T1-weighted images) that are shown. **A** and **B**, Coronal scans; **C** and **D**, axial scans.

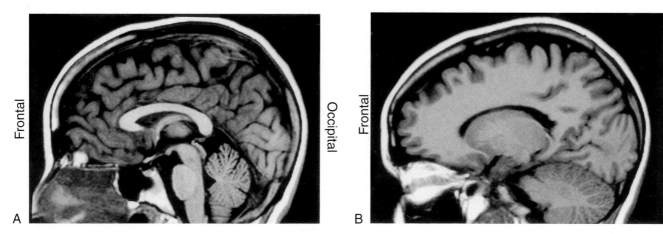

Figure 1-11. MRI of the brain in the median sagittal plane (**A**) and in the sagittal plane but off the midline (**B**). The frontal lobe is to the left, and the occipital lobe is to the right. Other directions within the brain in this plane are appreciated by a comparison with Figure 1-7.

to a certain molecule and is in solution for intravenous injection. The gadolinium causes an increase in signal by shortening the relaxation time for T1. Owing to a breakdown of the blood-brain barrier, intravascular gadolinium enters the pericellular spaces, where it increases the relaxation state of water protons and generates a bright signal on T1-weighted images.

Acute subarachnoid hemorrhage is poorly imaged by MRI on T1-weighted images but well imaged by CT (Table 1-2). Some MRI sequences are sensitive for detection of acute bleeding, but other factors may limit this method of examination. Special MRI techniques can also determine if a brain infarct or ischemia is acute (about 1 to 3 hours old) or subacute (about 4 hours old or more). Contraindications to MRI are cardiac pacemakers, cochlear implants, ferromagnetic foreign bodies in the eye, and certain aneurysm clips. Large metallic implants or ferromagnetic foreign bodies in the body may heat up. The general appearance of the brain and adjacent structures in health and disease on MRI and CT is summarized in Tables 1-1 and 1-2.

Imaging of the Brain and Skull

Patients lie on their back (supine) for imaging of the brain or spinal cord and the surrounding bony structures of the skull and vertebral column (Fig. 1-10). In this position, the posterior (dorsal) surface of the brainstem and spinal cord and the caudal aspect (occipital pole) of the cerebral hemispheres face down. The anterior (ventral) surface of the brainstem and spinal cord and the frontal pole are face up (Fig. 1-10).

Images of the brain are commonly made in *coronal, axial* (horizontal), and *sagittal* planes. To illustrate the basic orientation of the CNS in situ, we shall look at examples of images in all three of these planes, shown as they would appear in the clinical setting (Figs. 1-10 and 1-11). Coronal imaging planes are oriented perpendicular to the rostrocaudal axis of the forebrain but are nearly parallel to the rostrocaudal axis of the brainstem and spinal cord. Therefore, a coronal image obtained at a relatively rostral level of the cerebral hemispheres (Fig. 1-10A) will show only forebrain structures, and these structures will appear in cross section (perpendicular to their long axis). As the plane

of imaging is moved caudally, brainstem structures enter the picture (Fig. 1-10B), but the brainstem is cut nearly parallel to its rostrocaudal axis.

Axial images, in contrast, are oriented parallel to the rostrocaudal axis of the cerebral hemispheres but nearly perpendicular to the long axis of the brainstem and spinal cord. Consequently, an axial image obtained midway through the cerebral hemispheres (Fig. 1-10C) will show only forebrain structures, with the rostral end of the forebrain at the top of the image and the caudal end at the bottom. As the plane of imaging is moved farther anteriorly (ventrally) relative to the forebrain, the brainstem appears (Fig. 1-10D). The brainstem, however, is cut nearly in cross section and is oriented with the anterior (ventral) surface "up" (toward the top of the image) and the posterior (dorsal) surface "down."

Images made in the sagittal plane are at, or parallel with, the midsagittal plane of the brain or spinal cord. This is the plane running right through the middle (midline) of the head from rostral to caudal (along the frontal-to-occipital axis), or along the midline of the spinal cord in a rostrocaudal axis. Sagittal images of the brain, be they at the midline (Fig.1-11A) or in the sagittal plane but off the midline (Fig. 1-11B), are oriented such that the frontal area is to the left and the occipital area is to the right. The various directions within the brain can be appreciated by comparing the midsagittal MR image with a drawing in the comparable orientation (compare Fig. 1-7 with Fig. 1-11A).

A point also needs to be made about how the clinician looks at scans such as those in Figure 1-9. Coronal scans are viewed as though you are looking the patient in the face, whereas axial scans are viewed as though you are standing at the patient's feet looking toward his head while the patient lies supine in the machine. Axial scans, in other words, show the cerebral hemispheres from anterior (the more inferior portion of the hemisphere) to posterior (the more superior portion of the hemisphere), with the patient's frontal area and orbits at the top of the image and the occiput at the bottom. *In both coronal and axial views, the patient's left side is to the observer's right.* This is an absolutely essential concept to remember as one examines MRI and CT.

Synopsis of Clinical Points

- Muscle stretch reflexes are commonly tested in the neurologic examination (p. 4).
- Generally when a patient has a long tract deficit accompanied by a cranial nerve deficit, the cranial nerve deficit is the best localizing sign (pp. 6–7).
- Deficits (motor + sensory) on the same side of the body usually signify a lesion in the forebrain (p. 7).
- Alternating, or crossed, deficits (body on one side, head on the other side) are usually indicative of brainstem lesions (p. 7).
- Deficits of the body only usually signify a lesion of the spinal cord (p. 7).
- Symptoms are departures from normal structure/function that are experienced by the patient (p. 8).
- Signs are departures from normal structure/function that can be observed and evaluated by a physician (pp. 8–9).
- CT is especially useful in visualizing bone and acute and subacute hemorrhage (pp. 9–10).
- MRI is especially useful in visualizing anatomic detail in either T1- or T2-weighted images (pp. 10–12).
- CSF is black in T1-weighted MR images and white in T2-weighted MR images (p. 10).
- When viewing CT or MRI the observer's right is the patient's left and the observer's left is the patient's right (pp. 12–13).

Sources and Additional Reading

Grossman CB: Magnetic Resonance Imaging and Computed Tomography of the Head and Spine, 2nd ed. Baltimore, Lippincott Williams & Wilkins, 1996.

Jackson GD, Duncan JS: MRI Neuroanatomy: A New Angle on the Brain. New York, Churchill Livingstone, 1996.

Kirkwood JR: Essentials of Neuroimaging. New York, Churchill Livingstone, 1990.

Kretschmann HJ, Weinrich W: Cranial Neuroimaging and Clinical Neuroanatomy: Magnetic Resonance Imaging and Computed Tomography, 2nd ed. New York, Thieme Medical Publishers, 1992.

Osborn AG: Diagnostic Neuroradiology. St. Louis, Mosby, 1994.

Chapter 2

The Cell Biology of Neurons and Glia
J. P. Naftel, M. D. Ard, J. D. Fratkin, and J. B. Hutchins

The number of cells in the adult human central nervous system (CNS) has been estimated at 100 billion. All arise from a relatively small population of precursors, yet a diversity of cell types is seen in the adult. Their most basic classification is as *neurons* and *glia (glial cells)*.

Overview

Nerve cells (neurons) manipulate information. Doing so involves changes in the *bioelectrical* or *biochemical* properties of the cell, and these changes require a vast expenditure of energy for each cell. The nervous system, compared with other organs, is the greatest consumer of oxygen and glucose. These energy requirements arise directly from the metabolic demand placed on cells, which have a large surface area and concentrate biomolecules and ions against an energy gradient. Along with maintaining its metabolism, each neuron (1) *receives information* from the environment or from other nerve cells, (2) *processes information*, and (3) *sends information* to other neurons or effector tissues.

Unlike neurons, *glia* do not receive and transmit information with point-to-point specificity. Rather, their primary function is control of the environment within the CNS. They *shuttle nutritive molecules* from blood vessels to neurons, *remove waste* products, and *maintain the electrochemical* surroundings of neurons. Glial cells are also essential in the early development of the CNS for *guiding developing neurons* to their correct locations, and, in the adult, glia provide *structural support* for nerve cells.

For neurons to carry out the three tasks of receiving, processing, and sending information, they must have specialized structures that are designed to carry out each of these tasks. The basic parts of a neuron are shown in Figure 2-1. Additionally, specialized mechanisms and structures exist for some special problems faced by neurons. Two such problems are immediately apparent. First, the mix of ions inside neurons is quite different from the mix outside the cell. Maintaining this difference requires huge amounts of energy, since ions must be pumped against electrical and diffusion gradients. The large surface area of neurons compounds this problem. Second, those neurons that send information over long distances must have a way to supply these distant sites with macromolecules and energy. To fully understand the cell biology of neurons, it is important to see the biochemical, anatomic, and physiologic properties of neurons as part of an integrated whole, the machinery that permits the neuron to do its specialized functions. In the following sections, we examine how neuronal architecture and chemistry are designed to meet these special demands.

The Structure of Neurons

The archetypical neuron is bounded by a continuous plasma membrane and consists of a *cell body*, or *soma*, from which *dendrites* and an *axon* arise (Figs. 2-1 and 2-2). The cell body contains the nucleus surrounded by a mass of cytoplasm that contains the organelles necessary for protein synthesis and metabolic maintenance. Most neurons *(multipolar)* have several dendrites extending from the cell body (Figs. 2-1 and 2-2). These are usually relatively short processes that taper from a thick base and, in doing so, branch extensively. In contrast, there is a single axon, which is a relatively long process (extending from a few millimeters to more than a meter) with a uniform diameter. The axon has few, if any, branches along most of its length, branching extensively only near the distal end (the *terminal arbor*) (Figs. 2-1 and 2-2). In most neurons, information normally flows from the dendrites to the cell body to the axon (and its terminals), and then to the next neuron or effector tissue. These components of the neuron are described in the order in which information is processed.

Dendrites

Dendrites usually branch extensively in the vicinity of the cell body, giving the appearance of a tree or bush (Figs. 2-1 to 2-3A). They receive signals either from other neurons through contacts (*synapses*) made on their surfaces or from the environment via specialized receptors. Information travels from distal to proximal along dendrites to converge at the cell body.

Small bud-like extensions *(dendritic spines)* of a variety of shapes are frequently seen on the more distal branches of the dendritic tree (Figs. 2-1 and 2-3B, C). These are usually the sites of *synaptic contacts* (discussed later). The branches of dendrites increase in thickness as they anastomose in their course toward the cell body.

The only organelles seen in thin, distal dendritic branches are cytoskeletal elements, that is, *microtubules* and *neurofilaments* (the type of intermediate filament that occurs only in neurons). Thicker dendrites contain, in addition to cytoskeletal elements, *mitochondria*, some saccules of endoplasmic reticulum, and collections of polyribosomes and free ribosomes (Figs. 2-1 and 2-3D, E). In many nerve cells the distal dendrites collect into large, trunk-like *primary dendrites* that contain the same organelles as the cell body. The microtubular and neurofilamentous skeletons of the dendritic tree are continuous throughout its extent and help to maintain its branched structure.

Cell Body

The cell body of a neuron is also called the *soma* (plural, *somata*) or *perikaryon* (plural, *perikarya*) (Figs. 2-2 and 2-4). The perikaryon is the *metabolic center* of the nerve cell. Abundant mitochondria reflect the high energy consumption of the cell. Active protein synthesis is indicated by the large size of the nucleus and its content of diffuse chromatin (euchromatin) and at least one prominent nucleolus (the site of ribosomal RNA synthesis). In the cytoplasm, *ribosomes* are abundant, and the *rough endoplasmic reticulum* (rER) and *Golgi complex* are extensive (Fig. 2-1). The rER is basophilic (binds basic dyes) as a result of the large amount of ribosomal RNA attached to the endoplasmic membrane. These extensive, stacked layers of rER are seen as patches of basophilic staining (called *Nissl substance*) in histologic preparations of nerve cells.

Neurons are classified into three general types on the basis of the shape of the cell body and the pattern of processes emerging from it. These types are the multipolar, pseudounipolar, and bipolar cells (Table 2-1; see also Fig. 2-2).

The cell bodies of *multipolar* neurons vary widely in shape, so their profiles in tissue sections may appear fusiform, flask shaped, triangular, polygonal, or stellate (Fig. 2-2A-C). Variations of a stellate polygon are most common. This shape results from the presence of multiple, tapering dendrites that emerge from the cell body. The cell body also emits a single axon that generally appears thin relative to the dendrites because the axon does not taper (discussed in the following section). Multipolar neurons account for greater than 99% of all neurons, and the different kinds have characteristic patterns of processes, some of which are listed in Table 2-1.

The *pseudounipolar* (or *unipolar*) has a spherical cell body with a centrally placed (concentric) nucleus. The cell body emits a single process that courses only a short distance before bifurcating into a long peripheral branch and a long central branch (Fig. 2-2D). The peripheral branch courses as part of a peripheral nerve to convey sensory information from a somatic or visceral structure, such as skin, skeletal muscle, or wall of intestine. The distal end of the peripheral process is dendrite-like in the sense that its terminal branches receive information either by functioning as sensory receptors or by contacting other structures that function as receptors. The central branch courses as part of a nerve root to convey the sensory information to the

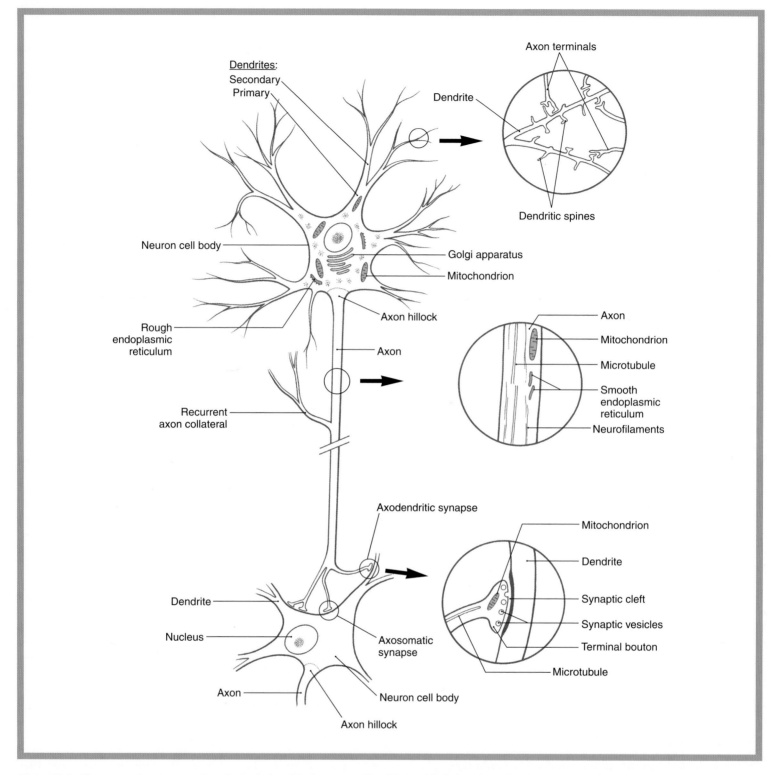

Figure 2-1. Diagrammatic representation of a typical multipolar neuron. Dendrites, with their variety of spines *(top inset)*, branch in the immediate vicinity of the cell body while the single axon, with its occasional recurrent collaterals, may travel great distances to the next neuron. The cell body contains the organelles essential for neuronal function. Microtubules *(middle and bottom insets)* are important structures for the transport of substances within the axon. The axon ends as a terminal arbor that forms many terminal boutons *(bottom inset),* each containing the necessary machinery for synaptic transmission.

CNS. In effect, the distal and central processes function together as a single axon. The cell bodies of pseudounipolar cells are found primarily in the sensory ganglia of cranial and spinal nerves.

Bipolar neurons have a round or oval perikaryon, with a single large process emanating from each end of the cell body (Fig. 2-2E, F). They are commonly found in structures associated with the special senses. In the retina, bipolar cells are interposed between receptor cells and the neurons that send long axons from the retina to the thalamus (output cells). In the olfactory system, they function as both the receptors and the output

neurons, with their axons projecting to the olfactory bulb; and in the vestibular and auditory systems, they are the output cells that send information to the brainstem.

Unless special staining methods are used, the cell body of a neuron has the appearance of being the entire cell when viewed in histologic sections. However, the volume of the cell body of a neuron constitutes only a small fraction, often less than 1%, of the volume of the axon and dendrites even though the cell body synthesizes and continually replaces all structural molecules of these processes.

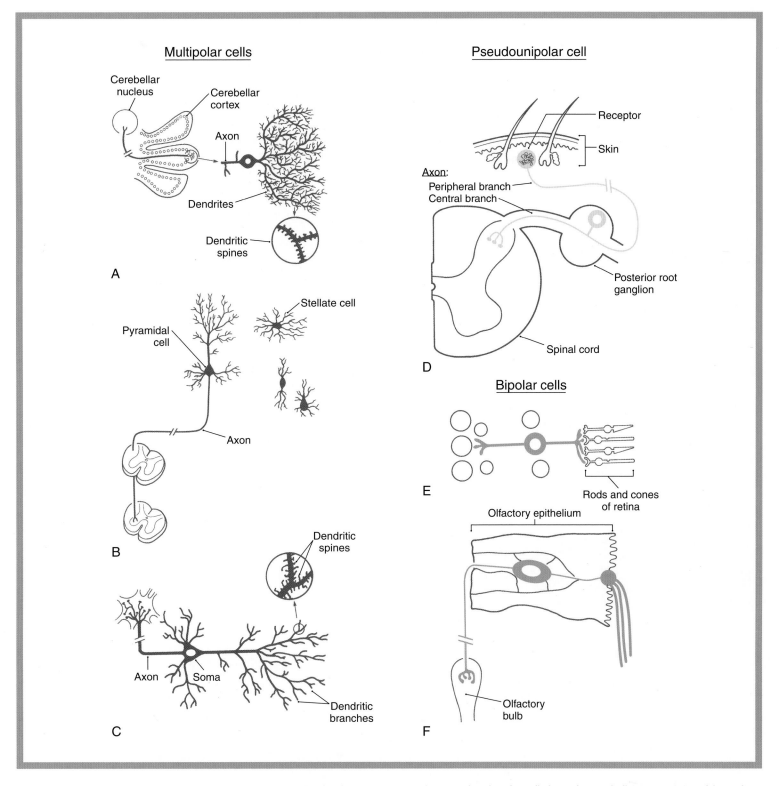

Figure 2-2. Examples of various types of neurons showing the dendrites, somata, and axons of multipolar cells from the cerebellar cortex (**A**) and from the cerebral cortex (**B** and **C**). Compare these with a pseudounipolar cell of the posterior root ganglion (**D**) and with bipolar cells from the retina (**E**) and olfactory epithelium (**F**).

Axons and Axon Terminals

The *axon* arises from the cell body at a small elevation called the *axon hillock*. The proximal part of the axon, adjacent to the axon hillock, is the *initial segment*. The cytoplasm of the axon (axoplasm) contains dense bundles of *microtubules* and *neurofilaments* (Figs. 2-1 and 2-5A, B). These function as structural elements, and they also play key roles in the transport of metabolites and organelles along the axon. Axons are typically devoid of ribosomes, a feature that distinguishes them from dendrites at the ultrastructural level.

In contrast to dendrites, axons may extend for long distances before branching and terminating. An extreme example is the length (about 1.5 meters) of the axon of a sensory neuron that conveys touch information from a toe of a tall individual. The axon of such a neuron accounts for approximately 99.8% of the total volume of the neuron. The surface area of an axon can be several thousand times the surface area of the parent cell body. Axons are sometimes referred to as *nerve fibers*, although strictly speaking a nerve fiber includes both the axon and a sheath that is provided by support cells (described in a subsequent section).

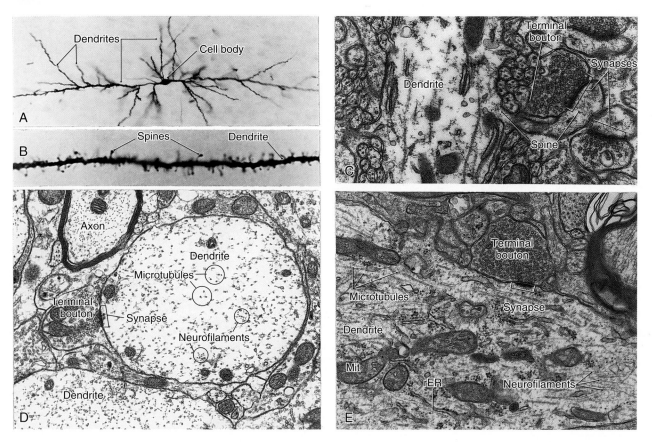

Figure 2-3. Elements of dendrite structure. Dendritic tree of a multipolar neuron (**A**) and dendritic spines (**B**), both in Golgi-stained cortical tissue. Ultrastructural features of dendrites, showing an axonal terminal bouton synapsing on a dendritic spine (**C**), a cross section of a dendrite with characteristic cytoskeletal elements and organelles (**D**), and a longitudinal section of a dendrite in the anterior horn of the spinal cord (**E**). (A and B courtesy of Dr. Jose Rafols; D courtesy of Dr. Alan Peters.)

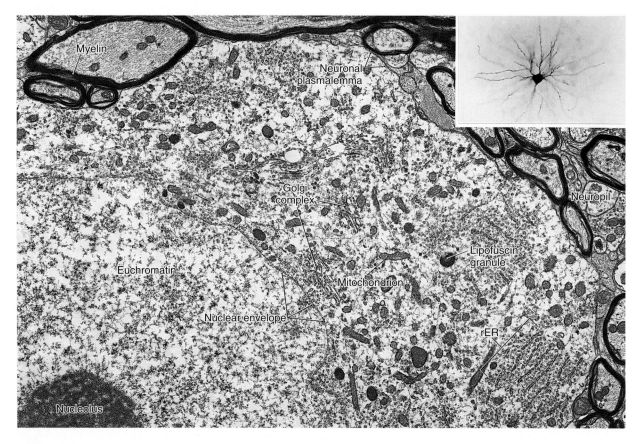

Figure 2-4. The cell body of a multipolar neuron as seen on electron micrograph and in a Golgi-stained preparation *(inset)*. *(Inset* courtesy of Dr. Jose Rafols.)

Table 2-1. A Few of the Neuronal Types Found in the Nervous System

Type of Neuron	Location of Cell Bodies
Pseudounipolar	Posterior root or cranial nerve ganglion
Bipolar	Retina
	Olfactory epithelium
	Vestibular ganglion
	Auditory (spiral) ganglion
Multipolar	
Stellate ("star-shaped")	Many areas of CNS
Fusiform ("spindle-shaped")	Many areas of CNS
Pyriform ("pear-shaped")	Many areas of CNS
Pyramidal	Hippocampus; layers II, III, V, and VI of cerebral cortex
Purkinje	Cerebellar cortex
Mitral	Olfactory bulb
Chandelier	Visual areas of cerebral cortex
Granule	Cerebral and cerebellar cortex
Amacrine ("axonless")	Retina

CNS, central nervous system.

Axons in the CNS often end in fine branches known as *terminal arbors* (Fig. 2-5C). In most neurons, each axon terminal is capped with small *terminal boutons* (*boutons termineaux*, terminal buttons) (Figs. 2-1 and 2-3C, E). These correspond to functional points of contact (synapses) between nerve cells.

In some cells, boutons are found along the length of the axon, where they are called *boutons en passant*. Other axons contain swellings, or *varicosities*, which are not button-like but still can represent points of cell-to-cell information transfer.

The site at which an axon terminal communicates with a second neuron, or with an effector tissue, is called a *synapse* (from the Greek word meaning "to clasp"). In general, the synapse can be defined as a contact between part of one neuron (usually its axon) and the dendrites, cell body, or axon of a second neuron. The contact can also be made with an effector cell such as a skeletal muscle fiber. Synapses are considered later in this chapter in the section "Neurons as Information Transmitters."

Axonal Transport

Nerve cells have an elaborate transport system that moves organelles and macromolecules between the cell body and the axon and its terminals. Transport in the axon occurs in both directions (Table 2-2; Fig. 2-6). Axonal transport from the cell body toward the terminals is called *anterograde* or *orthograde*; transport from the terminals toward the cell body is called *retrograde*.

Anterograde axonal transport is classified into *fast* and *slow* components. Fast transport, at speeds of up to 400 mm/day, is based on the action of a protein called *kinesin*. Kinesin, an adenosine triphosphatase (ATPase), moves macromolecule-containing vesicles and mitochondria along microtubules in much the same manner as a small insect crawling along a straw. Slow transport carries important structural and metabolic components from the cell body to axon terminals; its mechanism is less well understood.

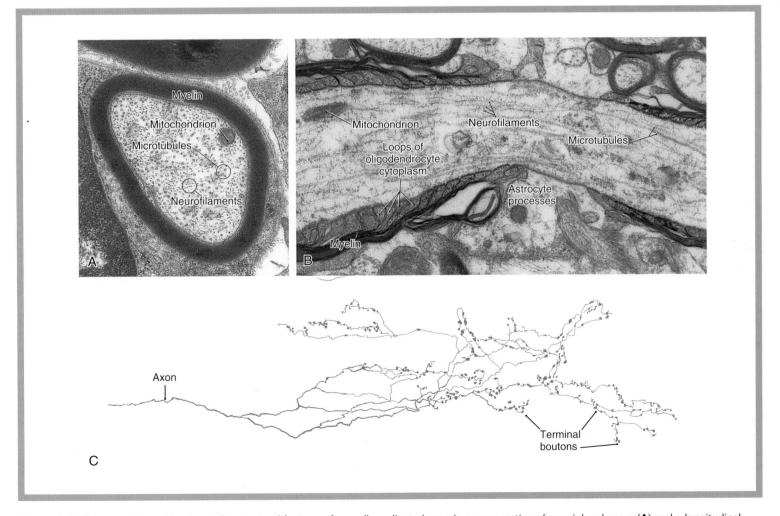

Figure 2-5. Elements of axon structure. Ultrastructural features of a small myelinated axon in a cross section of a peripheral nerve (**A**) and a longitudinal view at a node of Ranvier of a myelinated axon in the central nervous system (**B**). Drawing of the complete terminal arbor of an axon in the thalamus, reconstructed from serial sections (**C**). (**C** courtesy of Dr. Ed Lachica.)

Table 2-2. Characteristics of Axonal Transport

Direction of Transport	Speed of Transport	Proposed Mechanism	Substances Carried
Anterograde	Fast (100–400 mm/day)	Kinesin/microtubules	Proteins in vesicles
		Neurotransmitters in vesicles, mitochondria	
	Slow (~1 mm/day)	Unknown	Cytoskeletal protein components (actin, myosin, tubulin)
			Neurotransmitter-related cytosolic enzymes
Retrograde	Fast (50–250 mm/day)	Dynein/microtubules	Macromolecules in vesicles, "old" mitochondria
			Pinocytotic vesicles from axon terminal

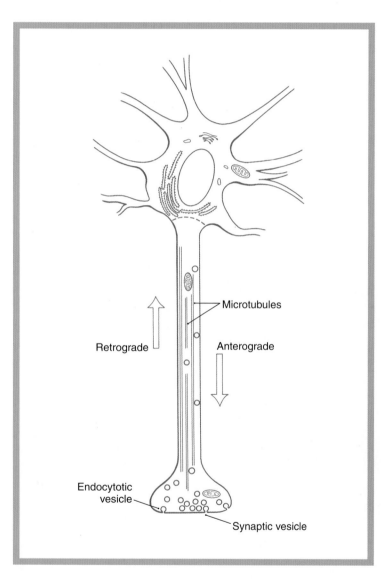

Figure 2-6. Anterograde and retrograde axonal transport.

Retrograde axonal transport allows the neuron to respond to molecules, for example, growth factors, which are taken up near the axon terminal by either *pinocytosis* or *receptor-mediated endocytosis*. In addition, this form of transport functions in the continual recycling of components of the axon terminal. Retrograde transport along axonal microtubules is driven by the protein dynein rather than by kinesin.

Axonal transport is important in the pathogenesis of some human neurologic diseases. The *rabies virus* replicates in muscle tissue at the site of a bite by a rabid animal and is then transported in a retrograde direction to the cell bodies of neurons innervating the muscle. The neurons produce and shed copies of the rabies virus, which, in turn, are taken up by the terminals of adjacent cells. In this way the infection becomes distributed throughout the CNS, causing the behavioral changes associated with this disease. From the CNS, the virus travels to the salivary glands by means of anterograde axonal transport in neurons innervating these glands. The infected salivary glands, in turn, shed the virus in the saliva.

The toxin produced by the bacterium *Clostridium tetani* is also transported in a retrograde direction in nerve cells whose axons terminate at the site of infection. *Tetanus toxin* is released from the nerve cell body and taken up by the terminals of neighboring neurons. However, unlike the rabies virus, which is replicated in the cell body, the tetanus toxin is diluted as it passes from cell to cell. In spite of this dilution effect, patients infected with C. *tetani* may suffer from a range of neurologic deficits.

Axonal Transport as a Research Tool

The ability of neurons to transport intracellular materials is exploited in investigations of neuronal connections. For example, when the enzyme *horseradish peroxidase* (HRP) or a *fluorescent substance* is injected into regions containing axon terminals, it is taken up by these processes and transported in a retrograde direction to the cell body. After histologic preparation, the cell bodies containing these retrograde tracers are visualized. The presence of the label in a cell body suggests that the neuron has axon terminals at the site of injection.

Tracer studies can also exploit the anterograde transport system of neurons. For example, if radioactively labeled amino acids are injected into a group of neuronal cell bodies, they will be incorporated into neuronal proteins and transported in an anterograde direction. The axons containing the labeled proteins can then be detected by autoradiography. Another commonly used anterograde tracer is HRP conjugated to the glycoprotein-binding molecule (lectin) *wheat germ agglutinin* (WGA-HRP). Anterograde tracers are used to identify the distribution patterns of axons arising from a specific population of neuronal cell bodies.

The fact that the cell body is the trophic center of the neuron provides two other methods of studying connections in the nervous system. If the cell body is destroyed, the axon undergoes *anterograde (wallerian)* degeneration. These degenerated axons can be visualized when neural tissue is impregnated with silver nitrate. Variations on this method make it possible to conduct studies on human material obtained at autopsy. Conversely, injury to the axon will result in a set of changes in the cell body that are referred to as *chromatolysis*. The cell body swells, the nucleus assumes an eccentric position, and the Nissl substance disperses. (This breakup of the dye-binding parts of the cell gives chromatolysis its name.) This technique has also been used in animal experimentation and in human autopsy material.

Classification of Neurons and Groups of Neurons

Functionally related nerve cell bodies and axons are often aggregated to form distinct structures in the nervous system. Table 2-3 lists the main terms used for such structures. In the CNS, a cluster of functionally related nerve cell bodies is most commonly called a *nucleus* (plural, *nuclei*), although cell bodies that are arranged in a layer may be called a *layer, lamina,* or *stratum* and columnar groups of cell bodies may be called *columns*. This last term is used for two types of structures. In the cerebral cortex it refers to a group of cells that are related by function and by the location of the stimulus that drives them. These functional groups form columns oriented perpendicular to the plane of the cortex. The second type of column is found in the spinal cord and refers to a longitudinal group of functionally related cells that extend for part or all of the length of the brainstem or spinal cord.

Bundles of axons in the CNS are called *tracts, fasciculi,* or *lemnisci*. These are typically composed of specific populations of functionally related fibers (as in the corticospinal tract and medial lemniscus). A group of several tracts or fasciculi is called a *funiculus* or, in certain cases, a *system*. In the peripheral nervous system (PNS), collections of cell bodies form a *ganglion* (plural, *ganglia*), which may be either *sensory* (dorsal root, cranial nerve) or *motor* (visceromotor or autonomic); and axons make up *nerves, rami,* or *roots*.

As noted previously, neurons can be classified into multipolar, pseudounipolar, or bipolar neurons on the basis of shape of the cell body and the number and arrangement of processes. Neurons may also be classified on the basis of functional characteristics. A neuron that conducts signals from the periphery toward the CNS is called *afferent;* one that conducts signals in the opposite direction is called *efferent*. Neurons with long axons that convey signals to a distant target are called *projection neurons,* whereas neurons that act locally (because their dendrites and axon are limited to the vicinity of the cell body) are called *interneurons* or *local circuit cells*.

Neurotransmitter specificity also can be used to describe neurons and their axons. For example, cells that contain the neurotransmitter *dopamine* are called *dopaminergic* neurons. The neurons whose axons form the corticospinal tracts produce the neurotransmitter *glutamate* and are called *glutamatergic*.

The distinctions among categories based on shape, projection type, or transmitter type are not as clear as those implied in the preceding discussion. For example, most neurons only vaguely resemble the "ideal" multipolar cell. In addition, neurons may overlap several categories of classification. In practice, reference to ganglia, nuclei, and tracts commonly uses a blend of these terms. For example, *posterior root ganglion* cells are *pseudounipolar* (their shape), *sensory* (type of input), and *afferent* (information conveyed toward the CNS), and many are *peptidergic* (they contain peptides such as substance P).

Electrical Properties of Neurons

The communicative function of neurons is carried out by fluctuations in their electrical potential. Chapter 3 explains the electrical properties of neurons in depth; at this point, only a brief introduction is needed.

Neurons carry a negative electrical charge relative to the extracellular fluid bathing them. The negative charge is due to the preponderance of negatively charged protein molecules and negative ions such as chloride within the cell. Outside the cell,

Table 2-3. Terms Used to Describe Groupings of Neuronal Components

Name	Description	Examples
CNS Structures Nucleus (plural, nuclei)	A group of functionally related nerve cell bodies in the CNS	Inferior olivary nucleus, nucleus, ambiguus, caudate nucleus
Column	In the cerebral cortex, a group of nerve cell bodies that are related in function and in the location of the stimulus that drives them and that form a column oriented perpendicular to the plane of the cortex	The ocular dominance and orientation columns of the visual cortex
	In the spinal cord, a group of functionally related nerve cell bodies that form a longitudinal column extending through part or all of the length of the spinal cord	Clarke's column
Layer, lamina (laminae), stratum (strata)	A group of functionally related cells that form a layer oriented parallel to the plane of the larger neural structure that includes it	Layer IV of cerebral cortex, the stratum opticum of superior colliculus
Tract, fasciculus (fasciculi), lemniscus (lemnisci) (*fasciculus* is Latin for "bundle")	A bundle of parallel axons in the CNS	Optic tract, corticospinal tract, medial longitudinal fasciculus, fasciculus gracilis, medial lemniscus
Funiculus (funiculi) (Latin for "cable")	A group of several parallel tracts or fasciculi	Anterior, posterior, and lateral funiculi of spinal cord
PNS Structures Ganglion (ganglia)	A group of nerve cell bodies located in a peripheral nerve or root; it forms a visible knot	Posterior root ganglia, trigeminal ganglion
Nerve, ramus (rami), root	A peripheral structure consisting of parallel axons plus associated cells	Facial nerve, ventral roots of spinal nerves, gray and white rami of spinal nerve roots

CNS, central nervous system; PNS, peripheral nervous system.

extracellular fluid is richer in positive ions, particularly sodium. The uneven distribution of charged particles is maintained by the neuronal plasma membrane, which limits passage of ions, permitting them to cross only when specific *ion channels* open. The plasma membrane is therefore referred to as *semi-permeable* because certain ions can cross at certain times but there is not a free exchange.

The opening and closing of specific ion channels can be controlled by chemical signals, including neurotransmitters. Channels in some sensory receptor neurons can be controlled by mechanical distortion of the membrane. Still other channels are controlled by voltage changes in the neuron. These allow for an explosive feed-forward amplification from a small, chemically induced voltage change to a much larger *action potential* that occurs with the simultaneous opening of a large number of channels at once. The small, chemically induced voltage changes are restricted to tiny local areas within the neuron. They result in *depolarization* of the neuron, if positive (sodium) ions enter the cell, reducing its net negative charge, or *hyperpolarization* if positive (potassium) ions exit, increasing the total negative charge inside the cell.

When the sum of all tiny, local depolarizations and hyperpolarizations reaches a threshold of depolarization at the initial segment of the axon, then the voltage-controlled sodium channels open, producing an action potential. The action potential is large enough that it does not remain local but is propagated anterogradely along the entire length of the axon and reaches all of the axon terminals. Arrival of the action potential at the axon terminals causes release of neurotransmitter at synapses, stimulating ion channel opening and local electrical voltage changes in the next neuron in the chain of communication, the postsynaptic neuron.

Neurons as Information Receivers

Neurons collect, transform, and transmit information. Collection of information by the nerve cell is the first step in this chain of events. Neurons can receive input from other neurons or directly from the environment. *Sensory information* enters the nervous system by the latter of the two routes.

Sensory Neural Information

Neurons that receive information from the environment are called *primary sensory neurons*. These include photoreceptors, chemoreceptors, mechanoreceptors, thermoreceptors, and nociceptors. Further information on these receptor types is found in the chapters describing sensory systems. For most receptors, a stimulus results in a graded depolarizing potential in the primary sensory neuron, called a *generator potential*.

The process of converting sensory input into a form interpretable by the nervous system is *transduction*. Each type of sensory receptor transduces a physical stimulus into electrical or chemical changes, which then can be transmitted as signals within the nervous system.

The rod and cone *photoreceptors* of the retina are specialized for transducing light energy in the form of *photons*. As few as three photons (possibly even a single photon!) can be detected by a trained human observer. As a photon strikes the photoreceptor, it sets in motion a complex chain of events culminating in the closing of a large number of sodium channels that normally are open. As a result, the photoreceptor cell becomes *hyperpolarized*. This makes the photoreceptor unique among sensory cells, in that the membrane potential becomes more negative on application of the stimulus, rather than more positive.

In humans, the taste and olfactory receptor cells mediate the two primary types of *chemoreception*. Both receptor types respond to the presence of specific chemicals dissolved in a solution. Also included in this category are receptors in the hypothalamus, which sense low blood glucose, low oxygen tension, or changes in blood pH; O_2 and pH receptors are also found in the aortic sinus and the carotid body.

Mechanoreceptors transduce various qualities of physical force into electrical signals that are transmitted by sensory neurons. Such receptors are found in the vestibular, auditory, and somatosensory systems.

Other types of sensory receptors include *nociceptors*, which transduce noxious (painful) stimuli, and *thermoreceptors*, which sense temperature changes in the skin and viscera. These receptors mediate what is commonly called "pain"; this is one of the most common complaints in clinical medicine.

Other Neural Information

Although sensory neurons transduce external stimuli, most nerve cells rely on other neurons for input. In general, the direction of information flow in a neuron is from dendrites to soma to axon, but most cells also receive information at their cell bodies, and many receive information at the axon terminal. In all these cases, the reception of information is mediated by synapses. Synapses are the points of information transfer from one neuron to another.

Neurons as Information Transmitters

Synapses

The synapse is the location at which a process of one neuron (usually an axon terminal) communicates with a second neuron or an effector (gland or muscle) cell. In general, there are two broad morphologic categories of synapses, *chemical* and *electrical* (or *electrotonic*). The vast majority of synapses in the mammalian CNS are of the chemical type.

Chemical Synapses

The most common type of CNS synapse comprises an axon terminal of one neuron that is apposed to a dendrite or dendritic spine of a second neuron. The prototypical chemical synapse consists of a *presynaptic element*, a *postsynaptic element*, and the intervening space (the *synaptic cleft*), which is 20 to 50 nm wide (Figs. 2-1 and 2-7). The presynaptic element typically takes the form of an axonal bouton. The bouton contains mitochondria, which supply energy for synaptic function, and also a prominent collection of *vesicles*, which contain the neurotransmitter that will be released into the synaptic cleft. These vesicles are often aggregated near sites on the presynaptic membrane called *active sites* (or *zones*), which are the sites of neurotransmitter release. Directly across the synaptic cleft is the postsynaptic membrane, which often appears thick and dark in electron micrographs (Figs. 2-1 and 2-7). Mitochondria are typically present in its vicinity.

As explained in detail in Chapter 4, communication across the synapse is mediated by the neurotransmitter stored in the presynaptic vesicles (Figs. 2-1 and 2-8). Neurotransmitter release is initiated by the arrival of an action potential, which depolarizes the presynaptic terminal. In the terminal, depolarization causes *calcium channels* to open. The resulting influx of Ca^{2+} into the cell initiates a sequence of events that cause synaptic vesicles to fuse with the presynaptic plasma membrane and release their neurotransmitter into the cleft (see Chapter 4 for more detail). The transmitter diffuses across the cleft to bind to specific *receptors* on the postsynaptic membrane, and this event triggers an electrochemical or biochemical change in the postsynaptic cell. This change represents the information as received by the postsynaptic cell.

Two functional properties of chemical synapses should be noted. First, they are *unidirectional*; that is, they transmit information only in the direction from the presynaptic cell to

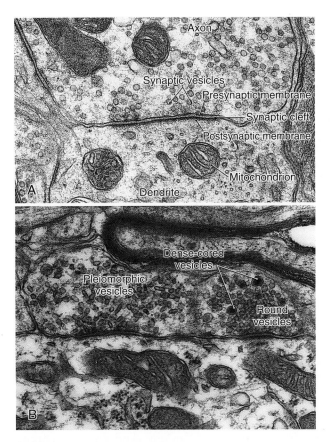

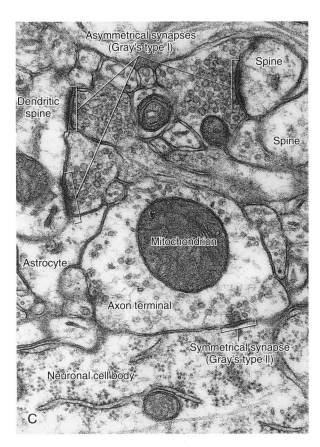

Figure 2-7. Ultrastructural elements of a chemical synapse (**A**) and three principal forms of synaptic vesicles (**B**). Examples of asymmetrical and symmetrical synapses in visual cortex (**C**). (**C** courtesy of Dr. Alan Peters.)

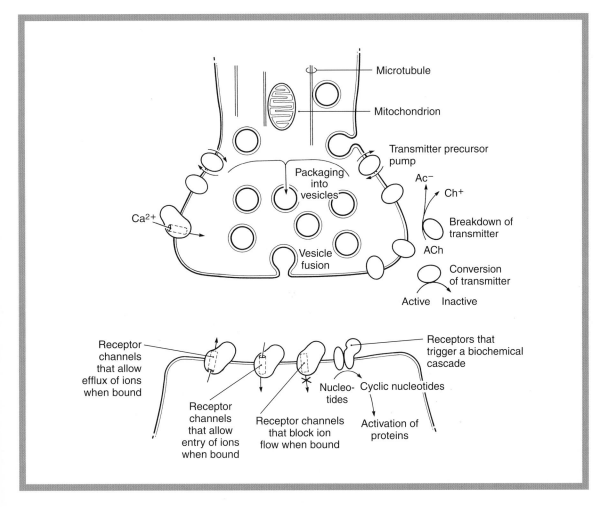

Figure 2-8. Diagrammatic representation of the events occurring at a generalized chemical synapse. Ac⁻, acetate; ACh, acetylcholine; Ch⁺, choline.

Table 2-4. Morphologic Characteristics of Gray Type I and Type II Synapses

Gray Type I Synapses
Dense material present on postsynaptic membrane but not presynaptic membrane (so that the synapse is visibly asymmetrical)
Synaptic cleft 30 nm wide
Synaptic vesicles round and large (30–60 nm), with clear centers
Synaptic region up to 1–2 μm long

Gray Type II Synapses
Dense material present on both the presynaptic and the postsynaptic membranes (so that the synapse appears symmetrical)
Synaptic cleft 20 nm wide
Synaptic vesicles oval, flattened, or pleiomorphic (variable) in shape
Synaptic region less than 1 μm long

the postsynaptic cell. This directionality results because only the presynaptic cell releases the neurotransmitter, and only the postsynaptic cell expresses the receptor protein that will elicit the normal postsynaptic response to the neurotransmitter. Second, the strength of the effect on the postsynaptic membrane is variable and depends partly on the amount of neurotransmitter released into the synapse. Each synaptic vesicle contains a fixed amount of neurotransmitter (called a *quantum*), so the amount of neurotransmitter released depends on the number of vesicles that fuse with the presynaptic membrane in response to Ca^{2+} influx.

With light microscopy, chemical synapses are visible only as the terminal boutons of an axon, but in the early years of electron microscopy, two basic morphologic types of synapse became apparent. They were named *Gray type I* and *type II* synapses. The characteristics of these synapse types are listed in Table 2-4 and illustrated in Figure 2-7C. At one time it was believed that type I synapses were excitatory in function and type II synapses were inhibitory. We now know that the excitatory or inhibitory function of a synapse depends on the nature of the receptors present on the postsynaptic membrane and cannot be reliably predicted from the ultrastructural characteristics of the presynaptic bouton. Nevertheless, the scheme is still a useful way to classify chemical synapses. For example, synapses using acetylcholine often have the Gray type I morphology, whereas those using γ-aminobutyric acid (GABA) usually resemble Gray's type II synapses.

Although the vesicles of Gray type I and type II synapses differ in size and shape, in both cases the centers of the vesicles appear clear (electron lucent). Vesicles with an electron-dense core are also seen in some synaptic endings; these dense-cored vesicles are generally thought to contain neuropeptides or serotonin as a neurotransmitter. This type of synapse is not included in the Gray classification.

Neurotransmitters

As we have seen, *neurotransmitters* are a means by which information is exchanged among nerve cells as well as between nerve cells and effector cells. Neurotransmitters are considered fully in Chapter 4 and are mentioned here briefly in relation to the structure of a typical neuron.

Some neurotransmitters appear to be consistently either excitatory (i.e., glutamate) or inhibitory (i.e., GABA), but the effect (excitation or inhibition) of a neurotransmitter on a responsive postsynaptic neuron is not due to any inherent property of the signaling molecule itself. Rather, the nature of the specific receptor dictates the response. For example, neurons that respond to the neurotransmitter dopamine can express either of

two types of dopamine receptors. Binding of dopamine to one of these, the D_1 receptor, results in activation of adenylate cyclase, whereas binding of dopamine to the other, the D_2 receptor, results in inhibition of adenylate cyclase activity.

Neurotransmitters may be *biogenic amines* (e.g., acetylcholine, dopamine, norepinephrine), *amino acids* (e.g., glutamate, GABA), *nucleotides* (e.g., adenosine), *neuropeptides* (e.g., substance P, cholecystokinin, somatostatin), or even *gases* (e.g., nitric oxide, carbon monoxide). Many of these neurotransmitters are stored in and released from synaptic vesicles in the axon terminal as described previously, but in other cases (e.g., nitric oxide) generation and release of the neurotransmitter does not involve vesicles.

Biogenic amines (acetylcholine) and amino acid neurotransmitters (GABA) are synthesized in the axon terminal, although the enzymes necessary for their synthesis are produced in the cell body and shipped to the terminal by axonal transport. The axon lacks the machinery to synthesize proteins (or membrane lipids) and thus must obtain these materials from the cell body. Thus, *axonal transport* is always necessary to support synaptic function.

Disorders of Neurotransmitter Metabolism

Disorders of neurotransmitter metabolism account for a large variety of neurologic and psychiatric illnesses, but in many cases the etiology is not well understood. This category of diseases is under intensive investigation, and four examples are briefly discussed here.

Parkinson disease affects dopamine-synthesizing neurons located in an area of the brainstem known as the *substantia nigra*. For unknown reasons, these dopaminergic cells begin dying at an accelerated rate. The loss of dopamine results in a characteristic tremor and inability to properly control movement. Originally, therapy involved administering supplements of L-dopa, a precursor for dopamine. This treatment increases dopamine synthesis by mass action but loses its effectiveness with time. Currently, therapy involves a combination of L-dopa with carbidopa, which inhibits the enzyme L-aromatic amino acid decarboxylase. Because carbidopa cannot cross the *blood-brain barrier* (defined later), it decreases the metabolism of L-dopa in peripheral tissues, making more L-dopa available to the CNS for dopamine synthesis in the remaining neurons.

Bipolar disorder affects several million Americans and appears to be caused by imbalances in the phosphatidyl inositol (PI)–linked neurotransmitter systems. An increase in PI turnover is a biochemical change triggered by some subcategories of acetylcholine, serotonin, norepinephrine, and histamine receptors. It is thought that a pathologic imbalance in PI turnover may result in mood changes. The drug lithium carbonate stabilizes PI turnover, thereby stabilizing the patient's mood.

Alzheimer disease affects more than 1 million Americans. Although the accuracy of diagnosis by psychological testing has improved, a definitive diagnosis can be made only by postmortem microscopic examination of brain tissue. Alzheimer disease is characterized by the degeneration of neurons in basal forebrain nuclei, the loss of synapses in the cerebral cortex and hippocampus, and the presence of pathologic structures called *neurofibrillary tangles* and *senile plaques*. Cortical cells normally receive terminals from *cholinergic* (acetylcholine-releasing) cells in the basal forebrain nuclei. In Alzheimer disease these terminals are lost and the activity of choline acetyltransferase (the enzyme responsible for acetylcholine synthesis) in the cortex and hippocampus of diseased patients is extremely low. Other neurotransmitter systems, particularly neuropeptides, are also affected by this disease.

In many cases of *myasthenia gravis*, the patient's immune system produces antibodies to the nicotinic acetylcholine receptor, a ligand-gated channel found at the synapse between primary motor neurons and skeletal muscle fibers. Binding of these antibodies to the receptor results in pathologic destruction of the neuromuscular junctions, which in turn causes the muscle weakness characteristic of this disease.

Glia

Unlike neurons, glial cells do not propagate action potentials. Rather, they provide neurons with structural support and maintain the appropriate microenvironment essential for neuronal function. In addition, astrocytes modulate synaptic activity in their vicinity by releasing small amounts of glutamate.

Glia account for most of the cells in the nervous system, and normal brain function requires them. The major types of glial cells in the CNS (Fig. 2-9; Table 2-5) are *astrocytes* and *oligodendrocytes*, derived from neuroectoderm, and *microglia*, derived from mesoderm. The analogous cell types in the PNS are the satellite cells, Schwann cells, and macrophages.

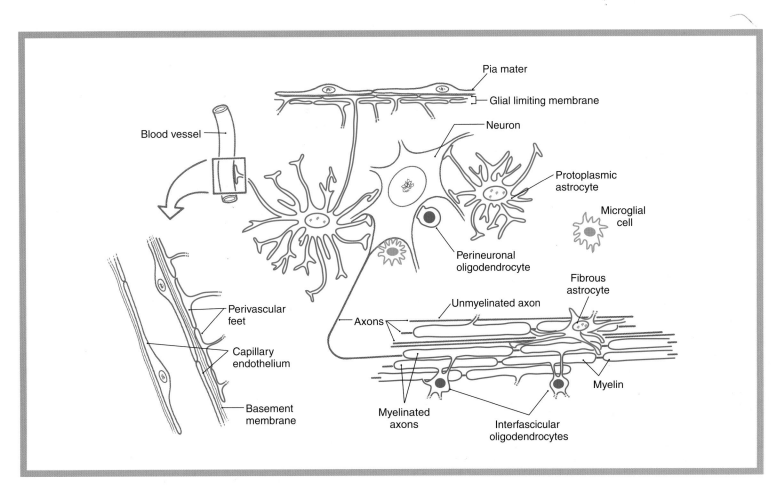

Figure 2-9. Relationships of central nervous system glial cells to neuronal cell bodies, axons, blood vessels, and pia mater.

Table 2-5. Types of Glial Cells and Their Locations and Functions

Cell Type	Location	Function(s)
CNS Astrocytes	Throughout the CNS; contact neuronal cells bodies, dendrites, and axons and form a complete lining around the external surfaces of the CNS and around CNS blood vessels; gray matter astrocytes are called *protoplasmic* and white matter astrocytes are called *fibrous*	Maintenance of extracellular ionic environment; secretion of growth factors; structural and metabolic support of neurons

Oligodendrocytes
  Myelinating
  Satellite cells
	Form myelin sheaths around CNS axons
	Surround CNS neuronal cell bodies
		Myelination
		Unknown

Microglia	Gray and white matter of CNS	Scavenging and phagocytosis of debris following cell injury and death; secretion of cytokines
PNS Schwann cells	Form myelin sheaths around myelinated axons and ensheath unmyelinated axons	Myelination; biochemical and structural support of myelinated and unmyelinated axons
Satellite cells	Surround neuronal cell bodies in PNS ganglia	Unknown

CNS, central nervous system; PNS, peripheral nervous system.

Astrocytes

Astrocytes occur throughout the CNS. They are highly branched cells with processes that contact most of the surfaces of neuronal dendrites and cell bodies, as well as some axonal surfaces. Other astrocyte processes end in expansions called *end-feet* (Fig. 2-9). Astrocyte end-feet join together to completely line the interfaces between the CNS and other tissues. The outer surface of the brain and spinal cord, where it meets the inner surface of the *pia mater* (the innermost of the meningeal membranes that enclose the CNS), is covered with a coating of several layers of joined end-feet called the *glia limitans* (or glial limiting membrane). Similarly, every blood vessel in the CNS is jacketed by a layer of end-feet that separates it from the neural tissue.

As shown in Figure 2-9, the astrocytes of gray matter, called *protoplasmic astrocytes,* differ in shape from the astrocytes of white matter, called *fibrous astrocytes* because of their greater content of intermediate filaments. Astrocytes can be distinguished immunohistochemically (for purposes of research and diagnosis) by the presence of intermediate filaments with a distinctive marker protein, *glial fibrillary acidic protein* (GFAP). The GFAP content of protoplasmic astrocytes increases in pathologic conditions.

Structural Support and Response to Injury

During development, astrocytes (in the form of radial glial cells) provide a pathway for neuronal migration. In the adult brain, astrocytes frame certain clusters of neurons, for example, the barrels of the somatosensory cortex of rodents. In white matter, they also enclose bundles of unmyelinated axons.

If injury to the CNS results in destruction of cells, the space created by the breakdown of debris is filled by proliferation or hypertrophy (or both) of astrocytes, resulting in the formation of an *astrocytic scar.* That astrocytes retain the ability to proliferate in the mature brain (and thus are susceptible to events that disrupt the control of cell division) explains why the majority of CNS tumors are of astrocytic origin.

Growth Factors and Cytokines

Current research on astrocytes indicates that they secrete growth factors vital to normal function of some neurons. They also secrete cholesterol and lipoproteins necessary for synaptic growth and plasticity. In disease processes, astrocytes may secrete cytokines and immune mediators such as interleukin (IL)-1, IL-6, and prostaglandin. Thus astrocytes as well as microglia contribute to the regulation of inflammatory processes in the CNS. Microglial cells, neurons, and neighboring astrocytes also both secrete and have receptors for cytokines such as IL-1.

Environmental Modulation

The ionic composition and pH of the extracellular fluid are buffered by astrocytes. These cells have ion channels in their membranes that are different from those in neurons. For example, potassium ions released from neurons during firing of an action potential are cleared from the extracellular space by astrocytes via plasma membrane ion channels. Astrocytes are connected to each other by gap junctions and act as syncytia through which excess potassium ions are shunted to perivascular spaces, restoring balance after heavy local activity. Astrocytes also propagate calcium waves, which spread through gap junctions between astrocytes to cover broad areas. Intracellular calcium levels in astrocytes, as in all cells, regulate secretory activity.

Metabolism

Astrocytes participate in neurotransmitter metabolism. Their membranes have receptors for some neuroactive substances and uptake systems for others. Astrocytic uptake systems serve to quickly terminate the postsynaptic effect of some neurotransmitters by removing them from the synaptic cleft. For example, the amino acid neurotransmitter glutamate is taken up by astrocytes and is then inactivated by the enzymatic addition of ammonia to produce glutamine (catalyzed by the enzyme *glutamine synthetase*). Glutamine released from astrocytes can be taken up and reconverted to glutamate in neurons. This astrocytic pathway also detoxifies ammonia in the CNS.

In addition to this metabolic support role, astrocytes modulate synaptic transmission by releasing small amounts of glutamate, a transmitter that binds to extrasynaptic glutamate receptors on nearby neurons (Fig. 2-10). Astrocytes release glutamate when their intracellular calcium rises in response to neuronal glutamate or other neurotransmitters or in response to inflammatory mediators such as prostaglandin from microglia.

Regional Heterogeneity

Astrocytes vary biochemically between gray matter (protoplasmic astrocytes) and white matter (fibrous astrocytes), and from one region of gray matter to another. White matter astrocytes differ from gray matter astrocytes in terms of their ion channels, neurotransmitter receptors and uptake systems, and other special properties. For unknown reasons, astrocyte tumors of particular types occur in characteristic distributions rather than with random frequency throughout the CNS. For example, the malignant tumor glioblastoma multiforme develops most frequently in the frontal or temporal lobe of the cerebral cortex.

Astrocytes at the Blood-Brain Barrier

In many tissues, solutes can pass freely between the capillary plasma and the interstitial space by diffusing through gaps between endothelial cells. In the CNS, vessels are induced by the surrounding jacket of astrocyte end-feet to form extensive tight junctions, so solutes can reach the neural tissue only by passing through the endothelial cells (Fig. 2-11). The resulting restricted exchange constitutes the *blood-brain barrier.* In a strict sense, the blood-brain barrier is formed by the tight junctions of the endothelium. However, many people refer to the blood-brain barrier more inclusively as the physical complex of endothelium, basal lamina, and astrocyte end-feet surrounding each CNS vessel (see also Chapter 8). Water, gases, and lipid-soluble small molecules can diffuse across the endothelial cells, but other substances must by carried across by transport systems, and their exchange is highly selective. This selectivity is further enhanced by a reduction in pinocytotic transport. In most tissues of the body, a high level of pinocytotic activity by endothelial cells transports solutes nonspecifically from the blood plasma to the perivascular space. In contrast, endothelial cells of capillaries in most parts of the CNS show little pinocytotic activity. The blood-brain barrier is of major clinical importance because it largely excludes many drugs from the CNS.

Oligodendrocytes

Oligodendrocytes, like astrocytes, occur in both gray matter and white matter (Fig. 2-9). The function of oligodendrocytes is *myelination,* that is, the provision of an electrochemically insulating sheath around all but the smallest axons in the white matter (Figs. 2-9 and 2-12). Other oligodendrocytes lie adjacent to and surround neuronal cell bodies in the gray matter, but they do not make myelin and the significance of this arrangement is not well understood.

A myelin sheath is a membranous wrapping around an axon that greatly increases the speed of conduction of action potentials along the axon. Large-diameter axons have thick myelin sheaths and high conduction velocities; smaller-diameter axons have thinner myelin sheaths and slower conduction velocities;

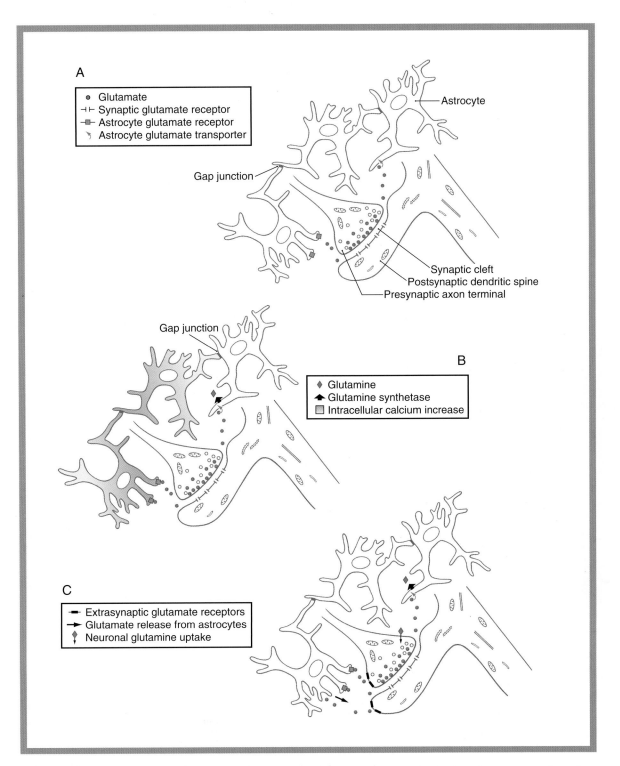

Figure 2-10. Astrocytes participate in neural transmission. Glutamatergic transmission is affected in two ways. First, glutamate *(red circles)* diffusing from active synapses is taken up by the astrocyte glutamate transporter (on uppermost astrocyte in **A**, **B**, and **C**) to be metabolized to glutamine (**B** and **C**, *green diamonds*). Glutamine in turn is transported into the presynaptic axon terminal for recycling into glutamate (**B** and **C**). Second, astrocyte cell surface receptors for glutamate *(blue squares)* also respond to the neurotransmitter, increasing intracellular calcium (indicated by *gray shading* of astrocytes in **B** and **C**; *darker gray* represents greater increase in calcium concentration, *lighter gray* indicates less increase). The calcium increase passes via gap junctions to neighboring astrocytes. The increase in intracellular calcium causes astrocytes to release small amounts of glutamate, affecting extrasynaptic glutamate receptors on neighboring neurons (**C**). Activation of extrasynaptic glutamate receptors on the presynaptic axon terminal modulates transmitter release, and on the postsynaptic neuron it modulates responses (EPSPs and IPSPs) to synaptic transmission.

and the smallest axons are unmyelinated and have the slowest conduction velocities.

Myelin is formed by a cell-cell interaction in which an axon destined for myelination is recognized by proteins on the oligodendrocyte surface. The oligodendrocyte responds by producing a flattened, sheet-like process that wraps repeatedly around the axon (Fig. 2-13). As the layers of membrane accumulate, all cytoplasm is excluded, so that the mature myelin sheath consists of layers of oligodendrocyte plasma membrane firmly pressed together. Cytoplasm remains only in the innermost and outermost turns of the oligodendrocyte process.

The myelin sheath surrounding an axon is not continuous along its entire length. Rather, the axon is covered by a series of myelin segments, each formed by an oligodendroglial cell. The interruptions between segments are called *nodes of Ranvier* (Fig. 2-5B). Morphologic specializations at the nodes include a dense undercoating of the axonal membrane, as seen at the initial segment of the axon, and contact by an astrocyte process. The

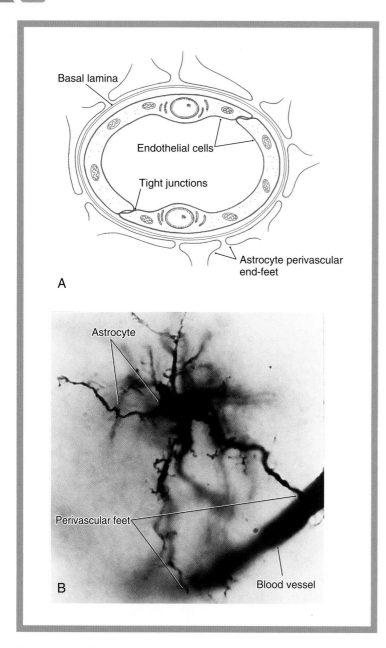

Figure 2-11. The relationship of astrocytes to CNS blood vessels. **A,** Perivascular end-feet cover blood vessels of the CNS. **B,** Golgi-stained astrocyte with end-feet apposed to a blood vessel. (**B** courtesy of Dr. Jose Rafols.)

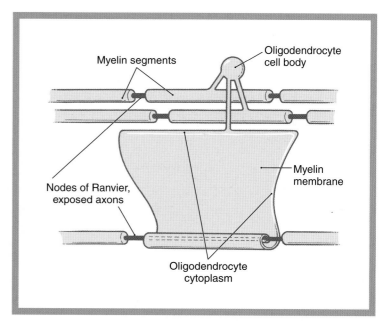

Figure 2-12. Myelin sheath formation by processes of an oligodendrocyte. The cytoplasm of the oligodendrocyte is trapped on the edges of the cell membrane as it wraps around the axon. (Based on data from Butt AM, Ransom BR: Visualization of oligodendrocytes and astrocytes in the intact rat optic nerve by intracellular injection of lucifer yellow and horseradish peroxidase. Glia 2:470-475, 1989.)

Microglia

Microglial cells are the immune effector cells of the CNS and are the predominant cells involved in CNS inflammation. The embryonic origin of the microglial cells is controversial, but the prevailing view is that they develop from hematopoietic cells of the monocyte-macrophage lineage, which migrate into the CNS during development. Microglia make up about 1% of the CNS cell population (Fig. 2-9). During health, they are considered to be at rest, or quiescent.

Like macrophages, microglia are able to become phagocytic scavengers. When the CNS suffers injury, activated microglial cells migrate to the site of damage, where they proliferate and phagocytose cell debris.

The cytokines IL-1β and tumor necrosis factor-α (TNF-α), as well as other cytokines and prostaglandins, are secreted by activated microglial cells. Some of the molecules secreted by activated microglial cells are neurotoxic (including glutamate, oxygen radicals, and TNF-α), and neurons may be directly damaged by inflammatory reactions in the CNS. Thus, microglial reaction may be a secondary cause of neuronal damage following *stroke* or *trauma*. Excessive secretion of IL-1β and TNF-α by microglial cells also induces endothelial cells to open the blood-brain barrier, allowing leukocyte infiltration into the brain parenchyma. CNS inflammation of such magnitude can be fatal in *bacterial meningitis*. For this reason, immunosuppressive drugs may be given with antibiotics to treat the infection.

Microglial cells are the CNS cells targeted by human immunodeficiency virus (HIV), the virus that causes *acquired immunodeficiency syndrome* (AIDS). The mechanism by which HIV infection of microglia leads to neuronal damage and dementia is not yet fully understood.

Inflammatory processes in the CNS can lead to oxidative damage to tissue due to release of oxygen radicals by microglia and astrocytes. Inflammatory processes can be both injurious and protective. For example, in multiple sclerosis, demyelination results from inflammatory signaling that allows T lymphocytes to extravasate and enter CNS tissue. However, animal experiments have shown that inflammatory signaling molecules are

rapid ionic exchanges across the axonal membrane essential for generating the action potential and propagating it down the axon occur at the nodes of Ranvier. The depolarization is then passively conducted along the axon (as a graded potential) to the next node. This method, *saltatory conduction*, is faster than having ionic exchanges occur continuously along the length of the axon.

The segments of myelin between adjacent nodes of Ranvier are called *internodal segments*, or *internodes*. Although the name *oligodendrocyte* means "cell with few branches," some of these cells give rise to myelinating processes forming internodal segments on as many as 40 axons.

In *demyelinating* diseases, such as *multiple sclerosis*, groups of oligodendrocytes and their corresponding myelin segments degenerate and are replaced by astrocytic plaques. This loss of myelin results in an interruption of the propagation of the action potential down these axons. Demyelinated axons survive temporarily, and some remyelination is possible by the growth of oligodendrocyte precursor cells that reside in the adult CNS. The particular array of motor, visual, or general sensory losses in a patient with multiple sclerosis reflects the locations of the demyelinating lesions.

also necessary for remyelination of axons by oligodendrocyte precursors.

Tumors of the Central Nervous System

Primary brain tumors arise from the cells that make up the structure of the brain and spinal cord, as well as its coverings. Individual cells belonging to any of the cell populations found in brain tissue or the leptomeninges can give rise to a brain tumor, provided that genetic and environmental stimuli favor cell proliferation.

Glia-Derived Tumors

Glial cells are a frequent source of primary brain tumors in adults and children, and, of these, astrocytomas are the glial tumors encountered most often. To help predict the outcome for the patient, astrocytomas are traditionally evaluated on the basis of how closely or how little the neoplastic cells resemble non-neoplastic astrocytes (degree of differentiation). This *grading* of astrocytomas is an attempt to better define the biologic aggressiveness of the tumor and to approximate the tumor's effect on the life span of the patient (prognosis).

Grade 1 astrocytomas are uncommon tumors that resemble differentiated astrocytes that react to an injury within brain tissue (Fig. 2-13A). Usually they arise from fibrillary astrocytes in the white matter, which have many stubby processes (Fig. 2-13E). They grow slowly, and gradual enlargement may be the main clue that a neoplasm does exist. Occasionally, proto-plasmic astrocytes, denizens of gray matter with fewer processes, may form tumors that contain fluid-filled cysts.

The astrocytes of *grade 2* astrocytoma, which have prominent processes filled with glial filaments, infiltrate between myelinated axons in white matter and increasingly cluster around neurons in cortical gray matter (Fig. 2-13B). Although commonly encountered in adult patients, years may elapse before these tumors are symptomatic. However, if they recur after surgery, these astrocytomas may become more aggressive, transforming into a higher grade. Generally grade 1 and 2 astrocytomas are slowly growing masses.

Grade 3 astrocytomas have nuclei that are often enlarged, with increased density of chromatin. Uniformity of nuclear appearance is lost. Mitotic figures, consisting of chromosomes on spindles (Fig. 2-13C), may be frequently noted in tumor cells and are one indicator of rapid cell proliferation. The density of blood vessels is increased. These are rapidly growing, malignant tumors.

Grade 4 astrocytomas are highly malignant tumors. The astrocytes of these tumors may be spindled, and the elongated nuclei may have many mitotic figures. They can invade the lepto-meninges, spreading from one contiguous gyrus to its neighbor. Also known as *glioblastoma multiforme* (GBM), this astrocytoma subtype characteristically extends from one hemisphere into the other as it marches through the corpus callosum. Complex neovascular structures (Fig. 2-13D), and sharp borders between living and dead tumor tissue (Fig. 2-13F), are intrinsic features of glioblastoma. Unfortunately, this "high grade" tumor is the most common astrocytoma encountered in middle-aged and elderly adult patients. After diagnosis, the survival time of some patients with a grade 4 tumor (GBM) may be measured in only weeks.

Oligodendroglia, which myelinate axons in the white matter, are also found in the gray matter, where they are neuronal "satellite" cells. These cells can produce slow-growing tumors, located in the lobes of the brain rather than in the diencephalon or in the basal ganglia. The oligodendroglia in these tumors have dark, round nuclei centered within clear cytoplasm, much like the yolk of a fried egg embedded in egg white. Tumor cells form sheets that are subdivided into geometric units by capillary twigs. Hallmarks of oligodendrogliomas are enlarged clusters around neurons (satellitosis) and nodules of tumor cells beneath the pia.

The ventricular spaces of the brain and the central canal of the spinal cord are lined by an epithelium of ependymal cells. Tumors of these cells are termed *ependymomas*. When ependymomas occur in children or adolescents, they are found in the fourth ventricle. In adults, they are located in the spinal cord, especially at the cervical level. These glial tumors are less infiltrative than astrocytomas. Because they are more circumscribed, they can be more easily dissected away from the surrounding spinal tissues and removed by a neurosurgeon.

Tumors that stem from the last member of the glial family, microglia, were first depicted as forming cellular aggregates around tiny arterioles. The modern interpretation is that these tumors are lymphomas, a large family of neoplasms consisting of bone marrow–derived (B lymphocytes) or thymus-derived cells (T lymphocytes). Unlike the lymph nodes in which these tumors predominate, there are no lymphatics in the brain. Current thinking suggests that the malignant cells reach the central nervous system by breaching the barrier between blood and brain tissue. Lymphomas of the brain are more frequent in patients who suffer from one of the various states of acquired immunodeficiency (e.g., HIV infection or immunodeficiency induced by medicines required after organ transplants). In addition, genetic footprints of another virus (Epstein-Barr virus) can frequently be detected when molecular genetic techniques are applied to microscopic sections of lymphomas. Some of the lymphomas can be successfully treated with medicines or radiation.

Tumors in Children

Tumors that primarily affect children may contain cells that function like stem cells. Medulloblastomas arise in the cerebellar hemispheres of children and consist of primitive "blue cells" that are capable of developing along several pathways. The initial cells can mature into members of the glial family, or into neurons, all of which may be found in the same tumor. Although the cells still appear as "blue cells," electron microscopy or immuno-histochemistry can demonstrate astrocytic or neuronal features of the incompletely differentiated cells. Most medulloblastomas retain the characteristic unrestrained growth of embryonal cells, without differentiation. They quickly spread along the surface of the brain and spinal cord and must be treated aggressively.

Benign Primary Brain Tumors

Benign primary brain tumors are often covered by a fibrous, vascularized capsule that discretely demarcates the tumor from surrounding normal brain. As a benign tumor enlarges, it pushes against brain tissue, rather than extending finger-like projections that invade white and gray matter for great distances. Benign primary brain tumors cause problems by compressing normal tissue as they grow. Frequently encountered benign primary tumors of the brain include *meningioma* (see Chapter 7) and *schwannoma*.

Metastatic Brain Tumors

Metastatic brain tumors arise from malignant cells that originate outside the nervous system. The growth pattern of metastatic tumors differs from primary tumors. Microscopic clumps of malignant cells break away from the initial growths and travel via the bloodstream to the brain. These cell aggregates become lodged at tiny arteriolar branch points, frequently located at the junction of gray and white matter. Using intracellular enzymes

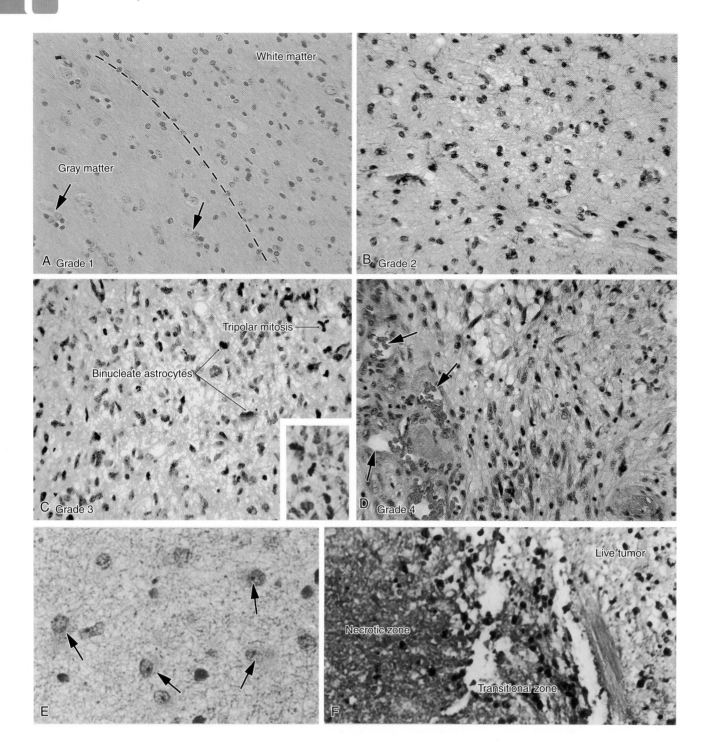

Figure 2-13. The *grades* of astrocytomas are 1/I (**A, E**), 2/II (**B**), 3/III (**C**), and 4/IV (**D, F**). *Grade 1*: The density of astrocytes, cells with vesicular chromatin and stubby processes, is increased in white matter when compared with gray matter (**A**, compare upper right with lower left). Within the gray matter these cells are clustered around neurons (**A**, *arrows*). These enlarged astrocytes have homogeneous nuclei, nucleoli, conspicuous cytoplasmic bodies, and stellate processes (**E**).
Grade 2: Astrocyte nuclei vary in shape; and the staining intensity, and cell density, is increased (**B**).
Grade 3: Heterogeneity of astrocyte size and shape (pleomorphism) is more apparent (**C**). Cells with enlarged nuclei or with two nuclei (binucleate astrocytes) are present. Abnormal tripolar mitotic figures and mitotic figures on spindles (**C**, *inset*) signify a heightened level of cell proliferation. The clear spaces between cells indicate microcystic edema.
Grade 4: Spindle-shaped, oval, elongated, and curved nuclei are abundant, indicating the extreme pleomorphism of this grade, which is also known as *glioblastoma multiforme* (**D**). Large, complex vascular structures with clusters of cells surrounding the lumina (**D**, *arrows*) are characteristic of glioblastoma. Another feature is the sharp border and the transitional zone between the live tumor and the necrotic zone (**F**).

that dissolve basement membranes, the malignant cells escape from the confines of the vasculature and start to grow in the brain. Some of the most prevalent malignant tumors that affect men and women frequently metastasize to the brain. *Lung carcinoma* is the most common primary tumor to secondarily involve the brain. *Breast carcinoma* may spread to the dura or to the brain substance. *Prostate carcinoma* can spread to the spinal cord through the veins of Batson's venous plexus.

Supporting Cells of the Peripheral Nervous System

The PNS contains supporting cells called *satellite cells* and *Schwann cells*, which are analogous to astrocytes and oligodendrocytes, respectively. Satellite cells surround the cell bodies of neurons in sensory and autonomic ganglia, and Schwann cells ensheath the axons in peripheral nerves (Fig. 2-14).

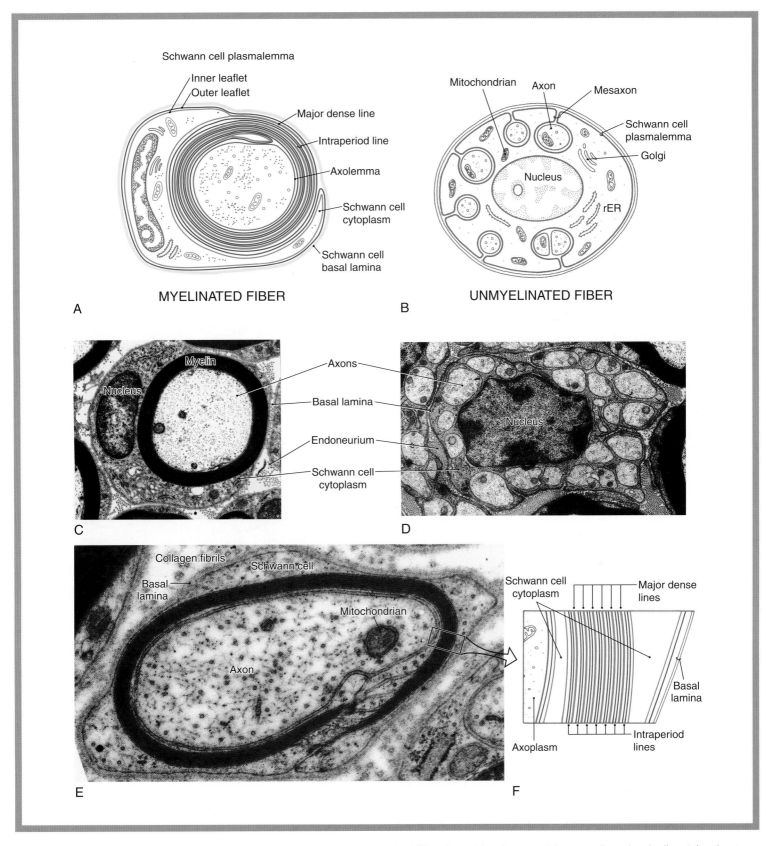

Figure 2-14. Diagrammatic representation of myelinated (**A**) and unmyelinated (**B**) fibers in peripheral nerves. Schwann cells ensheath all peripheral nerve axons. Multiple wraps of the plasmalemma of a Schwann cell fuse to form compact myelin (see also Fig. 2-13). The inner leaflet of the plasmalemma *(red)* fuses to form major dense lines, and the outer leaflets *(blue)* of each adjacent wrap contact each other to form intraperiod lines (**A**). In an unmyelinated fiber, small axons occupy troughs formed by invaginations of the Schwann cell plasmalemma (**B**). Electron micrographs of a myelinated fiber (**C**) and an unmyelinated fiber (**D**) composed of a single Schwann cell supporting more than 20 axons. A small myelinated fiber sectioned through part of a Schmidt-Lantermann cleft reveals the membrane composition of myelin (**E**). The layers of the boxed segment of myelin in **E** are diagrammed in **F**.

In the PNS, as in the CNS, large- and intermediate-diameter axons have myelin sheaths, and the smallest-diameter axons are unmyelinated. Schwann cells produce these myelin sheaths and also envelop the unmyelinated axons. The myelin sheaths are similar to the CNS type, consisting of a tight spiral wrapping of fused plasma membrane. They are also formed similarly by a Schwann cell that is attracted to an axon segment and wraps repeatedly around it to produce a compact sheath (Fig. 2-14). As in the CNS, cytoplasm remains only in the innermost and outermost layers of this wrapping (Fig. 2-14).

There are some differences between CNS and PNS myelin. Small pockets of cytoplasm known as *Schmidt-Lanterman clefts* are found at irregular intervals in PNS myelin. A *basal lamina* covers the external surface of the Schwann cell. The basal lamina is formed by the Schwann cell and may help to stabilize it during the process of myelin formation. In addition, each Schwann cell forms the myelin of only a single internode of a PNS axon, in contrast to the CNS, where oligodendrocytes send out numerous processes each of which forms a myelin internode. Unmyelinated axons in the PNS are enclosed in canals formed by invaginations in Schwann cells (Fig. 2-14). These Schwann cells also are covered by a basal lamina.

External to the Schwann cell basal lamina, peripheral nerve fibers are covered by three connective tissue sheaths (Fig. 2-15). The innermost of these, the *endoneurium*, consists of thin type III collagen fibrils and occasional fibroblasts between individual nerve fibers. At the second level, a distinctive sheath, the *perineurium*, surrounds each group (fascicle) of axons. The perineurium is composed of several concentric layers of flattened fibroblasts, which are unusual because they have a basal lamina and an abundance of pinocytotic vesicles (Fig. 2-15). Perineurial cells also are connected to each other by tight junctions. This arrangement forms a protective *blood-nerve* barrier against diffusion of substances into peripheral nerve fascicles. Last, the entire peripheral nerve is covered by *epineurium*, a dense connective tissue sheath of type I collagen and typical fibroblasts.

Tumors of peripheral nerve are usually of Schwann cell origin. The type called a *schwannoma* arises singly and, because it is encapsulated and does not include nerve fibers, is easily excised. The type known as a *neurofibroma* is usually multiple. Neurofibromas are generally difficult to remove because they are unencapsulated and infiltrate nerve bundles.

Degeneration and Regeneration

In the adult mammalian nervous system, neurons lost through disease or trauma are not replaced. Although the adult CNS retains a very small number of neural stem cells, neuronal proliferation is an almost immeasurably rare event outside the olfactory epithelium and hippocampus. In degenerative diseases, such as Parkinson or Alzheimer disease, death of neurons leads to eventual depopulation of the specific groups of neurons affected. However, if axons are damaged but the cell bodies remain intact, regeneration and return of function can occur in some circumstances.

The chance of axonal regeneration is best when a peripheral nerve is compressed or crushed but not severed. In milder lesions in which focal demyelination occurs without axonal degeneration (*neurapraxia*), there is loss of conduction in the nerve, but recovery is to be expected. When compression or crushing kills the axons distal to the site of injury, the neuronal cell bodies, which are in the spinal cord or in sensory or autonomic ganglia, usually survive. These cell bodies may undergo chromatolysis in response to the trauma. Days to weeks later, *axonal sprouting* starts at the point of injury, and the axons grow distally. Meanwhile, in the distal part of the nerve, axons die and are removed by macrophages, but the Schwann cells remain. They lose their myelin but keep their basal lamina. Within these tubes of basal lamina, Schwann cells proliferate, forming cordons called *bands of Büngner*. These Schwann cells and basal lamina tubes guide the distally growing axonal sprouts. Macrophages, which have been activated by phagocytosis of myelin debris, signal Schwann cells to secrete nerve growth factor, a neurotrophin that promotes axon growth. Regeneration depends on a variety of influences, including neurotrophins and the basal lamina. The growth rate of sprouting axons is about 1 mm/day.

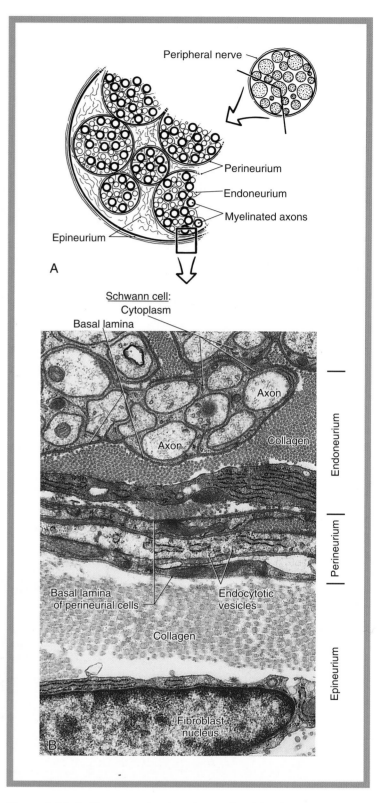

Figure 2-15. A, The connective tissue layers of peripheral nerves. **B**, An electron micrograph corresponding to the area enclosed by the box in **A** reveals ultrastructural elements characteristic of each of the three sheaths.

In a compression injury (*axonotmesis*), the proximal axon sprouts and distal bands of Schwann cells remain in their original orientation, so nerve fibers are lined up just as they were before the injury. Therefore, when the axons regenerate, they will find their original positions within the nerve and are more likely to accurately reconnect with their proper targets.

When a peripheral nerve is severed (*neurotmesis*) rather than crushed, regeneration is less likely to occur. Sprouting occurs at the proximal end of the axon, and the axon grows, but it may not reach its distal target. As axons grow from the proximal stump toward the distal stump, some may enter appropriate bands of Büngner and may be directed to their correct peripheral targets. These nerve fibers will become functional. Some axons may enter bands of Büngner that lead them to incorrect targets, so normal function does not return. Other axons may fail to enter the Schwann cell tubes, instead ending blindly in connective tissue to form a *neuroma*. Mechanical or chemical stimulation of these blindly ending sensory axons may be the cause of "phantom pain" in persons with amputated limbs.

In axon tracts of the CNS, little or no regeneration can be expected, and in humans there is no regeneration to a functional state. Basal lamina guides, such as those found in the PNS, are not available. When a CNS axon is severed, the neuron mounts a sprouting response. Astrocytes hypertrophy and proliferate at the site of injury and fill any space left by the injury or by degeneration of the damaged nerve tissue. The responding astrocytes grow in a random orientation and form a scar rather than a pathway. Furthermore, astrocytes may not secrete adequate growth factors to sustain regrowing axons. The astrocytic scar appears to be a barrier rather than a guidance mechanism for axonal sprouts. Moreover, specific molecules present in oligodendrocyte myelin may also inhibit axonal regrowth. Eventually the axonal sprouts are retracted, and the loss of function associated with the severed pathway is permanent.

Synopsis of Clinical Points

- Rabies viruses are transported retrogradely to the cell bodies of the axons innervating the muscle (p. 20).
- Rabies viruses replicate within the cell bodies of infected neurons and are taken up by the terminals synapsing on the cell body (p. 20).
- Tetanus toxin is transported retrogradely from the site of infection to the cell body of the neuron (p. 20).
- Tetanus toxin does not replicate but is diluted as it passes from neuron to neuron (p. 20).
- Anterograde and retrograde axonal transport is seen in a variety of neurologic diseases and is a powerful research tool (p. 20).
- Pain is one of the most common neurologic complaints encountered (p. 22).
- Neurologic diseases may alter the function of the synapse (p. 22).
- Disorders of neurotransmitter metabolism are seen in a variety of neurologic diseases (p. 24).
- Loss of the neurotransmitter dopamine is seen in Parkinson disease (p. 24).
- Imbalances in certain neurotransmitters may result in bipolar disorder (p. 24).
- In Alzheimer patients, acetylcholine-containing cells, and their terminals, are lost in important forebrain areas (p. 24).
- The nicotinic acetylcholine receptors are destroyed by antibodies in myasthenia gravis (pp. 24–25).
- Astrocytes are found in both gray and white matter and can be the source of tumors in either location (p. 26).
- Characteristics of the blood-brain barrier are important in the passage of certain medications into the nervous system (p. 26).
- Multiple sclerosis is a demyelinating disease (p. 28).
- The AIDS virus targets the microglial cell (p. 28).
- Astrocytomas are the most frequently encountered glial cell tumor (p. 29).
- Grade 1/I astrocytomas are slowly growing tumors that arise more often in the white matter (p. 29).
- Grade 2/II astrocytomas are also slowly growing but are more infiltrative (p. 29).
- Grade 3/III astrocytomas have mitotic figures; this is one indicator of rapid growth (p. 29).
- Grade 4/IV astrocytomas are also called glioblastoma multiforme (p. 29).
- Glioblastoma multiforme (grade 4/IV) are highly malignant, rapidly growing invasive tumors (p. 29).
- Oligodendrogliomas are slow growing tumors that are more frequently located in the lobes of the brain (p. 29).
- Ependymomas arise from the cells lining the ventricles and are good candidates for surgical removal (p. 29).
- Lymphomas are brain tumors that were once regarded as arising from microglia (p. 29).
- Medulloblastomas are brain tumors that are more commonly seen in children (p. 29).
- Meningioma and schwannoma are examples of benign primary brain tumors (p. 29).
- Metastatic brain tumors arise from malignant cells that originate outside the nervous system; examples are carcinoma of the lung, breast, and prostate (pp. 29–30).
- Axonotmesis is a compression injury (p. 32).
- Neurotmesis is a transection injury (p. 32).
- A neuroma that develops in an amputated limb may be called a traumatic neuroma (p. 33).
- Mechanical or chemical stimulation of blindly ending sensory axons in an amputated limb may cause phantom pain (p. 33).

Sources and Additional Reading

Araque A, Carmignoto G, Haydon PG: Dynamic signaling between astrocytes and neurons. Annu Rev Physiol 63:795-813, 2001.

Araque A, Parpura V, Sanzgiri RP, Haydon PG: Tripartite synapses: Glia, the unacknowledged partner. Trends Neurosci 22:208-215, 1999.

Butt AM, Ransom BR: Visualization of oligodendrocytes and astrocytes in the intact rat optic nerve by intracellular injection of lucifer yellow and horseradish peroxidase. Glia 2:470-475, 1989.

Casagrande VA, Hutchins JB: Methods for analyzing neuronal

connections in mammals. In Methods in Neurosciences, Vol 3, Quantitative and Qualitative Microscopy. San Diego, Academic Press, 1990, pp 188-207.

Dani JW, Chernjavsky A, Smith SJ: Neuronal activity triggers calcium waves in hippocampal astrocyte networks. Neuron 8:429-440, 1992.

Gehrmann J, Matsumoto Y, Kreutzberg GW: Microglia: Intrinsic immuneffector cell of the brain. Brain Res Rev 20:269-287, 1995.

Hertz L: Neuronal-astrocytic interactions in brain development, brain function and brain disease. Adv Exp Med Biol 296:143-159, 1991.

Kettenmann H, Ransom BR (eds): Neuroglia. New York, Oxford University Press, 1995.

Lopes MBS, Vandenberg SR, Scheithauer BW: Molecular Genetics of Nervous System Tumors. New York, Wiley-Liss, 1993.

Peters A, Palay SL, Webster H deF: The Fine Structure of the Nervous System, 3rd ed. New York, Oxford University Press, 1991.

Shepherd GM (ed): The Synaptic Organization of the Brain, 3rd ed. New York, Oxford University Press, 1990.

Stevens CF: The neuron. Sci Am 241:55-65, 1979.

Steward O, Banker GA: Getting the message from the gene to the synapse: Sorting and intracellular transport of RNA in neurons. Trends Neurosci 15:180-186, 1992.

Unwin N: Neurotransmitter action: Opening of ligand-gated ion channels. Cell 72:31-42, 1993.

Chapter 3

The Electrochemical Basis of Nerve Function

Terry M. Dwyer

The nervous system harnesses electrical and chemical forces in its efforts to gather information, analyze data, and encode meaning as a string of action potentials (AP's). This chapter begins with a discussion of the fundamental electrical and chemical properties of the solutions of small ions and large proteins that comprise the interior of the cell and its environs and shows how a neuron employs those forces to ensure its own integrity—and how bacteria and our own immune system broach these defenses to destroy neurons. Next are the electrical properties of the nerve that allow us to sense our environment and integrate neural data. This chapter then concludes with the active changes in the nerve cell membrane that generate AP's to encode data and bring about distant activity.

The Combined Forces of Chemical Gradients and Electrical Potentials

Membranes enclose all cells in the body. Since cell membranes are composed of a lipid bilayer, large molecules such as proteins can neither enter nor leave the cell by simple diffusion, while small molecules like water can diffuse with relative ease. These impermeant molecules exert an *osmotic force* that draws water into the cell, causing it to swell and ultimately burst. As a result, the very first task of the cell is to ensure its own physical integrity, both by minimizing osmotic flow of water and by removing that excess water that does enter the cell. The mechanisms that perform this feat have been further adapted by the nervous system to both generate specialized fluids necessary for its proper function (such as the cerebrospinal fluid and the perilymph and endolymph of the ear), as well as to detect stimuli, transport signals, and integrate information.

Forces Due to Concentration Gradients

Pure water has a concentration of 55.5 M (the molecular weight of water is 18 and the weight of a liter of water is a kilogram: $1,000 \div 18 = 55.5$). Any solute added to water takes up space, displacing water molecules and so reducing their concentration. Table 3-1 provides an example modeled on a peripheral nerve cell and its surrounding fluid; this neuron's cell water is more dilute than extracellular water because the cell protein content is 10-fold greater than that in the body's interstitium—and 100-fold greater than that in the cerebrospinal fluid, which is the brain's interstitial fluid. Since all substances spontaneously tend to move from regions of a higher concentration to regions of a lower concentration, water will tend to move into the cell from the interstitium, causing the cell to swell.

Maintaining proper cell volume is so important that a variety of systems have evolved to counter the presence of cell proteins and to adjust to changing interstitial conditions. Indeed, pathologists generally see abnormal swelling in metabolically compromised cells, when the processes that counter this tendency are no longer adequately functioning. The following sections explain the physical principles used by these systems.

Osmotic forces measure the tendency of water to move down its concentration gradient across a semipermeable membrane. (A semipermeable membrane allows the passage of water but not any other dissolved molecule.) Since it is the solute (sodium, potassium, chloride, sucrose—the dissolved substance) that is measured, we generally speak in terms of the solute, and not the water. As a result, we dissemble, saying that *osmotic forces tend to move water from a more dilute solution (of solute, that is) to a more concentrated one*. Regardless, the source of energy that moves the water is its very own concentration gradient.

Aquaporins (*AQP's*, Fig. 3-1) are the proteins in cell membranes that allow cells to reach osmotic equilibrium rapidly. AQP's contain transmembrane pores so specialized for the

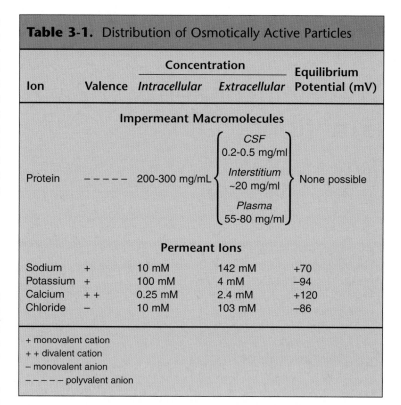

Table 3-1. Distribution of Osmotically Active Particles

Ion	Valence	Concentration Intracellular	Concentration Extracellular	Equilibrium Potential (mV)
Impermeant Macromolecules				
Protein	– – – – –	200-300 mg/mL	CSF 0.2-0.5 mg/ml; Interstitium ~20 mg/ml; Plasma 55-80 mg/ml	None possible
Permeant Ions				
Sodium	+	10 mM	142 mM	+70
Potassium	+	100 mM	4 mM	−94
Calcium	+ +	0.25 mM	2.4 mM	+120
Chloride	−	10 mM	103 mM	−86

+ monovalent cation
+ + divalent cation
− monovalent anion
– – – – – polyvalent anion

transport of water that they allow it to move almost as fast as in bulk solution—3×10^9 molecules per second for each pore—while excluding all other molecules. At least 10 distinct aquaporins are present in various cells in the human body, distributed in a tissue-specific manner. Congenital abnormalities result from the absence of specific AQP's: lack of AQP0 leads to cataracts; lack of AQP4 leads to deafness because it is needed for proper cochlear function; and AQP1 is required for adequate intraocular pressure.

Cells counter the osmotic force exerted by the *high intracellular concentrations of protein* by making a predominantly *extracellular particle* (sodium) impermeant as well. Consequently, sodium is generally more concentrated outside the cell (extracellular) than inside the cell (intracellular) (Table 3-1). The osmotic force exerted by this ionic gradient is proportional to the difference between the two concentrations and is given by the *van't Hoff* equation, which is analogous to the *ideal gas law*:

$$\Pi = (S_o - S_i) \times RT = (0.142 - 0.010) \times RT = 3.4 \text{ atmospheres}$$

Here the force is construed as the pressure (Π) that would be generated across a semipermeable membrane by this chemical gradient. The numerical value is the product of RT, a thermodynamic quantity that depends on temperature, times the difference between the intracellular and the extracellular molar concentrations of the substance S.

Electrical Forces

Cell proteins generally carry negative charges, and this large quantity of impermeant charge has important electrical consequences. In any solution, the number of positive and negative charges must be equal—the *principle of microscopic electroneutrality*. Since many of the cell's negative charges are on proteins, the remaining intracellular anions (like chloride) must be reduced relative to their extracellular concentration. In osmotic terms, this concentration gradient acts alongside that of sodium to minimize water flux across the cell membrane. In addition, chloride is also charged and so electrical forces (measured as voltages) must also come into play.

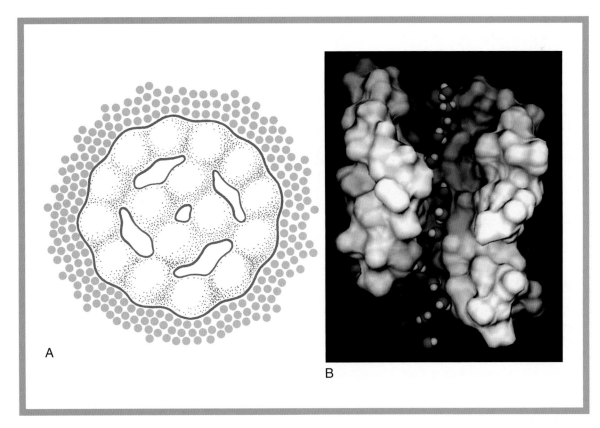

Figure 3-1. The tetrameric aquaporin channel has a fourfold symmetry that centers about rigid protrusions and a central dimple. The four pores are ringed by a highly mobile outer structure (**A**). A computer-simulated cutaway diagram shows the path for water flux (**B**). The narrowest part of the channel excludes larger molecules while the inner structure has a high dielectric that effectively substitutes for bulk water, allowing single water molecules to corkscrew through the channel. (**B** from deGroot BL, Grubmüller H: Water permeation across biological membranes: Mechanism and dynamics of aquaporins-1 and GlpF. Science 294:2353-2357, 2001.)

The best way to visualize the electrical forces involved in this chloride gradient is an approach that is analogous to the van't Hoff equation: calculate the force (in this case a voltage) that is generated by the ionic gradient:

$$V_s = z \cdot RT \cdot ln(S_o/S_i);$$
$$\text{for instance, } V_{Cl} = -1 \cdot 61 \cdot \log(10^3/4) = -86 \text{ mV}$$

where S is the concentration of the substance of charge z and V_s is the *Nernst potential* for that ion; *ln* is the natural logarithm, which is 2.303 times the more commonly used base-10 logarithm (log). There are three equivalent ways of saying this: 1) this voltage (V_{Cl}) is the potential at which Cl_o (chloride outside) is in equilibrium with Cl_i (chloride inside); 2) the concentration gradient (Cl_o/Cl_i) is just offset by electrical forces at V_{Cl}; and 3) at V_{Cl}, chloride movements into the cell are just equal to chloride movements out of the cell. This Nernst potential is also called the *equilibrium potential* for chloride, or simply the *chloride potential*.

Cations have the opposite valence as anions (the z term), and so (by the properties of the logarithm) the concentration gradient is inverted. Thus, for potassium, whose equilibrium potential is similar to chloride, the intracellular concentration exceeds the extracellular concentration (Table 3-1).

Returning to the case of sodium, the equilibrium potential is very different from potassium or chloride: $V_{Na} = 61 \cdot \log(142/10) = 70$ mV. This difference is easily tolerated since sodium is the effectively impermeant ion in most cells. Indeed, the steep sodium concentration gradient is used to great advantage in the effective transport of fluid and generation of AP's, as we shall soon see.

The Membrane Potential

In the long run, individual neurons exist at a steady state, with osmotic forces across the cell membrane balanced and with the concentration gradients of the permeant ions offset by a characteristic voltage (Fig. 3-2). The relationship among these electrochemical parameters was visualized by Goldman, and by Hodgkin and Katz, as being governed by the permeabilities of ions across the cell membrane:

$$V_m = 61 \, \log \left[\frac{P_K \times K_o + P_{Na} \times Na_o + P_{Cl} \times Cl_i}{P_K \times K_i + P_{Na} \times Na_i + P_{Cl} \times Cl_o} \right]$$

This relation is derived from the Nernst-Planck equation, with the algebraic contributions of individual ions being in proportion to P_s, their steady-state membrane permeability. While the P_s is itself difficult to measure and awkward to express, *relative permeabilities* are more straightforward concepts. For instance, it is easily demonstrated experimentally that the potassium permeability of a nonmyelinated nerve axon is 100 times that of sodium (and then easy to say that $P_{Na}/P_K = 1:100$). By using these relative permeabilities and postponing consideration of chloride until later, a more tractable form of the Goldman-Hodgkin-Katz voltage equation would be:

$$V_m = 61 \, \log \left[\frac{K_o + \frac{P_{Na}}{P_K} \times Na_o + \frac{P_{Cl}}{P_K} \times Cl_i}{K_i + \frac{P_{Na}}{P_K} \times Na_i + \frac{P_{Cl}}{P_K} \times Cl_o} \right] \cong 61 \, \log \left[\frac{4 + 1.42}{100 + .10} \right]$$
$$= -86 \text{ mV}$$

Potassium is now obviously the dominant ion in this calculation, with only a modest contribution from extracellular sodium.

This, then, is the reason for developing the concepts of electrical and concentration forces. The membrane potential is primarily due to the diffusion of potassium from the cell, withdrawing positive charges until the electrical potential across the membrane becomes approximately equal—but opposite—to the force generated by the potassium concentration gradient.

Cell chloride differs from cell calcium, sodium, and potassium because it is often in electrochemical equilibrium with its surroundings, which is to say that $V_{Cl} = V_m$. This is true in some nerve and muscle cells where chloride serves to stabilize the membrane potential. In these cases where the chloride equilibrium potential equals the membrane potential, V_{Cl} contributes nothing to the Goldman-Hodgkin-Katz calculation and can be safely omitted, as shown in the previous example. In other cells, chloride ions are pumped out, making V_{Cl} *more negative than V_m.* This is true in some postsynaptic nerve terminals, and when inhibitory neurotransmitters open chloride permeant channels, chloride ions diffuse passively into the neuron, transiently making the membrane potential more negative. Finally, chloride is actively accumulated in epithelial cells that secrete fluid, as will be explained in the next section.

Fluid Transport by Epithelia

The nervous system requires highly specialized fluids in the extracellular spaces of the brain, cochlea, and eye for the proper function of these organs. The brain is bathed in *cerebrospinal fluid* (CSF), a solution low in protein that is generated by the *choroid plexus* and removed through the *subarachnoid villi*. The cochlear *endolymph* is high in potassium, and the *ciliary body* of the eye is continuously producing a nutrient solution that flows past the lens and is taken up by specialized veins along the margin of the iris.

In each case, the specialized fluid is generated across an *epithelial layer* by the judicious placement of membrane pumps and channels (Fig. 3-2). Epithelial cells have two functionally distinct surfaces: the base and the sides (or *basolateral* surface), which are in contact with the interstitial fluid of the body, and the *apical* surface, which faces the lumen. Almost all epithelia restrict the *sodium pump* to the basolateral surface; the two exceptions are the choroid plexus and the retinal pigmented epithelium, where the sodium pump is exclusively in the apical membrane. Individual epithelia then distinguish themselves by distributing characteristic channels and transporters on their apical and basolateral surfaces.

The sodium pump (a *sodium-potassium adenosine triphosphatase [ATPase]*) is a molecule present in all cells that moves sodium out of the cell and potassium into the cell (Fig. 3-2). This exchange generates a steep concentration gradient for the two ions, fueled by the chemical energy stored in molecules of ATP (hence, *primary active transport*). We have already seen that

the potassium gradient determines the steady-state membrane potential. The sodium gradient is not only the basis of the AP, as we soon shall see, but it can also be harnessed to move large quantities of fluid. For instance, *Na/2Cl/K cotransport* pumps are present on the apical (ventricular) surface of the cells in the choroid plexus. The sodium electrochemical gradient provides the energy for this *secondary active transport mechanism* to drive potassium and chloride into the cell; specialized chloride channels on the apical surface then allow those ions to diffuse out of the cell. In addition, large quantities of carbonic *anhydrase* are present in the cells lining the choroid plexus, generating HCO_3^- ions that accompany chloride into the CSF. These chloride and bicarbonate ions are accompanied by passive movements of sodium and water molecules as dictated by electrical and osmotic forces. (Potassium channels on the basolateral surface recycle that ion back into the interstitium.) Other cotransport mechanisms move nutrients, antibiotics, and a wide variety of other organic molecules into the CSF, generating liters of CSF a week, all the time keeping an effective barrier to erythrocytes, leukocytes, and plasma proteins.

Modifying the placement and nature of the cell's pumps and channels alters the composition of the secreted fluid. For instance, cochlear endolymph is high in potassium because its epithelial cells have their potassium channels on the apical side, causing the potassium chloride pumped into the cell by the basolateral Na/2Cl/K cotransporter to exit the cell together into the scala media. Thus it can be seen that the large and effective concentration gradients, osmotic and electrical forces present in neurons require energy input by the sodium-potassium pump. However, the body has adapted these forces, each required for the physical integrity of the cell, to a wide variety of other purposes.

Ohm's Law

The resting membrane potential refers to the neuron at a steady state and is largely the result of the potassium, chloride, and sodium diffusion potentials; in addition, *membrane currents*—electrical charges carried by ions crossing the cell membrane—modify this voltage as described by *Ohm's law*:

$$V = I \times R \text{ or } V = I \div G$$

Thus current (I, in amperes) flowing through a conductance (G, in Siemens) or across a resistance (R, in ohms) will generate a voltage drop (Fig. 3-3). By a convention established by Benjamin

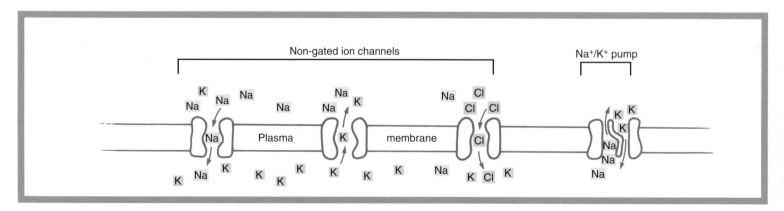

Figure 3-2. All membranes have pumps and channels. Channel proteins have water-filled pores that selectively allow small molecules to pass through the membrane. Illustrated here are three variations of those channels that are open continuously, one selective for sodium, one for potassium, and one for chloride. According to the concentration gradients diagrammed here, sodium will tend to enter the cell and potassium will tend to leave the cell, as will chloride. Pumps differ from channels because their water-filled cavity is open to only one side of the membrane at a time. Here the sodium pump is shown first accepting three intracellular sodium ions. After being phosphorylated by an ATP, the pump becomes closed to the interior and opens to the exterior, losing its affinity for the sodium ions, which consequently diffuse away. Next, two potassium ions enter the pump, and when the high-energy phosphate group is lost, the pump closes to the outside and opens to the inside, losing its affinity for the potassium ions; consequently, they diffuse away and the cycle is set to begin again.

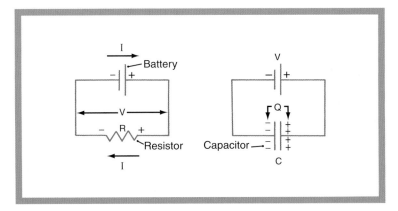

Figure 3-3. In a simple resistive electrical circuit, voltage (*V*) is imposed by a battery, much like an ionic concentration gradient across a cell membrane. Current (*I*) will flow through a resistor (*R*), which has a conductance (*G*). The conductance of resistors in parallel, such as channels in a membrane, sums algebraically. In a circuit where a voltage is impressed across a capacitor (*C*), such as the lipid bilayer of a membrane, a charge (*Q*, in coulombs) can be held by the capacitor, and is proportional to $V \times C$. Capacitors in series, such as found in the myelin sheath, add as their inverse:

$$\frac{1}{C_T} = \frac{1}{C_1} + \frac{1}{C_2} + \frac{1}{C_3} \ldots$$

Franklin, electrical current is the flow of positive charges: *positive charges leaving the cell are defined as a positive current.* Equivalently, negative charges entering the cell are also a positive current. Conversely, positive charges entering the cell are a negative current, as is the exit of negative charges. A familiar example is the sodium pump, which is *electrogenic* because it cycles three sodium ions out of the cell for every two potassium ions in; this net positive current removes positive charges from the cell interior, causing the membrane potential to be more negative than predicted by the Goldman-Hodgkin-Katz voltage equation. In a cell as large as a skeletal muscle fiber, this amounts to ~2 to 5 mV. In small nerve terminals, where the input resistance is much greater, this current can hyperpolarize the membrane by 15 mV or more.

Of even more interest is the flow of current through open membrane channels, because the number of open channels varies when the nerve is stimulated in any of a wide variety of ways. From Ohm's law, the magnitude and direction of the flow of an individual ion *S* through the cell membrane equals the driving force on that ion times its conductance:

$$I_s = (V_m - V_s) \times G_s$$

The electrical driving force on *S* is the difference between the voltage across the membrane (V_m) and that voltage where the ion is at electrochemical equilibrium (V_s, the Nernst potential). These relationships are summarized diagrammatically, for those familiar with electrical circuits, in Figure 3-4. Thus, the magnitude of the ionic flow will increase as the driving force—or the conductance—of the ion increases, and decrease as they decrease. In the face of an increasing conductance and a decreasing driving force, a situation that is described in the section on the AP, specific calculations are required to determine the final outcome.

Pain and a Syndrome of Periodic Paralysis

Pathologic conditions may alter the concentration of ions ordinarily seen in nerve cells (Table 3-1). For instance, tissue injury and death cause a local increase in the potassium concentration as cells release their contents. This increased extracellular potassium moves the steady-state membrane potential towards 0 mV, which generates AP's when done quickly enough. Thus, one source of pain is simply the direct stimulation of nerve endings by elevated potassium in the tissue interstitium.

In rare individuals who have certain genetic abnormalities, extracellular potassium can fall dramatically when epinephrine or insulin stimulates its uptake by muscle cells, leading to muscle weakness and even paralysis. This condition is called *hypokalemic periodic paralysis*. Surprisingly, the muscle membrane potentials are *less negative* than normal, just the opposite from what the Nernst equation predicts. For reasons not yet fully understood, the cell membrane loses its ability to select potassium over sodium, which is to say: P_{Na}/P_K declines markedly. The effect is so great that the cell is depolarized because the membrane potential moves away from V_K towards V_{Na}, as the Goldman-Hodgkin-Katz voltage equation predicts. This membrane potential change is slow, allowing the muscle fiber to undergo accommodation and so become inexcitable. (Accommodation is explained more fully in the section on AP's.)

Attack by the Immune System: Membrane Attack Complexes and Porins

The nervous system can be attacked by bacteria and even the body's own immune system in ways that short circuit membrane potentials and destroy the cell's integrity. Attack by the immune system depolarizes the cell membrane by inserting nonselective channels into cell membranes. This mechanism is one weapon of self defense employed by the human body's own cellular and humoral immune systems. The pore-forming elements of the body's immune system are the *porins*, from killer T lymphocytes;

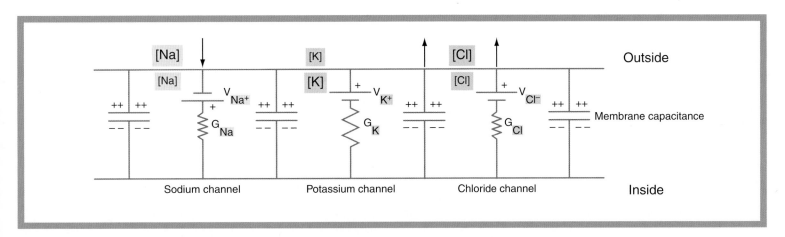

Figure 3-4. The cell membrane has conductive paths for sodium, potassium, and chloride, and so the concentration gradients of these ions exert electrochemical forces across the membrane. Since the conductance paths are in parallel, the driving forces of the ions combine in proportion to their relative permeabilities to generate a voltage across the membrane capacitance.

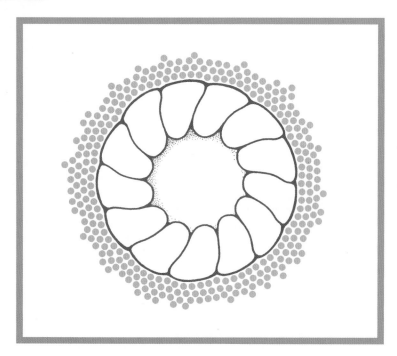

Figure 3-5. Membrane attack complexes are stable membrane structures formed by elements of the complement system—a polymerized ring of thirteen C9 monomers.

defensins, produced by phagocytes and epithelial cells; and two elements of the complement cascade, C8 and C9. C8 forms individual, <3 nm pores while C9 aggregates to form >10 nm pores, termed membrane attack complexes (*MACs*, Fig. 3-5). (MACs attack myelin sheaths of motor neurons, causing a paralysis discussed later in this chapter.) At 16 nm, porins are even larger.

The channels through MACs and porins are wide enough to easily pass sodium, potassium, chloride, and sucrose, discriminating little among them. The channels' conductances are correspondingly large: 2 nS (nanoSiemens) for the MAC and 6 nS for porin. As a consequence, the formation of just a single C9 aggregate or insertion of a single porin molecule results in a large flow of ions. Like all nonselective channels, the currents flowing through MAC and porin channels are carried primarily by sodium ions because the magnitude of the driving force for sodium is the greatest: $|V_m - V_{Na}| >> |V_m - V_{Cl}| > |V_m - V_K|$. If $V_m = -90$ mV (to take a simple example), the driving force on the sodium will be:

$$[(-90 \text{ mV}) - (+70 \text{ mV})] = -160 \text{ mV},$$

and the current flowing through the MAC is easy to calculate:

$$I = (-160 \text{ mV}) \times (2 \text{ nS}) = -320 \text{ pA}$$

Since one ampere is the flow of 6.3×10^{18} charges per second, the number of sodium ions flowing through a single MAC is 2×10^9 per second.

By following the movements of the various ions due to the electrical forces on them, it is possible to see that the cell gains osmotic particles, and so swells. For instance, because the net driving force on sodium is negative, it will enter the cell, with its positive charge tending to cancel the negativity of the membrane potential. In fact, the cell membrane potential will rapidly go to zero and remain there as long as the MACs are in the membrane. As a consequence, the driving force on chloride will increase; $(V_m - V_{Cl})$ being positive, the current will be positive, meaning that chloride is entering the cell along with the sodium. Thus, when sodium and chloride enter the cell, water follows, and the cell swells. Even more importantly, the MAC complexes are

so large that molecules the size of ATP can diffuse from the cell. Thus, attack by complement or killer T lymphocytes leads inexorably to cell swelling and lysis both because important metabolic contents are lost and because the osmotic pressures exerted by the remaining cell proteins cause cell swelling and death.

Microbial Attacks: Antibiotics
Inserting ion channels into cell membranes is also a weapon deployed by many microorganisms. Antibiotics such as *amphotericin* and *gramicidin*, and α-*staphylotoxins* from *Staphylococcus aureus*, lyse cells by broaching their membranes with large pores. When used clinically, amphotericin preferentially attacks fungal cells in fungal meningitis, but there is a narrow therapeutic range, as amphotericin also attacks cell membranes in the nervous system. In overwhelming sepsis, α-staphylotoxins attack all cells of the body, leading to multiple organ failure and cardiovascular collapse, primarily due to the loss of the integrity of cell membranes.

Graded Potentials

Electrical events underlie much of the nerve activity in our body. Indeed, many of our ordinary feelings and sensations begin with *graded potentials* that are due to changes in the ionic conductance of the sensory receptor's cell membrane and, consequently, the cell membrane potential itself. Similarly, nervous input is electrically integrated by the combined actions of excitatory and inhibitory synapses on nerve cell bodies. Finally, *AP's* are regenerative electrical signals that transmit the information to distant cells. The remainder of this chapter explains how the principles governing chemical and electrical forces contribute to the function of the nervous system.

Generator Potentials
All bodily sensations are graded, with transduction mechanisms generating bigger electrical signals—and consequently more AP's—for bigger stimuli. These graded responses are *generator potentials* that can be the direct result of the stimulus opening membrane channels or increasing the current through existing membrane channels. More often, intermediary chemical signals connect the initial sensation to the opening of membrane channels, the identity of which is just now being identified in experimental settings (Table 3-2).

Many sensations are transduced by more than one mechanism, depending on the importance of the sensation or the strength of the signal, for instance the sensing of changes in osmotic pressure by both visceral and hypothalamic receptors. Indeed, this ability is widespread throughout the body where many cells respond autonomously to the shrinking or swelling of their volume. Considering the fundamental importance of the maintenance of intracellular proteins, it is not surprising that osmosensors are present in lower animals as well. The best understood of these stretch activated channels (*MscL*, the *m*echanosensitive *c*hannel of *l*arge conductance [Fig. 3-6]) is tethered to the cytoskeleton and cell membrane and is closed off at its inner edge by loose coils of its C-terminal sequence. With stretch, the whole MscL molecule dilates as the cytoskeleton tugs on it, initially uncoiling the redundant structure at the channel's inner mouth and finally opening a 4-nm wide channel that spans the full width of the membrane. The action of the MscL gives an example of a transient, graded sensory system with negative feedback: if the extracellular osmotic pressure falls, the cell swells, opening MscL channels, resulting in the loss of osmotically active particles and thus water. As a consequence, the cell shrinks and the channels again close.

Table 3-2. Graded Potentials are Mediated by a Variety of Gene Families

Sensation	Chapter	Channel Family	Permeant Ion(s)	Channel Activity	Electrical Change
Vision	20	CNG	Na^+	↓ cGMP closes	Hyperpolarize
Hearing	21	TRP (N types)	K^+, Ca^{2+}	Stretch opens	Depolarize
Smell	23	CNG	Na^+, Ca^{2+}	↑ cAMP opens	Depolarize
Vomeronasal	23	TRP (C2)	Na^+, Ca^{2+}	↑ IP_3 opens	Depolarize
Touch	18	ENaC	Na^+	Stretch opens	Depolarize
Osmoregulation	19	TRP (V4)	Ca^{2+}, Mg^{2+}	Opens when cells swell	Depolarize
Taste					
Salt	23	ENaC	Na^+	Ion current	Depolarize
Sweet, Bitter, Umani (I)	23	TRP (M5)	Na^+	Phospholipase activity opens	Depolarize
Sweet, Bitter, Umani (II)	23	CNG	K^+	↓ cAMP closes	Depolarize
Sour	23	ENaC	H^+	Ion current	Depolarize
Nocioceptive					
Heat	18	TRP (vanilloid types)	Na^+, Ca^{2+}	Heat or capsaicin opens	Depolarize
Cold	18	TRP (M- and A-types)	Na^+, Ca^{2+}	Cold and menthol opens	Depolarize

CNG, cyclic nucleotide gated channel, a family of potassium channels (homotrimeric 6 transmembrane polypeptide subunits); ENaC, epithelial sodium channel, a family of sodium channels blocked by amiloride (heterotetrameric 2 transmembrane polypeptide subunits); TRP, transient receptor protein, six related families of cation-selective channel proteins (homo- and heterotetramers of six transmembrane polypeptide subunits).

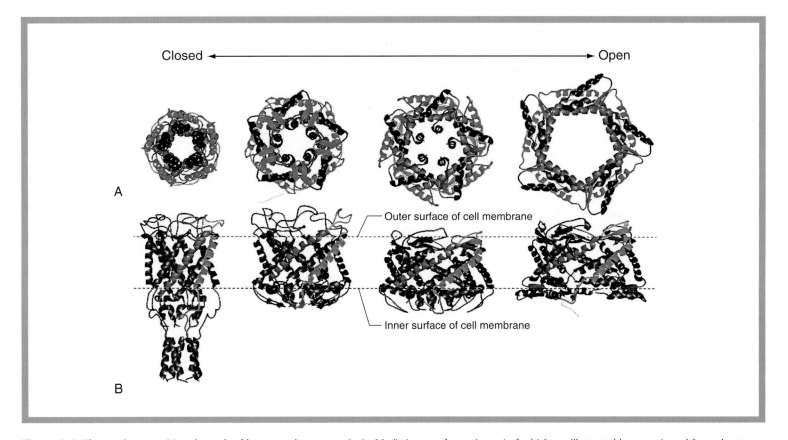

Figure 3-6. The mechanosensitive channels of large conductance exist in 11 distinct conformations, 4 of which are illustrated here as viewed from the top (**A**) or side (**B**). With the membrane at its most relaxed *(left)*, the MscL has its smallest diameter and an abundance of redundant structure gathered at the inner surface of the cell membrane. As the membrane is stretched *(right)*, the molecular diameter spreads and the cytoplasmic folds are pulled into the plane of the membrane. Finally, a pore opens *(right)* as the protein extends fully. (From Sukharev S, Durell SR, Guy HR: Structural models of the MscL gating mechanism. Biophys J 81:917-936, 2001.)

Synaptic Potentials

Vertebrate nervous systems use chemicals to communicate between cells, as already introduced in Chapters 1 and 2, and these signals alter the target nerve or effector cell by a combination of electrical and metabolic mechanisms, as is more fully described in Chapter 4. The most specialized structure supporting this chemical signaling is the *synapse*, and the best understood synapse is the *neuromuscular junction* (NMJ), in large part because it is readily accessible for experimental investigation (see Chapters 2, 4, and 24). For this reason, the NMJ will be used extensively to illustrate the nature of the synaptic potential.

As with generator potentials, neurotransmitters may act to open membrane channels either directly or via intermediary signals. For instance, *acetylcholine* (*ACh*) opens the *nicotinic receptor* at the NMJ directly. In contrast, the cholinergic *muscarinic receptor* is a *G protein*, in which case ACh acts indirectly by two mechanisms. The first is to release the Gβγ *subunit*, which opens certain potassium channels. The second is to stimulate or inhibit adenyl cyclase and various lipases, altering the concentrations of *cAMP*, the *inositol phosphates*, *diacylglycerol*, and *calcium*. Closely related structurally to the nicotinic AChR are the ligand-gated channels for GABA (the $GABA_A$ receptors), *serotonin*, and *glycine*, and the behavior and pharmacology of those channels are similar in many ways to the acetylcholine receptor. The *glutamate* and the *purinergic* receptors are evolutionarily and functionally distinct from this family, and from each other.

Synaptic Structure and Function: The Neuromuscular Junction

Motor nerve axons branch at their termini to innervate many muscle fibers, all of which contract together as a *motor unit*. The myelin sheath stops at each nerve terminal, exposing the naked axon to the muscle membrane at a specialized disk-shaped region called the *motor end plate* (Fig. 3-7). In this region, numerous transmitter-filled vesicles are gathered about release points, the *active zones*, which are stripes of docking proteins in close approximation to voltage-sensitive calcium channels. In electron microscopy, these aggregations of proteins are called *dense bars*. Such an arrangement allows for an efficient coupling of the motor nerve's AP, the resulting voltage-dependent calcium influx, and finally the calcium-dependent release of the transmitter vesicles' contents.

The membrane of the skeletal muscle fiber is thrown up into numerous *subjunctional folds* in the end plate region, with the tops of the folds situated immediately opposite the active zones of the nerve terminal. Clustered on the top of the folds are nicotinic *acetylcholine receptors (AChR)*, which respond to released neurotransmitter (acetylcholine) by increasing the

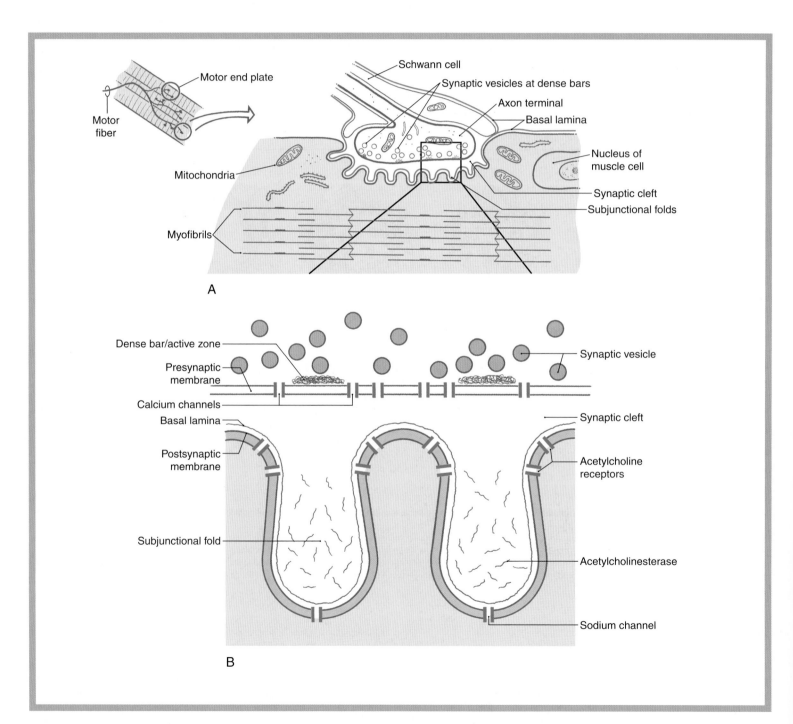

Figure 3-7. The neuromuscular junction (**A**) is the synapse between the motor nerve and a skeletal muscle that contains special structures in the nerve terminal that deliver the calcium signal release vesicles containing the neurotransmitter acetylcholine (**B**). The postsynaptic membrane contains receptors that recognize the transmitter signal and initiate an action potential, whereas the synaptic cleft holds acetylcholinesterase molecules that dispose of the transmitter by hydrolysis (**B**).

conductance of the muscle membrane to sodium and potassium. The released transmitter reaches the AChR's within tens of microseconds after release, ensuring a speedy transmission. Equally importantly, the transmitter will not have time to disperse, guaranteeing that the dense cluster of AChR's will be exposed to a high concentration of transmitter; consequently, almost all the released transmitter will be bound to, and act on, the receptors. Clustered at the base of the folds are large numbers of voltage-dependent sodium channels, guaranteeing that one muscle AP will fire for each AP in the motor nerve.

Between the nerve and the muscle lies a narrow but very deep *synaptic cleft*. The cleft matrix contains a *basal lamina with collagen* and *laminin* that combine to keep the nerve and muscle in close approximation and precise register during the active muscle activity. The depths of the synaptic cleft contain a high concentration of *acetylcholinesterase (AChE)* molecules that are held in place by their long collagen-like tail. Thus, one purpose of the synaptic cleft is to trap acetylcholine and to rapidly hydrolyze the transmitter into choline and acetate. This positioning ensures that little ACh diffuses out from under the nerve terminal and that the transmitter is present for only a brief (~1 ms) period of time.

Receptor Binding and Channel Gating

All synaptic receptor molecules have a distinct region that specifically binds the transmitter. In the case of the NMJ, one or two acetylcholine (ACh) molecules bind in a highly specific manner to the large extracellular portion of the AChR molecule (Fig. 3-8). The binding sites each span two subunits: the $\alpha\epsilon$ (or γ) and the $\alpha\delta$ interfaces. In the presence of the transmitter, three loops of the α subunit come together with a loop of the ϵ or δ subunit to form a box of nonpolar and aromatic amino acids, primarily tryptophanes and tyrosines. The open, conducting conformation is stabilized when ACh is in this box. Since there are two α subunits in the receptor complex, two ACh molecules must be bound before ion flow can begin. Once the first ACh leaves, its α subunit is free to close, at which time ion flow ceases.

The specificity of the AChR binding site has been utilized by pharmacologists to design molecules that specifically relax skeletal muscle fibers, for instance during surgery, but have no unwanted side effects on heart or vascular smooth muscle contractility. *Curare*, a plant product, was the first of these muscle relaxants; *succinylcholine* and many more have been designed for particular purposes. The duration of action and potency of effect are largely due to the affinity of the drug to the binding site, which in turn reflects how well the drug fits into the box-like geometry of the amino acids that comprise the $\alpha\epsilon$ and the $\alpha\delta$ interfaces.

Just as specific muscle relaxants bind to the AChR, other receptors also have characteristic activators and inhibitors. *Strychnine* binds to the glycine receptor, blocking its inhibitory activity and leading to a hyperexcitable state, a tool used long ago by medical students to remain alert for exams; this was effective but only within a very narrow range of dosing since slightly higher doses cause convulsions. *Benzodiazepines* bind to GABA$_A$ receptors, increasing the effectiveness of the endogenous GABA; *barbiturates* bind to GABA$_A$ receptors, inhibiting their activity. Thus, specificity of action within the nervous system reflects in part the different structures of receptor molecules in their transmitter-recognition region.

Specific Responses via Increases in Ionic Permeability

The specific recognition of a transmitter molecule is only one of the two necessary functions of a receptor molecule; the second is to effect a change in the target cell. The nicotinic AChR is an example of those receptors that open to expose a water-filled channel that spans the membrane and that selectively allows ionic currents to flow down their electrochemical gradients. The narrowest region of the AChR channel is girdled by the hydrophobic amino acids leucine and valine and forms a *gated* barrier to the movement of charged atoms (Fig. 3-8). When this gate is open, uncharged and positively charged molecules smaller than 0.65 nm × 0.65 nm can pass through; negative ions are excluded by multiple rings of negatively charged amino acids. Individual channel activity can be demonstrated electrically by the patch clamp technique (Fig. 3-9).

Since ACh activates cation-permeable receptors at the NMJ, this transmitter generates an end plate potential *(EPP)*, which is one specific type of excitatory postsynaptic potentials *(EPSP's)*, and which is explained in the following way. The conductance

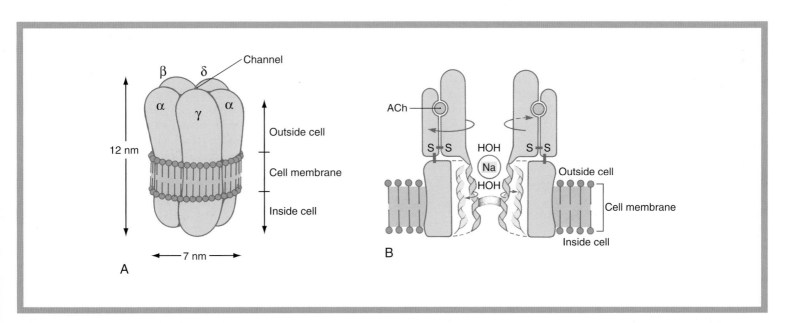

Figure 3-8. The acetylcholinesterase receptor (AChR) is a complex of five homologous subunits, two of which (the α-subunits) bind acetylcholine **(A)**. The extracellular domain of the AChR is formed of β-sheets and is where the transmitter binds. The membrane domain is composed of 20 α-helices (4 per subunit), 5 of which (1 per subunit) are mobile and form the ion pore. The remaining helices are hydrophobic and form a rigid pentagonal frame embedded in the membrane. With the binding of acetylcholine **(B)**, the mobile transmembrane α-helices are swung away from each other, pivoting around a disulfide bridge (S-S) to the outer rigid structure, enlarging the pore and allowing ion permeation.

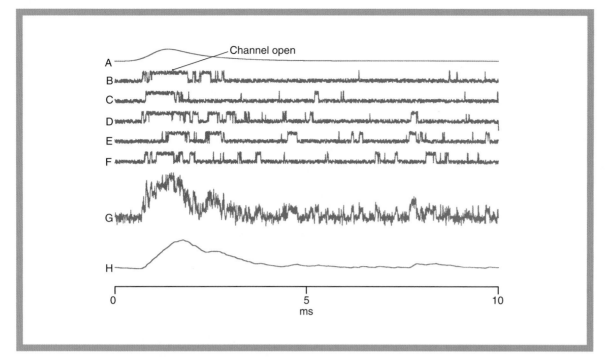

Figure 3-9. Simulated here are the events that comprise synaptic activity at a neuromuscular junction. The cleft transmitter (**A**) concentration rises within a millisecond as it diffuses from its release site, and then declines with time as it is hydrolyzed by cleft acetylcholinesterase. The postsynaptic current (**G**) is the sum of many single channels' activities (**B** through **F**), which together cause a depolarization in the surrounding muscle membrane (**H**).

of the postsynaptic membrane (ΔG) increases in proportion to the number of channels opened (n) and the conductance of an individual AChR (γ):

$$\Delta G_{EPP} = n \times \gamma$$

In the case of this AChR, the channel is permeable to both sodium and potassium, so the reversal potential (V_{ACh}) is approximately 0 mV. Consequently, the current flowing through this new conductance will be negative—or inward—and so will depolarize the muscle fiber (again assuming a resting membrane potential of –90 mV):

$$\Delta I_{EPP} = (V_M - V_{ACh}) \times \Delta G_{EPP}$$
$$= (-90 - 0) \times \Delta G_{EPP} = -90 \times \Delta G_{EPP}$$

Other synapses in the nervous system act to inhibit neuron activity. These include synapses activated by glycine and GABA, both of which open anion-selective *chloride channels* because chloride carries most of the synaptic current. Since the chloride equilibrium potential is slightly more negative than the steady-state membrane potential of most neurons, the current of the inhibitory postsynaptic potential *(IPSP)* will be positive and will tend to hyperpolarize the cell:

$$\Delta I_{IPSP} = (V_M - V_{IPSP}) \times \Delta G_{IPSP}$$
$$= [-90 - (-94)] \times \Delta G_{IPSP} = +4 \times \Delta G_{IPSIP}$$

Muscle Weakness: Failure of Transmission at the Neuromuscular Junction

Under normal circumstances, the EPSP at the NMJ is always large enough to provide an adequate stimulus for an AP to fire, and so there is a one-to-one correspondence between the firing of the motor nerve and the muscle's AP. Alcohols and local anesthetics interfere with NMJ transmission by preventing ion permeation: the vestibule of the AChR is large enough to admit local anesthetic molecules, which bind tightly and prevent ions from passing. The region behind the gating α-helix is also water filled and contains a specific site for alcohol and the binding of local anesthetics such as *lidocaine* (*arrow* in Fig. 3-8).

Toxins also specifically interfere with synaptic transmission at the NMJ. The three botulinum toxins are metalloproteinases that specifically attack the docking proteins syntaxin, synaptobrevin, and SNAP-25 on the presynaptic side of the NMJ. This effectively interrupts exocytosis and causes a paralysis that lasts until new docking proteins are synthesized. α-*Latrotoxin*, the toxin of the black widow spider, specifically binds to neurexin, another docking protein, first causing a massive emptying of the nerve terminal of neurotransmitter vesicles, followed by a loss of that end plate's function.

Acquired *myasthenias*—those diseases characterized by muscle weakness—can be due to the activity of the immune system. *Myasthenia gravis* is the most common syndrome, characterized by the fluctuating severity of the weakness, by the early involvement of ocular muscles, and by its response to cholinergic drugs. In myasthenia gravis, a small area of the extracellular region of the AChR—nanometers away from the transmitter binding site—is vulnerable to autoimmune attack. These amino acids form an epitope that is shared by peptides expressed during certain viral illnesses and by cells in the thymus that can activate antigen-specific T lymphocytes. Antibodies generated as a consequence of this activity may crosslink AChR's, increasing their rate of endocytosis and consequent lysosomal destruction, reducing their normal lifetime from a week to half that value. When the increased rate of loss becomes sufficient, the current generated during the end plate potential will be insufficient to trigger the nerve AP, and muscle weakness will ensue. In other individuals, the antibodies bind complement, leading to the formation of MAC's and lysis of the muscle cell. In still other individuals, the antibodies are of no pathologic consequence whatsoever, so a simple determination of antibody titer is not absolutely predictive of the severity of the disease. Over the longer term, the severity of the immune response is reduced by the use of corticosteroids or more even powerful immunosuppressive agents, or the thymus may be removed. The most direct treatment is the use of drugs that inhibit cholinesterase activity, such as the anticholinesterase pyridostigmine.

Anticholinesterase therapy is designed to increase and prolong the synaptic concentrations of ACh. An untoward consequence

The Electrochemical Basis of Nerve Function 45

of intensive anticholinesterase therapy is the *desensitization* of AChR's by the prolonged exposure to ACh. When the desensitization progresses too far, the loss of functional AChR's overtakes the benefit of the prolonged exposure to transmitter, and the patient becomes weaker. This condition is termed a *cholinergic crisis*, and is a therapeutic dilemma since any individual patient might become weaker because the immune disease worsens or because the number of AChR's is being reduced through desensitization. The test to distinguish between the two possibilities is the double-blind use of a short-acting cholinesterase inhibitor (with a ventilator nearby in case the patient becomes too weak to breathe): if the patient's strength is improved, then the immune disease is becoming worse and the anticholinesterase therapy must be increased; if the patient weakens, then he or she is in a cholinergic crisis, and the anticholinesterase therapy must be reduced.

Muscle weakness may also accompany small cell carcinoma of the lung, owing to the production of antibodies to calcium channels in the presynaptic nerve terminal. In this situation, the weakness is a *paraneoplastic process*—a syndrome that is associated with a primary neoplasm elsewhere in the body. Such a condition is variously called the *myasthenic syndrome* or the *Lambert-Eaton syndrome*. Characteristically, these patients gain strength with repeated muscle activity, unlike those with myasthenia gravis who fatigue more rapidly than normal. This improvement is because repeated firing of the nerve AP causes *potentiation* or *facilitation* of transmitter release as more calcium enters the nerve terminal with each succeeding action potential. With sufficient activity, many of the affected nerve terminals will

again have adequate calcium to release transmitter to generate a muscle AP.

Action Potentials in the Nerve and in the Neuron

Action potentials are brief electrical transients, visible when recorded as intracellular voltages or extracellular currents (Fig. 3-10). AP's occur throughout the body's tissues, regulating secretion of insulin from the islets of Langerhans and secretion of aldosterone from the *zona glomerulosa* and even signaling fertilization of the egg by the sperm. In the nervous system, AP's serve to integrate the generator potentials from sense organs and the synaptic input to cell bodies, with the magnitude of the result being sent down the neuron's axon encoded as a frequency. Axonal AP's can travel for a meter or more without decrement and without distortion, at speeds that can be maximized by increasing the axon diameter or by adding insulating layers of myelin. Such fidelity is possible because the AP is a self-regenerating electrical signal that is automatically produced by the inherent properties of specific membrane proteins.

Extracellular recordings of nerve activity monitor AP's in many nerve fibers at once (Fig. 3-10A). In this case, afferent nerve fibers from the carotid body baroreceptors are seen to fire rhythmically in response to the increase in arterial blood pressure during systole. These fibers have a low degree of *tonic* activity plus a superimposed *phasic* discharge proportional to the rate of change in blood pressure.

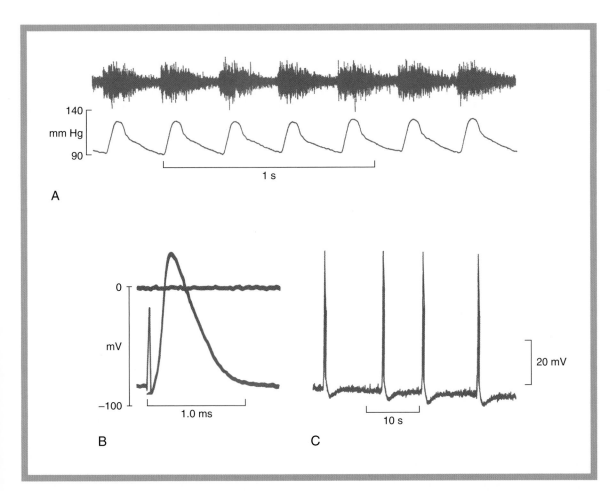

Figure 3-10. Action potentials take many forms. An extracellular recording of a small bundle of baroreceptor afferents (**A**) measures the electrical currents of action potentials that fire in response to changes in blood pressure, plotted in the lower trace. An intracellular recording from a myelinated nerve axon measures the voltages associated with an action potential (**B**): a 50-μs electrical stimulus at time zero, the rapid upstroke to a peak voltage greater than 0 mV, and a complete recovery by 1 ms. Intracellular recordings of action potentials in most other neurons have complex waveforms, such as hippocampal pyramidal cells that fire a burst of a half-dozen spikes that are terminated with a 1- or 2-second long afterhyperpolarization (**C**).

An understanding of the many varieties of AP's in individual nerve cells is made possible by intracellular recordings. At one extreme is the axon of a myelinated nerve (Fig. 3-10B), which is electrically silent except when an AP is triggered at the axon hillock of the cell body. The AP is complete within a millisecond and reflects the activity of a single active current. More complex AP's are seen in pyramidal cells of the hippocampus (Fig. 3-10C), which are entrained to the firing of other pyramidal cells. These AP's contain three to four spikes and end with a *hyperpolarizing afterpotential*. The remainder of this chapter will characterize these AP's more fully and describe the mechanisms that generate their complex waveforms.

Compound Action Potentials

Much of the nerve activity described in this book was demonstrated in experiments that used extracellular electrodes to record the combined firings of many individual nerve fibers (such as electroencephalograms [EEG's], which are recordings from regions of the brain, and electromyograms [EMG's], which are recordings from peripheral nerves, such as Figures 3-10A and 3-11). The electrical basis for these recordings lies in the membrane currents that flow during the AP's. As the sodium ions first enter the nerve cell, and then potassium ions leave, electrical charges are removed and then added to the extracellular fluid. Since the extracellular fluid is a solution of various

salts, it has electrical resistance, and so the flow of these ions is an electrical current that generates a voltage (Ohm's law).

While nerve axons vary in size from less than 1 μm to more than 20 μm, their sizes cluster generally into four groups (Fig. 3-11). The smaller axons conduct AP's more slowly than do the larger axons, so it is reasonable that any given nerve bundle or tract of nerves contains fibers that can be grouped by their conduction velocities. The four different groups each have a characteristic set of functions, which will be more fully described in Chapter 17.

In clinical practice, nerve conduction velocity measurements are often performed to determine if nerve transmission is slower than normal by stimulating a peripheral nerve with a pair of electrodes and recording the resulting compound AP at a distance away (Fig. 3-11B). For instance, an electrophysiologist might stimulate the median nerve at the elbow and record the compound AP in the volar aspect of the hand to test if there is a compression neuropathy in the carpal tunnel. At a low stimulus strength, only the Aα peak appears, as the largest fibers have the lowest thresholds. For a 30-cm separation between the stimulating and the recording electrodes, the delay should be 4 ms, since the expected conduction velocity is expected to be 80 m/s or more. In a diabetic or a compression neuropathy, the speed would decline, or conduction would fail altogether. With increasing stimulus intensity, smaller and smaller fibers are recruited, and additional peaks appear at longer latencies; they are later because they are slower. Significantly, the magnitude of the signal is not a good indicator of the number of fibers of a given group: the larger-diameter nerves have proportionately greater amounts of membrane, and so will contribute much larger signals than will small nerves. In fact, Figure 3-11A shows that there are many more C fibers than A or B fibers, yet the C fiber electrical signature is much smaller than the A fiber peak (Fig. 3-11B).

Cable Properties of Nerve Processes

Electrical events in real neurons are complicated by the fact that neuronal activity exists in time and over distance. Those familiar with electrical circuitry will recognize similarities between nerve cells and telephone or network cables laid in the ground: an electrical signal is transmitted down the length of a core conductor but tends to leak through an imperfect insulating sheath. Furthermore, there is often a shield around the cable that protects it electrically but that also degrades the signal due to the capacitative coupling between the two.

Because the lipid bilayer effectively separates charge, the cell membrane has a large capacitance, on the order of 0.9 μF/cm^2 (microfarads per square centimeter). Consequently, time is required for the currents to change the membrane capacitance (Fig. 3-12). As shown in Figure 3-9, synaptic currents charge the postsynaptic membrane, generating the postsynaptic potentials. The speed with which a current charges a membrane is characterized by τ (tau), its *time constant*, defined as the time required for a signal to decay to 1/e or 37% of its initial value (e being 2.71828..., the base of the natural logarithm). With a resistor (R) and a capacitor (C) in series, $\tau = RC$, and so increasing the access resistance or the membrane capacitance will slow the time constant.

The spatial properties of the neuron are characterized by its *length constant*, which is the distance required for a signal to decay to 1/e (37%) of its initial value and which varies according to the neuron's structure and activity. For instance, the length constant is dramatically increased by myelin, resulting in much faster nerve conduction due to the increased linear reach of any given node's depolarization. In contrast, the length constant of a nerve dendrite is reduced by inhibitory activity that increases the chloride conductance; in so doing, the resistance of the dendrite membrane declines, and its length constant is shortened.

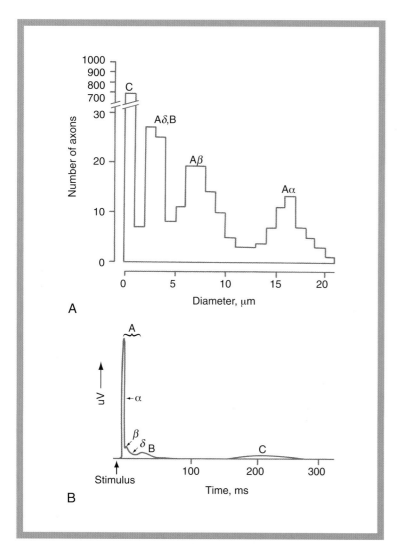

Figure 3-11. Peripheral nerves contain axons that vary widely in diameter but in a way that is grouped systematically according to function (**A**). The smaller C fibers are the most numerous, but they generate the smallest signal because of their small surface area (**B**). By contrast, the larger A fibers generate a much larger electrical signal even though they are fewer in number.

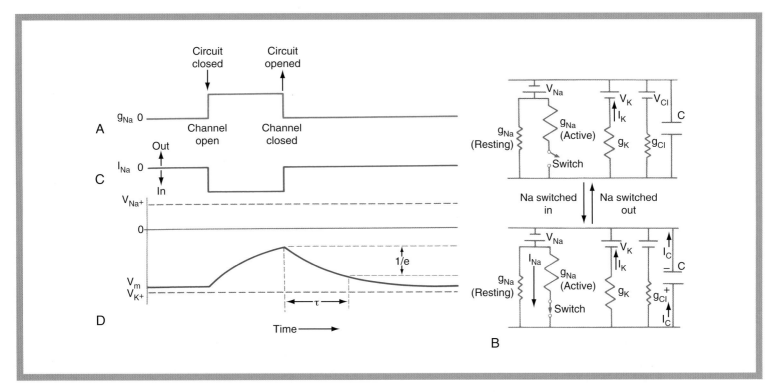

Figure 3-12. An electrotonic, or passive, change in membrane potential is simulated as the consequence of opening a sodium channel (**A**) for a brief period of time, allowing a current to flow (**C**) through an equivalent circuit of membrane (**B**). The resulting change in membrane voltage (**D**) is not instantaneous because of the membrane capacitance; the time constant of the membrane, τ, is that time required for the voltage transient to decay by 63%, or to 1/e of its peak.

As a consequence, any nearby excitatory input will decay rapidly, and so have diminished influence over whether an AP is triggered at the initial segment of the cell's axon (Fig. 3-13).

Nerve Conduction Velocity

The speed and precision of nerve conduction are very important for somatomotor activity, less so for visceromotor (autonomic) control of the body. Consequently, the nervous system has optimized some fibers for high velocity of nerve conduction and relaxed that requirement for other fibers. One way to speed conduction is to reduce the electrical resistance of the cytoplasm of the nerve. This is accomplished by increasing the cross-sectional surface area, which is proportional to the nerve diameter squared, in order to get more highly conductive ionic media per unit length. This comes at a cost, as more membrane is included in the larger diameter, whose capacitance slows the AP in proportion to the diameter; hence the speed of the AP increases simply as the diameter, averaging 1.7 m/s per micron of axon diameter for unmyelinated nerve fibers of the size found in humans. Invertebrates take this modification to extremes, with the giant motor axon of the squid reaching 100 to 500 μm in diameter in order to obtain the speeds necessary for rapid motor activity.

The alternative approach, which is more practical for the size limitations of the vertebral bony canal, is to insulate the axon with a myelin sheath. The insulation provided by the myelin greatly augments the resistance already provided by the nerve membrane as well as decreases its effective capacitance. Both changes work together to increase the length constant of the fiber, which reduces how quickly the electrical signal generated at the node decays away passively. Consequently, distant nodes reach threshold more rapidly, and conduction velocity is boosted. For example, a 10-μm myelinated fiber (axon plus its myelin sheath) has the same speed as a 500-μm unmyelinated axon (20 m/s at 20°C, comparing a frog motor nerve with a squid giant axon), but occupies only $(10/50)^2$ or 1/2500 of the space.

Thus, vertebrates always use myelinated nerves to achieve the fastest conduction times, averaging 6 m/s per micron diameter (see Chapter 17).

Regenerative Potentials Employing a Single Active Current

The simplest example of the AP mechanism occurs in the myelinated nerve. Much of this neuron's axon is well insulated by multiple lipid bilayers applied by oligodendrocytes in the CNS and Schwann cells in the periphery (see Chapter 2). Active currents are generated only in short intervals of naked axonal membrane—the *nodes of Ranvier*. Since the exposed axonal membranes at the nodes comprise no more than 0.05% of the total axon, it is economically possible to pack in a 100-fold more *voltage-activated sodium* and *always-open potassium channels* than would be found in nonmyelinated axons (Fig. 3-14).

A Sodium Channel Activated by Depolarization

The key to the self-regenerative nature of the AP was fully characterized by Hodgkin, Huxley, and Katz during the summer of 1951, after a dozen years of reflection during World War II and its aftermath. They simplified the complex nature of an AP—which involves the flow of various ions down their electrochemical gradient through conductances that change continuously—by studying the open and shut behavior of the sodium or potassium conductance at defined voltages by the method of the *voltage clamp*. In so doing, they could separate out the contribution of a single ion (sodium or potassium) and focus on its conductance as the membrane potential was varied in a controlled manner.

Two general principles emerged from these experiments that have been shown true for virtually all AP's. *First* is the notion of separate currents flowing through quite different and highly characteristic channels: the depolarization being due to the

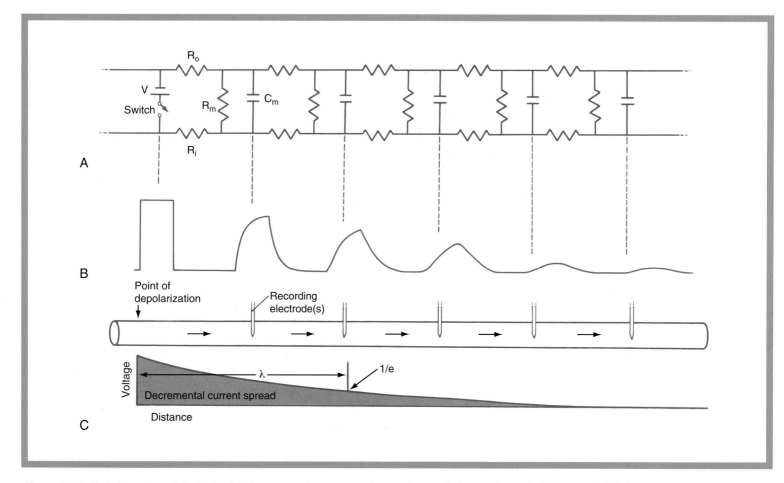

Figure 3-13. Periodic nerve activity is simulated as a repeating square voltage pulse, made by opening and closing a switch (**A**). Five recording electrodes are situated down the length of the nerve fiber (**C**) to record voltage transients (**B**). At each succeeding site, the amplitude is reduced and the signal slowed, with the length constant (λ) being that distance required for the signal to decay by 63%, or to 1/e of its peak.

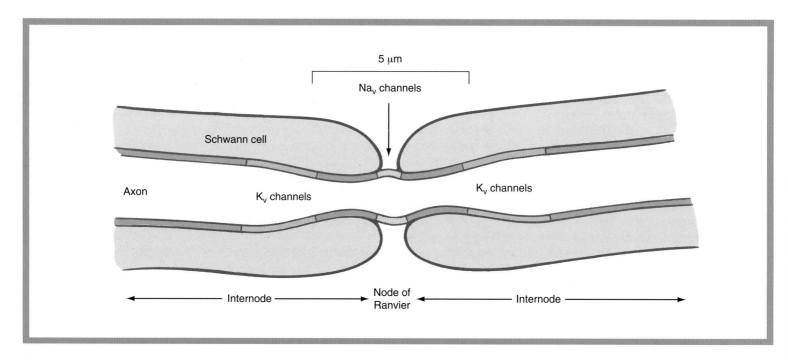

Figure 3-14. The myelinated nerve's voltage-dependent sodium channels are limited to nodal membrane, whereas the voltage-dependent potassium channels are only in the paranodal region.

influx of sodium or calcium ions and the repolarization being due to the efflux of potassium or influx of chloride ions. *Second* is the notion of multiple conformations, or states, for a channel. For instance, a *closed* sodium channel is stimulated to *open* when the cell membrane potential becomes more positive, that is, when it is depolarized. The open state does not last forever but

changes to a nonconducting *inactive* state over a time period measured in milliseconds (Fig. 3-15) and can return to the *closed* state only when the membrane potential is returned to a more negative value. The three states of the sodium channel—closed, open, and inactive—are the key to our understanding of almost all the known characteristics of the AP.

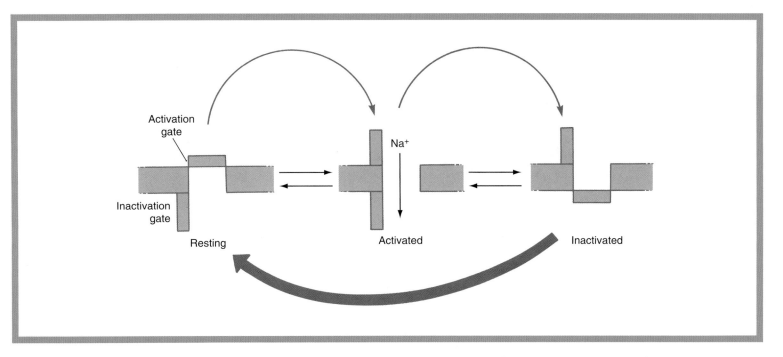

Figure 3-15. In the resting state, the sodium channel has (metaphorically) a closed activation gate and an open inactivation gate. When a neuron is depolarized, positive charges in the channel protein tend to move away from the inner surface of the membrane, which causes a transmembrane path to open for the passage of sodium ions. With time, the inactivation gate closes, blocking any further ion movement. Return to the resting state is possible only when the membrane voltage again becomes negative and these movements are reversed.

Regeneration

Opening sodium channels causes sodium current to flow, with the sodium ions moving down both an electrical gradient and a concentration gradient. The entrance of these positive ions causes the membrane potential to become less negative. This voltage change is exactly the stimulus for *opening more* sodium channels, resulting in more inward current, resulting in more depolarization, resulting in an even stronger stimulus for the remaining closed sodium channels to open. Such a process is a feed-forward system, which *repeatedly generates* a full-blown electrical signal that spreads down the entire length of an axon, using only the native characteristics of a node's sodium channel.

Repolarization

The lifetime of the *open* sodium channel is limited to a few milliseconds. Following this brief period, the sodium channel passes into the *inactive* state, a nonconducting state where it cannot return to the open state, regardless of the membrane potential. Without the voltage-dependent inward sodium current, and in the presence of a large resting potassium conductance, the membrane potential rapidly returns to the resting level, hence *repolarization*. Thus, not only is the regenerative upstroke of the AP an automatic feature of the nodal sodium channel, but so is its conclusion.

Threshold Voltage

Action potentials are initiated when generator potentials cross a narrowly defined range—the *threshold voltage*. A millivolt less and no AP will be triggered; a millivolt more and the AP abruptly takes off, all because three events are competing among themselves. The *closed* sodium channels are opening at a rate that becomes faster and faster as the membrane is depolarized; however, at the same time, the newly *opened* sodium channels do not last forever, as they undergo *inactivation*. Finally, the membrane conductances to potassium and chloride will tend to damp out the signal. These dynamic changes also mean that the rate of depolarization is also important, as will be described more completely in the section on accommodation. The outcome of these competing events is the basis of the Hodgkin-Huxley

formulation of the mechanism of the AP and is demonstrated in the teaching section of the *http://physiology.umc.edu/* website.

Refractory Period

It is not possible to elicit a second AP for a brief time after any given AP, and this is the *absolute refractory period* when the vast majority of the neuron's sodium channels are *inactivated* and cannot be opened (Fig. 3-16). With time, the *inactivated* channels do return to the *closed* state, but the entire process takes many

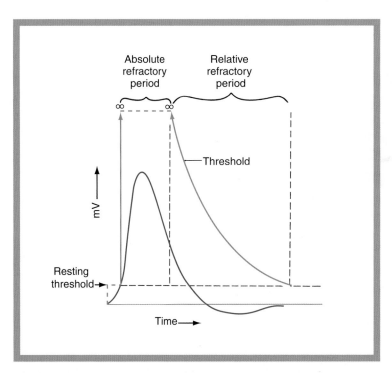

Figure 3-16. One action potential *(blue)* is triggered by a depolarization to the resting threshold voltage *(dotted line)*. It is not possible to elicit a second action potential during the absolute refractory period, when the threshold for a second action potential *(red)* is infinitely great. The threshold returns to normal during the relative refractory period, during which time it becomes progressively easier and easier to elicit a second action potential.

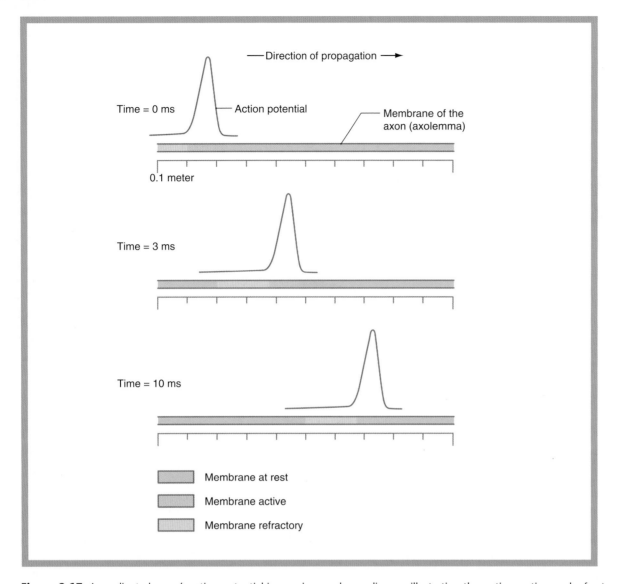

Figure 3-17. A myelinated nerve's action potential is superimposed on a diagram illustrating the resting, active, and refractory states of the nerve's membrane. If the conduction velocity is 60 m/s, the 1- to 2-ms duration of the action potential is spread over ~72 mm, or 36 nodes, with active membrane shaded *blue*. Trailing behind is the inactive, refractory membrane, shaded *pink* and extending for 150 mm or 75 nodes. The middle panel shows the nerve 3 ms later, with the action potential advancing 180 mm; and the bottom panel is later still.

milliseconds. During this time, it is relatively more difficult than normal to elicit a second AP—*the relative refractory period.*

Unidirectional Propagation

There are no echoes in the nervous system: once an AP is sent down a motor nerve, the job is done and the AP does not bounce back and forth across the length of the axon (Fig. 3-17). Again, it is the inactive state of the sodium channel that prevents the AP from changing its direction of propagation. This is because once the AP passes, the sodium channels left behind are in the *inactivated* state and are *refractory* to any further stimulation. The AP stops at the end of the axon because there are no more *closed* sodium channels to activate, neither ahead, because there is no more nerve, nor behind, because they are *inactivated.*

Saltatory Conduction

The AP of the myelinated nerve is said to jump (from Latin: *saltus*) from node to node, since active currents are possible only in the 1-μm node of the myelinated nerve; the adjacent ~2 mm of internode is well insulated by up to 300 layers of membrane laid down by the oligodendrocytes or Schwann cells (Fig. 3-14). This insulation is both resistive and capacitive. With each additional layer of membrane, the passive conductance to potassium and chloride is reduced by a factor of 2, 3, 4.... Equally

importantly, the capacitance is reduced by an equal factor. Thus, as the electrical signal generated at the nodes travels down the internal conductor of the axon—down the cytoplasm—little can leak through the internodal membrane by ionic flow and little is needed to charge the membrane capacitance, as it is so small. Quantitatively, while the internode is ~2,000 times the length of the node, the conductance and capacitance are each 600-fold less than at the node. Consequently, the whole of the internode requires approximately half the charge to depolarize it as would a single node $(2,000 \div [600 \times 600])$. In effect, the myelinated AP dances from node to node, being largely unencumbered by the intervening internodal membrane (the *saltator* and *saltatorix* being dancers of sometimes ill repute in ancient Rome).

A brief snapshot in time would show that the AP extends over many inches of axon. The speed at which the AP travels is great—60 m/s for a 10-μm axon at body temperature. Since the duration of the AP is ~1.2 ms, the linear extent of the AP is ~72 mm, or 36 nodes, at 2 mm per internode.

Gating, Selectivity, and the Structure of the Sodium Channel

A score of voltage-dependent sodium and calcium channels (Na_V's and Ca_V's) are known to exist in humans. These homologs appear globose and contain a surprisingly complex array of

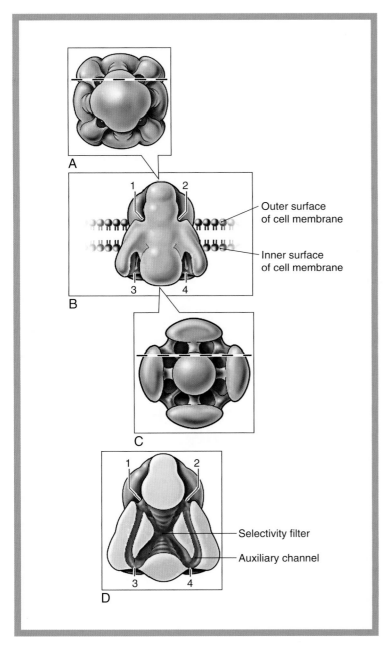

Figure 3-18. The sodium channel protrudes out from the cell membrane, as seen from the top (**A**), side (**B**), bottom (**C**), and in cross section (**D**). The ion pore has four vestibules toward the outside surface (two of which are numbered 1 and 2 in panels **B** and **D**) and eight vestibules toward the inside (labeled 3 and 4), that all join together at the transmembrane region to form the high field strength selectivity filter. Small auxiliary channels, no wider than a water molecule or a hydrogen ion, participate in the movement of the activation gate's voltage sensor. (From Caterall WA: A 30 view of sodium channels. Nature 409:988-990, 2001.)

membrane potentials move these gating charges toward the inside of the cell; depolarizations cause these amino acids to move outward and to open the pores to ion flow.

Modifiers of Excitability

Clinicians have long known that magnesium sulfate *stabilizes* nerve membranes, as do local and general anesthetics. Conversely, low levels of calcium increase membrane *excitability*, producing unwanted spontaneous activity in nerves that are ordinarily quiescent. With the knowledge that regenerative currents derive from specific voltage-dependent sodium channels, it is now possible to understand the molecular mechanisms by which clinical interventions easily modify excitability and how demyelinating diseases lead to loss of nerve function.

Accommodation

A slow but prolonged application of a subthreshold stimulus will cause a nerve to lose the ability to generate an AP; the nerve is said to *accommodate* to the stimulus. Again, knowing that the sodium channel can exist in one of three conformations, *closed*, *open*, and *inactive*, means that a subthreshold stimulus will stimulate channels to open, but at a rate that is too slow for there to be a sufficient number of *open* channels at any one time to fire an AP. Instead, the channels will *inactivate*. If the subthreshold stimulus lasts long enough, all sodium channels will be *inactivated* and no AP will be possible. This process causes nerves to "go to sleep" when pressure is applied for a long period of time.

Two distinct types of inactivation exist in all sodium channels: *fast* and *slow*. *Fast inactivation* was introduced earlier and is the process that terminates the AP within milliseconds and controls features such as the refractory period and unidirectional AP transmission. *Slow inactivation* requires depolarizations that last tens or hundreds of milliseconds, such as illustrated in Figure 3-10C, where the excitability of the hippocampal pyramidal cell declines over a 40-ms period as fewer and fewer sodium channels are in the *closed* state, and so available to generate a new AP. Slow inactivation also contributes to adaptation in the neocortex, in motor neurons, in neurons of the subthalamic nucleus, and in nociceptor cell bodies in the posterior (dorsal) root ganglion.

Anode Break

Action potentials can be triggered at the end of a hyperpolarizing pulse of current, as would have been delivered from the anode of an old-fashioned vacuum tube stimulator of the early 20th century. This is the opposite of the usual stimulus, a depolarizing pulse of current that sends the membrane potential positive to the threshold voltage. However, this observation led to understanding the behavior of nerves that fire spontaneously at a fixed rate (Fig. 3-10C). In these pacing neurons, each AP is followed by a deep hyperpolarization. As this hyperpolarization relaxes back to a more positive voltage, it triggers another AP when the threshold voltage is again crossed. While details vary from cell to cell, the basic mechanism relates to the three states of the sodium channel: during the hyperpolarizing pulse, more and more sodium channels switch over from the *inactive* to the *closed* state. The greater is the fraction of *closed* channels, the lower the threshold and the easier it is to trigger an AP. Hence, it is actually possible that the passive return to the normal resting potential is fast enough to be a sufficient stimulus to fire an AP while the vast majority of the sodium channels are still *closed*.

Tetany

Abnormal levels of calcium, magnesium, and hydrogen ions alter nerve activity. Increased concentrations *stabilize* nerve

water-filled passages (Fig. 3-18). Sodium ions enter Na_V only to find the interior lined with *aspartate-glutamate-lysine-alanine* sequences. These negatively charged amino acids create a *high field strength site* within the channel pore that closely mimics what had been the sodium ion's immediate surroundings in bulk water. Since the channel's interior is similar to the external solution, sodium enters the pore, sheds some of its surrounding water as it in turn displaces resident water molecules in the high field strength region, and then reenters bulk water on the far side with relative ease. Exclusion of large ions such as potassium is due to their weaker field strength, which cannot effectively dislodge water molecules from the high field strength sites within the pore.

A surprisingly mobile sequence of amino acids with a positive charge acts as the *voltage sensor*, not only for Na_V and Ca_V but also for voltage-dependent potassium channels. Negative

membranes, leading to fatigue, depression, anorexia, and constipation. Indeed, large infusions of magnesium sulfate have long been the accepted safe treatment for the life-threatening hypertension and seizures accompanying the eclampsia of pregnancy. Reduced levels of these ions *increase* excitability, causing tetany (a combination of tingling sensations and muscle spasms), mental irritability, and ultimately seizures. Metabolic or respiratory alkalosis exacerbates symptoms of low calcium or magnesium and can trigger overt symptoms in borderline or *latent* tetany, as will tapping the facial nerve in front of the ear (Chvostek sign) or causing a brief period of ischemia by inflating a blood pressure cuff (Trousseau sign).

Divalent cations like Ca^{2+} modify the excitability of nerves by binding to the negative *surface charges* on the phospholipids and on the oligosaccharide groups decorating membrane proteins. These negative surface charges are present in large numbers and create a voltage drop of ~30 mV across the last few nanometers immediately above the cell surface. Having this negative *surface potential* means that the cell's membrane potential is divided into two parts: one portion occurring across the surface charges on the membrane exterior and the remaining drop falling across the 3 nm lipid portion of the membrane bilayer. High concentrations of divalent cations neutralize the anionic surface charges, abolishing the negative surface potential and shifting the entire membrane potential onto the lipid interior of the bilayer. A transmembrane protein such as the voltage-dependent sodium channel would then experience a more negative voltage and have a reduced tendency to open: the neuron becomes *stabilized*. Conversely, when the concentrations of calcium or magnesium fall, divalents leave the membrane surface and more anionic charges are exposed. The surface potential becomes more negative and assumes a greater fraction of the membrane potential. Transmembrane proteins then experience a less negative voltage, the sodium channels become more likely to open, and an AP can be triggered by a much smaller stimulus: the neuron becomes *hyperexcitable*. When this condition is severe, the axons of sensory and motor nerves spontaneously fire volleys of action potentials, generating the signs and symptoms known as *tetany*.

Use-Dependent Block and the Treatment of Epilepsy

Seizures are excessive and paroxysmal neuronal activity, either locally in a small region of the brain or spreading across the entire cortex. Optimal drug treatment of epilepsy targets the high-frequency AP's of the seizure while preserving normal function as much as possible. Fortunately, sodium channels (like ACh receptors) have a binding site for *local anesthetics* like lidocaine and phenytoin. The site is inside the pore and is accessible only when the channel is open. As a consequence, local anesthetic block of sodium channels is *use dependent*—the more the channel is used, the more channels are plugged, and the more complete the block is. No more entry is possible once the channel is closed, but the local anesthetics can exit, releasing the block during periods of inactivity. Thus use-dependent block can augment the endogenous mechanisms that ordinarily bring a burst of nerve activity to an end (see Fig. 3-10C).

Genetic Defects, Toxins, and Venoms

The exact balance among the three states of the sodium channel is critical for proper function of the AP. This is readily apparent in a rare inherited cause of epilepsy *(generalized epilepsy with febrile seizures)*, two motor diseases *(hyperkalemic periodic paralysis* and *paramyotonia congenita)* and a cardiac arrhythmia *(long QT syndrome, type 3)*. In each case, slowed inactivation leads to repeated AP firing, and in some cases to a refractory state and paralysis. Toxins also interfere with sodium channel function, most famously tetrodotoxin (from the puffer fish

and a North American salamander) and saxitoxin (from diatoms that cause the red tide). These all bind to the closed sodium channel, preventing it from opening. Scorpion stings cause pain, spasms, and ultimately paralysis because their venom slows Na_V inactivation and causes activation to occur at more negative voltages.

Demyelinating Disease

The loss of the myelin sheath, as with multiple sclerosis, interrupts myelinated AP transmission for three reasons. *First*, the internodal membrane contains no sodium channels, so it cannot contribute to the regenerative currents needed for an AP. *Second*, the loss of the electrical insulation of the myelin means that the capacitance of the internode increases and the resistance of the internode decreases. *Third, voltage-activated potassium channels* are clustered in the internodal regions immediately adjacent to—but normally electrically insulated from—the nodes; once the myelin is lost, these potassium channels oppose the nodal sodium currents. All three factors act together to reduce the length constant of the nerve, causing the currents at the active nodes of Ranvier to have less of an effect at the distant resting nodes. With sufficient destruction, the length constant becomes less than the internodal distance. Transmission then ceases when it becomes impossible to reach threshold.

Potassium and the Variety of Neuronal Activity

Diverse patterns of activity are required of neurons, which in turn differ greatly in their geometries. Individual cells adapt to their particular functions by expressing sodium, calcium, potassium, and chloride channels drawn from scores of families and a multitude of transcripts. Three of these functions require particular potassium channels and will be discussed next: terminating the AP, controlling excitability, and pacing a rhythmic pattern.

Repolarizing the Neuron

Neurons use a variety of strategies to terminate their AP's. The nodes of Ranvier simply have a high resting potassium conductance. Unmyelinated axons are more ambitious in that they terminate their AP's promptly by opening potassium channels: the depolarization of the AP activates a potassium current through one or more K_V channels (Fig. 3-19). K_V's are normally gated shut, saving the neuron energy that would otherwise be spent to pump potassium out of a leaky cell, but open in response to the upstroke of an AP. The resulting pore sieves ions by *size*, allowing only the smallest hydrated monovalent cations to pass. Potassium is a large ion, so its charge density is not strong enough to attract as many waters as sodium; consequently its *hydrated radius* will be the smaller, and its passage will be the easier. K_V remains open as long as the membrane is depolarized; closing is guaranteed because I_{KV} will return the membrane potential towards V_K, the potassium equilibrium potential, repolarizing the membrane and allowing K_V to close. Thus, the AP is brought to a conclusion and the membrane returns to its high resistance state as well.

Controlling Excitability

Whereas the brief, definitive AP of the myelinated axon is well suited for a motor nerve, other nerve axons and cell bodies require signals that are more prolonged, by either extending the duration of a single AP or repeating the AP in bursts of 2, 6, 12, or more. Some of these needs are met by I_{NaV}, which can be carried by any one of the nine Na_V's. More often the task is performed by one or more of the 10 voltage-dependent calcium

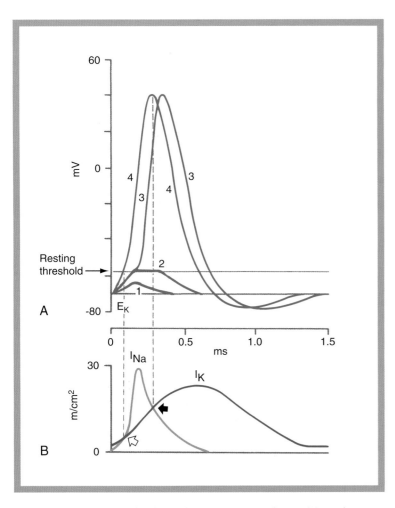

Figure 3-19. A subthreshold stimulus to a giant squid axon (1) produces a local response that quickly decays away because the potassium current remains larger than the sodium current (**A**). With a stimulus that is just below the threshold (2), the voltage remains depolarized for many microseconds before decaying back to rest; in this case, sodium channels opened in response to the depolarization but were insufficient in number to initiate the action potential. A slightly larger stimulus (3) brings the voltage above the threshold, causing a regenerative growth of the action potential (**A**). A superthreshold stimulus (4) causes the action potential to rise more quickly and to a greater amplitude, owing to the sodium channels opening faster at more positive potentials. The underlying sodium and potassium currents are both plotted as upward deflections (**B**). The *open arrow* points to the time when the sodium current becomes greater in magnitude than the potassium current, allowing the action potential to begin its regenerative phase. The *solid arrow* points to the time when the currents again cross, this time being at the peak of the action potential when there is no further depolarization owing to the equality of the inward and outward currents.

channels, Ca_V's, which are abundant throughout the nervous system and varied in their nature. Ca_V's ability to extend the duration of the AP is most dramatically seen in heart muscle but also apparent in Figure 3-10. They are also well adapted for firing bursts of AP's.

Neurons that fire calcium-dependent AP's (for instance the hippocampal pyramidal neuron in Fig. 3-10C) often have an additional current that repolarizes and stabilizes the cell membrane, which is due to the opening of the calcium-dependent potassium channel K_{Ca}. Both Ca_V and Na_V contribute to each of the AP's in the burst that is characteristic of isolated pyramidal cells. While the little bit of calcium that enters during a single AP is readily buffered by the cell, a train of AP's will effectively raise internal calcium, open K_{Ca} channels, drive the membrane potential to hyperpolarized potentials, and thence break off the train of AP's. In the intact hippocampus, networks of pyramidal cells fire single AP's rhythmically, entrained by the response of Na_V, Ca_V, and K_{Ca} to the cell's synaptic inputs. In this way,

the hippocampus can respond by altering the AP frequency while automatically limiting the number of AP's in a sequence, avoiding the excessive and uncontrolled activity characteristic of a seizure.

Simply changing the membrane potential by the action of one or more of the membrane channels may have highly complex consequences. While hyperpolarizing a membrane would seem to move the neuron away from its threshold, the opposite may actually be the case. AP's are more easily triggered at the more negative membrane potentials since more Na_V's are closed (versus inactivated). Other voltage-dependent channels are modified as well. Figure 3-20B illustrates the actions of the transient *A-current* due to K_A channels, which open at negative potentials. The experiment in this figure is one in which the neuron is first conditioned with a short hyperpolarization and then tested with a depolarizing stimulus. As illustrated, there is a delay before the stimulus is adequate to trigger a train of AP's. This delay is the time required for the K_A channels to close, and with longer or weaker hyperpolarizing conditioning, the delay is less. So a rhythmic pacing like Figure 3-20A is very complex and can be predicted in detail only by thorough computer simulations.

Pacing AP's

Individual nerve, muscle, and endocrine cell types differ widely in their need for rhythmic firing of AP's modulated by V_m, synaptic inputs, and metabolic conditions. Thalamocortical relay neurons fire action potentials in two distinct patterns: a train of single AP's much like shown in Figure 3-20B and a rhythmic pattern as in Figure 3-20A. A dozen channel types are involved in the specifics, with four Na_V and Ca_V channels contributing to the spike activity. As with the *solitary nucleus*, currents through K_A and K_{Ca} channels terminate the burst of AP's. However, it is current through the *HCN (hyperpolarization-activated cyclic nucleotide binding channels)* that is the pacing current that determines the rhythmicity of this neuron (and the sinoatrial node of the heart as well). Like cyclic nucleotide gated (CNG) channels (see Table 3-2), HCN channels are permeable to both sodium and potassium ions and are activated by cyclic nucleotides. Most importantly, HCN channels are activated at hyperpolarizing membrane potentials but inactivate with time. Thus, HCN channels are open at the end of the AP burst, joining with the currents through K_A and K_{Ca} to repolarize the neuron. HCN channels then slowly inactivate, allowing the membrane potential to drift towards 0 mV, away from V_K, and towards the AP threshold and a new burst of AP's.

Modifying a pacing neuron's frequency is key to controlling its signal. HCN channels, for instance, can bind cAMP, increasing the AP frequency. K_{ATP} is a current that increases when cell ATP levels fall, reducing the AP frequency. Finally, synaptic input can change the background sodium, potassium, or chloride currents, modifying the effectiveness of the HCN channels and increasing or decreasing AP frequency.

Neuronal Activity as Information

The neurons that were introduced in the preceding chapter, and that will be discussed throughout the remainder of the book, can be highly complex in structure, having a vast number of inhibitory and excitatory synaptic inputs on the dendrites and on the cell body (Fig. 3-21). Their information is encoded as AP's, and whether the neuron fires an axonal AP is determined by how synaptic activity modulates the cell's intrinsic electrical activity. Recall that synaptic potentials are graded in nature, spreading passively along the cell's membrane, decreasing in size with distance and time. Consequently, the geometry and timing of synaptic activity are crucial. For instance, as synaptic input

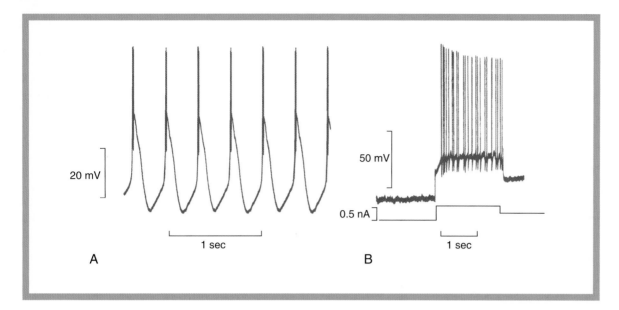

Figure 3-20. A, Thalamocortical relay neurons spontaneously fire bursts of action potentials. **B**, A hyperpolarizing prepulse experimentally applied to a neuron in the ventral part of the *solitary nucleus* introduced a pause of 0.25 second before the train of action potentials fired.

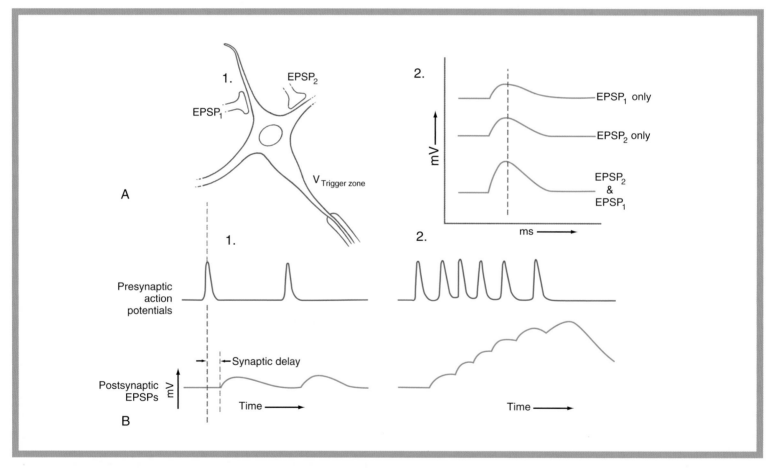

Figure 3-21. A, Two nearly simultaneous excitatory signals sum together to yield a larger electrical stimulus at the initial segment of the axon than would either one alone. **B**, Increasingly rapid excitatory inputs summate over time to yield larger and larger stimuli to the neuron.

increases in frequency, the resulting changes in membrane potential begin to add together and thus become more effective than any one single postsynaptic potential; this is called *temporal summation*. Similarly, as more and more excitatory synaptic inputs become active, the cell body is depolarized to a greater and greater extent; this is called *spatial summation*. Inhibitory synaptic inputs do the converse. It is the combined effects of all these factors that modulate the intrinsic electrical activity of the neuron cell body to determine whether the axon fires an AP—whether a bit of information is sent down the axon.

Synopsis of Clinical Points

- Loss of function mutations in aquaporin channels leads to congenital deafness and blindness (p. 36).
- In syndromes of periodic paralysis, muscle fibers are paralyzed when they are depolarized by elevations *or* reductions in potassium concentration (p. 39).
- Depolarization and nerve cell death follow insertion of large membrane channels derived from activated killer T lymphocytes, phagocytes, and elements of the complement system (p. 39).
- Microbes can kill nerve cells by insertion of pore-forming toxins (p. 40).
- Paralytic drugs act at neuromuscular junctional receptor proteins (p. 43).
- Botulinum toxins prevent transmitter release, whereas the toxin of the black widow spider empties the neuromuscular junctions of their transmitter (p. 44).
- Myasthenic syndromes may be due either to a reduction in transmitter release or to a loss of transmitter receptors (p. 44).
- Metabolic or traumatic damage slow nerve transmission (p. 46).
- The hyperexcitability of tetany results when alkalosis and hypocalcemia exaggerate the surface potential of a nerve cell membrane and reduce the fraction of the membrane potential sensed by a sodium channel (p. 51).
- Excessive rates of action potential firing are effectively treated with local anesthetics and antiepileptics that block open sodium channels in a use-dependent manner (p. 52).
- Gene mutations, toxins, and venoms interfere with the correct function of the nerve sodium channel, causing paralysis, myotonia, and seizures (p. 52)
- Demyelinating diseases interrupt nerve transmission because membrane insulation is lost and potassium channels are exposed (p. 52).

Sources and Additional Reading

Ashcroft FM: Ion Channels and Disease. San Diego, Academic Press, 2000.

Biesecker G, Lachmann P, Henderson R: Structure of complement poly-C9 determined in projection by cryo-electron microscopy and single particle analysis. Mol Immunol 30:1369-1382, 1993.

Blair NT, Bean BP: Role of tetrodotoxin-resistant Na^+ current slow inactivation in adaptation of action potential firing in small-diameter dorsal root ganglion neurons. J Neurosci 23:10338-10350, 2003.

Clapham DE: TRP channels as cellular sensors. Nature 426:517-524, 2003.

deGroot BL, Grubmüller H: Water permeation across biological membranes: Mechanism and dynamics of aquaporins-1 and GlpF. Science 294:2353-2357, 2001.

Dekin MS, Getting PA: In vitro characterization of neurons in the ventral part of the nucleus tractus solitarius: II. Ionic basis for repetitive firing. J Neurophysiol 58:215-228, 1987.

Hille B: Ion Channels of Excitable Membranes, 3rd ed. Sunderland, MA, Sinauer Associates, 2001.

Hoffman JF, Jamieson JD (eds): Handbook of Physiology, Section 14, Cell Physiology. Oxford, Oxford University Press, 1977.

Kaupp UB, Siefert R: Cyclic nucleotide-gated ion channels. Physiol Rev 82:769-824, 2002.

Kellenberger S, Schild L: Epithelial sodium channel/degenerin family of ion channels: A variety of functions for a shared structure. Physiol Rev 82:735-767, 2002.

Kozono D, Yasui M, King LS, Agre P: Aquaporin water channels: Atomic structure molecular dynamics meet clinical medicine. J Clin Invest 109:1395-1399, 2002.

Kunze DL, Andresen MC: Arterial baroreceptors: Excitation and Modulation. In Zucker IH, Gilmore JP (eds): Reflex Control of the Circulation. Boca Raton, FL, CRC Press, 1991.

Lambris JD, Reid KB, Volanakis JE: The evolution, structure, biology and pathophysiology of complement. Immunol Today 20:207-211, 1999.

McCormick DA, Huguenard JR: A model of the electrophysiological properties of thalamocortical relay neurons. J Neurophysiol 64:1384-1400, 1992.

Miyazawa A, Fujiyoshi Y, Unwin N: Structure and gating mechanism of the acetylcholine receptor pore. Nature 423:949-955, 2003.

Rasband MN, Shrager P: Ion channel sequestration in central nervous system axons. J Physiol 525:63-73, 2000.

Sato C, Ueno Y, Asal K, et al: The voltage-sensitive sodium channel is a bell-shaped molecule with several cavities. Nature 409:1047-1051, 2001.

Siegel GJ, Agranoff BW, Albers RW, Fisher SK, Uhler MD (eds): Basic Neurochemistry: Molecular, Cellular, and Medical Aspects, 6th ed. Philadelphia, Lippincott Williams & Wilkins, 1999.

Scheuring S, Muller DJ, Stahlberg H, Engel HA, Engel A: Sampling the conformational space of membrane protein surfaces with the AFM. Eur Biophys J 31:172-178, 2002.

Sukharev S, Durell SR, Guy HR: Structural models of the MscL gating mechanism. Biophys J 81:917-936, 2001.

Traub RD, Miles R, Wong RK: Model of the origin of rhythmic population oscillations in the hippocampal slice. Science 243:1319-1325, 1989.

Woodbury JW: Action potential: Properties of excitable membranes. In Rugh RC, Patton HD, Woodbury JW, Towe AL (eds): Neurophysiology, 2nd ed. Philadelphia, WB Saunders, 1965.

Chapter 4

The Chemical Basis for Neuronal Communication

R. W. Rockhold

Neurons in the human brain communicate primarily by the release of small quantities of *chemical messengers,* most of which are commonly called *neurotransmitters.* These chemicals alter the electrical activity of neurons after they interact with receptors on cell surfaces. Therapeutic alteration of brain function requires an understanding of the processes that regulate the synthesis and release of neurotransmitters, and the means by which receptors alter neuronal electrical activity and biochemical function.

Overview

The brain contains approximately 100 billion (10^{11}) neurons, each of which can make as many as 100,000 terminal contacts. Thus, it has been estimated that the human brain contains approximately 10^{16} connections between neurons. Communication at most of these connections is mediated by *chemical messengers.* The transfer of information between neurons takes place at structurally and functionally specialized locations called *synapses.* Most synapses use chemical messengers that are released in discrete units *(quanta)* from presynaptic axonic or dendritic terminals, in response to depolarization of the terminal.

Rapid diffusion of a chemical messenger across the *synaptic cleft* is followed by binding of this substance to receptors spanning the postsynaptic membrane. There is a resultant alteration in the electrical, biochemical, or genetic properties of that neuron. Less frequently, chemical messengers may also be released at sites without synaptic specializations. These messengers diffuse more widely than do neurotransmitters released at synaptic sites, and they influence receptors located at distant sites and on more than one neuron. Whether synaptic or nonsynaptic, chemical communication in the nervous system depends on (1) the nature of the presynaptically released *chemical messenger,* (2) the type of postsynaptic *receptor* to which it binds, and (3) the mechanism that couples receptors to effector systems in the target cell.

Western medicine is based fundamentally on modification of biologic function by drugs. Much of this alteration is focused on processes of chemical neurotransmission, whether in the central nervous system (CNS) or the periphery. The focus in this chapter is on basic elements of chemical neurotransmission. A model synapse, the noradrenergic synapse, is introduced, and a series of therapeutically important drugs is highlighted to illustrate potential medical targets in such a synapse.

Fundamentals of Chemical Neurotransmission

Neurotransmitters

Specific criteria that define whether a chemical messenger can be identified as a *neurotransmitter* are listed in Table 4-1. Although a wide variety of putative neurotransmitters have been identified, these criteria have been met for only a few chemical substances. Generally, these transmitters can be categorized as *small-molecule messengers* (having fewer than 10 carbon atoms) or larger *neuropeptides* (containing 10 or more carbon atoms).

Small-molecule chemical messengers are classed as amino acids, biogenic amines, and nucleotides or nucleosides (Table 4-2). *Amino acid* neurotransmitters include γ-aminobutyric acid (GABA), glycine, aspartate, and glutamate. The vast majority of signaling within the nervous system is carried by amino acid neurotransmitters, specifically GABA and glutamate. For example, it has been estimated that roughly every fifth nerve cell and one of every six synaptic contacts utilizes GABA as a neurotransmitter. The *biogenic amines* include the familiar neurotransmitters acetylcholine, dopamine, norepinephrine,

Table 4-1. Criteria Necessary to Define a Substance as a Neurotransmitter

I. Localization	A putative neurotransmitter must be localized to the presynaptic elements of an identified synapse and must be present also within the neuron from which the presynaptic terminal arises.
II. Release	The substance must be shown to be released from the presynaptic element upon activation of that terminal and simultaneously with depolarization of the parent neuron.
III. Identity	Application of the putative neurotransmitter to the target cells must be shown to produce the same effects as those produced by stimulation of the neurons in question.

Table 4-2. Substances Believed to Act as Chemical Messengers in the Central Nervous System

Small Molecules	Neuropeptides
Amino acids GABA Glycine Glutamate Aspartate Homocysteine Taurine	**Opioid peptides** Methionine enkephalin Leucine enkephalin β-Endorphin Dynorphin(s) Neoendorphins(s)

Biogenic amines
Acetylcholine
Monoamines
    Catecholamines
        Dopamine
        Norepinephrine
        Epinephrine
    Serotonin
    Histamine
	Posterior pituitary peptides
	Arginine vasopressin
	Oxytocin
	
	Tachykinins
	Substance P
	Kassinin
	Neurokinin A
	Neurokinin B
	Eledoisin

Nucleotides and nucleosides Adenosine ATP	**Glucagon-related peptides** Vasoactive intestinal peptide Glucagon Secretin Growth hormone–releasing hormone
Other Nitric oxide	**Pancreatic polypeptide–related peptides** Neuropeptide Y **Other** Somatostatin Corticotropin-releasing factor Calcitonin gene–related peptide Cholecystokinin Angiotensin II

ATP, adenosine triphosphate; GABA, γ-aminobutyric acid.

epinephrine, serotonin, and histamine. The nucleotide/nucleoside class includes adenosine and adenosine triphosphate (ATP). *Nitric oxide,* which functions as an endogenous *nitrovasodilator* in the cardiovascular system, has also been identified as a putative neurotransmitter.

More than 40 neuropeptides have been identified in brain tissue. These include methionine enkephalin (met-enkephalin) and leucine enkephalin (leu-enkephalin), as well as larger peptides, such as endorphins, calcitonin gene-related peptide

(CGRP), arginine vasopressin, cholecystokinin, and many others (Table 4-2).

With a few exceptions, one being nitric oxide, *the chemical messengers used by neurons are stored in secretory vesicles and released from them by exocytosis.* In the case of neurotransmitters, these vesicles are found mainly in the presynaptic nerve terminals.

Fast and Slow Synaptic Transmission

The diffusion of a chemical message across the synaptic cleft can be quite rapid. At the neuromuscular junction, for example, it takes only about 50 microseconds for acetylcholine to reach the postsynaptic membrane. Total *synaptic delay*, the time from presynaptic release of neurotransmitter to the activation or inhibition of the postsynaptic neuron, is variable. This variability is influenced by the transduction mechanisms in the postsynaptic neuron.

Transduction mechanisms can be divided into fast and slow types. *Fast chemical neurotransmission* operates with a total synaptic delay of only a few milliseconds, whereas *slow chemical neurotransmission* usually requires hundreds of milliseconds. In both cases, the receptors on the postsynaptic membranes are glycoproteins that span the lipid bilayer membrane and transduce an extracellular chemical signal into a functional change in the target neuron. The difference relates to the complexity of the transduction mechanism.

In *fast chemical neurotransmission* the postsynaptic receptor is itself an ion channel. This type of transmission is associated exclusively with *small-molecule neurotransmitters.* The binding of transmitter stimulates the channel to open, permitting a flux of ions across the membrane that alters the membrane potential. The process is fast because it is direct. Ion channels in this type of neurotransmission are called *ligand-gated* or *receptor-gated ion channels;* the ions normally involved are Na^+, K^+, Ca^{2+}, and Cl^-. Movement of these ions causes a change in the *transmembrane electrical potential,* which, if it exceeds threshold, may lead to generation of an action potential.

In *slow chemical neurotransmission* the signal is transduced by a mechanism involving G protein–coupled receptors. These proteins and their action are discussed later in the chapter. Briefly, the binding of the transmitter (frequently a *neuropeptide*) causes the receptor to activate a G protein, which in turn binds to and influences an effector protein, which elicits the cellular effect. In some cases, the effector protein is an ion channel, which is induced to open or close. Transduction in these cases can be almost as rapid as in fast neurotransmission. More often, the effector is an enzyme that produces an intracellular second messenger, such as cyclic AMP (cAMP), whose cytoplasmic concentration is altered in response to the reception of a signal (binding of the transmitter) at the cell surface and that elicits intracellular responses to the signal. Second messengers can produce a plethora of cellular responses, ranging from the opening or closing of membrane ion channels to alterations in gene expression. These effects are mediated by complex sequences of chemical events, which is why they are relatively slow.

Information Flow Across Chemical Synapses

Transmission of information at a chemical synapse involves the following general sequence of events (Fig. 4-1): (1) secretory vesicle synthesis and transport to the synaptic terminal; (2) for small-molecule neurotransmitters, loading of the transmitter into the vesicle (for neuropeptides, this step accompanies vesicle synthesis); (3) depolarization of the presynaptic terminal; (4) vesicle docking with the presynaptic membrane, exocytosis of its contents, and trans-synaptic diffusion of the transmitter; (5) binding of transmitter to, and activation of, the postsynaptic receptor; (6) transduction of the signal resulting in a postsynaptic

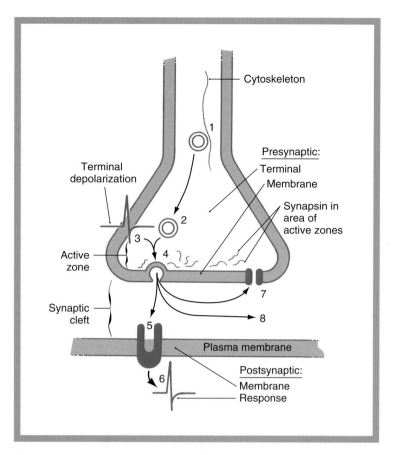

Figure 4-1. A generalized scheme for chemical synaptic transmission. The main steps are as numbered: (1) proximodistal axonal transport of a secretory vesicle; (2) synthesis and loading of small-molecule messengers in synaptic vesicles (neuropeptides are synthesized and loaded into large dense-cored vesicles in the soma); (3) depolarization of the presynaptic terminal by an arriving action potential, which causes (4) fusion of vesicles with the plasma membrane and exocytosis of the vesicle contents; (5) binding of transmitter with a postsynaptic receptor to produce (6) a postsynaptic response; and finally, elimination of the transmitter from the synapse by either (7) uptake into a cell (here, the presynaptic cell) or (8) enzymatic degradation in the synaptic cleft.

response and one or two terminal steps; and (7) active reuptake of the transmitter by the presynaptic terminals or by glia or (8) enzymatic degradation of the transmitter in the synaptic cleft. These final events eliminate transmitter from the synaptic cleft and thereby terminate its action.

In many synapses, the amount of transmitter that a presynaptic terminal releases in response to an action potential can be regulated from outside the cell. Two regulatory mechanisms are (1) *presynaptic receptor–mediated autoregulation* and (2) *retrograde transmission.* In presynaptic receptor–mediated autoregulation the neuron self-regulates the subsequent quantal release of its own chemical messenger. As a neurotransmitter enters the synaptic cleft, it stimulates not only postsynaptic receptors but also receptors located on the membranes of the terminal from which it was released. This constantly updates the presynaptic neuron concerning neurotransmitter synthesis, release, and the efficiency of information transfer. In most cases, autoregulation is inhibitory. Loss or reduction of this input is interpreted as a reduction in signaling ability and the presynaptic neuron increases the subsequent synthesis and release of stored neurotransmitter.

In *retrograde transmission* the postsynaptic neuron responds to synaptic activation by releasing a second chemical messenger. This messenger diffuses back across the synapse and alters the function of the presynaptic terminal. Nitric oxide is currently the best example of a mediator of retrograde transmission.

Synthesis, Storage, and Release of Chemical Messengers

Neuronal chemical messengers are stored in two types of vesicles: *small vesicles* (also called *synaptic vesicles*) and *large dense-cored vesicles*. Synaptic small vesicles (~50 nm in diameter) appear clear and empty in electron micrographs and contain small-molecule chemical messengers such as GABA, glutamate, and acetylcholine. A subset of these small vesicles, with electron-dense cores, are found in both central and peripheral neurons. These vesicles contain the catecholamine family of biogenic amines (dopamine, norepinephrine, and epinephrine). Synaptic vesicles cluster near the exocytotic surface of a presynaptic nerve terminal in regions called *active zones* (Fig. 4-1).

Large dense-cored vesicles (~75 to 150 nm in diameter) are less numerous and appear in other intraneuronal locations, as well as in the axon terminal. The electron-opaque, dense core is composed of soluble proteins that are mainly one or more neuropeptides. This core may also contain a small chemical messenger—often a biogenic amine, *co-stored* with a neuropeptide.

Neurons in certain hypothalamic nuclei contain a third type of vesicles called the *neurosecretory vesicles*. These vesicles are large (~150 to 200 nm in diameter), contain neurohormones, and are especially concentrated in axon terminals in the neurohypophysis (the posterior pituitary).

Composition of Vesicle Membranes

All vesicles are composed of a lipid bilayer membrane, spanned by a variety of proteins. Some proteins are common to both large dense-cored vesicles and synaptic vesicles, such as those that form *calcium channels*, and the proteins *synaptotagmin* and *SV2*. Other proteins are found in high concentrations only in synaptic vesicles; these include *synaptophysin* and *synaptobrevin*. The differences in protein content reflect the different roles that large dense-cored vesicles and synaptic vesicles play in neurons.

Vesicles also contain proteins that act to accumulate small chemical messengers. These take the form of membrane pumps or transporters, most of which are coupled to the transport of protons. Synaptic vesicles contain at least four classes of *proton-coupled transporters* for chemical messengers, each specific for a different type of messenger. One class, the vesicular monamine transporter (VAMT), drives the accumulation of biogenic amines, including the catecholamines dopamine, norepinephrine, and epinephrine, as well as the monoamine serotonin. Others are specific for acetylcholine, glutamate, and GABA/glycine. Large dense-cored vesicles can also accumulate small chemical messengers in addition to their neuropeptides. However, it is believed that the transporters involved are different from those used by synaptic vesicles.

Biosynthesis

In terms of biosynthesis, an important difference between synaptic vesicles and large dense-cored vesicles is that the former can be recycled and refilled in the axon terminal, whereas the latter are both made and filled in the neuronal soma and are not recycled. This reflects the fact that small-molecule neurotransmitters can be synthesized in axon terminals, whereas neuropeptides, because they are synthesized on ribosomes and processed through the endoplasmic reticulum and Golgi complex, can be made only in the soma (Fig. 4-2). The *cis* face of the Golgi complex (also called the proximal or forming face) is prototypically concave towards the nucleus of the cell, whereas the *trans* face (distal or maturation face) is convex (Fig. 4-2). Peptides from the endoplasmic reticulum enter the *cis* face of the Golgi complex and are sorted and packaged into vesicles that bud from its *trans* face.

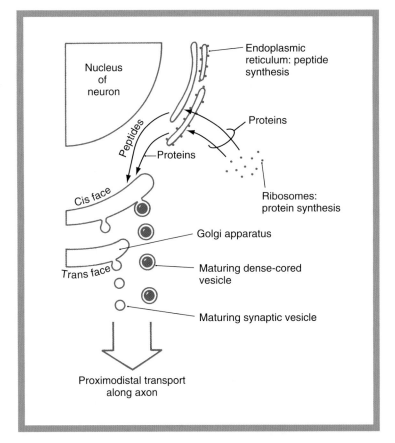

Figure 4-2. The synthesis of large, dense-cored vesicles and of synaptic vesicles in the neuron cell body. Synaptic vesicles are formed without existing stores of neurotransmitter; these are synthesized as the vesicles move into the nerve terminal. Large dense-cored vesicles are formed with existing stores of neuropeptide messengers as electron-dense cores.

Large, dense-cored vesicles contain neuropeptide messengers and are filled during the process of vesicle synthesis in the Golgi complex. These vesicles are translocated, by fast axonal transport (range 4 to 17 mm/hr), from the cell body to axonal or dendritic release sites (Fig. 4-3). Frequently, neuropeptides are synthesized in the form of large precursor peptides that may be cleaved to yield more than one secreted bioactive neuropeptide. Maturation of neuropeptides can require covalent chemical modification of amino acid side chains, often with the addition of small chemical groups. Examples of the types of chemical modifications include the addition of methyl groups (methylation), sugar moieties (glycosylation), and sulfate groups (sulfation). This process of maturation can occur within the endoplasmic reticulum, during packaging of peptides into large dense-cored vesicles within the Golgi complex, or during axonal transport.

In general, synaptic vesicles are formed initially by budding from the Golgi apparatus within the cell body (Figs. 4-2 and 4-4). After transport to and release from the presynaptic terminal, however, the lipoprotein membrane components of the synaptic vesicles are *recycled* in a continuous process that occurs within nerve terminals (Fig. 4-4). *Synthesis of the chemical messenger in a synaptic vesicle can occur while the vesicle is in the nerve terminal, rather than in the cell body.*

Some small-molecule neurotransmitters are synthesized in the cytosol of the axon and axon terminal and then transported into synaptic vesicles, whereas others are synthesized in the vesicle itself. The synthesis of acetylcholine is an example of the first of these mechanisms. The soluble enzyme *choline acetyltransferase (CAT)* catalyzes the acetylation of choline from acetyl coenzyme A (CoA) to yield the neurotransmitter acetylcholine.

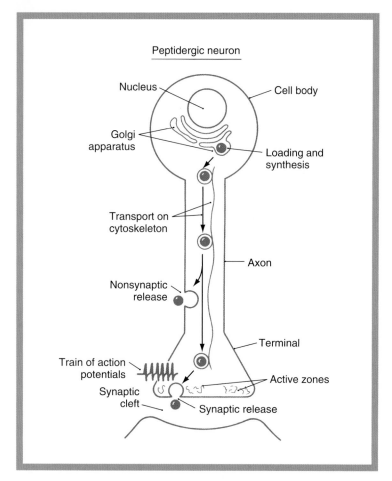

Figure 4-3. The formation, transport, and use of large dense-cored vesicles (containing neuropeptides) in a representative peptidergic neuron.

A high-affinity vesicular membrane transport protein concentrates this transmitter in cholinergic synaptic vesicles. Synthesis of the catecholamine norepinephrine is an example of the second mechanism. In the case of norepinephrine, synthesis occurs within the synaptic vesicle. The immediate precursor to norepinephrine, dopamine, is concentrated within the *noradrenergic* synaptic vesicle by a transporter specific for biogenic amines (the VAMT). Only then is dopamine converted to norepinephrine by the action of the enzyme *dopamine β-hydroxylase,* which is attached to the luminal border of the vesicular membrane.

Transporters for small chemical messengers concentrate compounds inside the vesicle to levels 10 to 1000 times higher than those found in the cytosol. The energy required for this transport is derived from an ATP-driven proton pump. The exchange of protons for the chemical messenger allows accumulation of the latter inside the vesicle.

Localization

As mentioned earlier, *synaptic vesicles* are preferentially concentrated in *active zones* of the nerve terminal (Figs. 4-4 and 4-5). These zones are biochemically and anatomically specialized for neurotransmitter release. Large numbers of voltage-sensitive calcium channels are clustered in the plasma membrane of active zones. Consequently, depolarization of the axon terminal (or in special cases the dendrites) results in a high local concentration of Ca^{2+}. This calcium causes synaptic vesicles to bind to the plasma membrane and stimulates exocytotic release of vesicle contents into the synaptic cleft. Active zones also contain high

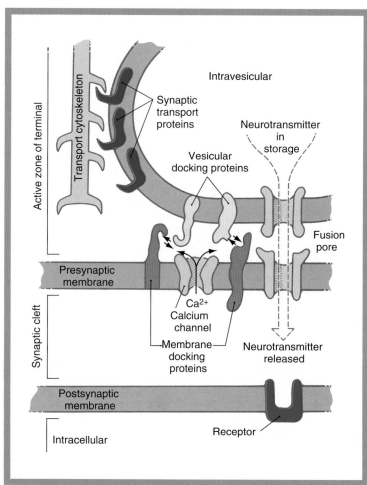

Figure 4-5. The protein components that mediate transport and docking of synaptic vesicles and the probable formation of the fusion pore.
Depolarization opens voltage-dependent calcium channels, allowing ingress of Ca^{2+}, which facilitates formation of the docking complex. Once docking is accomplished, additional proteins, under the influence of elevated intracellular Ca^{2+} levels, associate to form a fusion pore.

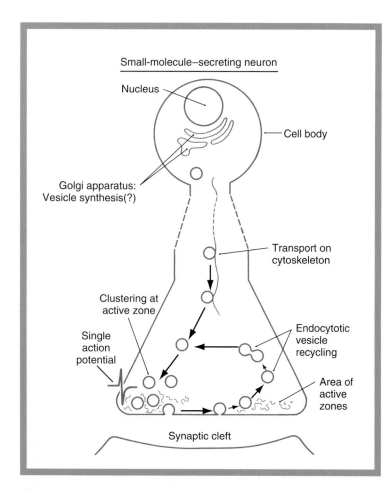

Figure 4-4. The formation, transport, and cycling of synaptic vesicles (containing small-molecule neurotransmitters) in a representative neuron.

concentrations of the filamentous protein *synapsin,* which aids in the clustering of synaptic vesicles.

Although *large dense-cored vesicles* may accumulate in active zones, they also bind to the plasma membrane and release their contents from other sites in the terminal and axon that lack active zones (Fig. 4-3). As with synaptic vesicles, exocytosis depends on a local increase in Ca^{2+} concentration. However, the release mechanisms for large dense-cored vesicles appear to be more sensitive to Ca^{2+} than those for synaptic vesicles. Therefore, sites of release do not require the high density of Ca^{2+} channels found in active zones. Release sites outside active zones (such as those associated with large dense-cored vesicles) also do not have anchoring proteins such as synapsins.

Release

The essential structural elements critical for synaptic vesicle release are depicted in Figure 4-5. Proteins in the vesicle wall interact with cytoskeletal proteins to propel vesicles into the active zone. The surface of the synaptic vesicle contains two groups of proteins that are crucial for exocytotic release: *docking proteins* and elements of the *fusion pore.* A rise in intracellular Ca^{2+} levels causes the vesicular docking proteins to interact with docking proteins on the cell membrane, creating a *docking complex* that brings the two membranes into apposition. Complementary proteins on both membranes then interact to form the *fusion pore,* and the lipid bilayers of the two membranes fuse at this site to form a rapidly expanding hole. Stored neurotransmitter in the vesicle begins to leak out through the fusion pore and exits in bulk (complete exocytosis) as the pore expands.

It is likely that large dense-cored vesicles use somewhat different proteins and mechanisms for docking and exocytosis than those used by synaptic vesicles. Also, while synaptic vesicles undergo exocytosis in response to single nerve impulses (Fig. 4-4), large dense-cored vesicles respond preferentially to high-frequency trains of impulses (Fig. 4-3). In experiments using peripheral nerves, a stimulation frequency of 10 Hz is often required to elicit neuropeptide release. Frequencies of that magnitude occur naturally in the autonomic nervous system under conditions of extreme behavioral or physiologic stress. Consequently, neuropeptides may play a role in stress responses.

Signal Transduction

Chemical messengers, once released from a presynaptic site, must interact with a postsynaptic neuron to transmit information. The postsynaptic membrane contains target molecules that exhibit an affinity for individual chemical messengers; these molecules are known as *receptors.* Most receptors are transmembrane glycoprotein chains. The binding of a messenger with its receptor precipitates a change in the architecture (*conformation*) of the glycoprotein chain that begins the process of information transfer. Some exceptions do exist. For example, there are *intracellular receptors* for testosterone. To be activated, drugs such as testosterone must first traverse the plasma membrane to gain access to the receptor.

Receptors and Receptor Subtypes

The *receptor* is capable of altering intracellular function in response to a change in the concentration of a specific chemical messenger in the environment. Thus, a receptor transduces a chemical signal (i.e., the concentration of a chemical messenger) into an intracellular event.

Receptors may be categorized by several means. One simplifying proposal identifies receptors into four general categories: (1) those termed *ligand-gated* channels (also called *transmitter-gated* channels), in which binding of a chemical messenger alters the probability of opening of transmembrane pores or channels; (2) those in which the receptor proteins are coupled to intracellular G proteins as transducing elements; (3) those consisting of single membrane-spanning protein units that have intrinsic enzyme activity (for example, having tyrosine kinase activity); and (4) those termed *ligand-dependent regulators of nuclear transcription* (including receptors for corticosteroids such as testosterone).

On a more specific level, it is common for receptors to be grouped according to the type of native chemical messenger to which they respond. Thus, all the receptors that respond to physiologically relevant concentrations of acetylcholine are called *acetylcholine receptors* (often termed *cholinergic receptors*). Similarly, *adrenoceptors* (often termed *adrenergic receptors*) respond to the catecholamine chemical messengers, epinephrine (previously called adrenaline) and norepinephrine (noradrenaline). Traditionally (and functionally), *receptors are identified by the response of a cell or tissue to a series of chemicals of different but closely allied molecular structures.* Each compound in the series produces identical cell or tissue responses. However, each compound will exhibit a distinct potency (i.e., the concentration required to elicit the desired response) at each different receptor. The rank order of potency for a series of chemicals at each receptor then defines that unique receptor. It is common to rank potencies in terms of the concentration of an agent that produces 50% of the maximal biologic response in the test cell or tissue, or the *effective concentration* (EC_{50}).

Agents that activate a receptor, whether they be native neurotransmitters or exogenous drugs, are termed receptor *agonists.* In contrast, receptor *antagonists* bind to a receptor but do not elicit any response. Rather, by preventing binding of an agonist to its receptor, the antagonist prevents any receptor-mediated signal from being produced. More recently, functional identification of a receptor has been complemented and amplified by molecular cloning techniques, which identify receptor similarities based on the primary amino acid sequence.

The receptors that respond to a given transmitter can often be divided into *subtypes* that elicit different biologic responses. For example, cholinergic receptors are divided into *nicotinic* and *muscarinic* subtypes. A cholinergic synapse with nicotinic receptors is commonly excitatory, whereas one with muscarinic receptors is commonly inhibitory. These receptor subtypes are named after plant compounds that stimulate them selectively and helped lead to their discovery. Nicotinic receptors are named after the nicotine of tobacco, and muscarinic receptors are named after muscarine, a substance found in the toxic mushroom *Amanita muscaria.*

The multiplicity of receptor subtypes can seem overwhelming at first. In the cholinergic system, both nicotinic and muscarinic receptors have subtypes of their own. For example, five different muscarinic receptor subtypes, termed M_1 to M_5, have been recognized. Adrenergic receptors (described in more detail elsewhere) are classified broadly into α-*adrenoceptor* and β-*adrenoceptor* subtypes, each of which is further delineated. Currently, six α-adrenoceptors (α_{1A}, α_{1B}, α_{1D}, α_{2A}, α_{2B}, α_{2C}) and four β-adrenoceptors (β_1, β_2, β_3, and β_4) are recognized. The serotonergic system is yet more complex, with 14 recognized receptor subtypes. Distinctions between subtypes are conferred by differences in coupling to intracellular second messenger systems, by changes in amino acid sequence of the receptor protein(s), or by insertion of different protein subunits (in receptors in which the integral ion channel is oligomeric, i.e., constructed of multiple, distinct protein subunits). The $GABA_A$ receptor is a good example of this last type of modification. This receptor, like the nicotinic acetylcholine receptor, is a pentamer that forms a transmembrane ion channel. Molecular studies have identified 19 related $GABA_A$ receptor subunits in mammals.

Regional differences in the subunit construction of the receptor, which are believed to confer subtle alterations in receptor function, are found in the brain and periphery.

Structure and Function

Transmembrane receptor proteins have a general structure that is based on glycoprotein chains that fold into the neural membrane in multiple loops (Fig. 4-6), although many of the receptors with intrinsic enzyme-associated activity consist of only a single transmembrane subunit. The protein is held in the membrane by several hydrophobic membrane-spanning segments (usually α *helices* but in specialized regions having a β-*pleated sheet* conformation), which are connected by loops that project into the aqueous environment on either side of the membrane. The N-terminal (NH_2-terminal) and C-terminal (COOH-terminal) segments also project into the aqueous environment; they are typically relatively straight. In some transmembrane receptors, such as the β-adrenergic receptor, the N-terminal segment projects extracellularly and the C-terminal segment projects intracellularly (Fig. 4-6). In contrast, in voltage-gated ion channels, the N-terminal and C-terminal segments usually both project intracellularly. G protein–coupled receptors are formed from a single polypeptide chain, whereas most ligand-gated ion pores are multisubunit structures.

In G protein–coupled receptors, the transmembrane segments of the protein (usually seven in number) form a cluster that contains the binding site or sites for chemical messengers. The site is usually in a relatively hydrophobic pocket in the cluster, although it is sometimes on the extracellular surface of the protein. The receptor binds with its G protein transducer through multiple cationic sites on intracellular hydrophilic regions. The β-adrenergic receptors are the best characterized of the G protein–coupled receptors; their functioning is discussed later in the chapter.

Ligand-Gated Ion Channels

Ligand-gated ion channels are formed by several structurally distinct protein subunits called *channel subunits* (Fig. 4-7). Each channel subunit is a transmembrane glycoprotein (as described previously) with membrane-spanning segments connected by intracellular and extracellular loops. The channel subunits complex to form a roughly cylindrical structure that encloses a water-filled transmembrane channel. As exemplified by the nicotinic cholinergic receptor, the external face of the channel is enlarged and cuplike (Fig. 4-7). The channel narrows as it crosses the membrane, reducing the inner diameter such that it can selectively pass small cations (Na^+, K^+, and Ca^{2+}) or anions (Cl^-). The internal face of the channel widens again as it emerges from the lipid bilayer. The inner surface of the pore is blocked at rest by amino acid residues that project into the aqueous lumen of the pore and prevent the conductance of charged ions. This part of the channel is termed the *gate. Binding sites*, which most commonly occur at relatively hydrophobic regions within the transmembrane region of the channel, are specific for a chemical messenger. When a binding site is filled, conformational changes occur within the channel protein to open the gate and permit selective passage of ions across the membrane.

Two gene superfamilies of ligand-gated ion channels have been identified. One contains nicotinic cholinergic, serotonin (5-hydroxytryptamine), GABA, and glycine receptors; the other encodes the receptors for the excitatory neurotransmitter glutamate. The segregation of receptors into different superfamilies is based on the degree of homology of amino acid sequences. The subunits of the various receptors in a superfamily have 20% to 40% sequence homology with each other. The subunits of any given receptor generally have sequence homology of greater than 40%.

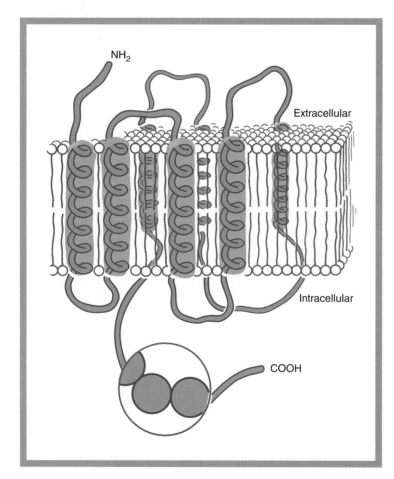

Figure 4-6. A membrane-linked receptor protein (human β-adrenergic receptor), embedded in a neuronal plasma membrane. Hydrophobic transmembrane amino acid sequences are coiled in an α-helical array and form a cluster of seven transmembrane columns. The G protein, although not shown here, would associate with intracellular loops of the receptor protein. The enlarged area denotes the fact that the protein is composed of linked amino acids.

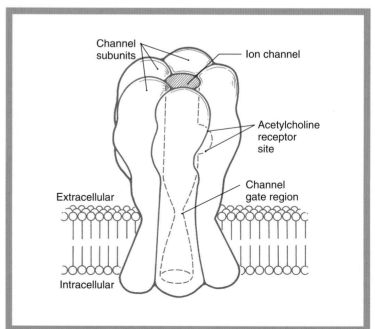

Figure 4-7. A typical ligand-gated ion channel, the nicotinic cholinergic receptor. This receptor is composed of five nonhomologous channel subunit proteins, each containing four hydrophobic membrane-spanning regions. Acetylcholine binds to the nicotinic receptor in the central core.

G Protein–Coupled Receptors

The G protein receptors introduce a further level of complexity to chemical transmission (Fig. 4-8). *About three fourths of all chemical messengers transmit their information through G protein–coupled receptors.* The basic elements of this system include a *receptor*, which must face the external surface of the membrane, the *guanosine triphosphate (GTP)-binding protein*, which consists of α, β, and γ subunits, and an *effector protein*, which may be an enzyme that alters the concentrations of intracellular *second messengers* (such as Ca^{2+}, inositol 1,4,5-trisphosphate, diacyl glycerol, or members of the eicosanoid family), or may be an ion channel (Fig. 4-8). The responses mediated by these receptors are generally slow (hundreds of milliseconds to minutes). The G protein–coupled receptor complex transduces an extremely wide range of chemical messages. About 100 different receptors have been identified that can link to a G protein, and at least 20 distinct G proteins have a similar number of effector proteins. The biogenic amines, bioactive peptides, eicosanoids, light (one of the first characterized G protein–coupled receptors was rhodopsin in the mammalian photoreceptor), and odorants all interact with G protein–coupled receptors.

The G protein functions to amplify a signal received by a transmembrane receptor, transmitting that message to effector proteins within a neuron. Each G protein exists as a complex (a *heterotrimer*) formed by α, β, and γ subunits (Fig. 4-8). The αβγ heterotrimer maintains a loose association with the receptor glycoprotein but is not covalently bound to the receptor. Within the heterotrimer, the α subunit determines the nature of the G protein. It has the ability to bind GTP, detach from the coupled βγ complex, and alter the activity of an effector protein. The effector proteins whose activity can be modulated by α subunits are diverse and include the enzyme adenylyl cyclase as well as ion channels for calcium and potassium. In contrast, the βγ complex anchors α subunits to membrane sites and inhibits the GTP-guanosine diphosphate (GDP) exchange that activates the α subunit.

The resting form of a G protein exists as the heterotrimer, with GDP bound to the α subunit and the α subunit bound by the βγ complex (Fig. 4-8A). When activated, the α subunit exchanges GDP for GTP and dissociates from the βγ complex. The α subunit is then free to bind with and alter the activity of the effector protein; in this example it is adenylyl cyclase (Fig. 4-8B, C). The α subunit has an integral slow GTPase activity, which eventually hydrolyzes the bound GTP to bound GDP (usually in 3 to 15 seconds). Reassociation of the α subunit–GDP complex with the βγ complex then completes the cycle (Fig. 4-8C, D).

The most completely characterized G protein–coupled receptor is the β_2-adrenergic receptor. The endogenous ligand for this receptor is the catecholamine epinephrine. Epinephrine is a neurotransmitter that is confined to a very small number of cell groups within the brain and to chromaffin secretory cells in the adrenal gland. It is used clinically in cardiopulmonary

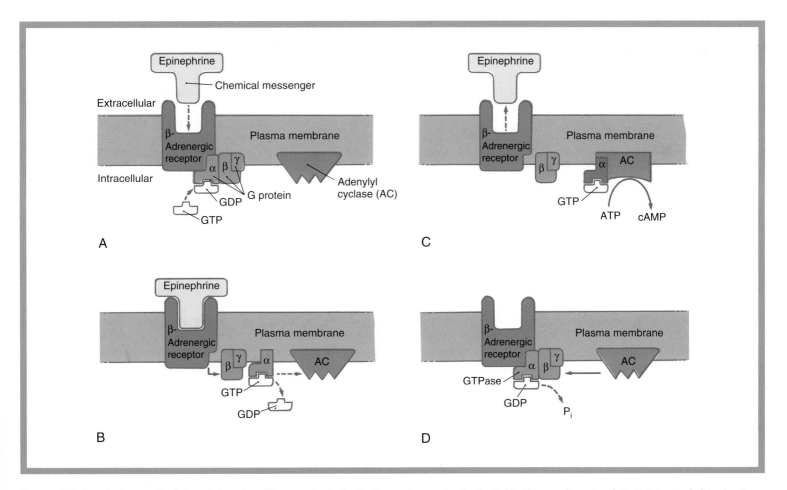

Figure 4-8. A typical example of G protein action. The receptor is the β-adrenergic receptor (activated in this case by epinephrine). It is coupled to the G_s type of G protein, which has a stimulatory action on the effector, adenylyl cyclase. When stimulated, adenylyl cyclase produces the second messenger cyclic adenosine monophosphate (cAMP) from adenosine triphosphate (ATP). The cycle of G protein action is as follows: (**A**) In the resting state, the G protein is in the form of an αβγ heterotrimer and the α subunit carries bound GDP. (**B**) Epinephrine binding to, and conformation change of, the receptor protein and the G protein. Guanosine diphosphate (GDP), which has been bound to the α subunit, exchanges for guanosine triphosphate (GTP) as the α subunit dissociates from the βγ complex and from the receptor. (**C**) Binding of the α subunit (with GTP attached) to adenylyl cyclase alters the conformation of the enzyme. This increases enzymatic catalysis of the substrate ATP to cAMP. (**D**) Slow enzymatic dephosphorylation of GTP to GDP by the GTPase allows the α subunit to return to its resting conformation. As this occurs, the α subunit dissociates from adenylyl cyclase and reassociates with the βγ subunit. The heterotrimeric G protein reestablishes a loose association with the receptor protein.

resuscitation during cardiac asystole and to treat anaphylactic reactions. The β_2-adrenergic receptor is coupled to a G protein that stimulates activity of adenylyl cyclase, catalyzing formation of cAMP from intracellular ATP stores (Fig. 4-8). The stimulatory G protein associated with the β_2-adrenergic receptor is called G_s.

Effector Proteins

As mentioned earlier, G proteins can interact with two main kinds of effector proteins: *ion channels* (called *G protein–coupled ion channels*) and *enzymes that alter the level of intracellular second messenger compounds*. The action of the G protein on its target may be positive or negative. That is, it may cause a channel to open or, more rarely, close, or it may stimulate or inhibit a target enzyme. Most synaptic G protein responses are mediated through second messenger systems. Second messengers can elicit a variety of cellular responses, including the opening or closing of ion channels in the cell membrane (note that this indirect mechanism is in addition to the mechanism by which G proteins can interact directly with ion channels), the release or reuptake of Ca^{2+} from intracellular storage sites, alterations in the activity of key cellular enzymes, and alterations in the expression of specific genes. Many of these effects are mediated by *protein kinases*, enzymes that regulate the activity of other proteins by phosphorylation. A given G protein–coupled receptor may activate more than one mechanism and produce multiple coordinated effects. G protein–coupled systems therefore have the capacity to mediate complex changes in neuronal function.

The best-known second messenger systems involve the enzymes *adenylyl cyclase* (Fig. 4-8) and *guanylate cyclase*. Adenylyl cyclase produces the second messenger cyclic GMP (cGMP) from cytoplasmic GTP. Another important second messenger system involves the enzyme phospholipase C, which hydrolyzes the membrane phospholipid *phosphatidylinositol 4,5-bisphosphate* to produce the second messengers *inositol 1,4,5-trisphosphate* (*IP_3*) and *diacylglycerol* (*DAG*). G proteins can also interact with *phospholipase A_2*, which stimulates the formation of members of the eicosanoid family, and with another enzyme called *phospholipase D*.

Receptor Regulation

The postsynaptic receptor is not static, either in terms of response to agonists or in the number of active receptors present on the membrane. The response of postsynaptic receptors to changes in the synaptic environment is a crucial element in neuronal communication. One of the most intensively studied postsynaptic receptor response systems is that of a G protein–coupled receptor, the β-adrenergic receptor—specifically, the β_2-adrenergic receptor subtype. Continuous or repeated exposure of the β_2-adrenergic receptor to an agonist will result in a diminution of the response of that agonist. The mechanisms by which this loss of response occur are characterized by the time frame over which they occur. Exposure to an agonist for seconds to minutes will result in a reduction in the agonist-induced response through processes called *desensitization*. The loss of receptor responsiveness is mediated by agonist-induced changes in the receptor conformation that permit binding of additional intracellular proteins to the receptor. These proteins cause *phosphorylation* (i.e., addition of phosphate moieties) of the intracellular portions of the receptor. Phosphorylation changes the affinity of the receptors to other intracellular proteins that uncouple activated receptors from their effector proteins.

Homologous desensitization occurs when stimulation of the receptor by an agonist evokes the phosphorylation. Desensitization can also be produced without direct stimulation of the receptor in question, which is termed *heterologous desensitization*.

In this latter case, intracellular phosphorylating enzymes are recruited by stimuli other than activation of the receptor. If the stimulus is maintained, the receptor protein may be subsequently sequestered into invaginations of the membrane that undergo internalization, effectively removing the receptor from the membrane surface. Once internalized, a receptor can be degraded or, in some circumstances, recycled back into the membrane as a fully sensitive, active receptor. Receptor *downregulation*, on the other hand, is caused by exposure to agonists for longer periods of time—hours to days—and is characterized by a reduction in the number of active receptors on the cell surface. Downregulation may be achieved by enhanced protein receptor degradation, decreased transcription of the messenger RNA (mRNA) for that receptor, or enhanced degradation of receptor mRNA.

Regulation of Neuronal Excitability

As we have seen, neurotransmitters cause the opening or closing of ion channels in the postsynaptic membrane. If the transmitter signal is transduced by a G protein mechanism, it also may have other effects. The result will be a transient, local change in the polarization of the postsynaptic membrane, called a *synaptic potential*. This potential consists of either a depolarization or a hyperpolarization of the membrane relative to the resting potential. (Membrane potentials and the electrical properties of neuronal cell membranes are discussed in more detail in Chapter 3.) Synaptic potentials are graded in amplitude, reflecting the varying strengths of the incoming synaptic signals that elicit them. They generally do not exceed 20 mV. Local potentials of this type spread passively over the membrane of the postsynaptic cell, gradually losing amplitude and dying out. However, if they reach a *trigger zone*—a locus at which action potentials can be initiated—they may contribute to the production or suppression of action potentials. An action potential is triggered whenever the membrane is depolarized beyond a certain threshold potential. Therefore, *depolarizing* synaptic potentials tend to promote action potentials and are called *excitatory postsynaptic potentials* (EPSPs). Conversely, *hyperpolarizing* synaptic potentials inhibit the production of action potentials and are called *inhibitory postsynaptic potentials* (IPSPs).

In the CNS, a neuron is constantly bombarded by neurotransmitters, each of which can generate or modify a synaptic potential. Neurotransmitters that move the membrane toward depolarization (by reducing the –70 mV resting potential), with the resultant production of an action potential, are commonly called *excitatory neurotransmitters*. Neurotransmitters that move the membrane away from depolarization (by making the resting membrane more negative, the membrane is hyperpolarized) are frequently referred to as *inhibitory neurotransmitters. Because the postsynaptic response is actually elicited by the receptor rather than by the transmitter, the postsynaptic receptor determines whether a given neurotransmitter will be excitatory or inhibitory.* Some neurotransmitters can have either effect, depending on the type of postsynaptic receptor present.

Excitatory neurotransmitters act by promoting the opening of channels selective for cations (either Na^+ or Ca^{2+}) that flux into the cell and depolarize the membrane. In some cases, as in that of certain glutamate receptor subtypes, the neurotransmitter binds directly to a stereospecific site on an associated ion channel. Glutamate receptor subtypes of this ilk are classified as *ionotropic*. Excitatory ionotropic glutamate receptors include the NMDA, AMPA, and kainate subtypes, each of which is named after a selective ligand for that subtype (NMDA, *N*-methyl-D-aspartate; AMPA, α-amino-3-hydroxy-5-methyl-4-isoxazole propionic acid). In other cases, opening of cation channels is accomplished indirectly, following alteration of an intracellular second messenger system or systems. Inhibitory neurotransmitters act by opening channels for K^+ or Cl^-. Important examples of inhibitory neurotransmitters are the amino acids *GABA* and *glycine*.

It is essential to recognize that *a single chemical messenger can evoke either an EPSP or an IPSP, depending on the receptor to which it binds*. A good example is the neurotransmitter norepinephrine. Like glutamate, norepinephrine binds to multiple receptor subtypes. In the CNS, receptors for norepinephrine fall into two categories: α-adrenergic and β-adrenergic receptors. Both types are G protein coupled. The G protein to which β-adrenergic receptors are coupled is of a type called G_s, which *stimulates* the activity of adenylyl cyclase and thus produces a rise in intracellular cAMP. This rise in cAMP leads to an EPSP. In contrast, the G protein to which the $α_2$-adrenergic receptor subtype is coupled, called G_i, *inhibits* the activity of adenylyl cyclase. The resulting fall in intracellular cAMP leads to an IPSP. In both cases, cAMP acts through enzymes called *cAMP-dependent protein kinases*. In the pathway under discussion, the final targets are membrane ion channels, which open or close in response to the phosphorylation of sites on their cytoplasmic domains. Consequently, norepinephrine can elicit either an excitatory or inhibitory response, depending on the receptor.

Maintenance of the Synaptic Environment

The concentration of a chemical messenger in the synaptic cleft is crucial to information transfer. However, the time frame during which a chemical message is active must be limited if a temporally discrete signal is to be produced. This is particularly true when neurons fire at rates of more than several depolarizations per second. Simple diffusion out of the synaptic cleft is rarely adequate to effectively terminate the postsynaptic signal. Accordingly, active mechanisms exist to reduce or eliminate chemical messengers in the synaptic cleft. The principal mechanisms are *enzymatic degradation of transmitter in the cleft* and *transporter-mediated uptake* across cell membranes.

Acetylcholine and the neuropeptides are examples of transmitters that are neutralized by enzymatic degradation in the cleft. Acetylcholine is cleaved by the enzyme *acetylcholinesterase*, which is synthesized by the neuron and inserted into the postsynaptic membrane near receptor sites. Neuropeptides are degraded through hydrolysis by the action of multiple *peptidases*, which are found in extracellular fluid.

The neurotransmitters whose action is terminated by uptake from the synaptic cleft include the monoamines (such as serotonin, histamine, and the catecholamines) and the amino acid neurotransmitters GABA, glycine, glutamate, and aspartate. This uptake is accomplished by the action of specific membrane-bound *transport proteins*. The monoamine class of biogenic amines (including the catecholamines, serotonin, and histamine) is avidly removed from the synaptic space by such transport proteins. Specificity for neurotransmitter uptake is provided by these transporters. Unique proteins have been identified that preferentially transport individual monoamines, the best identified of which are the *norepinephrine* (NET), *dopamine* (DAT), and *serotonin* (SERT) *transporters*.

In the case of norepinephrine, *reuptake* into the cytoplasm of the presynaptic terminal (a process known as *uptake 1*; subserved by the NET) is primarily responsible for terminating the action of the transmitter (Fig. 4-9). After reuptake, some norepinephrine is enzymatically degraded by the mitochondrial enzyme *monoamine oxidase* (MAO), whereas an additional fraction is retained in a cytoplasmic pool. The norepinephrine in this pool is an important target for drug action. Norepinephrine can also be removed through the action of a transporter on the postsynaptic membrane and in glia (*uptake 2*; subserved by the *extraneuronal monoamine transport*, EMT), although this process is usually less effective (Fig. 4-9). Norepinephrine transported into the postsynaptic neuron is degraded by the enzyme *catechol-O-methyltransferase* (COMT).

In the CNS, glial cells, primarily astrocytes, also express transporter proteins on their membranes and can remove transmitters from the synaptic cleft. The actions of the amino acids, GABA, glycine, glutamate, and aspartate are all terminated by active transport into neurons and glial cells. No active uptake mechanisms have been found that terminate the action of neuropeptides (see Chapter 2).

The mechanisms of termination of some other chemical messengers, such as adenosine, ATP, and nitric oxide, are less well understood. Nitric oxide is very labile; it undergoes redox reactions with membrane and cytoplasmic sulfhydryl moieties, reducing them and becoming oxidized itself. Specific ATPases may terminate the action of ATP functioning as a neurotransmitter.

Drug-Induced Parkinson Disease

A therapeutically relevant example of interaction with neurotransmitter transporters occurs in the substantia nigra, where the action of neurotransmitter dopamine is terminated, in part, by uptake into glia by means of the EMT (uptake 2). Glia normally metabolize dopamine to inactive products by means of an MAO isoform, MAO-B, that is confined largely to the CNS. However, in the early 1980s in California, several cases of idiopathic paralysis that resembled severe Parkinson disease were noted in young persons. Through insightful clinical investigation, a young neurologist, W. Langston, recognized a connection between the clinical symptoms and botched synthesis of an illicit analogue of meperidine (a potent opioid analgesic legally supplied under the trade name Demerol) that resulted in formation of MPTP (1-methyl-4-phenyl-1, 2, 3, 6-tetrahydropyridine). Subsequent study determined that MPTP is transported into glia and metabolized by MAO-B into a related neurotoxic compound, MPP+ (1-methyl-4-phenylpyridinium), that is released from glia and transported into nigral dopaminergic neurons by the DAT (uptake 1), selectively damaging them and producing a characteristic triphasic clinical syndrome that closely resembles Parkinson disease. The clinical hallmarks of this syndrome begin with intravenous injection of a contaminated meperidine analogue, which characteristically produces a burning sensation and a "high" that is more "spacey and giddy" than that usually experienced with heroin injection. Within 2 to 3 days, bradykinesia and rigidity of movement and awkward posture leading to inability to move begin to develop. These early responses may develop into a permanent parkinsonian syndrome with bradykinesia, rigidity, resting tremor, fixed stare, and loss of postural reflexes. The analysis of this tragedy has led to the use of MPTP as an extraordinarily helpful model of Parkinson disease.

Pharmacologic Modification of Synaptic Transmission

Drugs can alter virtually every level of neuronal and synaptic function. Therapeutic effects are most commonly achieved by actions of drugs on *neurotransmitter synthesis, vesicular uptake and storage, depolarization-induced exocytosis, neurotransmitter-receptor binding*, and *termination of neurotransmitter action*. Increasingly, drugs are being developed that modify neurotransmitter action through interaction with *postsynaptic effector systems*.

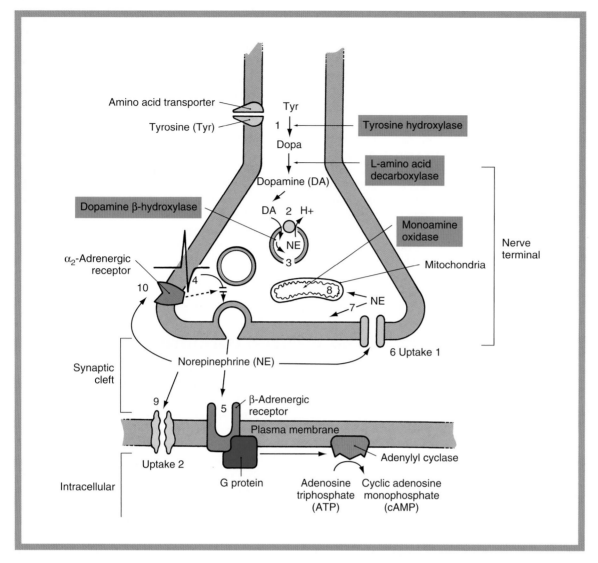

Figure 4-9. The noradrenergic β$_2$-adrenergic receptor synapse. Pharmacologic agents are identified by the numerals. Synthetic and degradative enzymes are shown in *red*; membrane receptors, transporters, and ion channels in *green*; and the postsynaptic effector G protein in *blue*. (1) α-*Methyltyrosine* competitively inhibits tyrosine hydroxylase; (2) *reserpine* irreversibly inhibits the monoamine-H$^+$ vesicular transport pump (the VAMT); (3) α-*methyldopa* acts as a false transmitter, displacing norepinephrine in the synaptic vesicle; (4) *guanethidine* blocks the ability of membrane depolarization to cause exocytotic release of vesicle contents; (5) *propranolol* is a competitive antagonist at β-adrenergic receptors; (6) *cocaine* blocks synaptic membrane reuptake of norepinephrine (Uptake 1; NET); (7) *tyramine* displaces norepinephrine from a cytoplasmic storage pool back into the synaptic cleft; (8) *tranylcypromine* blocks the degradation of norepinephrine by mitochondrial monoamine oxidase; (9) *corticosterone* prevents uptake of norepinephrine by the postsynaptic membrane (Uptake 2; EMT); (10) *yohimbine* is a competitive antagonist at presynaptic, autoinhibitory α$_2$-adrenergic receptors.

The Noradrenergic Synapse

The noradrenergic synapse is used to illustrate the range of pharmacologic agents that can modify synaptic transmission (Fig. 4-9). Noradrenergic synapses use the neurotransmitter norepinephrine, and their postsynaptic receptors fall into the two classes introduced earlier, the α-adrenergic and β-adrenergic receptors. In the peripheral nervous system, norepinephrine is a critical neurotransmitter in the regulation of the *sympathetic* division of the *autonomic nervous system*. In the CNS, norepinephrine is synthesized in neurons concentrated in several discrete brainstem regions; these areas send noradrenergic axons throughout the brain and exert widespread effects. The greatest single source of norepinephrine in the mammalian CNS is the locus ceruleus, a paired structure in the floor of the pontine fourth ventricle. In humans, cerulear noradrenergic neurons number only about 12,500/side yet influence brain function from the spinal cord to the cerebral cortex.

Norepinephrine is synthesized from the amino acid *tyrosine* in a sequence of three enzymatic reactions (Fig. 4-9). The first two occur in the cytoplasm; the final reaction takes place within the synaptic vesicle. Tyrosine is accumulated in the terminal by a membrane-bound amino acid carrier and is converted to dopa by *tyrosine hydroxylase* (step 1 in Fig. 4-9). The rate of this conversion makes it the rate-limiting step in norepinephrine synthesis. Regulation of tyrosine hydroxylase is accomplished by phosphorylation of the enzyme by intracellular protein kinases, which increases the rate of enzymatic catalysis. The drug α-*methyltyrosine* can limit noradrenergic function by acting as a competitive inhibitor of tyrosine hydroxylase, thereby reducing the rate of norepinephrine synthesis. This drug, also called *metyrosine* (Demser), is used clinically in management of patients who suffer from symptoms due to the excess production of catecholamines arising from tumors of adrenal chromaffin cell tissue, or *pheochromocytomas*.

Dopa is converted to *dopamine* (a neurotransmitter in its own right) by L-amino acid decarboxylase. Dopamine is transported into, and concentrated within, the synaptic vesicle by a monoamine-H$^+$ transporter (the VAMT; step 2 in Fig. 4-9). The accumulation of dopamine (and ultimately, norepinephrine) can be prevented by *reserpine*, a plant alkaloid that irreversibly inactivates the vesicular transporter (step 2 in Fig. 4-9). The inability to fill vesicles with neurotransmitter results in a progressive reduction in the level of transmitter in the axon terminal, which inhibits neurotransmission.

Reserpine, one of the earliest therapeutic agents available for the treatment of hypertensive cardiovascular disease, markedly reduces the ability of cardiac noradrenergic neurons to stimulate the heart to increase rate and contractility, thus lowering cardiac output. In addition, noradrenergic neurons that innervate arteriolar smooth muscle produce less norepinephrine, which results in less vasoconstriction and an overall reduction in blood pressure. Reserpine can precipitate parkinsonian symptoms that result from depletion of dopamine in nigrostriatal terminals as well as increased neurohypophyseal release of prolactin leading to galactorrhea as a result of deletion of tuberoinfundibular dopamine. Reserpine may also worsen clinical depression, a finding that contributed to the monoamine theory of depression. Today, reserpine is only rarely used to treat hypertension.

Within the vesicle, dopamine is converted to norepinephrine by *dopamine β-hydroxylase*. The accumulation of both dopamine and norepinephrine can also be reduced by administration of α-*methyldopa* (Aldomet). This dopa analogue is enzymatically converted in successive steps to α-methyldopamine and α-methylnorepinephrine, which takes the place of the normal synthetic products, resulting in reduction of noradrenergic transmission (Fig. 4-9). Elevated sympathetic nerve activity contributes to hypertensive cardiovascular disease. Clinically, α-methyldopa is an effective antihypertensive drug and is one of the most commonly used drugs for managing hypertension during pregnancy.

The drug *guanethidine* interferes with the coupling between excitation of the nerve terminal and exocytotic release of norepinephrine, thereby reducing the amount of norepinephrine released. In addition, guanethidine acts like reserpine to inactivate vesicular transport. Unfortunately, guanethidine causes such a profound inhibition of noradrenergic neuron function that its use is associated with undesirable and unpleasant adverse effects, including excessively reduced heart rate, nasal congestion, and *orthostatic hypotension* (a decline in blood pressure that occurs upon standing erect, owing to the effects of gravity causing pooling of blood in the lower extremities) (see Chapter 29).

Once released into the synaptic cleft, norepinephrine can bind to two sets of receptors: (1) postsynaptic α-adrenergic or β-adrenergic receptors, which elicit the postsynaptic response, or (2) presynaptic receptors, partially but not exclusively of the α$_2$-adrenergic subtype, which are involved in autoregulation. Eventually, the norepinephrine is removed from the synapse by reuptake into the presynaptic terminal or uptake into the postsynaptic cell. *Propranolol* (Inderal and others) is an example of a drug that interferes with the binding of norepinephrine to postsynaptic β-adrenergic receptors. This drug binds competitively to the receptor and prevents its activation, thereby blocking the postsynaptic response (in this case, the rise in intracellular cAMP mediated by G$_s$ activation of adenylyl cyclase). Propranolol and related β-adrenergic receptor antagonists are extremely effective and widely used in cardiovascular medicine.

Indications include, but are not limited to, management of hypertension, *angina pectoris* (chest pain due to cardiac ischemia), congestive heart failure, and myocardial infarction.

The autoregulatory presynaptic receptors for norepinephrine exert an inhibitory effect over the amount of norepinephrine released in response to an action potential. They influence both the synthesis of norepinephrine and its exocytotic release. The α$_2$-adrenergic receptors that are responsible for these effects can be blocked by the drug *yohimbine*. The resulting loss of autoinhibition increases the amount of norepinephrine released and enhances noradrenergic function.

Blockade of α$_2$-adrenergic receptors and reduction in norepinephrine release reduces postsynaptic effects of norepinephrine. In many peripheral tissues, the actions of the sympathetic (noradrenergic) component of the autonomic nervous system normally are finely balanced by those of the parasympathetic component (which, in most cases, releases acetylcholine) (see Chapter 29). Decline in the function of one component frequently leads to overexpression of the function of its opposing system. This is particularly true in the male urogenital tract, where erection has been linked both to activation of cholinergic nerves and to blockade of α$_2$-adrenergic receptors. Yohimbine (Yocon, Aphrodyne, and others) is chemically similar to reserpine and obtained from botanical sources. Present in many herbal preparations and beverages, yohimbine has a lengthy folk history as an aphrodisiac. Therapeutic use has, in recent years, proved modestly effective in promoting erectile function in male patients with impotence of vascular or diabetic origin or of psychogenic origin.

Many psychomotor stimulant drugs, including cocaine and *amphetamine*, enhance motor performance, relieve fatigue, and exert positive reinforcing effects by enhancing synaptic concentrations of monoamines. Cocaine does so by reversible inhibition of membrane monoamine transporters. The order of potency for inhibition of NET, SERT, and DAT is SERT > DAT > NET. The action of amphetamine is more diverse. As a substrate for the monoamine transporters, amphetamine is said to "reverse" the normal process of membrane transport. Thus, amphetamine promotes movement of cytoplasmic monoamines into the synapse. Amphetamine also enhances release of vesicular monoamine stores into the cytoplasmic pool and reduces intracellular degradation by inhibiting MAO. Monoamine oxidase has two isoforms, MAO-A and MAO-B. Monoamine oxidase-A is found in the periphery primarily and preferentially degrades norepinephrine and serotonin, whereas MAO-B is largely confined to the brain. Both MAO-A and MAO-B have similar affinities for dopamine. A variety of MAO inhibitors are used clinically. Nonselective inhibitors that block both MAO-A and MAO-B, such as *tranylcypromine* (Parnate) and phenelzine (Nardil and others) have utility in managing major depressive disease but suffer from frequent side effects. A selective inhibitor of MAO-B, selegiline (L-deprenyl; Eldepryl), preferentially blocks mitochondrial degradation of dopamine in the CNS and is useful in management of Parkinson disease. Agents such as *tyramine* displace norepinephrine from the cytoplasmic pool back into the synapse, also enhancing noradrenergic activity.

Sources and Additional Reading

Ballard PA, Tetrud JW, Langston JW: Permanent human parkinsonism due to l-methyl-4-phenyl-1,2,3,6-tetrahydropyridine (MPTP): Seven cases. Neurology 35:949-956, 1985.

Cooper JR, Bloom FE, Roth RH: The Biochemical Basis of Neuropharmacology, 8th ed. New York, Oxford University Press, 2002.

Cowan WM, Sudhof TC, Stevens CF: Synapses. Baltimore, John Hopkins University Press, 2001.

Danner S, Lohse MJ: Regulation of β-adrenergic receptor responsiveness, modulation of receptor gene expression. Rev Physiol Biochem Pharmacol 136:183-223, 1999.

Jessell TM, Kandel ER: Synaptic transmission: A bidirectional and self-modifiable form of cell-cell communication. Cell 72/Neuron 10(Suppl):1-30, 1993.

Katzung BG: Basic & Clinical Pharmacology. New York, McGraw-Hill, 2004.

Kelly RB: Storage and release of neurotransmitters. Cell 72/Neuron 10(Suppl):43-53, 1993.

Nestler EJ, Hyman SE, Malenka RC: Molecular Neuropharmacology: A Foundation for Clinical Neuroscience. New York, McGraw-Hill, 2001.

Raiteri L, Raiteri M, Bonanno G: Coexistence and function of different neurotransmitter transporters in the plasma membrane of CNS neurons. Prog Neurobiol 68:287-309, 2002.

Somogyi P, Tamás G, Lujan R, Buhl EH: Salient features of synaptic organization in the cerebral cortex. Brain Res Rev 26:113-135, 1998.

Chapter 5

Development of the Nervous System
O. B. Evans and J. B. Hutchins

The central nervous system (CNS) develops from primitive ectoderm, one of the three germ layers of the embryo. From a few dozen cells, which together weigh perhaps a microgram, the brain becomes an organ weighing about 800 g at birth, 1200 g at 6 years of age, and about 1400 g in the adult—about a billionfold increase. Most but not all neurons undergo their last cell division before birth. The development of a fully functional nervous system requires division and migration of nerve cells and the formation of synaptic connections.

Overview

In view of the complex embryology of the human CNS, it is remarkable that there are so few congenital CNS defects. Although 3% of births are associated with major malformations of the CNS, most fetuses and infants in this category do not survive. About 75% of spontaneously aborted fetuses and 40% of infants who die within the first year of life have major CNS malformations.

The basic form of the human CNS is complete by about the sixth week of gestation. The next phases, which include cellular proliferation and migration, are most prominent in the second trimester of gestation but continue until term. Myelination peaks during the third trimester but continues until adulthood. The development of synaptic connections between neurons and the response of the brain to its experiences result in its functional maturity. This developmental process continues throughout life.

From a few primordial cells, about 100 billion neurons develop, each with thousands of contacts with other neurons. Through this network of interconnecting neurons, the human brain is capable not only of directing the movement of the body and sensing the environment but also of thinking, reasoning, experiencing emotions, and dreaming.

Development of the Neural Tube: General Concepts

One of the first indicators of the developing nervous system to appear is the *neural groove* on the posterior aspect of the trilaminar embryo (Fig. 5-1A, B). The neural groove deepens and the *neural folds* at the lateral margins of the *neural plate* become obvious as they elevate and eventually join along the posterior midline to form the *neural tube* (Fig. 5-1C). This apposition and fusion of the neural folds and of the overlying ectoderm initially takes place at what will be the cervical levels of the spinal cord, then proceeds rostrally and caudally from this location (Fig 5-1D). The anterior and posterior neuropores, as described later, are the last points at which the neural tube closes. After formation of the neural tube, three layers, the *ventricular*, *marginal*, and *intermediate zones*, appear in rapid succession.

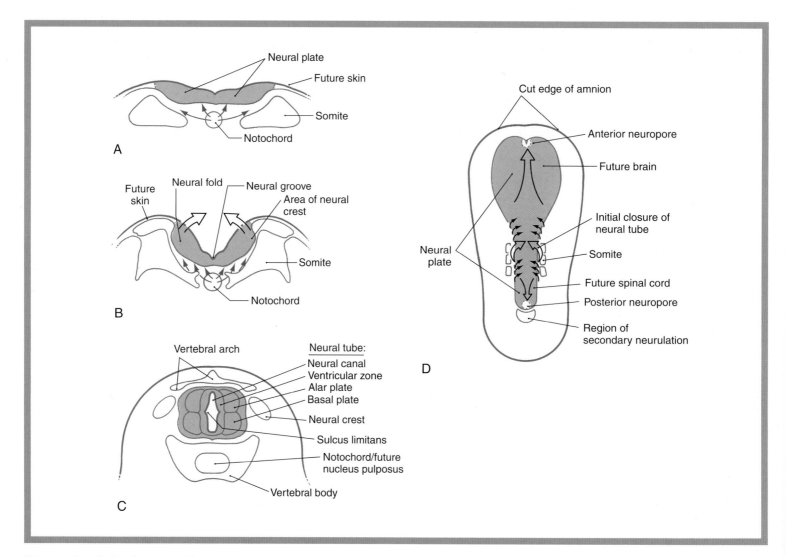

Figure 5-1. Early development of the nervous system. Cross sections (**A-C**) showing the transition from neural plate (**A**) to neural tube (**C**). A dorsal view (**D**) of the neural plate shows the point of initial closure and the direction of closure *(small arrows)* toward anterior and posterior neuropores. *Green arrows* (**A, B**) represent induction of neural tube formation.

Although transient in their embryonic form, these zones give rise to important adult derivatives.

In early stages this closing neural plate and tube consist of a single layer, the *ventricular zone*, composed of a pseudostratified layer of fusiform-shaped cells undergoing DNA replication and cell division (mitosis). The nuclei in the cells of this zone migrate in a to-and-fro manner within the cell as mitosis takes place (Fig. 5-2A). The progenitor cells of this layer will give rise to the neurons and some glial cells of the mature nervous system, and to the ependymal cells lining the ventricles.

Immediately after the ventricular zone is formed, the *marginal zone* appears (Fig. 5-2B). This zone is at the abluminal aspect of the neural tube and consists of the processes of cells located within the ventricular zone, but it does not contain their nuclei. The marginal zone contains almost no cell bodies. This zone will be invaded by axons of neurons that are located in the intermediate zone.

The third area to appear is the *intermediate zone*. The intermediate zone is formed between the ventricular and marginal zones as the progenitor cells from the ventricular zone give rise to immature postmitotic neurons (Fig. 5-2C). These immature neurons migrate into the area immediately external to the ventricular zone, where they set up residence. The processes of some intermediate zone neurons continue to grow into the marginal zone. Although the term is no longer appropriate, the intermediate zone generally corresponds to what was formerly called the mantle layer.

The *subventricular zone* forms at the interface of the ventricular and intermediate zones (Fig. 5-2D). Unlike the to-and-fro movement of nuclei in the cells of the ventricular zone, nuclei of subventricular zone cells generally do not migrate. The progenitor cells of the subventricular zone give rise to the macroglial cells of the CNS and to specific populations of developing neurons in the brainstem and forebrain.

The concept of *alar plate* and *basal plate* is best viewed by recognizing that the development of, as examples, the posterior horn (alar plate derivative) and anterior horn (basal plate derivative) is a dynamic process. The immature intermediate zone neurons that give rise to mature posterior or anterior horn neurons are the product of cell division in one zone with migration into, and further development in, a subsequently formed zone. It is helpful to think of the *alar and basal plates as consisting of the ventricular zone and adjacent intermediate zone*, which are, of course, dynamically changing as development occurs. The posterior part of the ventricular zone and adjacent intermediate zone represents the *alar plate*, whereas the corresponding layers in the anterior part of the developing neural tube represent the *basal plate*. As development proceeds, the ventricular zone will essentially disappear while the intermediate zone with its maturing neurons will progressively enlarge to form its adult derivatives. Consequently, the adult derivatives are the products of cell division in the ventricular zone, migration and formation of the intermediate zone, and maturation within this latter zone.

The three-zone configuration described previously—ventricular zone, intermediate zone, and marginal zone—is the basic organizational plan from which the brain and spinal cord will arise. To a large extent, the development of the brainstem and forebrain is just a more elaborate version of this basic plan. There are individual developmental events unique to these zones of the CNS. In the metencephalon, the basic plan of the neural tube is modified to accommodate development of the cerebellar cortex. In the forebrain the basic plan of the neural tube is modified to accommodate the development of the cerebral cortex.

The modification to accommodate the cerebral cortex is the appearance of the *cortical plate* and the *subplate* (Fig. 5-2D). The *cortical plate* forms at the interface of the marginal zone and the intermediate zone and it is composed of neurons that originate from the ventricular zone; these postmitotic immature neurons traverse the intermediate zone, using the radially oriented processes of *radial glia* as a scaffold, to take up their position as the cortical plate. (It is emphasized that cell migration on radial glia is characteristically seen in all portions of the developing nervous system.) The *subplate* is a narrow region located immediately internal to the cortical plate. The cerebral cortex develops from the cortical plate and the marginal zone. In those portions of the neural tube that form the cerebral cortex, the marginal zone gives rise to layer/lamina I of the cortex, the cortical plate to layers/laminae II to VI, and the subplate and intermediate zone to portions of the subcortical white matter. The histogenesis of the cerebellar cortex is a slight modification of this plan due to the presence of an external germinal layer. This layer originates from the rhombic lip (an alar plate derivative) and is located within the marginal layer. These relationships are described later in this chapter.

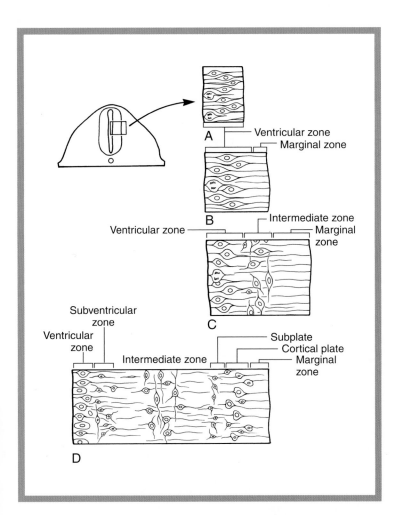

Figure 5-2. Histogenesis of the neural tube from early stages when there is just the ventricular zone (**A**) to later stages (**B, C**) when the marginal and intermediate zones appear external to the ventricular zone. Rostral to the spinal cord, the developing neural tube differentiates in a more complex manner (**D**) to accommodate more complex structures such as the cerebellar and cerebral cortices.

Brain Development

The first neural tissue appears at the end of the third week of embryonic development, when the embryonic disc is composed of *ectoderm, mesoderm,* and *endoderm.* A specialized part of the ectoderm, the *neuroectoderm,* gives rise to the brain, spinal cord, and peripheral nervous system (Fig. 5-1).

Induction

The *notochord* arises from axial mesoderm at about 16 days and is completely formed by the beginning of the fourth week. It defines the longitudinal axis of the embryo, determines the orientation of the vertebral column, and persists as the *nucleus pulposus* of the intervertebral discs. One important function of the notochord is *induction*: directing the overlying ectoderm to form the neural plate (Fig. 5-1A, B). Associated with this process is the production of *cell adhesion molecules* in the notochord. These molecules diffuse from the notochord into the neural plate and function to join the primitive neuroepithelial cells into a tight unit.

Within the neuroectoderm, some neuroepithelial cells elongate and become spindle shaped. This cellular elongation, also induced by the notochord, forms the *neural plate* and is completed by the end of the third week of gestation (Fig. 5-1A). The neural plate gives rise to most of the nervous system.

Primary Neurulation

The CNS develops from a hollow structure called the *neural tube*, which is produced by *neurulation*. There are two neurulation processes. Most of the neural tube forms from the neural plate by a process of infolding called *primary neurulation*. This part of the neural tube will give rise to the brain and to the spinal cord through lumbar levels. The caudal-most portion of the neural tube, which will give rise to sacral and coccygeal levels of the cord, is formed by a process called *secondary neurulation*. Secondary neurulation is described in the next section. By about day 18 after fertilization, the neural plate begins to thicken at its lateral margins (Fig. 5-1B). This thickening elevates the edges of the neural plate to form *neural folds*. At about 20 days, the neural folds first contact each other to begin the formation of the *neural tube*. This fusion initially takes place on the dorsal midline at what will become cervical levels of the spinal cord and proceeds, zipper-like, in rostral and caudal directions (Fig. 5-1C, D). During the process, the lumen of the neural tube, called the neural canal, is open to the amniotic cavity both rostrally and caudally (Fig. 5-1D). The rostral opening, the *anterior neuropore*, closes at about 24 days, and the caudal opening, the *posterior neuropore*, closes about 2 days later.

Neurulation is brought about by morphologic changes in the *neuroblasts*, the immature and dividing future neurons in the ventricular zone. As mentioned previously, these cells are elongated and are oriented at right angles to the dorsal surface of the neural plate, which will be the inner wall of the neural canal. Microfilaments in each cell form a circular bundle parallel to the future luminal surface, whereas microtubules extend along the length of the cell. The contraction of the circular bundle of microfilaments causes the microtubules to splay out like the rays of a fan. This forms an elongated conical cell with its apex at the neural groove and its base at the edge of the neural fold. Neurulation does not occur in embryos exposed to colchicine, which depolymerizes microtubules, or to cytochalasin, which inhibits microfilament-based contraction.

Congenital malformations associated with defective neurulation are called *dysraphic defects*. The process of induction also means that the proper development of a structure is dependent on the proper development of its neighbors. There is an intimate relationship of neural tissue to the surrounding bone, meninges, muscles, and skin. Because of this relationship, a failure of neurulation often impairs the formation of these surrounding structures.

Several well-controlled clinical trials have proved that supplementation with the vitamin *folic acid*, found in green, leafy vegetables, can reduce the incidence of neural tube defects. In the MRC Vitamin Study, carried out in Great Britain and published in 1991, women who had previously been delivered of a child with a dysraphic defect were assigned to either a folic acid supplementation group or a control group during a subsequent pregnancy. Folic acid supplementation reduced the incidence of neural tube defects by about 70% relative to that in untreated controls. The mechanism for this effect is not known at this time. It is thought that women who are delivered of infants with dysraphic defects have an inborn metabolic problem that is corrected by folate. One research group has suggested that the conversion of homocysteine to methionine, which requires folate as a cofactor, is the critical step. Because it is impossible to identify women at risk, and because the neural plate and tube develop so early in pregnancy, it is important that physicians recommend folic acid supplementation (400 µg/day) to all female patients who intend to have children, whether or not they are pregnant. Additionally, drugs taken for epilepsy, such as valproic acid or carbamazepine, can cause dysraphic defects.

Congenital Nervous System Defects of Primary Neurulation

Most dysraphic disorders occur at the location of the anterior or posterior neuropore. Failure of the anterior neuropore to close results in *anencephaly* (Fig. 5-3). In this defect, the brain is not formed, the surrounding meninges and skull may be absent, and there are facial abnormalities. The defect extends from the level of the *lamina terminalis*, the site of anterior neuropore closure, to the region of the *foramen magnum*. Anencephaly occurs in about 5 of every 10,000 live births. Neonatal death is inevitable.

An *encephalocele* is a herniation of intracranial contents through a defect in the cranium *(crania bifidum)* (Fig. 5-4A). The cystic structure may contain only meninges *(meningocele)*, meninges plus brain *(meningoencephalocele)*, or meninges plus brain and a part of the ventricular system *(meningohydroencephalocele)* (Fig. 5-4B-D). Encephaloceles are most common in the occipital region, but they may also occur in frontal or parietal locations.

A more subtle defect in the same area is thought to be the cause of the *Arnold-Chiari malformation*, a congenital herniation of the cerebellar vermis through the foramen magnum, which may cause pressure on the medulla oblongata and cervical spinal cord (Fig. 5-5). This defect may go unnoticed until early adulthood and is often associated with a cavitation of the spinal cord *(syringomyelia)* or of the medulla *(syringobulbia)*.

Defects in the closure of the posterior neuropore cause a range of malformations known collectively as *myeloschisis*. The defect always involves a failure of the vertebral arches at the affected levels to form completely and fuse to cover the spinal cord *(spina bifida)*. If that is the only defect, and the skin is

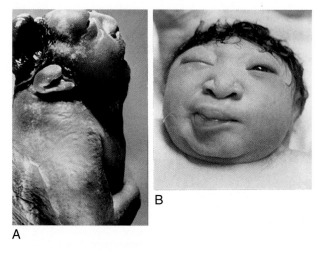

Figure 5-3. Lateral (**A**) and frontal (**B**) views of anencephaly. Note the associated cranial and facial abnormalities. (**A** courtesy of Dr. J. Fratkin.)

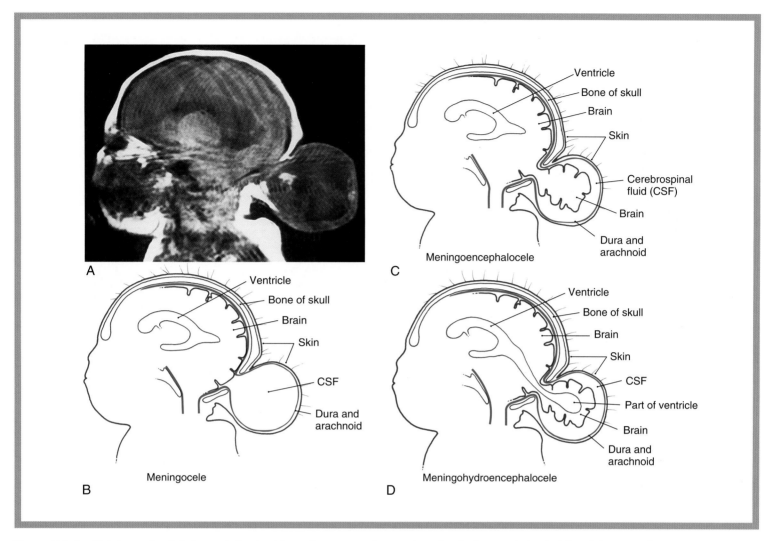

Figure 5-4. Sagittal views of occipital encephaloceles. Magnetic resonance image of meningohydroencephalocele (**A**) and drawings of meningocele (**B**), meningoencephalocele (**C**), and meningohydroencephalocele (**D**).

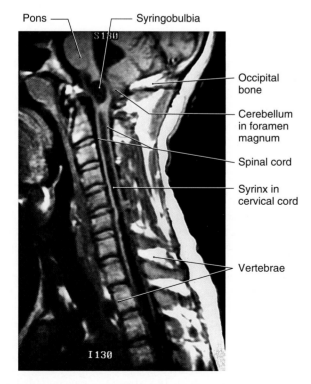

Figure 5-5. Sagittal MR image of a patient with Arnold-Chiari malformation and with cavitations in the medulla (syringobulbia) and cervical spinal cord (syringomyelia).

closed over it, the unseen condition is called *spina bifida occulta* (Fig. 5-6A, B). The site of the defect is usually marked by a patch of dark, coarse hairs. If the skin is not closed over the vertebral defect leaving a patent aperture, the malformation is called *spina bifida aperta.*

As with occipital encephaloceles, a cystic mass *(spina bifida cystica)* may also accompany spina bifida (Fig. 5-6C, D). This saccular structure may contain only meninges and cerebrospinal fluid (CSF) *(meningocele)* or meninges and CSF plus spinal neural tissue *(meningomyelocele).* In the latter case, the neural tissue may be the lower part of the spinal cord or, more commonly, a portion of the cauda equina. Infants with meningo-myelocele may be unable to move their lower limbs or may not perceive pain sensations from skin innervated by nerves passing through the lesioned area. These infants may also have other CNS malformations, such as *hydrocephalus* and the Arnold-Chiari malformation. The incidence of meningomyelocele is approximately 5 per 10,000 births.

Secondary Neurulation

The sacral and coccygeal segments of the spinal cord and their corresponding dorsal and ventral roots are formed by *secondary neurulation* (Fig. 5-1D). This process begins on day 20 and is complete by about day 42. A cell mass, the *caudal eminence,* appears just caudal to the neural tube and then enlarges and cavitates. The caudal eminence joins the neural tube, and its cavity becomes continuous with the neural canal.

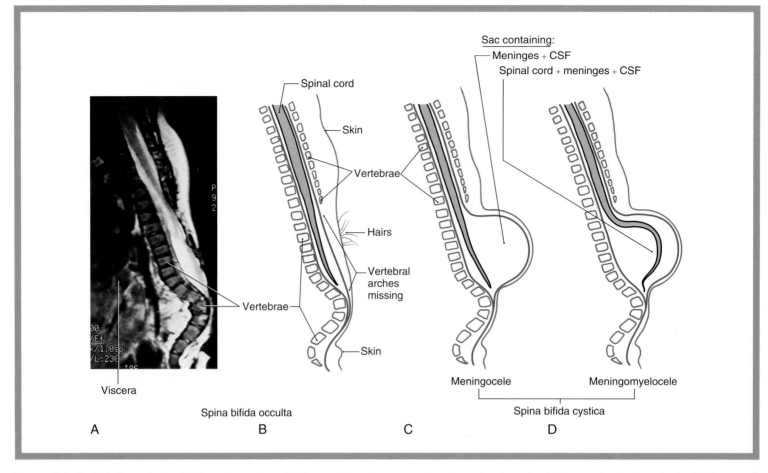

Figure 5-6. Sagittal views of spina bifida malformations. MR image (**A**) and corresponding views showing spina bifida occulta (**A, B**) and spina bifida cystica (**C**, meningocele; **D**, meningomyelocele). CSF, cerebrospinal fluid.

Congenital Nervous System Defects of Secondary Neurulation

Myelodysplasia refers to malformations of the parts of the neural tube formed by secondary neurulation. In most cases the malformation is covered with skin, but the site may be marked by unusual pigmentation, hair growth, *telangiectases* (large superficial capillaries), or a prominent dimple. A common abnormality is *tethered cord syndrome*, in which the conus medullaris and filum terminale are abnormally fixed to the defective vertebral column. The sustained traction damages the cord, with subsequent loss of sensations from the legs and feet and problems with bladder control.

Primary Brain Vesicles

During the fourth week after fertilization, in which the anterior neuropore closes, there is rapid growth of neural tissue in the cranial region. The three *primary brain vesicles* formed are *prosencephalon* (forebrain), *mesencephalon* (midbrain), and *rhombencephalon* (hindbrain) (Fig. 5-7A, B). At the rhombencephalon–spinal cord junction there is a slight bend in the developing neural tube; this is the *cervical flexure*. A second bend in the neural tube at the level of the mesencephalon is the *mesencephalic (or cephalic) flexure*.

Secondary Brain Vesicles

During the fifth week, the three primary brain vesicles are divided into five *secondary brain vesicles* (Fig. 5-7C, D). This requires two additional flexures. The *pontine flexure* divides the hindbrain into the *myelencephalon* caudally and the *metencephalon* rostrally. The mesencephalon does not partition further. The *telencephalic flexure* (shortened here from the longer term *diencephalic-telencephalic sulcus*) divides the forebrain into the *diencephalon* caudally and the *telencephalon* rostrally (Fig. 5-7C, D). The telencephalon (meaning "end-brain") forms as an outpocketing of the forebrain and expands enormously, with its complex lobes, gyri, and sulci, to become the largest part of the brain.

Diencephalon and Cerebral Hemispheres

The main structures of the forebrain develop during the second month of gestation. Because the mesoderm in this region is simultaneously forming facial structures, abnormalities of forebrain development are often associated with facial defects (Fig. 5-3). The process of forebrain development is referred to as *central induction*.

At about the end of the fifth week, the telencephalon gives rise to two lateral expansions called the *telencephalic (cerebral) vesicles* (Fig. 5-7C, D). These are the primordia of the cerebral hemispheres. Their adult derivatives include the cerebral cortex and the subcortical white matter (including the internal capsule), the olfactory bulb and tract, portions of the basal ganglia, the amygdala, and the hippocampus. The *diencephalon* develops into the thalamic nuclei and associated structures and also gives rise to the optic cup, which eventually forms the optic nerve and retina. By 10 weeks of development, the major structures of the CNS are clearly recognizable by their morphologic features, and immature versions of all structures in the brain are present by the end of the first trimester.

Defects of Prosencephalization

The sequence of events by which the primitive prosencephalon differentiates into the diencephalic and telencephalic vesicles

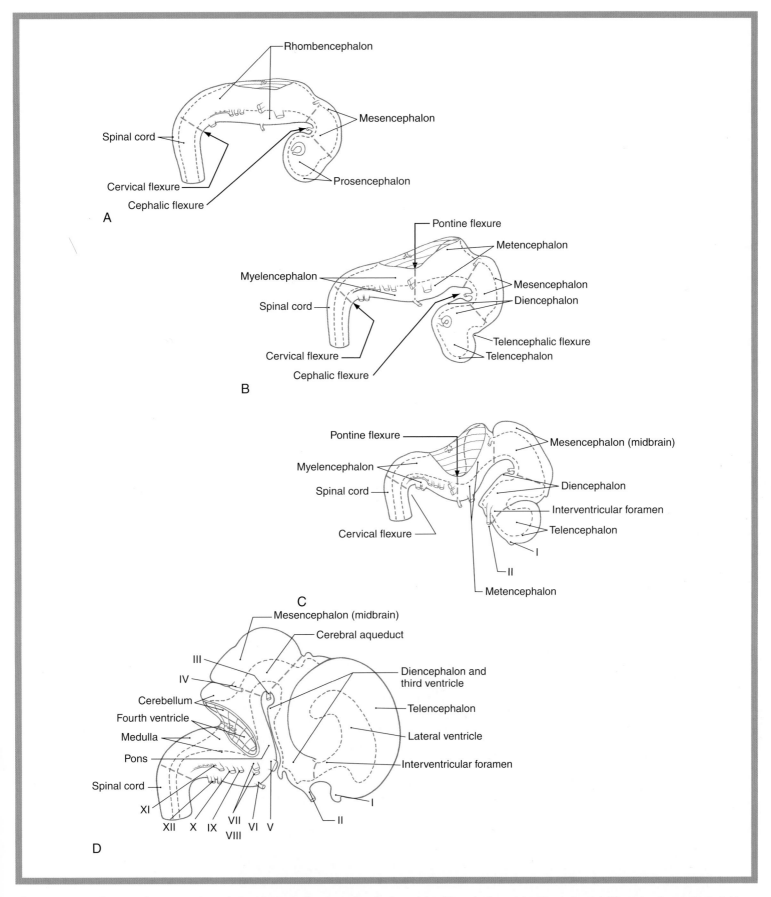

Figure 5-7. Developmental sequence from three primary to five secondary brain vesicles. Three brain vesicles (**A**, at about 4.75 weeks of gestation) divide into five vesicles (**B**, at about 6 weeks of gestation) with the appearance of additional flexures. In subsequent stages (**C**, at about 6.5 weeks of gestation; **D**, at about 8.5 weeks of gestation), there is rapid enlargement of forebrain regions, especially the telencephalon. Note that the ventricular spaces (*dashed lines,* **A-D**) follow the shape changes in the brain. Cranial nerves are indicated by Roman numerals.

is called *prosencephalization*. Failure of the prosencephalon to undergo cleavage results in a malformation called *holoprosencephaly* (Fig. 5-8A). In its most severe form *(alobar holoprosencephaly)*, no discernible lobes develop. There is a large single forebrain ventricle, the thalamus is poorly developed, and many structures (corpus callosum, longitudinal cerebral fissure and falx cerebri, olfactory structures) are lacking. In *semilobar holoprosencephaly* (Fig. 5-8B-D), there is some separation of the forebrain into two discernible lobes (more prominent in occipital areas) and partial development of the falx cerebri. The hemispheres have some visible lobes and gyri, and there are rudimentary but enlarged lateral and third ventricles. These large ventricles are continuous one with the other, and midline structures, such as the septum pellucidum, that normally separate the ventricles are missing (Fig. 5-8C, D). Most infants with holoprosencephaly also have facial malformations. These may be as subtle as mild *hypotelorism* (unusually close-set eyes) or as obvious as the presence of only a single, midline eye *(cyclops)* accompanied by a rudimentary nasal structure *(proboscis)*. In general, the more severe the brain malformation, the more severe the facial defect.

Infectious Diseases Causing Congenital Nervous System Defects

Fetal exposure to several common infectious diseases can cause congenital nervous system defects. The acronym "TORCH" is often used for the more common etiologic agents: *Toxoplasma*, Other (syphilis), Rubella, Cytomegalovirus, and Herpes simplex virus. Nervous system defects include cataracts, retinitis and blindness, deafness, cerebral calcifications, cerebral atrophy, and microcephaly. Infants actively infected at birth can also have rash, fever, anemia, bleeding, and other organ system disease.

Ventricular System

The ventricular system is an elaboration of the lumen of cephalic portions of the neural tube, and its development parallels that of the brain (Figs. 5-7 and 5-9A-D). This process, also discussed in Chapter 6, is summarized here. The cavities of the telencephalic vesicles become the *lateral ventricles*; the diencephalic cavity becomes the *third ventricle*; and the rhombencephalic cavity becomes the *fourth ventricle*. The cavity of the mesencephalon becomes the narrow *cerebral aqueduct (of Sylvius)* connecting

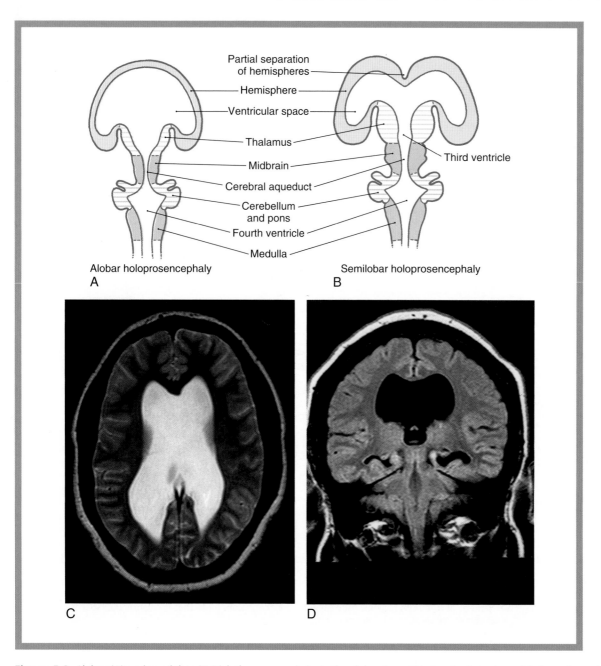

Figure 5-8. Alobar (**A**) and semilobar (**B-D**) holoprosencephaly. In the alobar form (**A**), the single brain vesicle has a horseshoe-shaped ventricle and many major brain structures are absent. Although ventricles are present in the semilobar form (**B, C**—axial MR image, T2 weighted, **D**—coronal MR image, T1 weighted), they are enlarged, and midline structures, such as the septum and fornix, are missing. Note the continuity of the lateral ventricles (**C**), the continuity of the lateral and third ventricles, and enlarged temporal horns of the lateral ventricles (**D**).

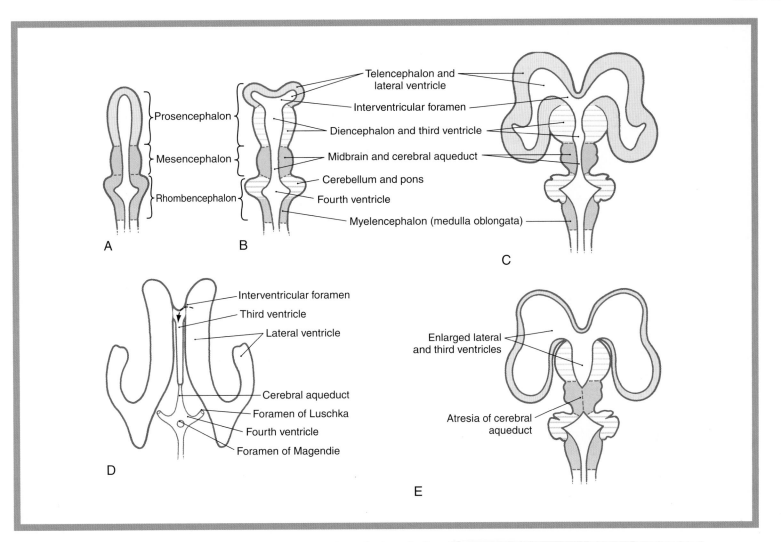

Figure 5-9. Development of the ventricular system and associated brain divisions (**A-C**) and the general adult pattern (**D**) as seen from the dorsal perspective. Failure of the cerebral aqueduct to form causes the third and lateral ventricles to enlarge (**E**).

the third and fourth ventricles, and the openings between the lateral ventricles and the third ventricle become the *intraventricular foramina (of Monro)*.

The ventricular system is lined with *ependymal cells*. Each ventricle originally has a thin roof composed of an internal layer of ependyma and an outer layer of delicate connective tissue *(pia mater)*. In each ventricle, blood vessels invaginate this membrane to form the *choroid plexus*.

Openings that arise in the caudal roof of the fourth ventricle during development form a communication between the ventricular system and the subarachnoid space. These are the midline *medial aperture (foramen of Magendie)* and the paired *lateral foramina of Luschka*. Although these foramina develop slowly, they are patent by the end of the first trimester. CSF is produced mainly by the choroid plexuses of the lateral and third ventricles. It escapes the ventricular system through foramina of the fourth ventricle and passes into the subarachnoid space. From there, it is absorbed into the venous system through the arachnoid villi located primarily in the superior sagittal sinus.

If the flow of CSF through the ventricles is obstructed during prenatal development, the ventricular system can become markedly dilated, a condition called *congenital hydrocephalus* (Fig. 5-10A). The cerebral aqueduct, only 0.5 mm in diameter, is a likely site for such a blockage. Congenital *atresia* (failure to form) of the aqueduct can occur as an isolated event, can be inherited, or can be associated with CNS deformities (Fig. 5-9E). *Stenosis*, or total obstruction, from cellular debris associated with an infection or from an *intraventricular hemorrhage*, may also occlude this narrow passage.

Enlarged ventricles are also seen in the *Dandy-Walker malformation*. Affected patients have a cystic dilation of the fourth ventricle accompanied by a variable degree of *aplasia* (absence or defective development) of the *cerebellar vermis* (Fig. 5-10B). In some cases, there is also obstruction of the foramina of the fourth ventricle.

Peripheral Nervous System

Neural Crest

The *peripheral nervous system* develops mostly from cells of the *neural crest* (Table 5-1; see also Fig. 5-1). These cells, which arise from the lateral edge of the neural plate, detach and move to locations lateral to the neural tube. The neural crest gives rise to most of the peripheral nervous system, as well as to a number of other structures (Table 5-1).

Placodes

Specialized epidermal cells called *placodes* are found in the developing head region. These will join neural crest cells, and together placodes and neural crest form the ganglia of cranial nerves V, VII, VIII, IX, and X.

Cranial Nerve Ganglia

Cranial nerves V (trigeminal nerve), VII (facial nerve), IX (glossopharyngeal nerve), and X (vagus nerve) have sensory ganglia that originate from neural crest and placode cells and contain pseudounipolar cell bodies. These are the *trigeminal* or *semilunar* (V) ganglion, the *geniculate* ganglion (VII), the *superior*

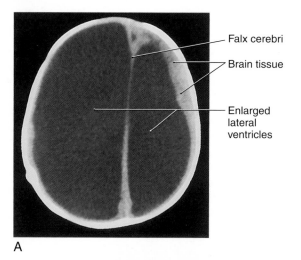

A

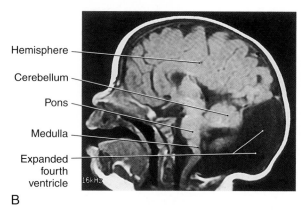

B

Figure 5-10. A, Axial MR image from a 9-month-old boy with congenital hydrocephalus. The brain is compressed and is visible as a thin rim on the inner surface of the skull and on the falx cerebri. **B,** Sagittal MR image from a 5-month-old boy with a Dandy-Walker malformation. In addition to aplasia of the cerebellum and a pronounced enlargement of the fourth ventricle, this patient has almost complete agenesis of the corpus callosum.

Table 5-1. Principal Structures Derived from Neural Crest Cells

Neural Elements
Neurons of:
    Posterior root ganglia
    Paravertebral (sympathetic chain) ganglia
    Prevertebral (preaortic) ganglia
    Enteric ganglia
    Parasympathetic ganglia of cranial nerves VII, IX, and X
    Sensory ganglia of cranial nerves V, VII, VIII, IX, and X*

Non-neural Elements
Schwann cells
Melanocytes
Odontoblasts
Satellite cells of peripheral ganglia
Cartilage of the pharyngeal arches
Ciliary and pupillary muscles
Chromaffin cells of the adrenal medulla
Pia and arachnoid of the meninges

*Some of the sensory cells in these ganglia arise from placodes.

and *inferior* (IX) ganglia of the glossopharyngeal nerve, and the *jugular* and *nodose* (X) ganglia of the vagus nerve. It is also common to refer to the jugular and nodose ganglia as, respectively, the *superior* and *inferior ganglia* of the vagus nerve. The distal processes of these cranial nerves travel as the sensory

components of the corresponding cranial nerve, whereas the proximal processes innervate the appropriate cranial nerve nuclei in the brainstem. A notable exception to this pattern is the *mesencephalic nucleus of the trigeminal nerve*. In this cranial nerve nucleus, pseudounipolar cells have failed to migrate with the neural crest and remain inside the CNS. They form, in essence, a "ganglion" ectopically trapped inside the mesencephalon.

The cell bodies of the ganglia of cranial nerve VIII (the *vestibulocochlear nerve*) arise primarily from the *otic placode*, with a small contribution from neural crest. These ganglion cells retain a bipolar shape in the adult.

Posterior (Dorsal) Root Ganglia

Pseudounipolar cells of *posterior*, or *dorsal*, *root ganglia* are derived from neural crest. Each spinal nerve and its corresponding ganglion are associated with a segment (or *somite*) of the developing embryo (Fig. 5-11). As the somites grow out to form portions of the body's connective tissue and musculature, the peripheral processes of the developing pseudounipolar cells of the corresponding dorsal root ganglia grow distally, using the extracellular matrix of the underlying tissue as a guide (Fig. 5-11).

The matrix molecules *fibronectin* and *laminin* contain the amino acid sequence arginine-glycine-aspartate (called the *RGD sequence* after the one-letter abbreviations for these amino acids). This sequence is recognized by proteins known as *integrins* on the surface of neural crest cells. The selective adhesion of the peripheral process of a neural crest cell to the RGD sequence of the extracellular matrix is probably involved in guiding the distal processes to their correct targets.

The segmental nature of the embryo is reflected in the segmental sensory innervation of the body surface (Fig. 5-11; see also Fig. 18-4). These segments, known as *dermatomes*, are important in the diagnosis of many neurologic disorders.

Visceral Motor System

The postganglionic sympathetic and parasympathetic neurons of the visceral motor system are also derived from the neural crests. Some of these cells remain near their site of origin to form the *sympathetic chain ganglia* adjacent to the vertebral column. Other cells migrate with branches of the aorta to form the sympathetic *prevertebral ganglia*.

Most of the autonomic (visceromotor) neurons of the digestive tract (*Auerbach* and *Meissner* plexuses) are formed by neural crest cells that migrate from the area of the rhombencephalon. Consequently these cells receive vagal innervation in the adult. Visceromotor (autonomic) neurons of the descending colon and pelvic structures are derived from neural crest cells that arise from sacral cord levels during secondary neurulation.

The human syndrome *congenital megacolon (Hirschsprung disease)* (Fig. 5-12) closely resembles an animal model in which excess extracellular matrix molecules are present in the colon. This results in aberrant migration of neural crest–derived cells. In this animal model, and in Hirschsprung disease in humans, neurons forming the enteric ganglia fail to migrate into the lower bowel. In the absence of these cells, no sensory signal indicating the presence of feces in the colon is sent to the CNS. Therefore, no motor signal is sent to control defecation.

Another clinical entity, *familial dysautonomia*, also reflects aberration in the development of neural crest derivatives. Patients with this disorder have both sensory symptoms (impaired pain and temperature perception) and autonomic symptoms (cardiovascular instability, gastrointestinal dysfunction).

Schwann Cells

The Schwann cells, which ensheathe and myelinate axons in the peripheral nervous system, are also derived from neural crest

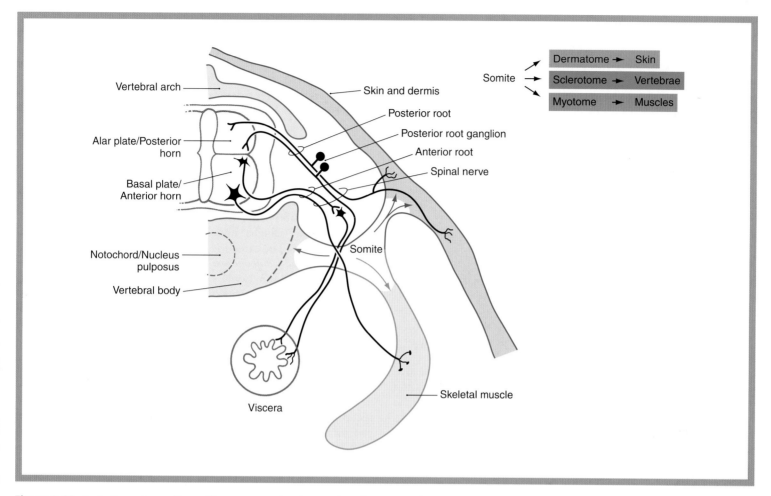

Figure 5-11. Derivatives of a somite and the corresponding innervation of structures that originate from the dermatome and myotome.

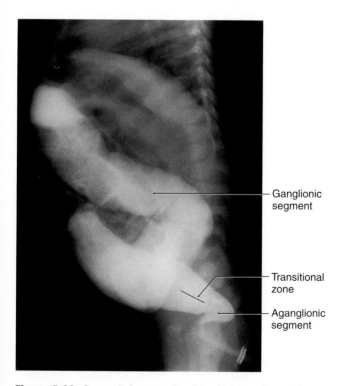

Figure 5-12. Congenital megacolon (Hirschsprung disease) in a neonate. The segment of the large bowel that is aganglionic (contains no ganglion cells) is constricted whereas the normal segment (containing ganglion cells) is enlarged. The transitional zone, in this patient, is a segment between the ganglionic and aganglionic portions that may contain some ganglion cells (hypoganglionic). (Courtesy of Dr. Richard C. Miller.)

cells (see Chapter 2). Schwann cells migrate in a segmental fashion, accompanying the growing processes of the peripheral nerve fibers they will eventually ensheathe.

Central Nervous System

Basic Features

In general, CNS neuroblasts arise at the ventricular surface of the developing brain (that is, the luminal surface of the neural tube). Just after the neural tube forms, there is no apparent cell differentiation in a cross section at any level. At this time, the neural tube is a pseudostratified columnar epithelium. As development proceeds and the wall of the neural tube thickens, however, dividing cells cluster at the ventricular surface, leaving a zone without cell bodies at the abluminal surface. This region, with few cell nuclei, is called the *marginal zone.*

As cells undergo their last division, they begin to migrate away from the luminal (ventricular) surface on transient glial cell guides called *radial glia.* As they migrate, they form a moving front of cell bodies between the marginal and ventricular zones called the *intermediate zone.* These features are common to all parts of the developing neuraxis; other elaborations are possible and are outlined in the following sections.

After cells migrate and take up their final positions in the developing brain, they begin to extend processes and form connections with other neurons or muscle cells. Dendritic processes begin to receive information from other developing cells. Meanwhile, an axonal process, tipped by a spade-like extension called the *growth cone,* begins to drive its way through intervening regions to reach distant targets.

Although the idea is controversial, both neurons and glia seem to originate from a single precursor cell population. Two main lineages arise: a *neuroblastic* lineage that generate neurons and a *glioblastic* lineage that includes precursors of radial glial cells, astroglial cells, and oligodendrocytes. The glioblastic lineage is believed to split into three main branches: (1) the *type 1 astrocyte* progenitor, (2) the *oligodendrocyte/type 2 astrocyte precursor* (called the *O2A progenitor*), and (3) the *radial glia* progenitor. Whereas all other cell types persist into adulthood, radial glial cells in most regions of the brain appear to be converted to astrocytes, *ependymal cells*, or *tanycytes*. There are two notable exceptions. In the cerebellum, radial glial cells retain most of their features as *Bergmann glial cells*, and in the retina, they are seen as *Müller cells*. Differentiation of glial cells is influenced by a variety of *growth factors*, such as platelet-derived growth factor, ciliary neurotrophic factor, and fibroblast growth factor, which are secreted by neighboring glia and neurons.

Spinal Cord

The adult spinal cord gray matter is butterfly shaped and consists of anterior (ventral) and posterior (dorsal) horns. At some levels of the spinal cord, an *intermediate zone* and a *lateral horn* of the gray matter lie halfway between posterior and anterior horns.

The spinal cord develops from caudal portions of the neural tube (Fig. 5-1). The neural canal in this region will become the central canal of the spinal cord (Fig. 5-7). Neuroblasts that give rise to spinal cord neurons are produced between the 4th and 20th weeks of development by a burst of proliferation in the ventricular layer lining the neural canal. These cells migrate peripherally to form four longitudinal *plates*, which will become the gray matter of the spinal cord: a pair of anteriorly located cell masses, which constitute the *basal plate*, and a pair of posteriorly located masses, which constitute the *alar plate*. The basal and alar plates on each side are separated by a longitudinal groove called the *sulcus limitans* in the lateral wall of the central canal. The *basal plate* develops into the *anterior (ventral) horn* of the spinal cord and the *alar plate* will become the *posterior (dorsal) horn* of the spinal cord (Fig. 5-11). Development in the basal plate somewhat precedes that in the alar plate; postmitotic neurons are clearly evident in the basal plate during week 20 of development. That portion of the adult spinal cord commonly called the intermediate zone (and the lateral horn) originates from the interface of the alar and basal plates.

As the basal plate develops, axons of nascent motor neurons form the developing anterior (ventral) roots that will innervate peripheral structures. Anterior horn motor neurons innervate skeletal muscle and are classified as *general somatic efferent* (GSE). The lateral horn motor neurons project to autonomic (visceromotor) ganglia and are classified as *general visceral efferent* (GVE). The categories GSE, GVE, and so on are referred to as *functional components*. The cord regions devoted to the GSE and GVE functional components can be thought of as constituting distinct longitudinal *cell columns* in the gray matter (Fig. 5-13). The GSE column runs the full length of the spinal cord. The GVE column extends from T1 through L2, where it is called the *intermediolateral cell column*, and from S2 through S4, where it is called the *sacral visceromotor nucleus*.

Neurons of the alar plate receive the central processes of developing posterior root ganglion (sensory) cells. Sensory neurons whose peripheral processes innervate the skin and receptors in joint capsules, tendons, and muscles are classified as *general somatic afferent* (GSA). Those that innervate receptors in visceral structures, such as the stomach, are classified as *general visceral afferent* (GVA). Like the GSE and GVE regions, the GSA and GVA functional components constitute separate columns (Fig. 5-13).

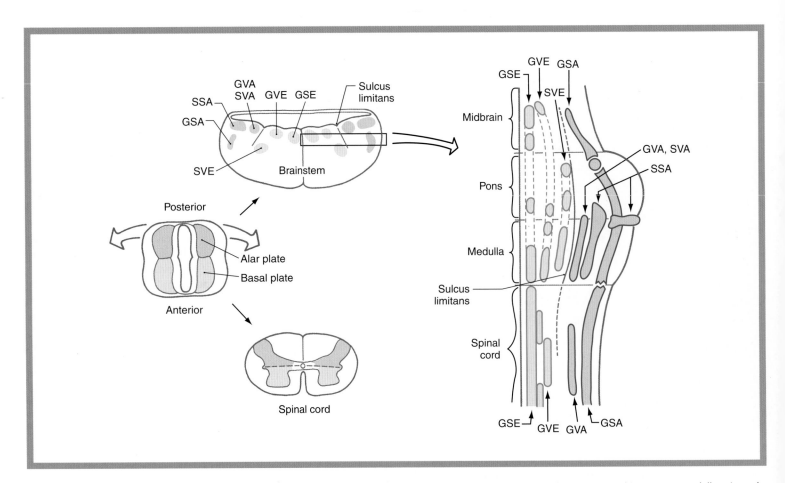

Figure 5-13. The derivatives of the alar (*in blue*) and basal (*in pink*) plates in the spinal cord and brainstem. Nuclei are grouped into rostrocaudally oriented cell columns that correspond to their functional components. GSA, general somatic afferent; GSE, general somatic efferent; GVA, general visceral afferent; GVE, general visceral efferent; SSA, special somatic afferent; SVA, special visceral afferent; SVE, special visceral efferent.

As each somite develops, it subdivides into a *sclerotome*, which forms vertebrae; a *dermatome*, which forms skin and dermis; and a *myotome*, which forms muscles (Fig. 5-11). The derivatives of the dermatomes and myotomes are innervated, respectively, by the axons of the posterior (sensory) and anterior (motor) roots of the corresponding spinal cord levels. These roots join at about the level of the future *intervertebral foramina* to form the *spinal nerves* (Fig. 5-11). The spinal nerves thus show the same segmental pattern as that for the dermatomes and myotomes they innervate. By contrast, the vertebrae develop between the spinal nerves and are thus *intersegmental* in position, even though they originate from the segmental sclerotomes. This situation comes about because the sclerotomes each split into cranial and caudal halves, and the vertebral rudiments are formed by the union of the caudal half of one sclerotome with the cranial half of the next posterior sclerotome.

Relationship of Spinal Cord to Vertebral Column

Although the spinal cord retains its general shape from the third trimester into adulthood, its physical relationship to the vertebral column alters dramatically (Fig. 5-14). By the end of the first trimester, the spinal cord, its meningeal coverings, and the surrounding vertebral arches are fully formed. The spinal nerves exit at about right angles to the spinal cord and pass through the intervertebral foramina. As development proceeds, the vertebral column and the spinal cord both grow caudally. However, the vertebral column grows slightly faster than does the spinal cord. The net result is that the cord seems to be drawn rostrally by its attachment to the brain. The intervertebral foramina, containing the spinal nerves, move caudally; and the posterior and anterior roots from lumbar, sacral, and coccygeal levels are significantly lengthened to form a bundle called the *cauda equina* (Fig. 5-14).

Brainstem

The brainstem consists of the *myelencephalon* (medulla oblongata), the *pons* (a part of the metencephalon), and the *mesencephalon* (midbrain). Although developmentally the cerebellum is a part of the metencephalon, it is considered a "suprasegmental" structure and not a part of the brainstem.

As one travels from the rostral part of the spinal cord to the caudal part of the brainstem *(medulla oblongata)*, two features are notable. First, the appearance of the cerebellum and the flaring open of the central canal into the fourth ventricle force the dorsal portion of the neural tube *(alar plate)* to rotate dorsolaterally (Fig. 5-13). This rotation results in a lateral-to-medial orientation of sensory *(alar plate)* versus motor *(basal plate)* areas of the developing brainstem, in contrast to their dorsoventral relationship in the spinal cord. Second, the *sulcus limitans*, which disappears in the spinal cord during development, is retained as an important landmark in the floor of the fourth ventricle (Fig. 5-13).

The basal plate in the brainstem give rise to motor cranial nerve nuclei, and the alar plate gives rise to sensory cranial nerve nuclei. As in the spinal cord, these portions of the basal and alar plates differentiate into rostrocaudally oriented cell columns, each of which is associated with a specific functional component. As shown in Figure 5-13, however, there are six cell columns and seven corresponding functional components in the brainstem, as compared with four in the spinal cord. This difference occurs because "special" functional components are unique to the head—special visceral efferent (SVE), special visceral afferent (SVA), and special somatic afferent (SSA). As development proceeds, some of these columns fragment into distinct, separate nuclei. The nuclei derived from a given cell column have the same functional component, and they generally remain aligned along the same rostrocaudal axis but may lie in different parts of the brainstem (Fig. 5-13).

Sensory neurons in the brainstem originate from the alar plate. They give rise to four sensory cranial nerve nuclei (Fig. 5-13; see also Fig. 10-7). The *spinal trigeminal nucleus* forms a continuous cell column from the cord-medulla junction to midpontine levels, whereas the *principal sensory trigeminal nucleus* is found in the rostral pons anterior to the spinal nucleus. Both of these nuclei receive GSA input via cranial nerves V, VII, IX, and X. The *solitary nucleus* extends the entire length of the medulla and receives GVA and taste (SVA) input via cranial nerves VII, IX, and X. Although the *vestibular* and *cochlear nuclei* also arise from the alar plate, the peripheral fibers projecting to these nuclei originate primarily from the *otic placode*. These fibers

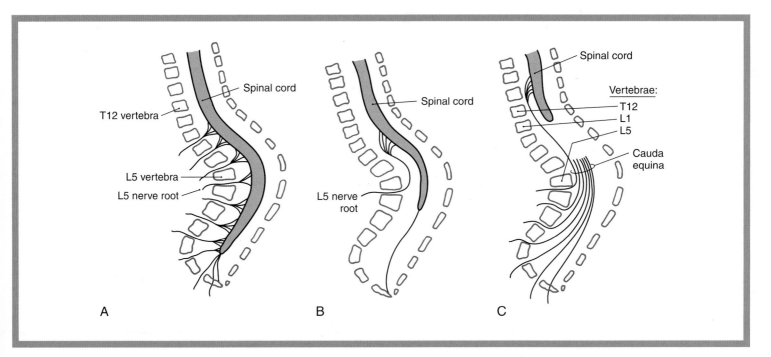

A   B   C

Figure 5-14. The differential growth of the vertebral column and spinal cord forms the cauda equina. The relationship of the cord to the vertebral column is shown diagrammatically at about 12 weeks of gestation (**A**), at 16 to 18 weeks of gestation (**B**), and at about 1 year of age (**C**).

are classified as SSA. The alar plate also gives rise to other brainstem cell groups, such as the inferior olivary nucleus of the medulla, the basilar pontine nuclei, and the substantia nigra of the midbrain.

Motor neurons in the brainstem originate from the *basal plate*. In contrast to cranial nerve nuclei derived from the alar plate, most of which form continuous cell columns, those cell groups that arise from the basal plate form separate nuclei (Fig. 5-13) stacked into discontinuous columns. There are three such broken columns: GSE, GVE, and SVE, taken from medial to lateral.

The nuclei of the most medial column have a GSE functional component and innervate muscles that originate from occipital somites (the tongue) or from mesoderm in the vicinity of the optic cup (the eye muscles). These are the *hypoglossal nucleus* (XII, in the medulla), the *abducens nucleus* (VI, pons), and the *oculomotor* and *trochlear nuclei* (III, IV) of the midbrain.

The next lateral column of nuclei has a GVE functional component and innervates visceral motor ganglia, which, in turn, innervate visceral structures. These nuclei are the *dorsal motor vagal nucleus* (X) and the *inferior salivatory nucleus* (IX) of the medulla, the *superior salivatory nucleus* (VII) of the pons, and the *Edinger-Westphal nucleus* (III) of the midbrain. These nuclei project via the vagal (X), glossopharyngeal (IX), facial (VII), and oculomotor (III) nerves, respectively.

The most lateral and ventral column of nuclei originating from the basal plate innervates muscles that arise from the mesoderm of the *pharyngeal arches*, and, consequently, it is designated as SVE. These cell groups are the *ambiguus nucleus* (IX, X) of the medulla and the *facial nucleus* (VII) and *trigeminal motor nucleus* (V) of the pons.

Along with the posterolateral-anteromedial division of brainstem into alar and basal plates, there is a rostral-caudal segmentation of the developing rhombencephalon into *rhombomeres*. These are clusters of immature neurons separated from each other by thin, transversely oriented bands of neuroepithelial cells. Cells in one rhombomere give rise to a specific motor nucleus (or nuclei) but will not migrate into adjacent rhombomeres. In general, the cell clusters forming the rhombomeres represent the rostral continuation of the alar and basal plates of the developing spinal cord. Indeed, motor nuclei originate from specific rhombomeres and input from the corresponding sensory ganglia enters the corresponding rhombomere.

Rhombomeres are also sites of *homeobox gene* expression. These genes (abbreviated *Hox*) are "master switches" that control the formation of large blocks of tissue. For example, the gene *Hox 2.1* is expressed only in the rhombomeres that give rise to cranial nerves X and XII; *Hox 2.9* is expressed only in the region of the developing facial nerve. There is considerable sequence similarity between homeobox genes from widely divergent species (such as flies and humans). This similarity implies that expression of homeobox genes is an essential element of neural development that has been preserved in evolution. One example of a congenital defect affecting developmental sequences within the rhombomeres is the *Möbius syndrome*. This syndrome is characterized by a variety of developmental defects, including (1) *aplasia* (poor development of, or absence of) of the abducens and facial motor nuclei, with the correlated motor deficits of facial and eye movement; (2) weakness of the muscles innervated by the oculomotor and trochlear nerves; (3) atrophy/weakness of the tongue and weakness of the masticatory muscles; and (4) a variety of skeletal defects affecting the face and body. These patients have *strabismus, dysarthria*, and difficulty closing their mouth or blinking and may have corneal abrasions.

Cerebellum

The cerebellum arises from the *rhombic lip*, an alar plate structure that forms part of the wall of the fourth ventricle. The rostral part of the rhombic lip forms the cerebellum, whereas the caudal part gives rise to the *inferior olivary, cochlear*, and *pontine* nuclei.

The rhombic lips join dorsal to the developing fourth ventricle to form the *cerebellar plate*. During the histogenesis of the cerebellar cortex, fissures appear that divide the cerebellum into its main lobes (Fig. 5-15A-C). The first, the *posterolateral fissure*, divides the cerebellar plate into the *flocculonodular lobe* and the *corpus cerebelli*. Despite its name, the *primary fissure* is the second to appear, and it divides the corpus cerebelli into *anterior* and *posterior lobes*. The advent of additional fissures divides the anterior and posterior lobes into the lobules characteristic of the adult brain.

The process of cerebellar cortical development involves the migration of immature neurons to form the cells characteristic of the adult brain (Fig. 5-15D). Initially the cerebellar primordium is composed of the *ventricular zone*, the *intermediate zone*, and the *marginal zone*. By the end of the first trimester, a second layer of immature neurons has appeared in the outer part of the marginal layer. This is called the *external germinal* (or *granular*) *layer*, and the intermediate zone is now called the *internal germinal* (or *granular*) *layer*.

Radial glial cells extend from the ventricular zone to the surface of the marginal layer and are necessary for the proper migration of developing neurons (Fig. 5-15D). Immature neurons of the internal germinal layer migrate outward along the radial glia to form the *cerebellar nuclei* and the *Purkinje cells, Golgi cells*, and the *unipolar brush cells* of the cerebellar cortex. Immature neurons of the external germinal layer migrate inward along the radial glia to form the *granule cells*. Other cells of the external germinal layer congregate just external to the Purkinje cell layer, where they will differentiate into the *stellate cells* and *basket cells* of the *molecular layer*.

Developing cerebellar neurons participate in other important cell interactions in addition to those with the radial glial cells. For example, as the granule cells migrate inward, they sprout axons that form synaptic contacts with the Purkinje cell dendrites that are growing into the molecular layer (Fig. 5-15E). Continued growth and development of Purkinje cell dendrites depend on these contacts with granule cell axons. Purkinje cell dendrites are stunted in the mutant mouse weaver, in which the granule cells die during development. These and other experimental mutant animals with cerebellar defects show the characteristic manifestations of cerebellar disease in humans: *ataxia, hypotonia*, and *tremor*.

Thalamus

The gray matter of the diencephalon develops from a continuation of the brainstem alar plates; there is no homolog of the basal plate in the diencephalon. This alar plate is recognizable at 4 weeks of gestation, and by 6 weeks of gestation it has differentiated into three main areas of the diencephalon: the *epithalamus, thalamus (dorsal thalamus)*, and *hypothalamus* (Fig. 5-16A, B). These structures are visible as swellings in the wall of the third ventricle, where they are separated from each other by the *epithalamic* and *hypothalamic sulci*. As development progresses, the epithalamic area remains quite small, whereas the hypothalamus and especially the thalamus enlarge. In about 80% of individuals, the two thalami fuse across the third ventricle to form the *interthalamic adhesion (massa intermedia)*.

The basic concepts of the development of the thalamus are the same as for other CNS regions. *Radial glia* extend from the third ventricle to the pial surface, and developing neurons migrate along this guide (Fig. 5-16B, C). The development of the thalamus occurs in an *"outside-first"* sequence. That is, the first neurons to undergo their final cell division migrate to the

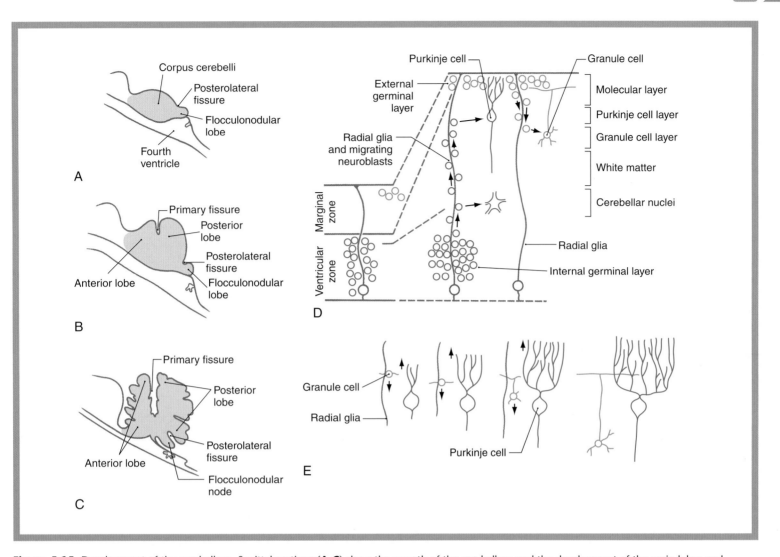

Figure 5-15. Development of the cerebellum. Sagittal sections (**A-C**) show the growth of the cerebellum and the development of the main lobes and fissures. Cytodifferentiation of the cerebellar cortex and nuclei (**D**). Note the migration of neuroblasts on radial glia and the formation of connections between granule cell axons and Purkinje cell dendrites (**E**). As granule cells migrate inward, they trail an axon that forms contacts with the dendrites growing outward from Purkinje cells. These axons become the parallel fibers of the cerebellar cortex.

outermost portion of the thalamus, where they mature. This means that the most lateral of the thalamic nuclei, such as the geniculate nuclei and the lateral and ventral nuclei, are generated first. The most medial thalamic nuclei, such as the dorsomedial nucleus, are the last to develop.

An important process in the development of the thalamic relay nuclei is the establishment of orderly maps of the sensory world. For example, a retinotopic (vision) map is formed in the lateral geniculate nucleus. As retinal ganglion cells send axons to the lateral geniculate nucleus, the arrangement of axonal contacts on cells in this visual relay center must accurately reflect the positions of ganglion cells in the retina. In this way, the map of visual space on the retina is maintained in the lateral geniculate nucleus and, ultimately, in the visual cortex. Similar maps are formed in the medial geniculate nucleus (tonotopic mapping) and ventral posterolateral nucleus (somatotopic mapping).

Cerebral Cortex

The cerebral cortex is generated using the basic mechanisms described previously for other regions. Except during mitosis and cytokinesis, cortical neuroblasts retain connections to both the ventricular and the pial surfaces of the developing brain and thus have a fusiform shape (Fig. 5-17). The nucleus engages in a peculiar cycle of migration within the cell, however. During the G_1 phase of the cell cycle (before DNA replication), the nucleus travels from near the ventricular pole of the cell to near the pial pole. During the G_2 phase (after DNA replication), it reverses direction and migrates back to a ventricular position. At the start of mitosis, the cell loses contact with the pial surface, but after cytokinesis the daughter cells grow processes that reconnect with the pial surface (Fig. 5-17). The cycle is then ready to repeat.

Unlike in other regions of the brain, in the cerebral cortex the first cells to migrate will disembark from the radial glial cells and take up positions close to the ventricular surface. Successive "waves" of immature neurons, migrating along radial glia, force their way through the differentiated cell layers to take up positions progressively closer to the pial surface. This sequence is called an "inside-out" pattern of development. These ranks of cells form the cortical plate as the axons of previously settled cells grow toward their targets.

The cerebral cortex proper is formed from expansion of the superficial part of the intermediate zone, the subplate and cortical plate (Fig. 5-18). Developing axons, originating in regions such as the thalamus that innervate the cortex, send out and form transient synaptic contacts in the subplate. The subplate is a transient structure that does not persist into adulthood. Neuronal cell bodies vacate the area between the subplate and the ventricular surface; most of the remaining cell bodies are glial cells. This region forms the white matter of the adult nervous system. The ventricular zone is reduced to a single layer of ependymal cells that line the lateral ventricles in the adult.

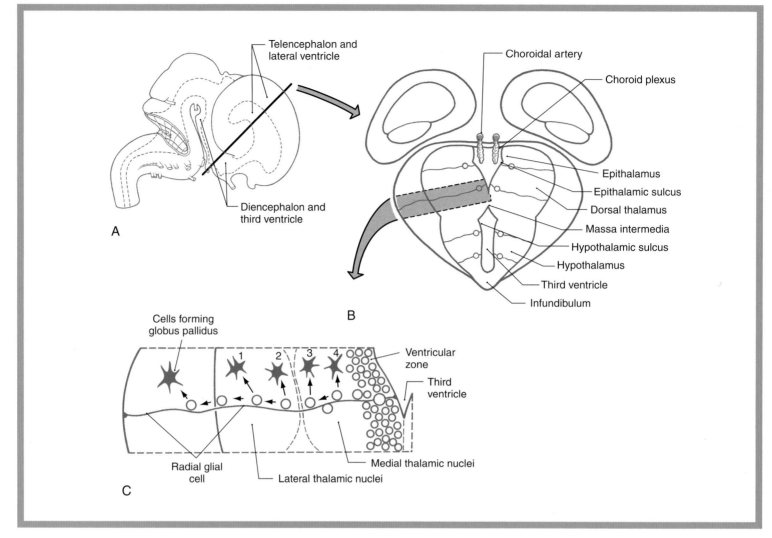

Figure 5-16. Development of the diencephalon. The diencephalon is shown in a lateral view (**A**) and in a coronal view (**B**, plane from **A**) at about 8 weeks of gestation. Details of cell migration (**C**, detail from **B**) show that lateral cell groups (**C**, 1) are formed first whereas more medial cell groups (**C**, 4) are formed last.

During peak periods of cellular migration the hemispheric fissures appear and mold the telencephalic surface into the gyri and sulci characteristic of the adult brain. By the end of the first trimester the *longitudinal cerebral, sylvian,* and *transverse cerebral fissures* are recognizable. The secondary sulci are completed by 32 weeks of development, with tertiary sulci completed during the last month of gestation.

Abnormalities of Cortical Development

Abnormal patterns of gyri and sulci may be caused by disorders of cell migration in the developing cerebral cortex (Fig. 5-19). If gyri fail to form, the cerebral cortex will have a smooth surface, a condition called *lissencephaly.* Unusually large gyri constitute *pachygyria,* and unusually small gyri constitute *microgyria.* Any of these conditions may affect the whole cerebrum or may be localized, and they may coexist in the same patient. For example, a young patient may have lissencephaly and pachygyria in different regions of the same cerebral hemisphere (Fig. 5-19).

The migration of immature neurons from the ventricular surface can be disrupted, causing mature neurons to take up residence in the intermediate zones. The term *heterotopia* is used to describe this defect. The degree of disruption varies from mild, microscopic clusters of neurons in the white matter and deeper cortical layers to large, macroscopic clusters of neurons that can be seen grossly and on neuroimaging (Fig. 5-20). In the most severe case, an entire cellular migration wave is disrupted.

This causes layers of gray matter alternating with layers of white matter (band heterotopia; Fig. 5-20A, B). In patients with band heterotopia the cellular layers of the cortex are excessively thick and disordered, the ventricles may be quite large, and the gyri/sulci patterns of the cortex are grossly abnormal (Fig. 5-20). Heterotopias can be found in isolation or associated with other congenital defects of the nervous system. For example, a brain may have heterotopia with lissencephaly and/or pachygyria. Heterotopias can be associated with epilepsy and developmental disorders.

Abnormal patterns of sulcal and gyral development are seen in *schizencephaly,* a condition in which there are unilateral or bilateral clefts in the cerebral hemispheres (Fig. 5-21A) of almost any size. Small defects may consist of a thin spot in the hemisphere where the pia and ependyma come abnormally close. In severe cases, the defect is large, resulting in a substantial loss of brain tissue and producing an open channel between the ventricular cavity and the subarachnoid space (Fig. 5-21B, C). One of the important characteristics of this type of developmental deficit is the continuity of cortex from the surface of the brain into the channel of the defect (Fig. 5-21B, *arrows*). In especially severe cases the schizencephaly may be bilateral with a significant loss of brain tissue (Fig. 5-21D). These patients have a variety of mental deficits. Schizencephaly may result from a profound failure of cell migration. An alternative explanation, which may apply particularly to severe cases, is that the affected

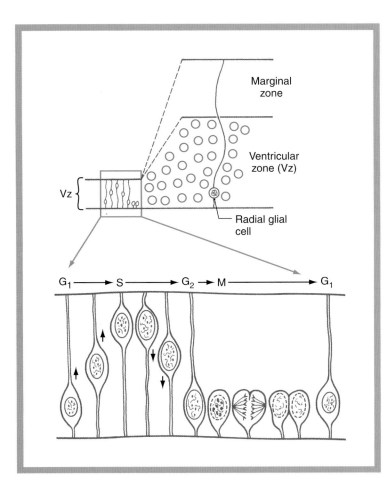

Figure 5-17. Early development of the cerebral cortex. The nuclei of the neuroblasts undergo a cycle of outward and inward migrations as the neuroblasts progress through their cell cycle. Phases of the cell cycle: G_1, first gap phase; S, DNA replication; G_2 second gap phase; M, mitosis.

region did not receive an adequate blood supply during development. The result would be a central area of necrosis, which would become a thin spot or an open channel, surrounded by a zone of abnormal neuroblast migration.

Cellular Events in Brain Development

The organization of the brain ultimately determines its function. Three important parameters in brain organization are (1) the density of neurons, (2) the pattern of axon and dendrite branching, and (3) the pattern of synaptic contacts. These characteristics begin to develop toward the end of the peak period of neuronal migration at the sixth month of gestation. Although neuronal density and the basic patterns of axonal and dendritic growth are determined within the first 2 to 3 years after birth, remodeling of synaptic connections continues throughout life.

Overproduction of Neurons and Apoptosis

Embryogenesis produces one and a half to two times more neurons than are present in the mature brain. By 24 weeks of gestation, almost all of these neurons have been produced. Subsequent to this, there is selective death of neurons.

Genetically programmed cell death *(apoptosis)* of neurons is a feature of cellular development in many areas of the brain. In contrast to necrosis (cell death resulting from injury), apoptosis requires protein synthesis and therefore is an active cellular process.

Some growth factors interrupt the normal process of apoptosis. *Nerve growth factor, brain-derived neurotrophic factor,* and *fibroblast growth factor* are known to limit cell death. This finding has led to the idea that the administration of growth factors may block the neuronal cell death that occurs in certain degenerative diseases.

Axonal Outgrowth

After neuroblasts complete their final cell division and migrate to their final location, they begin to extend a single axon with one or more distal elaborations known as *growth cones.* This spade-shaped extension of the growing axon is capable of driving through fields of developing nervous or mesenchymal tissue to reach distant targets. The guidance of growth cones is influenced by both *tropic factors* (which guide a cell toward a particular target) and *trophic factors* (which maintain the metabolism of a cell or its processes). As an axon grows, it may send out branches, each with its own growth cone. Some branches may terminate in sites that will not ultimately be innervated by the cell. For example, cells of the motor cortex that send axons

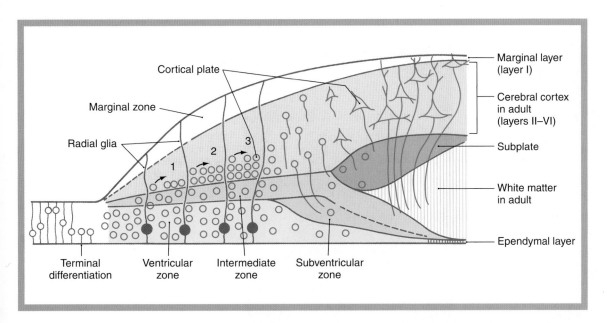

Figure 5-18. Later development of the cerebral cortex. Inner cellular layers (1) are formed first, and progressively more superficial layers (2, 3) are formed later.

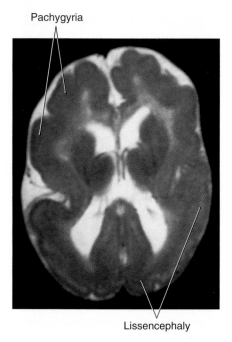

Pachygyria

Lissencephaly

Figure 5-19. Axial MR image of a 6-month-old female patient with malformations of the cerebral cortex that includes areas of lissencephaly and pachygyria in the same brain.

into the spinal cord to innervate motor neurons also send transient branches to structures of the brainstem; these ectopic connections are not normally maintained.

Synaptogenesis

Once an axonal growth cone arrives at its site of termination, it undergoes biochemical and morphologic changes to become a *presynaptic terminal*. Similarly, the area of the target neuron contacted by the presynaptic process begins expressing the characteristic postsynaptic machinery, such as neurotransmitter receptors and second messenger molecules.

One view of synapse development is that there is competition for the synaptic space available on target neurons. A synapse that forms will persist only if it exchanges the right cues with the target cell. Many synapses that form are subsequently lost and are replaced by other synapses that may be more successful.

Thus, only a subset of the large number of synapses that form are ultimately retained. This is the concept of *synaptic stabilization*, and it requires (1) a signal generated by the presynaptic cell, possibly the neurotransmitter to be used at the adult synapse; (2) a means for the postsynaptic cell to respond to the presynaptic signal; and (3) a "retrograde signal" from the postsynaptic cell to the presynaptic cell to indicate which contacts are to remain in maturity.

Plasticity and Competition

An important process related to the development of neuronal organization is *plasticity*. The developing brain is not as vulnerable to injury as is the mature brain. Infants who suffer significant cortical injury in the prenatal or early postnatal period may show surprising functional recovery, ending up with few or no obvious deficits. The mechanism of plasticity relates to alterations in selective neuronal death and axonal simplification and to the retention of transient axonal branches and synapses that would otherwise be lost, as discussed previously.

One example of plasticity and the competition for synaptic space is the development of visual cortical connections. Fibers conveying visual input from each eye arrive in overlapping territories in the visual cortex during the fetal period. Normally the synaptic space within this region is equivalently distributed to terminals carrying input from each eye. However, if the input from one eye is lost or if it is not functionally equivalent to the input from the other eye, the terminals from the "good" eye will experience a competitive advantage and occupy a larger share of the available synaptic space. The period of time during which these types of plastic changes can occur is called the *critical period*. Other areas of cortex have their own critical periods; the duration and time of occurrence of the critical period vary from region to region.

The concept of a critical period has clinical implications. If the input from one eye is dysfunctional during the critical period for visual system development (for example, if one eye is severely myopic), the axon terminals carrying information from that eye are at a disadvantage as they compete for synaptic space. If the causative disorder goes untreated, the "good" eye has exclusive access to visual cortex and input from the "bad" eye is ignored. This condition is called *amblyopia*. If the myopia is corrected later in life, no signals can pass from the retina to the visual cortex because the appropriate synaptic connections

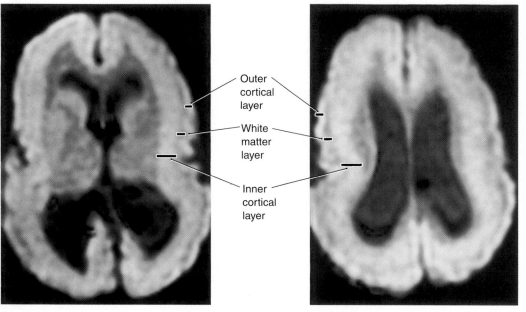

Outer cortical layer

White matter layer

Inner cortical layer

A

B

Figure 5-20. Band heterotopia in a female child (**A**, **B**, MRI flare). The brain is grossly abnormal, the ventricles are large, and the cortex is excessively thick. Note that there is (1) a superficial, but narrow, layer of cortex, (2) an equally narrow layer of white matter internal to this narrow cortical layer (compare the appearance of this white matter layer with the other white matter in the hemisphere), and (3) a wide band of gray matter internal to the white matter layer.

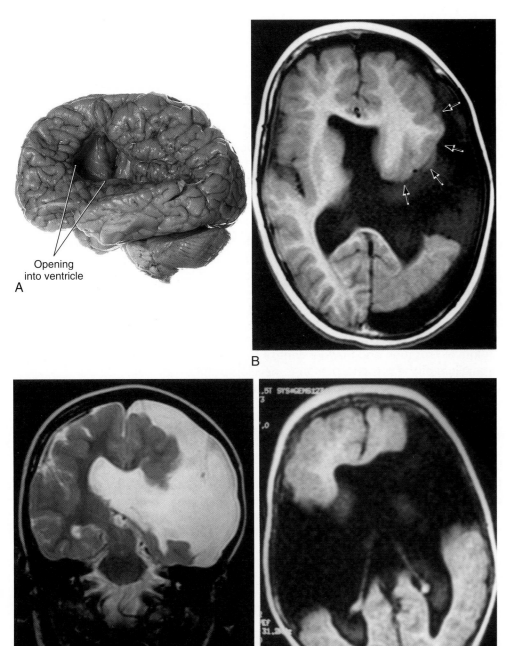

Figure 5-21. A to **D**, Examples of schizencephaly in the brains of young children. The defect may present as an open channel of varying size extending from the ventricular space into the subarachnoid space (**A-C**). Cortical tissue extends from the external surface of the hemisphere into, and through, the opening of this channel (**B**, *arrows*). In some patients the defect may be bilateral, in which case the loss of brain tissue may be profound (**D**).

Opening into ventricle

A

B

C

D

were not formed during the critical period. As a result, the eye remains functionally blind. This blindness can be avoided by implementing clinical interventions that equalize competition for synaptic territory during the critical period.

Synaptic development occurs in parallel with cellular proliferation and migration. Dendritic spines are the site of many synaptic contacts, especially in cortical neurons. The rate of spine formation varies in different parts of the brain but is usually maximal during the sixth month after birth. Many children with mental retardation, including those with *Down syndrome*, have fewer and less complex axonal and dendritic ramifications and fewer dendritic spines than in normal children. In some patients there is a disturbance of the cytoskeletal structure that supports the architecture of axonal processes. Axonal and synaptic development are especially vulnerable to *perinatal hypoxia, malnutrition,* and *environmental toxins.*

Myelination

Oligodendrocytes myelinate neuronal axons in the CNS. Myelination begins at about the sixth month of development and peaks between birth and the first year of life, but it continues into adulthood. A delay in myelination can result in a delay in functional development. The best example is a congenital cortical blindness that resolves during the first year of life.

There is a definite hierarchy in the regional maturation of myelin formation. The motor and sensory tracts throughout the nervous system mature early, whereas the association tracts mature relatively late.

Several neurodegenerative diseases *(leukodystrophies)* affect the formation of myelin. Many other inborn errors of amino and organic acid metabolism impair myelination, notably phenylketonuria. Finally, inadequate nutrition also can impair myelination.

Synopsis of Clinical Points

■ During development, immature neurons migrate using radial glia (pp. 71, 79, 82, 83).
■ Taking folic acid during pregnancy reduces the likelihood of a dysraphic defect (p. 72).
■ Certain medications may increase the likelihood of the occurrence of a dysraphic defect (p. 72).
■ Anencephaly is associated with a failure of the anterior neuropore to close (p. 72).
■ A developmental defect in the cranium through which cranial contents may herniate is a crania bifidum (p. 72).
■ An encephalocele is a sac-like structure resulting from a failure of the cranium to develop properly (p. 72).
■ An encephalocele containing only meninges is a meningocele (p. 72).
■ An meningoencephalocele is a cystic structure on the head containing meninges and brain (p. 72).
■ A cyst-like structure on the head containing meninges, brain, and a portion of the ventricular system is a meningohydroencephalocele (p. 72).
■ An Arnold-Chiari malformation is a congenital defect (p. 72).
■ Syringomyelia is a cavitation in the spinal cord, and syringobulbia is a cavitation of the medulla of the brainstem (p. 72).
■ A failure of the posterior neuropore to close results in malformation collectively known as myeloschisis (p. 72).
■ Spina bifida is a failure of the vertebral arches to fuse completely over the spinal cord (p. 72).
■ Spina bifida occulta is a failure of the vertebral arches to fuse, but the defect is covered by skin (p. 73).
■ A failure of the vertebral arches to form with a patent channel open to the surface is spina bifida aperta (p. 73).
■ A spina bifida cystica may contain meninges or meninges plus portions of the spinal cord or spinal roots (p. 73).
■ Myelodysplasia refers to developmental defects related to secondary neurulation (p. 74).
■ The tethered cord syndrome may result in loss of sensation and bladder control (p. 74).
■ Holoprosencephaly, in its various forms, is a failure of the prosencephalon to develop properly (p. 76).
■ Abnormally close-set eyes is hypotelorism; abnormally wide-set eyes is hypertelorism (p. 76).
■ Facial malformations in holoprosencephaly may include cyclops or a proboscis (p. 76).
■ Infectious diseases may cause developmental defects (p. 76).
■ Blockage of the cerebral aqueduct during development will cause hydrocephalus (p. 77).
■ A failure of the cerebral aqueduct to properly form is congenital atresia (p. 77).
■ Enlarged ventricles are seen in the Dandy-Walker malformation (p. 77).
■ Congenital megacolon (Hirschsprung disease) results from a failure of neural crest cells to properly migrate (p. 78).
■ Aberrant development of neural crest derivatives results in familial dysautonomia (p. 79).
■ Möbius syndrome is a congenital absence of correct innervation patterns of some cranial nerves (p. 82).
■ Abnormal migration of maturing neurons on radial glia, of the lack of such migration, results in a variety of defects in the arrangement of the cerebral cortex (p. 84).
■ Failure of gyri and sulci to form is lissencephaly (p. 84).
■ The presence of unusually large gyri is called pachygyria (p. 84).
■ Exuberant migration of maturing neurons on radial glia may result in microgyria (p. 84).
■ Aberrant development of the cerebral cortex results in patterns of gyri and sulci in which the normal landmarks are not seen (p. 84).
■ Waves of maturing neurons may fail to migrate into the cortex and may take up residence at intermediate locations; this is a heterotopia (p. 84).
■ Abnormal patterns of gyri and sulci may accompany unilateral or bilateral clefts in the brain; this is schizencephaly (p. 84).
■ Schizencephaly may be a thin spot in the hemisphere wall with ependyma and meninges intact or may be a large cleft with continuation between the ventricular space and the subarachnoid space (p. 84).
■ A lack of input from one eye during a critical developmental period may result in amblyopia (p. 86).
■ Amblyopia can be treated if caught early (p. 87).
■ Children with Down syndrome have less complex dendrites and fewer dendritic spines (p. 87).
■ Leukodystrophy is a loss of myelin; this disease may have a variety of causes (p. 87).

Sources and Additional Reading

Barkovich AJ: Pediatric Neuroimaging, 2nd ed. New York, Raven Press, 1995.

Boulder Committee: Embryonic vertebrate central nervous system: Revised terminology. Anat Rec 166:257-262, 1970.

Evans OB: Manual of Child Neurology. New York, Churchill Livingstone, 1987.

Jacobson M: Developmental Neurobiology, 3rd ed. New York, Plenum Press, 1991.

McConnell SK: The determination of neuronal fate in the cerebral cortex. Trends Neurosci 12:342-349, 1989.

Noden DM: Vertebrate craniofacial development: The relation between ontogenetic process and morphological outcome. Brain Behav Evol 38:190-225, 1991.

Purves D, Lichtman JW: Principles of Neural Development. Sunderland, MA, Sinauer Associates, 1985.

Rakic P: Principles of neural cell migration. Experientia 46:882-891, 1990.

Scott JM, Weir DG, Molly A, McPartlin J, Daly L, Kirke P: Folic acid metabolism and mechanisms of neural tube defects. Ciba Found Symp 181:180-191, 1994.

Shatz C: The developing brain. Sci Am 267:61-67, 1992.

Walsh C, Cepko CL: Clonally related cortical cells show several migration patterns. Science 241:1342-1345, 1988.

Section **2**

Regional Neurobiology

Chapters

6–16

Chapter 6

The Ventricles, Choroid Plexus, and Cerebrospinal Fluid

J. J. Corbett, D. E. Haines, M. D. Ard, and J. A. Lancon

The ventricular spaces of the brain are the adult elaborations of the neural canal of early developmental stages. These spaces, the choroid plexuses in them, and the cerebrospinal fluid (CSF) produced by the choroid plexus are essential elements in the normal function of the brain.

Overview

By about the third week of development, the nervous system consists of a tube closed at both ends and somewhat hook shaped rostrally (Fig. 6-1). The cavity of this tube, the *neural canal*, eventually gives rise to the *ventricles* of the adult brain and the *central canal* of the spinal cord. The former becomes quite elaborate as the various parts of the brain differentiate, whereas the latter becomes progressively smaller as the spinal cord differentiates into its adult pattern.

The choroid plexus, which secretes the CSF that fills the ventricles and the subarachnoid space, arises from tufts of cells that appear in the wall of each ventricle during the first trimester. These cells are specialized for a secretory function. The production of CSF is an active process that requires an expenditure of energy by the choroidal cells.

Any condition that causes CSF to accumulate, such as overproduction or an obstruction of its movement through the ventricle system, produces serious neurologic deficits. Perhaps the most widely recognized example is *hydrocephalus* as seen in a fetus or in a newborn. This condition is usually caused by an obstruction of CSF flow with resultant enlargement of the ventricular spaces upstream to the blockage. The bones of the developing skull move apart, and the head may enlarge significantly. In most of these cases some type of surgical diversion of CSF flow (a shunting procedure) is necessary.

Development

The *anterior (rostral)* and *posterior (caudal) neuropores* close at about 24 and 26 days, respectively. At this point, the neural tube is lined by the differentiating *neuroepithelial cells* of the ventricular zone, which are undergoing waves of cell division. Some of these precursor cells give rise to the *ependymal cells* that line the developing (and mature) ventricular system and the central canal.

The brain is initially composed of three primary brain vesicles—*rhombencephalon, mesencephalon,* and *prosencephalon*—each containing a portion of the cavity of the neural tube (Fig. 6-1A, D). The appearance of the *pontine flexure* in the rhombencephalon and a progressively deepening groove that separates the diencephalon from the telencephalon (the *diencephalic-telencephalic sulcus,* shortened here to *telencephalic flexure*) divides these three vesicles into the five brain vesicles (*myelencephalon, metencephalon, mesencephalon, diencephalon, telencephalon*) characteristic of the adult brain (Fig. 6-1B, E). With subsequent development, the telencephalic (cerebral) vesicles enlarge significantly (Fig. 6-1C, F). As the brain enlarges from three to five vesicles, each part pulls along a portion of the cavity of the primitive neural tube. These spaces in each brain vesicle form the ventricle of that part of the brain in the adult. Consequently, the shape of the ventricular system conforms, in

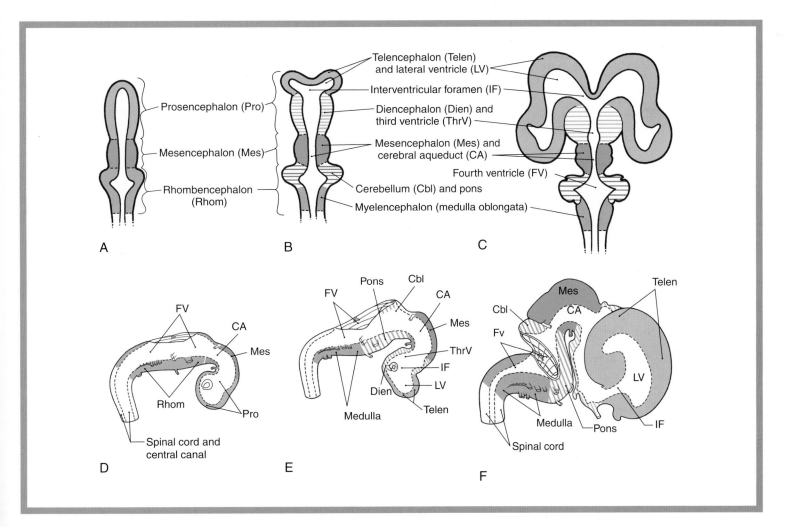

Figure 6-1. The early development of the brain and ventricular system, showing how brain growth and the configuration of the ventricles interrelate. Diagrammatic dorsal views (**A-C**) correlate in general with lateral views (**D-F**) at about 5 weeks (**D**), 6 weeks (**E**), and 8.5 weeks (**F**) of gestation. The outlines of the ventricles are shown in **D-F** as *dashed lines*.

general, to the changes in configuration of the surrounding parts of the brain.

The lateral ventricles follow the enlarging cerebral hemispheres, and the third ventricle remains a single midline space (Fig. 6-1A-C). The communications between the lateral ventricles and the third ventricle, the *interventricular foramina (of Monro)*, are initially large but become small, in proportion to the enlarging brain, as development progresses (Fig. 6-1C, F).

Proliferation of the neural elements of the mesencephalon results in a reduction in the size of the cavity of this vesicle to form the *cerebral aqueduct* of the adult brain (Fig. 6-1C, F). This creates a constricted region in the ventricular system and thus a point at which the flow of CSF may be easily blocked. Occlusion of the cerebral aqueduct during development may be the result of glial scarring *(gliosis)* due to infection or a consequence of developmental defects of the forebrain, a rupture of the amnionic sac in utero, or forking of the aqueduct. The last entity is a genetic sex-linked condition in which the aqueduct is reduced to two or more very small channels that do not properly meet. In addition, the cerebral aqueduct may be reduced to such a small channel that flow is reduced or essentially blocked. Whatever the cause, occlusion of the cerebral aqueduct results in a lack of communication between the third and fourth ventricles and blocks the egress of CSF from the third ventricle. Caudally, the cerebral aqueduct flares open into the fourth ventricle (Fig. 6-1B, C, E, F).

Foramina of the Fourth Ventricle

The ventricles and central canal of the spinal cord form a closed system when they first arise. However, in the second and third months of development, three openings form in the roof of the fourth ventricle, rendering the ventricular system continuous with the subarachnoid space surrounding the brain and spinal cord. The caudal part of the roof of the fourth ventricle consists of a layer of ependymal cells internally and a delicate layer of connective tissue externally (Fig. 6-2). The future apertures first appear in the form of small bulges in the caudal roof and at the lateral extremes of the fourth ventricle. The membrane forming the roof at these points becomes thinned and breaks down. The resultant openings are the medial *foramen of Magendie* (also called the *median aperture*) and the lateral *foramina of Luschka* (Fig. 6-2).

Formation of the Choroid Plexus

In the adult, the *choroid plexus* is found in both lateral ventricles and in the third and fourth ventricles (Fig. 6-4). The development of this structure is essentially the same in all of these spaces and is described here for the fourth ventricle.

The caudal roof of the fourth ventricle is composed of ependymal cells on the luminal surface and a delicate layer of connective tissue, the pia mater, on its external surface. These structures collectively form the *tela choroidea* (Fig. 6-3). Developing arteries in the immediate vicinity invaginate the

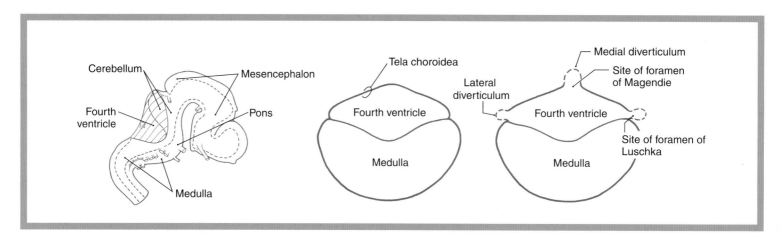

Figure 6-2. Development of the foramina of Luschka and Magendie in the fourth ventricle.

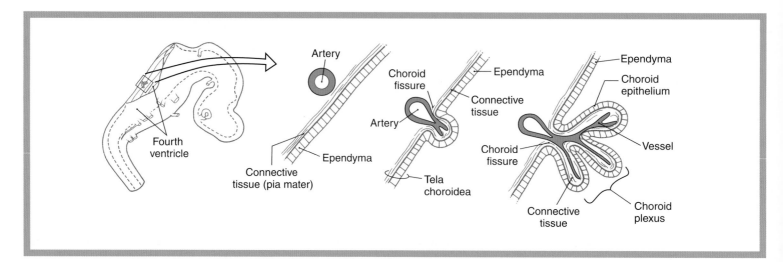

Figure 6-3. Development of the choroid plexus.

roof of the ventricle to form a narrow groove, the *choroid fissure*, in the tela choroidea (Fig. 6-3). These small developing arteries to the fourth ventricle are branches of what will become the posterior inferior cerebellar artery in the adult. The involuted ependymal cells, along with vessels and a small amount of connective tissue, represent the primordial choroid plexus inside the ventricular space. As development progresses, the choroid plexus enlarges, forms many small elevations called *villi*, and begins to secrete CSF (Fig. 6-3; see also Fig. 6-18). By about the end of the first trimester, the choroid plexus is functional, the openings in the fourth ventricle are patent, and there is circulation of CSF through the ventricular system and into the subarachnoid space.

The choroid plexuses of the third and lateral ventricles develop much in the same manner. A choroid fissure appears in the roof of the third ventricle and in the medial wall of the lateral ventricle, where the covering of each (the tela choroidea) is thin. The choroid plexus develops along these lines, bulges into the respective space, and is continuous from lateral to third

ventricles through the interventricular foramen (Fig. 6-4). The small arteries serving the choroid plexus of the third ventricle are branches of the medial posterior choroidal artery and those serving the choroid plexus of the lateral ventricles are branches of the lateral posterior choroidal artery and the anterior choroidal artery (see Chapter 8 for further information).

Ventricles

Lateral Ventricles

The cavities of the telencephalon are the *lateral ventricles*, of which there is one in each hemisphere (Fig. 6-4). As the development of the hemispheres creates the frontal, temporal, and occipital lobes, the lateral ventricles are pulled along and thus acquire their definitive adult shape of a flattened "C" with a short tail (Fig. 6-4). This shape is present by birth. The lateral ventricle consists of an *anterior horn*, a *body*, and *posterior* and *inferior horns* (Fig. 6-4). The junction of the body with the posterior and inferior horns constitutes the *atrium of the lateral*

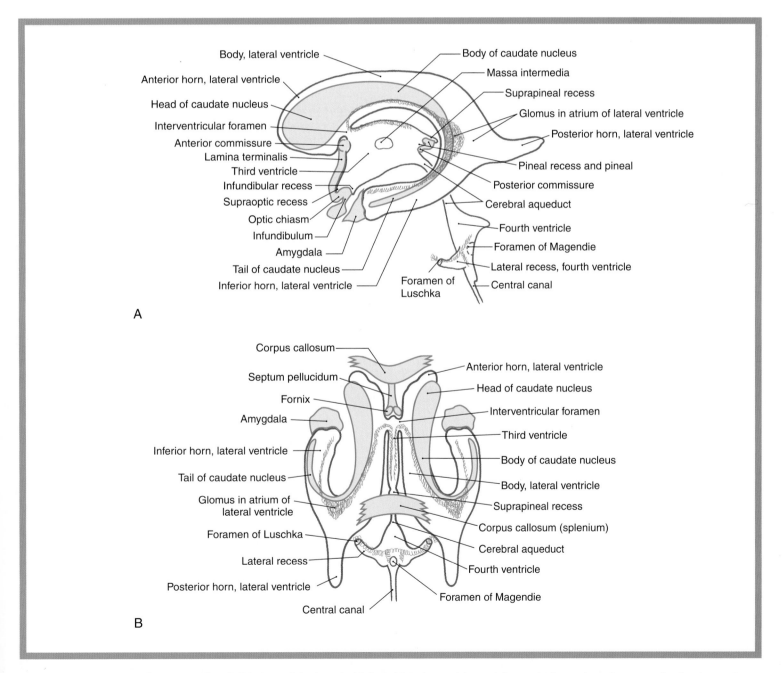

Figure 6-4. Lateral (**A**) and posterior (dorsal) (**B**) views of the lateral, third, and fourth ventricles and the cerebral aqueduct. Structures that border on the various parts of the ventricular system are shown in *green* and the choroid plexus is shown in *red*.

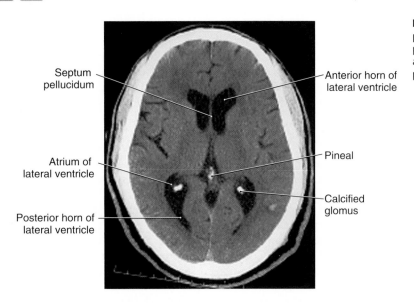

Septum pellucidum

Atrium of lateral ventricle

Posterior horn of lateral ventricle

Anterior horn of lateral ventricle

Pineal

Calcified glomus

Figure 6-5. CT scan showing a calcified glomus in a 66-year-old male patient. Note that calcifications are also present in the pineal in this patient. These calcifications form a triangle, the shape of which may be altered by changes in brain shape or by midline shift secondary to some pathologic process.

ventricle. An especially large clump of choroid plexus, the *glomus* (or *glomus choroideum*), is found in the atrium (Fig. 6-4). In adults and especially in elderly persons, the glomus may contain calcifications that are visible (as white spots) on radiographs or computed tomographic (CT) scans (Fig. 6-5). Shifts in the position of the glomus, usually accompanied by alterations in the volume or shape of the surrounding ventricle, may indicate some type of ongoing pathologic process or space-occupying lesion.

The elaborate shape of the lateral ventricle means that different structures border on different parts of this space. The anterior horn and body of the lateral ventricle are bordered medially by the *septum pellucidum* (at rostral levels) and by a bundle of fibers called the *fornix* (at caudal levels) and posteriorly (superiorly) by

the *corpus callosum* (Figs. 6-4 and 6-6). The floor of the body of the lateral ventricle is made up of the *thalamus*, and the *caudate nucleus* is characteristically found in the lateral wall of the lateral ventricle throughout its extent (Figs. 6-4 and 6-6). In the temporal lobe, the inferior horn of the lateral ventricle contains the tail of the *caudate nucleus* in its lateral wall, the hippocampal formation in its medial wall, and a large group of cells (the *amygdaloid complex*) in its rostral end (Figs. 6-4 and 6-6).

The openings between the lateral and third ventricles, the *interventricular foramina* (of Monro), are located between the column of the fornix and the rostral and medial end of the thalamus. There are two interventricular foramina, one opening from each lateral ventricle into the single midline third ventricle (Fig. 6-4B).

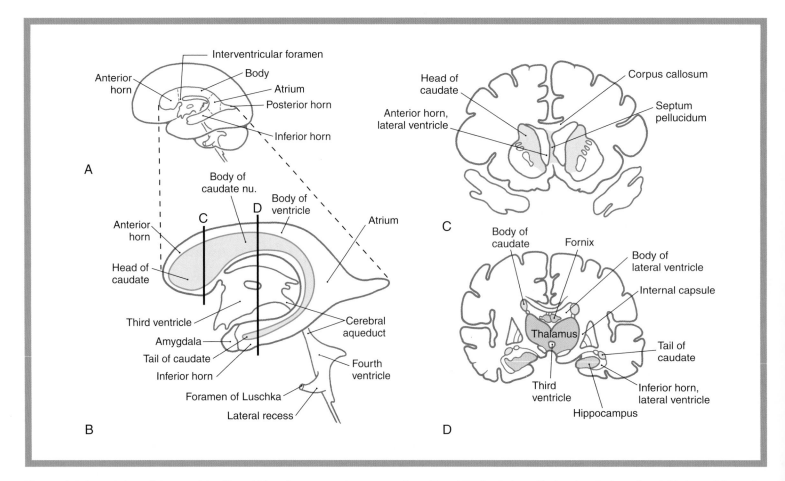

Figure 6-6. Lateral view of the ventricles (**A** and **B**) and representative cross sections (**C** and **D**, details from **B**) showing the lateral and third ventricles and the major structures that border on these spaces.

Third Ventricle

The *third ventricle*, the cavity of the diencephalon, is a narrow, vertically oriented midline space that communicates rostrally with the lateral ventricles and caudally with the *cerebral aqueduct* (Figs. 6-4 and 6-8). The third ventricle has an elaborate profile on a sagittal view (Fig. 6-4A), but it is quite narrow in the coronal and axial planes (Fig. 6-7).

The boundaries of the third ventricle are formed by a variety of structures, the most important being the dorsal thalamus and hypothalamus, and by structures that form small outpocketings called recesses (Figs. 6-4A and 6-8). These are the *supraoptic recess* (above the optic chiasm), the *infundibular recess* (in the infundibulum, the stalk of the pituitary), the *pineal recess* (in the stalk of the pineal), and the *suprapineal recess* (above the pineal). The rostral wall of the third ventricle is formed by a short segment of the *anterior commissure* and a thin membrane, the *lamina terminalis*, that extends from the anterior commissure anteriorly (ventrally) to the rostral edge of the optic chiasm (Figs. 6-4A and 6-8). The floor of the third ventricle is formed by the *optic chiasm* and *infundibulum* and their corresponding recesses, plus a line extending caudally along the rostral aspect of the midbrain to the cerebral aqueduct. The caudal wall is formed by the *posterior commissure* and the recesses related to the pineal, whereas the roof is the *tela choroidea*, from which the choroid plexus is suspended (Figs. 6-4A and 6-8).

Cerebral Aqueduct

The *cerebral aqueduct*, the extension of the ventricle through the mesencephalon, communicates rostrally with the third ventricle and caudally with the fourth ventricle (Figs. 6-4A

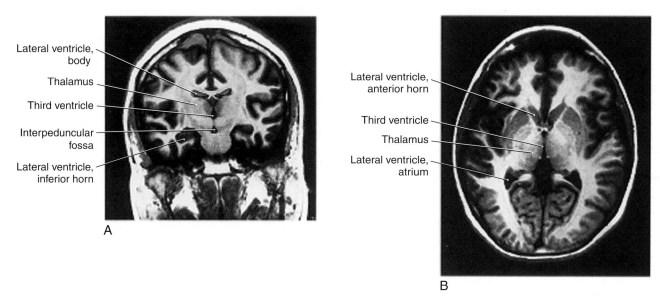

Figure 6-7. MR images of the third ventricle in coronal (**A**) and axial (**B**) views.

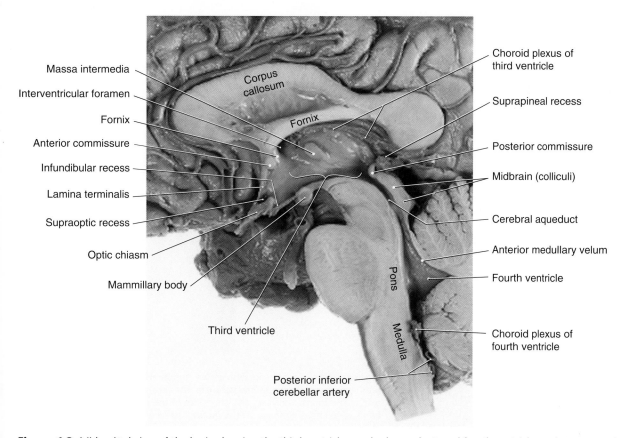

Figure 6-8. Midsagittal view of the brain showing the third ventricle, cerebral aqueduct, and fourth ventricle, and structures closely related to these spaces.

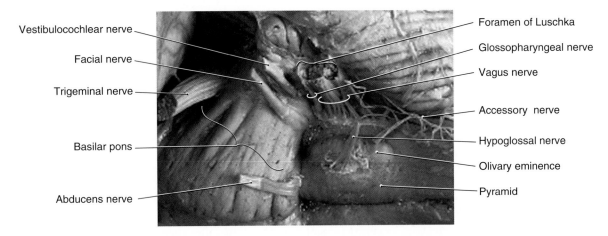

Vestibulocochlear nerve
Facial nerve
Trigeminal nerve
Basilar pons
Abducens nerve

Foramen of Luschka
Glossopharyngeal nerve
Vagus nerve
Accessory nerve
Hypoglossal nerve
Olivary eminence
Pyramid

Figure 6-9. Anterolateral view of the brainstem at the pons-medulla junction showing the foramen of Luschka and the principal structures located in this area. Note the tuft of choroid plexus in the foramen. This area of the subarachnoid space, into which the foramen of Luschka opens, is the lateral cerebellomedullary cistern.

and 6-8). This midline channel is about 1.5 mm in diameter in adults and contains no choroid plexus. Its narrow diameter makes it especially susceptible to occlusion. For example, cellular debris in the ventricular system (from infections or *hemorrhage*) may clog the aqueduct. Tumors in the area of the midbrain (such as *pinealoma*) may compress the midbrain and occlude the aqueduct. The result is a blockage of CSF flow and enlargement of the third and lateral ventricles at the expense of the surrounding brain tissue. This has been called *triventricular hydrocephalus* because it simultaneously involves the enlargement of three ventricles. The cerebral aqueduct is surrounded on all sides by a sleeve of gray matter that contains primarily small neurons; this is the *periaqueductal gray* or *central gray*.

Fourth Ventricle

The *fourth ventricle* is a roughly pyramid-shaped space that forms the cavity of the metencephalon and myelencephalon (Figs. 6-4 and 6-8). The apex of this ventricle extends into the base of the cerebellum, and caudally it tapers to a narrow channel that continues into the cervical spinal cord as the central canal. Laterally the fourth ventricle extends over the surface of the medulla as the *lateral recesses*, to eventually open into the area of the pons-medulla-cerebellum junction, the *cerebellopontine angle*, through the *foramina of Luschka* (Figs. 6-4 and 6-9). The irregularly shaped *foramen of Magendie* is located in the caudal sloping roof of the ventricle (Figs. 6-4 and 6-10). Although the roof of the caudal part of the fourth ventricle and the lateral recesses is composed of *tela choroidea*, the rostral boundaries of this space are formed by brain structures. These include the cerebellum (covering about the middle third of the ventricle) and the superior cerebellar peduncles and anterior medullary velum (covering the rostral third of the ventricle). The floor of the fourth ventricle, the *rhomboid fossa* (see Fig. 10-3), is formed by the pons and medulla (Fig. 6-8). *The only openings between the ventricles of the brain and the subarachnoid space surrounding the brain are the foramina of Luschka and Magendie in the fourth ventricle.*

Hemorrhage into the Ventricles

A variety of events may result in blood accumulating in the ventricular spaces in the brain (Fig. 6-11). These include hemorrhage into the substance of the brain (such as *cerebral hemorrhage*) that subsequently ruptures into the ventricular space, rupture of an intracranial aneurysm (especially those located immediately adjacent to the third or fourth ventricles), or severe head trauma. In this last case there may also be blood in the

subarachnoid space and/or in the substance of the brain depending on the degree of injury. Additional, but less frequent, causes are rupture, or bleeding, from an intraventricular arteriovenous malformation (AVM), or bleeding from a tumor located in, or invading, the ventricular space. Whatever the cause, blood in the ventricles, especially acute blood, is clearly seen on CT (Fig. 6-11). The white appearance of the blood characteristically outlines the ventricular spaces and is clearly distinguishable from blood at other intracranial locations. In fact, blood in the ventricular spaces can create an *in vivo cast* showing details of the ventricular spaces and their relationships (Fig. 6-11). Alterations of size, shape, or position of a ventricle containing blood may be indicative of further neurologic complications.

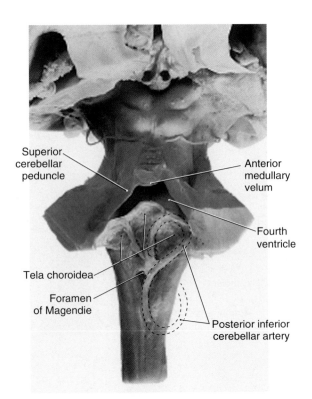

Superior cerebellar peduncle
Anterior medullary velum
Fourth ventricle
Tela choroidea
Foramen of Magendie
Posterior inferior cerebellar artery

Figure 6-10. Posterior (dorsal) view of the brainstem with the cerebellum removed to expose the fourth ventricle, the tela choroidea of the caudal roof of the fourth ventricle, and the route of the posterior inferior cerebellar artery. The choroid plexus on the internal surface of the tela is served by this vessel.

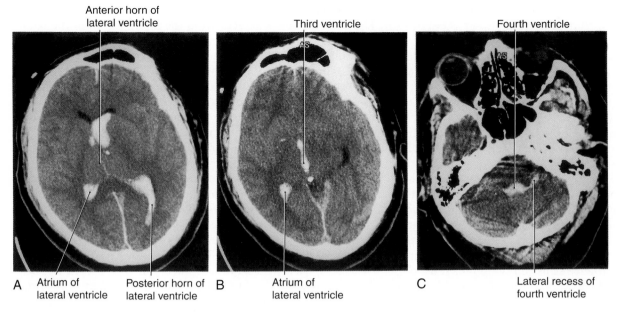

Anterior horn of
lateral ventricle

Third ventricle

Fourth ventricle

A   Atrium of   Posterior horn of   B   Atrium of   C   Lateral recess of
     lateral ventricle   lateral ventricle   lateral ventricle   fourth ventricle

Figure 6-11. CT scans showing examples of blood in various parts of the lateral (**A, B**), third (**B**), and fourth (**C**) ventricles. Acute blood appears white in CT. Note that the blood clearly outlines the characteristic shape of the ventricular spaces.

Ependyma, Choroid Plexus, and Cerebrospinal Fluid

Ependyma

The ventricles of the brain and the central canal of the spinal cord are lined by a simple cuboidal epithelium, the *ependyma*. Ependymal cells contain abundant mitochondria and are metabolically active. Their luminal surfaces are ciliated and have microvilli, and the bases contact the subependymal layer of astrocytic processes. There is not a continuous basal lamina between ependymal cells and the subjacent glial cell processes (Fig. 6-12). Ependymal cells are attached to each other by *zonulae adherens* (desmosomes).

In some regions, particularly the third ventricle, there are patches of specialized ependymal cells called *tanycytes* (Fig. 6-12). Tanycytes have basal processes that extend through the layer

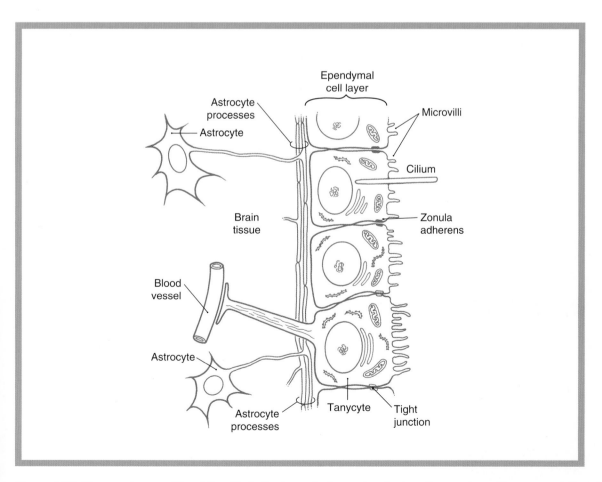

Ependymal
cell layer

Astrocyte
processes

Astrocyte

Microvilli

Cilium

Brain
tissue

Zonula
adherens

Blood
vessel

Astrocyte

Astrocyte   Tanycyte   Tight
processes   junction

Figure 6-12. The ependyma and its relationship to the layer of subependymal astrocytic processes, with a representation of a tanycyte.

of astrocytic processes to form end-feet on blood vessels and in the neuropil. They may function to transport substances between the ventricles and the blood. In contrast to ependymal cells, tanycytes are attached to each other and to immediately adjacent ependymal cells by tight junctions. Desmosomes are also present between tanycytes.

Ependymomas

This tumor, which constitutes 5% to 6% of all glial cell neoplasms, originates from the ependymal cells lining the ventricles (Fig. 6-13). Although these tumors may appear in any ventricle, the majority (60% to 75%) are located in the spaces of the posterior fossa. Ependymomas may also be found within the spinal cord or in the region of the cauda equina. These neoplasms are seen most frequently in children younger than 5 years of age. In general, the location of the ependymoma determines the symptoms experienced by the patient. Lesions in supratentorial locations (Fig. 6-13) may produce signs and symptoms reflecting their location, for example, hydrocephalus in the case of blocked CSF flow or seizure activity. Lesions in infratentorial locations frequently cause nausea and vomiting, headache, other signs and symptoms related to hydrocephalus, and cranial nerve signs and symptoms indicative of compression of, or tumor infiltration into, the brainstem.

The histologic appearance of ependymomas may vary, even from place to place within the same tumor. Generally these tumors are characterized by clusters of various sizes that are composed of polygonal or columnar cells arranged in a circle facing a lumen *(true rosettes)* (Fig. 6-14A, B) or a small blood vessel *(perivascular* or *pseudorosettes)* (Fig. 6-14C). These configurations are made up of long cell processes impinging on a vessel with cell bodies and nuclei located somewhat distal to these processes. Less commonly seen are *ependymal rosettes* consisting of cell clusters surrounding lumina of varying sizes. The cell apexes in these clusters may contain a *basal body (blepharoplast)* associated with the *cilium of the ependymal cell.* The blepharoplast is visualized with stains for glial fibrillary proteins. The presence of this basal body, in a stained section, is one feature that differentiates this tumor from a choroid papilloma as described later. The tissue septa between cell rosettes are usually thick and contain layers of neuroglial cell processes.

Treatment for patients with ependymoma is primarily with surgical removal followed by focal irradiation. Incomplete removal, for example, in cases with tumor infiltration into the brainstem, reduces survival rates even with radiation therapy and chemotherapy.

Choroid Plexus

The choroid plexus extends from the inferior horn of the lateral ventricle into the atrium, where the glomus choroideum is located, along the floor of the body of the lateral ventricle, continues through the interventricular foramen, and attaches to the roof of the third ventricle (Figs. 6-4, 6-15, and 6-16). A tumor of the choroid plexus at the point where it is continuous through the interventricular foramen (Fig. 6-16) may result in an enlargement of the lateral ventricle on that side with signs and symptoms of increased intracranial pressure (vomiting, lethargy, headache, possible papilledema). Such lesions are candidates for surgical removal. The choroid plexus of the fourth ventricle is attached to the caudal roof and extends laterally into the foramen of Luschka (Figs. 6-4 and 6-9).

The choroid plexus in each ventricle is thrown into a series of folds called *villi* (singular, *villus*). These are covered on their ventricular (luminal) surfaces by a continuum of dome-shaped structures, each with numerous microvilli (Fig. 6-17A, B). Each dome represents the luminal surface of one *choroid epithelial cell,* and the shallow grooves between domes are the points of contact between adjacent *choroid* cells (Fig. 6-17B, C). Each villus consists of a core of highly vascularized connective tissue derived from the pia mater and a simple cuboidal covering (the *choroid epithelial cell layer*), which is derived from ependymal cells (Figs. 6-3 and 6-17B, C). The abundant capillaries in the connective tissue core of each villus are surrounded by a *basal lamina*. The endothelial cells of these capillaries have numerous *fenestrations,* which allow a free exchange of molecules between blood plasma and the extracellular fluid in the connective tissue core (Fig. 6-18). The connective tissue core itself consists of fibroblasts and collagen fibrils. Another basal lamina is formed at the interface between the connective tissue core and the choroid epithelial cells that form the surface of each villus (Figs. 6-17 and 6-18). These choroid cells have microvilli on their apical (ventricular) surface, interdigitating cell membranes on their sides, and irregular bases. Each is attached to its neighbor by continuous *tight junctions (zonulae occludentes)* that seal off the subjacent extracellular space from the ventricular space (Figs. 6-17C and 6-18). This represents the *blood-CSF barrier.* Choroid epithelial cells contain a nucleus, numerous mitochondria, rough endoplasmic reticulum, and a small Golgi apparatus (Figs. 6-17C and 6-18). Thus, they are specialized to control the flow of ions and metabolites into the CSF.

Although choroid epithelial cells are joined by tight junctions, ependymal cells are not (Fig. 6-18). Therefore, fluid exchange occurs freely between CSF and the extracellular fluid of the

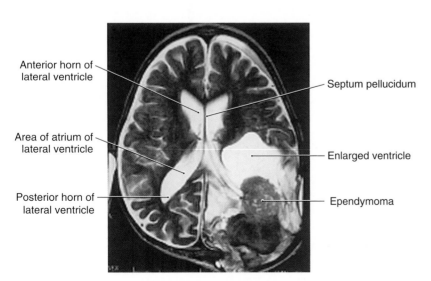

Figure 6-13. MR (T2-weighted) image of an ependymoma in a 1-year-old male patient. Note that the tumor has extensively invaded the parietal and occipital lobes of the cerebral hemisphere.

Anterior horn of lateral ventricle

Septum pellucidum

Area of atrium of lateral ventricle

Enlarged ventricle

Posterior horn of lateral ventricle

Ependymoma

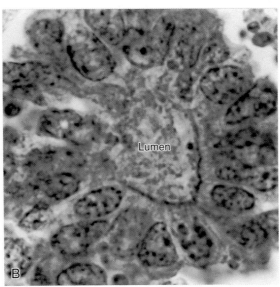

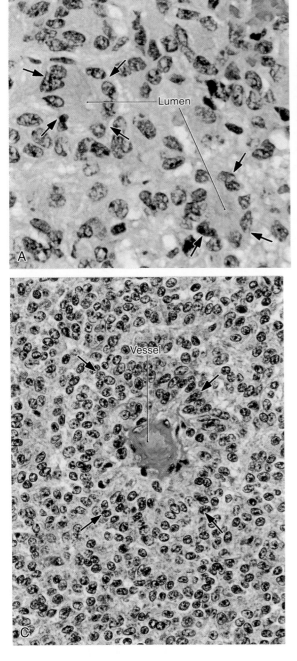

Figure 6-14. Histologic section showing the characteristics of a true rosette (**A, B**) and a perivascular rosette (or pseudorosette—**C**). In the true rosette (**A, B**) the cells cluster around a small lumen; the apparently incomplete lumen in **B** is due to the plane of the section. In a perivascular rosette (**C**) the cells cluster (arrows) around the lumen of a small vessel.

brain parenchyma. The composition of CSF can thus sometimes reflect disease processes occurring in brain tissue. For example, catabolites of catecholamines are reduced in quantity in the CSF of patients with Parkinson disease, a neurodegenerative disorder involving loss of dopaminergic neurons.

In humans the blood supply to the choroid plexuses is via the *choroidal arteries* and the *posterior cerebellar arteries*. Choroid plexus in the inferior horn, atrium of the lateral ventricle, and body of the lateral ventricle is served by the *anterior choroidal artery* (a branch of the internal carotid) and the *lateral posterior choroidal artery* (a branch of P_2). The *medial posterior choroidal artery* (also a branch of P_2) serves the choroid plexus of the third ventricle. The choroid plexus located inside the fourth ventricle is served by branches of the *posterior inferior cerebellar artery* (Figs. 6-8 and 6-10), and the tuft that extends out of the foramen of Luschka into the subarachnoid space (Fig. 6-9) is served by the *anterior inferior cerebellar artery*.

Tumors of the Choroid Plexus
Tumors of the choroid plexus are relatively rare, comprising somewhat less than 1% of all intracranial tumors. In general

these lesions are classified as *choroid plexus papillomas* (Fig. 6-19), which are benign and the more frequently seen, or as *choroid plexus carcinomas*, which are malignant and rarely seen. Although these tumors may be seen in patients of any age, they are more common between birth and 10 years. They more often occur in the fourth ventricle (50% to 60%) but may also be found in the lateral and third ventricles. These patients present with signs and symptoms of increased intracranial pressure (headache, nausea, vomiting, lethargy), hydrocephalus (excessive production of CSF), or deficits of eye movement due to pressure on the roots of III, IV or VI. The treatment of choice for the more commonly seen tumor, a *choroid plexus papilloma*, is surgical removal. The more rarely seen, and more virulent, *choroid plexus carcinoma* is treated more aggressively, first with chemotherapy, followed by surgery, then with a combination of chemotherapy and radiation.

Histologically, these tumors are characterized by clusters of cuboidal or columnar cells that are strikingly similar to normal choroid plexus epithelium (Fig. 6-19). These cell clusters are insinuated between comparatively thin areas containing small vessels and loose connective tissue. This is one important difference between this tumor and an ependymoma, which has thick

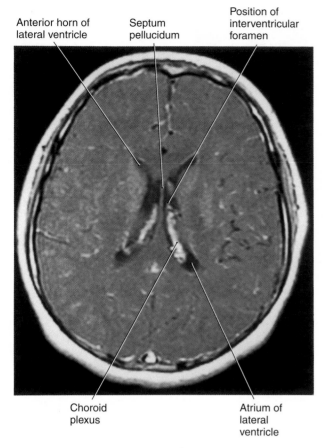

Anterior horn of
lateral ventricle

Septum
pellucidum

Position of
interventricular
foramen

Choroid
plexus

Atrium of
lateral
ventricle

Figure 6-15. Axial MR image showing the choroid plexus in the body of the lateral ventricle between the atrium and the point where it passes through the interventricular foramen.

Table 6-1. A Comparison of the Constituents of Cerebrospinal Fluid (CSF) with Blood Plasma*

	CSF	Plasma
Chloride (Cl⁻)	125.0 mEq/L	100.0 mEq/L
Magnesium (Mg²⁺)	2.7 mEq/L	1.3 mEq/L
Sodium (Na⁺)	143.0 mEq/L	138.0 mEq/L
Creatinine	1.1 mg/dL	1.2 mg/dL
Potassium (K⁺)	2.9 mEq/L	4.5 mEq/L
Calcium (Ca²⁺)	2.4 mEq/L	5.0 mEq/L
Glucose	60.0 mg/dL	90.0 mg/dL
Proteins	34.0 mg/dL	6,500.0 mg/dL
Albumin	155.0 mg/L	35,000.0 mg/L
Uric acid	0.7 mg/dL	4.0 mg/dL

*These are general averages that approximate the center of a range.

intervening areas that are composed of glial cell processes (compare Figs. 6-14 and 6-19). Mitotic figures are infrequently seen but when present may indicate that the tumor is malignant.

Cerebrospinal Fluid in Health and Disease

Choroid epithelial cells secrete CSF by selective transport of materials from the connective tissue extracellular space (Fig. 6-18). Sodium chloride is actively transported into the ventricles, and water passively follows the concentration gradient thus established. Other materials, including large molecules, are transported in pinocytotic vesicles from the basal to the apical surface of the epithelium and exocytosed into the CSF. *Compared with blood plasma, CSF has higher concentrations of chloride, magnesium, and sodium; similar concentrations of creatinine; and lower concentrations of potassium, calcium, glucose, proteins, albumin, and uric acid* (Table 6-1). Deviation from these normal values is indicative of a pathologic state or ongoing pathologic process.

Normal CSF is clear and colorless and contains very little protein (15 to 45 mg/dL), little immunoglobulin, and only one to five cells (leukocytes) per milliliter. Changes from these normal values are useful in the diagnosis of a variety of disease processes (Table 6-1).

Lumbar puncture is used to collect a sample of CSF for analysis and to measure CSF pressure. A needle is inserted between the third and fourth (or fourth and fifth) lumbar vertebrae into the dural sac, the spinal fluid pressure is measured, and a few milliliters of fluid is withdrawn. Because the average volume of CSF in the adult is about 120 mL, and the rate of production is about 450 to 500 mL/day, the sample removed is quickly replaced. When there is evidence of blood in the retrieved sample of CSF, it is important to establish if this observation is due to subarachnoid hemorrhage or due to damage to a vessel during the procedure: a *traumatic tap*. What is commonly called the *three-tube test* provides the answer. Three successive tubes of CSF are drawn. If the first tube contains blood, the second little or none, and the third none, it was most likely a traumatic tap. If all three tubes contain bloody CSF that is also xanthochromic, it most likely means that there is bleeding into the subarachnoid space.

The numbers and types of cells found in CSF vary according to the type of disease. In bacterial meningitis or brain abscesses, neutrophils predominate and may reach concentrations of 1000 to 20,000/mL and the CSF is cloudy. In syphilitic meningitis, by contrast, 200 to 300 cells/mL would be typical, and most of these would be lymphocytes. Lymphocytes are also the predominant cell type found in active multiple sclerosis, even though there are usually fewer than 50 cells/mL of CSF. The diagnosis of multiple sclerosis also rests on specific changes in the immunoglobulin G content of CSF and a slight increase in the number of mononuclear cells; immunoglobulin G is both derived from the blood and produced by lymphocytes in the CSF, where it is released during an autoimmune reaction attack.

In marked contrast to the elevated numbers of white blood cells seen in central nervous system (CNS) infections, numerous red blood cells are present in the CSF of patients who have bleeding into the *subarachnoid space (subarachnoid hemorrhage)*. For example, this condition may result from rupture of an intracranial aneurysm or arteriovenous malformation. Patients with subarachnoid hemorrhage or those with primary CNS tumors usually have elevated protein levels in their CSF. Elevated CSF protein is also seen in patients with syphilis or meningitis and in cancer patients in whom the disease has spread (metastasized) into the CSF. The CSF of cancer patients may also contain malignant cells characteristic of their primary lesions.

Cerebrospinal Fluid Production and Circulation

The CSF produced by the choroid plexuses passes through the ventricular system to exit the fourth ventricle through the foramina of Luschka and Magendie (Fig. 6-20). At this point, the CSF enters the subarachnoid space, which is continuous around the brain and spinal cord. The CSF in the subarachnoid space provides the buoyancy necessary to prevent the weight of the brain from crushing nerve roots and blood vessels against the internal surface of the skull. The weight of the brain, about 1400 g in air, is reduced to about 45 g when it is suspended in CSF. Consequently, the tethers formed by delicate connective tissue strands traversing the subarachnoid space, the *arachnoid trabeculae* (Fig. 6-20), are adequate to maintain the brain in a stable position within its CSF envelope.

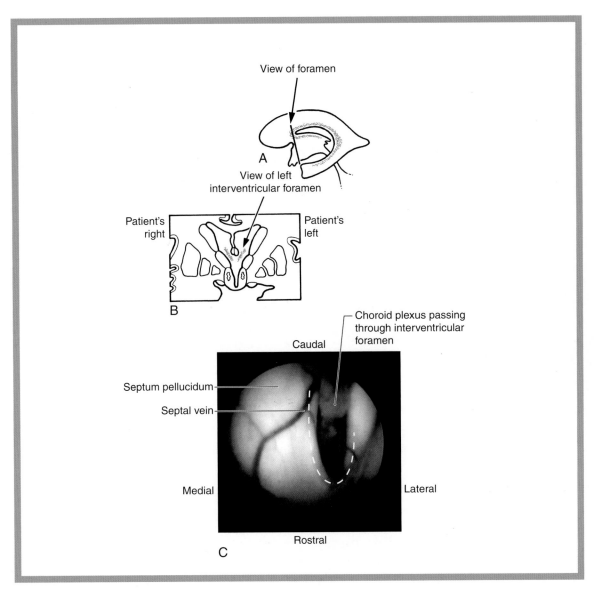

Figure 6-16. Lateral (**A**) and coronal (**B**) views showing the position of the interventricular foramen (**C**) in an intraoperative photograph. When looking down into the lateral ventricle (**C**), note that the choroid plexus passes from the lateral ventricle through the foramen and into the third ventricle. The *dashed line* represents the position of the fornix.

The movement of CSF through the ventricular system and the subarachnoid space is influenced by two major factors. First, there is a subtle pressure gradient between the points of production of CSF (choroid plexuses in brain ventricles) and the points of transfer into the venous system (arachnoid villi). Because CSF is not compressible, it tends to move along this gradient. Second, CSF is also moved in the subarachnoid space by purely mechanical means. These include gentle movements of the brain on its arachnoid trabecular tethers during normal activities and the pulsations of the numerous arteries found in the subarachnoid space.

After passing through the subarachnoid space, the CSF reaches the arachnoid villi that extend into the superior sagittal sinus and into the venous lakes *(lateral lacunae* or *lateral lacunae of the superior sagittal sinus)* lateral to the superior sagittal sinus (Fig. 6-20). The subarachnoid space and the CSF it contains extend into the core of each villus. At this point CSF enters the venous circulation through two routes. A limited amount passes between the cells making up the arachnoid villus, whereas most is transported through these cells in membrane-bound vesicles (see also Chapter 7). About 330 to 380 mL of CSF enters the venous circulation per day, and about 120 mL is present in ventricles and subarachnoid space at any given time.

Hydrocephalus and Related Conditions

Blockage of CSF movement or a failure of the absorption mechanism will result in the accumulation of fluid in the ventricular spaces or around the brain (Fig. 6-21). The results, commonly called *hydrocephalus*, are characterized by an increase in CSF volume, enlargement of one or more of the ventricles, and, usually, an increase in CSF pressure. Dilation of the cerebral ventricles may result from a blockage of CSF flow through the system, as in *obstructive hydrocephalus;* from factors not related to impaired flow, as in *communicating hydrocephalus;* or from brain atrophy, as in *hydrocephalus ex vacuo.* Ventricular dilation may also be a sequela to trauma, meningitis, or subarachnoid hemorrhage. Typically there is a moderate to severe increase in intracranial pressure in patients with hydrocephalus.

Obstructive Hydrocephalus
Obstructive hydrocephalus may result from an obstruction somewhere within the ventricular system or within the subarachnoid space. Common intraventricular sites of potential obstruction are the interventricular foramen (or foramina), cerebral aqueduct, caudal portions of the fourth ventricle, and

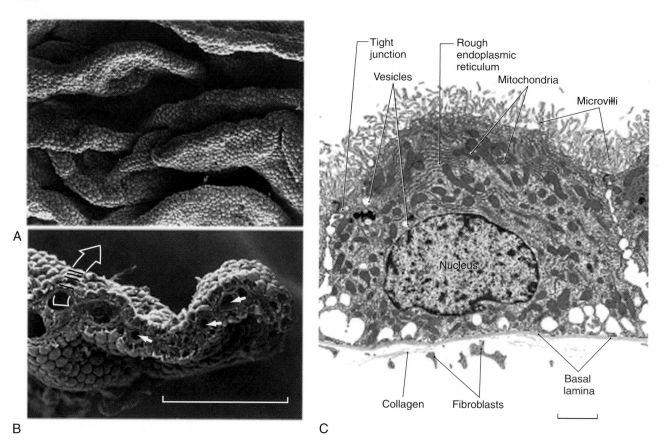

A

B

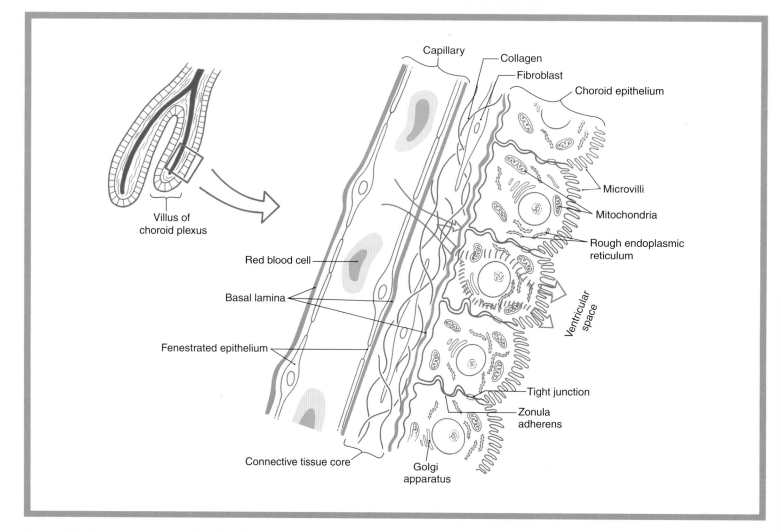

C

Tight junction

Vesicles

Rough endoplasmic reticulum

Mitochondria

Microvilli

Nucleus

Collagen   Fibroblasts

Basal lamina

Figure 6-17. Elements of the choroid plexus. Scanning electron micrographs of the surface (**A**) of several villi of the choroid plexus and the cut surface (**B**) of one villus. The characteristic appearance of the luminal surface of the choroidal cells is seen in both micrographs. The *arrows* in **B** mark vessels in the core of the villus *(solid arrows)* and the route of fluid movement from the vessels into the ventricular space *(broken arrow)*. Transmission electron micrograph (**C**) showing the internal structure of one choroid epithelial cell. Primate; scale = 100 μm for **A** and **B** and 2 μm for **C**.

Capillary

Collagen

Fibroblast

Choroid epithelium

Microvilli

Mitochondria

Rough endoplasmic reticulum

Ventricular space

Tight junction

Zonula adherens

Villus of choroid plexus

Red blood cell

Basal lamina

Fenestrated epithelium

Connective tissue core

Golgi apparatus

Figure 6-18. The basic structure of the choroid plexus and the route of fluid transport (shown in *green*) through the choroid epithelium to produce cerebrospinal fluid.

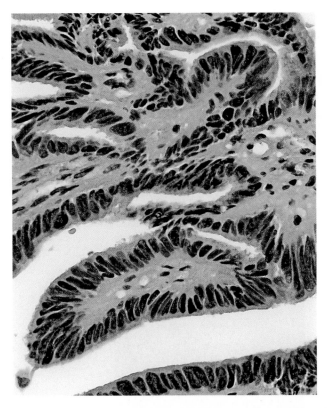

Figure 6-19. Histologic features of a choroid plexus papilloma. Although this tumor has similarities to normal choroid plexus, note the proliferation of elongated and cuboidal cells, the thickened stroma, and the tongue-shaped (or papillary) appearance of portions of the tumor.

foramen of the fourth ventricle. Extraventricular obstruction may occur at any place in the subarachnoid space but is more common around the base of the brain, at the tentorium cerebelli and tentorial notch, over the convexity of the hemisphere, and at the superior sagittal sinus.

Aqueductal Stenosis

Aqueductal stenosis may be caused by a tumor in the immediate vicinity of the midbrain (as in *pineoblastoma* or *meningioma*) that compresses the brain and occludes the cerebral aqueduct. This channel may also be occluded by the cellular debris seen following *intraventricular hemorrhage*, by bacterial or fungal infections, or by ependymal proliferation due to viral infections of the CNS (especially mumps). One major sequela of aqueductal blockade is enlargement of the third and both lateral ventricles (Fig. 6-21). This is sometimes called triventricular hydrocephalus because three ventricles simultaneously enlarge as a result of one lesion or occlusion. Unilateral obstruction of one interventricular foramen, for example by a colloid cyst in one interventricular foramen, results in enlargement of the lateral ventricle on that side. Blockage of both interventricular foramina will produce enlargement of both lateral ventricles. Obstruction of the exit channels of the fourth ventricle, the foramina of Magendie and Luschka, will result in enlargement of all parts of the ventricular system.

Communicating Hydrocephalus

In *communicating hydrocephalus*, the flow of CSF through the ventricular system and into the subarachnoid space is not

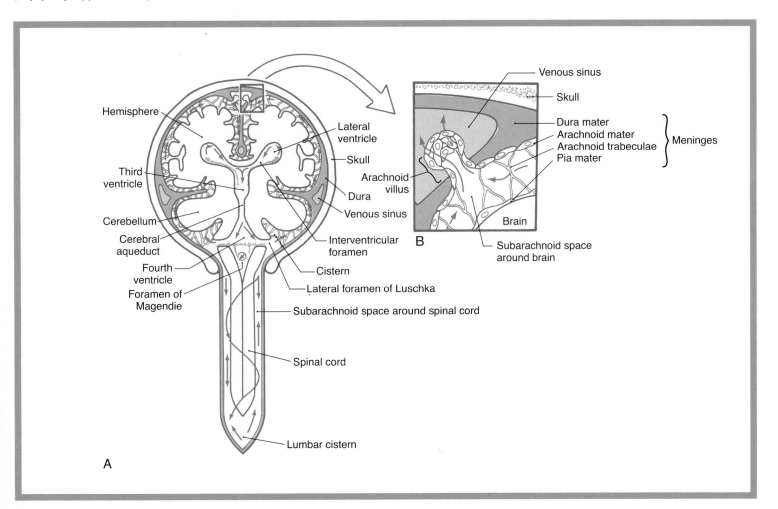

Figure 6-20. Representation of the brain and spinal cord (**A**) showing the locations of choroid plexus *(red)* and the routes of flow taken by cerebrospinal fluid (CSF) *(green)* through the ventricles and the subarachnoid space around the central nervous system. The detail (**B**) shows the relationship of an arachnoid villus to the subarachnoid space and the venous sinus. Although not shown here, the venous sinus is lined by an endothelium. CSF enters the venous system primarily by transport through cells of the arachnoid villus (**B**, *dashed green arrows*), although some fluid moves between these cells (**B**, *solid green arrow*).

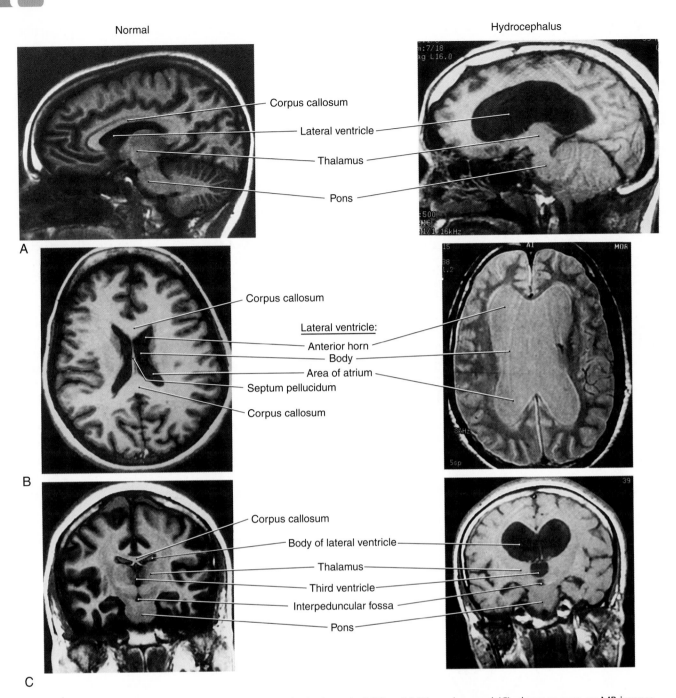

Figure 6-21. Comparison of normal and hydrocephalic brains in sagittal (**A**), axial (**B**), and coronal (**C**) planes as seen on MR images.

impaired. However, movement of CSF through the subarachnoid space and into the venous system is partially or totally blocked. This block may be caused by a congenital absence (agenesis) of the arachnoid villi. Alternatively, these villi may be partially blocked by red blood cells subsequent to a subarachnoid hemorrhage. An exceedingly high level of protein in the CSF (above 500 mg/dL), as seen in patients with CNS tumors or inflammation, may also contribute to communicating hydrocephalus. The high CSF pressure is due partially to the sequestering of protein in the arachnoid villi and subsequent blockage of CSF transport into the venous system.

Additional causes of communicating hydrocephalus include the interruption of CSF movement through the subarachnoid space caused by either subarachnoid hemorrhage or a major CNS infection, such as leptomeningitis, and the subsequent inflammatory response. Overproduction of CSF in patients with *papilloma of the choroid plexus* may also be a factor. In all of these situations there is an enlargement of all parts of the ventricular system. Although rare, hydrocephalus may also be seen in patients with impaired venous flow from the brain.

Hydrocephalus ex Vacuo

This is actually not a true hydrocephalus but rather a generalized atrophy of the brain resulting in ventricles that are relatively larger owing to the loss of white matter. There is no increase in intracranial pressure, there are no neurologic deficits other than those that may be related to brain atrophy, and treatment is not indicated. Ex vacuo changes may also refer to atrophy with a change in ventricular size that may follow, by several years, an event such as a stroke.

Idiopathic Intracranial Hypertension

Idiopathic intracranial hypertension (pseudotumor cerebri) is an enigmatic condition most commonly seen in obese women of child-bearing age and in persons with chronic renal failure; it is possibly related to vitamin A toxicity. There is an increase in intracranial pressure (>25 cm H_2O), with little evidence of pressure increase on CT or magnetic resonance imaging studies, such as ventricular enlargement or effacement of sulci or cisterns. These patients usually experience headache and a variety of visual deficits (up to blindness) due to papilledema (swelling of the optic disc). Treatment includes a program of weight loss, medication, and, if needed, shunting (lumboperitoneal) or surgical fenestration, which consists of making a window in the optic sheath to relieve pressure on the optic nerve. These modalities are usually effective in preserving and/or improving vision.

Normal Pressure Hydrocephalus
The cause of this form of hydrocephalus is unclear. The name is a misnomer since CSF pressure is elevated episodically when measured over time. Affected patients are usually elderly. In most cases the cause is unknown. Although intracranial pressure may initially be elevated and the ventricles enlarged, the pressure may wax and wane over time or even subside to a high-normal level; however, the effects of the increased pressure remain.

Patients with normal-pressure hydrocephalus experience a diagnostic triad consisting of urinary problems (frequency, urgency, or incontinence), impaired gait that is most obvious on stepping up as on a curb, and dementia. In some patients the combination of a difficult shuffling gait and dementia may mimic the clinical picture in degenerative disease such as Alzheimer and Parkinson diseases. Treatment is a shunting procedure to reduce CSF pressure and volume. In some cases there is general clinical improvement with lessening of all symptoms including those related to mental status.

Synopsis of Clinical Points

- A blockage of CSF flow may result in hydrocephalus (p. 91).
- Points of potential blockage of CSF flow within the ventricular system are the interventricular foramina, cerebral aqueduct, and foramina of the fourth ventricle (p. 92).
- Blood in the ventricles may originate for several sources, create casts of the ventricular space, and is clearly distinguished from blood in other locations (pp. 96–97).
- Ependymomas arise from ventricular lining cells, have a characteristic histologic appearance, and are treated by excision and radiation (p. 98).
- A choroid plexus tumor blocking the interventricular foramen may result in increased intracranial pressure (p. 99).
- Symptoms of increased intracranial pressure include nausea and headache (p. 99).
- Signs of increased intracranial pressure include vomiting and papilledema (p. 99).
- Choroid plexus (CP) tumors may be classified as CP papilloma or CP carcinoma, may result in excessive CSF production, and are usually treated surgically (pp. 99–100).
- Variations in the constituents of CSF are a valuable diagnostic tool (p. 100).
- The three-tube test can determine if there is a traumatic tap (p. 100).
- Obstructive hydrocephalus occurs when there is an obstruction in the CSF pathway (pp. 101–103).
- Tumors compressing the midbrain or cellular debris occluding the aqueduct may result in aqueductal stenosis and hydrocephalus (pp. 95–96, 103).
- Obstruction to CSF flow in the subarachnoid space or movement into the venous sinuses may result in communicating hydrocephalus (pp. 101–103).
- Hydrocephalus ex vacuo may be seen in elderly patients or in victims of stroke (p. 104).
- Deficits characteristic of idiopathic hypertension are seen in obese women of child-bearing age (pp. 104–105).
- Patients with hydrocephalus ex vacuo may have no obvious neurologic deficits (p. 104).

Sources and Additional Reading

Davson H, Welch K, Segal MB: Physiology and Pathophysiology of the Cerebrospinal Fluid. Edinburgh, Churchill Livingstone, 1987.

Fishman RA: Cerebrospinal Fluid in Diseases of the Nervous System. Philadelphia, WB Saunders, 1992.

Kida S, Yamashima T, Kubota T, Ito H, Yamamoto S: A light and electron microscopic and immunohistochemical study of human arachnoid villi. J Neurosurg 69:429-435, 1988.

North B, Reilly P: Raised Intracranial Pressure: A Clinical Guide. Oxford, Heinemann, 1990.

Pardridge WM (ed): Introduction to the Blood-Brain Barrier. Cambridge, Cambridge University Press, 1998.

Peters A, Palay SL, Webster H deF: The Fine Structure of the Nervous System, Neurons and Their Supporting Cells, 3rd ed. New York, Oxford University Press, 1991.

Russell DS: Observations on the Pathology of Hydrocephalus. London, Her Majesty's Stationery Office, 1949.

Segal MB (ed): Barriers and Fluids of the Eye and Brain. Boca Raton, FL, CRC Press, 1992.

Upton ML, Weller RO: The morphology of cerebrospinal fluid drainage pathways in human arachnoid granulations. J Neurosurg 63:867-875, 1985.

Wood JH (ed): Neurobiology of Cerebrospinal Fluid, vols 1 and 2. New York, Plenum Press, 1980 and 1983.

Yamashima T: Functional ultrastructure of cerebrospinal fluid drainage channels in human arachnoid villi. Neurosurgery 22:633-641, 1988.

The Meninges
D. E. Haines

The human nervous system is extremely delicate and lacks the internal connective tissue framework seen in most organs. For protection, the brain and spinal cord are each encased in a bony shell, enveloped by a fibrous coat, and delicately suspended within a fluid compartment. In the living state, the nervous system has a gelatinous consistency, but when treated with fixatives, it becomes firm and easy to handle.

Overview

The brain and spinal cord are surrounded by the skull and vertebral column, respectively. With the exception of the intervertebral foramina, through which the spinal nerves and their associated vessels pass, and the foramina in the skull, which serve as conduits for arteries, veins, and cranial nerve roots, this bony encasement is complete. The membranous coverings of the central nervous system (CNS), the *meninges*, are located internal to the skull and vertebral column. The meninges (1) protect the underlying brain and spinal cord; (2) serve as a support framework for important arteries, veins, and sinuses; and (3) enclose a fluid-filled cavity, the *subarachnoid space*, which is vital to the survival and normal function of the brain and spinal cord.

The presence of this bony and meningeal encasement of the CNS is a double-edged sword. Although these structures offer maximum protection, in the case of trauma or in a disease process they can be very unforgiving. For example, growth of a tumor creates a mass that will increase intracranial pressure and compress or displace various portions of the brain. Something has to give inside the skull when a space-occupying lesion develops, and it is the delicate tissue of the brain that gives. The neurologic deficits that result depend on the location of the mass, the rapidity with which it enlarges, and which parts of the brain are damaged.

Development of the Meninges

The meninges develop from cells of the *neural crest* and *mesenchyme* (mesoderm), which migrate to surround the developing CNS between 20 and 35 days of gestation (Fig. 7-1A–C). Collectively, these neural crest and mesodermal cells form the *primitive meninges (meninx primitiva)*. At this stage no obvious spaces (venous sinuses, subarachnoid space) are present in the meninges. Between 34 and 48 days of gestation, the primitive meninges differentiate into an outer, more compact layer called the *ectomeninx* and an inner, more reticulated layer called the *endomeninx* (Fig. 7-1D). As development progresses (45 to 60 days of gestation), the ectomeninx becomes more compact and spaces appear in this layer that correlate with the positions of the future venous sinuses. Concurrently, the endomeninx becomes more reticulated and the spaces that appear in its inner part correspond to the subarachnoid spaces and cisterns of the adult. In general, the ectomeninx will become the *dura mater* of the adult brain and the endomeninx will form the *arachnoid mater* and *pia mater* (the *leptomeninges*) of the adult nervous system (Fig. 7-1D). By the end of the first trimester the meninges have generally reached the overall plan as seen around the adult brain and spinal cord.

One developmental defect associated with closure of the neural tube and formation of the meninges in the lumbosacral area is the *congenital dermal sinus* (also called just *dermal sinus*) (Fig. 7-1E). This defect is caused by a failure of the ectoderm (future skin) to completely pinch off from the neuroectoderm and the primitive meninges that envelop it. As a result, the meninges are continuous with a narrow, epithelium-lined channel that extends to the skin surface (Fig. 7-1E). Dermal sinuses are sometimes discovered in young patients who have recurrent,

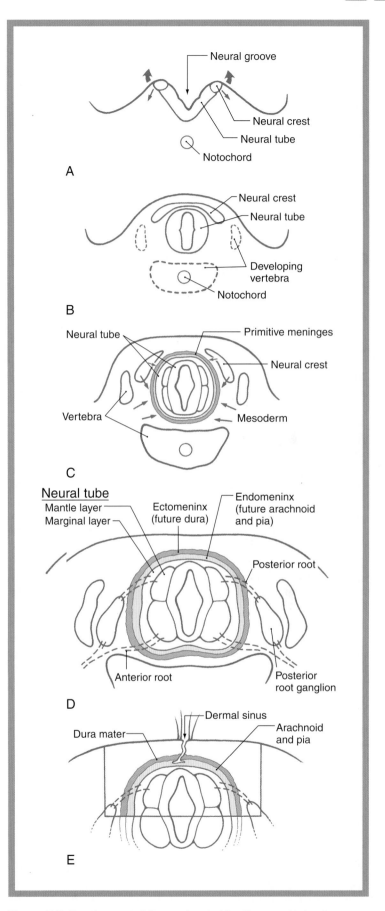

Figure 7-1. Development of the meninges. After the neural tube closes (**A, B**), cells from the neural crest and mesoderm (**C**, *arrows*) migrate to surround the neural tube and form the primordia of the dura and of the arachnoid and pia (**D**). A dermal sinus (**E**) is a malformation in which there is a channel from the skin into the meninges.

but unexplained, bouts of meningitis. These lesions are surgically removed, and recovery is usually complete.

The ectomeninx around the brain is continuous with the skeletogenous layer that forms the skull. This relationship is maintained in the adult, where the dura is intimately adherent to the inner surface of the skull. In the spinal column, the ectomeninx is also initially continuous with the developing vertebrae. However, as development proceeds, the spinal ectomeninx dissociates from the vertebral bodies. A layer of cells remains on the vertebrae to form the periosteum, and the larger part of the ectomeninx condenses to form the spinal dura. The intervening space becomes the spinal *epidural space* (Fig. 7-2). This space is essential for the administration of *epidural anesthetics*.

Overview of the Meninges

In general, the meninges consist of fibroblasts and varying amounts of extracellular connective tissue fibrils. The structural features of each meningeal layer reflect the fact that the fibroblasts of that particular layer are modified to serve a particular function.

The human meninges are composed of the *dura mater,* the *arachnoid mater,* and the *pia mater* (Figs. 7-2 and 7-3). The outermost portion, the *dura mater,* also called the *pachymeninx,* is adherent to the inner surface of the skull but is separated from the vertebrae by the *epidural space* (Fig. 7-2). Around the brain the inner portions of the dura give rise to infoldings or septa, such as the *falx cerebri* or *tentorium cerebelli* (Fig. 7-2), which separate brain regions from each other. Major venous sinuses are found at the points where these septa originate. Spinal and cranial nerves, as they enter or exit the CNS, must pass through a cuff of the dura that is continuous with the connective tissue of the peripheral nerve. Blood vessels traverse the dura in similar fashion. Rostrally the dura sac is attached to the rim of the foramen magnum. Caudally the sac ends at about the level of the second sacral vertebrae and is attached to the coccyx by the *filum terminale externum* (or *dural part of the filum terminale*) (Fig. 7-2).

The inner two layers of the meninges, the arachnoid mater and the pia mater (Figs. 7-2 and 7-3), are collectively known as the *leptomeninges.* This term is also commonly used in clinical medicine (as in *leptomeningeal cysts* and *leptomeningitis*). The arachnoid is a thin cellular layer that is attached to the overlying dura but, with the exception of the arachnoid trabeculae, is separated from the pia mater by the *subarachnoid space.* The arachnoid around the brain is directly continuous with the arachnoid lining the inner surface of the spinal dura (Fig. 7-2). Consequently, the spinal and cerebral subarachnoid spaces are also directly continuous with each other at the foramen magnum. The *subarachnoid space* contains cerebrospinal fluid (CSF) and vessels and is bridged by fibroblasts of various sizes and shapes that collectively form the *arachnoid trabeculae.* The arachnoid is avascular and does not contain nerve fibers.

The *pia mater* is located on the surface of the brain and spinal cord and closely follows all their various grooves and elevations (Figs. 7-2 and 7-3). Around the spinal cord the pia mater contributes to the formation of the *denticulate ligaments* and the *filum terminale internum* (or *pial part of the filum terminale*) (Fig. 7-2).

Dura Mater

Periosteal and Meningeal Dura

The *dura mater (pachymeninx)* is composed of elongated fibroblasts and copious amounts of collagen fibrils (Fig. 7-3). This membrane contains blood vessels and nerves and is generally

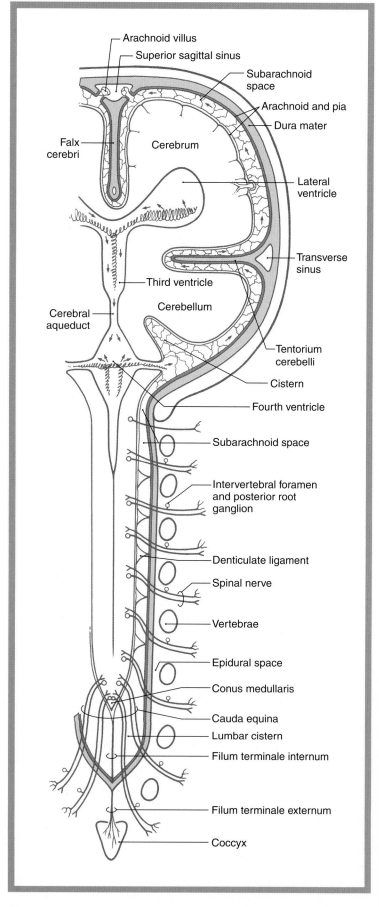

Figure 7-2. The relation of the meninges to the brain and spinal cord and to their surrounding bony structures. The dura is represented in *blue,* the arachnoid in *red.* (From Haines DE: Neuroanatomy: An Atlas of Structures, Sections, and Systems, 5th ed. Baltimore, Lippincott Williams & Wilkins, 2000.)

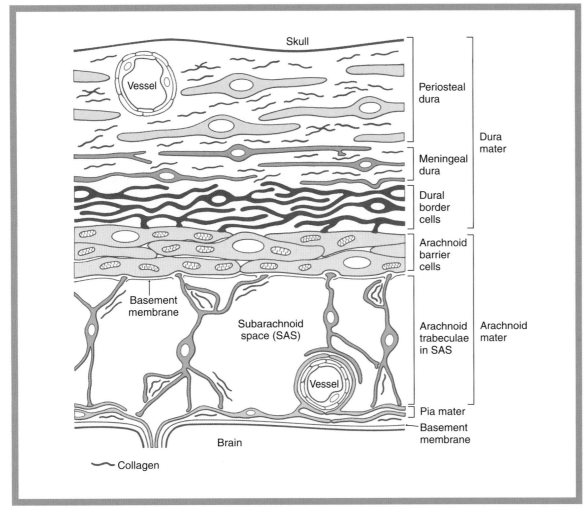

Figure 7-3. The structure of the meninges. Layers of the dura are shown in shades of *gray,* the arachnoid in shades of *pink,* and the pia in *green.* (From Haines DE: On a question of a subdural space. Anat Rec 230:3:21, 1991.)

divided into outer *(periosteal),* inner *(meningeal),* and *border cell* portions. There is no distinct border between periosteal and *meningeal* portions of the dura (Fig. 7-3). Fibroblasts of the *periosteal dura* are larger and slightly less elongated than other dural cells. This portion of the dura is adherent to the inner surface of the skull, and *its attachment is particularly tenacious along suture lines and in the cranial base.* In contrast, the fibroblasts of the *meningeal dura* are more flattened and elongate, their nuclei are smaller, and their cytoplasm may be darker than in periosteal cells. Although cell junctions are rarely seen between dural fibroblasts, the large amounts of interlacing collagen in periosteal and meningeal portions of the dura give these layers of the meninges great strength.

Dural Border Cell Layer
The innermost part of the dura is composed of flattened fibroblasts that have sinuous processes. Collectively, these cells form the *dural border cell layer* (Fig. 7-3). The extracellular spaces between the flattened cell processes of dural border cells contain an amorphous substance but no collagen or elastic fibers. Cell junctions (desmosomes, gap junctions) are occasionally seen between dural border cells and cells of the underlying arachnoid.

Because of its loose arrangement, enlarged extracellular spaces, and lack of extracellular connective tissue fibrils, *the dural border cell layer constitutes a plane of structural weakness at the dura-arachnoid junction.* This layer is externally continuous with the meningeal dura and internally continuous with the arachnoid. Consequently, *bleeding into this area of the meninges will disrupt and dissect open the dural border cell layer* rather than invade

the overlying dura or the underlying arachnoid. *In the normal (and healthy) human there is not a naturally occurring, or preexisting, space at the dura-arachnoid interface* (Fig. 7-3). We shall consider meningeal hemorrhages after discussing the arachnoid.

Blood Supply
The arterial supply to the dura of the anterior cranial fossa originates from the *cavernous portion of the internal carotid,* the *ethmoidal arteries* (via the ethmoidal foramina), and branches of the ascending pharyngeal artery (via the foramen lacerum). The *middle meningeal artery* serves the dura of the middle cranial fossa and may be compromised when there is trauma to the skull. It is a branch of the maxillary artery and enters the skull through the foramen spinosum. The accessory meningeal artery (via the foramen ovale) and small branches from the lacrimal artery (via the superior orbital fissure) also serve the dura of the middle fossa. The dura of the posterior fossa is served by small meningeal branches of ascending pharyngeal and occipital arteries and by minute branches of the vertebral arteries.

The spinal dura is served by branches of major arteries (such as vertebral, intercostal, and lumbosacral) that are located close to the vertebral column. These small meningeal arteries enter the vertebral canal via the intervertebral foramina to serve the dura and adjacent structures.

Nerve Supply
The nerve supply to the dura of the anterior and middle fossae is from branches of the *trigeminal nerve. Ethmoidal nerves* and

branches of the *maxillary* and *mandibular nerves* innervate the dura of the anterior fossa, whereas the dura of the middle fossa is served mainly by branches from the *maxillary* and *mandibular nerves*. The dura of the posterior fossa receives sensory branches from dorsal roots C2 and C3 (and from C1 when this root is present) and may have some innervation from the vagus nerve. The *tentorial nerve*, a branch of the ophthalmic nerve, courses caudally to serve the tentorium cerebelli. Autonomic fibers to the vessels of the dura originate from the superior cervical ganglia and gain access to the cranial cavity by simply following the progressive branching patterns of the vessels on which they lie.

Nerves to the spinal dura originate as recurrent branches of the spinal nerve located at that level. These delicate strands pass through the intervertebral foramina and distribute to the spinal dura and to some adjacent structures.

Dural Infoldings and Sinuses

As noted previously, the dura has *periosteal* and *meningeal* parts. The *periosteal dura* lines the inner surface of the skull and functions as its periosteum. The meningeal dura is continuous with the periosteal dura but draws away from it at specific locations to form the *dural infoldings* (or *reflections*). The largest of these is the *falx cerebri* (Figs. 7-4 and 7-5A). It is attached to the crista galli rostrally, to the midline of the inner surface of the skull, and to the surface of the tentorium cerebelli caudally. The falx cerebri separates the right hemisphere from the left. The *superior sagittal sinus* is found where the falx cerebri attaches to the skull, the *straight sinus* where it fuses with the *tentorium cerebelli*, and the *inferior sagittal sinus* in its free edge (Fig. 7-4). Many large superficial veins located on the surface of the cerebral hemispheres empty into the superior sagittal sinus.

The *tentorium cerebelli* is the second largest of the dural infoldings (Figs. 7-4 and 7-5B, C). Rostrally, it attaches to the clinoid processes, rostrolaterally to the petrous portion of the temporal bone (location of the *superior petrosal sinus*), and caudolaterally to the inner surface of the occipital bone and a small part of the parietal bone (location of the *transverse sinus*) (Figs. 7-4 and 7-5B, C). The tent shape of the tentorium divides the cranial cavity into *supratentorial* (above the tentorium) and *infratentorial* (below the tentorium) compartments (Fig. 7-5B; see also Fig. 7-11). The supratentorial compartment is divided into right and left halves by the falx cerebri (Fig. 7-5A, B). The sweeping edges of the right and left tentoria, as they arch from the clinoid processes to join at the straight sinus, form the *tentorial notch* (Fig. 7-6). The occipital lobe is above the tentorium, the cerebellum is below it, and the midbrain passes through the tentorial notch.

Located below the tentorium cerebelli on the midline of the occipital bone is the *falx cerebelli* (Fig. 7-4). This small dural infolding extends into the space found between the cerebellar hemispheres and usually contains a small *occipital sinus* that communicates with the *confluence of sinuses*.

The smallest of the dural infoldings, the *diaphragma sella* (Figs. 7-4 and 7-6), forms the roof of the hypophyseal fossa and encircles the stalk of the pituitary. The *cavernous sinuses* are found on either side of the sella turcica, and the *anterior* and *posterior intercavernous sinuses* are found in their respective edges of the diaphragma sella.

The relationships of venous sinuses are discussed in Chapter 8. It should be emphasized, however, that *venous sinuses are endothelium-lined spaces* that communicate with each other. In addition, large veins from the surface of the brain empty into the venous sinuses. As they enter the sinus, these veins are

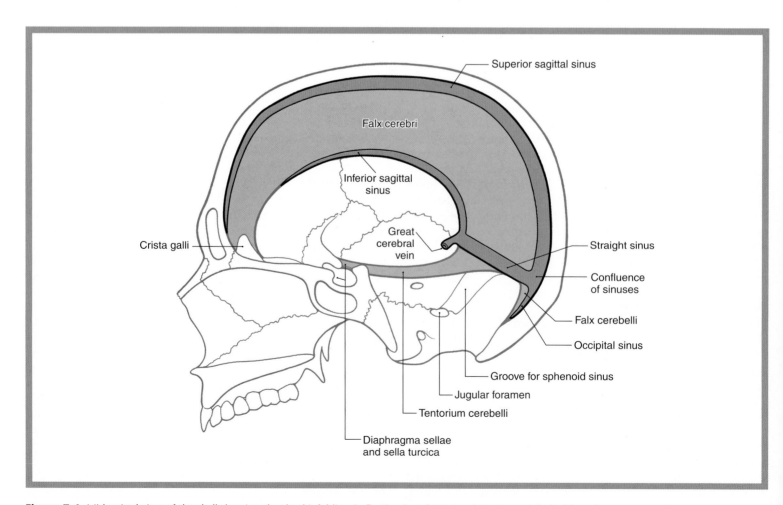

Figure 7-4. Midsagittal view of the skull showing the dural infolding (reflections) and venous sinuses associated with each. (From Haines DE, Fredrickson RG: The meninges. In Al-Mefty O [ed]: Meningiomas. New York, Raven Press, 1991.)

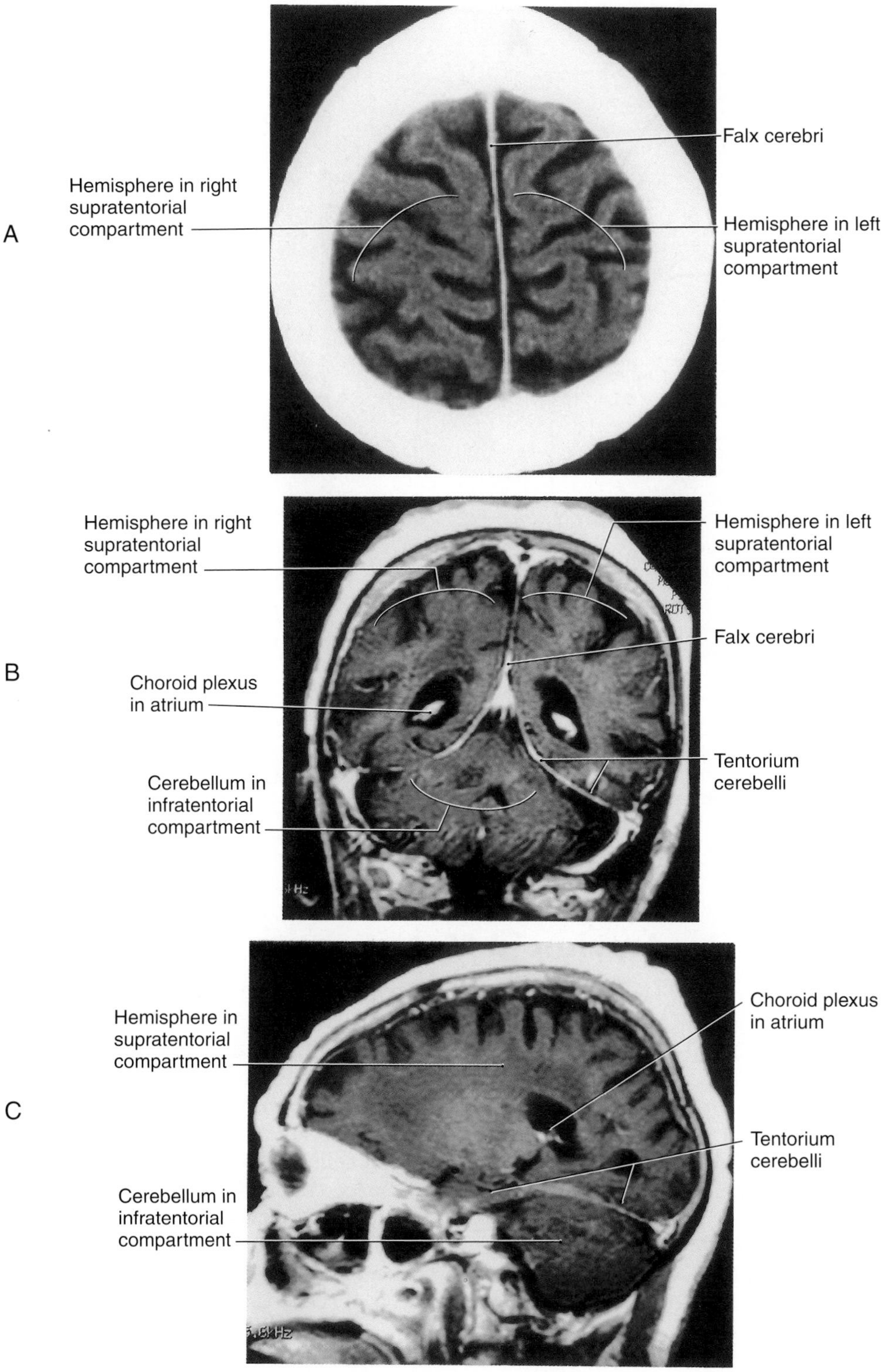

Figure 7-5. Axial (**A**), coronal (**B**), and sagittal (**C**) T1-weighted MR images showing the relationships of the falx cerebri (**A, B**) and the tentorium cerebelli (**B, C**). Note the positions of the right and left supratentorial compartments and the infratentorial compartment in relation to these large dural reflections in all three planes.

attached to a cuff of dura. Consequently, a blow to the head (or a minor bump to the head in an aged person) may cause the brain to shift just enough in the subarachnoid space to tear a vein at the point where it enters the sinus. This tear may allow venous blood to enter the subarachnoid space or may create a hematoma at the dura-arachnoid interface.

Compartments and Herniation Syndromes

The interior of the cranial cavity is divided into a *supratentorial compartment* located superior to the *tentorium cerebelli* and consisting of *right and left halves* (separated by the *falx cerebri*), and a single *infratentorial compartment* located inferior to the *tentorium cerebelli* (Fig. 7-5). The concept of supratentorial and infratentorial compartments, and understanding their contents and relationships, is an essential element in the diagnosis of what are commonly called *herniation syndromes*. In general, a

herniation syndrome occurs when there is an intracranial event (hemorrhage, rapid tumor growth, traumatic brain injury) that causes an increase in intracranial pressure forcing the comparatively gelatinous brain over the edge of a dural reflection. These syndromes are described only briefly here and are considered in more detail in later chapters.

The following are examples of herniation syndromes related to the *supratentorial compartments*. A lesion in one cerebral hemisphere may expand toward the midline, deform the falx cerebri, and force the cingulate gyrus under the edge of the falx into the opposite hemisphere; this is a *subfalcine* or *cingulate herniation*. In this example, the deficits may reflect occlusion of the adjacent anterior cerebral artery. *Central* (or *transtentorial*) *herniation* is the situation in which the diencephalon is forced downward through the tentorial incisure or notch. This is a neurologic emergency, and in about 90% of patients there is

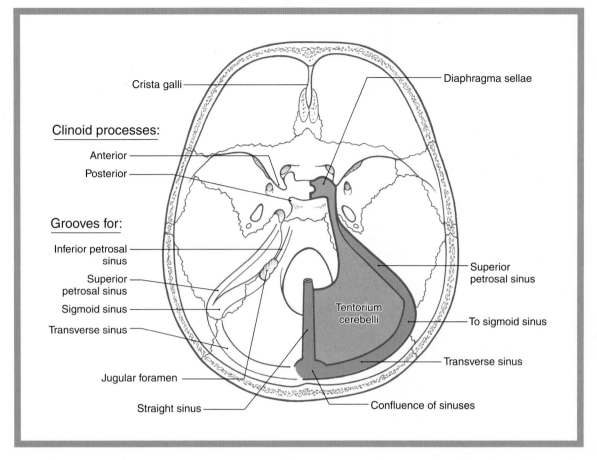

Figure 7-6. View of the cranial base from the dorsal aspect showing the tentorium cerebelli (and its associated sinuses) and the diaphragma sellae. Also indicated are the positions of grooves formed by some of the major sinuses.

serious disability or death. *Uncal herniation* is the case when a rapidly expanding lesion, usually a hematoma, forces the uncus, a medial structure of the temporal lobe, over the edge of the tentorium cerebelli with resultant damage to the midbrain. The most common deficits are (1) a decreased level of consciousness, (2) dilation of the pupil and a loss of most eye movement reflecting damage to the ipsilateral oculomotor nerve, and (3) a contralateral hemiplegia reflecting damage to the descending corticospinal fibers. However, this early stage is likely to be followed by serious complications or death.

Examples of herniation syndromes related to the *infratentorial compartment* include *upward cerebellar herniation* and *tonsillar herniation*. In the former, a mass or pressure increase in the posterior fossa may force the cerebellum upward through the tentorial incisura, inflicting damage to the midbrain. In the latter, the tonsils of the cerebellum are forced downward into, and possibly through, the foramen magnum. The resulting pressure on the medulla may damage respiratory centers and result in sudden death. All of the herniation syndromes are potentially serious, and all measures should be taken to avoid their occurrence.

Cranial Versus Spinal Dura

At the margin of the foramen magnum, the *periosteal dura* essentially stops, but the *meningeal dura* continues caudally in the vertebral canal to eventually attach to the inner aspect of the coccyx as the *filum terminale externum (dural part of the filum terminale or coccygeal ligament)* (Fig. 7-2). The *spinal dural sac* is anchored rostrally and caudally and is separated from the adjacent vertebrae by an *epidural space* that contains venous channels, some lymphatics, and fat deposits. There are no dural infoldings around the cord; consequently, there are no venous sinuses in the spinal dura.

Arachnoid Mater

The *arachnoid mater* is located internal to the dural border cell layer and is regarded as having two parts (Fig. 7-3). The portion of the arachnoid directly apposed to the dural border cells is the *arachnoid barrier cell layer*, and the spindly cells that traverse the subarachnoid space constitute the *arachnoid trabeculae*.

The *subarachnoid space* is located between the arachnoid barrier cell layer and the pial cells located on the surface of the brain or spinal cord. This space contains CSF, many superficial vessels, and the roots of cranial and spinal nerves as they enter or exit the nervous system. Enlarged regions of the subarachnoid space are called *subarachnoid cisterns;* these are discussed later in the chapter.

Arachnoid Barrier Cell Layer

Fibroblasts of this layer are more plump than the flattened cells of the dura (Fig. 7-3). The arachnoid barrier cell layer is tenuously attached to the dural border cell layer by occasional cell junctions. In contrast, arachnoid barrier cells have closely apposed cell membranes and are joined to each other by *numerous tight (occluding) junctions*—hence the "barrier" characteristic of this layer. This close apposition of cell membranes excludes any significant extracellular space; consequently, no collagen is found in this layer of the meninges. The tight junctions between these arachnoid cells not only serve as a barrier against the movement of fluids or other substances but also impart strength to the membrane. In the human, a basement membrane (basal lamina) is found on the surface of the barrier cell layer that faces the subarachnoid space.

Arachnoid Trabeculae and the Subarachnoid Space

The *arachnoid trabeculae* are composed of flattened, irregularly shaped fibroblasts that bridge the subarachnoid space in a random fashion (Fig. 7-3). Trabecular cells attach to the barrier layer and may attach to each other, to pial cells, or to blood vessels in the subarachnoid space. Although much of the extracellular collagen associated with trabecular cells is confined in the folded processes of these cells, some may be found free in the subarachnoid space. The attachments of the trabecular cells and their framework of collagen fibrils give added strength to the arachnoid mater.

The *subarachnoid space* is located internal to the barrier cell layer and external to the pia mater (Figs. 7-2 and 7-3). It contains CSF, trabecular cells and collagen fibrils, arteries and veins, and the roots of cranial nerves. Although some vessels may lie free in the subarachnoid space, most are covered by a thin layer of the leptomeninges (Fig. 7-3). These large vessels in the subarachnoid space may be damaged from trauma or may rupture spontaneously, resulting in the spread of blood around the brain; this event is a *subarachnoid hemorrhage*. CSF is produced by the *choroid plexuses* of the lateral, third, and fourth ventricles. It exits the ventricular system via the foramina of Magendie and Luschka to enter the subarachnoid space (*arrows* in Fig. 7-2). After circulating around the brain and spinal cord, CSF reenters the vascular system primarily through the *arachnoid villi*. The subarachnoid space around the spinal cord is the route used to administer *spinal anesthesia*.

Although it is common to refer to the brain as "floating" in the CSF of the subarachnoid space, it is actually *suspended within this space*. The structural basis for this fact is as follows. The dura is adherent to the skull, the arachnoid to the dura, the arachnoid trabeculae to the pia, and the pia to the surface of the brain. Consequently, the brain is suspended, through this chain, within the fluid milieu of the subarachnoid space by the numerous delicate strands of the arachnoid trabeculae. This is possible because the brain loses about 97% of its weight when it is suspended in CSF. For example, a brain that weighs about 1400 g in air will weigh only about 45 to 50 g in fluid.

Because the arachnoid trabeculae are not rigid, the brain may move within the fluid-filled subarachnoid space. In a closed-head injury, the brain may move on its trabecular tethers in response to a sudden blow and be subjected to minor damage *(concussion or contusion)*. This injury may result in no, or only momentary, loss of consciousness. Such a minor injury may be found at the point of the blow or at a site opposite the contact *(contrecoup injury)*.

Arachnoid Villi

The small specialized portions of the arachnoid that protrude into the superior sagittal sinus through openings in the dura form the *arachnoid villi* or *arachnoid granulations* (Figs. 7-7 and 7-8). If they are especially large or calcified (as in older persons), they may be called *pacchionian bodies*.

Arachnoid villi extend into the sinus through tight cuffs in the meningeal dura and are found just off the midline or in cul-de-sacs (the *lateral* or *venous lacunae*) of the sinus (Figs. 7-7 and 7-8). The vast majority of arachnoid villi are located in the lateral lacunae of the superior sagittal sinus (Fig. 7-12). The space in the center of each villus is continuous with the subarachnoid space around the brain. This space is enclosed in a layer of cells that are markedly similar to arachnoid barrier cells, and these arachnoid cells, in turn, are surrounded by a capsule of cells that are essentially the same as dural border cells. These two layers are continuous with their respective meningeal layers through the stalk of the villus (Fig. 7-7). The *endothelial lining of the sinus* is reflected onto the villus and may cover this structure entirely or may leave a few arachnoid cells exposed; the exposed

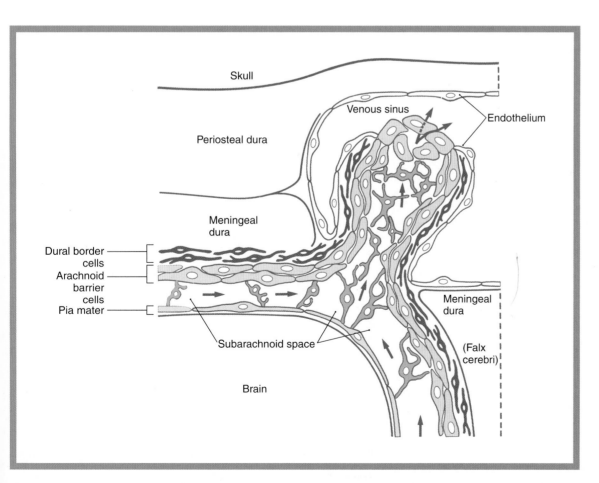

Figure 7-7. Structure of the arachnoid villi. Note the continuity of the cell layers of the villus with those of the meninges. Cerebrospinal fluid *(arrows)* passes from the subarachnoid space into the villus and then into the venous sinus. (From Haines DE, Fredrickson RG: The meninges. In Al-Mefty O [ed]: Meningiomas. New York, Raven Press, 1991.)

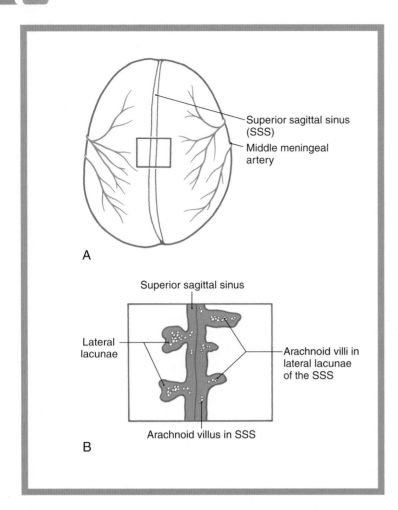

Figure 7-8. A superior view of the superior sagittal sinus (**A**) and a detail (**B**) showing the sinus and the arachnoid granulations, which are found primarily in the lateral lacunae.

cells are called *arachnoid cap cells*. The endothelium covering the villus sits on a basement membrane beneath which some extracellular collagen may be found.

Arachnoid villi are structurally adapted for the transport of CSF from the subarachnoid space into the venous circulation (Fig. 7-7). CSF moves only from the villus into the sinus. The two routes of fluid movement are through small intercellular channels located between cells and by way of a vacuole-mediated transport of fluid and other elements (bacteria, blood cells) through villus cells. As CSF traverses the villus, it moves down a pressure gradient from a point of higher pressure (the subarachnoid space) to a point of lower pressure (the venous sinus). If the pressure on the venous side exceeds that on the subarachnoid space side, the flow of CSF will slow or stop. Venous blood, however, never flows from the sinus into the subarachnoid space.

Meningioma

Tumors of the meninges, collectively called *meningiomas*, are *primary intracranial tumors but not primary tumors of the brain*. This means that these tumors originate from structures that are intimately associated with the CNS (indeed, portions of the meninges arise from the neural crests that are derived from the neural plate) but do not originate from the brain substance itself.

Origins and Locations

Meningiomas arise from arachnoid cells found in the villi, at points where blood vessels and cranial nerves traverse the dura, and along the base of the skull. In clinical parlance, these specific cells are called *arachnoid cap cells*. As one would expect, most

meningiomas (about 90%) are found in the cranial cavity or in association with the spinal cord (about 9%). *Ectopic meningiomas* are tumors with the histologic features of meningiomas that are found outside the brain and spinal cord (about 1%).

In descending order of occurrence meningiomas are found in the following locations: *parasagittal, convexity, sphenoid ridge,* and *tuberculum sellae* or *suprasellar* (Fig. 7-9). When found at these points it is common to refer to these tumors as a *parasagittal meningioma,* a *convexity meningioma,* and so on, as illustrated in Figure 7-9. Meningiomas are also found at the cribriform plate of the ethmoid bone (*olfactory groove meningioma,* Fig.7-10), attached to the falx cerebri *(falcine meningioma),* and at locations such as the optic nerve, along the petrous part of the temporal bone, or the clivus, attached to the tentorium cerebelli *(tentorial meningioma,* Fig. 7-11) and at the foramen magnum. Based on their position, convexity meningiomas impinge on an identifiable portion of the hemisphere. Consequently, convexity meningiomas may also be designated by the lobe of the brain involved, such as a *frontal lobe meningioma* (Fig. 7-12). On rare occasions, meningiomas may also be found within the ventricular system.

Patients presenting with meningioma are typically in the range of 40 to 60 years (peak incidence at about 45 years) and, by a small margin, are more likely to be female (ratio of 3:2). These tumors are usually single, but some patients may have more than one. Multiple meningiomas may be seen in patients with

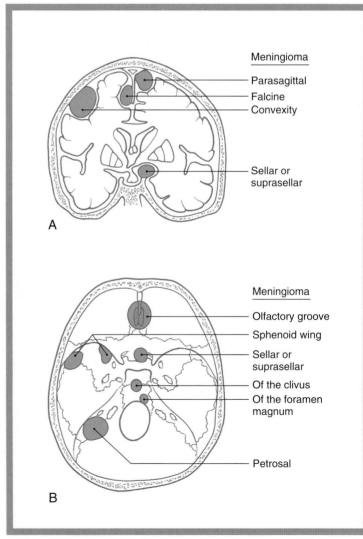

Figure 7-9. Coronal view of the brain (**A**) and a view of the base of the skull (**B**) illustrating the locations of meningiomas. In these examples note that the name of this tumor usually signifies its position in relation to a meningeal reflection or bony landmark.

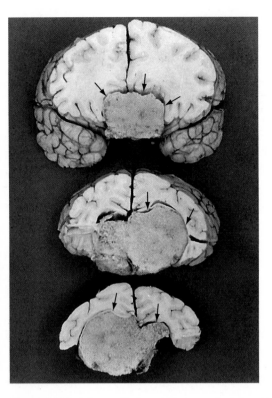

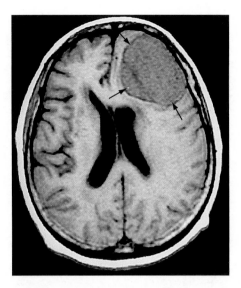

Figure 7-12. Axial MR (T1-weighted) image of a meningioma in the frontal lobe of a 62-year-old female patient. Note the sharp interface between the tumor and the brain *(arrows)* and the midline shift. The tumor is clearly external to the brain substance.

Figure 7-10. A large olfactory groove meningioma. Note that this tumor has significantly compressed *(arrows)* but not invaded the brain in these sequential slices through the frontal lobe. (Courtesy of Dr. Jonathan Fratkin, University of Mississippi Medical Center.)

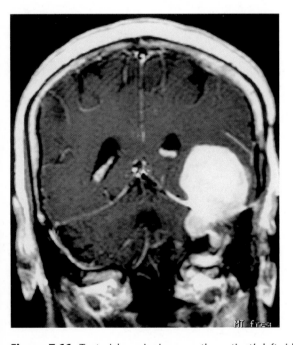

Figure 7-11. Tentorial meningioma on the patient's left side. This tumor extends into the supratentorial and infratentorial compartments and, although relatively large, has not displaced the brain or ventricular system to any noticeable degree. This is a testament to its slow growth.

neurofibromatosis (of the central type); these patients may also have bilateral vestibular schwannomas.

General Histologic Features

The majority of meningiomas are slow-growing benign tumors that do not invade the substance of the brain. Malignant meningiomas are relatively rare, but when they occur they may invade brain tissue and/or the dura, thereby significantly complicating their treatment. These tumors contain many mitotic figures and may metastasize to distant sites.

Based on their histologic characteristics, meningiomas can be divided into three general types. While there are variations on these types, these variations are beyond the scope of this book. *Meningotheliomatous* (or *syncytial*) *meningiomas* are composed of polygon-shaped cells with large centrally located nuclei that contain nucleoli and sometimes vacuoles (Fig. 7-13A). These cells are arranged in sheets and some cells form small concentric aggre-gations suggesting whorls. In many areas of these tumors the borders between cells are obscured, giving the tumors the appearance of a syncytium. *Transitional meningiomas* have an appearance intermediate between syncytial and fibrous meningiomas and are characterized by cells arranged in tight concentric whorl formations separated by thin septa of spindle-shaped cells (Fig. 7-13B). These whorls may form around a centrally located cell or a small blood vessel. Psammoma bodies (Greek for "grains of sand"), made up of concentric layers of calcium, are also seen in this type of meningioma. *Fibroblastic* (or *fibrous*) *meningiomas* contain layers of long spindle-shaped cells with elongated nuclei; in some areas the sheets are many cells thick and contain large amounts of collagen (Fig. 7-13C). Whorl formations and psammoma bodies may also be present in this tumor.

Symptoms and Treatment

Since meningiomas are slow growing, symptoms may appear very slowly or not at all. It is not uncommon to see meningioma as an incidental finding in patients who have died of other causes or who have been subjected to imaging studies for some other problem, such as trauma or stroke. Contrast medium–enhanced computed tomography (CT) and magnetic resonance imaging (MRI) are especially valuable in the *evaluation* of this tumor; edema surrounding the lesion is especially evident in MRI. A *diagnosis* requires histologic confirmation.

Neurologic symptoms or signs in patients with meningioma are generally due to compression of brain structures or involvement of cranial nerves, or to secondary causes such as edema. In addition, these patients may present with seizures or with slowly developing personality or behavioral changes that may (or may not) accompany specific deficits related to cranial nerve or long-tract involvement.

The treatment of choice for meningioma is surgical removal. The location of the mass may dictate the ease, or difficulty, of its removal. A convexity meningioma is rather straightforward,

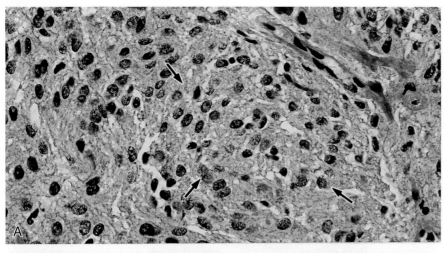

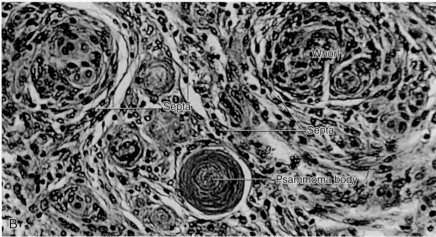

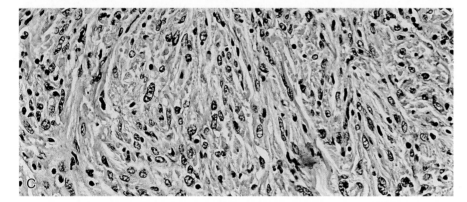

Figure 7-13. Histologic features of a meningotheliomatous (syncytial) meningioma (**A**), a transitional meningioma (**B**), and a fibroblastic meningioma (**C**). Sheets of elongated cells and structures suggesting whorls *(arrows)* are seen in the syncytial tumor (**A**). Thin septa of elongated fibroblasts are insinuated between obvious whorl formations in the transitional tumor (**B**); note the psammoma body. The fibroblastic tumor contains many elongated cells forming sheets of various sizes (**C**).

whereas a parasagittal tumor is more complex, owing to its potential involvement of the superior sagittal sinus. In like manner, meningiomas in the region of the cavernous sinus may involve branches of cranial nerves III, IV, V, and VI and/or the internal carotid artery while a tumor of the sella may envelop optic structures. Radiation therapy may be used to treat specific types of meningiomas, but chemotherapy has not proven to be effective at the present time.

Meningeal Hemorrhages

At this point, it is appropriate to consider meningeal hemorrhages that are *specifically related to the dura-skull interface and to the arachnoid-dura interface*. These lesions share the common feature of being most likely caused by trauma.

Extradural and "Subdural" Hemorrhages

If we exclude, for the moment, subarachnoid hemorrhages, which are considered later in this chapter, *meningeal hemorrhages* can be generally described as *extravasated blood that strips the dura from the skull or dissects open the dural border cell layer* (Fig. 7-14). The most common cause in both situations is an injury to the head, with or without skull fracture. In a head injury, the periosteal dura may be loosened from the skull with consequent damage to a major artery; the middle and accessory meningeal arteries are common victims. Extravascular blood dissects the periosteal dura from the skull and collects to form an *extradural (epidural) hematoma* (Figs. 7-14 and 7-15). These lesions tend to be lenticular shaped and appear "short and wide" owing to the fact that they do not cross the dural attachment at suture lines (Fig. 7-15). The neurologic deficits seen in patients

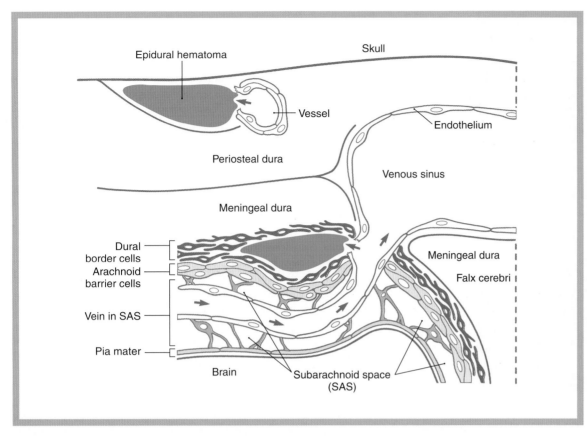

Figure 7-14. The relationship of extravasated blood to the meninges. The epidural hematoma is located between the dura and the skull. Bleeding into the dura-arachnoid interface, classically called a "subdural" hematoma, is actually into a structurally weak cell layer at this juncture.

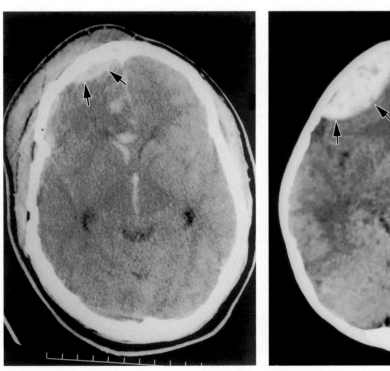

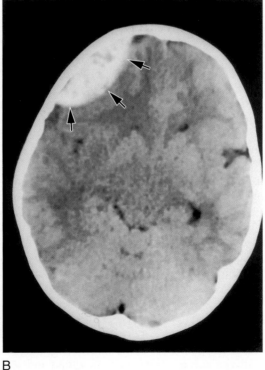

A   B

Figure 7-15. Examples (**A**, **B**—*arrows*) of epidural hematomas in CT scans on the patient's right side. The smaller lesion in **A** is obviously of traumatic origin; this patient has soft tissue damage, a fractured skull, blood in the substance of the brain, and blood in the anterior horn of the lateral ventricle and in the third ventricle. The cause of the larger lesion (**B**) is not obvious. Compare the shape of these lesions with that of a "subdural" hematoma in Figure 7-16.

with epidural hemorrhage are usually those characteristic of increased intracranial pressure. These deficits are, in order of occurrence, headache, confusion and disorientation, lethargy, and finally a state of unresponsiveness. In some cases of head trauma, the patient may initially be rendered unconscious followed by a lucid interval (the patient is wide awake and conversant), then subsequently deteriorate rapidly and die; this is called *talk*

and die. Keeping this in mind, it is essential to follow these patients closely.

In contrast to extradural hemorrhages, bleeding into the meninges at the junction of the arachnoid with the dura originates mainly from venous structures. A common cause is the tearing of "bridging veins" as they pass through the subarachnoid space and enter a dural venous sinus (Fig. 7-14). Although these lesions

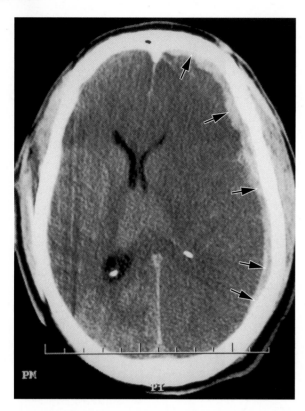

Figure 7-16. An example of a so-called subdural hematoma *(arrows)* in CT scan on the patient's left side. This lesion is long and thin and extends for considerable distance over the surface of the hemisphere by dissecting through the dural border cell layer: note the shift in the midline. Compare the shape of this lesion with that of the epidural hematomas in Figure 7-15.

are commonly called "subdural," as noted previously, there is *no naturally occurring space at the arachnoid-dura junction.* Hematomas at this junction are usually caused by *extravasated blood that splits open the dural border cell layer* (Figs. 7-14 and 7-16). In contrast to epidural lesions, so-called *subdural hematomas* appear "long and thin" because they are not constrained by any dural attachments (Fig. 7-16). This extravascular blood does not collect within a preexisting space but rather creates a space at the dura-arachnoid junction. Because these so-called *subdural hematomas* are usually found *within a specific layer of cells,* they actually constitute *"dural border"* hematomas. These lesions generally contain blood in their central area and myofibroblasts, fibroblasts, mast cells, proliferating blood vessels, and dural border cells in the surrounding capsule.

Hygroma

Trauma to the skull may also result in tearing of the arachnoid membrane. In such instances, CSF, which is under pressure (100 to 150 mm H_2O in a recumbent position), also may dissect open and collect with the dural border cell layer. These lesions are called *hygromas.*

Pia Mater

The *pia mater* consists of flattened cells with long, equally flattened processes that closely follow all the surface features of the brain and spinal cord (Fig. 7-3). The pia and arachnoid together constitute the *leptomeninges.* Vessels in the subarachnoid space (Fig. 7-3) may be covered by a single layer of pial cells, may be enveloped by several layers of leptomeningeal cells, or may lie free in this space. The pia is separated from the brain surface by a *glial basement membrane* and by occasional places where pial cells pull away from the brain to form a small *subpial space.* Pial cells at the brain surface may be arranged in a single layer or in several layers. Single pial cell processes and their subjacent collagen correspond to the *pia intima;* these closely

follow surface features of the brain and spinal cord. When there are several tiers of pial cell processes, the outer layers correspond to the *epipial layer.* In general, the pia is thicker on the spinal cord than on the brain.

Where small vessels penetrate the surface of the brain and spinal cord, they pull along a small envelope of pial cell processes and extracellular space. These *perivascular spaces (Virchow-Robin spaces)* extend for varying distances into the parenchyma of the nervous system and may serve as conduits for the movement of extracellular fluid between the subarachnoid space and the minute spaces around neurons and glial cells.

The spinal cord is anchored in the subarachnoid space by three structures: two pial modifications plus a reticulated septum of arachnoid cell processes that attaches to the posterior midline of the cord. The first of the pial structures, the *denticulate ligaments,* run longitudinally along each side of the spinal cord about midway between the posterior and anterior roots and attach to the inner surface of the arachnoid-lined dural sac (Fig. 7-2). From each ligament a series of 20 to 22 structures, shaped much like shark's teeth, extend laterally to attach to the inner surface of the arachnoid-lined dural sac. Second, extending caudally from the conus medullaris is a tough strand composed primarily of pia; this is the *filum terminale internum (pial part of the filum terminale).* The filum terminale internum attaches to the caudal end of the dural sac, which in turn attaches to the coccyx as the *filum terminale externum (dural part of the filum terminale or coccygeal ligament)* (Fig. 7-2). Together, these anchoring structures serve a function analogous to that of the arachnoid trabeculae around the brain.

The large space caudal to the conus medullaris, which contains CSF, posterior and anterior roots (constituting the *cauda equina*), and the filum terminale internum, is the *lumbar cistern* (Fig. 7-2). The retrieval of CSF is an important diagnostic tool for evaluating a variety of CNS disorders. A needle introduced into the lumbar cistern *(spinal tap or lumbar puncture)* through the third to fourth or fourth to fifth lumbar interspace is the primary method used to collect a sample of CSF from this cistern (see Fig. 9-2).

Cisterns, Subarachnoid Hemorrhages, and Meningitis

The *subarachnoid space* is the thin envelope of space located between the arachnoid and pia (Figs. 7-2 and 7-7). This space has a number of naturally enlarged regions called *subarachnoid cisterns,* which contain CSF, arteries and veins, and in some cases, cranial nerve roots (Fig. 7-17; Table 7-1). Cisterns occur where the brain draws away from the skull as part of its natural variation in shape, thus enlarging the subarachnoid space. In addition to discussing cisterns we shall consider subarachnoid hemorrhage and meningitis at this point, as these clinical problems are most specifically related to the leptomeninges.

Cisterns

Cisterns are usually named according to the structures on which they border. For example, the *interpeduncular cistern* is found in the interpeduncular fossa, the *dorsal cerebellomedullary cistern (cisterna magna)* is found between the cerebellum and the medulla, and so on (Fig. 7-17). Typically, the shapes of cisterns, as seen on MRI and computed tomography (CT), are determined by the corresponding shapes of surrounding brain structures (Fig. 7-18); this characteristic relationship is useful in diagnosis. The *cisterna magna* is a potential source of CSF if the lumbar cistern is not accessible. In a *cisternal puncture,* a needle is carefully introduced into the cisterna magna through the atlanto-occipital membrane and a sample of fluid is withdrawn.

Cisterns are bordered by particular brain structures, contain segments of major vessels, and may also contain cranial nerve roots or other structures (Table 7-1). Consequently, a progressively

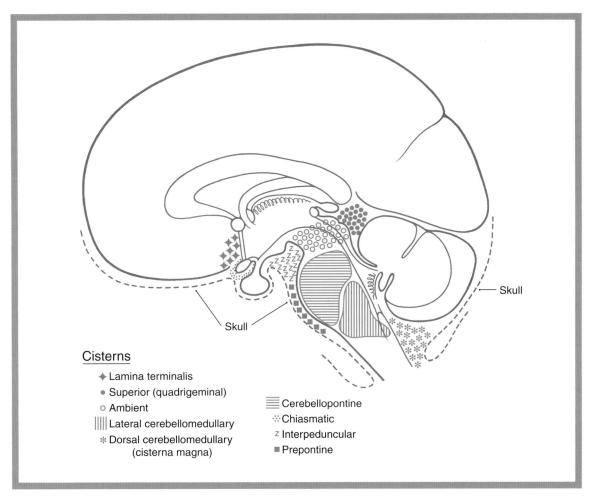

Cisterns

- ✦ Lamina terminalis
- ● Superior (quadrigeminal)
- ○ Ambient
- ||||| Lateral cerebellomedullary
- ✳ Dorsal cerebellomedullary (cisterna magna)

- ≣ Cerebellopontine
- ⁘ Chiasmatic
- ᴢ Interpeduncular
- ■ Prepontine

Figure 7-17. The locations of the major subarachnoid cisterns in relation to brain structures. Although the cerebellopontine, lateral cerebellomedullary, and ambient cisterns are located on the lateral aspect of the brainstem, their approximate positions are indicated on this midsagittal view. Compare with Table 7-1. (From Haines DE, Fredrickson RG: The meninges. In Al-Mefty O [ed]: Meningiomas. New York, Raven Press, 1991.)

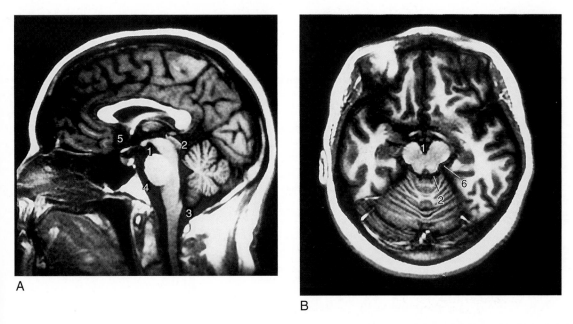

Figure 7-18. MR images in sagittal (**A**) and axial (horizontal, **B**) planes with some of the major cisterns indicated: 1, interpeduncular; 2, superior (quadrigeminal); 3, cisterna magna (dorsal cerebellomedullary); 4, prepontine; 5, of the lamina terminalis; 6, ambient.

enlarging aneurysm or a slow hemorrhage into a particular cistern may result in signs or symptoms related to the structures found in, or next to, the cistern. For example, an aneurysm protruding into the interpeduncular cistern may affect the oculomotor nerve (Table 7-1) and, consequently, eye movements or pupil size.

Subarachnoid Hemorrhage

A subarachnoid hemorrhage is an extravasation of blood (usually arterial) into the subarachnoid space (Figs. 7-19 and 7-20). The most common cause of subarachnoid hemorrhage is trauma, whereas the most common cause of nontraumatic (or spontaneous)

Table 7-1. Some Principal Cisterns and the Main Arteries, Veins, Cranial Nerves, and Other Structures Associated with Them

Cistern	Artery(ies)	Vein(s)	Cranial Nerve(s)	Structure(s)
Ambient	Portions of posterior cerebral, quadrigeminal, and superior cerebellar arteries	Basal vein (of Rosenthal)	Trochlear	Lateral aspect of crus cerebri
Cerebellopontine (inferior – also called lateral cerebellomedullary)	Vertebral artery and proximal branches of PICA	Retro-olivary and lateral medullary veins	Glossopharyngeal, vagus, spinal accessory, and hypoglossal	Pyramid, inferior olivary eminence, and choroid plexus
Cerebellopontine (superior)	Distal branches of anterior inferior cerebellar, labyrinthine, and basilar arteries	Pontomesencephalic and petrosal veins	Trigeminal, facial, and vestibulocochlear	
Chiasmatic	Ophthalmic artery and small branches to chiasm and hypophysis		Optic nerve and optic chiasm	
Cisterna magna (also called dorsal cerebellomedullary)	Distal branches of PICA, posterior spinal artery, and branches to choroid plexus of fourth ventricle	Tonsillar and dorsal medullary veins		Roots of C1, C2
Interpeduncular	Rostral end of basilar artery and portions of posterior cerebral, choroidal, and thalamogeniculate arteries	Portions of basal vein (of Rosenthal)	Oculomotor root	Mammillary body, medial edge of crus cerebri
Prepontine	Basilar artery and its branches	Pontine veins	Abducens	
Quadrigeminal	Portions of posterior cerebral, quadrigeminal, and choroidal arteries	Great cerebral vein (of Galen)	Trochlear root	Pineal, superior and inferior colliculi

PICA, posterior inferior cerebellar artery.
Data from Yasargil MG: Microneurosurgery, Vol I, Neurosurgical Anatomy of the Basal Cisterns and Vessels of the Brain, Diagnostic Studies, General Operative Techniques and Pathological Considerations of the Intracranial Aneurysms. Stuttgart, Georg Thieme, 1984.

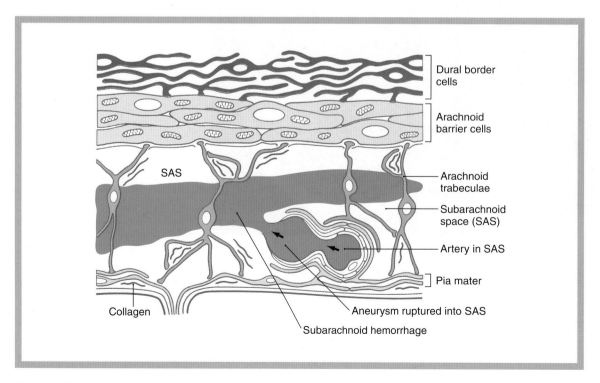

Figure 7-19. Bleeding into the subarachnoid space (subarachnoid hemorrhage) after rupture of an aneurysm into the subarachnoid space.

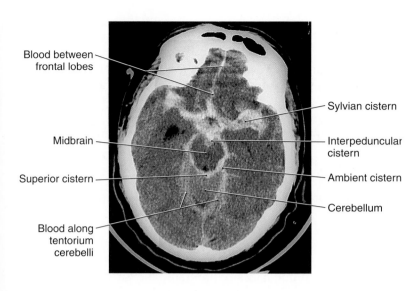

Blood between frontal lobes

Midbrain

Superior cistern

Blood along tentorium cerebelli

Sylvian cistern

Interpeduncular cistern

Ambient cistern

Cerebellum

Figure 7-20. CT scan showing subarachnoid hemorrhage from a ruptured aneurysm in a 64-year-old male patient. Note the blood in the cisterns and also outlining the midbrain and tentorium cerebelli.

subarachnoid hemorrhage is rupture of an intracranial aneurysm. In traumatic subarachnoid hemorrhage, the source of the blood may be due to damage to large veins. In either case, blood is extruded into the subarachnoid space and may be sequestered in cisterns or migrate through the subarachnoid space and subsequently may be seen on imaging studies to outline structures such as brain divisions or dural reflections (Fig. 7-20). Aneurysms are clearly defined dilations in the walls of arteries (Fig. 7-19). Although many aneurysms are thought to be congenital, they may also be caused by an ongoing pathologic process or by trauma or may be secondary to a general systemic problem such as hypertension. Subarachnoid hemorrhage from a ruptured aneurysm is most common in persons between 40 and 65 years of age. Rupture of an intracranial aneurysm is a potentially catastrophic event. About one third of affected patients die before or soon after admission to a medical facility, about one third have permanent and significant disabilities (cognitive, motor), and about one third may recover with minimal neurologic sequelae.

The occurrence of a subarachnoid hemorrhage may be signaled by a sudden excruciating headache, neck stiffness, vomiting or nausea, and a depression or loss of consciousness. Patients who do not become unconscious at the time of the hemorrhage may describe the headache as "explosive and awful," "the absolutely worst headache I have ever had." Bloody CSF obtained by lumbar or cisternal puncture is diagnostic for subarachnoid hemorrhage, and blood can be clearly identified in the subarachnoid space on CT examination (Fig. 7-20). In some cases a patient may have warning signs and symptoms of an impending subarachnoid hemorrhage (leaking aneurysm). These include intermittent headache, nausea or vomiting, and fainting spells *(syncope)*. In persons with neurologic signs that can be traced to an aneurysm, the treatment of choice is to clip the aneurysm or its stalk, thereby separating it from the cerebral circulation.

Meningitis

Meningeal infection may be of either bacterial or viral origin. With *bacterial meningitis*, the meningeal infection is most often located in the subarachnoid space and involves the arachnoid and pia, hence the designation *leptomeningitis*. Such infections may result from a variety of causes, including trauma (which may introduce bacteria into the head or spine), septicemia, and metastasis from another site of infection in the body. Bacterial meningitis is generally classified as acute or subacute, depending on how rapidly the disease progresses. The most common causative agents are *Streptococcus pneumoniae* and *Neisseria meningitidis* (accounting for about 70% to 75% of cases).

Signs of acute bacterial meningitis include elevated temperature, alternating chills and fever, and headache; the patient is acutely ill and may have a depressed level of consciousness. These signs and symptoms seen in concert with increased CSF pressure and cloudy CSF containing many white blood cells, increased protein, and bacteria are diagnostic of the disease. The inflammatory process may result in thickening of the leptomeninges with consequent partial obstruction of CSF flow and signs of hydrocephalus. Although the death rate is low in acute cases with proper treatment, the patient may become ill suddenly and may die within 2 days in rapidly advancing cases.

Subacute bacterial meningitis is usually seen in patients with tuberculosis (tuberculous meningitis) or may be due to mycotic infections. The course of the disease is longer (encompassing weeks rather than days), and the onset is slow and characterized by headache, fever, irritability, and wakefulness at night. In both acute and subacute meningitis, the prognosis is excellent (with about a 90% cure rate) with early diagnosis and proper treatment.

Viral meningitis is caused by a range of viral agents, is most commonly seen in younger patients (younger than 25 years of age), and is a disease for which no antiviral medications are available. The patient becomes ill over a period of days and experiences fever, headaches of increasing intensity, and confusion and possibly an altered level of consciousness. In a minority of cases, more serious signs and symptoms may be seen, such as seizures, rigidity, or cranial nerve palsies. Treatment in mild cases is supportive and generally focuses on medications for fever, pain, and general discomfort. After an acute period of 1 to 2 weeks, the signs and symptoms moderate, and generally the patient recovers without permanent deficits.

Synopsis of Clinical Points

- An infant or child suffering recurrent bouts of meningitis may have a congenital dermal sinus (pp. 107–108).
- Attachments of the dura to the skull are especially strong at suture lines; this directly relates to the shape and extent of epidural lesions (p. 109).
- In the normal adult there is no subdural space but there is a subdural hematoma (p. 109).
- The intracranial space is divided into supratentorial and infratentorial compartments; herniation syndromes directly relate to arrangement of these compartments (pp. 111–112).
- Meningiomas are primary intracranial tumors, named according to their location, arise from arachnoid cells, have characteristic histologic appearances, and are candidates for surgery (pp. 114–116).
- Epidural hemorrhages are lenticular shaped, short and wide, and do not cross suture lines (pp. 116–117).
- Patients with epidural hemorrhage may "talk and die" (p. 117).
- So-called subdural hemorrhages are actually in the dural border cell layer, are long and thin, and are not constrained by dural attachment (pp. 117–118).
- The most common cause of subarachnoid blood is trauma (p. 119).
- The second most common cause of subarachnoid blood, or the most common cause of nontraumatic (or spontaneous) subarachnoid blood, is aneurysm rupture (pp. 119–120).
- Subarachnoid hemorrhage can be signaled by "the worst headache I have ever had" (p. 121).
- A patient with bacterial meningitis may become ill suddenly with fever, chills, and headache and die if not treated quickly and properly (pp. 121–122).
- CSF is a valuable tool in the diagnosis of bacterial meningitis (p. 121).
- Patients with viral meningitis become sick over days, are moderately ill for about 2 weeks, and almost always recover without deficits (p. 122).

Sources and Additional Reading

Alcolado R, Weller RO, Parrish EP, Garrod D: The cranial arachnoid and pia mater in man: Anatomical and ultrastructural observations. Neuropathol Appl Neurobiol 14:1-17, 1988.

Al-Mefty O: Meningiomas. New York, Raven Press, 1991.

Frederickson RG: The subdural space interpreted as a cellular layer of meninges. Anat Rec 230:38-51, 1991.

Haines DE: On the question of a subdural space. Anat Rec 230:3-21, 1991.

Haines DE, Harkey LH, Al-Mefty O: The "subdural space": A new look at an outdated concept. Neurosurgery 32:111-120, 1993.

Nabeshima S, Reese TS, Landis DMD, Brightman MW: Junctions in the meninges and marginal glia. J Comp Neurol 164:127-170, 1975.

Nicholas DS, Weller RO: The fine anatomy of the human spinal meninges. J Neurosurg 69:276-282, 1988.

Orlin JR, Osen K, Hovig T: Subdural compartment in pig: A morphologic study with blood and horseradish peroxidase infused subdurally. Anat Rec 230:22-37, 1991.

Peters A, Palay SL, Webster HD: The Fine Structure of the Nervous System: The Neurons and Supporting Cells, 3rd ed. Philadelphia, WB Saunders, 1991.

Schachenmayr W, Friede RL: The origin of subdural neo-membranes: I. Fine structure of the dura-arachnoid interface in man. Am J Pathol 92:53-68, 1978.

Van Denabeele F, Creemans J, Lambrichts I: Ultrastructure of the human spinal arachnoid mater and dura mater. J Anat 189:417-430, 1996.

Williams PL (ed): Gray's Anatomy, 38th ed. New York, Churchill Livingstone, 1995.

Yasargil MG: Microneurosurgery, Vol I, Microsurgical Anatomy of the Basal Cisterns and Vessels of the Brain, Diagnostic Studies, General Operative Techniques and Pathological Considerations of the Intracranial Aneurysms. Stuttgart, Georg Thieme, 1984.

Chapter 8

A Survey of the Cerebrovascular System

D. E. Haines and J. A. Lancon

About 50% of the problems that occur inside the cranial cavity and result in neurologic deficits are vascular in origin. Consequently, a good understanding of cerebrovascular patterns is absolutely essential to establish an accurate diagnosis of the neurologically compromised patient. The brain is a voracious consumer of oxygen and therefore requires a great deal of oxygenated blood. Although it makes up only about 2% of total body weight in adults, the brain receives 15% to 17% of the total cardiac output and consumes about 20% of the oxygen used by the entire body!

An ongoing flow of oxygenated blood is essential for continued brain function. The average person will lose consciousness if the brain is deprived of blood for 10 to 12 seconds; after 3 to 5 minutes, irreparable brain damage or death may result. There are exceptions, however. Individuals who become hypothermic with a subsequent decrease in arterial blood flow to the brain, as in a winter near-drowning, may be revived after 10, 15, or even 20 minutes with little or no permanent damage. In these cases, the reduction in body temperature protects the brain against the consequences of reduced blood flow.

Overview

Blood is supplied to the brain by the *internal carotid* and *vertebral arteries*. The internal carotid arteries enter the skull and then divide into the *anterior* and *middle cerebral arteries*. The vertebral arteries pass through the foramen magnum and join to form the *basilar artery*; hence, the term *vertebrobasilar* is frequently applied to this part of the cerebral circulation. The basilar artery branches into right and left *posterior cerebral arteries*.

Venous outflow from the brain travels through superficial and deep veins, which drain into the dural venous sinuses. Blood in the sinuses, in turn, enters the internal jugular vein. Superficial veins in the scalp and veins in the orbit also may communicate with the dural sinuses, but these are not major conduits for venous drainage from the brain.

This chapter presents an overview of the cerebrovascular system, with emphasis on the distribution pattern of vessels on the surface of the brain and spinal cord. Details of the distribution of blood vessels to internal structures are covered when we consider nuclei and tracts within the central nervous system (CNS).

Causes of Vascular Compromise

Intracranial hemorrhage originates from arteries or veins and may result from diseases, trauma, developmental defects, or infections. Such bleeding is classified according to its location. *Meningeal hemorrhages* are found in relation to the coverings of the brain (see Chapter 7), whereas bleeding into the subarachnoid space is called *subarachnoid hemorrhage*. Hemorrhage may occur into the ventricular spaces *(intraventricular)* or into the substance of the brain *(parenchymatous)*. Although many events can lead to cerebrovascular problems with resultant dysfunction, only three examples—aneurysm, cerebral embolism, and arteriovenous malformation (Fig. 8-1)—are considered here.

Aneurysm

An *aneurysm* is the dilation of a vessel wall (Fig. 8-1A), usually an artery, that extends from the lumen to the vessel surface and includes all layers of the vessel wall. Aneurysms located inside the skull, *cerebral aneurysms*, may range from small *(berry or saccular aneurysms)* to very large *(giant aneurysms* are greater than 2 cm in diameter), or they may involve an elongated portion of the vessel *(fusiform aneurysm)*. Larger aneurysms may cause signs or symptoms by compression of adjacent structures such as cranial nerve roots. The second most common cause of blood in

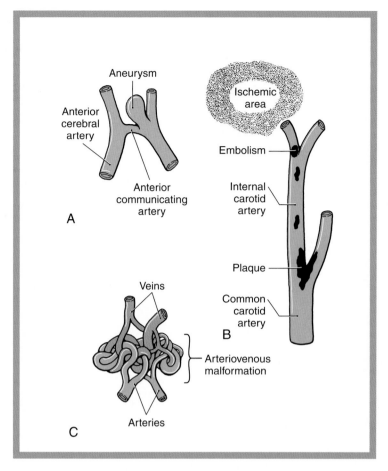

Figure 8-1. Representation of an aneurysm (**A**), an embolism (**B**), and an arteriovenous malformation (**C**).

the subarachnoid space *(subarachnoid hemorrhage)* is rupture of a cerebral aneurysm, the first most common cause being trauma.

Most *intracranial* (or *cerebral*) *aneurysms* (about 85%) are found on the branches of the internal carotid artery system (Fig. 8-2). On this portion of the vascular tree, aneurysms are most frequent on the anterior communicating artery or at its junction with the anterior cerebral artery, on the internal carotid artery or at its junction with the posterior communicating artery, or at the bifurcation of the M1 segment of the middle cerebral artery (Fig. 8-2). About 10 to 15% of intracranial aneurysms are located on branches of the vertebrobasilar system (Fig. 8-2). When present on these vessels, aneurysms are more likely to be located at the bifurcation of the basilar artery, on the basilar artery, or on the posterior inferior cerebellar artery or at its junction with the vertebral artery. Regardless of where they may occur, *intracranial aneurysms are frequently located at branch points of vessels or at points where the vessels may make an abnormally sharp abrupt turn in their course.* The treatment of choice is to clip the stalk of the aneurysm so as to separate its friable sac from the cerebral circulation.

Cerebral Embolism

A *cerebral embolism* is the occlusion of a cerebral vessel by some extraneous material (such as clot, tumor cells, clump of bacteria, air, plaque fragments). This occlusion leads to *ischemia* (a localized anemia) and, if prolonged, ultimately to *infarction* (a localized vascular insufficiency resulting in necrosis) of the area served by the vessel (Fig. 8-1B). In many cases the deficits seem in the patient reflect the loss of function of the damaged area of the brain or spinal cord. An embolus made up exclusively of blood products is called a *thrombus*.

The size of the embolus determines where it lodges. Very small emboli may temporarily occlude small cerebral vessels

Although small in diameter, the spinal cord is the most important conduit between the body and the brain. It conveys sensory input from the arms, trunk, legs, and most of the viscera and contains fibers and cells that control the motor elements found in these structures. Consequently, injury to the spinal cord, especially at cervical levels, may cause permanent and catastrophic deficits, or even death.

Overview

The spinal cord participates in four essential functions. First, it receives primary sensory input from receptors in skin, skeletal muscles, and tendons *(somatosensory fibers)* and from receptors in thoracic, abdominal, and pelvic viscera *(viscerosensory fibers)*. Through multisynaptic relays in the spinal cord, much of this sensory input is conveyed to higher levels of the neuraxis.

Second, the spinal cord contains *somatic motor neurons* that innervate skeletal muscles and *visceral motor neurons* that, after synapsing in peripheral ganglia, influence smooth and cardiac muscle and glandular epithelium. Any disease process that damages the somatic motor neuron (as in *poliomyelitis*) or compromises its ability to elicit a response in the skeletal muscle (as in *myasthenia gravis*) will result in weakness or paralysis.

Third, somatosensory fibers enter the spinal cord and influence anterior horn motor neurons either directly or indirectly through interneurons. These activated motor neurons, in turn, produce rapid involuntary contractions of skeletal muscles. The sensory fiber, the associated motor neuron, and the resultant involuntary muscle contraction constitute the circuit of the *spinal reflex*. Reflexes are essential to normal function and can be used as diagnostic tools to assess the functional integrity of the spinal cord.

Fourth, the spinal cord contains descending fibers that influence the activity of spinal neurons. These fibers originate in the cerebral cortex and brainstem, and damage to them adversely influences the activity of spinal motor and sensory neurons. In many cases the position of a lesion in the brainstem or spinal cord may give rise to a predictable or characteristic series of deficits, such as in *decorticate rigidity* or an *alternating hemianesthesia*.

Although not the specific topic of this chapter, it should also be noted that injury to peripheral nerves will result in motor or sensory deficits distal to the lesion. These are most noticeable in the extremities and may present as motor deficits *(flaccid paralysis)*, a loss of sensation *(anesthesia)*, or abnormal sensations *(paresthesia)*.

Development

Neural Plate

As is explained in more detail in Chapter 5, the spinal cord arises from the caudal portion of the embryonic *neural plate* and from the *caudal eminence*. The neural plate gives rise to the cervical, thoracic, and lumbar levels, whereas the caudal eminence gives rise to the sacral and coccygeal levels. The neural plate appears as a specialized area of ectoderm *(neuroectoderm* or *neuroepithelial cells)* posterior to the notochord at about 18 days (Fig. 9-1A, B). By 20 days of gestation, the neural plate is an oblong structure that is larger at its rostral area (future brain) and tapered caudally (future spinal cord).

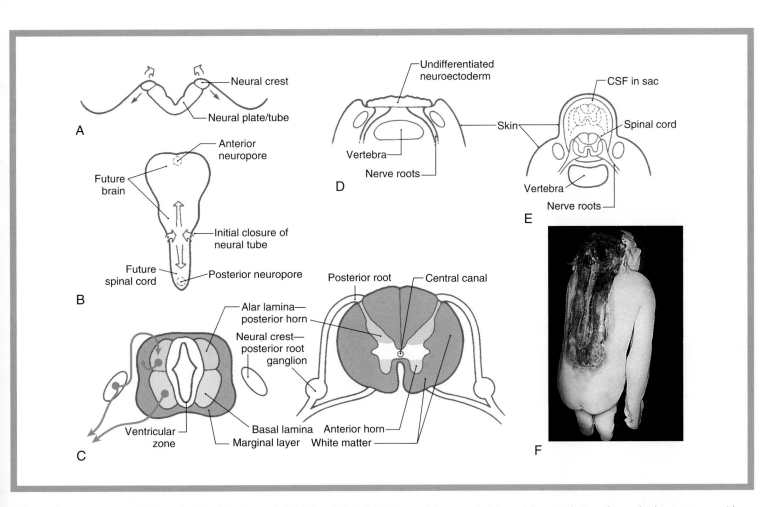

Figure 9-1. Development of the spinal cord. Cross-sectional (**A**) and dorsal (**B**) views of the neural plate and the correlation of neural tube structures with the adult cord (**C**). The *white area* between the *blue* (posterior horn) and *pink* (anterior horn) of the adult spinal cord represents the approximate position of the intermediate gray. Malformations involving defects of the nerve tissue and/or surrounding bone include rachischisis (**D**), meningocele (**E**, *solid cord*) or meningomyelocele (**E**, *dashed cord*), and anencephaly with rachischisis (**F**). CSF, cerebrospinal fluid. (Photograph courtesy of Dr. Jonathan Fratkin.)

Beginning on day 21, the edges of the neural plate *(neural folds)* enlarge posteromedially to meet on the midline (Fig. 9-1B, C). The initial apposition of the neural folds to form the *neural tube* takes place at what will become, in the adult, cervical levels of the spinal cord. This closure simultaneously proceeds in rostral and caudal directions, ultimately creating small openings at either end, between the *cavity of the neural tube* and the surrounding amniotic cavity. These openings are the *anterior* and *posterior neuropores*. The anterior and posterior neuropores close at 24 and 26 days of gestation, respectively.

Neural Tube

That portion of the neural tube that will differentiate into the spinal cord initially consists of the *ventricular zone* and the *marginal zone* (see Chapter 5 for more detail). The ventricular zone contains cells, *neuroblasts* and *glioblasts*, that are undergoing mitosis (cell division) and the precursor cells that will form the *ependymal cell* layer lining the central canal. The marginal zone is initially narrow and contains the processes of cells of the ventricular zone but does not contain their cell bodies or nuclei.

Following their final cell division, postmitotic neurons (as well as glial cells) migrate out of the ventricular zone and form the laterally adjacent *intermediate zone*. This establishes the basic three-layered structure, *ventricular zone*, *intermediate zone*, and *marginal zone*, of the neural tube. As development progresses, the intermediate zone enlarges and the processes arising from the maturing neurons of this zone enter the marginal zone. The *neural crests* detach from the lateral edge of the neural plate and assume a location anterolateral to the neural tube.

Structures of the developing neural tube can be correlated with their adult counterparts (Fig. 9-1C). *Neural crest cells* differentiate into cells of the *posterior root ganglia*, among other structures. The intermediate zone (the term preferred instead of mantle zone) contains four rostrocaudally oriented columns of maturing neurons, forming the paired *alar plates posteriorly* and the paired *basal plates anteriorly*. The alar plate and basal plate are separated from each other by the *sulcus limitans*. Maturing neurons of the alar plate differentiate into the tract neurons and interneurons of the *posterior horn* of the adult, and those of the basal plate become the motor neurons and interneurons of the *anterior horn*. The axons of basal plate neurons, which become somatic motor neurons, extend distally as parts of peripheral nerves. The intermediate gray (Fig. 9-1D, white area between blue and pink), an important region of the spinal cord insinuated between the posterior and anterior horns in the adult, originates from portions of both alar and basal plates.

The marginal zone is invaded by processes of maturing neurons located in the ventricular zone (Fig. 9-1C) and by the descending axons of neuroblasts found in the developing brainstem or cerebral cortex. These axons, most of which become myelinated, form the various tracts of the white matter of the adult spinal cord.

Neural Tube Defects

A variety of defects result from the failure of the neural tube to properly close (Fig. 9-1). *Rachischisis* occurs when the neural folds do not join at the midline and the undifferentiated neuroectoderm remains exposed. In its extreme form, *rachischisis totalis* (or *holorachischisis*), the entire spinal cord remains open. *Rachischisis partialis* (or *merorachischisis*) is the situation in which the spinal cord is partially closed and partially flayed open.

A failure of the anterior neuropore to close results in a failure of the skull and the underlying brain to properly develop. While commonly called *anencephaly* (meaning without brain) the term *meroanencephaly* (meaning without part of brain) is actually more accurate since the brainstem may be fairly intact but the forebrain and cerebellum are largely absent. Rachischisis and meroanencephaly are catastrophic developmental defects that, in most cases (particularly the latter), are not compatible with life.

In other cases the neural tube may develop normally, but the surrounding vertebrae may not form properly, resulting in *spina bifida occulta* or *spina bifida cystica*. The former is characterized by partially missing vertebral arches; the area of the defect may be indicated by a patch of dark hairs. The latter is seen as enlargements that may contain only meninges and cerebrospinal fluid (CSF) *(meningocele)* or meninges, CSF, and portions of the spinal cord *(meningomyelocele)*. These are described in greater detail in Chapter 5.

Spinal Cord Structure

The adult spinal cord is composed of a butterfly-shaped central area of neuron cell bodies, the *gray matter*, and a surround of myelinated fibers, the *white matter*. Although the cavity of the neural tube was prominent during development, this space is reduced to a small ependyma-lined *central canal* in the adult spinal cord (Fig. 9-1C).

Surface Features

The human spinal cord extends from the *foramen magnum* to the level of the first or second lumbar vertebra. It consists of 8 cervical, 12 thoracic, 5 lumbar, and 5 sacral levels plus 1 coccygeal level. *Each level (or segment) of the spinal cord is specified by the intervertebral foramina through which the posterior and anterior roots attached to that segment exit the vertebral canal* (Fig. 9-2). Although generally cylindrical, the cord has *cervical* (C4 to T1) and *lumbosacral* (L1 to S2) *enlargements*, which serve, respectively, the upper and lower extremities.

There are eight cervical roots (and spinal cord levels) but only seven cervical vertebrae. So how do the roots relate to their corresponding vertebrae? The C1 root is located between the base of the skull and the C1 vertebra (Fig. 9-2). Therefore, roots C1 through C7 are located above (rostral to) their respectively numbered vertebrae, and the C8 root is located between the C7 and T1 vertebrae. Beginning with the T1 vertebra and extending caudally, all roots are located caudal to their respectively numbered vertebrae (Fig. 9-2). It is also important to remember that *the level of the spinal cord is determined by the intervertebral foramen through which the posterior and anterior roots originating from that cord level exit*.

There are few superficial markings on the spinal cord (Fig. 9-3). The *posterior median sulcus* separates the posterior portion of the cord into two halves and contains a delicate layer of pia, the *posterior median septum*. The *posterolateral sulcus*, which runs the full length of the cord, represents the entry point of posterior root (sensory) fibers. This area is frequently called the *posterior (dorsal) root entry zone*. In cervical and upper thoracic regions, a *posterior intermediate sulcus* and *septum* are found between the posterolateral and posterior median sulci. This sulcus and septum are insinuated between the medially located *gracile fasciculus* and the laterally located *cuneate fasciculus* (Figs. 9-3 and 9-12). Due to the organization of the gracile and cuneate fasciculi, the posterior intermediate septum is only present in upper thoracic and cervical cord levels.

On the anterolateral surface of the spinal cord, the *anterolateral sulcus* is the exit point for anterior root (motor) fibers (Fig. 9-3). Because the anterior roots exit in a somewhat irregular pattern this sulcus is not as distinct as the posterolateral sulcus.

The *anterior median fissure* is a prominent space dividing the anterior part of the cord into halves (Fig. 9-3). This fissure contains delicate strands of pia and, more importantly, the *sulcal branches* of the *anterior spinal artery*.

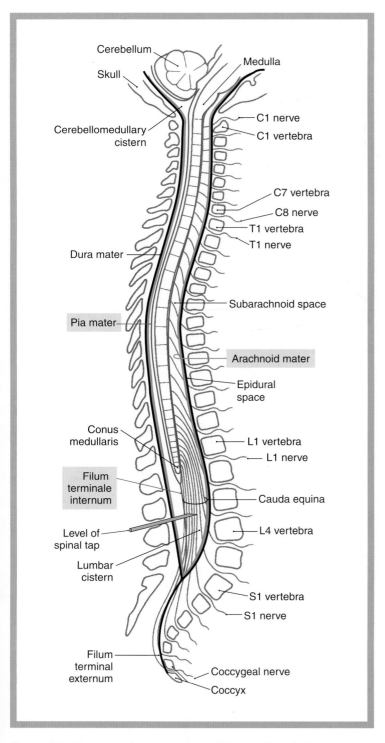

Figure 9-2. Diagrammatic representation of the spinal cord, the meninges, and other adjacent structures. Note the location for a lumbar puncture (spinal tap).

Spinal Meninges

The tubular dural sac that encloses the spinal cord is attached cranially to the rim of the foramen magnum, and its closed caudal end is anchored to the coccyx by the *filum terminale externum* (Figs. 9-2 and 9-3). This dural sac is separated from the vertebrae by the epidural space. The spinal cord, in turn, is attached to the dural sac by the laterally placed *denticulate ligaments* and by the *filum terminale internum*. This latter structure extends caudally from the end of the spinal cord, the *conus medullaris*, and terminates in the attenuated (closed) portion of the dural sac, which is located adjacent to the S2 vertebrae. The filum terminale externum extends caudally from

the closed dural sac to its attachment on the inner aspect of the coccyx (Fig. 9-2).

The arachnoid mater adheres to the inner surface of the dura mater, and the pia mater is intimately attached to the surface of the cord. The subarachnoid space between these layers is continuous with the subarachnoid space around the brain and is likewise filled with cerebrospinal fluid. In adults the conus medullaris is located at the level of the L1 or L2 vertebral body. Extending caudally from this point to the end of the dural sac is an enlarged part of the spinal subarachnoid space, the lumbar cistern (Fig. 9-2). This cistern contains the posterior and anterior roots from spinal segments L2 to Coc1 as they sweep caudally. Collectively, these roots form the *cauda equina*. The method of choice for obtaining a sample of CSF for diagnostic purposes is the lumbar puncture (spinal tap), in which a large-bore needle is introduced between the L3 and L4 or L4 and L5 vertebral arches into the lumbar cistern (Fig. 9-2).

White Matter

The white matter of the spinal cord is divided into three large regions, each of which is composed of individual *tracts* or *fasciculi*. The *posterior funiculus* is located between the posterior median septum and the medial edge of the horn (Fig. 9-3). At cervical levels this area consists of the *gracile* and *cuneate fasciculi*; collectively, these are commonly referred to as the *posterior columns*.

The *lateral funiculus* is the area of white matter located between the posterolateral and anterolateral sulci (Fig. 9-3). This region of the cord contains clinically important ascending and descending tracts, the locations of which are shown in Figure 9-12. Those most important in diagnosing the neurologically impaired patient are the *lateral corticospinal tract* and the *anterolateral system* (ALS).

Located between the anterolateral sulcus and the ventral median fissure is a comparatively small region, the *anterior funiculus* (Fig. 9-3). This area contains *reticulospinal* and *vestibulospinal fibers*, portions of the ALS, the *anterior corticospinal tract*, and a composite bundle called the *medial longitudinal fasciculus* (MLF).

Two small but important components of the white matter are the *anterior white commissure* and the *posterolateral (dorsolateral) tract* (Fig. 9-3). The former is located on the anterior midline and is separated from the central canal by a narrow band of small cells. The posterolateral tract is frequently called the *tract of Lissauer*. It is a small bundle of lightly myelinated and unmyelinated fibers capping the posterior horn.

Gray Matter

The gray matter of the spinal cord is composed of neuron cell bodies, their dendrites and the initial part of the axon, the axon terminals of fibers synapsing in this area, and glial cells. Because this area has few myelinated fibers, it appears distinctly light and has a characteristic shape in myelin-stained sections (Figs. 9-3 and 9-5).

The spinal gray is divisible into a *posterior (dorsal) horn*, an *anterior (ventral) horn*, and the region where these meet, commonly called the *intermediate zone* (or *intermediate gray*). Based on the shape, size, and distribution of neurons located in these areas, the gray matter is divided into *laminae (Rexed laminae) I to IX* and an *area X* around the central canal (Fig. 9-3). These laminae are also characterized by the input they receive and the trajectory of axons arising therein.

The posterior horn is composed of laminae I to VI (Fig. 9-3). The most distinct structure in the posterior horn, the *substantia gelatinosa* (lamina II), is capped by cells of the *posteromarginal nucleus* (lamina I). Laminae III to VI are arranged in a series

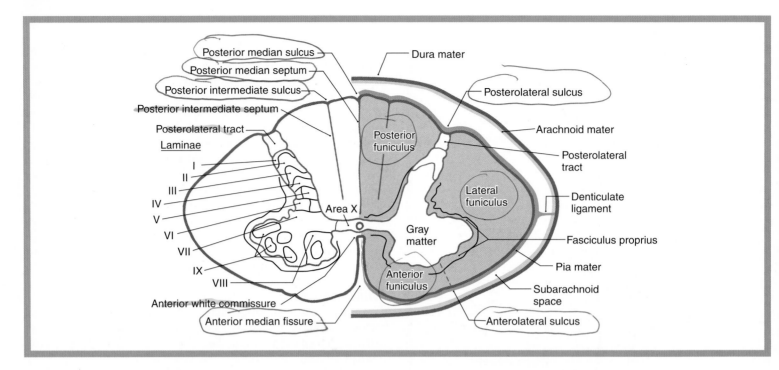

Figure 9-3. The spinal cord at C7 showing the basic organization of the gray and white matter and the meninges (shown only on the *right*). The lamination pattern of the gray matter is shown only on the *left.*

internal to the substantia gelatinosa. Laminae III and IV may also be called the *nucleus proprius (posterior* or *dorsal proper sensory nucleus);* their cells have elaborate dendrites that extend into lamina II. Laminae V and VI, which form the base of the posterior horn, are usually divided into medial and lateral portions.

The intermediate zone, lamina VII, extends from the area of the central canal to the lateral edge of the spinal gray and varies in shape at different levels. Particularly characteristic of lamina VII at thoracic levels are the *posterior thoracic nucleus (dorsal nucleus of Clarke)* and the *intermediolateral nucleus;* the latter is frequently called the *intermediolateral cell column.*

The anterior horn is made up of laminae VIII and IX (Fig. 9-3). The former contains a population of smaller cells that are interneurons and tract cells. The latter consists of several distinct clusters of large motor neurons whose axons directly innervate skeletal muscle.

Blood Supply

The blood supply to the spinal cord is derived from the *anterior* and *posterior spinal arteries* and from branches of segmental arteries (Fig. 9-4). The segmental branches that serve the posterior and anterior roots and the posterior root ganglia are

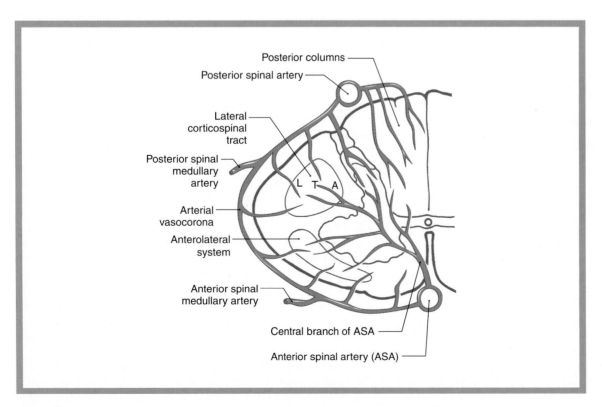

Figure 9-4. Blood supply to the spinal cord. Note that the lateral corticospinal tract and the anterolateral system receive a dual blood supply; also note the topographic arrangement of corticospinal fibers. L, leg/lower extremity; T, trunk; A, arm/upper extremity.

the *radicular arteries*, and the branches that largely bypass the roots to supplement the blood supply to the cord are the *spinal medullary arteries*. One especially large spinal medullary artery, the *artery of Adamkiewicz*, is most often seen at L2 on the left. This vessel is an important source of blood supply to the cord and must be preserved during surgery in this area; damage to this artery may result in an infarct at lower thoracic and upper lumbar levels of the cord. At each level, terminal branches of the spinal medullary arteries join together to form an arterial network, the *arterial vasocorona*, on the surface of the spinal cord (Fig. 9-4).

The posterior columns and peripheral parts of the lateral and anterior funiculi are served by the posterior spinal arteries and arterial vasocorona. Most of the gray matter and the adjacent parts of the white matter are served by the *central branches* of the *anterior spinal artery* (Fig. 9-4). These central branches tend to alternate: one serves the left side of the cord; the next serves the right side.

Trauma, as in hyperextension of the cervical spine, may cause occlusion or spasm of the anterior spinal artery or mechanical injury to the cord. The result is bilateral damage to the cervical cord *(central cervical cord syndrome)*. The characteristic features of the syndrome are bilateral weakness of the extremities, primarily evident in the arms, forearm, and hands; a patchy loss of sensation below the lesion; and possible urinary retention.

Regional Characteristics

Although all spinal levels have posterior, lateral, and anterior funiculi and posterior and anterior horns, their shapes and proportions vary between major spinal regions (Fig. 9-5). For example, cervical (C4 to T1) and lumbosacral (L1 to S2) cord levels have prominent posterior and anterior horns because of the extensive sensory input from, and motor outflow to, the upper and lower extremities. In contrast, the posterior and anterior horns at thoracic levels are small; sensory input is less dense, and there is no appendicular musculature at these levels.

When viewing the spinal cord in the *clinical setting*, as in magnetic resonance imaging (MRI) or computed tomography (CT), it is important to note that anterior and posterior are reversed when compared with the orientation commonly used in the anatomic setting (Fig. 9-5). Both have their advantages, but it is absolutely essential to remember the orientation and consequent location of tracts in the spinal cord in CT and/or MRI since these images are used in the evaluation of the neurologically compromised patient. In short, *anterior is up in the image and posterior is down* (Fig. 9-5). In addition, the right and left sides of the patient are standardized; *the observer's right is the patient's left and the observer's left is the patient's right.*

Cervical Levels

The cervical cord is round to oval and proportionately larger than at other spinal levels (Fig. 9-5). There is a large amount of white matter because a full complement of ascending and descending fiber tracts is present. The gracile and cuneate fasciculi are especially obvious structures at cervical levels.

At cervical levels C1 to C3 the posterior and anterior horns are comparatively small, which results in the shape of the upper cervical spinal cord as being more round than oval. The horns at C3 to C4 are becoming larger as part of the cervical enlargement, thus the shape of the spinal cord is transitioning from more round to more oval. At cervical levels C4 to C8 the posterior and anterior horns are quite large, reflecting the sensory input from and motor innervation to the upper extremity. At these levels the spinal cord is distinctly oval (Fig. 9-5). The oval shape of the spinal cord is also quite obvious in a myelogram at lower cervical levels (Fig. 9-5).

Thoracic Levels

In general, the thoracic cord is round and the posterior and anterior horns are small (Fig. 9-5). From upper to lower thoracic levels there is a progressive decrease in the amount of white matter. Although both the gracile and cuneate fasciculi are present at upper thoracic levels (above T6), only the gracile fasciculus is present at lower thoracic levels (below T6). However, the small size of the posterior and anterior horns makes the white matter in thoracic levels appear proportionately large. As seen in a myelogram at about midthoracic levels, there is more space around the spinal cord than at lower cervical levels (Fig. 9-5).

Two structures especially obvious in the gray matter at thoracic levels are the *posterior thoracic nucleus (dorsal nucleus of Clarke)* and the *lateral horn* (Fig. 9-5). The former, a prominent cell group in medial parts of lamina VII, contains neurons whose axons project to the cerebellum. The latter, also part of lamina VII, is a protrusion into the lateral funiculus formed by underlying the *intermediolateral cell column*. These cells are preganglionic sympathetic neurons whose axons will terminate in either paravertebral or prevertebral ganglia.

Lumbar Levels

At lumbar levels the cord is also round (Fig. 9-5). The posterior and anterior horns are quite large, and there is considerably less white matter than at higher levels. Therefore, the posterior and anterior horns appear proportionately large, the reverse of the situation at thoracic levels. In parallel with the situation at cervical levels, the proportionately large size of the posterior and anterior horns at lumbar levels accommodates, respectively, the significant sensory input from and motor outflow to the lower extremity. The posterior thoracic nucleus (dorsal nucleus of Clarke) is usually obvious at L1 and possibly L2 levels.

As the posterior and anterior roots descend in the more caudal portions of the dural sac, they form fascicles around the lower lumbar levels of the spinal cord. A myelogram at this level clearly illustrates not only the position of the rootlets in relation to the spinal cord but also the expanse of the subarachnoid space at these levels (Fig. 9-5). The roots surrounding the lumbar spinal cord form the upper portions of the cauda equina, which is much more obvious at slightly lower levels (Fig. 9-5).

Sacral Levels

At sacral levels, the spinal cord is round and is smaller than at lumbar levels (Fig. 9-5). It consists mainly of gray matter, with the white matter forming a relatively thin shell. The intermediate gray matter at levels S2, S3, and S4 contains preganglionic parasympathetic cell bodies (the *sacral visceromotor nucleus*). The substantia gelatinosa (lamina II) is especially obvious at sacral levels.

At sacral levels of the spinal cord the cord its self is quite small and is surrounded by the posterior and anterior roots that are descending in the dural sac (Fig. 9-5). At this point the roots, as they pass the sacral and coccygeal cord to enter the lumbar cistern, form the *cauda equina*. The subarachnoid space around the lumbar, sacral, and coccygeal cord is continuous with the space of the lumbar cistern; a myelogram through the lumbar cistern reveals the roots forming the cauda equina but no spinal cord (Fig. 9-5).

Spinal Nerves

The spinal nerves are formed by the junction of the posterior and anterior roots of the spinal cord (Fig. 9-6). As there are 31 spinal cord levels (8 cervical, 12 thoracic, 5 lumbar, 5 sacral, 1 coccygeal), so are there 31 corresponding pairs of spinal nerves. Each spinal nerve contains afferent fibers that convey sensory

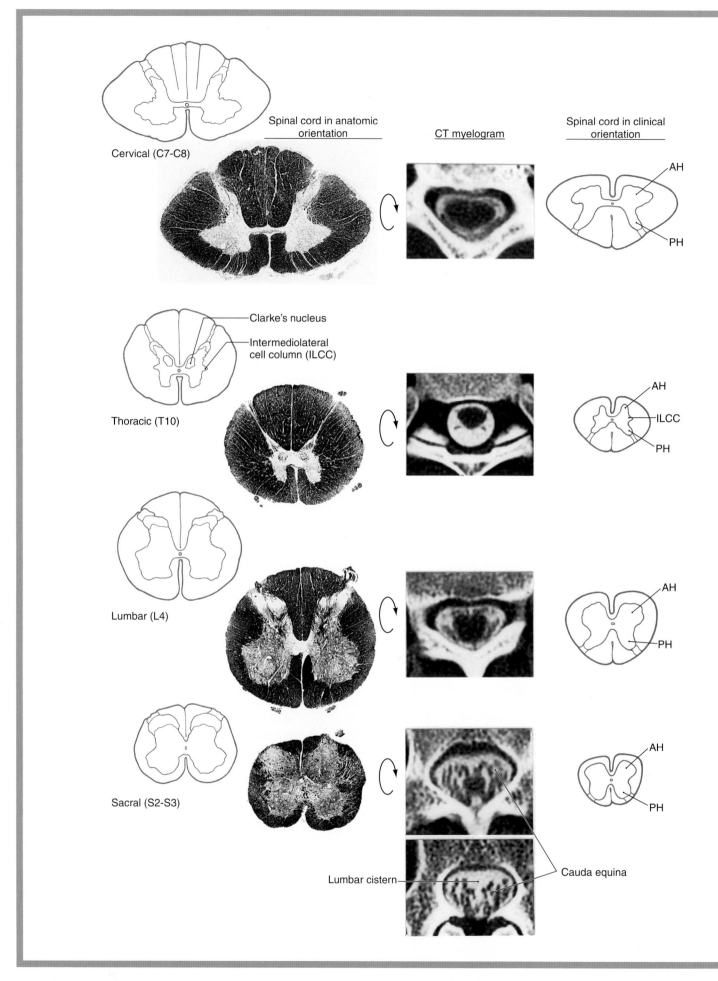

Figure 9-5. Representative levels of the spinal cord in anatomical *(left two columns)* and clinical *(right two columns)* orientations. The overall shape of the spinal cord at each level is clear in the myelogram and essentially identical to the corresponding anatomic section. Note that in CT, as shown here, or in MRI, the anterior and posterior horns (AH and PH) in the clinical orientation are the reverse of those seen in the anatomic orientation (compare far right and left columns). (CT myelogram from Haines DE: Neuroanatomy: An Atlas of Structures, Sections, and Systems, 6th ed. Baltimore, Lippincott Williams & Wilkins, 2004.)

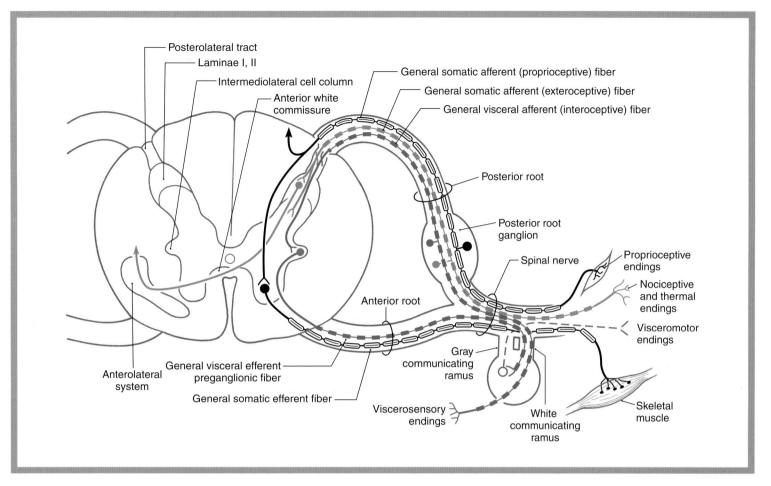

Figure 9-6. The spinal nerve shown on a representative cord level. The relative thickness of the various types of fibers is indicated. The narrow-diameter fiber passing through the gray communicating ramus and terminating in visceromotor endings represents a general visceral efferent (GVE) postganglionic fiber.

input from the periphery and efferent fibers arising from spinal motor neurons. These fibers, plus circuits in the spinal gray, are the structural basis for the *spinal reflexes* routinely tested in the neurologic examination (see Chapter 33).

The spinal nerve may contain up to four types of fibers. Two of these are sensory and have their cell bodies in the posterior root ganglion, and two are motor and have their cell bodies in the spinal cord gray matter (Figs. 9-6 and 9-7).

Sensory Components of the Spinal Nerve

Sensory information is brought to the spinal cord by neuronal processes whose cell bodies reside in the posterior root ganglia. The central processes of these neurons penetrate the spinal cord, and the peripheral processes pass outward in the spinal nerves to innervate body structures. Sensory input originates from (1) the body surface; (2) deep structures such as muscles, tendons, and joints; and (3) internal organs. Fibers conveying input from the first two areas are classified as *general somatic afferent* (GSA), whereas sensory fibers from the gut and other visceral structures are classified as *general visceral afferent* (GVA). The GSA fibers are further classified as either *exteroceptive* or *proprioceptive* (Figs. 9-6 and 9-7).

Exteroceptive (GSA) fibers arise from (1) receptors that are sensitive to mechanical, thermal, or chemical stimuli that may cause tissue damage or (2) receptors sensitive to discriminative touch or vibratory stimuli. The former fibers (Aδ and C) are slowly conducting (0.5 to 30 m/s) and unmyelinated, or lightly myelinated, and they enter the cord via the *lateral division of the posterior root* (Fig. 9-6). These fibers may ascend or descend (or both) in the *posterolateral tract (tract of Lissauer)* before entering the posterior horn to terminate primarily in laminae I to V. The latter fibers (Aβ) are rapidly conducting (30 to 70 m/s)

and heavily myelinated, and they enter the cord through the *medial division of the posterior root* (Fig. 9-6). After entering the posterior funiculus, these fibers may give rise to ascending or descending collaterals.

Proprioceptive (GSA) fibers originate from receptors located in muscles, tendons, or joints that are sensitive to stretch or pressure; some vibratory sense is also conveyed by these fibers (Figs. 9-6 and 9-7). These are rapidly conducting (70 to 120 m/s; Ia, Ib, Aα and Aβ), heavily myelinated fibers that also enter the *medial division of the posterior root*. The central processes of these proprioceptive fibers (and of the heavily myelinated exteroceptive fibers) may directly enter, and ascend in, the posterior columns, or they may branch into the spinal gray to synapse in relay nuclei (such as the posterior nucleus of Clarke) or on cells in the anterior horn that participate in spinal reflexes.

The spinal nerve also conveys sensory information from thoracic, abdominal, and pelvic viscera. This *interoceptive* input originates primarily from receptors that are sensitive to nociceptive stimuli and is conveyed via GVA fibers (Figs. 9-6 and 9-7). These fibers travel through (for example) the *splanchnic nerves* and traverse the sympathetic chain and *white communicating ramus* to enter the spinal nerve. Their central processes enter the lateral division of the posterior root and terminate in laminae I and V to VII. These GVA fibers are also lightly myelinated and slowly conducting (1 to 20 m/s).

Neurotransmitters of Primary Sensory Neurons

Although several neuroactive substances have been implicated as transmitters in primary afferent fibers, those having an important role are *substance P* (SP), *calcitonin gene–related peptide* (CGRP), and *glutamate*. Small-diameter (A-δ and C) fibers arising from visceral and somatic structures—that is, GVA

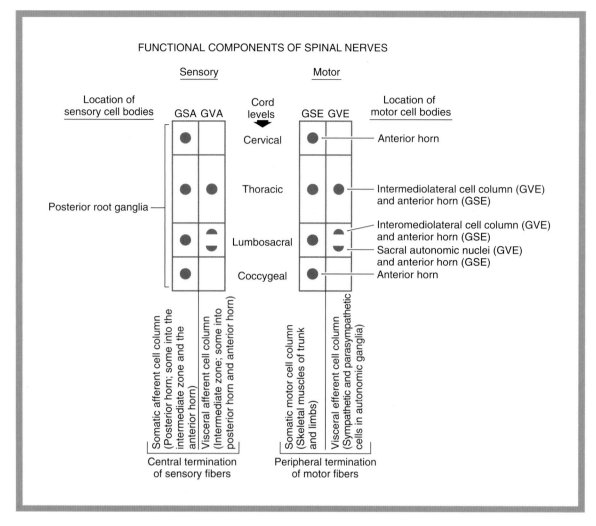

Figure 9-7. Functional components of the spinal nerve: The locations of sensory cell bodies and the targets of their central processes and the locations of the motor cell bodies and their peripheral targets. GSA, general somatic afferent; GVA, general visceral afferent; GSE, general somatic efferent; GVE; general visceral efferent.

and small-diameter GSA fibers—use one or more of these three neurotransmitters, and it is probable that some large-diameter, heavily myelinated GSA fibers use glutamate. Specifically, SP and CGRP can be found in small-diameter GVA and GSA fibers, and these peptides plus glutamate are also found in the smaller cell bodies of the posterior root ganglion, from which these fibers arise. Centrally, fibers and terminals containing these three neurotransmitters can be found in laminae I, II, and V, where the small-diameter axons synapse with cells that relay the information to higher levels of the neuraxis. Conversely, some of the large bodies in posterior root ganglia, which give rise to large-diameter GSA fibers, contain glutamate. This transmitter is also found in the posterior columns in large-diameter, heavily myelinated fibers, indicating that it may function in the relay of proprioceptive information.

Deafferentation Pain and the Posterior Root Entry Zone Procedure

In general, the phenomenon of *deafferentation pain* occurs when the anatomic pathways for pain perception, that being intact nerve rootlets, tracts and nerves themselves, are partially or entirely disrupted. This condition may develop, for example, following amputation (traumatic or otherwise), peripheral nerve injury, lesions of central tracts resulting in hemiplegia, quadriplegia or paraplegia, or damage to the posterior rootlets at the rootlet-cord interface. Deafferentation pain may be perceived as dull and aching, pins-and-needles (sharp pain), searing, or burning sensations. The mechanism for the pain is likely due to a combination of an increased sensitivity of the central (disconnected/

damaged) neurons, plasticity changes in the damaged cell groups, and a decrease in central inhibition at the lesion site.

An especially instructive example of cause, treatment, and potential complication is seen in *avulsion of the posterior rootlets*. This injury, commonly seen in accidents involving motorcycles, is the forceful separation (*avulsion*, a pulling or tearing out) of the posterior roots from the spinal cord, more often in the brachial plexus. The pain is in the distribution of the damaged posterior roots.

One treatment for this intractable pain is the DREZ (for dorsal root entry zone) procedure, although PREZ (for posterior root entry zone procedure) has a nice ring. In this procedure a small electrode is placed into the posterior horn at the entry zone (hence the name of the procedure) and radiofrequency lesions are made at the levels of the avulsed roots. Significant, or total, relief from pain is seen in 80% to 90% of these patients. Interestingly enough, complications may include deficits related to the laterally adjacent corticospinal tract or the medially adjacent cuneate fasciculus. These are, respectively, a weakness of the upper and/or lower extremity on the same side and the loss of proprioceptive and vibratory sensations on the ipsilateral upper extremity. Some patients will describe the proprioceptive problem as a buzzing sensation on the upper extremity on the side of the procedure.

Motor Components of the Spinal Nerve

The spinal cord gives rise to two types of motor fibers: (1) those that directly innervate skeletal (striated) muscle and (2) visceromotor (autonomic) fibers that synapse on a second neuron, usually located in a peripheral visceromotor ganglion. The latter (or postganglionic) neurons innervate smooth muscle, cardiac muscle, or glandular epithelium (Figs. 9-6 and 9-7).

The motor cells that innervate skeletal muscle are located in the anterior horn; these cells and their peripheral processes are classified as *general somatic efferent* (GSE) (Fig. 9-7). GSE cells from the anterior horn also supply motor innervation to the specialized *intrafusal* muscle fibers of the *muscle spindles* (neuromuscular spindles), sensory structures in muscles that detect muscle length, and various aspects of contraction dynamics. Large motor neurons in the anterior horn are organized in two general but overlapping patterns (Fig. 9-8). First, cells innervating proximal muscles are located medially and cells innervating more distal muscles are located progressively more laterally. This explains why the anterior horn is smaller and narrower at thoracic than at cervical and lumbar levels. At thoracic levels the anterior horn contains motor neurons innervating the axial muscles of the trunk, whereas at cervical and lumbar levels it also contains the more lateral groups of motor neurons that innervate the limbs. Second, within the anterior horn at C4 to T1 and L1 to S2, motor neurons innervating extensors tend to be more anteriorly located in the horn, whereas those innervating flexors tend to be found more posteriorly located.

The visceromotor (autonomic) motor neurons of the spinal cord are classified as *general visceral efferent* (GVE) and have their cell bodies in lamina VII (Figs. 9-6 and 9-7). At cord levels T1 to L2, these cells belong to the *intermediolateral cell column* (sympathetic cells), whereas at sacral levels S2 to S4, they belong to the parasympathetic system and form the *sacral visceromotor nucleus* located in the lateral part of lamina VII. Unlike the single-neuron GSE projection, visceromotor pathways consist of two neurons in series (Fig. 9-6). The spinal cord neuron projects to a visceromotor ganglion and is therefore classified as *GVE-preganglionic*. In the ganglion, it synapses with a *GVE-postganglionic neuron, which innervates the target structure.*

Motor fibers (GSE and GVE) exit in the anterior root and pass into the spinal nerve (Fig. 9-6). GSE fibers continue through the spinal nerve and are conveyed by the progressive branching of peripheral nerves to the skeletal muscles of the body. In contrast, GVE-preganglionic fibers leave the spinal nerve to join the sympathetic trunk via the *white communicating ramus* (Fig. 9-6). Once they have entered the sympathetic trunk, these preganglionic fibers follow any of several routes, which are considered in detail in Chapter 29. Suffice it to say, GVE-postganglionic fibers from cells of the sympathetic chain ganglia rejoin the spinal nerves via the *gray communicating ramus*, whereas those of the prevertebral ganglia distribute only to the gut. Also, GVE-preganglionic parasympathetic neurons are present at S2 to S4 levels. Their axons leave the spinal cord in the anterior roots to eventually join branches of the ventral primary rami that form the pelvic nerve.

Neurotransmitters of Spinal Motor Neurons and Myasthenia Gravis

The three populations of spinal motor neurons are (1) large anterior horn cells (*α motor neurons*) that innervate extrafusal skeletal muscle cells, (2) smaller cells (*γ motor neurons*) that innervate only the intrafusal fibers of the muscle spindles, and (3) cells that give rise to preganglionic sympathetic (T1 to L1) or parasympathetic (S2 to S4) fibers, which terminate in peripheral visceromotor (autonomic) ganglia. All three of these cell populations use *acetylcholine* as their neurotransmitter. Consequently, acetylcholine is abundant in axon terminals at the *neuromuscular junction*, and numerous *nicotinic acetylcholine receptors* are present on the postsynaptic junctional folds of the muscle membrane.

Myasthenia gravis, a neurologic disease characterized by moderate to profound muscle weakness, is closely correlated with the presence of circulating antibodies directed against nicotinic receptor sites on the postsynaptic membrane. The result is a blockage of transmission at the neuromuscular junction. A characteristic of this disease in muscle fatigability; as the day progresses muscle fatigue becomes progressively worse.

This disease is most frequently seen in patients between 20 and 40 years of age, although younger patients may exhibit symptoms. There are three characteristics of myasthenia gravis. First, muscle weakness may wax and wane over periods of minutes or hours, one day, or several days or weeks. Second, muscles controlling eye movement are frequently involved first (in about 40% of patients), resulting in *diplopia* and *ptosis*, and are ultimately involved in about 85% of all patients. Muscles of the pharynx or larynx, face, and extremities may eventually be involved, but almost always in concert with ocular muscles. These patients exhibit *dysarthria* and *dysphagia*. Third, the weakness responds to the administration of drugs that enhance cholinergic transmission.

Spinal Reflexes

Afferent fibers in spinal nerves may synapse on tract cells that relay information to higher levels of the neuraxis, or they may terminate on motor neurons or interneurons, both of which may participate in reflex circuits. Reflexes require an afferent fiber, interneurons and/or motor neurons, and a target tissue, usually skeletal muscle. Reflexes may be relatively simple and confined to a single cord level (*intrasegmental*) or complex, involving multiple cord segments (*intersegmental*). Certain disease or central nervous system lesions can affect spinal reflexes, resulting in reflexes that are greatly exaggerated (*hyperreflexia*), diminished (*hyporeflexia*), or absent (*areflexia*). Numerous reflexes are part of the standard neurologic examination (see Chapter 33); only a few examples are given here.

Muscle Stretch Reflex

Although this is sometimes called a *tendon reflex* or *deep tendon reflex*, it is more correctly called a *muscle stretch reflex* because

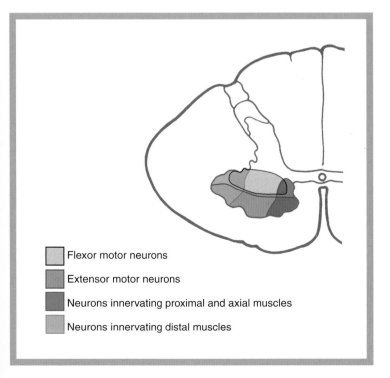

Flexor motor neurons

Extensor motor neurons

Neurons innervating proximal and axial muscles

Neurons innervating distal muscles

Figure 9-8. Representation of the general organization of motor neurons in the anterior horn.

the stimulus is stretch of a muscle spindle located within the muscle. This reflex may be elicited by tapping any large tendon (such as the triceps or Achilles); a common example is the *knee-jerk* or *quadriceps stretch reflex* (Fig. 9-9). A brisk tap on the patellar tendon stretches the primary sensory endings in muscle spindles located in the quadriceps femoris muscle, sending an impulse toward the posterior root ganglion via heavily myelinated, rapidly conducting group Ia fibers. The central processes of these afferent axons synapse on and excite motor neurons in the anterior horn that innervate the quadriceps femoris muscle. The result is a sudden contraction of these muscles and an extension (dorsiflexion) of the leg at the knee. Because this reflex requires only one synapse and is a response to muscle stretch, it also may be called a *monosynaptic stretch reflex* or a *myotatic reflex.*

An extension of the simple stretch reflex is seen in *reciprocal inhibition* and *autogenic inhibition* (also called the *inverse myotatic reflex*). In reciprocal inhibition, one group of muscles is excited and the antagonistic group is inhibited (Fig. 9-9). In this situation, the muscle spindle is stretched by a tap on the patellar tendon, and the impulse enters the spinal cord via a group Ia primary sensory fiber. This fiber branches and has excitatory terminations on quadriceps femoris motor neurons and on group Ia inhibitory (glycinergic) interneurons. As a result, the quadriceps (extensor) contracts, whereas the interneurons inhibit spinal motor neurons innervating the hamstring (flexor) muscles, which remain passive. This action enhances the effectiveness of the reflex.

The receptor involved in *autogenic inhibition* is the *Golgi tendon organ* (Fig. 9-9). This receptor responds to relatively high tension (higher than that needed to activate the muscle spindles). Activation causes an increase in the rate of firing of the group Ib sensory fibers that arise from this receptor. In the spinal cord, these fibers terminate on group Ib inhibitory (glycinergic) interneurons, which inhibit motor neurons that innervate the muscle attached to the tendon from which the afferent volley originated.

Flexor Reflex

A further level of complexity in spinal reflexes is seen in the *flexor reflex (withdrawal reflex or nociceptive reflex)* (Fig. 9-10). This type of reflex is initiated by cutaneous input, is frequently a response to nociceptive stimuli, and represents an attempt to protect a body part by extricating it from the source of injury. Lightly myelinated or unmyelinated primary sensory fibers (A-δ or C fibers) conveying nociceptive input enter the posterolateral tract (of Lissauer) where they may branch and ascend or descend for short distances. Many of these fibers enter the spinal gray, where they form excitatory synaptic contacts with ascending tract cells and with both excitatory and inhibitory interneurons (Fig. 9-10). While tract neurons relay this nociceptive information to higher levels of the neuraxis, the excitatory glutaminergic interneurons synapse on flexor motor neurons, resulting in activation of the ipsilateral flexor muscles of the thigh

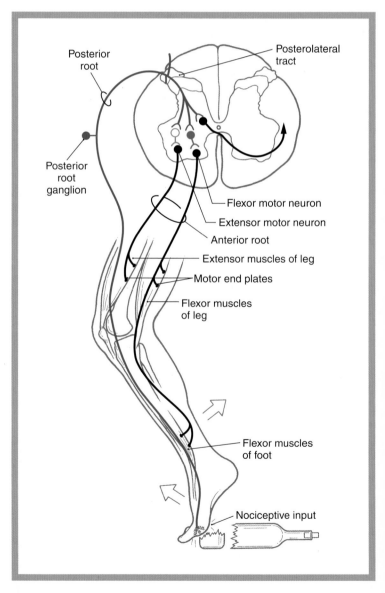

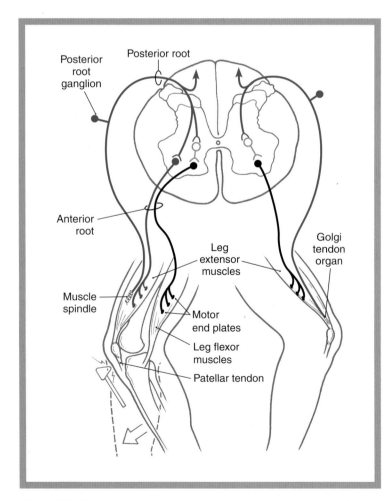

Figure 9-9. Pathway for the patellar tendon reflex and reciprocal inhibition *(left)* and autogenic inhibition *(right)*. The inhibitory glycinergic interneurons are represented by the *red* open cell bodies.

Figure 9-10. Pathway for the flexor reflex. The inhibitory glycinergic interneuron is represented by the *red* open cell and the excitatory glutaminergic interneuron by the *green* closed cell. In addition to being involved in reflexes, this nociceptive input is also relayed to higher levels of the neuraxis via the anterolateral system (ascending *black* fiber).

(iliopsoas), leg (hamstring muscles), and foot (tibialis anterior) and withdrawal of the extremity. This action is enhanced by the synapse of inhibitory interneurons on extensor (antagonistic) motor neurons and the resultant decreased activity (inhibition) of extensor muscles, for example, the quadriceps femoris muscles. The flexor reflex, considering its afferent and efferent limbs, involves several spinal segments.

Crossed Extension Reflex
The *crossed extension reflex* builds on the basic circuits of the flexor reflex but also involves musculature of the contralateral side of the body (Fig. 9-11). By way of interneurons, nociceptive input on A-δ or C fibers excites ipsilateral leg flexor motor neurons and inhibits ipsilateral leg extensor motor neurons. Consequently, the flexors contract, the extensors relax, and the extremity is withdrawn from the painful stimulus. If the reflex occurs during standing or walking, however, the opposite leg must participate in the response to keep the person from falling. The same nociceptive input that resulted in withdrawal on the ipsilateral side is conveyed to interneurons that project to the contralateral anterior horn (Fig. 9-11). These fibers excite motor neurons polysynaptically, innervating contralateral extensor muscles and inhibiting motor neurons that innervate contra-lateral flexor muscles. Thus, there is an ipsilateral flexion and

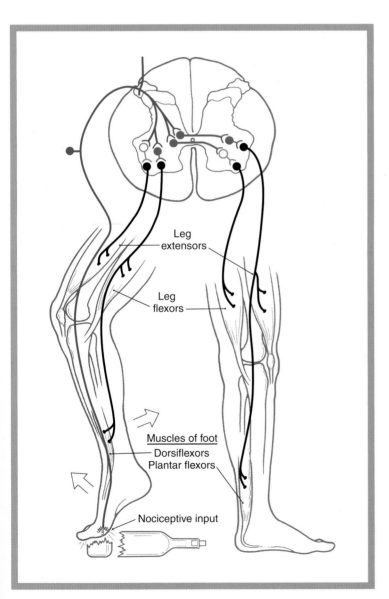

Figure 9-11. Pathway for the crossed extension reflex. Glycinergic interneurons (inhibitory) are represented by the open *red* cell bodies and glutaminergic interneurons (excitatory) by the closed *green* cells.

withdrawal from the stimuli accompanied by an extension of the contralateral leg to support the body.

Peripheral Nerve Lesions

The posterior and anterior roots from one level of the spinal cord join to form a single spinal nerve, which, in turn, combines with other spinal nerves to form the peripheral nerves of the body. Peripheral nerves usually contain both motor and sensory fibers, but some nerves contain only one or the other. Consequently, damage to peripheral nerves may give rise to motor deficits, sensory deficits, or to a combination of these. The etiology and types of peripheral nerve disease are numerous, and only general examples are discussed here.

Radiculopathy
Radiculopathy (*radix* is Latin for "root") is the result of damage to a nerve root. The most common cause is *spondylolysis* or *intervertebral disc disease* with resultant damage to one, or more, nerve roots. Due to the overlap of dermatomes on the body, compression of a single root may not cause a significant sensory loss. However, the main symptom experienced by these patients is the perception of a sharp, burning pain (patients will frequently describe these as a "shooting pains") in the dermatomal distribution of the damaged spinal nerve. Cervical disc disease may result in pain in the base of the neck, over the shoulder, or down the upper extremity, while lumbar disc problems may result in low back pain or in pain radiating down the lower extremity, as in *sciatica*.

Mononeuropathy
The most common cause of *mononeuropathy* (deficits reflecting the distribution of a single anatomically defined peripheral nerve) is trauma. Other causes include entrapment or compression syndromes (such as the *carpal tunnel syndrome*). Characteristic examples of *traumatic mononeuropathy* deficits and the damaged nerve are as follows: deviation of the tongue on protrusion/ hypoglossal nerve; loss of flexion adduction and extension of the fingers/ulnar nerve; loss of dorsiflexion of the foot and toes/deep peroneal nerve; loss of pronation of the forearm and movements of the fingers/median nerve; and loss of flexion of the toes/tibial nerve.

One of the more common entrapment mononeuropathies is the *carpal tunnel syndrome*. Basically the median nerve is compressed by fluid accumulation in the synovial sheaths of the carpal tunnel, creating a largely sensory deficit (although weakness of some finger muscles may occur). The symptoms are numbness, tingling, and pain from the thumb, index, and middle finger; treatment is to section the transverse carpal ligament and relieve the pressure on the median nerve.

Polyneuropathy
As its name implies, a *polyneuropathy* includes motor and sensory deficits that reflect damage to multiple peripheral nerves. Although there are a variety of diseases that may affect multiple peripheral nerves, one of the most common is *diabetes mellitus*. In diabetes the more distal portions of the fibers are affected first *(distal axonopathy)*, starting in the lower extremity and then progressing to the upper extremity. The small-diameter myelinated and unmyelinated fibers are affected first followed by larger-diameter fibers as the disease progresses.

Patients may experience numbness and a loss of pain and thermal sensations in the feet (affecting the longest fibers first), progressing up to about the knees, then the same deficits are perceived in the hands progressing up the forearm. As the disease progresses, larger-diameter fibers become involved and the vibratory and position sensations are diminished or lost.

Since this sensory loss starts with the feet/legs and jumps to the hand/forearm it is common to describe this pattern as a *stocking/glove sensory loss*. While seen as primarily a sensory loss, these patients may also exhibit weakness of distal portions of the extremities and have hyporeflexia.

Two other examples of lesions that result in loss of function related to peripheral nerves are *sensory neuronopathy* and *motor neuronopathy*. The former is a loss of cell bodies in the posterior root ganglion that results in a sensory loss that involves both *distal and proximal portions of an extremity* and may include most or all sensory modalities. The latter is seen in a loss of anterior horn motor neurons with resultant *flaccid weakness, muscle fasciculations, and eventual muscle atrophy*.

Pathways and Tracts of the Spinal Cord

The spinal cord white matter consists of (1) long *ascending* and *descending fibers* or *tracts*, which link the spinal cord to higher levels of the neuraxis, and (2) *propriospinal fibers* that project from one spinal level to another (Fig. 9-12; Table 9-1). Ascending

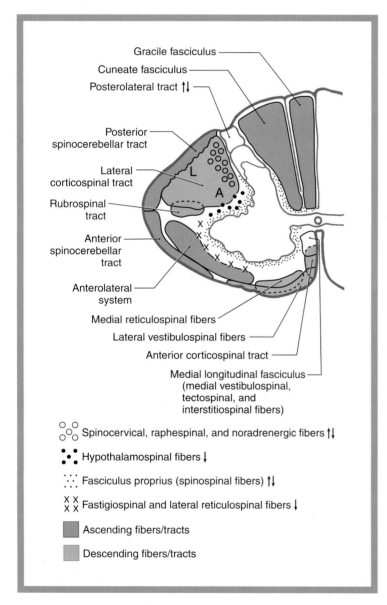

Figure 9-12. Ascending and descending pathways of the spinal cord shown in cross section as they are organized at cervical levels. Corticospinal fibers from the lower extremity region of the motor cortex (L) are located in lateral portions of the tract, whereas fibers from the arm-upper extremity regions of the cortex (A) are medially located in the tract. ↓, descending fibers; ↑, ascending fibers.

fibers convey information to higher levels of the neuraxis. Some descending fibers modulate the transmission of nociceptive information in the posterior horn, whereas others influence the activity of motor neurons. Propriospinal fibers form the basis for a wide variety of intraspinal reflexes.

Many tracts or fibers in the nervous system are *named according to the location of their cell body of origin and the area where their axons terminate.*

For example, the *corticospinal* fibers originate in the cerebral cortex *(cortico-)* and end in the spinal cord *(-spinal)*. These are descending fibers because the *cortex* is a more rostral part of the neuraxis than is the *spinal* cord. Likewise, the term *spinothalamic fiber* indicates that the cell of origin is in the spinal cord and the termination is in the thalamus; these are ascending fibers. In many situations *the name of the tract or group of fibers indicates three important facts about that fiber population:* (1) whether they are ascending or descending (corticospinal versus spinocerebellar); (2) the location of the cell body of origin (cortex versus spinal cord); and (3) the place where the axons in the tract terminate (spinal cord versus cerebellum). Keeping these basic principles in mind will expedite learning many tracts and pathways.

Functions of Ascending Tracts

The *gracile* and *cuneate fasciculi*, collectively called the *posterior columns*, are composed of the central processes of heavily myelinated primary sensory fibers that convey proprioceptive, tactile, and vibratory information from the ipsilateral side of the body (Fig. 9-12 and Table 9-1). Fibers in the gracile fasciculus originate from sacral, lumbar, and lower thoracic (below T6) levels; those in the cuneate fasciculus originate from upper thoracic (above T6) and cervical levels. Injury to the posterior columns on one side results in an *ipsilateral loss of proprioception, discriminative touch, and vibratory sense below the level of the lesion.*

The *posterior (dorsal) spinocerebellar* and *anterior (ventral) spinocerebellar* tracts are located on the lateral surface of the cord, meeting at approximately the level of the denticulate ligament (Figs. 9-3 and 9-12 and Table 9-1). The fibers of the former tract arise from the posterior thoracic nucleus (of Clarke) in lamina VII at T1 to L2, and the fibers of the latter tract arise primarily from cells of laminae V to VIII and from large ventral horn neurons called *spinal border cells*, both at lumbosacral levels. The information conveyed on spinocerebellar fibers influences, through synaptic stations in the cerebellum, thalamus, and motor cortex, the efficiency of motor activity.

In the anterolateral area of the spinal cord there is a large composite bundle called the *anterolateral system* (ALS) (Fig. 9-12 and Table 9-1). This system encompasses those regions of the white matter that were classically divided into anterior and lateral spinothalamic tracts. The ALS contains *spinothalamic, spinomesencephalic* (spinotectal, spinoperiaqueductal), *spinohypothalamic,* and *spinoreticular* fibers. The fibers of the ALS originate primarily from posterior horn cells, but it is now known that some arise from neurons in the anterior horn. Those fibers that coalesce to form the ALS cross in the *anterior white commissure*, ascending about two levels as they do so.

In general, fibers of the ALS convey nociceptive, thermal, and poorly localized (crude) touch information to higher levels of the neuraxis. Consequently, *injury to the spinal cord that involves ALS fibers will result in a loss of pain, temperature, and crude touch sensations on the contralateral side of the body beginning about one or two segments below the lesion.* The ALS is somatotopically organized; this means that in the spinal cord, lower portions of the body are represented more posterolaterally and upper levels are represented anteromedially.

Nociceptive input and some discriminative touch are also carried by *postsynaptic posterior column fibers* and by the *spinocervicothalamic tract.* The former originate from laminae III to

Table 9-1. Synopsis of the Principal Tracts and Fibers Located in the Funiculi, Their Laterality in the Cord, Origin, and Termination

Funiculus	Tract/Fibers	Laterality in Cord	Original	Termination
Posterior	Gracile fasciculus (↑)	—	Posterior root ganglia ↓ T$_6$	Medulla (gracile nuc.)
	Cuneate fasciculus (↑)	—	Posterior root ganglia ↑ T$_6$	Medulla (cuneate nuc.)
	Postsynaptic post. col. syst. (↑)	—	Lamina IV (III-VII)	Medulla
Lateral	Lateral corticospinal (↑)	X	Cerebral cortex	Laminae IV-IX
	Posterior spinocerebellar (↑)	—	Clarke's nucleus (lamina VII)	Cerebellum
	Anterior spinocerebellar (↑)	X, —	Laminae VII-IX	Cerebellum
	ALS (↑)	X	Laminae I-VII	
	(spinothalamic)	X		Thalamus
	(spinomesencephalic)	X		Midbrain
	(spinoreticular)	X, —		Ret. formation
	(spinohypothalamic)	X		Hypothalamus
	Spinocervical (↑)	—	Lamina IV (III-V)	Lateral cervical nucleus
	Rubrospinal (↓)	X	Red nucleus	Laminae V-VIII
	Lateral reticulospinal (↓)	X, —	Gigantocellular ret. nuc.	Laminae VII (VI-IX)
	Raphespinal (↓)	—	Raphe magnus	Laminae I, II, V
	Hypothalamospinal (↓)	X	Hypothalamus	Intermediolateral cell. col.
	Fastigiospinal (↓)	X	Fastigial nucleus	Laminae VII-IX
	Lateral vestibulospinal (↓)	—	Lateral vestibular nucleus	Laminae VII-VIII
	Cuneocerebellar (↑)	—	Lateral cuneate nucleus	Cerebellum
Anterior	Anterior corticospinal (↓)	—	Cerebral cortex	Laminae VI-IX
	Med. reticulospinal (↓)	—	Pontine ret. nuc. (oralis, caudalis)	Laminae VIII (VII, IX)
	MLF (↓)			
	(med. vestibulospinal)	—,X	Medial vestibular nucleus	Laminae VII-VIII
	(reticulospinal)	—	Medullary ret. form.	Laminae VI-VIII
	(tectospinal)	X, —	Tectum (midbrain)	Laminae VI, VIII

VIII (mainly IV) and ascend ipsilaterally in the dorsal columns. The latter fibers arise from the same laminae but ascend as a diffuse population in the posterior part of the lateral funiculus to end in the lateral cervical nucleus at levels C1 to C3. The existence of these minor fiber populations in humans may explain the recurrence of pain perception in some patients who have had an *anterolateral cordotomy* for intractable pain.

Other, more diffusely arranged, ascending fibers include *spino-olivary*, *spinovestibular*, and *spinoreticular fibers*. These are discussed in later chapters in relation to the functional systems they serve.

Functions of Descending Tracts

The lateral funiculus (Figs. 9-3 and 9-12 and Table 9-1) contains the *lateral corticospinal* and *rubrospinal* tracts, as well as other fiber populations that are more diffuse in their distribution (*reticulospinal, fastigiospinal, raphespinal, hypothalamospinal*). Corticospinal fibers arise from the cerebral cortex and descend through the brainstem. At the medulla–spinal cord junction, most fibers cross to form the *lateral corticospinal tract* but some remain uncrossed as the *anterior corticospinal tract*. Lateral corticospinal fibers are somatotopically arranged; fibers that originate from lower extremity areas of the cerebral cortex and project to lumbosacral levels are lateral, whereas those traveling to cervical levels from upper extremity areas of the cortex are medial (Fig. 9-12). One important function of this tract is to influence spinal motor neurons, *especially those controlling fine movements of the distal musculature*. Consequently, lesions of lateral corticospinal fibers on one side of the cervical cord result in *ipsilateral paralysis of the upper and lower extremities on that side (hemiplegia)*. In contrast, a lesion of corticospinal fibers above (rostral to) the spinal cord–medulla junction, and therefore above the decussation of these fibers, will result in *hemiplegia on the opposite (contralateral) side of the body*.

Rubrospinal fibers arise from the red nucleus of the midbrain, cross at that level, and descend in the spinal cord with lateral corticospinal fibers (Fig. 9-12). In general, rubrospinal fibers, as well as lateral corticospinal fibers, excite flexor motor neurons and inhibit extensor motor neurons.

Although diffusely arranged, other descending fibers in the lateral funiculus serve important functions (Fig. 9-12 and Table 9-1). *Reticulospinal fibers* in this area originate from the medullary reticular formation, and *fastigiospinal fibers* originate from the fastigial nucleus of the cerebellum. At spinal levels, the former are uncrossed and the latter are crossed. Because their function is to help maintain posture, these fibers tend to excite extensor motor neurons and inhibit flexor motor neurons. *Raphespinal fibers* originate mainly from the nucleus raphe magnus of the brainstem, descend bilaterally in posterior areas of the lateral funiculus, and function to modulate the transmission of nociceptive information at spinal levels. The activity of GVE motor neurons of the intermediolateral cell column is influenced by *hypothalamospinal fibers*, which descend through lateral areas of the brainstem and spinal cord. Lesions in the brainstem or cervical spinal cord that interrupt these fibers result in ipsilateral *ptosis, miosis, anhidrosis,* and *enophthalmos (Horner syndrome)*.

The *anterior funiculus* (Fig. 9-12 and Table 9-1) contains *reticulospinal* and *vestibulospinal* fibers, the *anterior corticospinal tract*, and the *medial longitudinal fasciculus* (MLF). Reticulospinal fibers in this area arise in the pontine reticular formation of the brainstem, whereas vestibulospinal fibers originate from the vestibular nuclei. *Lateral vestibulospinal fibers* arise from the lateral vestibular nucleus, and *medial vestibulospinal fibers* originate primarily from the medial vestibular nucleus. Reticulospinal and vestibulospinal fibers of the anterior funiculus function in postural mechanisms through their general excitation of extensor motor neurons and inhibition of flexor motor neurons. Fibers of the *anterior corticospinal tract* are uncrossed, but most of these fibers cross in the ventral white commissure before terminating on medial motor neurons that innervate axial muscles.

The MLF, although quite small, is generally regarded as a composite bundle containing *medial vestibulospinal fibers* (from the medial vestibular nucleus), *tectospinal fibers* (from the superior colliculus of the midbrain), *interstitiospinal fibers* (from the interstitial nucleus of the rostral midbrain), and some *reticulospinal fibers* (Fig. 9-12 and Table 9-1). Tectospinal and vestibulospinal fibers are found only at cervical levels; the other fibers extend to lower cord levels. These fibers terminate primarily in laminae VII and VIII but ultimately influence motor neurons innervating primarily axial and neck musculature.

The comparatively simple structure of the spinal cord belies its functional importance. Although the cord is smaller in diameter than the little finger, descending motor control of the body below the neck and all sensory input from the same areas must traverse it. Consequently, lesions in the spinal cord that would be considered of little consequence in larger parts of the brain may cause global deficits or death. As the cord merges into the brainstem, the organization and function of the central nervous system become progressively more complex.

Deficits Characteristic of Spinal Cord Lesions

The functional and clinical characteristics of ascending and descending tracts of the spinal cord are described in later chapters. However, it is appropriate at this point to touch on some general features that correlate with the structure of the spinal cord.

Syringomyelia
Cavitation of the central regions of the spinal cord, as in a small *syringomyelia,* will frequently damage fibers crossing in the anterior white commissure (Fig. 9-3). This bundle conveys fibers from the posterior horn across the midline to enter the ALS on the opposite side (Fig. 9-6). Consequently, a lesion of this structure will damage fibers coursing in both directions, resulting in a bilateral loss of pain and thermal sensations that correlate with the damaged levels of the spinal cord. For example, if the lesion is in mid-to-low cervical levels the pain and thermal sensory deficits will fall over the shoulders and arm in a "cape distribution." A large *syrinx* that involves the anterior white commissure and extends into the anterior horn results in a bilateral sensory loss, as noted earlier, and weakness of the corresponding extremity. Because these lesions are usually in the cervical levels, extension of the syrinx into one anterior horn results in an ipsilateral weakness of the upper extremity; if both anterior horns are involved, the weakness is bilateral. In *syringomyelia,* the cavity that develops in the central areas of the spinal cord does not have a lining of ependymal cells and, therefore, is not an enlargement of the central canal. Sometimes this is called a *noncommunicating syringomyelia* to differentiate it from a cystic structure that may connect with the central canal *(communicating*

syringomyelia). On the other hand, a cavitation of the central canal is called a *hydromyelia* (or *hydrosyringomyelia).*

Brown-Séquard Syndrome
A functional *hemisection of the spinal cord (the Brown-Séquard syndrome)* results in a clinical picture that reflects damage to the lateral corticospinal tract, the ALS, and the posterior columns. A lesion on the right at C4 to C5 will result in muscle weakness or paralysis *(hemiparesis, hemiplegia)* on the right side (corticospinal damage), loss of pain and thermal sensations on the left side (ALS damage—these fibers cross in the anterior white commissure), and a loss of proprioception, vibratory sense, and discriminative touch on the right (gracile and cuneate fasciculi injury). These lesions are frequently called *functional hemisections* in recognition of the fact that the cord is not perfectly cut halfway across but may be injured/deformed by, for example, pieces of a damaged vertebrae. The net result is a loss of function on one half of the spinal cord.

High Cervical Cord Lesion
Injury to high cervical levels of the spinal cord is, in general, a catastrophic event. In addition to the potential for a total loss of sensation for the body below the lesion and of voluntary motor control below the lesion, there is another important complicating factor. The *phrenic nucleus* is located in the central regions of the anterior horn at levels C3 to C7. This cell group innervates the diaphragm and in high cervical lesions is disconnected from the centers of the medulla that control breathing. Consequently, in patients with high cervical lesions, preserving the ability to breathe becomes a major factor in care.

Acute Central Cervical Spinal Cord Syndrome
The *acute central cervical spinal cord syndrome,* commonly called the *central cord syndrome,* is an incomplete spinal cord injury. This may result from hyperextension of the neck (sometimes in a patient with bony spurs on the vertebrae) that momentarily occludes blood supply to the cord via the anterior spinal artery. Consequently, the deficits reflect the territory served by the branches of this vessel. The results are bilateral weakness of the extremities, more so of the upper than the lower, varying degrees and patterns of pain and thermal sensation loss, and bladder dysfunction. Many of these patients recover most or all of their function within 4 to 6 days. In general, function of the lower extremities returns first, bladder function next, and function of the upper extremities last. Pain and thermal sensations may return at any time, and posterior column sensations are not affected in these patients.

Variations on these main themes may occur. For example, a spinal cord hemisection at T8 would affect the body below that level but would spare the upper trunk and upper extremity. A lesion involving the posterior columns bilaterally would result in proprioceptive and discriminative touch losses below the level of the lesion but would spare pain and thermal sensations. In our study of systems neurobiology we shall explore these and other examples of dysfunction resulting from spinal cord lesions.

Synopsis of Clinical Points

- Rachischisis occurs when the neural folds do not join and neuroectoderm remains exposed (p. 144).
- Failure of the vertebral column to develop properly around the spinal cord may result in spina bifida occulta or spina bifida cystica (p. 144).
- The spinal cord is a narrow-diameter structure conveying all ascending and descending information between the body and the brain; damage to the spinal cord may result in catastrophic deficits or death (pp. 143–144).
- Fibers conveying pain and thermal sensations enter the lateral division of the posterior root (pp. 144, 149).
- Fibers conveying proprioception, position sense, and vibratory sense enter the medial division of the posterior root (pp. 144, 149).
- Damage to, or avulsion of, the posterior roots may result in deafferentation pain consisting of dull aching, pins-and-needles, or burning sensations from the affected extremity (p. 150).
- Deafferentation pain may be relieved in most patients by a posterior root entry zone procedure (p. 150).
- Myasthenia gravis is a disease of the neuromuscular junction with characteristic signs and symptoms (p. 151).
- Myasthenia gravis presents as a triad: fluctuating muscle weakness, eye muscle weakness, and rapid response to certain medications (p. 151).
- Muscle stretch reflexes test the integrity of afferent and efferent fibers of the spinal nerve (pp. 151–152).
- Spinal reflexes are valuable measurers of the viability of the spinal nerve and of the spinal cord (p. 152–153).
- Intervertebral disc disease is the most common cause of radiculopathy (p. 153).
- Mononeuropathy is damage to an anatomically defined peripheral nerve; carpal tunnel syndrome is an entrapment mononeuropathy (p. 153).
- Polyneuropathy is damage to multiple peripheral nerves; a common cause of polyneuropathy is diabetes mellitus (pp. 153–154).
- A polyneuropathy may produce a stocking/glove sensory loss (p. 153–154).
- A Brown-Séquard syndrome (spinal cord hemisection) results in alternating sensory losses and an ipsilateral paralysis below the lesion (p. 156).
- A small syringomyelia damages the fibers of the anterior white commissure and results in a bilateral loss of pain and thermal sensations (p. 156).
- Trauma to high cervical cord levels may damage the phrenic nucleus and nerve, resulting in paralysis of the diaphragm (p. 157).
- Acute central cervical cord injury may result in deficits that eventually resolve with few or no deficits (p. 157).

Sources and Additional Reading

Brown AG: Organization in the Spinal Cord: The Anatomy and Physiology of Identified Neurons. Berlin, Springer-Verlag, 1981.

Dado RJ, Katter JT, Giesler GJ: Spinothalamic and spino-hypothalamic tract neurons in the cervical enlargement of rats: I. Locations of antidromically identified axons in the thalamus and hypothalamus. J Neurophysiol 71:959-980, 1994.

Quencer RM, Bunge RP, Egnor M, Green BA, Puckett W, Naidich TP, Post MJD, Norenberg M: Acute traumatic central cord syndrome: MRI-pathological correlations. Neuroradiology 34:85-94, 1992.

Rexed B: The cytoarchitectonic organization of the spinal cord in the cat. J Comp Neurol 96:415-495, 1952.

Rexed B: A cytoarchitectonic atlas of the spinal cord in the cat. J Comp Neurol 100:297-379, 1954.

Schoenen J, Faull RLM: Spinal cord: Cytoarchitectural, dendroarchitectural, and myeloarchitectural organization. In Paxinos G (ed): The Human Nervous System. San Diego, Academic Press, 1990, pp 19-53.

Willis WD: The pain system, the neural basis of nociceptive transmission in the mammalian nervous system, vol 8. In Gildenberg PL (ed): Pain and Headache. Basel, S Karger, 1985.

Willis W, Coggeshall RE: Sensory Mechanisms of the Spinal Cord, 2nd ed. New York, Plenum Press, 1991.

Yezierski RP: Spinomesencephalic tract: Projections from the lumbosacral spinal cord of the rat, cat, and monkey. J Comp Neurol 267:131-146, 1988.

Chapter 10

An Overview of the Brainstem

D. E. Haines and G. A. Mihailoff

The term *brainstem* (sometimes written *brain stem*) is used in two ways: it can mean either the portion of the brain that consists of the medulla oblongata, pons, and midbrain or the portion that consists of these structures plus the diencephalon. This book follows the former convention. For our purposes, therefore, *the brainstem consists of the rhombencephalon (excluding the cerebellum) and the mesencephalon*. These regions of the brainstem all share a basic organization, which is the topic of this chapter. The medulla, pons, and midbrain are discussed in detail in Chapters 11 to 13.

Basic Divisions of the Brainstem

Medulla Oblongata
At about the level of the foramen magnum, the spinal cord merges into the most caudal portion of the brain, the *medulla oblongata* or *myelencephalon*, commonly called the medulla. The foramen magnum marks the approximate location of the *motor (pyramidal) decussation of the medulla* (Fig. 10-1A). The medulla is slightly cone shaped and enlarges in diameter as it extends rostrally from the medulla–spinal cord junction toward the pons-medulla junction. On the posterior (dorsal) aspect of the medulla-pons continuum, this junction is represented by the caudal edge of the middle and inferior cerebellar peduncles, whereas anteriorly (ventrally), this border is formed by the caudal edge of the basilar pons (Fig. 10-1).

The cranial nerves associated with the medulla include the *hypoglossal* (XII, motor) and parts of the *accessory* (XI, motor), *vagus* (X, mixed), and *glossopharyngeal* (IX, mixed) *nerves* (Fig. 10-1A). The nuclei of the hypoglossal, vagal, and glossopharyngeal nerves are located in the medulla as well as portions of the nuclei of the trigeminal nerve.

The *abducens* (VI, motor), *facial* (VII, mixed), and *vestibulocochlear* (VIII, sensory) *nerves* are frequently called the *cranial nerves of the pons-medulla junction* because they exit the brainstem at this particular location (Fig. 10-1A).

Although the medulla does not have regions that are specifically regarded as tegmental or basilar (as is the case for the pons and midbrain), it does have regions that function in the same way and are rostrally continuous with these respective regions of the pons (Fig. 10-2). For example, the central regions of the medulla contain all the cranial nerve nuclei affiliated with the medulla and this medullary area is rostrally continuous with the tegmental area of the pons, which contains all of the cranial nerve nuclei associated with this latter portion of the brainstem. In similar manner, the pyramids of the medulla (containing corticospinal fibers) are located on the anterior ("basal") aspect of the medulla and are rostrally continuous into the basilar pons (Fig. 10-2).

Pons
The pons (the anterior part of the *metencephalon*) extends from the pons-medulla junction to an imaginary line drawn from the exit of the trochlear nerve posteriorly to the rostral edge of the basilar pons anteriorly (Fig. 10-1). What we commonly call the pons is actually composed of two portions, the *pontine tegmentum* (located internally; see Fig. 10-1) and the *basilar pons*. This latter structure is bulbous and quite characteristic of the anterior aspect of the pons. The pontine tegmentum contains portions of the trigeminal nuclei and the vestibular nuclei and, just rostral to the pons-medulla junction, the facial motor nucleus, superior salivatory nucleus, and abducens nucleus. The *trigeminal nerve* (V, mixed) emerges from the lateral aspect of the pons, and *abducens* (VI), *facial* (VII), and *vestibulocochlear* (VIII) nerves exit at the pons-medulla junction (Fig. 10-1A).

The cerebellum, although part of the metencephalon, is *not* part of the brainstem. It is joined to the brainstem by three large, paired bundles of fibers called the *cerebellar peduncles*. These are the *inferior cerebellar peduncle*, the *middle cerebellar peduncle* (or *brachium pontis*), and the *superior cerebellar peduncle* (or *brachium conjunctivum*), connecting the cerebellum to the medulla oblongata, basilar pons, and midbrain, respectively.

Midbrain
The *midbrain (mesencephalon)* extends rostrally from the pons-midbrain junction to join the diencephalon (thalamus). This latter interface is usually described as a line drawn from the posterior commissure posteriorly to the caudal edge of the

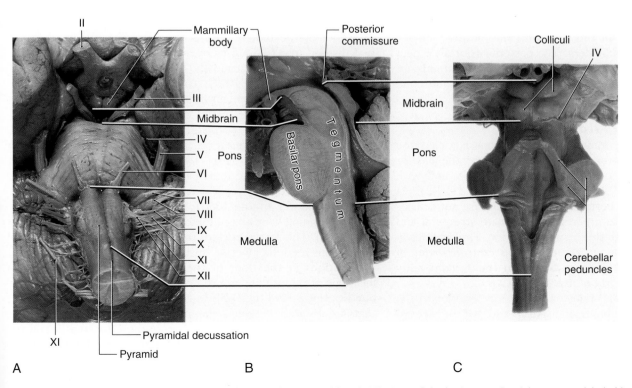

Figure 10-1. Anterior (ventral) (**A**), midsagittal (**B**), and posterior (dorsal) (**C**) views of the brainstem. Cranial nerves are labeled by their corresponding Roman numerals. In **C**, the cerebellum is removed to expose the posterior surface of the brainstem and the fourth ventricle.

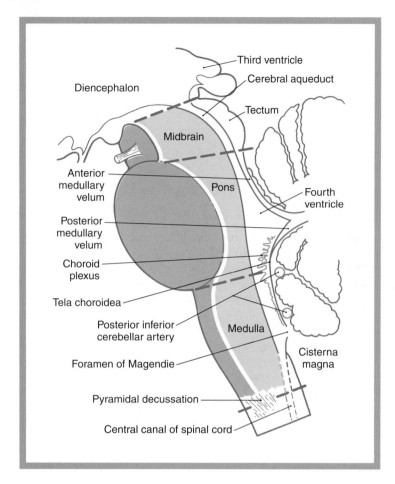

Figure 10-2. Midsagittal drawing of the brainstem. Ventricular spaces of the brainstem are outlined in *green*. The *tegmental* and *basilar areas* and *contiguous areas of the medulla* are shown in *light and dark gray,* respectively. Compare with Figure 10-1*B*.

mammillary bodies anteriorly (Fig. 10-1B). The *oculomotor nerve* (III, motor) exits the anterior aspect of the midbrain, whereas the *trochlear nerve* (IV, motor) exits its posterior aspect (Fig. 10-1A, C). The exit of the trochlear nerve is generally regarded as the junction of the pons with the midbrain on the posterior aspect of the brainstem. The posterior (dorsal) aspect of the midbrain is characterized by the *superior and inferior colliculi* and the anterior (ventral) aspect by the *crus cerebri* and *interpeduncular fossa.*

Tegmental and Basilar Areas
The central core of the midbrain and the pons is called the *tegmentum,* and their anterior (ventral) parts are the *basilar areas.* These regions are continuous with each other and with comparable areas of the medulla (Figs. 10-1B and 10-2). As noted earlier, the central portions of the medulla are not considered part of the tegmentum per se but do share structural and functional similarities with this brainstem region. The *tegmentum of the pons and midbrain* and the *contiguous central portion of the medulla contain ascending and descending tracts, many relay nuclei, and the nuclei of cranial nerves III to XII.*

The basilar part of each brainstem division is anterior to the tegmentum (of the midbrain and pons) and to the central portion of the medulla (Fig. 10-2). Consequently, these basilar structures also form a rostrocaudal continuum. Basilar structures of the brainstem include the descending fibers of the *crus cerebri* (midbrain), *basilar pons,* and *pyramid* (medulla) and specific populations of neurons in the midbrain and pons that originate from the alar plate of the embryonic brain.

Ventricular Spaces of the Brainstem

The ventricular spaces of the brainstem are the cerebral aqueduct in the mesencephalon and the fourth ventricle in the rhombencephalon (Fig. 10-2). The *cerebral aqueduct* is a narrow channel, 1 to 3 mm in diameter, that connects the third ventricle (the cavity of the diencephalon) with the fourth ventricle (the rhomboencephalic cavity). The cerebral aqueduct contains no choroid plexus; its walls are formed by a continuous mantle of cells collectively called the *periaqueductal gray.* The roof of the midbrain is the *tectum.*

The *fourth ventricle* is the cavity of the *rhombencephalon.* Its rostral portion lies between the pons and cerebellum, and its caudal part is located in the medulla (Fig. 10-2). The fourth ventricle is continuous rostrally with the cerebral aqueduct and caudally with the central canal of the caudal medulla and cervical spinal cord. It also communicates with the subarachnoid space via three openings: the midline *foramen of Magendie* and the two lateral *foramina of Luschka.* The foramen of Magendie is located in the caudal roof of the ventricle and opens into the *dorsal cerebromedullary cistern (cisterna magna)* (Fig. 10-2). The foramina of Luschka are located at the ends of the lateral recesses of the fourth ventricle and open into the subarachnoid space at the cerebellopontine angles (see Fig. 6-9). The *lateral recesses* are funnel-shaped portions of the fourth ventricle that extend around the brainstem at the pons-medulla junction (Fig. 10-4; see also Fig. 6-9).

The roof of the fourth ventricle is formed mainly by the *anterior* (or *superior*) *medullary velum* rostrally, by the thin membranous *tela choroidea* caudally, and by a small part of the cerebellum in the middle (Figs. 10-1B and 10-2). From rostral to caudal, the walls of the fourth ventricle are formed by the superior cerebellar peduncles, the middle and inferior cerebellar peduncles, and the attachment of the tela choroidea to the medulla (Figs. 10-3 and 10-4). The tela arises from the inferior surface of the cerebellum and sweeps caudally to attach to the "V"-shaped edges of the medullary portion of the ventricular space. The choroid plexus of the fourth ventricle is suspended from the inner surface of the tela, and parts of it protrude outward through the foramina of Luschka (see Figs. 6-4 and 6-9).

Rhomboid Fossa
The floor of the fourth ventricle is called the *rhomboid fossa.* It is divided into two halves by a deep *median sulcus,* and each half is traversed rostrocaudally by a groove called the *sulcus limitans* (Figs. 10-3 to 10-6). There are two slight depressions along the course of the sulcus limitans, somewhat like deep spots within this sulcus. The rostral depression, the *superior fovea,* is laterally adjacent to the *facial colliculus,* and the caudal depression, the *inferior fovea,* is laterally adjacent to the *vagal and hypoglossal trigones* (Figs. 10-3 and 10-4). In some surgical procedures involving the fourth ventricle or medulla, the sulcus limitans and foveae represent important landmarks. The *striae medullares* of the fourth ventricle are a series of fiber bundles running from the midline laterally into the lateral recess (Fig. 10-4). The rostral edge of these fibers is generally regarded as the pons-medulla junction in the floor of the fourth ventricle.

Elevations in the floor of the fourth ventricle indicate the locations of underlying cranial nerve nuclei and associated fiber bundles (Figs. 10-4 to 10-6). In general, the cranial nerve nuclei that are located between the median sulcus and the sulcus limitans are motor in function whereas those located lateral to the sulcus are sensory in function (Figs. 10-5 and 10-6). Medial to the sulcus limitans, the *hypoglossal* and *vagal trigones* represent the underlying *hypoglossal* and *dorsal motor vagal nuclei.* In the caudal pontine region, the *facial colliculus,* located medial to the sulcus limitans, marks the location of the underlying

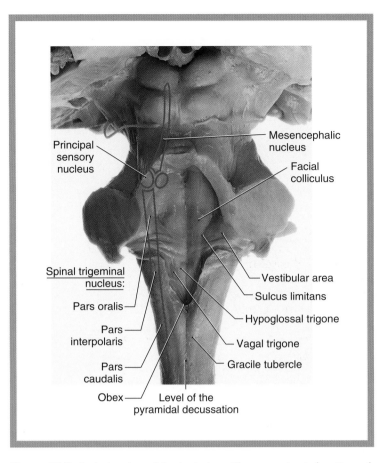

Figure 10-3. Posterior view of the brainstem. The approximate locations of the trigeminal nuclei are shown. The cerebellum is removed to expose the posterior aspect of the medulla and midbrain and the rhomboid fossa. The trigeminal motor nucleus, located medial to the principal sensory nucleus, is not labeled.

abducens motor nucleus and the *internal genu* of the facial nerve. Lateral to the sulcus limitans in the medulla and caudal pons is a flattened region called the *vestibular area*, which marks the location of the *vestibular nuclei.*

Cranial Nerve Nuclei and Their Functional Components

Cranial nerves, like spinal nerves, contain sensory or motor fibers or a combination of these fiber types. These various fibers are classified on the basis of their embryologic origin or common structural and functional characteristics. Primary sensory fibers, somatic motor neurons, and preganglionic and postganglionic visceromotor neurons that exhibit "... like anatomical and physiological characters so that they ... act in a common mode..." (Herrick) are classified as having a specific *functional component.* For example, fibers conveying sharp pain, a specific type of input, from widely separated body parts (the foot, hand, and face) have the same functional component. This principle, already introduced in relation to spinal nerves (see Chapter 9), is also directly applicable to cranial nerves.

Early in development, the rostrocaudally oriented cell columns forming the alar and basal plates of the spinal cord essentially extend throughout the brainstem. As development progresses, maturing neurons in alar and basal plates begin to migrate to form their adult structures, and the caudocephalic continuity of the cell columns may be disrupted. In this respect, *the primitive cell column retains its relative position as it differentiates, but it may become discontinuous as the individual nuclei derived from the same column are formed* (Figs. 10-5 and 10-7). Motor nuclei of cranial nerves arise from basal plate neurons, whereas the nuclei that receive primary sensory input via cranial nerves originate from the alar plate.

In the caudal medulla, the rostral continuation of the central canal is small; therefore, basal and alar plates are located anterior and posterior, respectively, to this space (Fig. 10-5). As the fourth ventricle flares open *at the level of the obex,* the alar plate shifts laterally and the basal plate retains an anterior (and now

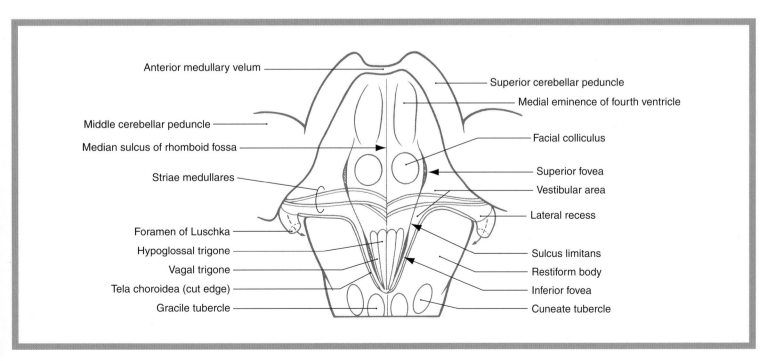

Figure 10-4. The rhomboid fossa (floor of the fourth ventricle), elevations and depressions in the floor, and structures bordering on the fossa. Compare with Figures 10-1C and 10-3. (From Haines DE: Neuroanatomy: An Atlas of Structures, Sections, and Systems, 5th ed. Baltimore, Lippincott Williams & Wilkins, 2000.)

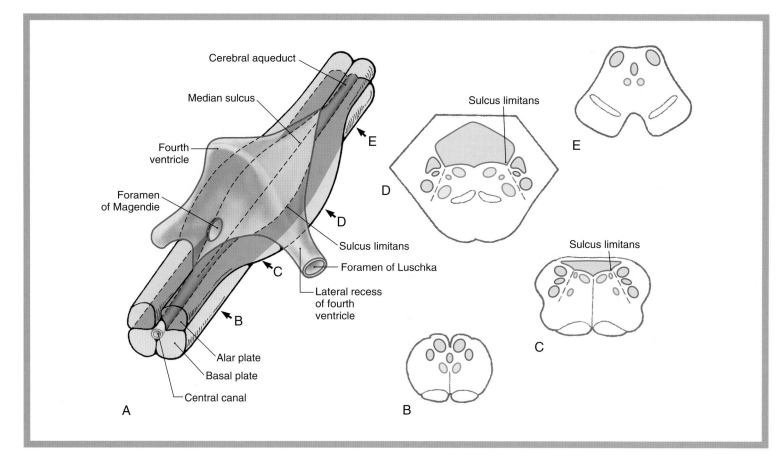

Figure 10-5. Diagram showing the alar and basal plates in relation to the ventricular spaces. The alar plates shift laterally (**A**), where the fourth ventricle flares open at the obex, and then shift back to a posterior position, where the ventricle funnels into the cerebral aqueduct. The position of structures derived from the alar and basal plates in relation to the sulcus limitans and the ventricular space is shown for the medulla (**B, C**), the pons (**D**), and the midbrain (**E**).

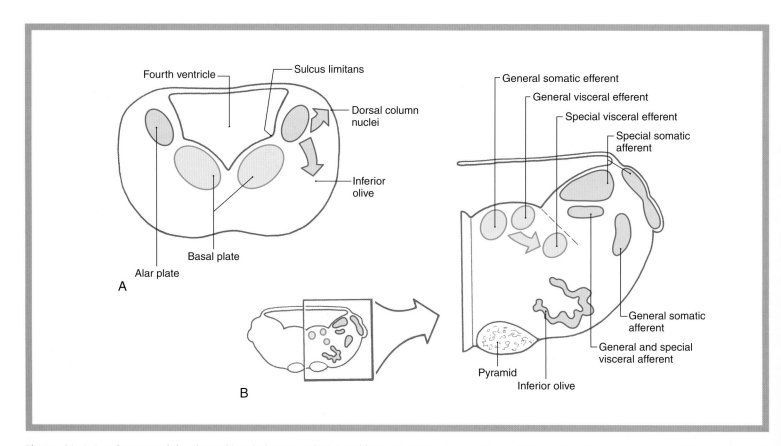

Figure 10-6. Development of the alar and basal plates at early (**A**) and later (**B**) stages, showing their relation to functional components of the cranial nerve nuclei in the brainstem.

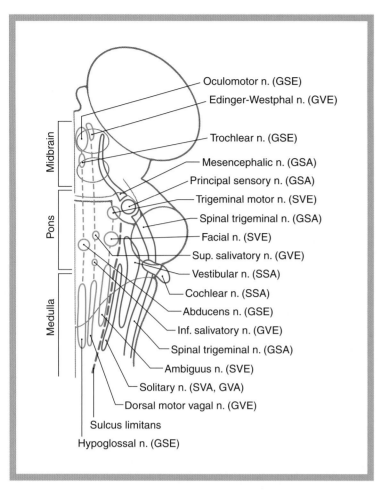

Figure 10-7. Diagram showing the cranial nerve nuclei of the brainstem and their functional components in the brainstem. The various nuclei are unrolled onto a single plane (see also Fig. 10-5B) with basal plate derivatives *(red)* and alar plate derivatives *(blue)* located medially and laterally, respectively, to the sulcus limitans. GSE, general somatic efferent; GVE, general visceral efferent; SVE, special visceral efferent; GSA, general somatic afferent; SSA, special somatic afferent; GVA, general visceral afferent; SVA, special visceral afferent.

and 10-7). The skeletal muscles innervated by these motor neurons originate from occipital myotomes (tongue musculature) and from mesenchyme in the immediate area of the orbit (extraocular muscles); therefore, their functional component is *general somatic efferent* (GSE) (Fig. 10-8). In addition, maturing neurons in the cervical spinal cord innervate muscles that originate from mesenchyme caudal to the fourth arch. These neurons form the accessory nucleus, and the mesenchyme differentiates into the trapezius and sternocleidomastoid muscles. The functional component of these cells is also *general somatic efferent* (GSE) (Fig. 10-8).

Lateral to the GSE cell groups, a second population of neuroblasts forms the *dorsal motor vagal nucleus, inferior salivatory nucleus, superior salivatory nucleus,* or the *Edinger-Westphal (visceromotor) nucleus* (Figs. 10-6 and 10-7). Because the axons of these cells synapse in peripheral ganglia that, in turn, innervate smooth muscle, cardiac muscle, or glandular epithelium, the functional component of these motor neurons is *general visceral efferent* (GVE) (Fig. 10-8).

The third set of cranial nerve motor nuclei to originate from the basal plate is represented by neuroblasts that migrate anterolaterally in the brainstem to form the *nucleus ambiguus,* the *facial nucleus,* or the *trigeminal motor nucleus* (Figs. 10-6 to 10-8). These motor neurons innervate skeletal muscles that originate from the pharyngeal arches rather than from occipital myotomes or head mesenchyme. Consequently, their functional component is *special visceral efferent* (SVE). An easy way to relate a specific pharyngeal arch with its appropriate cranial nerve and motor nucleus and with the muscles that are derived from that specific arch is shown in Table 10-1. Basically, *arches 1, 2, 3, and 4 correlate respectively with cranial nerves 5, 7, 9, and 10 (and their respective motor nuclei);* the specific muscles, having been mastered in gross anatomy, easily fall into this plan. These muscles are listed in Table 10-1.

Simultaneous with these developments in the basal plate, the alar plate gives rise to cell groups within the brainstem that receive sensory input via cranial nerves. Taste (*special visceral afferent* [SVA]) and *general visceral afferent* (GVA) sensations, such as pain from the gut, enter the brainstem with cranial nerves VII, IX, and X. The central processes of these sensory fibers form the *solitary tract* and end in the surrounding *solitary nucleus* (Figs. 10-7 and 10-8). Consequently, the functional components SVA and GVA are associated with these sensory fibers, which enter the solitary nucleus and tract. In a very real sense, the solitary tract and nucleus represent *the visceral center of the brainstem.* Regardless of which cranial nerves (VII, IX, X) convey visceral afferent information into the brainstem, that information terminates in the solitary nucleus.

The eighth cranial nerve, the vestibulocochlear, transmits signals concerned with balance, equilibrium, and hearing. These sensory fibers end in the *vestibular* and *cochlear nuclei* of the

medial) position (Figs. 10-5 and 10-6). Rostrally, as the fourth ventricle funnels into the cerebral aqueduct of the midbrain, the alar plate rotates back to a posterior position and the basal plate again assumes an anterior position (Fig. 10-5). The *sulcus limitans,* an embryologic landmark that persists in the medulla and pons of the adult, separates structures derived from the basal plate from those derived from the alar plate.

These points are clearly illustrated by first considering the basal plate. Some of these maturing neurons retain their position adjacent to the midline but become segmented into the *hypoglossal, abducens, trochlear,* or *oculomotor nuclei* (Figs. 10-6

Table 10-1. The Branchial Arches and Associated Cranial Nerves, Motor Nuclei, and Muscles as Related to the Special Visceral Efferent (SVE) Functional Component of the Brainstem

Arch	Cranial Nerve	Nucleus	Muscle(s) Innervated
1	Trigeminal (V)	Motor of the trigeminal nr.	Masticatory mus., tensor tympani, tensor veli palatini, mylohyoid, anterior belly of digastric
2	Facial (VII)	Motor of the facial nr.	Muscles of facial expression, stapedius, stylohyoid, posterior belly of digastric
3	Glossopharyngeal (IX)	Nucleus ambiguus	Stylopharyngeus
4	Vagus (X)	Nucleus ambiguus	Muscles of the pharynx (constrictors), palatopharyngeus, salpingopharyngeus, larynx (including the vocalis muscle, a medial portion of the thyroarytenoid mus.), striated muscle in upper two thirds of esophagus, and muscles of soft palate except tensor veli palatini

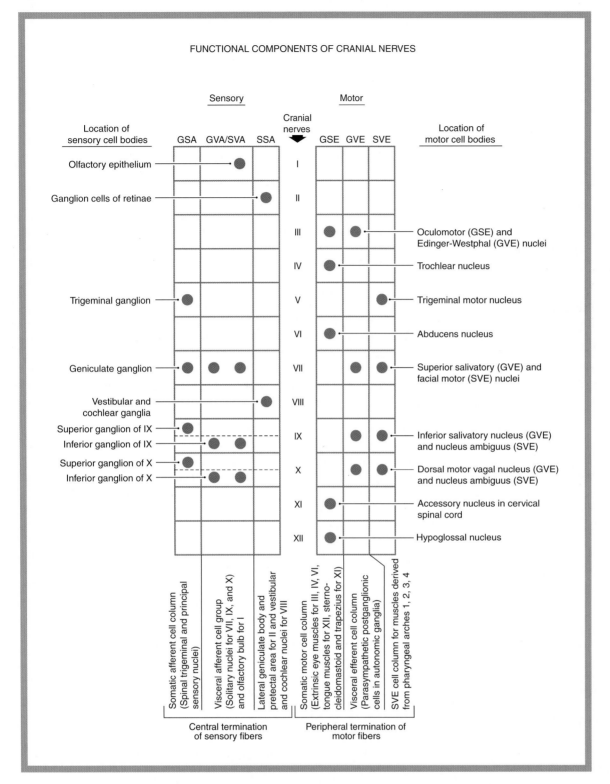

Figure 10-8. Functional components of the cranial nerves: The locations of sensory cell bodies and the targets of their central processes and the locations of the motor cell bodies and their peripheral targets.

medulla and pons, respectively (Figs. 10-6 and 10-7). Because of the unique embryologic origin of the peripheral receptors of these nerves, the functional component associated with these fibers and nuclei is *special somatic afferent* (SSA) (Figs. 10-7 and 10-8).

Sensory input from the face, oral cavity, and scalp to the apex of the head enters the brainstem via the trigeminal nerve. Centrally, many of these fibers enter the pons, turn caudally to form the *spinal trigeminal tract*, and synapse in the medially adjacent *spinal trigeminal nucleus* of the medulla. Others end in the *principal* sensory nucleus or ascend to form the *mesencephalic tract*. In the latter case the cell bodies form the immediately adjacent *mesencephalic nucleus*. Because these cell groups receive general sensory input, the functional component associated

with these fibers and nuclei is *general somatic afferent* (GSA) (Figs. 10-6 to 10-8). Just as the solitary tract and nucleus form the *visceral afferent center* of the brainstem, the spinal trigeminal tract and nucleus represent the main *somatic sensory center* of the brainstem. Even though four different cranial nerves (V, VII, IX, X) convey somatic sensory input into the brainstem, all of this type of information terminates in the spinal nucleus of V. The pattern of general somatic afferent information conveyed on these four nerves is especially useful in the diagnosis of the neurologically compromised patient.

The spinal trigeminal nucleus extends caudally from about midpontine levels to the spinal cord–medulla junction. On the basis of its cytoarchitecture and connections, the *spinal trigeminal nucleus* is divided into a *pars caudalis* (between the level of the cervical spinal cord and obex), a *pars interpolaris* (between the level of the obex and the rostral end of the hypoglossal nucleus), and a *pars oralis* (rostral to the level of the hypoglossal nucleus) (Fig. 10-3).

The blood supply to the brainstem originates from branches of the *vertebral* and *basilar arteries*. As we shall see in the next three chapters, branches of the vertebrobasilar system serve not only the medulla, pons, and most of the midbrain but also the entire cerebellum.

Herniation Syndromes Related to the Brainstem

The brainstem contains the nuclei of most of the cranial nerves, important nuclei that influence the spinal cord, heart rate and respiration, and all the ascending and descending tracts that connect the forebrain with the spinal cord. In this respect there are numerous clinical events that may arise in which damage to the brainstem causes deficits that may vary from mild to severe or may cause death, in some cases quite suddenly. These lesions will be explored in more detail in later sections in this text. At this point we briefly consider four herniation syndromes that are specifically related to the brainstem.

Herniation is best described as the protrusion of one anatomic structure into the territory of another (Figs. 10-9 and 10-10) with the result of causing *displacement, damage, destruction, and neurologic deficits*. In the case of the central nervous system, the causes of herniation are usually related to an increase in intracranial pressure (mass lesion—tumor; edema—brain swelling; large infarcts).

Central Herniation
Central herniation (also called *transtentorial herniation*) is the case in which a space-occupying lesion in the hemisphere (supratentorial compartment) elevates intracranial pressure and forces the diencephalon downward through the tentorial notch and into the brainstem (Fig. 10-9). Initially there may be a change in respiration, eye movements are irregular, and the pupils may be moderately dilated. As the damage progresses downward (caudally) into the brainstem there is significant change in

respiration (Cheyne-Stokes respiration with intermittent *tachypnea* and *apnea*), a profound loss of motor and sensory functions, and a probable loss of consciousness. This is a serious neurologic event and immediate measures should be taken to decrease intracranial pressure.

Uncal Herniation
The most common cause of *uncal herniation*, the movement of the rostromedial edge of the temporal lobe (the *uncus*) downward over the edge of the tentorium cerebelli (Fig. 10-10), is typically an expanding hemorrhagic lesion in the hemisphere. Uncal herniation initially compresses the midbrain, but if unchecked the damage may extend into lower brainstem levels. Early signs include a dilated pupil and abnormal eye movements (oculomotor nerve involvement) with double vision ipsilateral to the herniation followed by weakness of the extremities (corticospinal fiber involvement) opposite to the dilated pupil. As the herniation progresses, respiration is affected, abnormal reflexes appear, and there is a potentially rapid decline.

Upward Cerebellar Herniation
A mass in the posterior fossa may force portions of the cerebellum upward through the tentorial notch *(upward cerebellar herniation)* and compress the midbrain (Fig. 10-9). The result may be occlusion of branches of the superior cerebellar artery with resultant infarction of cerebellar structures and/or obstruction of the cerebral aqueduct and hydrocephalus. The latter is seen as signs characteristic of an increase in intracranial pressure (vomiting, headache, lethargy, decreased levels of consciousness).

Tonsillar Herniation
Pressure in the posterior fossa may force the cerebellar tonsils downward into, and possibly through, the foramen magnum; this is *tonsillar herniation* (Fig. 10-9). This may result in rapid compression of the medulla with a potentially catastrophic neurologic outcome. The medulla is damaged by mechanical compression/distortion and the vessels serving the medulla are simultaneously compressed and occluded. This vascular insult results in infarction of essential respiratory and cardiac centers in the medulla; there may be a rapid loss of respiration and a failure of medullary cardiac activity.

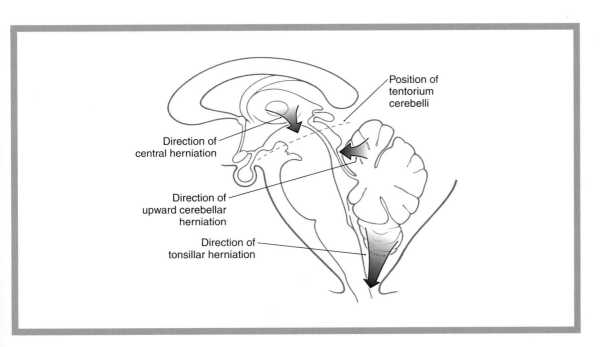

Figure 10-9. Median sagittal view of the thalamus, cerebellum, and brainstem, showing the general directions of central, upward cerebellar, and tonsillar herniations.

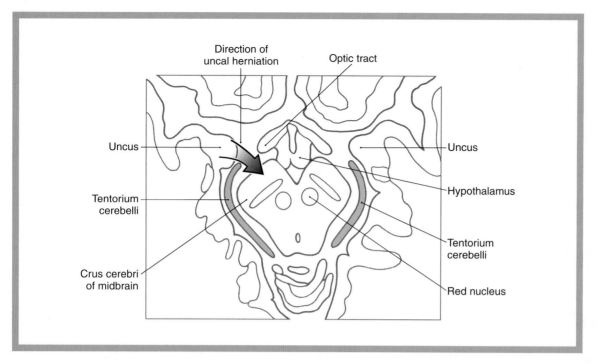

Figure 10-10. Axial view of the midbrain and its relationship to surrounding structures showing the direction of a herniation of the uncus over the edge of the tentorium cerebelli with consequent damage to the midbrain. Drawn from an MR image.

Synopsis of Clinical Points

- Most of the brainstem is located in the posterior cranial fossa and subject to tumors located in this confined area (pp. 159, 160).
- Nuclei of 9 of the 12 cranial nerves are located in the brainstem; brainstem lesions usually have cranial nerve signs/symptoms (pp. 159, 163).
- The ventricular spaces of the brainstem are the cerebral aqueduct and fourth ventricle (p. 160).
- Central herniation is the extrusion of portions of the forebrain downward through the tentorial notch; this is an extremely serious neurologic event (p. 165).
- Uncal herniation is when the uncus is forced over the tentorial edge and into the midbrain; if this is untreated it may result in a rapid decline (p. 165).
- Extrusion of the cerebellum through the tentorial notch is upward cerebellar herniation; this may damage the midbrain and result in hydrocephalus (p. 165).
- Tonsillar herniation is when the cerebellar tonsil is forced into the foramen magnum; compression of cardiac and respiratory medullary centers may be catastrophic (p. 165).

Sources and Additional Reading

Readings for the brainstem chapters are listed at the end of
   Chapter 13.

Chapter 11

The Medulla Oblongata
D. E. Haines and G. A. Mihailoff

The medulla oblongata, or *myelencephalon*, is the most caudal segment of the brainstem. It extends rostrally from the level of the foramen magnum to the pons. The cavity of the medulla consists of a narrow, caudal part, which is the continuation of the central canal of the cervical spinal cord, and a flared, rostral portion, which is the medullary part of the *fourth ventricle*. The modest size of the medulla (0.5% of total brain weight) belies its importance. All the tracts passing to or from the spinal cord traverse the medulla, and 7 of the 12 cranial nerves (VI to XII) are associated with the medulla or the pons-medullary junction. Also, the medullary reticular formation contains cell groups that influence heart rate and respiration. The blood supply to the medulla arises from branches of the *vertebral arteries*.

Development

The basic structural plan of the medulla is an elaboration of that seen in the spinal cord (Figs. 11-1 and 11-2). The basal and alar plates give rise to specific nuclei, and the surrounding mantle layer is invaded by axons originating from other levels. Beginning in the medulla, however, the basic derivatives of the primitive neural tube are augmented by the appearance of other structures that characterize each brainstem level.

Basal and Alar Plates

Maturing neurons of the *basal plate* of the medulla give rise to the *hypoglossal nucleus* (general somatic efferent [GSE] cells), the *dorsal motor vagal nucleus* and the *inferior salivatory nucleus* (both contain general visceral efferent [GVE] cells), and the nucleus ambiguus (special visceral efferent [SVE] cells) (Fig. 11-2). Caudal to the obex, the hypoglossal and dorsal motor vagal nuclei are quite small and are found in the central gray surrounding the central canal. Rostral to the obex, all of these nuclei are located medial to the sulcus limitans (Fig. 11-2B).

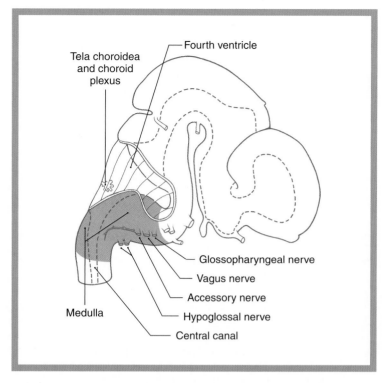

Figure 11-1. Lateral view of the brain at about 7 weeks of gestational age. The medulla is highlighted.

The cranial nerve nuclei derived from the *alar plate* in the medulla, and their corresponding functional components, include the *vestibular* and *cochlear nuclei* (special somatic afferent [SSA]), the *solitary nucleus* (general visceral afferent [GVA] and special visceral afferent [SVA]), and the *spinal trigeminal*

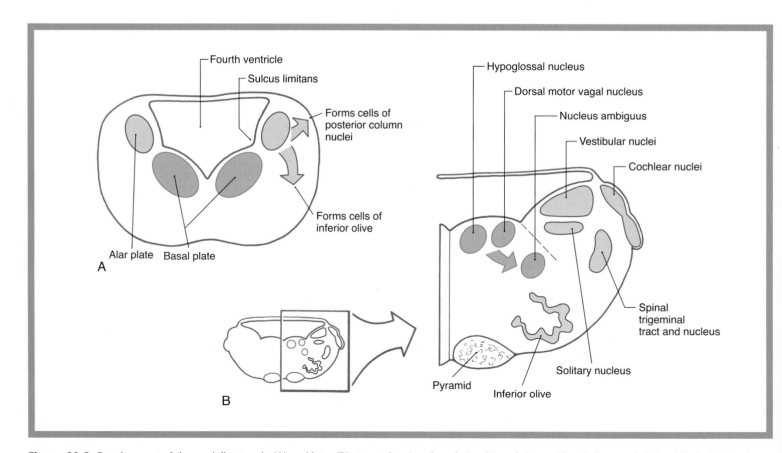

Figure 11-2. Development of the medulla at early (**A**) and later (**B**) stages showing the relationships of alar and basal plates and their adult derivatives in the medulla.

nucleus (general somatic afferent [GSA]) (Fig. 11-2). Alar plate neuroblasts caudal to the obex give rise to the *gracile* and *cuneate nuclei*. Rostral to the obex, some alar plate cells migrate ventromedially to form the nuclei of the *inferior olivary complex*.

Concurrent with these developmental events, ascending and descending fibers are traversing the medulla. An especially prominent bundle of axons collects on the anterior (ventral) surface of the medulla to form the *pyramids* (Fig. 11-2B).

External Features

Anterior Medulla

The anterior (ventral) aspect of the medulla is characterized by an *anterior median fissure*, two laterally adjacent longitudinal ridges, the *pyramids*, and the *olive (inferior olivary eminence)* (Fig. 11-3). The pyramids issue from the basilar pons and extend caudally to the *motor (pyramidal) decussation*, where about 90% of their fibers cross the midline. Most of the fibers that form the pyramid arise in the motor cortex as *corticospinal fibers*, consequently their crossing is frequently called the *motor decussation*. Rootlets of the *hypoglossal nerve* (cranial nerve XII) exit the medulla via the *preolivary sulcus*, a shallow groove located between the pyramid and the olive. The *abducens nerve* (cranial nerve VI) emerges at the pons-medullary junction, generally in line with the rootlets of cranial nerve XII.

Lateral Medulla

On the lateral aspect of the medulla, a shallow trough, the *postolivary sulcus*, is located between the *restiform body* and the large eminence formed by the underlying *inferior olivary nucleus* (Fig. 11-4A, B). Cranial nerves IX *(glossopharyngeal)*, X *(vagus)*, and the so-called medullary part of XI *(accessory)* emerge from the postolivary sulcus. In actuality the accessory nerve is made up of axons that arise from cells in the upper levels of the cervical spinal cord, ascend through the foramen magnum,

and then exit the skull via the jugular foramen along with the glossopharyngeal and vagus nerves. The *facial nerve* (VII), along with the *intermediate root* of the facial nerve (VIIi; see Chapter 12), and the *vestibulocochlear nerve* (VIII) emerge from the posterolateral medulla at the pons-medulla interface. The general region of the exit of the facial and vestibulocochlear nerves is clinically regarded as the *cerebellopontine angle*. Indeed, a *vestibular schwannoma* (sometimes, and incorrectly, referred to as an acoustic neuroma) is a tumor of the vestibular portion of the eighth cranial nerve and is a lesion located at the cerebellopontine angle. On the lateral medullary surface caudal to the level of the obex, fibers of the spinal trigeminal nucleus and tract assume a superficial location and form the *trigeminal tubercle (tuberculum cinereum)* (Fig. 11-4B, C). Rostral to the obex, these trigeminal fibers are located internal to a progressively enlarging *restiform body*.

Posterior Medulla

At and caudal to the level of the obex, the posterior surface of the medulla is characterized by the *gracile* and *cuneate fasciculi* and their respective *tubercles* (Fig. 11-4C). These tubercles are formed by the underlying *gracile* and *cuneate nuclei*. Rostro-lateral to the *gracile* and *cuneate tubercles* and forming a prominent elevation on the posterolateral aspect of the medulla is the *restiform body*. This structure contains a variety of afferent cerebellar fibers and becomes progressively larger as it extends toward the pons-medulla junction. In the caudal pons, fibers of the restiform body join with a much smaller bundle, the *juxtarestiform body*, to form the *inferior cerebellar peduncle*.

Vasculature

In general, the blood supply to the entire medulla and to the choroid plexus of the fourth ventricle arises from branches of the *vertebral arteries* (Fig. 11-16). The exceptions are the portion of the choroid plexus that extends out of the foramen of Luschka and the adjacent cochlear nuclei; these are served by branches

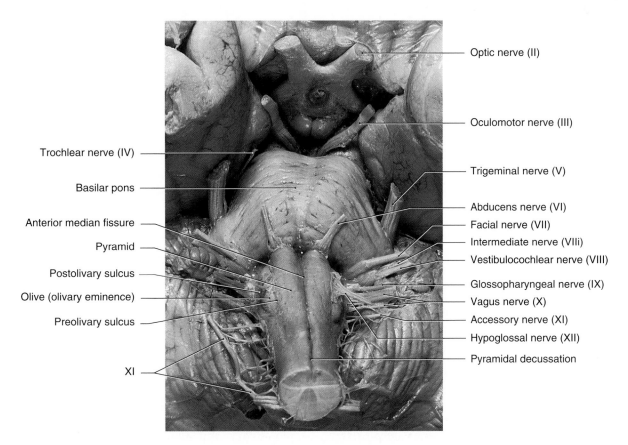

Figure 11-3. Anterior (ventral) view of the brainstem with emphasis on structures of the medulla.

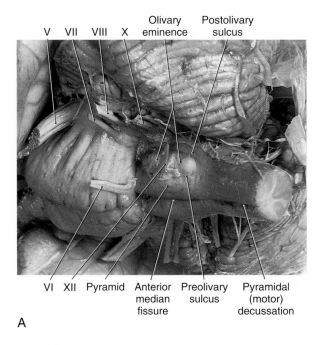

A

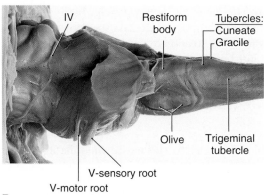

B

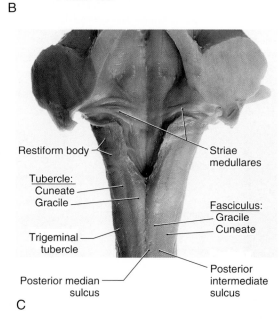

C

Figure 11-4. Anterolateral (**A**), lateral (**B**), and posterior (**C**) views of the medulla. Cranial nerves are indicated by Roman numerals, and the cerebellum has been removed from **B** and **C**. The same specimen is used in **B** and **C**.

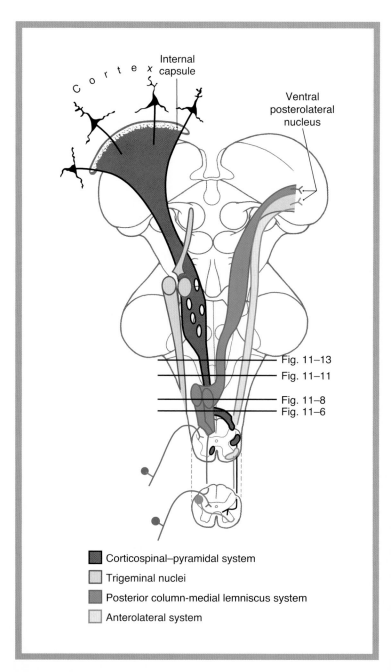

Corticospinal–pyramidal system

Trigeminal nuclei

Posterior column-medial lemniscus system

Anterolateral system

Figure 11-5. Diagram of the brain showing the location and trajectory of three important pathways and the trigeminal nuclei. The color coding for each is continued in Figures 11-6, 11-8, 11-11, and 11-13.

Internal Anatomy of the Medulla

Summary of Ascending Pathways

The ascending tracts that originate from the spinal cord gray matter (*anterolateral system, posterior* and *anterior spinocerebellar tracts*, and so on) and from posterior root ganglion cells (*gracile and cuneate fasciculi*) continue into the medulla (Fig. 11-5). Some anterolateral system fibers terminate in the medulla, as *spinoreticular fibers*, and others convey pain and temperature input to more rostral levels, including the thalamus as *spinomesencephalic* and *spinothalamic fibers*. Posterior column fibers synapse in the medulla, but the tactile and vibratory information carried by these fibers continues rostrally via the *medial lemniscus* (Fig. 11-5). Spinocerebellar axons enter the cerebellum through the restiform body (posterior tract) or the superior cerebellar peduncle (anterior tract). Other ascending bundles, such as *spino-olivary* and *spinovestibular* fibers, terminate in the medulla.

of the *anterior inferior cerebellar artery*, a branch of the basilar artery. In general, the medial medulla is served by the *anterior spinal artery*, the anterolateral medulla by small branches from the *vertebral artery*, and the posterolateral medulla rostral to the obex by the *posterior inferior cerebellar artery*. Caudal to the obex, the posterior medulla is served by the *posterior spinal artery*. The internal distribution of these vessels is discussed next.

Summary of Descending Pathways

The descending tracts that originate from the cerebral cortex (*corticospinal*; see Fig. 11-5) and from the midbrain (*rubrospinal, tectobulbospinal*), and pons (*reticulospinal, vestibulospinal*) traverse the medulla en route to the spinal cord. The medulla contributes additional fibers to the latter two fiber systems. At this level, the *medial longitudinal fasciculus* contains only descending fibers. The majority of these descending axons influence, either directly or indirectly through interneurons, the discharge patterns of motor neurons in the spinal cord gray matter.

Spinal Cord–Medulla Transition

The spinal cord–medulla transition is characterized by changes that begin at the caudal level of the *motor decussation* (Figs. 11-6 and 11-7). The spinal cord gray matter is replaced by the motor (crossing of corticospinal fibers) decussation; the central gray matter enlarges; the posterolateral tract (dorsolateral fasciculus) and substantia gelatinosa of the spinal cord merge, respectively, into the spinal trigeminal tract and nucleus; and nuclei characteristic of the medulla appear. The caudal medulla is described in the following sections beginning at the levels of the motor and sensory decussations.

Caudal Medulla: Level of the Motor Decussation

At the level of the *motor decussation (pyramidal decussation)*, about 90% of corticospinal fibers cross the anterior midline to form the contralateral *lateral corticospinal tract* of the cord (Figs. 11-5 to 11-7). Posteriorly, at this level the *gracile* and *cuneate nuclei* first appear in their respective fasciculi (Figs. 11-6 and 11-7). Because the *gracile* and *cuneate fasciculi* are collectively called the *posterior* (or *dorsal*) *columns*, their respective nuclei are frequently referred to as the *posterior column nuclei*. Laterally, the *spinal trigeminal tract* (visible on the surface of the medulla as the *trigeminal tubercle* or *tuberculum cinereum*) is located on the medullary surface. Internal to the spinal trigeminal tract is the *spinal trigeminal nucleus, pars caudalis* (Fig. 11-6).

The spinal trigeminal tract is composed of central processes of primary sensory fibers that enter the brain mainly in the trigeminal nerve. This tract also receives fibers that originate from cranial nerves VII, IX, and X. These primary sensory fibers terminate on cells of the spinal trigeminal nucleus, which, in turn, projects to the contralateral thalamus as the *anterior (ventral) trigeminothalamic tract*.

In the lateral medulla, the anterolateral system and *rubrospinal tract* are found medial to the superficially located *posterior* and *anterior spinocerebellar tracts* (Figs. 11-6 and 11-7). It is important to emphasize that anterolateral system fibers (conveying pain and temperature input from the contralateral side of the body) and spinal trigeminal tract fibers (conveying pain and temperature from the ipsilateral face) are located adjacent to each other throughout the lateral area of the medulla.

The anterior medulla contains the most rostral part of the *accessory nucleus* (cranial nerve XI), remnants of the medial motor cell column of C1, and the *medial longitudinal fasciculus* and *tectobulbospinal system*. The most rostral remnants of the *accessory nucleus* (cranial nerve XI) and the medial motor cell column of C1 are seen at the spinal cord/medulla junction but do not extend into the medulla. Immediately adjacent to these cell groups are the small fiber bundles of the *medial longitudinal fasciculus* and the *tectobulbospinal system* (Figs. 11-6 and 11-7). At this level, the tectospinal fibers in the tectobulbospinal system are incorporated into the medial longitudinal fasciculus. These small bundles are displaced laterally by the motor decussation compared with their medial positions at more rostral levels.

The *central gray* surrounds the central canal of the medulla and contains the caudal extremes of the hypoglossal (XII) and dorsal motor vagal nuclei (X) (Fig. 11-6). When the ventricle flares open at the level of the obex, these nuclei occupy the medial floor of the ventricular space.

Caudal Medulla: Level of the Sensory Decussation

Cells of the posterior column nuclei (gracile and cuneate nuclei) give rise to axons that swing anteromedially, as *internal arcuate fibers*, to cross the midline immediately rostral to the motor decussation (Fig. 11-5). This crossing of fibers at the midline constitutes the *sensory decussation*, so named because it is the point at which a major ascending sensory pathway (posterior column–medial lemniscus) crosses the midline.

At this level the posterior columns (gracile and cuneate fasciculi) are largely replaced by the *gracile* and *cuneate nuclei* (Figs. 11-8 and 11-9). Fibers conveying tactile and vibratory sensations from lower and upper levels of the body terminate,

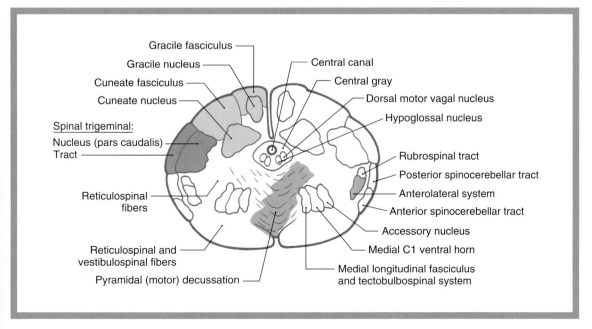

Figure 11-6. Cross section of the medulla at the level of the motor decussation. Correlate with Figure 11-5.

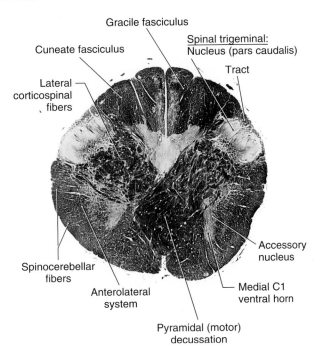

Figure 11-7. A fiber (myelin)-stained cross section of the medulla at the level of the motor decussation. Compare with Figure 11-6. (From Parent A: Carpenter's Human Neuroanatomy, 9th ed. Philadelphia, Lippincott Williams & Wilkins, 1995.)

The *spinal trigeminal tract* and *nucleus (pars caudalis)* maintain their position in the lateral medulla. The pars caudalis is that portion of the spinal trigeminal nucleus located caudal to the level of the obex. At this level, however, posterior spinocerebellar fibers have migrated posteriorly to cover the spinal tract, heralding the beginnings of the *restiform body* (Figs. 11-8 and 11-9). Just medial to the spinal trigeminal nucleus, a small column of motor neurons, the *nucleus ambiguus*, appears (Fig. 11-8). The axons of these SVE cells travel in the glossopharyngeal (IX) and vagus (X) nerves. Fibers of the *anterolateral system* and *rubrospinal tract* are located in the anterolateral medulla (Fig. 11-8). The *lateral reticular nucleus*, a distinct cell group adjacent to the anterolateral system, receives spinal input and projects to the cerebellum.

Structures characteristic of the anterior surface of the medulla at this level include the *pyramid*, fibers of the *hypoglossal nerve*, and the caudal end of the inferior olivary complex (Figs. 11-8 and 11-9). The inferior olivary nuclei (internal to the olivary eminence), which become larger at more rostral levels, receive input from a variety of areas and project primarily to the cerebellum. The inferior olivary nuclei are sometimes described as the *inferior olivary complex* since they collectively consist of *principal, medial accessory, and posterior accessory nuclei*. Internal to the pyramid, and along the midline from anterior to posterior, are the *medial lemniscus, tectobulbospinal fibers*, and *medial longitudinal fasciculus* (Fig. 11-8). At this level, medial longitudinal fasciculus fibers are characteristically found adjacent to the midline and anterior to structures of the central gray.

The *central gray* is larger than at the level of the motor decussation, and caudal parts of the *hypoglossal* and *dorsal motor vagal nuclei* and the *solitary nucleus* and *tract* can be clearly identified along its perimeter (Figs. 11-8 and 11-9). Hypoglossal (GSE) motor neurons innervate the ipsilateral half of the tongue. These fibers course anterolaterally along the lateral edge of the medial lemniscus and pyramid and share a common blood supply with these structures. The GVE cells of the dorsal motor vagal nucleus provide preganglionic parasympathetic fibers to visceromotor ganglia (autonomic ganglia), the postganglionic fibers of which innervate viscera in the thorax and abdomen. The *solitary tract* and *nucleus* receive GVA and SVA (taste) input from cranial nerves VII, IX, and X. At this caudal level of

respectively, in the gracile and cuneate nuclei. The axons of these cells, in turn, form the *internal arcuate fibers*, which cross the midline as the *sensory decussation* and collect to form the *medial lemniscus* on the contralateral side (Figs. 11-5, 11-8, and 11-9). Information from lower extremities (gracile cell axons) is conveyed in the anterior part of the medial lemniscus, and information from the upper extremities (cuneate cell axons) is conveyed in the posterior part of the medial lemniscus (see Fig. 12-13). The *accessory cuneate nucleus* is located lateral to the cuneate nucleus (Fig. 11-8). Its cells receive primary sensory input via cervical spinal nerves and project to the cerebellum as *cuneocerebellar fibers*. In doing so, they represent the upper extremity equivalent of the posterior spinocerebellar tract.

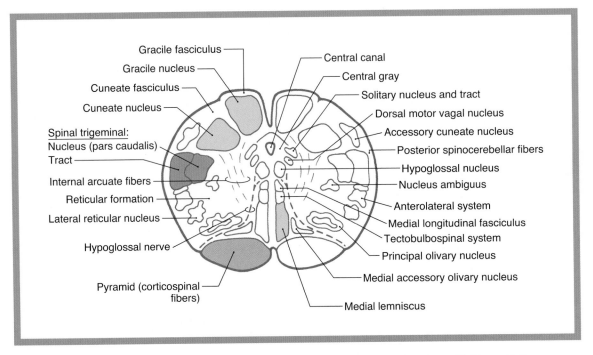

Figure 11-8. Cross section of the medulla at the level of the sensory decussation. Correlate with Figure 11-5.

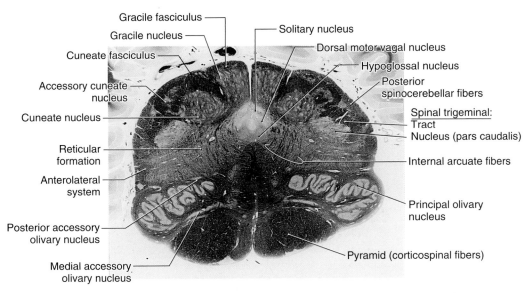

Figure 11-9. A fiber (myelin)-stained cross section of the medulla at the level of the sensory decussation. Compare with Figure 11-8.

the medulla, input to the solitary nucleus is primarily GVA in nature and originates mainly from thoracic and abdominal viscera (via cranial nerve X) and the carotid sinus (via cranial nerve IX).

The fourth ventricle flares open at the level of the *obex* (Fig. 11-10). The *area postrema* is an emetic (vomiting) center located in the wall of the ventricle at this level. Especially noticeable changes at this point compared with more caudal levels include enlargement of the inferior olivary complex and restiform body.

Midmedullary Level
Rostral to the obex, the structures in the medial floor of the fourth ventricle are the *hypoglossal* and *dorsal motor vagal nuclei* and, lateral to the *sulcus limitans*, the *vestibular nuclei* (Figs. 11-11 and 11-12). The latter cell groups consist, at this level, of *medial* and *inferior* (or *spinal*) *vestibular nuclei*. They receive input from cranial nerve VIII and interconnect with areas of the brain concerned with balance and eye movement. The *solitary tract* and *nucleus* occupy their characteristic position immediately inferior to the vestibular nuclei.

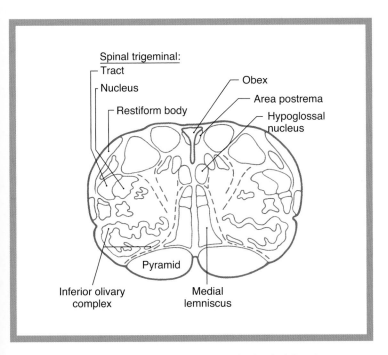

Figure 11-10. Cross section of the medulla at the level of the obex.

Laterally, the *restiform body* forms a prominent elevation on the posterolateral aspect of the medulla (Figs. 11-11 and 11-12). This structure contains *posterior spinocerebellar, cuneocerebellar, olivocerebellar, reticulocerebellar,* and other cerebellar afferents. In the base of the cerebellum, these fibers join with the *juxtarestiform body* to form the *inferior cerebellar peduncle*.

The *spinal trigeminal tract* and *nucleus (pars interpolaris)* are internal to the restiform body (Figs. 11-11 and 11-12). The pars interpolaris is the part of the spinal trigeminal nucleus located between the levels of the obex and the rostral end of the hypoglossal nucleus. Other structures in the lateral medulla are comparable to those seen more caudally. These include the *nucleus ambiguus* and the *lateral reticular nucleus* as well as the *anterolateral system, anterior spinocerebellar tract,* and *rubrospinal tract* (Fig. 11-11). At all medullary levels, neurons of the nucleus ambiguus contribute axons to cranial nerves IX and X, which innervate pharyngeal and laryngeal muscles, including those of the vocal folds.

Anterolaterally, the inferior olivary complex is prominent at midmedullary levels and is composed of a large, saccular *principal olivary nucleus* and diminutive *medial* and *posterior accessory olivary nuclei* (Figs. 11-11 and 11-12). These cell groups receive input from a variety of central nervous system nuclei and project primarily to the contralateral cerebellum (as *olivocerebellar fibers*) through the restiform body. Anteriorly and medially, the orientation of the *pyramid, medial lemniscus, medial longitudinal fasciculus,* and *tectobulbospinal system* remains essentially the same as at more caudal levels (Figs. 11-11 and 11-12).

Rostral Medulla and Pons-Medulla Junction
Comparison of Figures 11-11 and 11-13 shows that many of the structures seen in the mid medulla are present in essentially the same locations in the rostral medulla. Therefore, we shall emphasize the features that are different in the rostral medulla.

In the floor of the fourth ventricle, the positions occupied by the hypoglossal and dorsal motor vagal nuclei at more caudal levels are taken by the *prepositus (hypoglossal) nucleus* and the *inferior salivatory nucleus* (Fig. 11-13). The prepositus nucleus is a small, somewhat flattened cell group that is easily distinguished from the hypoglossal nucleus. The GVE cells of the inferior salivatory nucleus are located immediately inferior to the medial vestibular nucleus and medial to the solitary tract and nucleus. Axons of these salivatory nucleus cells distribute to the otic ganglion via peripheral branches of the glossopharyngeal nerve.

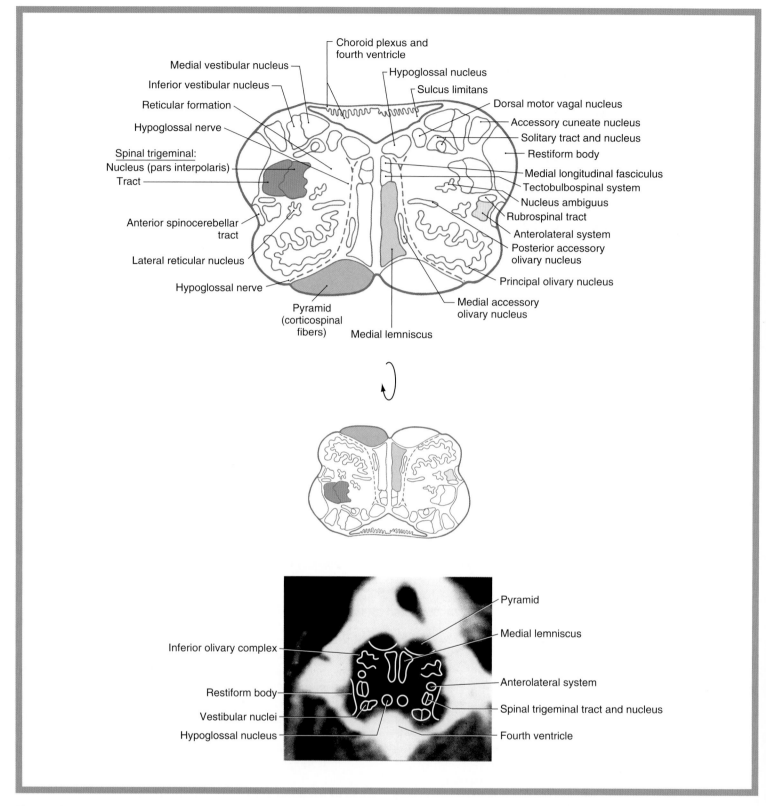

Figure 11-11. Cross section of the medulla at midolivary levels. Correlate with Figure 11-5. The anatomic orientation is flipped to illustrate internal structures in a clinical orientation; the clinically important tracts and nuclei are shown on a T2-weighted MR image at a comparable level of the mid medulla.

The *medial* and *inferior* (or spinal) *vestibular nuclei* are prominent at this level and are joined, in this plane of section, by the *posterior* and *anterior cochlear nuclei* (Figs. 11-12 and 11-13). The latter nuclei are located on the posterior and lateral aspects of the restiform body at the pons-medullary junction. The medial vestibular nucleus appears homogeneous in fiber-stained sections, and the inferior vestibular nucleus has a salt-and-pepper appearance (Fig. 11-12). This appearance results because small descending bundles of myelinated fibers (pepper) are intermingled with cells (salt) in the inferior nucleus. Medial to the restiform body is the spinal trigeminal tract and the *pars oralis* of the *spinal trigeminal nucleus* (Fig. 11-13). The pars oralis is that part of the nucleus located rostral to the level of the hypoglossal nucleus.

At this rostral level of the medulla, the *solitary tract and nucleus* retain their positions immediately inferior to the medial and inferior vestibular nuclei. However, in contrast to the more caudal parts of this nucleus (which receives mainly GVA input originating mainly from cranial nerves IX and X), this rostral portion of the nucleus receives primarily SVA (taste) input

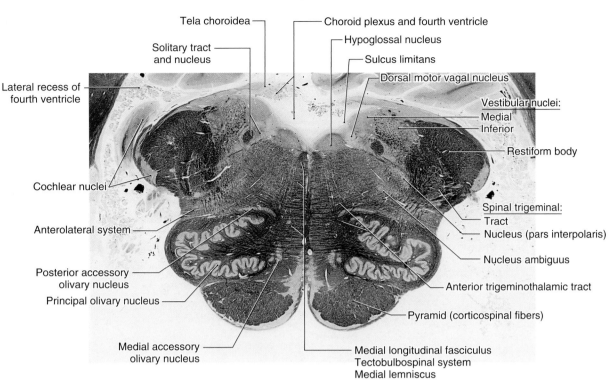

Tela choroidea
Choroid plexus and fourth ventricle
Hypoglossal nucleus
Solitary tract and nucleus
Sulcus limitans
Dorsal motor vagal nucleus
Lateral recess of fourth ventricle
Vestibular nuclei:
Medial
Inferior
Restiform body
Cochlear nuclei
Spinal trigeminal:
Tract
Nucleus (pars interpolaris)
Anterolateral system
Nucleus ambiguus
Posterior accessory olivary nucleus
Anterior trigeminothalamic tract
Principal olivary nucleus
Pyramid (corticospinal fibers)
Medial accessory olivary nucleus
Medial longitudinal fasciculus
Tectobulbospinal system
Medial lemniscus

Figure 11-12. A fiber (myelin)-stained cross section of the medulla at midolivary levels. This section is between the levels represented in Figures 11-11 and 11-13.

from nerves VII and IX. The solitary tract and nucleus do not extend craniad to the root of the facial nerve as this is the most rostral of the cranial nerves to contribute to these structures.

Although structures in anterior and medial areas of the medulla are unchanged from those at midmedullary levels, some changes take place at the pons-medullary junction that merit comment (Fig. 11-14). Fibers of the *restiform body* arch posteriorly to enter the cerebellum, where they are joined by fibers of the *juxtarestiform body* to form (collectively) the *inferior cerebellar peduncle*. The *facial motor nucleus* (SVE cells) appears anterolaterally, and the *trapezoid body* and *superior olivary nucleus* (both conveying auditory information) appear adjacent to the facial nucleus and the spinal trigeminal tract and nucleus (Fig. 11-14). The inferior olivary complex disappears, and the *central tegmental tract,* one source of input to the inferior olive, appears about where the latter cell group was located (Fig. 11-14). Finally, the *medial lemniscus* begins to shift anterolaterally and to rotate from a posteroanterior orientation, which it exhibits in the medulla, toward a horizontal orientation more characteristic of the pons (Fig. 11-14). At the pons-medulla junction, the cross section of the medial lemniscus is oriented obliquely (posteromedial to anterolateral); by the level of the mid pons, it is horizontal.

Reticular and Raphe Nuclei

The word *reticulum* is Latin for "little net" (diminutive of *rete,* "net") and denotes mesh-like structures. The *reticular nuclei* of the brainstem are diffuse and ill defined and have little apparent internal organization. Collectively, they make up the *reticular formation,* which may be thought of simply as including all of the cells that are interspersed among the more compact and named structures of the brainstem.

Raphe is a Greek word for "suture" or "seam." Thus, the *raphe nuclei* are bilaterally symmetrical cell groups in the brainstem that are located directly adjacent to the midline.

The *medial medullary reticular area* consists of the *central nucleus of the medulla* at caudal medullary levels and the *gigantocellular reticular nucleus* rostrally; the latter cell group extends

into the pons (Fig. 11-15). The *lateral medullary reticular area* contains a compact column of cells, the *lateral reticular nucleus,* and a diffuse population of cells that forms the *parvocellular nucleus* and the *ventrolateral reticular area* (area reticularis superficialis ventrolateralis) (Fig. 11-15). The latter cells function in the control of heart rate and respiration. Consequently, a sudden onset of *central apnea,* indicating damage to these respiratory areas, is often a prime early sign of medullary compression. The raphe nuclei of the medulla are the *nucleus raphes pallidus* and *nucleus raphes obscurus* and, at rostral levels, the *nucleus raphes magnus* (Fig. 11-15). The nucleus pallidus and nucleus obscurus are located at mid- to rostral medullary levels along the posterior and anterior midline, respectively. The nucleus raphes magnus begins in the rostral medulla and extends into the caudal pons (Fig. 11-15). In general, the raphe nuclei of the medulla and medulla-pons junction (magnus, pallidus, obscurus) project caudally to spinal cord targets. Cells of these raphe nuclei receive input from several areas, including the central gray of the mesencephalon, and project to the spinal cord. *Raphespinal* fibers from the raphe magnus are especially important for the inhibition of pain transmission in the posterior horn of the spinal cord. The principal neurotransmitter associated with these nuclei and their fibers is *serotonin,* although cholecystokinin-containing cells are also found in all three of these raphe nuclei and *enkephalin* is found in magnus neurons.

Internal Vasculature of the Medulla and Medullary Syndromes

The blood supply to the medulla arises from branches of the *vertebral arteries* (Fig. 11-16). These branches are the *anterior spinal artery* and the *posterior inferior cerebellar artery* (PICA). The *posterior spinal artery* is usually a branch of the PICA.

Medial structures of the medulla at all levels, including the pyramid, medial lemniscus, and hypoglossal nucleus and roots, are served by penetrating branches of the *anterior spinal artery* (Fig. 11-16). The branches of the anterior spinal artery that

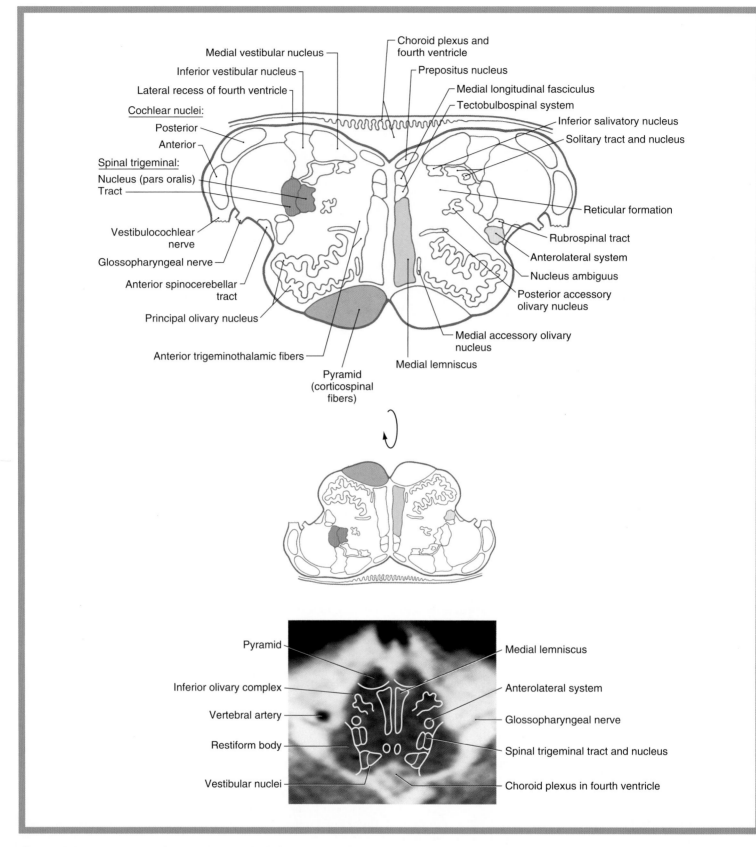

Figure 11-13. Cross section of the medulla at rostral olivary (and medullary) levels. Correlate with Figure 11-5. The anatomic orientation is flipped to illustrate internal structures in a clinical orientation; the clinically important tracts and nuclei are shown on a T2-weighted MR image at a comparable level of the rostral medulla.

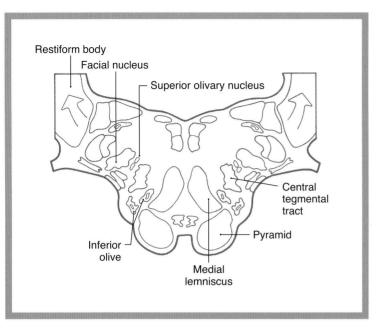

Figure 11-14. Cross section of the medulla at the pontomedullary junction. Fibers of the restiform body sweep up *(arrows)* into the cerebellum at this level.

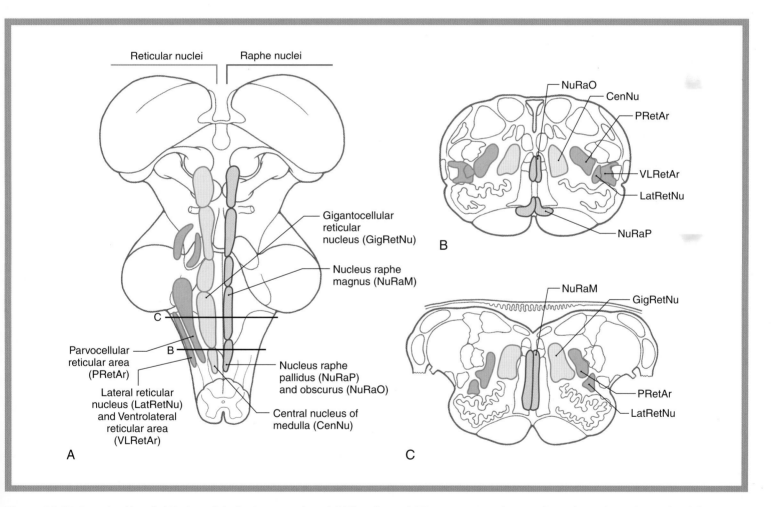

Figure 11-15. Posterior (dorsal) (**A**) view of the brainstem and caudal (**B**) and rostral (**C**) cross sections showing the raphe and reticular nuclei of the medulla.

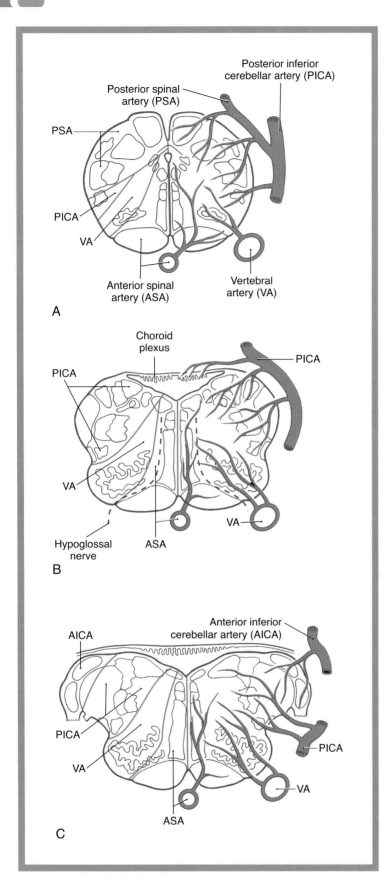

A

B

C

Figure 11-16. Blood supply of the medulla caudal to the obex (**A**), at midmedullary (**B**) and rostral medullary (**C**) levels. Arteries are shown on the *right,* and the territories served by each are indicated on the *left.*

penetrate into medial portions of the medulla tend to alternate to the right and left. Occlusion of these penetrating branches to one side of the medial medulla may result in a pattern of deficits characteristic of the *medial medullary syndrome.* This is also known as the *Dejerine syndrome.* The deficits and corresponding structures damaged in this syndrome include a contralateral hemiparesis (pyramidal and corticospinal damage), contralateral loss of proprioception and vibratory sense (medial lemniscus), and a deviation of the tongue to the ipsilateral side when protruded (hypoglossal root or nucleus injury). On the other hand, occlusion of the anterior spinal artery would result in bilateral deficits reflecting damage to both pyramids, both medial lemnisci, and both of the hypoglossal nuclei and/or their exiting roots.

The posterior medulla caudal to the obex is served by branches of the *posterior spinal artery* (Fig. 11-16A). Major structures in this area include the posterior column (gracile and cuneate) nuclei and the spinal trigeminal tract and nucleus. Although vascular lesions of the posterior spinal artery are rare, they may produce an ipsilateral loss of proprioception and vibratory sense on the body (damage to posterior columns and nuclei) coupled with an ipsilateral loss of pain and temperature sensation from the face (spinal trigeminal tract).

Rostral to the obex, the entire posterolateral medulla is served by branches of the *posterior inferior cerebellar artery* (PICA) (Figs. 11-16B, C and 11-17). Included in the territory served by this vessel are the anterolateral system, spinal trigeminal tract and nucleus, vestibular nuclei, solitary tract and nucleus, and nucleus ambiguus. Vascular insufficiency of the PICA (or blockage of one vertebral artery) gives rise to a characteristic set of sensory and motor deficits commonly called the *lateral medullary syndrome, PICA syndrome,* or *Wallenberg syndrome* (Fig. 11-17). The deficits seen and the corresponding structures involved are (1) contralateral loss of pain and temperature sensation from the body (anterolateral system), (2) ipsilateral loss of pain and temperature sensation from the face (spinal trigeminal tract and nucleus), (3) some vertigo and nystagmus (vestibular nuclei), (4) loss of taste from the ipsilateral half of the tongue (solitary tract and nucleus), and (5) hoarseness and dysphagia (nucleus ambiguus or roots of cranial nerves IX and X) (Fig. 11-17C). Patients with the lateral medullary syndrome may also have the *Horner syndrome,* owing to injury to hypothalamospinal fibers descending through the lateral areas of the medulla. We shall further explore the details of these clinical syndromes in later chapters.

In addition to this broad expanse of the medulla, branches of the PICA also serve the choroid plexus of the fourth ventricle. At the pons-medulla junction, the cochlear nuclei and a small adjacent part of the restiform body are served by branches of the *anterior inferior cerebellar artery* (Fig. 11-16C).

Tonsillar Herniation

Although the tonsil is a portion of the cerebellum, when this structure herniates (Fig. 11-18) it may have a profoundly negative impact on the medulla. The causes of tonsillar herniation vary, but examples include an expanding mass in the posterior fossa (tumor, hemorrhage), lumbar puncture in a patient with a mass lesion in a supratentorial or infratentorial location, or as a complication of surgery in the posterior fossa. In many cases *there is a rapid increase in intracranial pressure, or a shift in pressure, with an extrusion of the cerebellar tonsil downward into, and through, the foramen magnum.* This action impinges on the medulla (Fig. 11-18) and causes damage by two mechanisms. First, the medulla is rapidly compressed and distorted, causing mechanical injury. Second, concomitant with this compression,

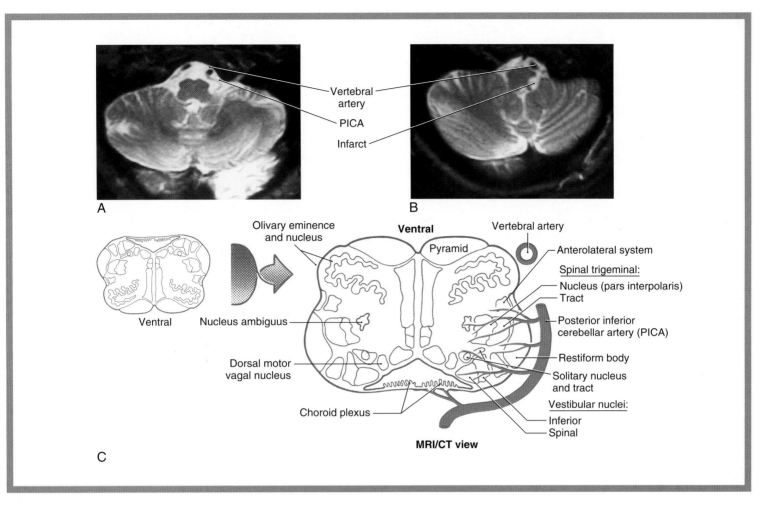

Vertebral artery

Figure 11-17. Lateral medullary (Wallenberg) syndrome. A normal MR image (**A**) shows the vertebral and posterior inferior cerebellar (PICA) arteries in relation to the medulla. The patient whose MR image is shown in **B** had an occlusion of the PICA, which resulted in an infarct of the territory of the medulla served by this vessel. The structures damaged in this lesion are shown in **C**. Compare with Figure 11-16.

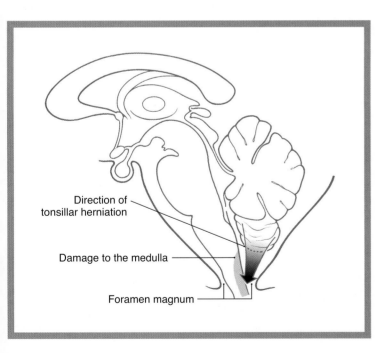

Figure 11-18. The principal herniation syndrome for the medulla is tonsillar herniation; the extrusion of the cerebellar tonsil into/through the foramen magnum. The *large arrow* indicates the route taken by the tonsil as it descends and the *shaded portion* of the medulla represents damage to this part of the brainstem.

the blood vessels serving the medulla are occluded, the medulla is deprived of oxygenated blood, and the affected area will become infarcted.

The major concern in acute herniation is damage to the *ventrolateral reticular area* of the medulla, which contains neurons that influence and control heart rate and respiration. The signs and symptoms include a sudden change in heart rate and respiration *(Cheyne-Stokes* with intermittent *apnea)*, increase in blood pressure *(hypertension)*, hyperventilation, rapidly decreasing levels of consciousness, and death. In some (chronic) cases the herniation may proceed slowly and while the medulla is deformed the patient suffers minimal neurologic consequences.

Synopsis of Clinical Points

- Six of the 12 cranial nerves exit from the medulla or medulla-pons junction; tumors in this confined space usually affect these nerves (pp. 168, 169).
- Lesions of the motor (pyramidal) decussation may result in bilateral weakness of the extremities (pp. 167, 171, 178).
- Deficits in the medial medullary (or Dejerine) syndrome reflect damage to the structures in this area; these deficits are ipsilateral deviation of the tongue, contralateral weakness of the extremities, and contralateral loss of proprioception/position sense (p. 178).
- Occlusion of the penetrating branches of the anterior spinal artery, or of the artery itself, may result in different patterns of deficits (p. 178).
- Deficits characteristic of the lateral medullary (or Wallenberg) syndrome may be seen following occlusion of the vertebral artery or of its major branch, the posterior inferior cerebellar artery (pp. 171, 178).
- Deficits in the lateral medullary syndrome reflect damage to structures in this area; these are an alternating hemianesthesia, vertigo, nystagmus, dysarthria, and dysphagia (p. 178).
- A rapidly expanding lesion in the fourth ventricle or lumbar puncture in a patient with a supratentorial mass may result in tentorial herniation (pp. 178, 179).
- Tonsillar herniation compresses the medulla and damages cardiac and respiratory centers (pp. 175, 178, 179).
- Cheyne-Stokes respiration and apnea are seen in patients with tonsillar herniation (pp. 175, 178, 179).

Sources and Additional Reading

Readings for the brainstem chapters are listed at the end of Chapter 13.

Chapter 12

The Pons and Cerebellum

G. A. Mihailoff and D. E. Haines

The *metencephalon* consists of the pons and cerebellum. The pons is the middle segment of the brainstem, the caudal part being the medulla and the rostral portion being the midbrain. Although comprising only about 1.3% of the brain by weight, the pons has many important functions. The motor and sensory nuclei and the exit points of cranial nerves V to VIII are associated with the pons. The *cerebellum is not part of the brainstem* but rather is considered a suprasegmental structure because it is located posterior to the brainstem. The cerebellum is comparatively large, comprising about 10.5% of the total brain weight. Functionally, the cerebellum is part of the motor system. The blood supply to the pons and cerebellum arises from branches of the basilar and cerebellar arteries.

Development

The pons and cerebellum are considered together in this chapter because they arise from the same region of the developing neural tube. The metencephalon extends from the pontine flexure to the mesencephalic isthmus (Fig. 12-1). At this level, the cavity of the neural tube is enlarged, forming the parts of the fourth ventricle associated with the pons and cerebellum.

Basal and Alar Plates

The *basal* and *alar plates* of the brainstem extend from the medulla rostrally into the developing pons. The cranial nerve *motor* nuclei found in the pons (trigeminal, abducens, facial, and superior salivatory) originate from the basal plate and are located medial to the sulcus limitans (Fig. 12-2A, B). The functional components of these motor neurons include *special visceral efferent* (SVE) (trigeminal and facial), *general somatic efferent* (GSE) (abducens), and *general visceral efferent* (GVE) (superior salivatory).

The cranial nerve *sensory* nuclei located in the pons include portions of the trigeminal and vestibulocochlear nuclei and the rostral tip of the solitary nucleus. These nuclei originate from the alar plate and are found lateral to the sulcus limitans (Fig. 12-2A, B). Their functional components are *general somatic afferent*

(GSA) for the trigeminal nucleus, *special somatic afferent* (SSA) for vestibular and cochlear nuclei, and *special* and *general visceral afferent* (SVA, GVA) for the solitary nucleus. The portion of the posterior pons that contains these motor and sensory nuclei, as well as the reticular formation and several ascending and descending tracts, is the *pontine tegmentum* (Fig. 12-2B).

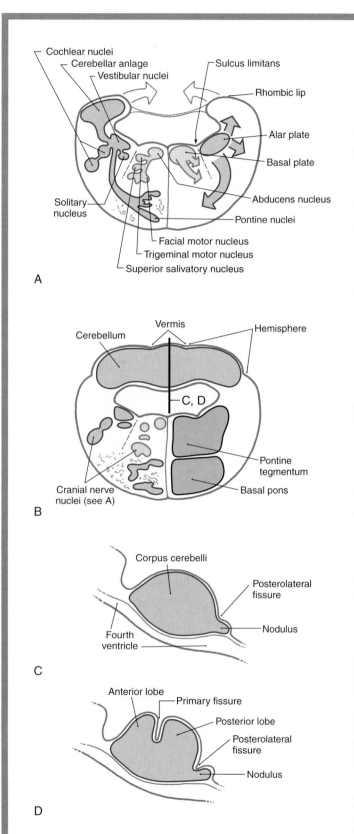

Figure 12-2. Development of the pons and cerebellum. The pontine alar and basal plates give rise to cranial nerve nuclei and the pontine nuclei, and the cerebellum originates from the rhombic lips (**A**, **B**). Sagittal views of the cerebellum (**C**, **D**; plane of section from **B**) show the relationships of posterolateral and primary fissures.

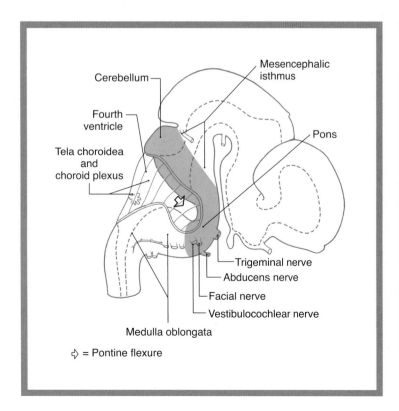

Figure 12-1. Lateral view of the brain at about 7 weeks of gestational age. The pons and cerebellum are highlighted.

The anterior area of the developing pons is invaded by large numbers of descending cortical fibers. Although some will terminate here, others pass through to more caudal targets. Immature neurons of the *alar plate* also migrate into this anterior pontine region to form the *basilar pontine nuclei*. These nuclei, their axons, and the descending fibers passing to and through this area collectively form the *basilar pons* (Fig. 12-2B).

Cerebellum
The cerebellum develops from the *rhombic lips* of the pontine alar plates. These lips expand posteromedially toward each other until they meet at the midline and fuse to form the *cerebellar plate* (Fig. 12-2A, B), which is the rudiment of the cerebellum. As development progresses, the cerebellum is divided by transverse fissures into lobes and lobules. The first of these fissures to appear is the *posterolateral fissure*, which separates the *flocculonodular lobe* caudally from the *corpus cerebelli* rostrally. The *primary fissure*, the second groove to appear, divides the corpus cerebelli into the *anterior* and *posterior lobes* (Fig. 12-2B-D). Internal changes, such as development of the cerebellar cortex and nuclei, take place concurrently with these external events.

External Features

Basilar Pons
The portion of the brainstem lying between the midbrain rostrally and the medulla caudally is the pons (*pons* is the Latin word for "bridge"). Anteriorly and laterally (Fig. 12-3), the pons consists of a massive bundle of transversely oriented fibers that enter the cerebellum as the *middle cerebellar peduncle (brachium pontis)*. The exit of the trigeminal nerve marks the transition from the basilar pons, which is anterior to the trigeminal root, to the middle cerebellar peduncle, which lies posterior to the exit of the trigeminal nerve (Figs. 12-3 and 12-4). Rostrally, the large axonal bundles forming the *crus cerebri* of the midbrain extend into the basilar pons. Caudally, some of these descending axons emerge to form the *pyramids* of the medulla (Fig. 12-4A).

The cranial nerves that emerge from the pons are the *trigeminal* (V), *abducens* (VI), *facial* (VII), and *vestibulocochlear* (VIII) nerves. The trigeminal nerve exits laterally and is composed of a large sensory root (the *portio major*) and a small motor root (the *portio minor*); these roots are seen in Figure 12-4A. The portion of the trigeminal nerve that traverses the subarachnoid space between the pons and the trigeminal ganglion forms a landmark that is visible on magnetic resonance images at this level (Fig. 12-4B). The abducens, facial, and vestibulocochlear nerves emerge in medial to lateral sequence along the pons-medulla junction (Fig. 12-3). Although cranial nerve VII is commonly called the facial nerve, it is actually composed of two roots, the *facial nerve* (SVE fibers) and the *intermediate nerve* (SVA, GVE, and GSA fibers). The *vestibulocochlear nerve* (SSA fibers) emerges posterolaterally and, with the facial and intermediate nerves and *labyrinthine artery*, occupies the internal acoustic meatus.

Rhomboid Fossa of the Pons
The *rhomboid fossa* forms the floor of the fourth ventricle. Its caudal portion is located in the medulla, and its larger, more rostral area is in the pons. The posterior surface of the *pontine tegmentum*, which forms the floor of the fourth ventricle, is visible only when the cerebellum is detached from the brainstem (Fig. 12-5). This part of the ventricular floor is characterized by an elevation called the *facial colliculus* located between the median fissure and the *superior fovea* of the *sulcus limitans* and by an area called the *vestibular area* located lateral to the sulcus limitans. The facial colliculus is formed by the underlying abducens nucleus and internal genu of the facial nerve (see later), and the vestibular area marks the location of the vestibular nuclei. The *brachium pontis* and the *brachium conjunctivum* form the lateral walls of the fourth ventricle in the pons; the roof is formed by the anterior medullary velum, by a small part of the cerebellum, and by a portion of the tela choroidea (Fig. 12-6).

Cerebellum
The cerebellum is located posterior to the brainstem and fills much of the posterior fossa. It is attached to the brainstem by three pairs of cerebellar peduncles *(superior, middle, and inferior)*. In sagittal section, the human cerebellum appears wedge shaped (Fig. 12-6), with its superior surface apposed to the tentorium cerebelli and its inferior surface curving toward the foramen magnum.

The cerebellum consists of *anterior, posterior,* and *flocculonodular lobes;* each lobe, in turn, is composed of lobules (Figs. 12-6 and

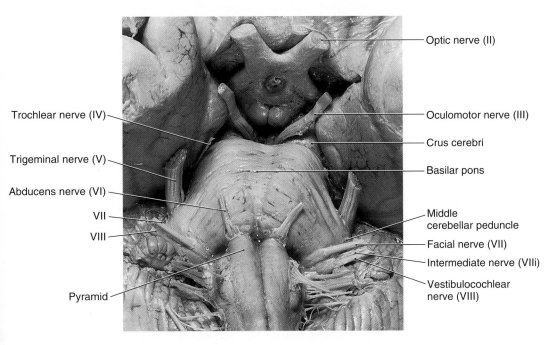

Figure 12-3. Anterior (ventral) view of the brainstem with emphasis on the pons.

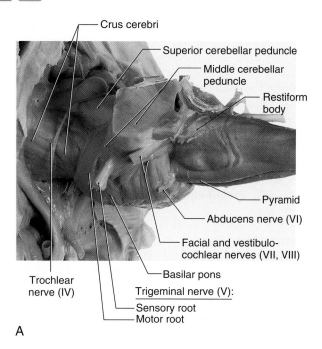

A

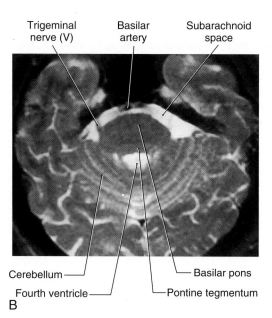

B

Figure 12-4. A dissection with the cerebellum removed showing the cranial nerves and relationships of the pons (**A**) and an MR image of the pons and root of the trigeminal nerve (**B**).

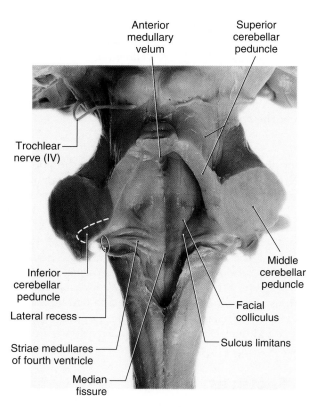

Figure 12-5. Pontine part of the fourth ventricle and rhomboid fossa. Also see Figure 10-4 for further details of the rhomboid fossa.

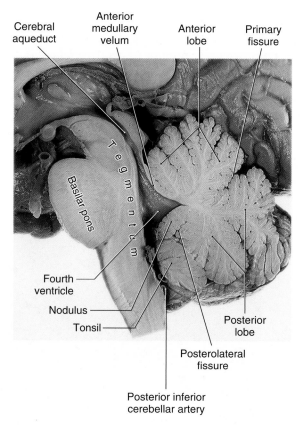

Figure 12-6. Sagittal view of the brainstem (with emphasis on the pons) and cerebellum.

12-7). Lobes and lobules are separated from each other by *fissures*. Lobules are made up of yet smaller folds of cerebellar cortex called *folia* (singular, *folium*). Cerebellar folia, lobules, and lobes can often be followed across the midline from one side of the cerebellum to the other.

Each cerebellar lobe (and lobule) is also divided into rostrocaudally oriented regions of cortex commonly called the *vermis* (medial), *intermediate* (paravermis), and *hemisphere* (lateral) *zones* (Fig. 12-7). The vermal zone is approximately 1.0 cm across at its widest point. The hemisphere is expansive in the human cerebellum and is separated from the vermis by a somewhat ill-defined intermediate zone.

Four *cerebellar nuclei* are located in the white matter core of each hemisphere. From medial to lateral, they are the *fastigial, globose, emboliform,* and *dentate* nuclei (Fig. 12-7). These cells receive input from branches of cerebellar afferent fibers and from Purkinje cells located in the cerebellar cortex. In turn, axons of cerebellar nuclear cells provide the main output signals of the cerebellum. The structure, function, and connections of the cerebellar cortex and nuclei are considered in greater detail in Chapter 27.

Vasculature of the Pons and Cerebellum

The *basilar artery* and its branches serve basilar and tegmental areas of the pons. The internal distribution of the basilar artery

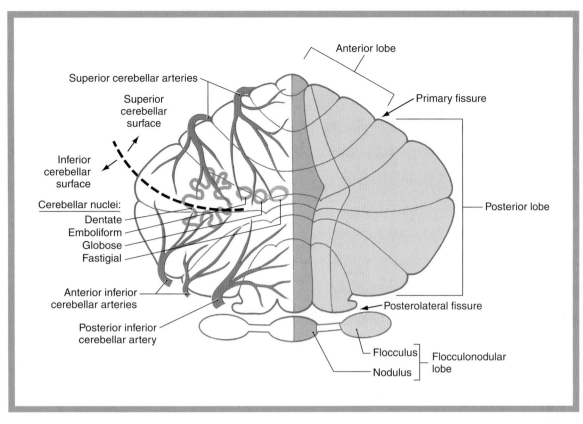

Figure 12-7. Unfolded view of the cerebellar surface with lobes and fissures labeled on the right side and the blood supply to the various lobes and their underlying nuclei indicated on the left. The colors of the rostrocaudal regions (zones) of the lobules correlate with the cerebellar nuclei to which they are related; *gray,* medial (vermis) area; *green,* intermediate (paravermis) area; *blue,* lateral (hemisphere) area.

and its branches is discussed later in this chapter. The *superior cerebellar artery*, through its *medial* and *lateral branches*, distributes to the superior surface of the cerebellum and most of the cerebellar nuclei; the inferior surface of the cerebellum is served by *anterior* and *posterior inferior cerebellar arteries* (Fig. 12-7).

Internal Anatomy of the Pons

Summary of Ascending Pathways
The major ascending pathways seen in the medulla continue into the pons (Fig. 12-8). These include the *medial lemniscus, anterolateral system, anterior trigeminothalamic fibers,* and the *anterior spinocerebellar tract.* Although most of these fibers continue through the pons, some anterolateral system fibers terminate in the pontine reticular formation (as *spinoreticular* fibers), and anterior spinocerebellar axons enter the cerebellum on the surface of the superior cerebellar peduncle. The *restiform body,* a prominent structure in the rostral medulla, sweeps posteriorly into the cerebellum in the caudal pons as the largest part of the inferior cerebellar peduncle.

Summary of Descending Pathways
The most prominent groups of descending fibers arise from cells located in the midbrain or forebrain and therefore traverse the pons (Fig. 12-8). These include the *corticospinal fibers,* the *central tegmental* and *rubrospinal tracts,* and the *tectobulbospinal system.* The *medial longitudinal fasciculus* occupies a characteristic position near the midline in the floor of the fourth ventricle. At the pons-medullary junction, this bundle contains mainly descending fibers; in the rostral pons it is made up primarily of ascending fibers.

Caudal Pontine Level
As noted earlier, the pons is divided into a posterior part, the *tegmentum,* and an anterior region, the *basilar pons.* This section

and the following two sections describe the anatomy of the pons at three levels: caudal pontine, midpontine, and rostral pontine. Each level is described from posterior to anterior beginning with the tegmentum and proceeding to the basilar pons.

At caudal pontine levels, the *facial colliculus* is formed by the underlying *abducens nucleus* and fibers comprising the *internal genu* of the facial nerve (Figs. 12-10 and 12-12). Axons from the GSE cells of the abducens nucleus course anteriorly through the tegmentum, pass adjacent to the corticospinal fibers in the basilar pons, and exit the brainstem at the pons-medullary junction as the abducens nerve (Figs. 12-10 and 12-12). The internal genu of cranial nerve VII is composed of the axons of SVE cells from the facial nucleus. These axons loop around the abducens nucleus from caudal to rostral, as the internal genu, then course anterolaterally to exit the brainstem (Fig. 12-12). Anterolateral to the abducens nucleus these SVE fibers are surrounded by cells of the *superior salivatory nucleus,* the axons of which exit the brainstem as the GVE component of the intermediate nerve (Fig. 12-12).

Medial to the abducens nucleus is the *medial longitudinal fasciculus* and the *tectobulbospinal system* (Fig. 12-11). As in the medulla, these bundles are internal to the ventricular space and adjacent to the midline.

The posterolateral tegmentum contains the vestibular nuclei and the solitary tract and nucleus (Figs. 12-9 and 12-11). The *lateral, medial,* and *inferior vestibular nuclei* are present at this level, whereas the *superior vestibular nucleus* becomes prominent more rostrally. The small bundles of fibers coursing between the vestibular nuclei and the cerebellum in the wall of the fourth ventricle form the *juxtarestiform body* (Figs. 12-10 and 12-11). This structure is composed of vestibulocerebellar and cerebellovestibular fibers and, along with *the laterally adjacent restiform body,* constitutes the *inferior cerebellar peduncle.* The rostral portions of the *solitary tract* and *nucleus* are located anterior to the vestibular nuclei and consist of a core of primary sensory

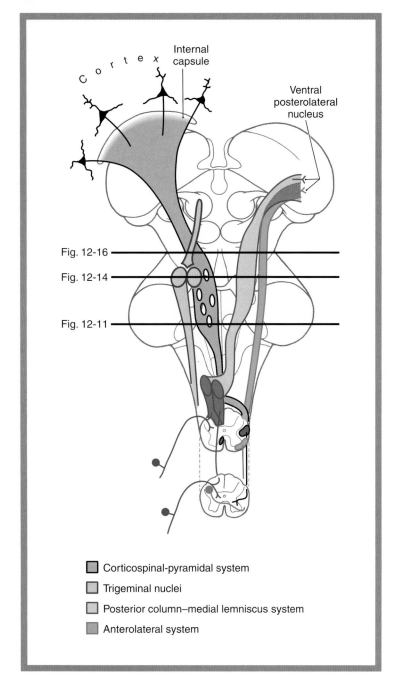

Internal
capsule

Ventral
posterolateral
nucleus

Cortex

Fig. 12-16

Fig. 12-14

Fig. 12-11

■ Corticospinal-pyramidal system

■ Trigeminal nuclei

■ Posterior column–medial lemniscus system

■ Anterolateral system

Figure 12-8. Diagrammatic representation of the brain showing the location and trajectory of three important pathways and the trigeminal nuclei. The color coding for each is continued in Figures 12-11, 12-14, and 12-16.

fibers (tract) surrounded by cell bodies (nucleus). This part of the solitary complex receives mainly taste input (SVA fibers) and is sometimes called the *gustatory nucleus*.

The central portion of the pontine tegmentum at caudal levels contains, from medial to lateral, the *central tegmental tract*, the *superior olivary nucleus*, the *facial motor nucleus*, and the *spinal trigeminal tract* and *nucleus* (Figs. 12-9, 12-11, and 12-12). A major part of the central tegmental tract includes fibers coursing from the red nucleus of the midbrain to the inferior olive of the medulla *(rubro-olivary fibers)*. Cells of the superior olive receive input from the anterior cochlear nucleus and send their axons into the lateral lemniscus on both sides. The route followed by motor facial fibers is shown in Figure 12-12; these axons innervate the ipsilateral muscles of facial expression. The spinal trigeminal tract is composed of general sensory (GSA) fibers from the ipsilateral half of the face, oral cavity, and much

of the scalp. Although most of this input is via the trigeminal nerve (hence the name of the tract), cranial nerves VII, IX, and X also make modest contributions to the spinal trigeminal tract and nucleus. Axons of the spinal trigeminal tract synapse in the spinal trigeminal nucleus, the cells of which project to the contralateral thalamus as *anterior trigeminothalamic fibers*.

The *anterolateral system*, *rubrospinal tract*, and *trapezoid body* are located in the anterolateral tegmentum (Fig. 12-11). Although pain and temperature signals from the contralateral side of the body are conveyed by anterolateral system fibers, some of these axons end in the pontine reticular formation as *spinoreticular fibers*. The trapezoid body is composed of decussating axons from the cochlear nuclei. After crossing, these fibers ascend to form the *lateral lemniscus* and convey auditory signals to the midbrain.

The *medial lemniscus* was oriented vertically in the medulla, but in the caudal pons it begins to shift to a horizontal position (Fig. 12-13; see also Fig. 12-9). At this level, the anterior part of the medial lemniscus (lumbosacral representation) shifts somewhat laterally, and its posterior portion (cervicothoracic representation) assumes a more medial location. The anterior surface of the medial lemniscus forms the border between the tegmentum and basilar pons.

The anterior pons contains the *basilar pontine nuclei*, longitudinally running *corticospinal* and *corticopontine fibers*, and transversely oriented *pontocerebellar fibers* (Figs. 12-9 and 12-11). On each side of the midline, the corticospinal fibers located in the pyramid of the medulla are, in the basilar pons, completely surrounded by the *basilar pontine nuclei*. These pontine cells receive input from diverse regions of the neuraxis. In turn, most of their axons cross the midline and enter the cerebellum via the *middle cerebellar peduncle (brachium pontis)* as pontocerebellar fibers.

Midpontine Level

Prominent features of the tegmentum at this level are the *principal* (or *chief*) *sensory trigeminal nucleus*, the *trigeminal motor nucleus*, and the *mesencephalic tract* and *nucleus* (Figs. 12-14 and 12-15). The principal sensory and motor trigeminal nuclei are located in the lateral tegmentum, and the mesencephalic tract and nucleus extend rostrally in the lateral wall of the central gray. Cells of the principal sensory nucleus receive GSA input from the ipsilateral trigeminal nerve and project to the thalamus via *posterior trigeminothalamic* (uncrossed) and *anterior trigeminothalamic* (crossed) *fibers*. The SVE cells of the trigeminal motor nucleus innervate the masticatory muscles on the ipsilateral side. Last, the unipolar cell bodies of the mesencephalic nucleus and their laterally adjacent processes, the mesencephalic tract, convey proprioceptive input to a variety of nuclei, including the trigeminal motor nucleus.

The *nucleus (locus) ceruleus* is located in the lateral floor of the fourth ventricle at this level (Fig. 12-14). Ceruleus neurons contain pigment (hence the alternative name *nucleus pigmentosus pontis*) and constitute the largest single location of noradrenaline/norepinephrine-containing cells in the central nervous system. Axons arising in the nucleus ceruleus project to widespread targets throughout the cerebral cortex, most of the diencephalon, limbic system, brainstem, cerebellar cortex and nuclei, and spinal cord. This extensive projection arises from a cell group containing only about 15,000 cell bodies, which indicates that these fibers branch profusely. When the activity level of the neurons in this nucleus is low, a state of quiescence is promoted, as in sleep. When there are sudden changes in the patient's environment, such as waking unexpectedly or if facing a threatening situation, activity of the nucleus ceruleus is high, noradrenaline/norepinephrine is released throughout the nervous system, and

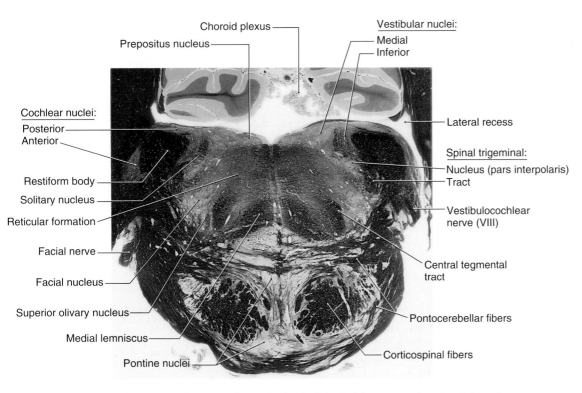

Figure 12-9. A fiber (myelin)-stained cross section at the level of the facial motor nucleus (caudal pons).

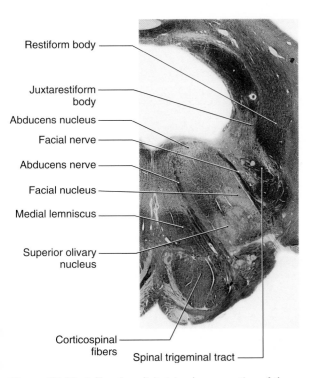

Figure 12-10. A fiber (myelin)-stained cross section of the pons at the level of the facial colliculus. Compare with Figure 12-11.

the individual is able to attend to the emergency or disruption. During times of normal non-stress and non-sleep activity these neurons have an intermediate level of activity. However, when the activity of nucleus ceruleus neurons fluctuates outside of levels that are correlated with normal life activities, the patient may experience behavior problems that require medical and/or psychiatric intervention.

A comparison of Figures 12-11 and 12-14 reveals that most major tracts in the pontine tegmentum (*medial longitudinal fasciculus, tectobulbospinal system, medial lemniscus, antero-*

lateral system, and anterior trigeminothalamic fibers) occupy positions comparable to those seen at more caudal levels. Consequently, this section emphasizes only the features that are new at midpontine levels. The medial lemniscus is oriented horizontally at this point (Figs. 12-13 and 12-15), and the *rubrospinal fibers* have shifted medial to the anterolateral system. Most auditory fibers are now concentrated in the *lateral lemniscus*, and rostral parts of the *superior olivary nucleus* appear just lateral to the central tegmental tract. *Anterior spinocerebellar fibers* migrate posteriorly and enter the cerebellum by coursing over the surface of the superior cerebellar peduncle. The *brachium conjunctivum (superior cerebellar peduncle)* arises from the cerebellar nuclei, sweeps rostrally, forming the lateral wall of the fourth ventricle (Figs. 12-14 and 12-15), and enters the caudal midbrain tegmentum, where it decussates.

Neurons in the ventral tegmentum close to the midline extend into posterior portions of the basilar pons and constitute the *reticulotegmental nucleus* (Figs. 12-14 and 12-15). This cell group is continuous with the basilar pontine nuclei, and its axons enter the cerebellum through the contralateral *brachium pontis*. These cells also share similar cytologic features and afferent projections with neurons of the basilar pons.

Rostral Pontine Level

The only cranial nerve structures present in the pontine tegmentum at rostral levels are the *mesencephalic nucleus* and *tract*. These structures are located in the lateral aspect of the periaqueductal gray and remain in this position into the midbrain (Fig. 12-16; see also Fig. 12-14). Anterior to the mesencephalic tract and nucleus is the *locus (nucleus) ceruleus;* this noradrenergic cell group also extends into the caudal midbrain.

The *brachium conjunctivum (superior cerebellar peduncle)* converges toward its decussation in the caudal midbrain, and most other major tracts in the tegmentum occupy positions comparable to those seen at midpontine levels (compare Fig. 12-14 with Fig. 12-16). The rubrospinal tract is shifted even more medially, and the *lateral lemniscus* is close to the posterolateral surface of the brainstem at this point. Also, the composition

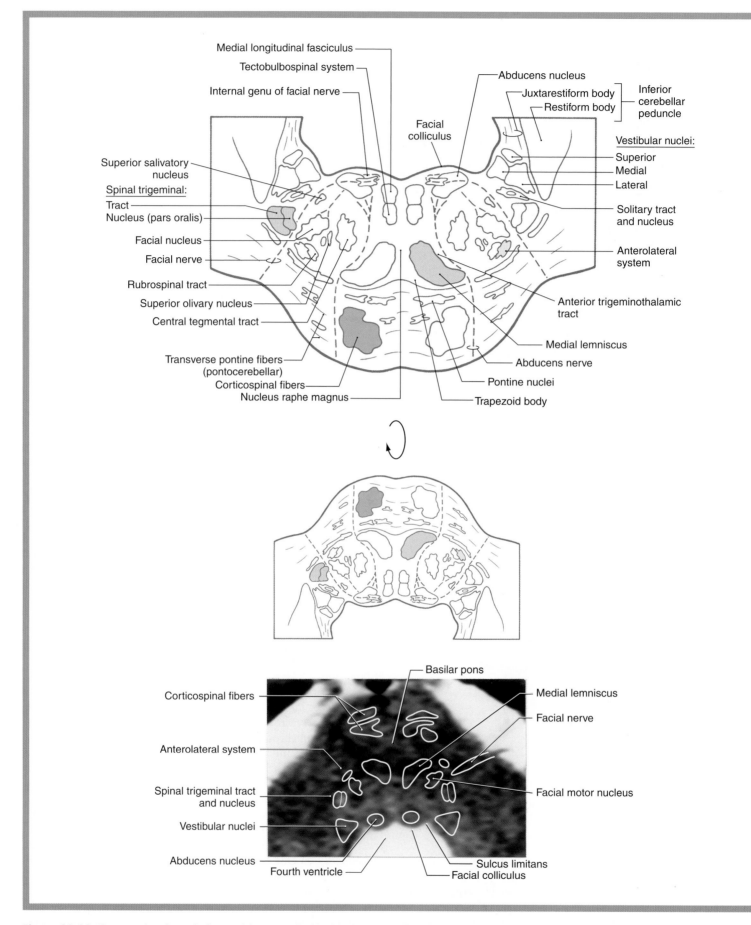

Figure 12-11. Cross section through the caudal pons at the level of the facial colliculus. Correlate with Figure 12-8. The anatomic orientation is flipped to illustrate internal structures in a clinical orientation; the clinically important tracts and nuclei are shown on a T2-weighted MR image at a comparable level of the facial colliculus in the caudal pons.

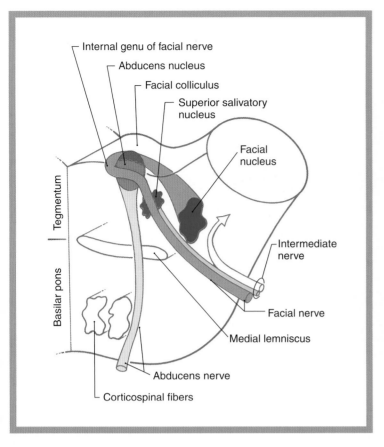

Figure 12-12. Diagrammatic representation of the left side of the pons, as viewed from rostral to caudal, showing the relationships of the abducens and facial nerves. The *arrow* indicates the general somatic afferent and special visceral afferent parts of the intermediate nerve; these fibers course caudally to enter the spinal trigeminal and solitary tract and nuclei, respectively.

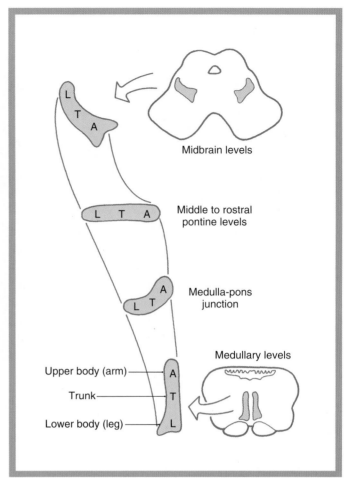

Figure 12-13. The orientation of the medial lemniscus at all brainstem levels. In this illustration, "arm" denotes the upper extremity, and "leg" denotes the lower extremity.

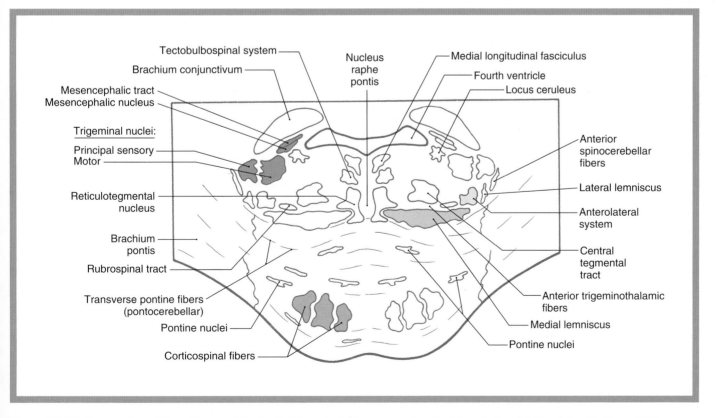

Figure 12-14. Cross section of the mid pons at the level of the principal sensory and motor trigeminal nuclei. Correlate with Figure 12-8.

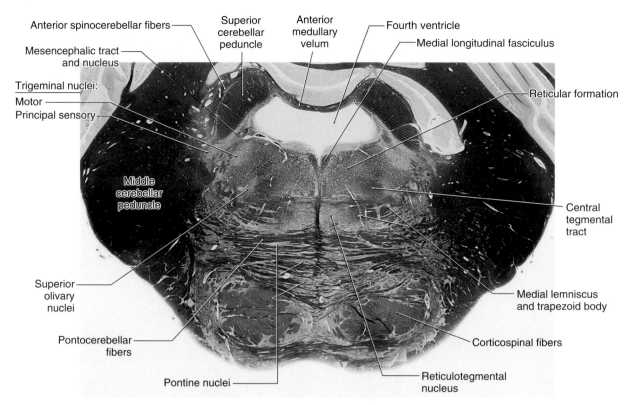

Anterior spinocerebellar fibers — Superior cerebellar peduncle — Anterior medullary velum — Fourth ventricle — Medial longitudinal fasciculus

Mesencephalic tract and nucleus

Trigeminal nuclei:
Motor
Principal sensory

Reticular formation

Middle cerebellar peduncle

Central tegmental tract

Superior olivary nuclei

Medial lemniscus and trapezoid body

Pontocerebellar fibers

Corticospinal fibers

Pontine nuclei

Reticulotegmental nucleus

Figure 12-15. A fiber (myelin)-stained cross section at the level of the principal sensory and motor trigeminal nuclei. Compare with Figure 12-14.

of the *basilar pons* is essentially the same as that seen at midpontine levels (Figs. 12-14 and 12-16).

Reticular and Raphe Nuclei

Much of the pontine tegmentum is occupied by the reticular formation. This central core is generally divided into a medial area of primarily large neurons (magnocellular region) and a lateral area of mainly small neurons (parvocellular region) (Fig. 12-17). The magnocellular reticular nuclei of the pons are, from caudal to rostral, the *gigantocellular reticular nucleus* and the *caudal* and *oral pontine reticular nuclei*. The parvocellular area nuclei of the pons contain a diffuse *lateral reticular formation* at caudal and midpontine levels and include the *medial* and *lateral parabrachial nuclei* at rostral levels. The latter cell groups are located adjacent to the brachium conjunctivum.

The *raphe nuclei* are symmetrically distributed on either side of the midline (Fig. 12-17). Next to the medial lemniscus at caudal pontine levels is the *nucleus raphes magnus* (the *raphe magnus*). This cell cluster extends caudally into the rostral medulla and is an important synaptic station for signals involved in the inhibition of pain at medullary and spinal levels. In the caudal one third of the tegmental pons, this cell group is replaced by the *nucleus raphes pontis*, which extends a little beyond midpontine levels. The *superior central nucleus* and *posterior (dorsal) raphe nucleus* are found in the rostral pons; the latter extends into the caudal midbrain (see Fig. 13-16). The more caudal of the pontine raphe nuclei (magnus) project primarily to the spinal cord while the more rostral (pontis, superior central) project primarily rostrally to innervate a variety of forebrain targets. Although the main neurotransmitter associated with the pontine raphe nuclei is *serotonin*, there are some *enkephalin-containing* cells in the raphe magnus.

Internal Vasculature of the Pons

Internal areas of the tegmental and basilar pons are served by branches of the *basilar artery* (Fig. 12-18). *Paramedian branches* distribute to medial areas of the basilar pons, including

corticospinal fibers and the exiting fibers of the abducens nerve. The lateral part of the basilar pons is served by *short circumferential branches*, and the entire tegmental area plus a wedge of the middle cerebellar peduncle receives blood via the *long circumferential branches*. At caudal levels (levels of the facial colliculus), the long circumferential supply is supplemented by branches of the *anterior inferior cerebellar artery*. Rostrally, beginning at about the level of the principal sensory and motor trigeminal nuclei, the blood supply to the pontine tegmentum is supplemented by branches of the *superior cerebellar artery*.

Vascular Syndromes of the Pons

At caudal pontine levels (Figs. 12-11 and 12-18) the territory of the *paramedian branches* of the basilar artery includes the exiting fibers of the *abducens nerve*, *corticospinal fibers*, and, most likely, portions of the *medial lemniscus*. Occlusion of the paramedial branches at this level results in an ipsilateral abducens nerve paralysis and a contralateral hemiparesis (the *Foville syndrome*) with a variable contralateral sensory loss reflecting various degrees of damage to the medial lemniscus. If the lesion in the Foville syndrome extends into the pontine tegmentum the patient may have additional deficits, such as an ipsilateral horizontal gaze paralysis, indicating damage to the medial portions of the pontine reticular formation. If the area of damage is shifted somewhat laterally to involve *corticospinal fibers* and the root of the *facial nerve*, the patient has a contralateral hemiparesis and an ipsilateral paralysis of the facial muscles (the *Gubler* or *Millard-Gubler syndrome*).

At midpontine levels occlusion of paramedial and short circumferential branches results in the *syndrome of the midpontine base*. The main structures damaged and their respective deficits are *corticospinal fibers* (contralateral hemiparesis), *sensory and motor trigeminal roots* (ipsilateral loss of pain and thermal sense in the face and paralysis of masticatory muscles), and *ataxia* (fibers of the middle cerebellar peduncle). Lesions within the pontine tegmentum may also combine cranial nerve

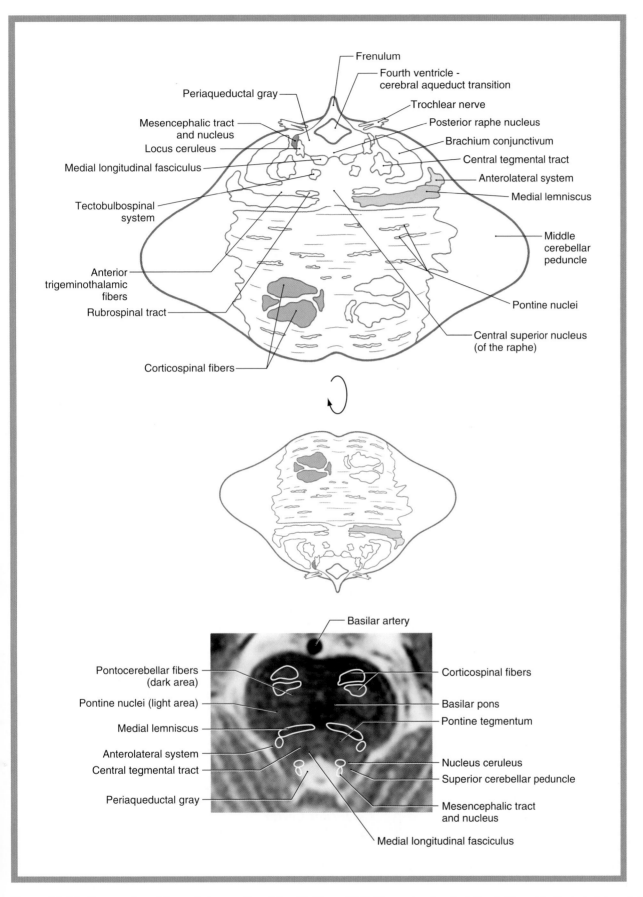

Figure 12-16. Cross section of the rostral pons. Correlate with Figure 12-8. The anatomic orientation is flipped to illustrate internal structures in a clinical orientation; the clinically important tracts and nuclei are shown on a T2-weighted MR image at a comparable level of the rostral pons.

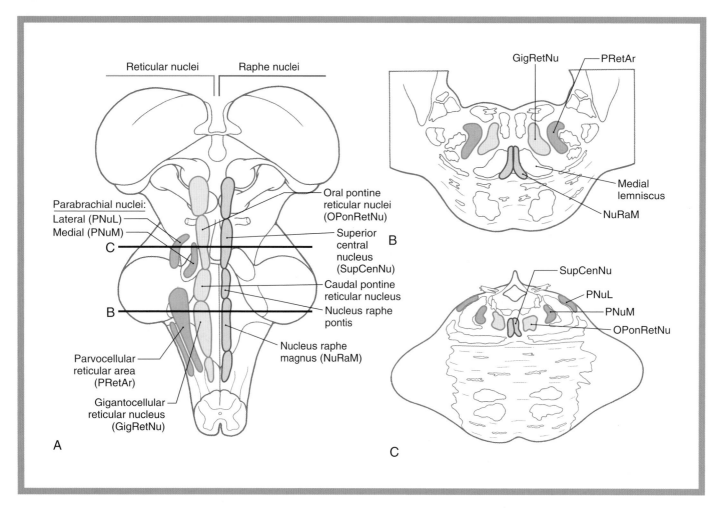

Figure 12-17. Posterior (dorsal) view of the brainstem (**A**) and caudal (**B**) and rostral (**C**) cross sections showing the raphe and reticular nuclei of the pons.

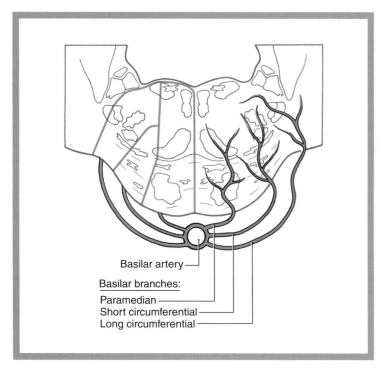

Figure 12-18. Blood supply of the pons. Arteries are shown on the right, and the general territories served by each are shown on the left.

signs and long tract signs. For example, a lesion in the caudal pontine tegmentum may damage the *abducens* and *facial nuclei* (paralysis of the ipsilateral lateral rectus muscle and facial musculature) and the *anterolateral system* (contralateral loss of pain and thermal sense on the body) (Fig. 12-11). At mid to more rostral pontine levels (Fig. 12-14), damage to the tegmentum may involve the *anterolateral system* in combination with the *trigeminal motor nucleus* and/or the *sensory and motor roots of the trigeminal nerve*. All of these examples illustrate a hallmark of brainstem vascular lesions, that is, an *ipsilateral cranial nerve sign coupled with a contralateral long tract sign*.

Internal Anatomy of the Cerebellum

Cerebellar Cortex

Each folium of the cerebellum is organized into three layers oriented parallel to the cortical surface. From external to internal, these are the *molecular, Purkinje cell,* and *granular layers* (Figs. 12-19 and 12-20). Internal to the granular layer, and forming the core of each folium, is a layer of subcortical white matter composed of all fibers arriving (afferents to the cortex) or leaving (efferents of the cortex) the cerebellar cortex.

The *molecular layer* contains *stellate cells, basket cells,* and the expansive dendrites of *Purkinje cells* (Fig. 12-19). In addition, the molecular layer contains two other major fiber populations: *climbing fibers* and *parallel fibers*. The former originate from the contralateral inferior olive and the latter from the granule cells (Fig. 12-19).

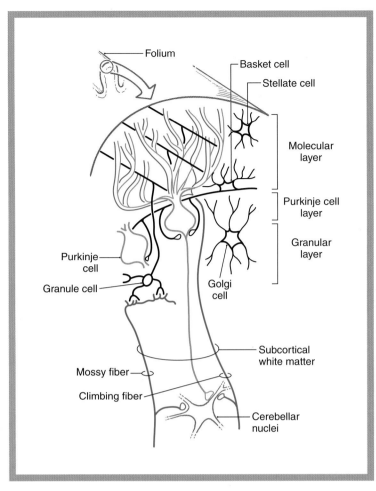

Figure 12-19. Diagrammatic representation of the cells and fibers of the cerebellar cortex.

to the long axis of the folium. Axons of Purkinje cells pass through the subcortical white matter to end in the cerebellar and vestibular nuclei.

The granular layer contains *granule cells*, *Golgi cells*, and *mossy fibers* (Figs. 12-19 and 12-20). The latter fibers originate from cells located in many nuclei throughout the brainstem and spinal cord. Traversing the granular layer are climbing fibers, en route to the molecular layer, and Purkinje cell axons leaving the cortex.

Cerebellar Nuclei

The cerebellar nuclei are, from medial to lateral, the *fastigial*, *globose*, *emboliform*, and *dentate* (Fig. 12-7). They receive input from Purkinje cell axons and from collaterals of cerebellar afferent fibers. In general, Purkinje cells of the vermis relate to the underlying fastigial nucleus, those of the intermediate cortex to the globose and emboliform nuclei, and those of the lateral cortex to the dentate nucleus (Fig. 12-7). Some Purkinje cells of the vermis and the flocculonodular lobe send axons directly to the vestibular nuclei. Cerebellar nuclear cells project to a variety of cell groups throughout the neuraxis, primarily via the brachium conjunctivum.

Vasculature of the Cerebellum

The blood supply to the cerebellar cortex and nuclei arises via branches of the *superior cerebellar artery* and the *anterior* and *posterior inferior cerebellar arteries* (Fig. 12-7). The superior cerebellar artery serves the superior surface of the cerebellum and, by way of penetrating branches, the fastigial, globose, and emboliform nuclei and most areas of the dentate nucleus. This vessel also distributes to the superior and middle cerebellar peduncles.

Branches of the anterior inferior cerebellar artery distribute to the more lateral areas of the inferior cerebellar surface, including the flocculus (Fig. 12-7). They also serve parts of the middle cerebellar peduncle, caudal regions of the dentate nucleus, and the choroid plexus in the subarachnoid space at the cerebellopontine angle.

The posterior inferior cerebellar artery (PICA) branches to more medial regions of the inferior cerebellar surface and to the nodulus (Fig. 12-7). The choroid plexus of the fourth ventricle receives branches from the PICA. This vessel is also an important source of blood to posterolateral regions of the medulla.

Purkinje cells are the efferent neurons of the cerebellar cortex. Their large somata form a single layer at the molecular layer–granular layer interface (Figs. 12-19 and 12-20). Each Purkinje cell has a complex dendritic tree that extends into the molecular layer and exhibits a fan-like orientation that is perpendicular

---

Synopsis of Clinical Points

- The root of the trigeminal nerve is the largest of the brainstem, a mixed nerve, and an important landmark in magnetic resonance imaging (p. 185).
- A tumor of the fourth ventricle impinging on the facial colliculus may result in weakness of the facial muscles and of the lateral rectus muscle on the ipsilateral side (p. 185).
- Low levels of activity in nucleus ceruleus neurons are correlated with vegetative activities (p. 186).
- Fluctuating levels of activity in nucleus ceruleus neurons may be seen in patients experiencing behavioral crises (p. 187).
- Lesion in the medial pons at caudal levels results in a contralateral hemiparesis and ipsilateral weakness of the lateral rectus muscle (Foville syndrome) (p. 190).
- Lesion in the medial pons at caudal levels may also result in a contralateral loss of proprioception, position, and vibratory sense if the medial lemniscus is involved (p. 190).
- Medial pontine lesions that extend laterally to include the facial nerve result in a Gubler or Millard-Gubler syndrome (p. 190).
- Lesions within the pontine tegmentum at midpontine to more rostral levels result in a variety of deficits reflecting damage to cranial nerve nuclei, long tracts, and other structures (p. 190).

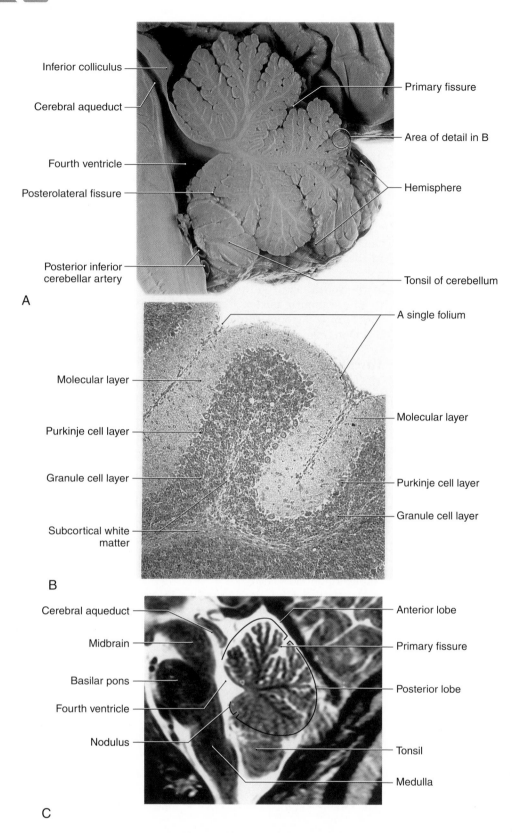

Inferior colliculus

Cerebral aqueduct

Fourth ventricle

Posterolateral fissure

Posterior inferior cerebellar artery

A

Primary fissure

Area of detail in B

Hemisphere

Tonsil of cerebellum

A single folium

Molecular layer

Purkinje cell layer

Granule cell layer

Subcortical white matter

Molecular layer

Purkinje cell layer

Granule cell layer

B

Cerebral aqueduct

Midbrain

Basilar pons

Fourth ventricle

Nodulus

Anterior lobe

Primary fissure

Posterior lobe

Tonsil

Medulla

C

Figure 12-20. Midsagittal view (**A**), a detail of the histology of the cerebellar cortex (**B**—the *arrowheads* point to the soma of representative Purkinje cells), and a midsagittal T2-weighted MR image of the cerebellum (**C**) that correlates with the view in **A**. (From Haines DE: Neuroanatomy: An Atlas of Structures, Sections, and Systems, 5th ed. Baltimore, Lippincott Williams & Wilkins, 2000.)

Sources and Additional Reading

Readings for the brainstem chapters are listed at the end of Chapter 13.

The Midbrain

G. A. Mihailoff, D. E. Haines, and P. J. May

The *mesencephalon*, or midbrain, is the most rostral portion of the brainstem. It gives rise to cranial nerves III and IV, conducts ascending and descending tracts, and contains nuclei that are essential to motor function. Caudally, the midbrain is continuous with the pons, and rostrally it joins the diencephalon. The *cerebral aqueduct*, the cavity of the midbrain, is continuous rostrally with the third ventricle and caudally with the fourth ventricle. The blood supply to the mesencephalon is primarily from proximal branches of the posterior cerebral arteries (P_1 or P_2) and from small penetrating branches of the posterior communicating artery.

Development

The mesencephalon (Fig. 13-1) arises early in development as one of the three primary brain vesicles. Immature neurons that arise from the *ventricular zone* to enter and form the *intermediate zone* give rise to *alar* and *basal plates*, which are continuous with the alar and basal plates of the rhombencephalon (Fig. 13-2). These cell groups are the rostral continuations of the same primitive cell columns described for the metencephalon. The surrounding *marginal layer* contains the developing axons of cells located in other levels of the neuraxis. The *cerebral aqueduct* is narrow relative to the fourth ventricle; therefore, the basal and alar plates lie anterior and posterior to it as in the spinal cord and caudal medulla.

Basal and Alar Plates

The immature neurons of the *alar plate* give rise to the quadrigeminal plate, from which the *superior* and *inferior colliculi* arise (Fig. 13-2A, *upper arrow*). In humans, the superior colliculus consists of alternating layers of cells and fibers, whereas the inferior colliculus appears more homogeneous but consists of a large central nucleus and several small, peripherally located nuclei. Immature alar plate neurons also migrate into anterior areas of the developing midbrain to form the *red nucleus* and the *substantia nigra* (Fig. 13-2A, *lower arrow*).

Immature neurons of the *basal plate* give rise to the *general somatic efferent* (GSE) neurons of the *oculomotor* and *trochlear*

nuclei. In addition, the *general visceral efferent* (GVE) cells of the *Edinger-Westphal nucleus*, a visceral motor cell group associated with the oculomotor complex, also arise from the basal plate (Fig. 13-2).

As the basal and alar plates differentiate, the marginal layer is invaded by axons originating from cells located outside the midbrain. These fibers collect in the anterolateral area of the developing mesencephalon to form an especially prominent bundle, the *crus cerebri* (plural, *crura cerebri;* see Fig. 13-2B).

External Features

Anterior (Ventral) Midbrain

The presence of a pair of large axon bundles, the crura cerebri, is a characteristic feature of the anterior aspect of the midbrain. These bundles emerge from the cerebral hemispheres caudal to the optic tracts, converge slightly toward the midline as they course through the midbrain, and disappear into the basilar pons (Fig. 13-3). The *oculomotor nerves* exit the medial edge of each crus and pass through the space between the crura, which

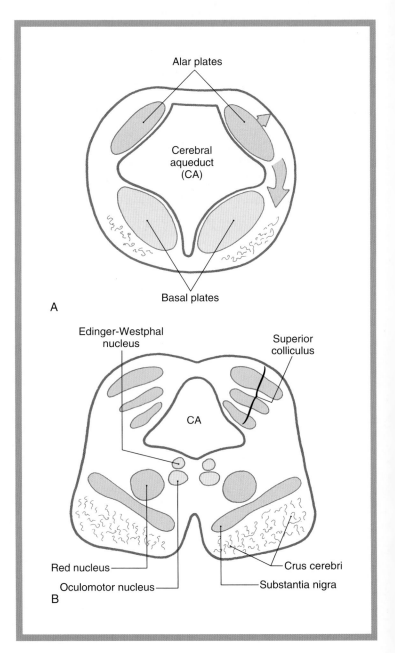

Figure 13-2. Development of the midbrain at early (**A**) and later (**B**) stages showing the alar and basal plates and the structures derived from each. The level shown at **B** is diagrammatic of the rostral (superior colliculus) midbrain.

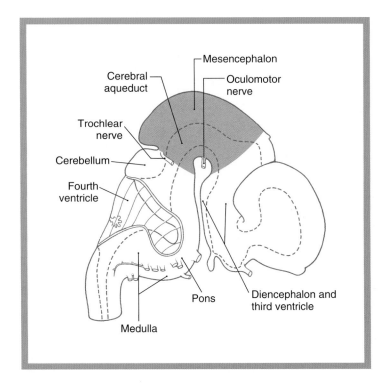

Figure 13-1. Lateral view of the human brain at about 7 weeks of gestation. The midbrain is highlighted.

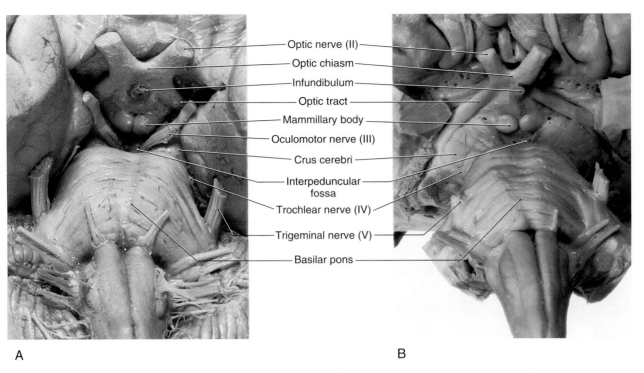

Figure 13-3. Anterior (ventral) views (**A**, undissected; **B**, dissected) of the brainstem with emphasis on the midbrain.

is called the *interpeduncular fossa* (Fig. 13-3). Anteriorly, the rostral limit of the midbrain is marked by the exit of the crura cerebri from the cerebral hemispheres and by the caudal edge of the mammillary bodies. The caudal border of the midbrain is formed where each crus enters the basilar pons.

The subarachnoid space of the interpeduncular fossa is called the *interpeduncular cistern.* This cistern contains the oculomotor nerves and the upper part of the basilar artery, including its bifurcation and proximal branches. Numerous vessels penetrate the roof of this fossa and create many small perforations (Fig. 13-3B). Consequently, this area is frequently called the *posterior perforated substance.*

Posterior (Dorsal) Midbrain

The posterior surface of the adult midbrain is characterized by four elevations collectively called the *corpora quadrigemina* (Fig. 13-4). The rostral two elevations are the *superior colliculi,* and the caudal two are the *inferior colliculi.* Just caudal to the inferior colliculus, the exit of the trochlear nerve marks the pons-midbrain junction on the posterior surface of the brainstem, whereas the midbrain-diencephalic boundary is formed by the posterior commissure (Fig. 13-5).

Rostrolaterally, the inferior colliculus is joined to the *medial geniculate body* of the diencephalon by a fiber bundle called the *brachium of the inferior colliculus* (Fig. 13-4). The inferior colliculus and the medial geniculate body are part of the auditory system. The *brachium of the superior colliculus* extends from the optic tract to the superior colliculus in a groove located between the *medial geniculate body* and *pulvinar* of the diencephalon (Figs. 13-4 and 13-14). The superior colliculus, pulvinar, and lateral geniculate body are parts of the visual and visual-motor systems.

On the midline, the *pineal gland,* a diencephalic structure, extends posteriorly above and between the superior colliculi (Fig. 13-5). Tumors of the pineal produce noncommunicating (obstructive) hydrocephalus because of compression of the colliculi of the midbrain and resulting occlusion of the cerebral aqueduct.

The subarachnoid space immediately posterior (dorsal) to the colliculi is the *quadrigeminal cistern.* This cistern contains

the exiting trochlear nerves, the great vein of Galen, and distal branches of the posterior cerebral arteries.

Vasculature of the Midbrain

The primary blood supply to the mesencephalon arises via branches of the *basilar artery,* with smaller branches from the *superior cerebellar, anterior choroidal, medial posterior choroidal,* and *posterior communicating arteries.* An important source of blood to the posterior portion of the midbrain is the *quadrigeminal*

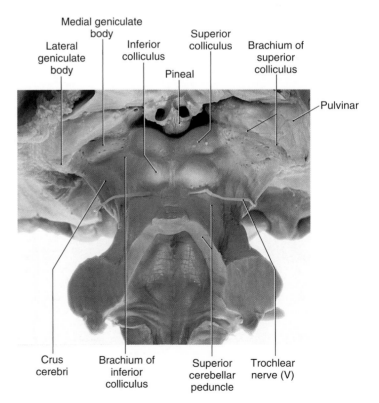

Figure 13-4. Posterior (dorsal) view (dissected) of the brainstem with emphasis on the midbrain and its junction with the diencephalon. (From Haines DE: Neuroanatomy: An Atlas of Structures, Sections, and Systems, 6th ed. Philadelphia, Lippincott Williams & Wilkins, 2004.)

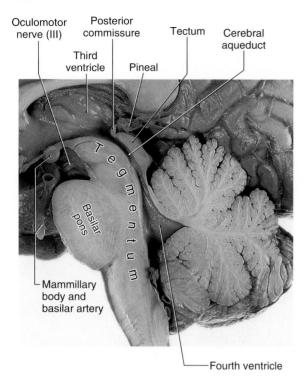

Figure 13-5. Sagittal view of the brainstem with emphasis on midbrain structures.

artery, a branch of the posterior cerebral artery (P$_1$ segment). Also, the *superior cerebellar artery* gives rise to branches that serve caudal parts of the posterior midbrain and adjacent regions of the pons.

Internal Anatomy of the Midbrain

General Regions: Tectum, Tegmentum, and Basis Pedunculi

The midbrain is divisible into three regions, which can be appreciated best in cross section. Posterior to the cerebral aqueduct is the *tectum* (roof) of the midbrain (Figs. 13-5 and 13-6). The characteristic structures of this area are the superior and inferior colliculi. The *periaqueductal gray (central gray)* is a sleeve of

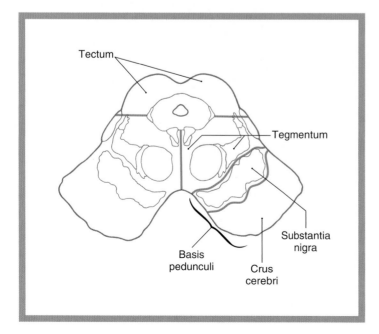

Figure 13-6. Major subdivisions of the midbrain.

neuron cell bodies that completely surrounds the cerebral aqueduct. The *tegmentum of the midbrain* extends from the base of the tectum to, but does not include, the substantia nigra. The anterolateral portion of the midbrain on either side is formed by the *basis pedunculi*, which consists of the *substantia nigra* and the *crus cerebri* (Fig. 13-6). In turn, the *crus cerebri* is composed primarily of descending fibers. The term *cerebral peduncle* is sometimes used for the crus cerebri but actually represents the entire midbrain below the tectum (tegmentum + basis pedunculi).

Summary of Ascending Pathways

The long ascending pathways that traverse the pons and medulla continue through the midbrain (Fig. 13-7). These include the *medial lemniscus, the anterolateral system*, and the *posterior and anterior trigeminothalamic tracts*. The *lateral lemniscus* is also prominent in the caudal midbrain. Other, smaller bundles, such

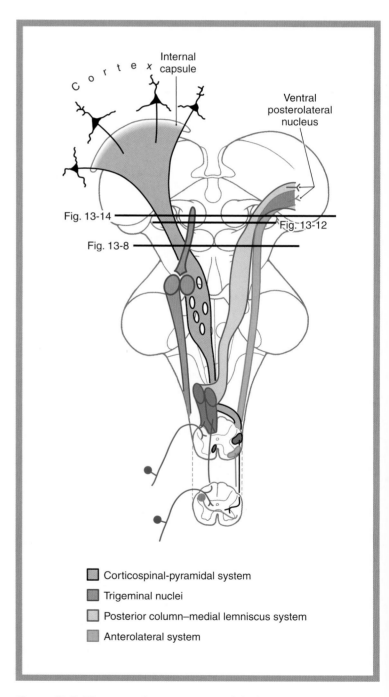

■ Corticospinal-pyramidal system

■ Trigeminal nuclei

■ Posterior column–medial lemniscus system

■ Anterolateral system

Figure 13-7. Diagrammatic representation of the brain showing the location and trajectory of three important pathways and the trigeminal nuclei. The color coding for each is continued in Figures 13-8, 13-12, and 13-14.

as the *medial longitudinal fasciculus*, are also present and occupy positions comparable to those seen in lower levels of brainstem.

Summary of Descending Pathways

Descending fibers from the cerebral cortex pass through the midbrain and, as we have seen, are also prominent features of the pons, medulla, and spinal cord (Fig. 13-7). At midbrain levels these *corticospinal, corticonuclear (corticobulbar)*, and *corticopontine* fibers are parts of the crus cerebri. Some of the descending fiber bundles that were discussed in the pons and medulla, such as the *tectobulbospinal system* and the *rubrospinal* and *central tegmental tracts*, originate from nuclei of the midbrain.

The following sections describe the anatomy of the midbrain at caudal and rostral brain levels and at the level of the midbrain-diencephalon junction. The anatomy is presented from posterior to anterior at each level, starting with the tectum and proceeding through the tegmentum to the basis pedunculi.

Caudal Midbrain Levels

Transverse sections through the caudal midbrain are characterized by the presence of the *inferior colliculus, trochlear nucleus*, and *decussation of the superior cerebellar peduncle* (Figs. 13-8 to 13-10). The inferior colliculus is composed of a large *central nucleus* bordered posteriorly by a smaller *pericentral (dorsal) nucleus* and laterally by an *external (lateral) nucleus*. Lateral lemniscus fibers enter the inferior colliculus from an anterior direction and give this area a goblet-like appearance (Figs. 13-8 and 13-9). The lateral lemniscus provides auditory input to the nuclei of the inferior colliculus, which then transmit this information to the medial geniculate body via fibers of the *brachium of the inferior colliculus*. A complete tonotopic representation (frequency map) of the cochlea is found in several of the central auditory nuclei (see Chapter 21).

The *periaqueductal gray*, or *central gray*, is a prominent collection of small neurons surrounding the cerebral aqueduct at all midbrain levels (Figs. 13-8 to 13-10, 13-12, and 13-13). It receives somatosensory input, is interconnected with the hypothalamus and thalamus, and projects caudally to brainstem nuclei. Its connections and the presence of a high level of opiate receptor binding activity indicate that the periaqueductal gray plays an important role in the brain mechanisms responsible for the suppression and modulation of pain (analgesia). The cell bodies of the *mesencephalic nucleus* and their laterally adjacent fibers, the *mesencephalic tract*, are located in the lateral edge of the periaqueductal gray, and the *posterior (dorsal) raphe nucleus* is located anteriorly on the midline, adjacent to the trochlear nucleus and medial longitudinal fasciculus (Fig. 13-8).

The central area of the tegmentum at the level of the inferior colliculus is occupied by the decussating fibers of the *superior cerebellar peduncle* (Figs. 13-8 and 13-9). From this point, the majority of these cerebellar efferent axons pass rostrally as *cerebellothalamic fibers* to targets in the midbrain and thalamus, although some turn caudally and enter the pons and medulla. Many of these cerebellar efferent fibers that turn caudally descend as a component of the *central tegmental tract*; this tract also contains other connections such as those from the *red nucleus* to the ipsilateral *inferior olivary complex (rubro-olivary fibers)*. At the level of this decussation, the *general somatic efferent* (GSE) cell bodies of the *trochlear nucleus* form an oval-shaped cell group nestled in the fibers of the *medial longitudinal fasciculus* (Figs. 13-8 and 13-10). The axons of trochlear motor neurons pass laterally and posteriorly around the periaqueductal gray to cross the midline before exiting the brainstem just caudal to the inferior colliculus. They innervate the superior oblique muscle. *Tectobulbospinal fibers* are ventral to the *medial longitudinal fasciculus*, and, as their name states, the fibers of the

central tegmental tract occupy the center of the tegmentum (Figs. 13-8 to 13-10).

Immediately anterior to the decussation of the superior cerebellar peduncle are the *interpeduncular nucleus* and *rubrospinal fibers* (Fig. 13-8). The interpeduncular nucleus is related to the limbic system, a part of the brain that functions in the control of emotional behavior.

Located in the anterolateral and lateral portions of the midbrain tegmentum are fibers of the *anterolateral system* and *medial lemniscus* (Fig. 13-8). The anterolateral system conveys pain and temperature signals from the contralateral side of the body. Most of its fibers terminate in the dorsal thalamus and therefore pass through the midbrain, but it also contains *spinomesencephalic fibers* that end in the midbrain. Some of these fibers synapse in the reticular nuclei of the midbrain and pons *(spinoreticular fibers)*, some synapse in the tectum *(spinotectal fibers)*, and some synapse in the periaqueductal gray. The latter fibers represent an important link in the pathways involved in the inhibition of pain at medullary and spinal levels. Medial lemniscal fibers have shifted from a horizontal position, characteristic of the rostral pons, to the anteromedial to posterolateral orientation of the midbrain. The somatotopy of fibers in the medial lemniscus follows accordingly (Fig. 13-11).

Posterior and *anterior trigeminothalamic tracts* are located adjacent to the central tegmental tract and the medial lemniscus, respectively (Figs. 13-8 and 13-9). These bundles are somewhat diffusely arranged and convey crossed (anterior) and uncrossed (posterior) somatosensory information from the face.

The base of the midbrain on either side is formed by the *basis pedunculi*, which consists of the *substantia nigra* and the *crus cerebri* (Fig. 13-8). The substantia nigra is related to motor function and is considered in the next section of this chapter. The crus cerebri contains *corticospinal, corticonuclear (corticobulbar)*, and *corticopontine* fibers. The former two fiber populations are found in the middle third of the crus cerebri. Corticospinal fibers projecting to lumbosacral cord levels (lower extremity representation) are found laterally, and corticonuclear (corticobulbar) fibers that project to cranial nerve nuclei (face representation) are located more medially. Corticospinal fibers projecting to cervical cord levels (upper extremity representation) occupy an intermediate position. Corticopontine fibers in the medial third of the crus arise from the frontal lobe *(frontopontine)*, whereas those in the lateral third originate from parietal, occipital, and temporal lobes *(parietopontine, occipitopontine, and temporopontine)*.

Rostral Midbrain Levels

Transverse sections through the rostral midbrain are characterized by the presence of the *superior colliculus, red nucleus*, and *oculomotor nuclei* (Figs. 13-12 and 13-13). The paired *superior colliculi* are composed of alternating layers of gray matter (cells) and white matter (fibers). The "superficial" three layers (I to III) receive input from the retina and visual cortices and project to the thalamus. The "deep" four layers (IV to VII) subserve gaze changes including eye movements and project to the thalamus, brainstem, and spinal cord. Descending crossed projections from the tectum pass to a variety of brainstem areas (as *tectoreticular* and *tecto-olivary fibers*) and—although this element is minor in humans—to the cervical spinal cord as *tectospinal fibers*. Together, these fibers constitute the *tectobulbospinal system* of the brainstem; the name "tectobulbospinal" reflects the diversity of the fibers in this bundle. *Rubrospinal fibers* originate from the contralateral red nucleus; these fibers descend to medullary and spinal levels, where they influence the activity of motor neurons innervating skeletal muscles.

Anterior to the periaqueductal gray, the oculomotor complex forms a "V"-shaped region between the medial longitudinal

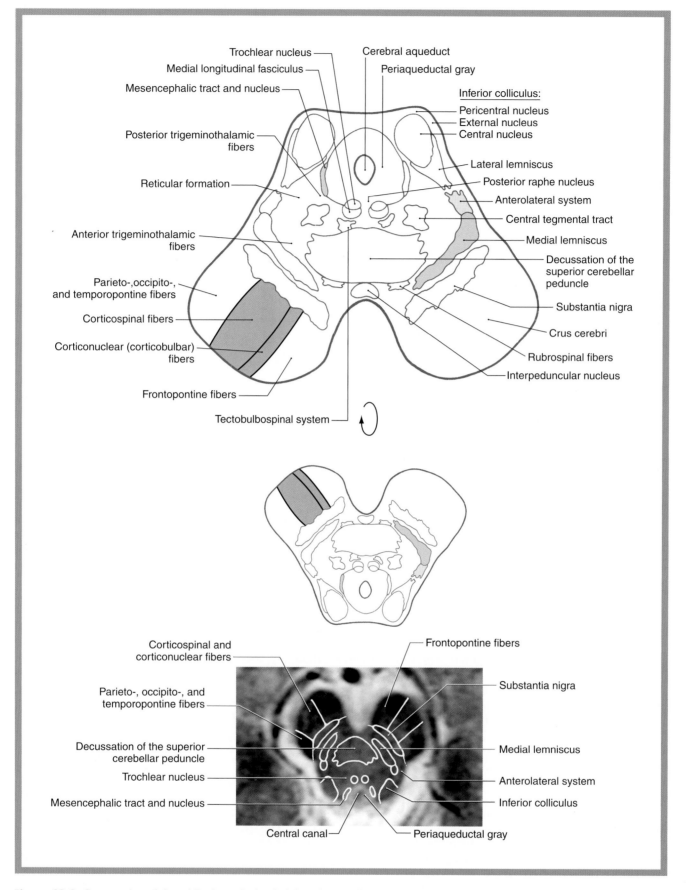

Figure 13-8. Cross section of the midbrain at the level of the inferior colliculus. Correlate with Figure 13-7. The anatomic orientation is flipped to illustrate internal structures in a clinical orientation; the clinically important tracts and nuclei are shown on a T2-weighted MR image at a comparable level of the inferior colliculus.

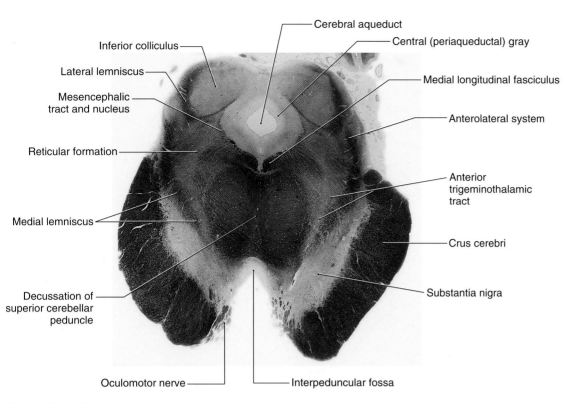

Figure 13-9. A fiber (myelin)-stained cross section of the midbrain at the level of the inferior colliculus. Compare with Figure 13-8.

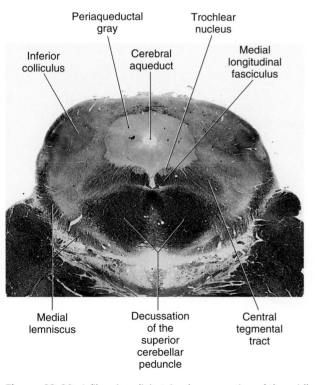

Figure 13-10. A fiber (myelin)-stained cross section of the midbrain at an intercollicular level showing the trochlear nucleus. Compare with Figure 13-8.

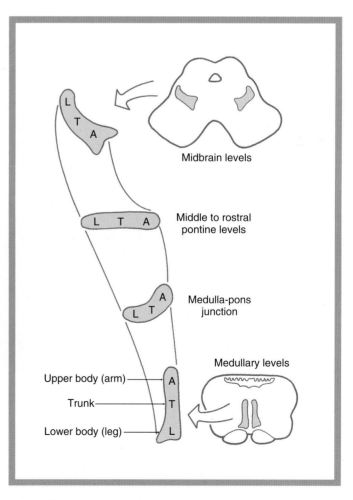

Figure 13-11. The orientation of the medial lemniscus in the midbrain as compared with that in the pons and medulla. In this illustration, "arm" denotes the upper extremity and "leg" denotes the lower extremity.

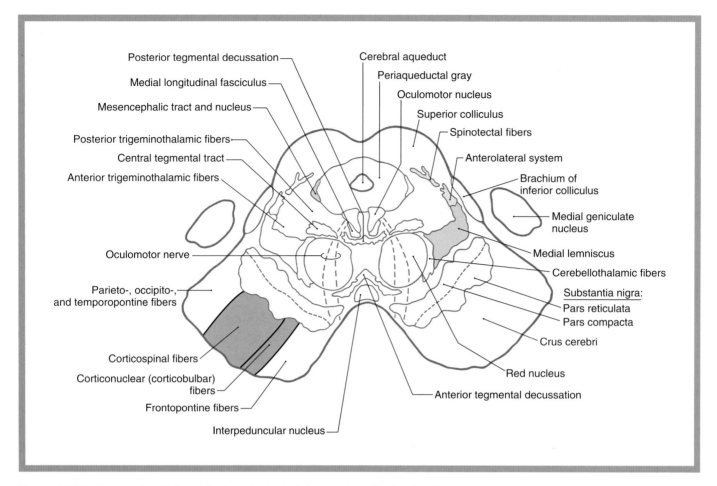

Figure 13-12. Cross section of the midbrain at the level of the superior colliculus. Correlate with Figure 13-7.

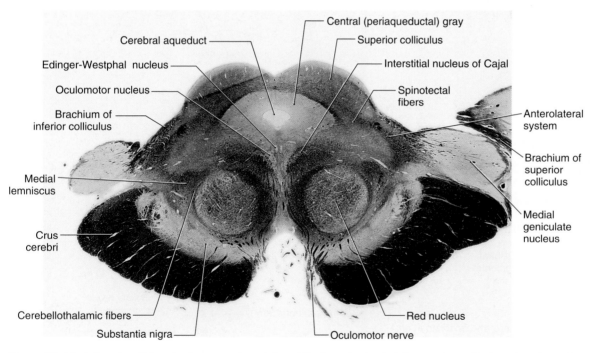

Figure 13-13. A fiber (myelin)-stained cross section of the midbrain at the level of the superior colliculus. This plane of section is between those illustrated in Figures 13-12 and 13-14.

fasciculi (Figs. 13-12 and 13-14). This complex consists of the *general somatic efferent* (GSE) cells of the oculomotor nucleus and the *general visceral efferent* (GVE) cells of the Edinger-Westphal nucleus. Oculomotor fibers arch through and medial to the red nucleus, emerge from the brainstem at the medial edge of the basis pedunculi, and innervate four of the six extraocular muscles. The *Edinger-Westphal nucleus* (Figs. 13-13 and

13-14) lies posterior to the oculomotor nucleus and provides the preganglionic parasympathetic fibers that travel to the ciliary ganglion via the oculomotor nerve. These parasympathetic fibers are located on the perimeter of the oculomotor nerve and, consequently, are the first to be affected in a compression injury to this nerve. The postganglionic fibers from the ciliary ganglion innervate the sphincter pupillae and ciliary muscles.

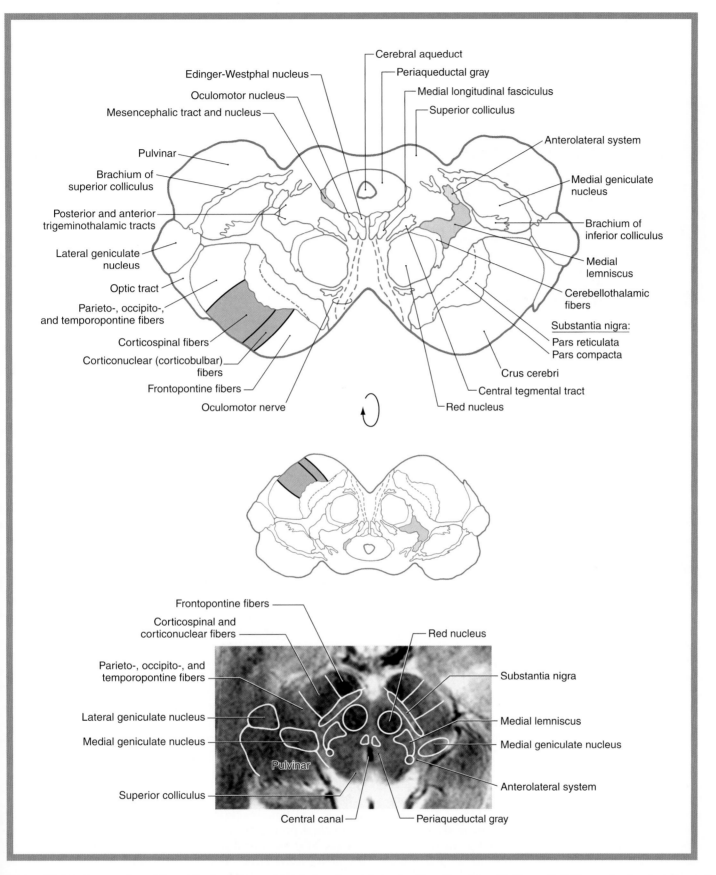

Figure 13-14. Cross section of the midbrain at the mesencephalon-diencephalon junction. Correlate with Figure 13-7. The anatomic orientation is flipped to illustrate internal structures in a clinical orientation; the clinically important tracts and nuclei are shown on a T2-weighted MR image at a comparable level of the superior colliculus and the mesencephalon-diencephalon junction. This MR image, as also shown in the corresponding drawing, contains midbrain structures as well as caudal diencephalic structures.

Several other cell groups are located close to the main oculomotor nucleus (Figs. 13-13 and 13-15). These include (1) the *interstitial nucleus of Cajal* located adjacent to the fibers of the medial longitudinal fasciculus (MLF), (2) the *nucleus of Darkschewitsch* situated within the ventrolateral border of

the periaqueductal gray, and (3) the *nucleus of the posterior commissure,* which is one of the *pretectal nuclei.* Most of these nuclei are involved in the control of eye movements.

The *red nucleus,* a prominent structure in the midbrain tegmentum at this level (Figs. 13-12 to 13-15), is so named

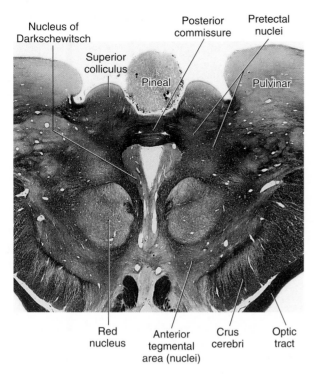

Nucleus of
Darkschewitsch

Superior
colliculus

Pineal

Posterior
commissure

Pretectal
nuclei

Pulvinar

Red
nucleus

Anterior
tegmental
area (nuclei)

Crus
cerebri

Optic
tract

Figure 13-15. A fiber (myelin)-stained cross section of the midbrain at the mesencephalon-diencephalon junction, showing the pretectal area. (From Haines DE: Neuroanatomy, An Atlas of Structures, Sections, and Systems, 6th ed. Philadelphia, Lippincott Williams & Wilkins, 2004.)

because in the unfixed brain the dense vascularity of the region gives it a pink color. It is composed of *caudal magnocellular* (large-celled) and *rostral parvocellular* (small-celled) regions, but these subdivisions are less distinct in primates and humans than in most other animals. The red nucleus is involved in motor function and has extensive connections throughout the neuraxis. Its efferents include the *rubrospinal tract*, which travels to the contralateral spinal cord, and *rubro-olivary fibers*, which descend in the *central tegmental tract* to the ipsilateral inferior olivary complex. Rubrospinal fibers arise from the magnocellular portion of the red nucleus and rubro-olivary fibers from its parvocellular portion. Afferents to the red nucleus arise primarily from the contralateral cerebellar nuclei and the ipsilateral cerebral cortex.

The major tracts of the caudal midbrain tegmentum are present in similar locations at rostral midbrain levels (Fig. 13-12). *Posterior* and *anterior tegmental decussations* cross the midline at the levels of the posterior and anterior limits of the red nuclei, respectively. The posterior decussation carries tectobulbospinal fibers, and the anterior decussation carries rubrospinal fibers. Immediately lateral to the red nucleus are *cerebellorubral* and *cerebellothalamic* fibers. These are crossed ascending fibers from the decussation of the superior cerebellar peduncle. *Posterior (dorsal)* and *anterior (ventral) trigeminothalamic fibers* and the *medial lemniscus* occupy central and more lateral areas of the tegmentum (Fig. 13-12). Fibers of the *anterolateral system* are located at the lateral extreme of the medial lemniscus and, at this level, *spinotectal fibers* enter the deep layers of the superior colliculus (Fig. 13-13).

The structure of the *basis pedunculi* and the organization of fibers in the *crus cerebri* are the same in the rostral midbrain as more caudally (Fig. 13-12). The *substantia nigra* is functionally associated with the basal nuclei and is commonly divided into a *compact part* (pars compacta) and a *reticular part* (pars reticulata) (Figs. 13-12 and 13-14). Cells of the reticular part project to the superior colliculus, thalamus, and pontine reticular formation, whereas those of the compact part project diffusely to

the *caudate nucleus* and *putamen*, where their synaptic terminals release dopamine. Parkinson disease, a deficit characterized by tremor and difficulty in initiating or terminating movement, is associated with the loss of dopamine-containing cells in the compact part.

Midbrain-Diencephalon Junction

The major tracts and nuclei seen at the level of the superior colliculus are still present in their same locations, at the mesencephalic-diencephalic interface. A comparison of Figures 13-12 and 13-14 reveals these similarities.

Groups of cells related primarily to the visual system and collectively referred to as the *pretectal nuclei* are located at the rostral extent of the superior colliculus laterally adjacent to the posterior commissure (Fig. 13-15). Indeed, the nucleus of the posterior commissure is one of the pretectal nuclei. The pretectal nuclei include a controlling center for the *pupillary light reflex*. Neurons involved in this reflex receive bilateral retinal inputs and project bilaterally to visceral motor (parasympathetic) neurons in the Edinger-Westphal nucleus.

Several structures appear at this junction that signal the transition from midbrain to thalamus (Fig. 13-14). Laterally, a small part of the *pulvinar* (a thalamic nucleus) is present, and portions of the *medial* and *lateral geniculate nuclei* also appear in the same plane. Fibers of the *brachium of the inferior colliculus* convey auditory signals to the *medial geniculate nucleus*. The optic tract contains visual fibers, some of which terminate in the lateral geniculate nucleus, while others continue into the superior colliculus and pretectal area via the *brachium of the superior colliculus* (Figs. 13-4 to 13-15). The *anterior (ventral) tegmental nucleus (of Tsai)* is a diffuse cell group located anteromedially to the red nucleus and rostrally continuous with the lateral hypothalamic area. Many of the cells of this nucleus utilize dopamine as a neurotransmitter and receive input from, and project to, hypothalamic and limbic structures that function in emotional behavior.

Reticular and Raphe Nuclei

The reticular formation of the midbrain tegmentum is composed of the *cuneiform* and *subcuneiform nuclei* (Fig. 13-16). The midbrain reticular formation participates in the ascending systems that regulate states of consciousness. Many of these neurons project to the thalamus, especially the thalamic reticular nucleus, and the hypothalamus. This ascending fiber system is largely responsible for maintaining an alert, wakeful state and thus forms part of the *ascending reticular activating system*. Lesions involving the midbrain reticular formation can result in *hypersomnia*, which is characterized by slow respiration and an electroencephalographic pattern (large-amplitude slow waves) indicative of a sleep state.

Located in anterior parts of the periaqueductal gray, the *posterior (dorsal) raphe nucleus* extends from the rostral pons into the caudal midbrain (Fig. 13-16). The serotoninergic cells of this nucleus project to wide areas of the cerebral cortex, where they modulate neuronal activity involved in sleep/dream cycles. *Serotonin-*, *enkephalin-*, and *cholecystokinin-containing* cells are also found in the central (periaqueductal) gray and, indeed, some neuroscientists consider the periaqueductal gray to function in concert with the raphe nuclei.

Internal Vasculature of the Midbrain

The blood supply to the midbrain originates from the *basilar artery* and its major branches (the *quadrigeminal* and *superior cerebellar arteries*) and from the *anterior choroidal artery*, which is a branch of the internal carotid, and the *medial posterior choroidal artery*, which is usually a branch of P$_2$ (Fig. 13-17). Medial regions of the midbrain receive numerous small branches

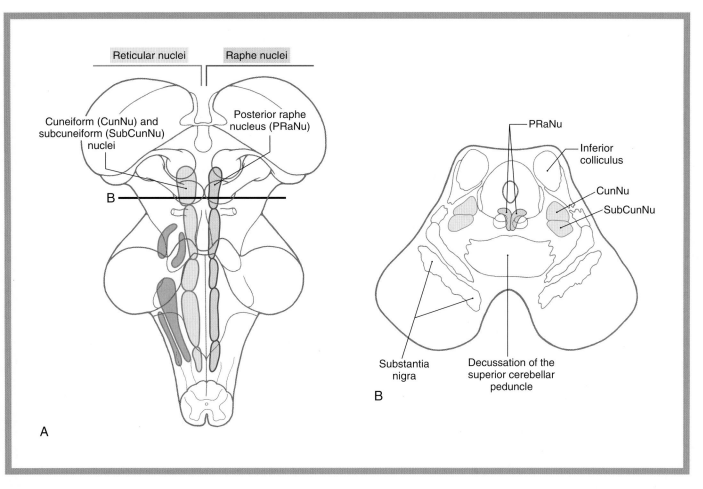

Figure 13-16. Posterior (**A**) view of the brainstem and a cross section (**B**) at the level of the inferior colliculus showing the raphe and reticular nuclei of the brainstem.

from the P₁ segment of the posterior cerebral artery and from the *posterior communicating artery*. These paramedian branches constitute the *posteromedial group* of branches from the circle of Willis. Included in their territory are the oculomotor, trochlear, and Edinger-Westphal nuclei; the exiting oculomotor fibers; the red nucleus; and medial aspects of the substantia nigra and crus cerebri (Fig. 13-17).

Ventrolateral regions of the midbrain are served by penetrating branches of the *quadrigeminal artery* (Fig. 13-17), the *anterior choroidal artery*, and the *medial posterior choroidal artery*. The region served by these branches includes the lateral parts of the crus and substantia nigra and the medial lemniscus.

The posterior midbrain is served primarily by the *quadrigeminal artery* (*collicular artery*), which typically arises from P₁ (Fig. 13-17). Much of the periaqueductal gray, the nuclei of the superior and inferior colliculi, the anterolateral system, and the brachium of the inferior colliculus are served by quadrigeminal branches. Additional blood supply to the area surrounding the exit of the trochlear nerve and the inferior colliculus arises from medial branches of the *superior cerebellar artery*.

Vascular Syndromes of the Midbrain

Occlusion of vessels serving the medial portions of the midbrain may result in the *Weber syndrome* (Fig. 13-18A). This results in an ipsilateral paralysis of all extraocular muscles except the lateral rectus and superior oblique, reflecting damage to the exiting root of the oculomotor nerve, and a paralysis of the contralateral extremities, indicating damage to corticospinal fibers in the crus cerebri. The ipsilateral pupil is also dilated. This lesion also includes damage to corticonuclear fibers in the crus, resulting in a weakness of the facial muscles of the lower half of

the face and a deviation of the tongue when protruded, both on the side contralateral to the lesion (see Chapter 25 for additional information).

If the vascular lesion is located in the more central area of the midbrain, the structures damaged include the fibers of the oculomotor nerve, the red nucleus, and the cerebellothalamic fibers. Collectively, the deficits seen following a lesion in this area constitute the *Claude syndrome* (Fig. 13-18B). Deficits include an ipsilateral paralysis of most eye movements: the eye is directed down and out with a dilated pupil (oculomotor nerve) and a contralateral ataxia, tremor, and incoordination that results from the damage to the red nucleus and cerebellothalamic fibers (see Chapters 24 and 25).

A large lesion that includes the territories of both the *Weber + Claude syndromes* results in a constellation of deficits called the *Benedikt syndrome* (Fig. 13-18C). These include an ipsilateral paralysis of most eye movements, contralateral weakness of the extremities, and contralateral tremor and ataxia. In each of these lesions it is possible that the GVE preganglionic parasympathetic fibers arising in the Edinger-Westphal nucleus may be damaged. Thus the pupil on the side of the lesion will be dilated due to the action of the intact sympathetic input to the dilator muscle of the iris.

Herniation Syndromes Related to the Midbrain

The midbrain lies at the intersection of the right and left supratentorial compartments with the infratentorial compartment. In this position it traverses the tentorial notch, extending from the caudal diencephalon to the rostral pons. The herniation

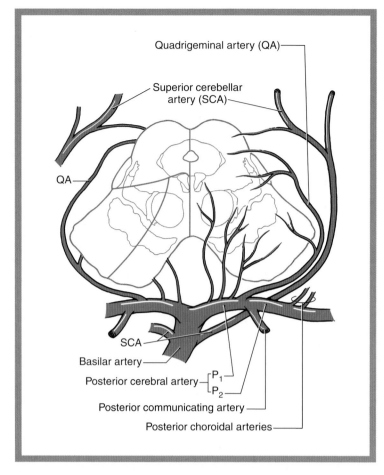

Figure 13-17. Blood supply of the midbrain. Arteries are shown mainly on the right and the territories served by each on the left. The anterior choroidal artery, which is a branch of the internal carotid and follows the general route of the optic tract (Fig. 13-3B), also sends branches to the lateral portions of the midbrain.

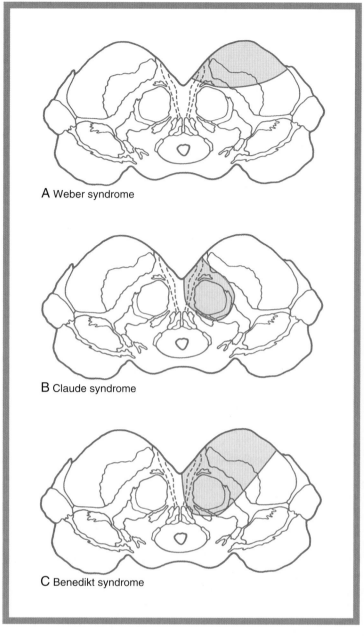

Figure 13-18. The location of midbrain lesions that result in deficits seen in the Weber (**A**), Claude (**B**), and Benedikt (**C**) syndromes; these lesions may result from vascular complications. These are illustrated in a clinical orientation (as is seen in MRI or CT); consequently, the observer's right is the patient's left and the observer's left is the patient's right. The laterality of the deficits follows accordingly.

syndromes related to the midbrain are *central* or *transtentorial herniation, upward cerebellar herniation,* and *uncal herniation.*

Central (or *transtentorial*) *herniation* (Fig. 13-19) may follow a large hemorrhage into the hemisphere or a large rapidly growing tumor. Essentially the enlarging mass (be it hemorrhage or tumor) forces the diencephalon downward through the tentorial incisure and into the midbrain. Prior to the herniation the patient is less alert (decreased level of consciousness) and may have altered respiratory patterns and eye movements. The patient responds to noxious stimuli but will have hyperactive muscle stretch reflexes. As intracranial pressure increases, the patient may become *decorticate* (lower extremities, trunk, and neck extended; upper extremities flexed). The herniation traverses the tentorial notch and impinges on the midbrain, beginning a series of catastrophic events. The patient is comatose, pupils are dilated and fixed, and respiration is irregular with changes in depth and rate (Cheyne-Stokes) or periods of *tachypnea* and eventual *apnea;* the patient becomes *decerebrate* with all four extremities extended (see Chapter 24 for more information). As the cone of ischemia extends into, and through, the midbrain the deficits are exacerbated and the likelihood of survival is greatly diminished.

Upward cerebellar herniation (Fig. 13-19) may result from an expanding mass in the posterior fossa. In this situation medial portions of the cerebellum pass upward through the tentorial notch and compress the midbrain. There is the eventual possibility of cerebellar infarction from compression of the superior cerebellar arteries and *hydrocephalus* from obstruction of the

cerebral aqueduct. If the primary cause of the herniation is treated in a timely manner there is usually a good outcome.

Uncal herniation results from an expanding lesion (usually a hematoma) in the hemisphere, frequently the temporal lobe, that forces the *uncus* over the edge of the tentorium and into the midbrain (Fig. 13-20). The initial finding is a dilated pupil (pressure on the third nerve) on the side of the herniation followed by a paralysis of most eye movement in the eye with the dilated pupil. As the herniation progresses, corticospinal fibers in the crus cerebri are compressed, resulting in a weakness of the contralateral upper and lower extremities. In addition, cranial nerve signs such as a *central seven* (lower facial muscles contralaterally), difficulty swallowing, and deviation of the tongue contralaterally on protrusion may also appear as a result of damage to corticonuclear fibers in the crus cerebri. If the cause of the uncal herniation is not treated, the deficits may escalate into those described earlier for central herniation with similar consequences.

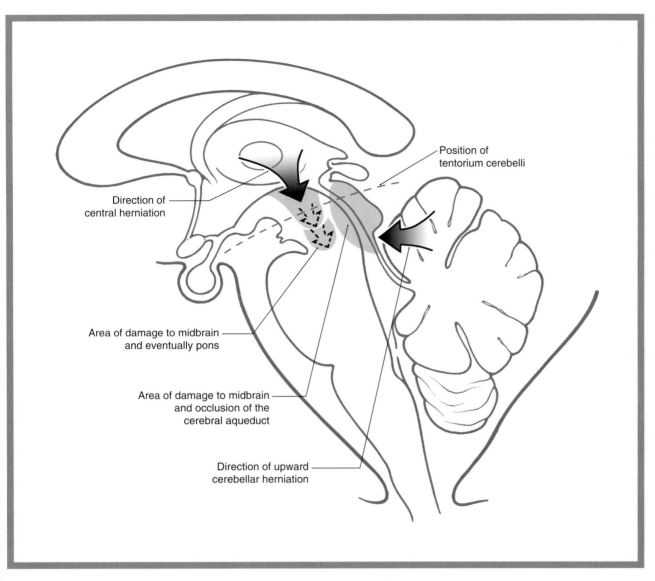

Figure 13-19. Two of the three important herniation syndromes related to the midbrain are central (or transtentorial) herniation and upward cerebellar herniation. The former proceeds downward through the tentorial notch whereas the latter proceeds upward through the notch.

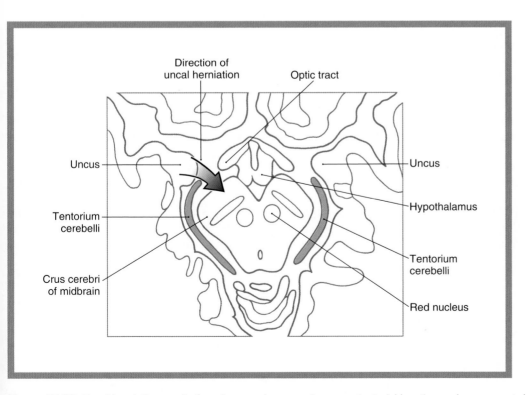

Figure 13-20. Uncal herniation results from increased pressure in a supratentorial location and consequent downward extrusion of the uncus over the edge of the tentorium and against the midbrain. This may produce many of the features of the Weber syndrome.

Synopsis of Clinical Points

- Aneurysm of the basilar bifurcation may impinge on the exiting root of the oculomotor nerve in the interpeduncular fossa (p. 197).
- Tumors of the pineal gland may impinge on the tectum of the midbrain, compress the aqueduct, and cause obstructive hydrocephalus (p. 197).
- The periaqueductal (central) gray contains opiate receptors and plays a role in pain modulation (p. 199).
- Lesions of the crus cerebri result in motor deficits related to the face and oral cavity and the body (p. 199).
- Loss of dopamine cells of the substantia nigra, the pars compacta, results in Parkinson disease (p. 204).
- The Weber syndrome is an ipsilateral paralysis of most eye movement and a contralateral hemiparesis (p. 205).
- The Claude syndrome is an ipsilateral paralysis of most eye movement and a contralateral ataxia and tremor (p. 205).
- The Claude + Weber syndromes = the Benedikt syndrome (p. 205).
- Central (or transtentorial) herniation may result in the patient becoming decorticate, then decerebrate with a significantly decreased probability of survival (p. 206).
- A rapidly expanding mass in the cerebellum may result in upward cerebellar herniation with possible cerebellar infarction and hydrocephalus (p. 206).
- Uncal herniation may compress the midbrain (and crus), resulting in characteristic motor weakness (p. 206).

Sources and Additional Reading

Bobillier P, Seguin S, Petitjean F, Salvert D, Tovret M, Jouvet M: The raphe nuclei of the cat brain stem: A topographical atlas of their efferent projections as revealed by autoradiography. Brain Res 113:449-486, 1976.

Bogerts B: A brainstem atlas of catecholaminergic neurons in man, using melanin as a natural marker. J Comp Neurol 197:63-80, 1981.

Brodal A: The Reticular Formation of the Brainstem, Anatomical Aspects and Functional Correlations. Springfield, IL, Charles C Thomas, 1958.

Brodal A: Neurological Anatomy, 3rd ed. New York, Oxford University Press, 1981.

Crosby EC, Humphrey T, Lauer EW: Correlative Anatomy of the Nervous System. New York, Macmillan, 1962.

Duvernoy HM: Human Brainstem Vessels. Berlin, Springer-Verlag, 1978.

Duvernoy H: The Human Brain Stem and Cerebellum, Surface, Structure, Vascularization, and Three-Dimensional Sectional Anatomy with MRI. Vienna, Springer-Verlag, 1995.

Haines DE: Neuroanatomy: An Atlas of Structures, Sections, and Systems, 6th ed. Philadelphia, Lippincott Williams & Wilkins, 2004.

Hobson JA, Brazier MAB (eds): The Reticular Formation Revisited: Specifying Function for a Nonspecific System. Int Brain Res Organization Monogram Series, vol 6. New York, Raven Press, 1980.

Hubbard JE, DiCarlo V: Fluorescence histochemistry of monoamine-containing cell bodies in the brain stem of the squirrel monkey (Saimiri sciureus): III. Serotonin-containing groups. J Comp Neurol 153:385-398, 1974.

Jenkins TW, Truex RC: Dissection of the human brain as a method for its fractionation by weight. Anat Rec 147:359-366, 1963.

Kretschmann H-J, Weinrich W: Cranial Neuroimaging and Clinical Neuroanatomy, Magnetic Resonance Imaging and Computed Tomography, 2nd ed. New York, Thieme Medical Publishers, 1992.

Larsell O, Jansen J: The Comparative Anatomy and Histology of the Cerebellum, The Human Cerebellum, Cerebellar Connections, and Cerebellar Cortex. Minneapolis, University of Minnesota Press, 1972.

Leblanc A: The Cranial Nerves: Anatomy, Imaging, Vascularisation. New York, Springer, 1995.

Nieuwenhuys R: Chemoarchitecture of the Brain. Berlin, Springer-Verlag, 1985.

Nieuwenhuys R, Voogd J, van Huijzen CHR: The Human Central Nervous System, A Synopsis and Atlas, 3rd ed. Berlin, Springer-Verlag, 1988.

Olszewski J, Baxter D: Cytoarchitecture of the Human Brain Stem, 2nd ed. Basel, S Karger, 1982.

Palay SL, Chan-Palay V: Cerebellar Cortex, Cytology and Organization. New York, Springer-Verlag, 1974.

Parent A: Carpenter's Human Neuroanatomy, 9th ed. Baltimore, Williams & Wilkins, 1996.

Paxinos G (ed): The Human Nervous System. San Diego, Academic Press, 1990, chapters 7-14.

Taber E, Brodal A, Walberg F: The raphe nuclei of the brain stem in the cat: I. Normal topography and cytoarchitecture and general discussion. J Comp Neurol 114:161-187, 1960.

Tatu L, Moulin T, Bogousslavsky J, Duvernoy H: Arterial territories of human brain: Brainstem and cerebellum. Neurology 47:1125-1135, 1996.

Weber JT, Martin GF, Behan M, Huerta MF, Harting JK: The precise origin of the tectospinal pathway in three common laboratory animals: A study using the horseradish peroxidase method. Neurosci Lett 11:121-127, 1979.

Chapter 14

A Synopsis of Cranial Nerves of the Brainstem

D. E. Haines and G. A. Mihailoff

Although the brainstem is quite small, comprising only about 2.6% of total brain weight, the size of this structure belies its importance. First, all ascending and descending tracts linking the spinal cord and the forebrain traverse the brainstem. Second, there are important ascending fibers (e.g., spinoreticular, spino-periaqueductal gray) and descending fibers (e.g., rubrospinal, vestibulospinal, reticulospinal) that interconnect the brainstem with the spinal cord. These tracts, and the more expansive connections they make, are essential to the successful function of the nervous system. Third, the nuclei and the exit and entrance points of 10 of the 12 cranial nerves are associated with the brainstem.

Lesions of the brainstem, regardless of their origin (vascular, tumor, trauma), frequently involve cranial nerves. Indeed, in patients with brainstem lesions who have long tract signs, the accompanying cranial nerve deficits usually represent excellent localizing signs.

Overview

In general, the exit of a cranial nerve from the brainstem ("exit" is used here with reference to both efferent and afferent fibers of the nerve) is associated with the same brainstem area in which the nuclei of that nerve are found. The obvious exception is the trigeminal nerve, the sensory nuclei of which form a continuous cell column from rostral regions of the midbrain to the spinal cord-medulla interface.

This chapter reviews cranial nerves of the brainstem from caudal (hypoglossal) to rostral (oculomotor) and presents a number of clinical examples. The goal here is not simply to review the information covered in the last three chapters but to *consider the cranial nerves in a somewhat broader perspective. Structure, function, and dysfunction are described in an integrated manner because this is how cranial nerves are evaluated in the clinical setting.*

Motor Cell Columns and Nuclei

Early in development the derivatives of the *basal plate* that form motor nuclei of the cranial nerves in the brainstem tend to form rostrocaudally oriented cell columns. As the brainstem enlarges, these cell columns become discontinuous. That is, they are in line with, but are separated from, each other in the adult brain (see Figs. 10-5 to 10-7). As we have seen, and shall review here, those nuclei that are in line with each other, and that have arisen from the same original cell column, have developmental, structural, and functional characteristics in common.

The most medial cranial nerve motor nuclei in the brainstem are the *hypoglossal* (XII), *abducens* (VI), *trochlear* (IV), and *oculomotor* (III) nuclei (Fig. 14-1). These nuclei share three characteristics. First, they are located adjacent to the midline and anterior to the ventricular space of their particular brain division. Second, the motor neurons in these nuclei innervate skeletal muscle that originates from head mesoderm in the occipital region (tongue muscles) and in the area of the orbit (extraocular muscles). Third, the functional component of the lower motor neurons in these nuclei is general somatic efferent (GSE), reflecting the fact that these motor neurons innervate skeletal muscles that originate from head mesoderm *not* located in a pharyngeal arch.

Laterally adjacent to the GSE cell column are the nuclei that collectively constitute the cranial part of the craniosacral division (parasympathetic) of the visceromotor nervous system. These nuclei—with the cranial nerves on which the preganglionic fibers travel—are (1) the *dorsal motor vagal nucleus*—vagus nerve; (2) the *inferior salivatory nucleus*—glossopharyngeal nerve; (3) *the superior salivatory nucleus*—the facial nerve-intermediate

part; and (4) the *Edinger-Westphal nucleus*—oculomotor nerve (Fig. 14-1; see also Fig. 10-7). These nuclei share the following characteristics. First, they form a discontinuous column located slightly lateral to the GSE nuclei. Second, the neurons in these nuclei give rise to preganglionic axons that terminate in a peripheral ganglion, the cells of which give rise to postganglionic fibers that innervate a visceral structure. Third, because these motor neurons are part of a pathway that innervates a visceral structure (tissue composed of smooth muscle, glandular epithelium, or cardiac muscle or a combination of these), they are classified as general visceral efferent (GVE). They can most accurately be identified as *GVE–preganglionic parasympathetic, as this term completely identifies their structural and functional relationships.*

The most lateral motor cell column in the medulla and in the pontine tegmentum is formed by the *nucleus ambiguus*, the efferents of which travel on the vagus and glossopharyngeal nerves, and by the *facial motor nucleus* and the *trigeminal motor nucleus*, related to facial and trigeminal nerves, respectively (Fig. 14-1; see also Fig. 10-7). These motor nuclei also share common characteristics. First, they form a discontinuous column in the more lateral part of the medulla and pontine tegmentum. Their position, as is the case for the GSE and GVE cell columns, reflects the differentiation of the basal plate in the brainstem. Second, the muscles innervated by these lower motor neurons originate from mesenchyme specifically located within the pharyngeal arches. The *muscles of mastication* (trigeminal nerve innervation) originate in arch I; the *muscles of facial expression* (facial nerve innervation), in arch II; the *stylopharyngeus muscle* (glossopharyngeal nerve innervation), in arch III; and the *constrictors of the pharynx, intrinsic laryngeal muscles, palatine muscles (except the tensor veli palatini), and the vocalis* (vagal nerve innervation), in arch IV. Third, owing to the fact that these lower motor neurons innervate a unique population of muscles, *skeletal muscles arising within pharyngeal arches*, they are classified as special visceral efferent (SVE).

Sensory Cell Columns and Nuclei

The derivatives of the *alar plate* that give rise to cranial nerve sensory nuclei of the brainstem are located lateral to the sulcus limitans (see Figs. 10-5 and 10-6). In contrast to the motor nuclei, which form rostrocaudally oriented but discontinuous cell columns, all three of the sensory nuclei in the brainstem form what can arguably be described as continuous cell columns in the adult. These sensory nuclei–cell columns are located in the lateral aspects of the brainstem.

The most medial of these cell columns is the *solitary tract and nucleus*, which is the visceral afferent center of the brainstem (Fig. 14-1; see also Fig. 10-7). *No matter what cranial nerve returns visceral afferent information to the brainstem, the central processes of these primary afferent fibers contribute to the solitary tract, the fibers of which terminate in the solitary nucleus* (Fig. 14-2). Visceral afferent information is conveyed centrally on the facial, glossopharyngeal, and vagus nerves and consists of taste fibers (special visceral afferent [SVA]) and fibers conveying general visceral sensation (general visceral afferent [GVA]). The majority of taste input reaches rostral portions of the solitary nucleus (sometimes called the *gustatory nucleus*), whereas most general visceral sensation enters the caudal portion of the solitary nucleus (sometimes referred to as the *cardiorespiratory nucleus*) (Fig. 14-2). Because the most rostral cranial nerve that contributes to the solitary tract and nucleus is the facial nerve (a nerve of the pons-medulla junction), the solitary tract and its nucleus are found throughout the medulla but do not extend rostrally beyond the pons-medulla junction.

Immediately and posteriorly adjacent to the solitary tract and nucleus are the *medial and spinal vestibular nuclei*. These

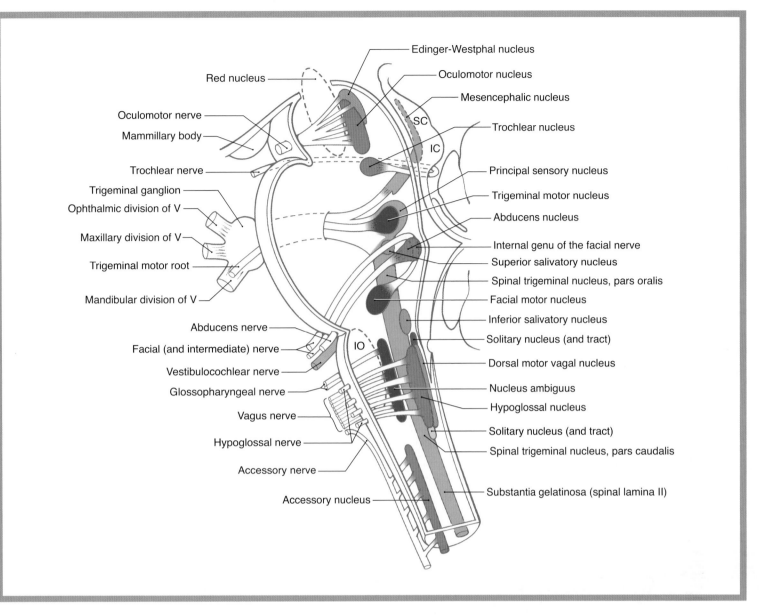

Figure 14-1. The location of cranial nerve nuclei and the course of their fibers within the brainstem. The functional component associated with each nucleus and with the fibers to or from that nucleus are color coded in this figure and in other figures showing connections in this chapter as follows: general somatic efferent (GSE), *red;* general somatic afferent (GSA), *light red;* special visceral efferent (SVE), *blue;* general visceral efferent (GVE), *light blue;* special visceral afferent (SVA), *green;* general visceral afferent (GVA), *light green;* and special somatic afferent (SSA), *gray.* (Modified with permission from Carpenter MB, Sutin J: Human Neuroanatomy, 8th ed. Baltimore, Williams & Wilkins, 1983.)

continue rostrally, are joined by the *anterior and posterior cochlear nuclei* at the pons-medulla junction, and interface in the caudal pons with the *superior and lateral vestibular nuclei* (Fig. 14-9). This cell column receives sensory input from the vestibulocochlear nerve (cranial nerve VIII) only and subserves the sense of hearing (SSA, exteroceptive functional component) and balance and equilibrium (SSA, proprioceptive functional component).

The nuclei of the trigeminal sensory system form a continuous cell column extending from the spinal cord-medulla junction to the rostral midbrain (Fig. 14-1; see also Fig. 10-7). The trigeminal sensory nuclei are divided into (1) the *spinal trigeminal nucleus* (consisting of a *pars caudalis, pars interpolaris,* and *pars oralis*), located in the lateral medulla and extending into the caudal pons; (2) the *principal sensory nucleus,* located at the mid-pontine level; and (3) the *mesencephalic nucleus,* extending rostrally into the midbrain at the lateral aspect of the periaqueductal gray (Fig. 14-1; see also Fig. 13-8). As is the case for the solitary tract and nucleus (the visceral receiving center of the brainstem), the principal sensory nucleus and especially the

spinal trigeminal nucleus constitute the general sensory receiving center of the brainstem. *Although general somatic afferent (GSA) pain and thermal sensations enter the brainstem on four different cranial nerves (trigeminal, facial, glossopharyngeal, and vagus), the central processes of these primary afferent fibers enter the spinal trigeminal tract and terminate in the medially adjacent spinal trigeminal nucleus.* This theme is revisited in the review of individual nerves later in the chapter.

Cranial Nerves of the Medulla Oblongata

The cranial nerves that are commonly identified as exiting the medulla are the hypoglossal nerve (cranial nerve XII) through the abducens nerve (cranial nerve VI) (Figs. 14-3 and 14-4). However, in the subsequent discussion, the abducens (VI), facial (VII), and vestibulocochlear (VIII) nerves are considered as the nerves of the pons-medulla junction. Consequently, the cranial nerves that are generally associated with *only* the medulla are the

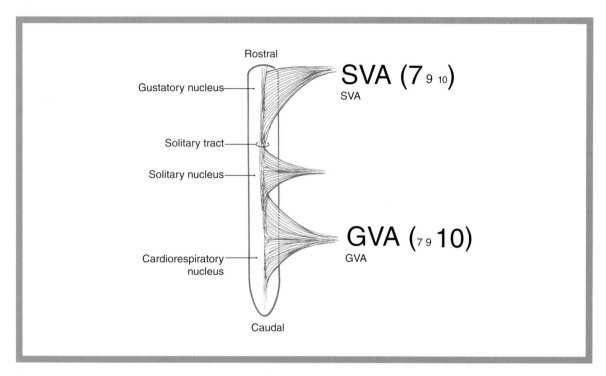

Rostral

Gustatory nucleus

SVA (7 9 10)
SVA

Solitary tract

Solitary nucleus

GVA (7 9 10)
GVA

Cardiorespiratory
nucleus

Caudal

Figure 14-2. Diagrammatic representation of the solitary tract and nucleus. The functional components associated with rostral versus caudal portions of the tract and nucleus, and the cranial nerves conveying this input, are shown in letters and numbers of proportionate size for each area.

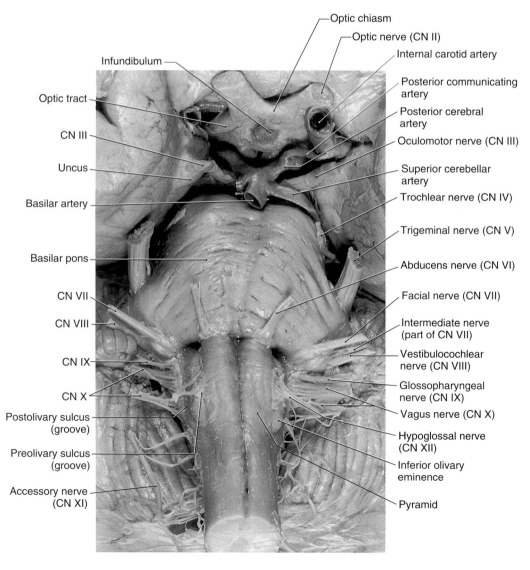

Infundibulum

Optic tract

CN III

Uncus

Basilar artery

Basilar pons

CN VII

CN VIII

CN IX

CN X

Postolivary sulcus
(groove)

Preolivary sulcus
(groove)

Accessory nerve
(CN XI)

Optic chiasm

Optic nerve (CN II)

Internal carotid artery

Posterior communicating
artery

Posterior cerebral
artery

Oculomotor nerve (CN III)

Superior cerebellar
artery

Trochlear nerve (CN IV)

Trigeminal nerve (CN V)

Abducens nerve (CN VI)

Facial nerve (CN VII)

Intermediate nerve
(part of CN VII)

Vestibulocochlear
nerve (CN VIII)

Glossopharyngeal
nerve (CN IX)

Vagus nerve (CN X)

Hypoglossal nerve
(CN XII)

Inferior olivary
eminence

Pyramid

Figure 14-3. An anterior (ventral) view of the brainstem with particular emphasis on cranial nerves (CNs).

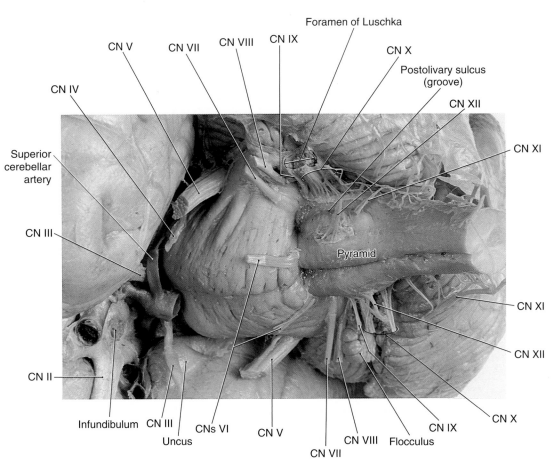

Foramen of Luschka

CN V   CN VII   CN VIII   CN IX

CN X

Postolivary sulcus (groove)

CN XII

CN IV

CN XI

Superior cerebellar artery

CN III

Pyramid

CN XI

CN XII

CN II

CN X

Infundibulum   CN III   CNs VI   CN V   CN IX

Uncus   CN VIII   Flocculus

CN VII

Figure 14-4. An anterolateral (ventrolateral) view of the brainstem with special emphasis on cranial nerves (CNs). Note the position and relationships of the foramen of Luschka.

hypoglossal (XII), *accessory* (XI), *vagus* (X), and *glossopharyngeal* (IX) nerves (Figs. 14-3 and 14-4). The unique situation of the accessory nerve is addressed further on.

Hypoglossal Nerve

The *hypoglossal nucleus* is located internal to the hypoglossal trigone. Axons of hypoglossal motor neurons pass anteriorly in the medulla along the lateral aspect of the medial lemniscus and the pyramid (see Fig. 11-11) to exit as a series of rootlets from the preolivary fissure as the *hypoglossal nerve* (Figs. 14-3 and 14-5). They continue through the *hypoglossal canal* and distribute to the intrinsic muscles of the tongue plus the hypoglossus, palatoglossus, and genioglossus muscles (Fig. 14-6). In addition to the hypoglossal nerve, the hypoglossal canal may also contain an emissary vein and a small meningeal branch to the dura of the posterior fossa from the ascending pharyngeal artery.

The blood supply to the hypoglossal nucleus and its exiting fibers is via penetrating branches of the *anterior spinal artery*. Occlusion of these branches (as in the medial medullary

syndrome) may result in paralysis of the genioglossus muscle with *deviation of the tongue toward the side of the lesion (the weak side) on protrusion*. In addition, the patient experiences a *contralateral hemiparesis* (corticospinal tract involvement) and a *contralateral loss of position sense, vibratory sense, and two-point discrimination* (medial lemniscus involvement), because the anterior spinal artery also serves these structures.

Other lesions that may affect hypoglossal function include a lesion of the root of the nerve only (causing tongue deviation to the side of the lesion with no other deficits) or injury to the internal capsule. In the latter case, corticonuclear (corticobulbar) fibers to hypoglossal motor neurons innervating the genioglossus muscle are predominantly crossed. Consequently, internal capsule lesions may result in a deviation of the tongue to the contralateral side (side opposite the lesion) on protrusion, in concert with other deficits such as a contralateral hemiplegia and a drooping of the facial muscles in the lower quadrant of the contralateral side of the face. See Chapter 25 for examples of lesions that result in hypoglossal nerve dysfunction.

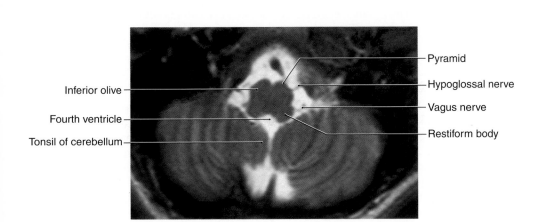

Inferior olive

Fourth ventricle

Tonsil of cerebellum

Pyramid

Hypoglossal nerve

Vagus nerve

Restiform body

Figure 14-5. Axial T2-weighted MR image of the medulla showing the roots of the hypoglossal (from the preolivary fissure) and the vagus (from the post- or retro-olivary fissure) nerves. Compare the shape of the medulla at this level with Figures 14-3 and 14-4.

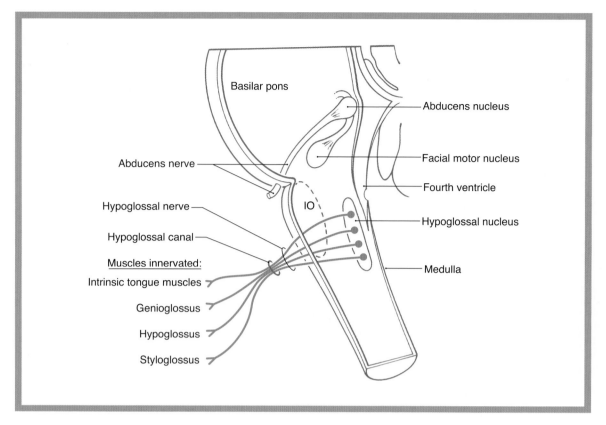

Figure 14-6. The central origin and peripheral distribution of the hypoglossal nerve (cranial nerve XII).

Accessory Nerve

This so-called cranial nerve was historically described as having a *cranial part* (from the medulla) and a *spinal part* (from the cervical spinal cord). However, experimental studies have shown that the neurons that innervate the sternocleidomastoid and trapezius muscles are located in the *cervical cord* only; these muscles are not innervated by motor neurons located in the medulla. However, for consistency, and in recognition of wide usage, the accessory nerve is considered here as a cranial nerve of the medulla.

The *accessory nerve* originates from motor neurons in the cervical spinal cord (Fig. 14-7). The axons of these neurons exit the lateral aspect of the cord, coalesce to form the nerve (Fig. 14-3), ascend to enter the cranial cavity via the foramen magnum, and exit the posterior fossa through the jugular foramen (Fig. 14-8). En route through the posterior fossa these fibers briefly join the caudal portions of the vagus nerve (Fig. 14-7) and then leave the vagus to exit the skull as the accessory nerve. It is this temporary apposition of vagus fibers to the intracranial portion of the accessory nerve that was originally interpreted as the so-called cranial part of the accessory nerve.

The relationship of the accessory nerve to the vagus nerve is very similar to the relationship of the seventh nerve to the trigeminal nerve via the chorda tympani. In the latter case the taste fibers from the anterior two thirds of the tongue travel on the trigeminal nerve and then join the seventh nerve via the chorda tympani. However, throughout their extent, these taste fibers are considered as part of the seventh nerve, not the fifth. In like manner, fibers of the accessory nerve temporarily join the vagus and then leave it to exit the skull (Fig. 14-7). These accessory nerve fibers do not originate from the medulla, do not distribute peripherally with the vagus, and have their cells of origin in the cervical spinal cord. What has classically been called the cranial part of the accessory nerve is actually a misnomer; these fibers are the caudal portions of the vagus nerve to which the accessory nerve temporarily relates. Reflecting the fact that the sternocleidomastoid and trapezius muscles in the human

originate from mesoderm caudal to the fourth arch (not *in* the fourth arch), the functional component associated with these motor neurons is GSE.

Lesions of the root of the accessory nerve result in *drooping of the shoulder* (trapezius paralysis) on the ipsilateral side and *difficulty in turning the head* to the contralateral side (sternocleidomastoid paralysis) against resistance. Weakness of these muscles is not especially obvious in cervical cord lesions, because a hemiplegia (indicating damage to corticospinal fibers) is the overwhelmingly obvious deficit. However, a lesion of the internal capsule may also result in deficits similar to those described previously, owing to interruption of the corticonuclear (corticobulbar) fibers to the accessory nucleus; these corticonuclear fibers are primarily uncrossed.

Vagus Nerve

The *vagus nerve* is located at an intermediate position between the midline and lateral aspect of the medulla, exits the postolivary sulcus (Figs. 14-3 to 14-5 and 14-9), and contains both motor and sensory components. This cranial nerve exits the cranial cavity via the jugular foramen (Fig. 14-8) and exhibits two ganglia immediately external to the foramen. The *superior ganglion* contains the cell bodies of GSA fibers, whereas the *inferior ganglion* contains the cell bodies of GVA and SVA fibers.

The motor cells in the medulla that distribute their axons on the vagus nerve are located in the *dorsal motor nucleus of the vagus* (GVE–parasympathetic preganglionic) and in the *nucleus ambiguus* (SVE) (Fig. 14-7). Preganglionic parasympathetic GVE cells of the dorsal motor nucleus send their axon, via branches of the vagus nerve, to end in *terminal (intramural) ganglia* located adjacent to, or within, visceral structures of the trachea and bronchi of the lungs, the heart, and the digestive system to a level just proximal to the splenic flexure of the colon (Fig. 14-7). In general, vagal influence causes constriction of the bronchioles, decreases heart rate, and increases blood flow, peristalsis, and secretions in the gut (see Chapter 29 for details). Axons of SVE motor neurons in the *nucleus ambiguus* distribute

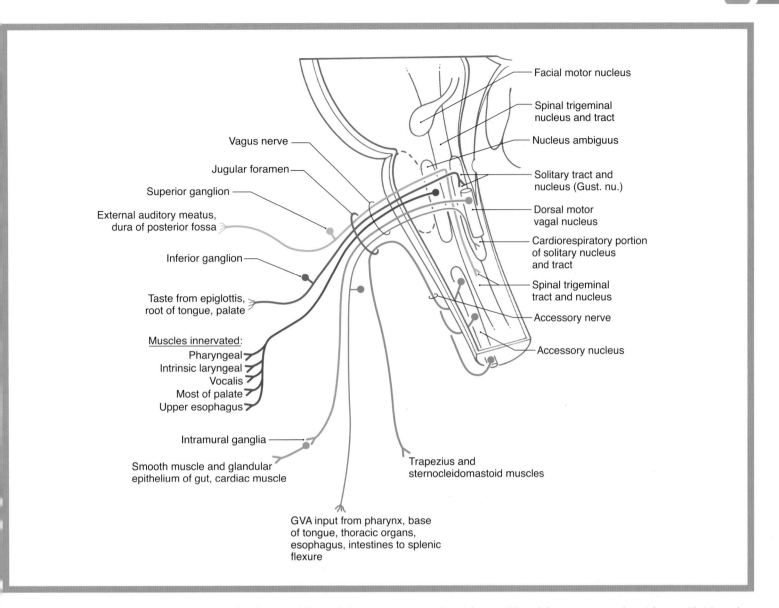

Figure 14-7. The central nuclei and peripheral distribution of fibers of the accessory nerve (cranial nerve XI) and the vagus nerve (cranial nerve X). Visceral afferent cell bodies (SVA, GVA) collectively form the inferior ganglion, and GSA cell bodies collectively form the superior ganglion of cranial nerve X. Gust. nu., rostral portions of solitary nucleus-gustatory nucleus.

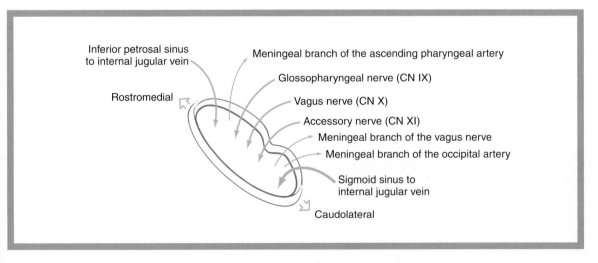

Figure 14-8. The right jugular foramen and its contents as viewed from the inside floor of the cranial cavity. The direction and size of the arrows indicate the relative size of structures entering or exiting the foramen. CN, cranial nerve.

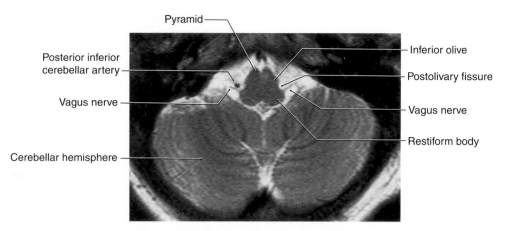

Figure 14-9. Axial T2-weighted MR image of the medulla showing the root of the vagus nerve (from the post- or retro-olivary fissure). Note the location of a portion of the posterior inferior cerebellar artery.

on branches of the vagus nerve to the constrictor muscles of the pharynx, the intrinsic laryngeal muscles (including the vocalis muscle), the palatine muscles (except the tensor veli palatini, which is innervated by the fifth nerve), and the skeletal muscle in about the upper half of the esophagus (Fig. 14-7). These muscles originate within the fourth pharyngeal arch, hence their innervation by neurons with an SVE functional component.

The sensory fibers conveyed on the vagus nerve relay general somatic, general visceral, and special visceral sensations. The general somatic sensations are represented by GSA input (recognized as pain and thermal sensations) from a small area on the ear and part of the external auditory meatus and from the dura of the posterior cranial fossa (Fig. 14-7). These fibers have their cell bodies in the superior ganglion of the vagus nerve and enter the medulla as part of the vagus, but the central processes of these GSA primary afferent fibers enter the *spinal trigeminal tract* and synapse in the medially adjacent *spinal trigeminal nucleus*.

The general and special visceral sensations conveyed by the vagus are represented by GVA and SVA fibers (Fig. 14-7). General visceral sensations from the heart, aortic arch, pharynx and larynx, lungs, and gut to about the level of the splenic flexure are conveyed by these GVA fibers. Their cell bodies are in the inferior ganglion of the vagus nerve, whereas the central processes of these GVA fibers enter the *solitary tract* and terminate in the surrounding *solitary nucleus*. The same trajectory is also followed by taste fibers (SVA fibers) on the vagus. These fibers originate from scattered taste buds on the epiglottis and base of the tongue, have their cell bodies in the inferior ganglion, enter the brainstem on the vagus nerve, and centrally distribute to the solitary tract and nucleus.

Both general sensory (GSA, GVA) and taste (SVA) information conveyed on the vagus nerve is eventually relayed to the sensory cortex, where it is interpreted as, for example, pain from the external auditory meatus (GSA), a sense of fullness from the gut (GVA), or taste (SVA). Details of these central pathways are described in later chapters.

A lesion of the root of the vagus nerve will result in *dysphagia*, owing to a unilateral paralysis of pharyngeal and laryngeal musculature, and *dysarthria*, owing to a weakness of laryngeal muscles and the vocalis muscle. There are, however, no lasting demonstrable symptoms specifically related to visceromotor (autonomic) dysfunction. Taste loss is not detectable and cannot be tested, and the small somatosensory (GSA) loss involving the external auditory meatus and canal is usually of no consequence.

Unilateral injury inside the medulla, as with tumors, vascular lesions, or syringobulbia, may give rise to similar deficits (as described earlier) due to damage to the nucleus ambiguus. Bilateral lesions of the medulla, although rare, result in *aphonia*, *aphagia*, *dyspnea*, or *inspiratory stridor*. Such lesions may be life threatening, especially if they involve the dorsal motor nucleus. Dysarthria may also be seen in patients after thyroid surgery if the recurrent laryngeal nerve has been damaged.

Glossopharyngeal Nerve

The *glossopharyngeal nerve* exits the medulla at the postolivary sulcus (Fig. 14-10) immediately rostral to the vagus nerve (Figs. 14-3 and 14-4) and leaves the skull via the jugular foramen (Fig. 14-8), along with the vagus and accessory nerves. Like the vagus, the glossopharyngeal nerve has two ganglia: an *inferior ganglion* containing visceral afferent cell bodies (for GVA and SVA fibers) and a *superior ganglion* containing GSA cell bodies.

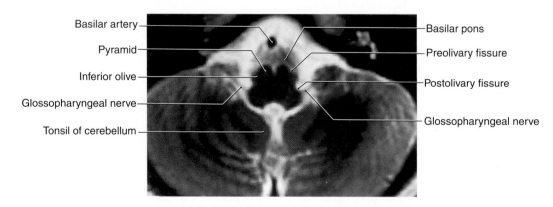

Figure 14-10. Axial T2-weighted MR image at the medulla-pons junction showing the root of the glossopharyngeal nerve (from the postolivary fissure). Note the distinct shape of the medulla at this level and the caudal aspect of the basilar pons.

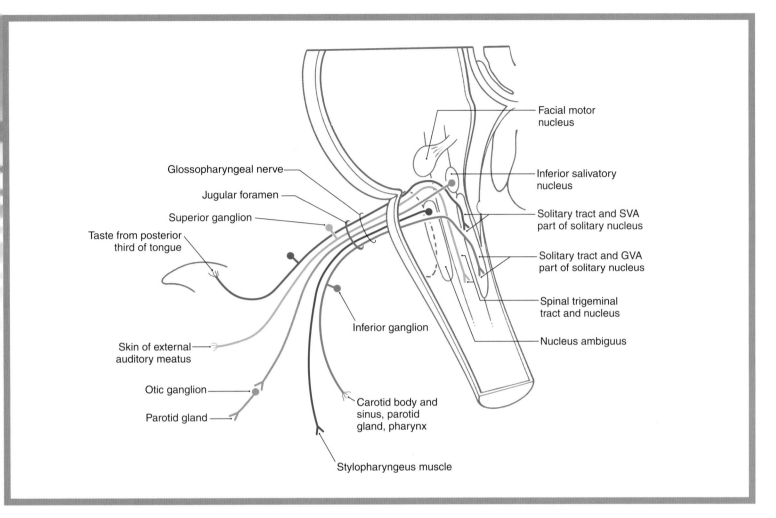

Figure 14-11. The central nuclei and peripheral distribution of fibers of the glossopharyngeal nerve (cranial nerve IX). Visceral afferent cell bodies (SVA, GVA) collectively form the inferior ganglion, and GSA cell bodies collectively form the superior ganglion of cranial nerve IX.

Motor fibers that distribute on the glossopharyngeal nerve originate from the *inferior salivatory nucleus* (GVE–preganglionic parasympathetic fibers) and from the *nucleus ambiguus* (SVE fibers) (Fig. 14-11). Axons of cells of the inferior salivatory nucleus exit on the glossopharyngeal nerve and join the tympanic nerve and then the lesser petrosal nerve to synapse with GVE-postganglionic neurons in the otic ganglion. These postganglionic parasympathetic cells supply secretomotor input to the parotid gland. The contribution of the nucleus ambiguus to the glossopharyngeal nerve serves to innervate the *stylopharyngeus muscle* (Fig. 14-11). This muscle assists in swallowing and participates in the efferent part of the *gag reflex*.

Again, as with the vagus nerve, the sensory fibers of the glossopharyngeal nerve are general sensory (GSA) and general and special visceral (GVA, SVA) (Fig. 14-11). The GSA fibers originate from cutaneous receptors on part of the pinna and the external auditory canal and have their cell bodies in the *superior ganglion*, and their central processes join the *spinal trigeminal tract* before terminating in the medially adjacent *spinal trigeminal nucleus*. The general visceral (GVA) fibers convey information from the parotid gland and the oropharynx, with an especially important input from the carotid body. The carotid body contains chemoreceptors that are sensitive to changing levels of oxygen and carbon dioxide in the blood. The primary afferent GVA fibers have their cell bodies in the inferior ganglion of the glossopharyngeal nerve, and centrally they enter the *solitary tract* to terminate in the *solitary nucleus*. Taste from the posterior one third of the tongue (Fig. 14-11) is conveyed centrally by SVA fibers that also have their cell bodies of origin in the inferior ganglion of the glossopharyngeal nerve. As is the case for all taste

fibers, the central processes of these afferent fibers enter the solitary tract and terminate on cells of the surrounding solitary nucleus. All afferent inputs on the glossopharyngeal nerve (GSA, GVA, SVA) are transmitted to relay nuclei of the thalamus and on to the sensory cortex, where the information is fully appreciated and interpreted.

Lesions of the ninth cranial nerve are relatively rare but may occur in combination with the vagal and accessory roots at the jugular foramen (Fig. 14-8). Deficits related only to glossopharyngeal nerve damage are largely restricted to a loss of taste from the posterior one third of the tongue and a loss of the gag reflex on the side of the lesion. In the latter case, both the sensory and motor limbs of the reflex are affected. In addition, the ninth nerve is subject to *glossopharyngeal neuralgia*. This disorder is characterized by attacks of intense idiopathic pain arising from the GVA sensory distribution of the nerve (pharynx, caudal parts of the tongue, tonsil, and possibly areas of the middle ear). The attacks may be spontaneous or may result from artificial stimulation of the back of the oral cavity or from swallowing or even talking. Glossopharyngeal neuralgia may be quite severe and can be seriously disabling.

Jugular Foramen

In addition to containing cranial nerves IX, X, and XI, which pass through approximately its middle third, the jugular foramen also serves as a conduit for other important structures (Fig. 14-8). In general, the foramen can be divided into a rostral and slightly medial area, a middle portion (containing cranial nerves IX, X, and XI), and a caudal and somewhat lateral portion.

The rostromedial portion (Fig. 14-8) contains the continuation between the *inferior petrosal sinus* and the *internal jugular vein*. The inferior petrosal sinus, although small, represents a communication between the cavernous sinus and the internal jugular vein. In addition the rostromedial portion of the jugular foramen also contains a *meningeal branch of the ascending pharyngeal artery*. This small vessel is one source of arterial blood to the meninges of the posterior fossa.

The caudolateral portion of the jugular foramen (Fig. 14-8) is the point at which the *sigmoid sinus* is continuous with the *internal jugular vein*. The sigmoid sinus is large and represents an important route for venous drainage from the brain. This part of the jugular foramen also contains the *meningeal branch of the occipital artery*, another source of arterial blood to the meninges of the posterior fossa. The *meningeal branch of the vagus nerve* enters the cranial cavity through this part of the foramen and serves as one of the nerves for the sensory innervation of the dura of the posterior fossa.

Syndromes of the Jugular Foramen

The deficits seem in *jugular foramen syndromes* reflect damage to the contents of the foramen or to structures immediately external to the foramen. The *syndrome of the jugular foramen* (also known as the *Vernet syndrome*) is usually caused by a lesion at, or immediately internal to, the foramen. These deficits are a loss of sensation (including taste) in the caudal third of the tongue (IXth nerve), loss of sensations in the larynx and pharynx, *dysarthria* and *dysphagia* resulting from paralysis of the vocal fold and muscles of the throat on the ipsilateral side (Xth nerve), and weakness of the ipsilateral sternocleidomastoid and trapezius muscles (XIth nerve). Lesions immediately external to the jugular foramen (as in the *Collet-Sicard syndrome*) result in deficits characteristic of damage to IX, X, and XI plus weakness of the tongue on the side of the lesion; this is because the exit of the hypoglossal nerve (via the hypoglossal canal) is adjacent to the jugular foramen and the root of this nerve is recruited into the lesion. The most inclusive syndrome of the jugular foramen is the *Villaret syndrome*, which includes deficits that are indicative of damage to the IXth, Xth, and XIth nerves, the hypoglossal nerve, and sympathetic fibers of the superior cervical ganglion, the last producing a *Horner syndrome* on the ipsilateral side of the head.

Cranial Nerves of the Pons-Medulla Junction

The cranial nerves of the pons-medulla junction are the *vestibulocochlear nerve* (the most lateral and, for the purposes of this discussion, exclusively sensory), the *facial nerve* (intermediate in location and a mixed nerve), and the *abducens nerve* (the most medial and exclusively motor) (Figs. 14-3 and 14-4).

There are three reasons why cranial nerves VI, VII, and VIII are considered as nerves of the pons-medulla junction. First, the abducens motor nucleus and the facial motor nucleus are located at the pons-medulla junction (Fig. 14-1; see also Figs. 12-9 and 12-10). Second, in humans the exit of all three of these nerves is located at the caudal edge of the pons (Fig. 14-3). Indeed, two of the three (facial and vestibulocochlear) nerves exit the skull via the same foramen. Third, in a broader comparative sense, cranial nerves VI, VII, and VIII do not exit from the medulla. For example, in animals with a more modest cerebral cortex and cerebellum (and consequently a smaller pons), these cranial nerves exit the brain in association with the trapezoid body, which is exposed on the surface of the brainstem. In humans, because of the larger size of the pons, the trapezoid body is located internally *but still* at the pons-medulla junction. For these reasons it is appropriate to consider these three cranial nerves in the manner presented here.

Vestibulocochlear Nerve

The eighth cranial nerve is the most lateral (Fig. 14-3) of the cranial nerves of the brainstem and is centrally related to the *posterior* and *anterior cochlear nuclei* (SSA, exteroception—hearing) and to the *medial, spinal (inferior), superior,* and *lateral vestibular nuclei* (SSA proprioception—balance and equilibrium). The two portions of cranial nerve VIII originate from highly specialized receptors that are well protected in the petrous portion of the temporal bone. These receptors are described in Chapters 21 and 22. Although the vestibular and cochlear nerve roots form separate fascicles at their origin, they move to form essentially a combined nerve root as they enter the brainstem. The vestibulocochlear nerve and the facial nerve enter the cranial cavity by passing through the internal acoustic meatus (Figs. 14-12 to 14-14).

The cochlear portion of cranial nerve VIII originates from cells in the spiral ganglion located in the cochlea (Fig. 14-13). This ganglion is made up of bipolar cells, the central processes of which travel on the cochlear division through the internal acoustic meatus to terminate in the *posterior* and *anterior cochlear nuclei*. The cochlear nuclei, in turn, project to several brainstem relay nuclei, which ultimately convey auditory information to the medial geniculate nucleus and from here to the auditory cortex and participate in auditory reflexes. These central pathways are described in Chapter 21.

Although the cochlear part of cranial nerve VIII is classically described as exclusively afferent (sensory), it is appropriate to note that cholinergic cells adjacent to the principal and accessory olivary nuclei give rise to axons that exit the brainstem on the cochlear nerve. These small bundles are called the *olivocochlear tract* (sometimes also called the *efferent cochlear bundle*). These efferent fibers of the cochlear nerve synapse in relation to the inner and outer hair cells and function to inhibit (dampen) the ability of the hair cell to respond to stimuli.

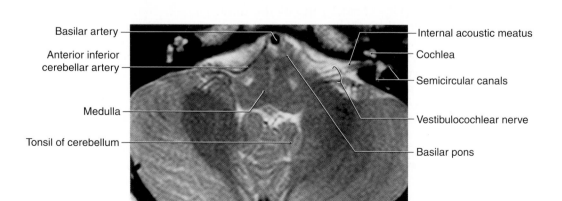

Basilar artery

Anterior inferior
cerebellar artery

Medulla

Tonsil of cerebellum

Internal acoustic meatus

Cochlea

Semicircular canals

Vestibulocochlear nerve

Basilar pons

Figure 14-12. Axial T2-weighted MR image at the pons-medulla junction through the internal auditory meatus and the exit of the vestibulocochlear nerve. The facial nerve also traverses this opening. Note the characteristic appearance of the brainstem at this level and the cochlea and semicircular canals. The labyrinthine artery arises from the anterior inferior cerebellar artery and serves the inner ear.

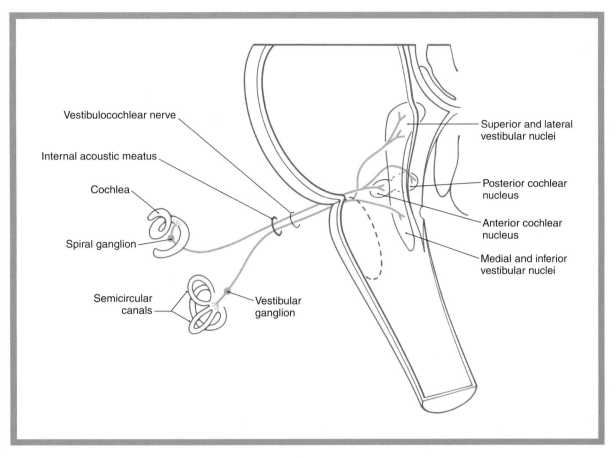

Figure 14-13. The peripheral origin and central termination of the primary sensory fibers of the vestibulocochlear nerve (cranial nerve VIII).

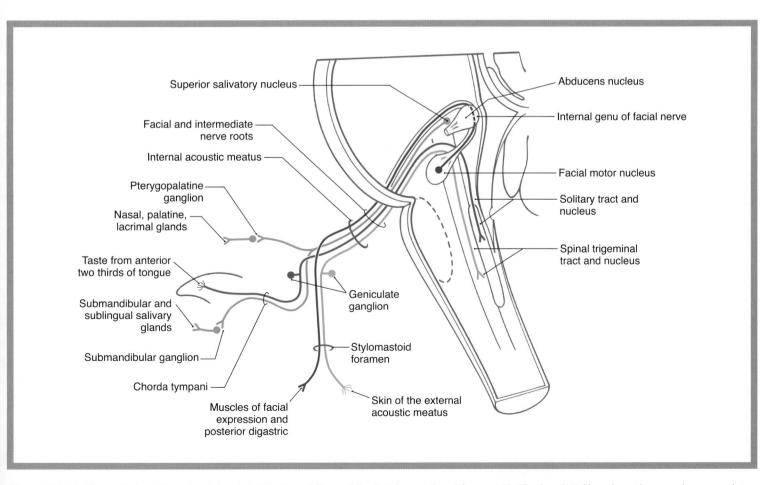

Figure 14-14. The central nuclei and peripheral distribution of fibers of the facial nerve (cranial nerve VII). The few GVA fibers from the nasopharynx, palate, and submandibular and sublingual salivary glands are not shown here; they have cell bodies of origin in the geniculate ganglion and project to more caudal regions of the solitary nucleus.

The vestibular division of cranial nerve VIII originates from the bipolar cells of the *vestibular ganglion* located medial to the *semicircular canals* (Fig. 14-13, see Chapter 22). The central processes of these cells travel on the root of the nerve, traverse the internal acoustic meatus, enter the brainstem at the pons-medulla junction, and distribute centrally to the *vestibular nuclei* located in the medulla and caudal pons (Fig. 14-13). *The internal acoustic meatus houses not only the vestibulocochlear nerve but also the facial nerve (including its intermediate part) and the labyrinthine artery.* After receiving input from the ampullae of the semicircular canals and the utricle and saccule, the vestibular nuclei have important central connections to the cerebellum, to oculomotor nuclei (nuclei of cranial nerves VI, IV, and III), and to other brainstem centers related to balance, position sense, equilibrium, and the coordination of eye movements with head movements. Specific information related to these central pathways is described in Chapter 22.

Lesions of the vestibulocochlear nerve may result from a wide range of causes. The clinical manifestations include *hearing loss, tinnitus, vertigo, dizziness,* and related problems such as *ataxia.* Injury to the cochlea, spinal ganglion, or cochlear fibers in cranial nerve VIII results in loss of hearing on the side of the lesion; this type of hearing loss is *sensorineural hearing loss.* Lesions within the brainstem (or at higher levels) may affect the patient's ability to precisely interpret or to localize a sound in space, but such lesions do not result in deafness in one ear. *Conductive hearing loss* results from a failure of conduction through the middle ear, usually involving the ossicles. *Tinnitus* is a ringing, hissing, or roaring sensation perceived by the patient. It is related to the auditory part of cranial nerve VIII and may result from injury to the peripheral part of the nerve or may follow central lesions that damage auditory fibers or structures. Injury to the vestibular fibers of cranial nerve VIII results in *vertigo* (a perception of movement) and nystagmus that may be accompanied by *nausea* and *vomiting.* The vertigo may be *subjective* (the patient perceives that his or her body is moving) or *objective* (the patient perceives that objects in the environment are moving). *Nystagmus* (rhythmic oscillatory movements of the eyes) results from the interruption of vestibular influence over the brainstem motor neurons controlling eye movement, and the nausea and vomiting are a natural consequence of the disconnection between body or eye movements and the environment.

Lesions of the vestibular nuclei and their main central connections, especially the cerebellum, result in a sensation of spinning called *vertigo* (*subjective vertigo*—the patient senses that he or she is moving; *objective vertigo*—the patient perceives that objects in the environment are moving), *ataxia* and unsteady gait (the patient feels that his or her "balance is off"), and *nystagmus.* These signs and symptoms may range from mild to severe and may be accompanied by nausea and vomiting. Signs and symptoms of vestibular dysfunction may result from a wide range of causes such as toxicity from certain medications, trauma, diabetes, cerebellar lesions, and acoustic neuroma. *Ménière syndrome* is characterized by hearing loss and sound distortion as well as vertigo and a sensation of dizziness or unsteadiness on walking or standing. The cause is unknown, but there seems to be an increase in endolymphatic pressure with an increase in size of the utricle, saccule, and cochlear duct.

Lesions in the Cerebellopontine Angle

This could rightfully be called "tumors of the cerebellopontine angle" since the vast majority of lesions found at this site are *vestibular schwannomas* (about 85%), *meningiomas* (5% to 10%), or *epidermoid tumors* (about 5%). Vestibular schwannomas are sometimes incorrectly called acoustic neuromas; this is incorrect because they are specifically tumors originating from Schwann

cells of the vestibular root not the "acoustic" root. The deficits associated with this specific tumor are initially *tinnitus, unsteady gait,* and *progressive loss of hearing in that ear* (as the tumor enlarges and impinges on the acoustic root), with a *weakness of ipsilateral facial muscles* appearing in later stages. If very large (usually greater than 3 cm), these tumors may impinge on the root of the trigeminal nerve and also produce sensory deficits and/or pain sensations similar to tic douloureux.

Meningiomas, in contrast, may arise from the margins of the internal acoustic meatus (frequently the anterior or superior edges) and result in a *facial weakness* early followed later by hearing loss and pain related to involvement of the trigeminal root. While a meningioma may erode and slightly enlarge the internal acoustic meatus, significant enlargement of this opening is a feature more commonly seen in the computed tomographic scan of patients with a vestibular schwannoma.

Epidermoid tumors (also called *epidermoid cysts* or *cholesteatoma*) arise from clusters of epidermis that are entrapped during development and give rise to a benign slow-growing lesion. These tumors are commonly lined with an epithelium and contain cellular debris, proteins, and cholesterol. Spillage of the cyst contents may cause recurrent bouts of aseptic meningitis. Although relatively rare, these lesions may be found anywhere in the central nervous system. When found at the cerebellopontine angle they cause deficits reflecting damage to the Vth, VIIth, and VIIIth cranial nerves.

Facial Nerve

The *facial motor nucleus* is located in the pons just rostral to the pons-medulla transition (Figs. 14-1 and 14-14). Axons from the SVE motor neurons of the facial nucleus course posteromedially to arch around the abducens nucleus from caudal to rostral before turning anterolaterally to exit the brainstem (Fig. 14-14). In their passage through the anterolateral pons these fibers are joined by GVE–preganglionic parasympathetic axons from neurons of the superior salivatory nucleus. These GVE fibers, along with SVA taste fibers from the anterior two thirds of the tongue, GSA fibers from the pinna, and a few GVA fibers, form the intermediate nerve (Fig. 14-14). The facial nerve fibers and intermediate nerve fibers are intermingled within the pons but emerge from the brainstem as two separate nerve bundles. For all practical purposes both of these nerve roots form what is commonly called the facial nerve; this nerve enters the internal acoustic meatus along with the vestibulocochlear nerve (Fig. 14-12).

After exiting the brainstem into the cerebellopontine angle, the facial and intermediate nerves merge and are joined by the vestibulocochlear nerve. These nerve trunks enter the petrous portion of the temporal bone through the *internal acoustic meatus* (Fig. 14-14) accompanied by the *labyrinthine artery.* Coursing posterolaterally through the facial canal in the petrous temporal bone, the facial nerve approaches the middle ear cavity, where it turns (*internal genu*) sharply posteriorly and continues superior and posterior to the middle ear cavity to eventually exit the temporal bone via the *stylomastoid foramen.* The *geniculate ganglion* (Fig. 14-14) of the facial nerve is located at the internal genu, and it is here that the *greater petrosal nerve* is formed by GVE–preganglionic parasympathetic fibers that leave the facial nerve. The greater petrosal nerve courses anteromedially through and on the petrous temporal bone to reach the area just superior to the foramen lacerum, where it joins the *deep petrosal nerve* to form the *nerve of the pterygoid canal.* From here, preganglionic parasympathetic axons enter the *pterygopalatine ganglion.* Postganglionic parasympathetic fibers from this ganglion supply the mucous membrane of the hard and soft palates, nasal cavity, and paranasal sinuses (Fig. 14-14). Other postganglionic parasympathetic fibers join the maxillary division (V₂) of the trigeminal nerve and continue on branches that enter the orbit to provide parasympathetic innervation of the lacrimal gland.

En route through the temporal bone, the facial nerve gives off a small branch containing SVE motor fibers that supply the stapedius muscle and a larger branch, the *chorda tympani* (Fig. 14-14). The latter nerve enters the middle ear cavity, passes across the inner surface of the tympanic membrane, and then exits the middle ear through the petrotympanic fissure to reach the infratemporal fossa. Here it joins the lingual branch of V₃ to distribute preganglionic parasympathetic fibers to the *submandibular ganglion* and to collect SVA taste afferent fibers from the anterior two thirds of the tongue (Fig. 14-14). Postganglionic fibers from the submandibular ganglion innervate the submandibular and sublingual salivary glands and portions of the mucosal surfaces of the tongue and oral cavity.

Upon exiting the stylomastoid foramen, the fibers of the facial nerve pass through, and around, the parotid gland as the nerve divides into its five terminal branches. Most of the fibers that remain in the facial nerve at this point provide motor innervation (SVE) to the muscles of facial expression (Fig. 14-14), the posterior belly of the digastric muscle, and the stylohyoid muscle. In addition, the facial nerve contains a relatively small number of cutaneous fibers (GSA) that supply portions of the external ear and external auditory canal.

The facial nerve includes three varieties of sensory fibers. The first, taste fibers (SVA), pass centrally from the anterior two thirds of the tongue first on the lingual branch of V₃. These SVA fibers then leave the lingual nerve via the chorda tympani to join the facial nerve to reach their cell bodies in the geniculate ganglion (Fig. 14-14). The central processes of these primary afferent fibers continue with the facial nerve, pass into the cranial cavity through the internal acoustic meatus, and enter the brainstem in the intermediate nerve. These SVA fibers enter the *solitary tract* and *terminate in rostral portions of the solitary nucleus*, the central receiving area for all taste sensory signals (Fig. 14-2).

The second variety of sensory fibers in the facial nerve is relatively small in number. Cutaneous sensory fibers (GSA) from regions of the external ear and external auditory canal course centrally on the facial nerve (Fig. 14-14). Moreover, it appears that the muscles of facial expression contain relatively few muscle spindles; therefore, the contingent of muscle afferent fibers normally found within the GSA population is small or nonexistent in the facial nerve. The cutaneous fibers reach their cell bodies in the geniculate ganglion (with SVA and GVA sensory neurons), and their central processes course into the brainstem with the intermediate nerve. In the brainstem, these GSA fibers enter the *spinal trigeminal tract* and terminate in the *spinal trigeminal nucleus* (Fig. 14-14); these signals are transmitted rostrally to the thalamus or used in local reflex circuits.

The third variety of sensory fibers is equally small in number. Receptors in the mucous membranes of the palate and nasopharynx give rise to primary sensory fibers (GVA) that have their cell bodies in the geniculate ganglion and enter the brainstem on the intermediate nerve. These fibers convey general sensory information from caudal regions of the oral cavity and will enter the more *caudal portions of the solitary tract and terminate in the adjacent nucleus*.

Corticonuclear (corticobulbar) fibers used in the performance of voluntary movements involving the muscles of facial expression distribute to the facial nuclei in a bilateral manner. The ipsilateral face motor cortex distributes *bilaterally* to those facial motor neurons that control muscles in the upper face (i.e., frontalis, orbicularis oculi). In contrast, the face motor cortex projects **only** *contralaterally* to those facial motor neurons that control the lower facial expression muscles, such as those located near the angle of the mouth that are used to smile voluntarily. *Lesions of the efferent fibers from the face motor cortex or of the internal capsule (supranuclear) result in drooping or sagging of the corner of the mouth contralateral to the lesion when the patient is asked to smile voluntarily.* Such lesions are referred to as *central seven* lesions. Of interest, although some patients cannot smile when asked to do so by the neurologist, they can sometimes smile "involuntarily" or spontaneously in response to an amusing comment or situation.

Signs and symptoms due to peripheral lesions of the facial nerve *(infranuclear; lower motor neuron)* depend on the location of the damage. If the injury occurs proximal to the geniculate ganglion (Fig. 14-14) and the origin of the greater petrosal nerve, the patient exhibits a *loss of voluntary control of ipsilateral facial expression muscles in the upper and lower portions of the face.* This motor (the *Bell palsy*) deficit is accompanied by decreased mucosal secretion in the nasal and oral cavities and decreased tear fluid production and salivary gland output, all on the ipsilateral side. Cutaneous sensation of the external ear and external auditory canal is also diminished, but innervation of this territory is difficult to assess because cranial nerves IX and X contribute as well. In addition, there is *decreased taste sensation (SVA) on the anterior two thirds of the tongue* (but general sensation on the face, GSA, is preserved—why?) and *hyperacusis* on the side ipsilateral to the lesion.

If the lesion occurs distal to the ganglion (Fig. 14-14) but proximal to the origin of the chorda tympani and stapedial nerve, decreased salivation and taste and hyperacusis may be present in conjunction with decreased facial expression throughout the ipsilateral side of the face. However, tear fluid production and the mucosal surfaces of the nasal and oral cavities are unaffected because the greater petrosal nerve is intact. It follows, then, that decreased function of all facial expression muscles on one side of the face in combination with the *absence of any deficits involving parasympathetic function or the sense of taste* serves to localize the lesion at, or distal to, the stylomastoid foramen (Fig. 14-14).

The SVE fibers originating in the facial nucleus also form the efferent limb of the *corneal reflex*. The afferent limb of this reflex travels via the ophthalmic division of cranial nerve V. The central processes of these fibers have their cell bodies in the trigeminal ganglion, enter the spinal trigeminal tract, and terminate in the spinal nucleus. Trigeminothalamic fibers originating in the spinal nucleus send collaterals into the facial motor nucleus and then continue rostrally to the thalamus; this collateral connection completes the reflex circuit.

Additional deficits reflecting involvement of the facial nerve are seen in *facial diplegia* and in *hemifacial spasm*. Bilateral paralysis of the facial muscles, *facial diplegia*, may be seen in congenital conditions, such as in myotonic muscular dystrophy or in the *Möbius syndrome*. In this latter syndrome there are complex congenital defects that affect movements of the face and eyes (due to partial agenesis of these respective nuclei) and cause defects of the extremities and skeleton. The bilateral facial weakness in the Möbius syndrome frequently affects the upper portions of the face more than the lower portions or the whole face. Facial diplegia is also seen in patients with *Lyme disease* (characteristic of the disease), in those with the *Guillain-Barré syndrome* (about 50% of fatal cases will have this feature), or in patients who may have botulism poisoning or infection with *Corynebacterium diphtheriae*. Hemifacial spasms are irregular, and sometimes painful, contractions of the facial muscles that may be triggered by voluntary movements of the facial muscles. While the etiology is unknown in some cases, hemifacial spasms may follow an episode of Bell palsy or result from compression of the root of the facial nerve by a lesion or vessel. In this latter case aberrant branches of the anterior inferior cerebellar artery are the likely candidates.

Abducens Nerve

The *abducens nucleus* is located internal to the facial colliculus (Fig. 14-1). This structure, in turn, is found in the floor of the rhomboid fossa just lateral to the median sulcus and rostral to the striae medullares of the fourth ventricle. *The abducens nucleus contains motor neurons and interneurons.*

The axons of the GSE motor neurons of the *abducens nucleus* course through the tegmental and basilar pons, exit at the pons-medulla junction generally in line with the preolivary sulcus as the *abducens nerve* (Figs. 14-3, 14-4, 14-10, 14-15, and 14-16), and enter the dura just caudal to the cavernous sinus. After the abducens nerve exits the brainstem at the pons-medulla junction, it courses rostrad along the surface of the basilar pons closely adjacent to the midline in the prepontine cistern (Figs. 14-15 and 14-16). These axons then enter and pass through the lumen of the sinus in close association with the cavernous portion of the internal carotid artery (see Fig. 8-21) and enter the orbit via the superior orbital fissure. The abducens nerve innervates the ipsilateral lateral rectus muscle (Fig. 14-16).

The interneurons in the abducens send their axons into the contralateral *medial longitudinal fasciculus*, where they ascend to the oculomotor nucleus on that side (Fig. 14-16). These crossed ascending fibers form excitatory synapses on oculomotor neurons that innervate the medial rectus muscle on that side. The connection thus formed is such that when, for example, the patient looks to the right (in the horizontal plane), the right lateral rectus contracts (this eye abducts) and the left medial rectus contracts (this eye adducts). Lesions that involve this pathway lead to the clinical condition known as *internuclear ophthalmoplegia*.

Lesions of the abducens nerve, the abducens nucleus, or the internuclear axons in the medial longitudinal fasciculus have similar, yet individually unique features. Injury to abducens fibers in the pons (as in a *medial pontine syndrome*) or in its course outside the brain results in a flaccid paralysis of the ipsilateral lateral rectus muscle; the affected eye is slightly introverted and does not abduct on attempted lateral gaze to that side. However, the opposite eye adducts because the internuclear neurons are intact.

A lesion of the abducens nucleus, such as a fourth ventricle tumor invading the facial colliculus, damages both the motor neurons and the internuclear neurons. The result is paralysis of

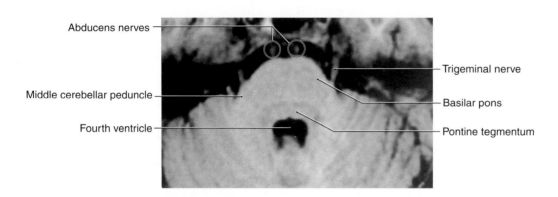

Figure 14-15. Axial T1-weighted MR image of the pons showing the exit of the trigeminal nerve and the abducens nerves *(in circles)* in the prepontine cistern.

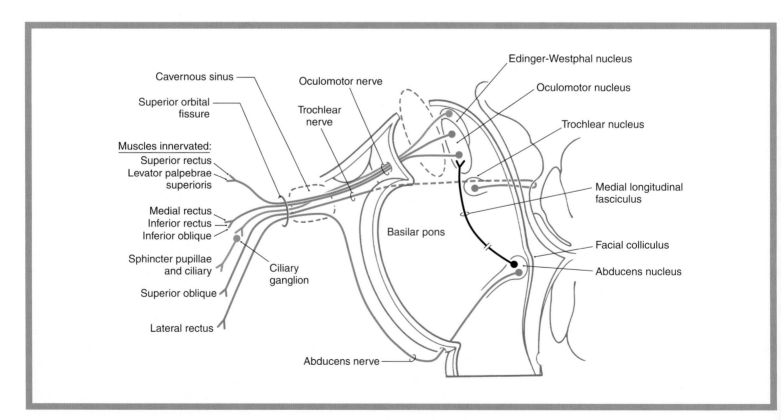

Figure 14-16. The central nuclei and peripheral distribution of fibers of the abducens nerve (cranial nerve VI), trochlear nerve (cranial nerve IV), and oculomotor nerve (cranial nerve III) nuclei. Interneurons in the abducens nucleus *(black)* enter the contralateral medial longitudinal fasciculus and distribute to medial rectus motor neurons in the nucleus of cranial nerve III. Disruption to this pathway results in internuclear ophthalmoplegia.

the lateral rectus muscle on the side of the lesion accompanied by failure of the opposite medial rectus muscle to contract on attempted gaze *toward the side of the lesion*. This particular example combines a lower motor neuron lesion of the lateral rectus on the side of the lesion with an internuclear ophthalmoplegia— a paralysis of the medial rectus on the opposite side seen in attempted gaze toward the side of the lesion.

Damage only to internuclear axons in the left medial longitudinal fasciculus (as in *multiple sclerosis*) results in an inability to adduct the left eye on attempted gaze to the right. In contrast, with lesions of the left abducens nucleus or nerve, the right eye can abduct, because the motor neurons in the right nucleus (and their axons) are intact. An extension of a lesion involving the abducens nucleus (resulting in weakness of the ipsilateral lateral rectus muscle and the contralateral medial rectus muscle) is seen in a lesion that involves the abducens nucleus and fibers of the immediately adjacent medial longitudinal fasciculus, resulting in the *one-and-a-half syndrome*. This syndrome is discussed in Chapter 25.

One important source of cerebral cortical influence over abducens motor neurons originates from cells in the frontal eye field (see Chapter 28). This area of cortex projects bilaterally to the paramedian pontine reticular formation (PPRF), also called the *horizontal gaze center*, and to the ipsilateral superior colliculus, which in turn projects to the contralateral PPRF. The PPRF, in turn, projects to the ipsilateral abducens nucleus. Sudden cortical damage (such as stroke or trauma) involving the frontal eye field results in an involuntary conjugate deviation of the eyes to the side of the lesion.

Cranial Nerve of the Pons

The largest of the cranial nerves of the brainstem, the *trigeminal nerve*, exits the lateral aspect of the pons (Figs. 14-3, 14-4, and 14-17). It consists of a large sensory root *(portio major)*, which is attached to the *trigeminal ganglion*, and a small motor root *(portio minor)*, which bypasses the ganglion (Fig. 14-18). The exit point of this nerve is also the border between the *basilar pons* and the *middle cerebellar peduncle*, which are located anterior (ventral) and posterior (dorsal), respectively, to the nerve roots (Fig. 14-17).

At the most general level of organization the trigeminal nerve consists of *ophthalmic* (V_1), *maxillary* (V_2), and *mandibular* (V_3) divisions; these are the large sensory branches originating from the trigeminal ganglion (Fig. 14-18). These branches serve the upper eyelid, forehead, and scalp to a point just beyond the vertex of the skull (V_1); the upper eyelid, upper lip and teeth, maxillary aspect of the face, and a lateral strip in the temporal area (V_2); and the lower lip and teeth, much of the oral cavity,

and the skin over the mandible and continuing as a band up the lateral side of the head rostral to the ear (V_3) (see Chapter 18). The ophthalmic division exits the cranial cavity via the *superior orbital fissure* (Fig. 14-18) and distributes to the orbit, with some branches exiting the orbit through the *supraorbital notch* (or foramen). The maxillary division exits the cranial cavity through the *foramen rotundum* (Fig. 14-18) and then immediately passes through the *pterygopalatine fossa* and the *inferior orbital fissure* into the orbit; some of these branches exit the orbit via the *infraorbital foramen* onto the maxillary region of the face. The mandibular division exits the cranial cavity through the *foramen ovale* (Fig. 14-18), as does the motor root of the fifth nerve.

Trigeminal Nerve

The *trigeminal nerve* is a mixed nerve, having sensory and motor components. The sensory nuclei form a continuous cell column that extends from the spinal cord–medulla junction to rostral levels of the mesencephalon. The motor nucleus is located medially adjacent to the principal sensory nucleus at about midpontine levels.

The sensory nuclei of the trigeminal nerve are the *spinal trigeminal nucleus*, extending from caudal to rostral throughout the lateral medulla and into the caudal pons; the *principal sensory nucleus*, located in the lateral parts of the pontine tegmentum at about midpontine levels at the rostral end of the spinal nucleus; and the *mesencephalic nucleus* and *mesencephalic tract*, which extend rostrally from the principal sensory nucleus into the midbrain along the lateral aspect of the periaqueductal gray (Fig. 14-18). The spinal trigeminal nucleus consists of a *pars caudalis* (from the spinal cord–medulla junction to the obex), a *pars interpolaris* (from the obex to the rostral end of the hypoglossal nucleus), and the *pars oralis* (to the caudal aspect of the principal sensory nucleus).

The trigeminal nerve, along with small contributions from cranial nerves VII, IX, and X from the external ear, conveys sensory input from the entire face from the posterior border of the mandibular ramus to just caudal to the vertex of the head, the cornea and conjunctiva, the mucosa of the nasal cavity and sinuses, the upper and lower teeth, the lining of the oral cavity including the tongue, and the lining of the pharynx and larynx (cranial nerves IX and X) and proprioceptive inputs from the muscles of mastication and extraocular muscles. The sensory information relayed on the fifth nerve is concerned with pain and thermal sensations, discriminative sensations, and proprioception.

Primary afferent fibers conveying pain, thermal sense, and nondiscriminative touch (GSA exteroception) from the head have their cell bodies in the trigeminal ganglion and in the geniculate ganglion (cranial nerve VII) and superior ganglia of

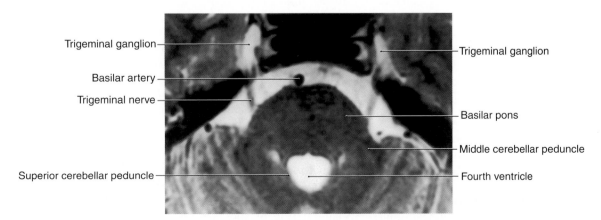

Trigeminal ganglion
Basilar artery
Trigeminal nerve
Superior cerebellar peduncle

Trigeminal ganglion
Basilar pons
Middle cerebellar peduncle
Fourth ventricle

Figure 14-17. Axial T2-weighted MR image of the pons showing the exit of the trigeminal nerve, its course across the subarachnoid space, and the trigeminal ganglion. The exit of this nerve represents the boundary between the basilar pons and the middle cerebellar peduncle.

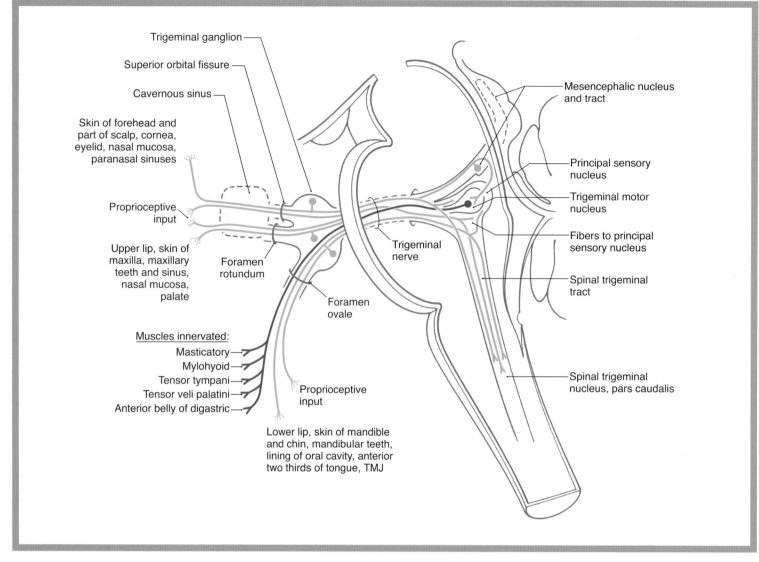

Figure 14-18. The central nuclei and peripheral distribution of fibers of the trigeminal nerve (cranial nerve V). Collaterals to the trigeminal motor nucleus from mesencephalic fibers connect the afferent and efferent limbs of the pathway underlying the jaw jerk reflex. TMJ, temporomandibular joint.

cranial nerves IX and X (the lateral three are related to the external ear only) (Figs. 14-7, 14-11, 14-14, and 14-18). Their central processes form the spinal trigeminal tract and terminate in the medially adjacent nucleus. Fibers conveying discriminative touch from the face and oral cavity (GSA exteroception) follow a similar trajectory, but centrally these fibers terminate in the principal sensory nucleus. Those fibers conveying GSA proprioceptive information from the masticatory muscles, extraocular muscles, and periodontal ligament receptors enter the brainstem via the trigeminal nerve. However, in clear contrast to other primary sensory fibers, these fibers have their cell bodies in the *mesencephalic nucleus, not in the trigeminal ganglion*. Sensory inputs to the spinal trigeminal nucleus and to the principal sensory nucleus are relayed to the thalamus via the *anterior* and *posterior trigeminothalamic tracts* and from the thalamus to the somatosensory cortex, where the sensations are perceived and interpreted.

The motor nucleus of the trigeminal nerve innervates muscles that originate from the first pharyngeal arch, hence their SVE functional component. The motor root of the trigeminal nerve exits the skull via the foramen ovale, along with V_3 (Fig. 14-18). These motor neurons innervate the muscles of mastication (including the medial and lateral pterygoid muscles), the tensor tympani, the tensor veli palatini, the mylohyoid, and the anterior belly of the digastric, all on the ipsilateral side (Fig. 14-18).

The motor nucleus receives afferent fibers involved in the *jaw jerk reflex*.

The most commonly tested reflexes that are associated with the trigeminal nerve are the *jaw jerk reflex* and the *corneal reflex*. The afferent limb of the *jaw jerk reflex* originates at receptors in the muscles of mastication, courses centrally on the mandibular division, and has its cell bodies in the mesencephalic nucleus. Collaterals from these afferent fibers project bilaterally to the trigeminal motor nucleus, the neurons of which give rise to the efferent limb of the reflex. The afferent limb of the *corneal reflex* originates from pain and touch receptors in the cornea. These fibers travel on the ophthalmic division of cranial nerve V, have their cell bodies in the trigeminal ganglion, and terminate centrally in the ipsilateral spinal trigeminal nucleus. Trigeminothalamic fibers en route to the thalamus send collaterals bilaterally into the facial motor nucleus, which is the origin of the efferent limb of this reflex; in response to a stimulus that touches the cornea, the eyes blink.

The primary deficits in patients with lesions of the trigeminal nerve, or its central nuclei, are sensory symptoms in the peripheral distribution of the nerve (or its individual division) and paralysis of the masticatory muscles. The sensory deficits are a complete loss of pain, thermal, and tactile sensations on the ipsilateral side of the face and much of the scalp; a loss of the same sensations in the oral cavity (and from the teeth) on the same side; and a loss of the corneal reflex occurring in response to corneal touch, also on the same side. However, because the efferent limb of the corneal reflex travels via the facial nerve, touching the cornea on the side opposite a trigeminal root lesion results in a blink on that side as well as a blink on the side of the root lesion. An injury to one trigeminal nerve does not cause a loss of the jaw jerk reflex.

Another sensory disorder associated with the trigeminal nerve is *tic douloureux (trigeminal neuralgia)*. This condition is characterized by severe, unexpected, lancinating pain restricted to one or more of the divisions of the nerve. Paroxysms of intense pain may result from stimulation of a trigger zone frequently located around the lip or nose or on the cheek. A wide variety of stimuli such as shaving, putting on makeup, talking, chewing, eating, a breeze on the face, or a sudden facial expression may precipitate an attack. Indeed, some patients may become malnourished because they avoid eating, chewing, and swallowing for fear of an attack. Trigeminal neuralgia is seen more frequently in patients older than 35 years of age, usually involves the maxillary division more often than the mandibular (second most commonly involved) or ophthalmic (rarely involved) division, and can severely compromise the quality of life. Trigeminal neuralgia may be seen in patients with multiple sclerosis, degenerative changes in the trigeminal ganglion, or vascular malformations. Compression of the trigeminal nerve root by aberrant vessels, usually branches of the *superior cerebellar artery*, is one known cause of trigeminal neuralgia. Having said this, it is also known that at autopsy some patients have what appears to be compression of the trigeminal root but did not exhibit symptoms of trigeminal neuralgia.

Motor deficits resulting from trigeminal root lesions result in paralysis of the masticatory muscles on that side. The patient has difficulty chewing food, and the jaw deviates toward the side of the lesion (the weak side) on closing. This deviation occurs because of the unopposed action (pull of the mandible toward the midline) of the pterygoid muscles on the opposite (undamaged) side. Although relatively rare, some patients with trigeminal neuralgia also experience *status trigeminus*, which are tic-like contractions of the masticatory muscles.

Sensory or motor deficits related to the trigeminal nerve can also occur from central lesions. Such lesions include, but are not limited to, tumors or vascular lesions in the medulla or pons, metastatic lesions, and the obstruction of vessels. A well-known example of a lesion due to vascular obstruction is the *lateral medullary syndrome* (also called the *posterior inferior cerebellar artery syndrome* or *Wallenberg syndrome*), in which there is an alternating sensory loss. This lesion (see Chapter 18) results in an ipsilateral loss of pain and thermal sense on the face (spinal trigeminal tract involvement) and a contralateral loss of the same sensations on the body (anterolateral system involvement), in concert with motor deficits most frequently related to damage to the nucleus ambiguus or vestibular nuclei.

Cranial Nerves of the Midbrain

The cranial nerves of the midbrain are the trochlear nerve (cranial nerve IV) and the oculomotor nerve (cranial nerve III) (Figs. 14-3 and 14-4). The nuclei of both nerves are located adjacent to the midline just ventral to the periaqueductal gray, both nerves are exclusively motor, and, like other exclusively motor nerves, they exit the midbrain just lateral to the midline. These two nerves, along with cranial nerve VI, innervate extraocular muscles.

Trochlear Nerve

The trochlear nerve is the only motor cranial nerve formed entirely by axons that cross the midline before their exit. For example, axons arising from the left trochlear nucleus arch caudally along the lateral edge of the periaqueductal gray to decussate in the most anterior aspect of the anterior medullary velum and then exit the brainstem immediately caudal to the right inferior colliculus (see Chapters 10 and 28).

The trochlear nucleus is situated posteriorly adjacent to the medial longitudinal fasciculus (MLF) at a cross-sectional level through the inferior colliculus (Fig. 14-16). After arching around the periaqueductal gray, decussating, and exiting from the posterior surface of the midbrain, the axons of these GSE motor neurons have a long intracranial course. They exit into the superior cistern and then course laterally and anteriorly through the ambient cistern on the lateral aspect of the midbrain (Fig. 14-19). The nerve then enters the dura, courses rostrally within the lateral wall of the cavernous sinus, and enters the orbit via the superior orbital fissure (Fig. 14-16). Cranial nerve IV innervates the superior oblique muscle, which normally functions to direct the eye inferolaterally, that is, downward and outward.

It is important to remember that trochlear motor neurons innervate the contralateral superior oblique muscle, as the clinical findings may reflect this innervation. For example, a lesion at the root of the nerve in the ambient cistern or cavernous sinus, or at the superior orbital fissure, results in paralysis of the superior oblique muscle on that side. If the lesion is on the left side, the left eye cannot rotate slightly downward and outward. On the other hand, in a patient with multiple sclerosis involving the MLF, the damage to which has extended to the trochlear nucleus, a variation on this theme may be seen. In this situation, a lesion in the right MLF with trochlear nucleus involvement results in paralysis of the left superior oblique muscle, and the left eye cannot rotate downward and outward to the left. In addition, and in clear contrast to the trochlear nerve root lesion, the patient also has internuclear ophthalmoplegia on the right; on attempted lateral gaze to the left, the right medial rectus muscle does not adduct the eye on that side.

An important source of cerebral cortical input to the trochlear nucleus is from neurons located in the frontal eye field. These projections pass to the rostral interstitial nucleus of the medial

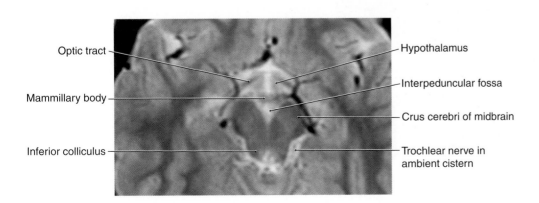

Optic tract — Mammillary body — Inferior colliculus — Hypothalamus — Interpeduncular fossa — Crus cerebri of midbrain — Trochlear nerve in ambient cistern

Figure 14-19. Axial T2-weighted MR image showing the position of the trochlear nerve in the ambient cistern.

longitudinal fasciculus (riMLF), also called the *vertical gaze center*, and to the superior colliculus, which also projects to the riMLF. The riMLF sends a large projection to the ipsilateral trochlear nucleus and a smaller projection to the nucleus on the contralateral side. Sudden cortical damage (such as from stroke or trauma) involving the frontal eye field results in an involuntary conjugate deviation of the eyes to the side of the lesion.

Oculomotor Nerve

The oculomotor nucleus is located within the ventral portion of the periaqueductal gray just posterior to the medial longitudinal fasciculus and is present in about the rostral half of the midbrain (Fig. 14-16). It is divided into several smaller subnuclei that contain GSE motor neurons that innervate all the extraocular muscles except the superior oblique and lateral rectus. This innervation involves ipsilateral muscles except for the superior rectus motor neurons, whose axons decussate within the nucleus to enter the contralateral oculomotor nerve. Although seemingly significant, this crossed pathway is typically ignored in the clinical setting, because the effect of losing the innervation to the (contralateral) superior rectus muscle is usually masked by the actions of the functionally intact muscles in that orbit.

Also located in the midbrain periaqueductal gray matter immediately posterior to the oculomotor complex is the Edinger-Westphal nucleus (Fig. 14-16). This group of visceral motor cells is composed of preganglionic parasympathetic GVE neurons whose axons project to the ciliary ganglion via the oculomotor nerve.

Oculomotor nerve fibers pass anteriorly (ventrally) through and around the red nucleus to eventually exit the midbrain in the interpeduncular fossa (Fig. 14-20). Emerging from the midbrain, the nerve passes between the posterior cerebral and superior cerebellar arteries, enters the interpeduncular cistern, and then penetrates the dura lateral to the sella turcica to course within the lateral wall of the cavernous sinus (see Chapter 8). The nerve then exits the dura and passes through the superior orbital fissure, along with cranial nerves IV, VI, and V_1, to enter the orbit (Figs. 14-16 and 14-18). In the orbit the oculomotor nerve divides into superior and inferior divisions, each division forming a few small communicating branches to the ciliary ganglion in addition to their muscular branches. The ciliary ganglion then gives off several small, short ciliary nerves, which reach the posterior aspect of the globe of the eye, where they penetrate the sclera to eventually reach the sphincter pupillae and ciliary muscles (Fig. 14-16).

There are four smooth muscles related to each orbit that require visceromotor innervation. The GVE fibers in the oculomotor nerve enter the *ciliary ganglion*, the postganglionic parasympathetic fibers of which innervate the *sphincter pupillae* and *ciliary muscles*. In contrast, the dilator pupillae muscle and the *superior tarsal muscle* are activated by sympathetic innervation. Postganglionic sympathetic fibers exit the superior cervical ganglion and course, via the internal carotid plexus, to join the ophthalmic artery. Coursing into the orbit with the latter artery via the optic canal, sympathetic postganglionic fibers may join the ciliary ganglion directly, may join the nasociliary nerve (a branch of V_2 from which the *long ciliary branches* originate), or may join the oculomotor nerve and then enter the ciliary ganglion. Once in the ciliary ganglion, the sympathetic fibers continue, *without synapsing*, into the *short ciliary nerves* to reach the *dilator pupillae muscle*. Some of the sympathetic postganglionic fibers that travel via the oculomotor nerve continue beyond the ciliary ganglion and levator palpebrae superioris to reach the superior tarsal muscle.

Although it is known that the extraocular muscles contain muscle spindles, the oculomotor, trochlear, and abducens nerves are regarded as purely motor nerves. The spindle afferent fibers

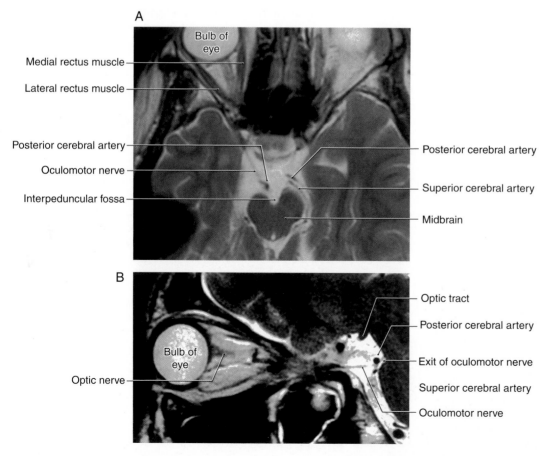

Figure 14-20. Axial (**A**) and sagittal (**B**) T2-weighted MR images of the midbrain and related structures showing the exit of the oculomotor nerve. Note the apposition of this nerve root to the superior cerebellar artery and the posterior cerebral artery. The oculomotor nerve passes through the superior orbital fissure along with the abducens and trochlear roots.

appear to join sensory nerves in the orbit, such as the frontal and nasociliary nerves, and eventually pass through V₁ to reach their cell bodies in the trigeminal ganglion. From here, sensory information enters the brainstem via the large sensory root of the trigeminal nerve.

The oculomotor nucleus does not receive direct cortical projections via the corticonuclear (corticobulbar) system. The cortex of the frontal eye field exerts its control over oculomotor neurons via projections to the rostral interstitial nucleus of the medial longitudinal fasciculus (riMLF, the vertical gaze center) and the superior colliculus. This part of the tectum also projects to the riMLF, which, in turn, sends numerous fibers to the ipsilateral oculomotor nucleus and a smaller contingent to the contralateral side. Consequently, cortical and capsular lesions have an effect on the actions of muscles innervated by the oculomotor nerve, but this effect is indirect and results from the loss of cortical input to the brainstem gaze control centers. *Cortical damage (such as from stroke or trauma) involving the frontal eye fields produces an involuntary conjugate deviation of the eyes toward the side of the injury. One easy way to remember this correlate is that the patient "involuntarily looks to the lesioned side." If the cortical lesion is large enough to involve corticospinal fibers, the deviation of the eyes is toward the side of the cortical damage but away from the side of the resulting hemiparesis.*

Lesions involving the oculomotor nucleus, the oculomotor nerve in the interpeduncular cistern, or the nerve in the lateral wall of the cavernous sinus all generally have the same result. Loss of the GSE motor fibers paralyzes all of the extraocular muscles in the ipsilateral orbit except the superior oblique and lateral rectus muscles. As a result, the ipsilateral eye assumes an *abducted and depressed position* (down and out), owing to the unopposed action of the lateral rectus and superior oblique

muscles. The patient also experiences *diplopia (double vision)* because the image seen by each eye cannot be directed to corresponding portions of each retina, as most of the extraocular muscles in one eye are not functional. Furthermore, interruption of the preganglionic parasympathetic fibers in the oculomotor nerve results in characteristic signs and symptoms in the ipsilateral eye. First, the pupil is dilated *(mydriasis)* and nonreactive to light because the sphincter pupillae muscle is denervated (the dilator pupillae muscle, innervated by sympathetic fibers, is intact). Second, the lens in the ipsilateral eye cannot accommodate because the ciliary muscle is also denervated. Third, although the innervation to the superior tarsal muscle is intact because the course of the sympathetic fibers does not involve the oculomotor nerve outside the orbit, the upper eyelid exhibits *ptosis* (droop) because the levator palpebrae has been denervated by the oculomotor nerve lesion.

Because the parasympathetic fibers are located near the periphery (outer surface) of the oculomotor nerve, visceromotor signs and symptoms such as a subtle ptosis or mildly diminished pupil reactivity can appear before the onset of, or in the absence of, any extraocular muscle dysfunction with external compressive injury to the oculomotor nerve. The external compression affects the superficially located, smaller-diameter visceromotor fibers first. In contrast, in diabetic patients, the onset of an eye movement disorder may not be accompanied by visceromotor signs or symptoms. This is because diabetes is a vascular problem and the larger vessels inside the nerve are compromised first, thereby affecting the internally located, larger-diameter GSE motor axons but sparing the smaller and more superficially located visceromotor fibers. Isolated lesions of the oculomotor nerve distal to its passage through the superior orbital fissure are relatively rare and produce variable symptoms depending on the location of the lesion.

Synopsis of Clinical Points

- An extramedullary hypoglossal root lesion results in a deviation of the tongue to the ipsilateral side upon protrusion (p. 213).
- An intramedullary lesion involving hypoglossal fibers (usually vascular) results in ipsilateral deviation of the tongue on protrusion and a contralateral hemiparesis usually accompanied by sensory losses (p. 213).
- Damage to the accessory nerve results in weakness of the ipsilateral sternocleidomastoid and trapezius muscles and difficulty turning the head to the contralateral side or elevating the ipsilateral shoulder, both against resistance (p. 214).
- The efferent limb of the gag reflex traverses the glossopharyngeal nerve (p. 217).
- The most noticeable deficits associated with a lesion of the vagal root are dysphagia and dysarthria (p. 216).
- Central lesions, such as the lateral medullary syndrome, may also result in dysphagia and dysarthria (p. 216).
- Syndromes of the jugular foramen result in deficits indicative of damage to the roots of IX, X, and XI (or combinations thereof); in more inclusive cases the XIIth nerve and sympathetic postganglionic fibers are involved (p. 218).
- Glossopharyngeal neuralgia is an intense idiopathic pain arising primarily from the pharynx, caudal tongue, and tonsils (p. 217).
- Lesions of the vestibular portion of the vestibulocochlear nerve result in vertigo, nystagmus, dizziness, and ataxia (p. 220).
- Lesions of the cochlear root of the vestibulocochlear nerve result in partial or total hearing loss and tinnitus (p. 220).
- Lesions of the vestibulocochlear nerve result in deficits reflecting damage to both portions of the nerve (p. 220).
- A tumor on the vestibular root is a vestibular schwannoma, not an acoustic neuroma (p. 220).
- Tumors in the cerebellopontine angle result in deficits characteristic of eighth nerve lesions; in cases of larger tumors the facial root and the trigeminal nerve may be involved (p. 220).
- Deficits seen following a lesion of the facial root include weakness of the muscles of facial expression and loss of taste on the anterior two thirds of the tongue, both on the ipsilateral side (p. 221).
- A "central seven" is a capsular lesion that produces weakness of the facial muscles on the lower portion on the contralateral side (p. 221).
- Facial diplegia is a bilateral weakness of the facial muscles (p. 221).

Continued

Synopsis of Clinical Points *(Continued)*

■ Hemifacial spasms are irregular contractions of the facial muscles that sometimes are painful and may be triggered by compression of the facial root (p. 221).

■ Damage to the abducens root results in paralysis on the ipsilateral lateral rectus muscle (p. 222).

■ Small lesions in the MLF on one side may result in internuclear ophthalmoplegia (p. 222).

■ Pontine lesions that involve the abducens nucleus (abducens lower motor neurons and interneurons) and the adjacent MLF (containing axons of abducens interneurons) may result in a one-and-a-half syndrome (p. 223).

■ A lesion of the root of the trigeminal nerve results in paralysis of the muscles of mastication and loss of sensation on the face and in the oral cavity, both on the ipsilateral side (pp. 224–225).

■ In cases of lesions of the trigeminal motor root, the jaw deviates toward the weak side on closing owing to the unopposed action of the pterygoid muscles on the healthy side (p. 225).

■ The corneal reflex and the jaw jerk reflex have their afferent and efferent limbs on the trigeminal nerve (p. 224).

■ Trigeminal neuralgia (tic douloureux) is an intense pain arising from the face usually from the corner of the mouth, cheek, or nose (p. 225).

■ Causes of tic douloureux include trigeminal root compression by aberrant vessels (p. 225).

■ Lesions of the oculomotor root result in paralysis of most eye movement and dilation of the pupil, both on the ipsilateral side (p. 228).

■ Damage to the trochlear root in the quadrigeminal (superior) cistern results in paralysis of the ipsilateral superior oblique muscle (p. 225).

■ Cortical lesions of the frontal eye fields result in conjugate deviation of both eyes toward the lesioned side (pp. 225–226).

■ Compression of the oculomotor nerve may result in subtle ptosis or diminished papillary activity first, followed by extraocular muscle dysfunction (p. 228).

Sources and Additional Reading

Carpenter MB, Sutin J: Human Neuroanatomy, 8th ed. Baltimore, Williams & Wilkins, 1983.

Crosby EC, Humphrey T, Lauer EW: Correlative Anatomy of the Nervous System. New York, Macmillan, 1962.

Duvernoy H: The Human Brain Stem and Cerebellum: Surface, Structure, Vascularization, and Three-Dimensional Sectional Anatomy with MRI. New York, Springer-Verlag, 1995.

Greenberg MS: Handbook of Neurosurgery, 5th ed. New York, Thieme, 2001.

Haerer AF: DeJong's The Neurologic Examination. Philadelphia, JB Lippincott, 1993.

Haines DE: Neuroanatomy: An Atlas of Structures, Sections, and Systems, 6th ed. Philadelphia, Lippincott Williams & Wilkins, 2004.

Kretschmann H-J, Weinrich W: Cranial Neuroimaging and Clinical Neuroanatomy: Magnetic Resonance Imaging and Computed Tomography, 2nd ed. New York, Thieme Medical Publishers, 1992.

LeBlanc A: The Cranial Nerves: Anatomy, Imaging, Vascularisation. New York, Springer-Verlag, 1995.

Moore KL, Dalley AF: Clinically Oriented Anatomy, 4th ed. Philadelphia, Lippincott Williams & Wilkins, 1999.

Nieuwenhuys R, Voogd J, van Huijzen CHR: The Human Central Nervous System: A Synopsis and Atlas, 3rd ed. Berlin, Springer-Verlag, 1988.

Parent A: Carpenter's Human Neuroanatomy, 9th ed. Baltimore, Williams & Wilkins, 1996.

Pryse-Phillips W: Companion to Clinical Neurology, 2nd ed. New York, Oxford University Press, 2003.

Rowland LP: Merritt's Neurology, 10th ed. Philadelphia, Lippincott Williams & Wilkins, 2000.

Victor M, Ropper AH: Adams and Victor's Principles of Neurology, 7th ed. New York, McGraw-Hill, 2001.

The Diencephalon

G. A. Mihailoff and D. E. Haines

Although considered by some investigators to be part of the brainstem, the diencephalon is treated here as a portion of the forebrain. The diencephalon includes the *dorsal thalamus, hypothalamus, ventral thalamus,* and *epithalamus,* and it is situated between the telencephalon and the brainstem. In general, the diencephalon is the main processing center for information destined to reach the cerebral cortex from all ascending sensory pathways (except those related to olfaction) and numerous other subcortical cell groups. The right and left halves of the diencephalon, for the most part, contain symmetrically distributed cell groups separated by the space of the *third ventricle.*

Overview

The *dorsal thalamus,* or *thalamus* as it is commonly called, is the largest of the four principal subdivisions of the diencephalon and consists of pools of neurons that collectively project to nearly all areas of the cerebral cortex. Some of the thalamic nuclei receive somatosensory, visual, or auditory input and transmit this information to the appropriate area of the cerebral cortex. Other thalamic nuclei receive input from subcortical motor areas and project to those parts of the overlying cortex that influence the successful execution of a motor act. A few thalamic nuclei receive a more diffuse input and accordingly relate in a more diffuse way to widespread areas of cortex.

The *hypothalamus* is also composed of multiple nuclear subdivisions and is connected primarily to portions of the forebrain, brainstem, and spinal cord. This part of the diencephalon is involved in the control of visceromotor (autonomic) functions. In this respect, the hypothalamus regulates functions that are "automatically" adjusted (such as blood pressure and body temperature) without our being aware of the change. In contrast, conscious sensation and some aspects of motor control are mediated by the dorsal thalamus.

The *ventral thalamus* and *epithalamus* are the smallest subdivisions of the diencephalon. The former includes the subthalamic nucleus, which is linked to the basal nuclei of the forebrain and functions in the motor sphere; lesions in the subthalamus give rise to very characteristic involuntary movement disorders. The epithalamus is functionally related to the limbic system.

Development of the Diencephalon

The cell groups that give rise to the diencephalon form in the caudomedial portion of the prosencephalon, bordering on the space that will become the third ventricle. The developing brain at this level consists initially of a roof plate and the two alar plates; it lacks a well-defined floor plate and basal plates.

A shallow groove appears in the wall of the third ventricle and extends rostrally from the developing cerebral aqueduct to the ventral edge of the interventricular foramen (Fig. 15-1A, B). This groove, the *hypothalamic sulcus,* divides the alar plate into a superior (dorsal) area, the future *dorsal thalamus,* and an inferior (ventral) portion, the future *hypothalamus.* The third ventricle, which is the vertically oriented, midline space of the diencephalon, is continuous with the paired lateral ventricles via the *interventricular foramina (foramina of Monro)* (Figs. 15-1B and 15-2). The dorsal thalamus on each side of the third ventricle increases rapidly in size and, in many brains, will partially fuse across the space of the third ventricle to form the *massa*

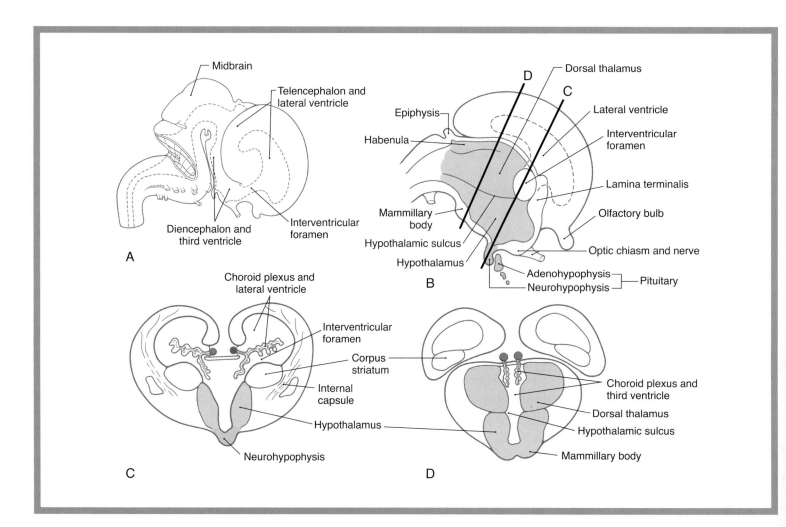

Figure 15-1. Development of the diencephalon. Lateral (**A**) and midsagittal (**B**) views of the forebrain at about 8 to 9 weeks of gestational age. The cross-sectional views (**C, D**) are taken from the planes shown in **B** and emphasize diencephalic structures.

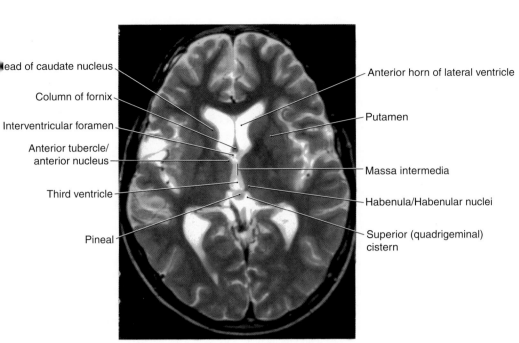

Figure 15-2. Axial T2-weighted MR image showing the interventricular foramen, massa intermedia, area of the habenula, and the pineal in the superior cistern. The interventricular foramen is the space (containing a small portion of choroid plexus) located between the column of the fornix and the anterior tubercle of the thalamus. The major nuclei of the dorsal thalamus in an axial plane are shown in Figure 15-10.

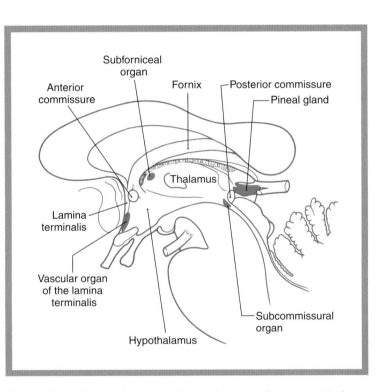

Figure 15-3. Midsagittal view showing the locations of circumventricular organs.

intermedia, or *interthalamic adhesion* (Figs. 15-2 to 15-4). This structure is present in about 80% of the general population.

The epithalamus develops from the caudal portion of the roof plate (Fig. 15-1B). By the seventh week, a small thickening of the roof plate forms. It gradually increases in size and evaginates to form the *epiphysis*, which develops into the *pineal gland* of the adult (Figs. 15-2 to 15-4). The portion of the roof plate immediately rostral to the epiphysis gives rise to the *habenula*, a small thickening in which the habenular nuclei will develop (Figs. 15-2 and 15-4).

Just anterior to the habenular region, the roof plate epithelium and adjacent pia mater give rise to the choroid plexus of the third ventricle, which, in the adult, remains suspended from the roof of this space (Fig. 15-1B-D). This choroid plexus is continuous through the interventricular foramina with that of the lateral ventricles. Elsewhere, in locations around the perimeter of the third ventricle, specialized patches of ependyma lie on the midline and form unpaired structures called the *circumventricular organs*. These structures include the subfornical organ, the organum vasculosum of the lamina terminalis, the subcommissural organ, and the pineal gland (Fig. 15-3). These cellular regions are characterized by the presence of fenestrated capillaries, which implies an absence of the blood-brain barrier. These structures are thought to release metabolites and neuropeptides into the cerebrospinal fluid or into the cerebrovascular system.

The development of the pituitary gland during the third week is linked to that of the diencephalon (Fig. 15-1B, C). A downward extension of the floor of the third ventricle, the *infundibulum*, meets the *Rathke pouch*, an upward outpocketing of the stomodeum, the primitive oral cavity. By the end of the second month, the Rathke pouch loses its connection with the developing oral cavity but maintains its attachment to the infundibulum. As development continues, the Rathke pouch gives rise to the *anterior lobe (adenohypophysis)* and *pars intermedia* of the pituitary gland, whereas the infundibulum differentiates into the *posterior lobe* of the pituitary gland, or *neurohypophysis* (Fig. 15-1B; see Chapter 30 for further information). A *craniopharyngioma* (Rathke pouch tumor) can arise from a portion of the Rathke pouch that fails to undergo proper migration and apposition to the infundibulum. These tumors mimic lesions of the pituitary and may cause visual problems, diabetes insipidus, and increased intracranial pressure.

Basic Organization

The junction between the diencephalon and midbrain lies along a line extending from the posterior commissure to the caudal edge of the mammillary body on the medial aspect of the hemisphere (Fig. 15-4). On the surface of the hemisphere, this interface is represented by a line starting at the caudal aspect of the mammillary body, extending anterolaterally over the edge of the crus cerebri, and following the caudal edge of the optic tract (Fig. 15-5). The boundary between the diencephalon and surrounding telencephalon is less distinct and is represented laterally by the internal capsule (discussed later) and rostrally by the interventricular foramen, lamina terminalis, and optic chiasm (Fig. 15-4).

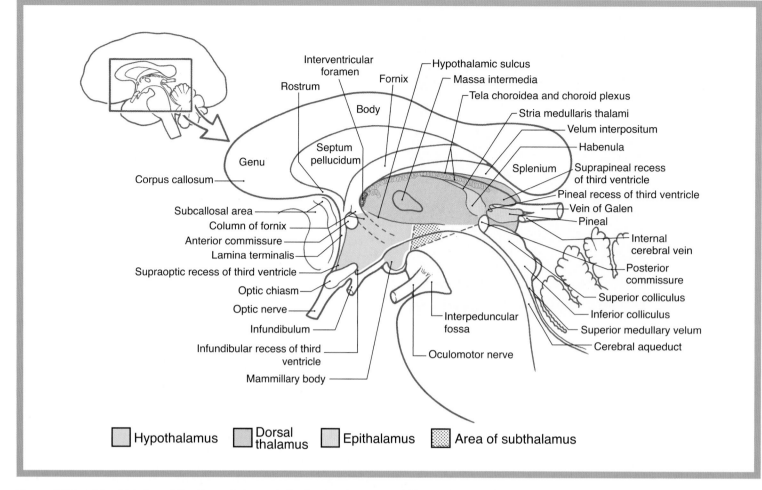

Figure 15-4. Midsagittal view of the diencephalon and closely related structures. This is a drawing of the specimen shown in Figure 15-6.

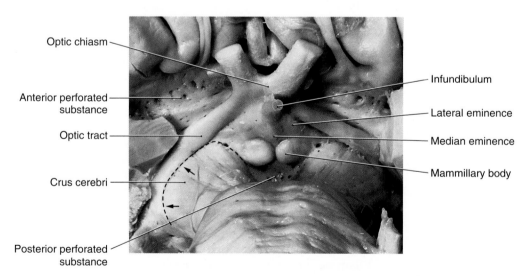

Figure 15-5. Anterior (ventral) view of the hemisphere emphasizing diencephalic structures visible on the surface and showing the diencephalic-mesencephalic interface as represented by the caudal edge of the optic tract *(arrows)*.

The cavity of the diencephalon, the *third ventricle,* is a narrow, vertically oriented midline space located between the paired dorsal thalami and hypothalami of the two sides (Figs. 15-6 and 15-7). In addition to its connections with the lateral ventricles and the cerebral aqueduct, the third ventricle has small evaginations or *recesses* associated with the optic chiasm *(supraoptic recess),* the infundibulum *(infundibular recess),* and the pineal gland *(pineal and suprapineal recesses)* (Figs. 15-1 and 15-4).

All four diencephalic subdivisions can be approximated in a midsagittal section of the forebrain (Figs. 15-4 and 15-6). The *dorsal thalamus* is located superior to the hypothalamic sulcus and extends from the interventricular foramen caudally to the

level of the splenium of the corpus callosum. The *hypothalamus* lies inferior to the hypothalamic sulcus and is bordered rostrally by the lamina terminalis and caudally by a line that extends from the posterior aspect of the mammillary body superiorly to intersect with the hypothalamic sulcus. The only diencephalic structures visible on the inferior surface of the hemisphere are those related to the hypothalamus, including the optic chiasm, infundibulum, medial and lateral eminences, and mammillary bodies (Fig. 15-5). The *ventral thalamus (subthalamus)* does not border on the ventricle; rather, it occupies a position caudal to the hypothalamus, rostral to the diencephalon-midbrain junction, and *lateral to the midline* (Figs. 15-4 and 15-7B). *Epithalamic*

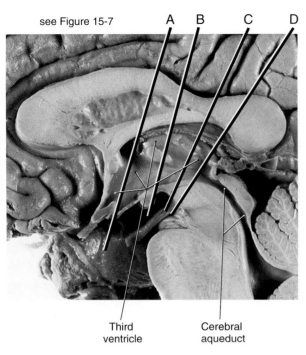

see Figure 15-7   A   B   C   D

Third   Cerebral
ventricle   aqueduct

Figure 15-6. Midsagittal view of the diencephalon. This view correlates with the drawing in Figure 15-3. Lines A through D indicate the planes of the stained sections in Figure 15-7.

structures are located posteriorly and caudally, in close apposition to the posterior commissure, and include the pineal gland, the habenular nuclei, and the main afferent bundle of these nuclei, the stria medullaris thalami.

Dorsal Thalamus (Thalamus)

The *dorsal thalamus* (or *thalamus*) (Figs. 15-4 and 15-7 to 15-9) is a massive collection of neuronal cell groups that participate in a widely diverse array of functions involving motor, sensory, and limbic systems. Typically, thalamic output neurons project to the cerebral cortex; in fact, very little information reaches the cerebral cortex without first being processed by thalamic neurons. As a result, the thalamus is often regarded as the functional "gateway" to the cerebral cortex. In turn, nearly all regions of the cerebral cortex give rise to reciprocal projections that return to the thalamic region from which they originally received input.

The thalamus is covered on its lateral aspect by a layer of myelinated axons, the *external medullary lamina*, which includes fibers that enter or leave the subcortical white matter (Fig. 15-7B, C). Within the external medullary lamina are clusters of neurons that form the *thalamic reticular nucleus*. The medial surface of the thalamus borders the third ventricle, and the external medullary lamina and thalamic reticular nucleus blend with the thalamic fasciculus and zona incerta, respectively, to form an interface between dorsal and ventral thalami (Fig. 15-7B).

An *internal medullary lamina*, also consisting of myelinated fibers, extends into the substance of the thalamus, where it forms partitions or boundaries that divide the thalamus into its principal cell groups (Figs. 15-9 and 15-10): the *anterior, medial, lateral,* and *intraluminar nuclear groups*. The latter are located in the portion of the internal medullary lamina that separates the lateral and medial nuclear groups. In addition, there are *midline thalamic nuclei* located just superior to the hypothalamic sulcus.

Finally, attached to the caudolateral portion of the thalamus are the *medial* and *lateral geniculate bodies* (and their *nuclei*)

(Figs. 15-7D, 15-8D, and 15-10). Although considered here as components of the lateral nuclear group, the geniculate nuclei are sometimes considered as a separate part of the thalamus, the *metathalamus*.

Anterior Thalamic Nuclei

This group of cells consists of a large principal nucleus and two smaller nuclei; collectively, these cell groups form the *anterior nucleus of the thalamus* (Figs. 15-7A, 15-8B, 15-9, and 15-10). The anterior nucleus forms a prominent wedge on the rostral aspect of the dorsal thalamus just caudolateral to the interventricular foramen; this wedge is the *anterior thalamic tubercle*. Rostrally, the internal medullary lamina divides to partially encapsulate the anterior nucleus. The cells of this nucleus receive dense limbic-related projections from (1) the mammillary nuclei via the mammillothalamic tract and (2) the medial temporal lobe (hippocampus) via the fornix. The output of this nucleus is primarily directed to the cingulate gyrus through the anterior limb of the internal capsule (Fig. 15-11).

Medial Thalamic Nuclei

This region of the dorsal thalamus comprises the *dorsomedial nucleus* (Figs. 15-8C and 15-9). This expansive group of neuronal cell bodies is composed of large *parvicellular* (located caudally) and *magnocellular* (located rostrally) parts and a small paralaminar part adjacent to the internal medullary lamina (Figs. 15-7B-D and 15-10). The two larger portions are linked to parts of the frontal and temporal lobes and to the amygdaloid complex (Fig. 15-11). Cells of the paralaminar subdivision receive input from the frontal lobe and substantia nigra and may play a role in the control of eye movement.

Lateral Thalamic Nuclei

This large collection of thalamic neurons is grouped into *dorsal* and *ventral tiers*. The relatively small group of *dorsal tier* nuclei includes the *lateral dorsal* and *lateral posterior nuclei* along with the much larger *pulvinar nucleus* (pulvinar) (Figs. 15-7B-D, 15-8D, 15-9, and 15-10). The connections of the lateral dorsal and lateral posterior nuclei are formed with the cingulate gyrus and parietal lobe, respectively (Fig. 15-10). The large *pulvinar nucleus* consists of anterior, medial, lateral, and inferior subdivisions. The inferior division receives input from the superior colliculus and projects to the visual association cortex. Other portions of the pulvinar project to areas of the temporal, parietal, and frontal lobes that are especially concerned with visual function and eye movements (Fig. 15-11).

The large *ventral tier* of the lateral group consists of three separate nuclei (Figs. 15-7, 15-8B, C, and 15-9). The *ventral anterior nucleus* (VA) and the slightly more caudal *ventral lateral nucleus* (VL) are important motor-related nuclei, whereas the *ventral posterior nucleus*, consisting of *ventral posterolateral* (VPL) and *ventral posteromedial* (VPM) *nuclei*, conveys somatosensory information to the cerebral cortex. The VA is composed of a large parvocellular portion and a small magnocellular part. The former receives input from the medial segment of the globus pallidus, and the latter receives afferents from the reticular portion of substantia nigra. The efferent projections from the VA are diffuse and appear to include selected parts of the frontal lobe (Fig. 15-11).

The VL (Figs. 15-7B and 15-10) is also composed of three subdivisions: a pars oralis, a pars medialis, and a pars caudalis. The largest of these, the pars oralis, receives a dense projection from the internal segment of the ipsilateral globus pallidus; some of these afferents enter the caudal subdivision. In contrast, the pars caudalis subdivision of the VL receives its main input from the contralateral cerebellar nuclei. Consequently, pallidal and

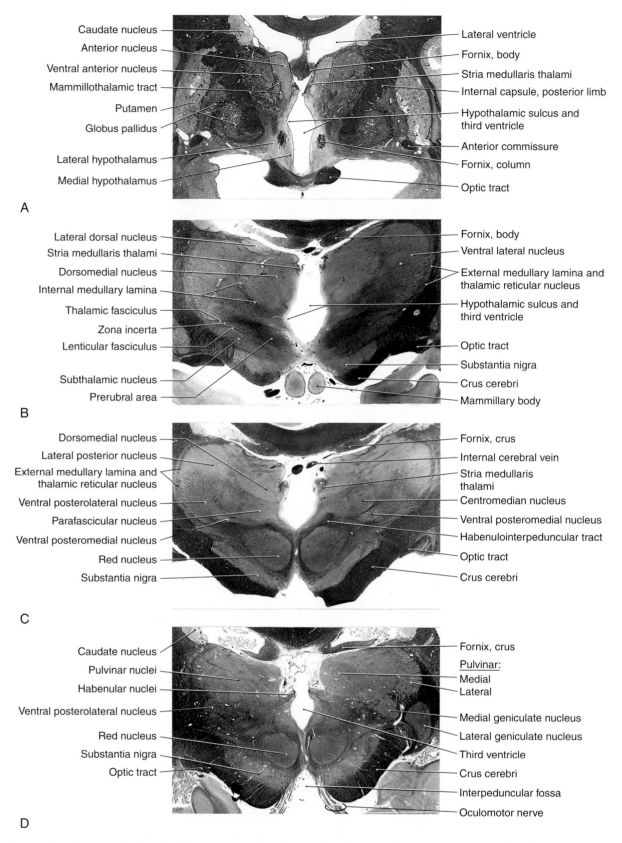

Caudate nucleus
Anterior nucleus
Ventral anterior nucleus
Mammillothalamic tract
Putamen
Globus pallidus
Lateral hypothalamus
Medial hypothalamus

Lateral ventricle
Fornix, body
Stria medullaris thalami
Internal capsule, posterior limb
Hypothalamic sulcus and third ventricle
Anterior commissure
Fornix, column
Optic tract

A

Lateral dorsal nucleus
Stria medullaris thalami
Dorsomedial nucleus
Internal medullary lamina
Thalamic fasciculus
Zona incerta
Lenticular fasciculus
Subthalamic nucleus
Prerubral area

Fornix, body
Ventral lateral nucleus
External medullary lamina and thalamic reticular nucleus
Hypothalamic sulcus and third ventricle
Optic tract
Substantia nigra
Crus cerebri
Mammillary body

B

Dorsomedial nucleus
Lateral posterior nucleus
External medullary lamina and thalamic reticular nucleus
Ventral posterolateral nucleus
Parafascicular nucleus
Ventral posteromedial nucleus
Red nucleus
Substantia nigra

Fornix, crus
Internal cerebral vein
Stria medullaris thalami
Centromedian nucleus
Ventral posteromedial nucleus
Habenulointerpeduncular tract
Optic tract
Crus cerebri

C

Caudate nucleus
Pulvinar nuclei
Habenular nuclei
Ventral posterolateral nucleus
Red nucleus
Substantia nigra
Optic tract

Fornix, crus
Pulvinar:
Medial
Lateral
Medial geniculate nucleus
Lateral geniculate nucleus
Third ventricle
Crus cerebri
Interpeduncular fossa
Oculomotor nerve

D

Figure 15-7. Four levels of the forebrain from rostral (**A**) to caudal (**D**) showing the internal structure of the hemisphere with emphasis on the diencephalon. These levels correlate with those shown in Figure 15-5 and with the planes represented in the exploded view in Figure 15-10. Weil stain.

cerebellar projections are largely *segregated* within this nucleus. The output of the VL reflects its segregated input in that the oral and caudal parts project to largely separate areas of the frontal lobe (Fig. 15-11).

The larger and more laterally located VPL nucleus and the comparatively smaller and more medially located VPM nucleus both receive somatosensory input from the contralateral side of the body (Figs. 15-7C and 15-10). The medial lemniscus and spinothalamic fibers terminate in a somatotopic manner (cervical

fibers medial, sacral fibers lateral) within the VPL, whereas trigeminothalamic fibers from the spinal trigeminal nucleus and the principal trigeminal sensory nucleus terminate in the VPM. Both the VPL and VPM project to the somatosensory cortex of the parietal lobe (Fig. 15-11).

A small group of cells called the *ventral posterior inferior nucleus* is situated ventrally between the VPL and VPM. These cells process vestibular input and project to lateral areas of the postcentral gyrus that are located in the depths of the central

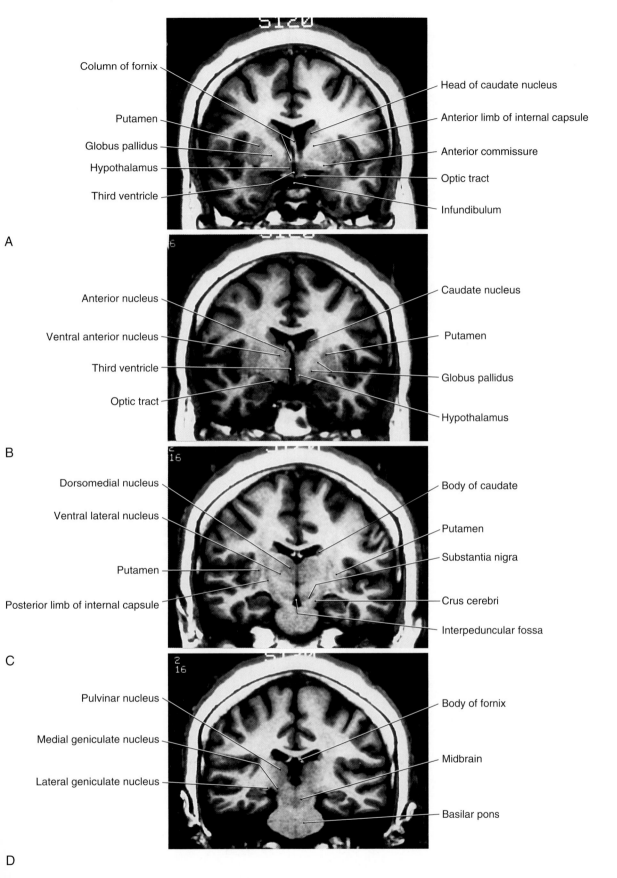

Column of fornix
Putamen
Globus pallidus
Hypothalamus
Third ventricle

Head of caudate nucleus
Anterior limb of internal capsule
Anterior commissure
Optic tract
Infundibulum

A

Anterior nucleus
Ventral anterior nucleus
Third ventricle
Optic tract

Caudate nucleus
Putamen
Globus pallidus
Hypothalamus

B

Dorsomedial nucleus
Ventral lateral nucleus
Putamen
Posterior limb of internal capsule

Body of caudate
Putamen
Substantia nigra
Crus cerebri
Interpeduncular fossa

C

Pulvinar nucleus
Medial geniculate nucleus
Lateral geniculate nucleus

Body of fornix
Midbrain
Basilar pons

D

Figure 15-8. MR images of the cerebral hemisphere in the coronal plane from rostral (**A**) to caudal (**D**). Although many structures are clearly seen, emphasis in the labeling is placed on diencephalic structures. All images are T1 weighted.

sulcus. Similarly, a small group of cells forming the rostral (oral) portion of the VPL receives cerebellar input and projects to the precentral gyrus of the frontal lobe; this nucleus probably represents a few cells that have been displaced from the slightly more rostrally located VL. This cell group is also called the *ventral intermediate nucleus* because of its location between the VL and VPL.

The *lateral* (LGB) and *medial* (MGB) *geniculate nuclei* are considered parts of the lateral thalamic nuclear group (Figs. 15-7D, 15-8D, and 15-10). The medial geniculate nucleus receives ascending *auditory* input via the brachium of the inferior colliculus and projects to the primary auditory cortex in the temporal lobe. The lateral geniculate nucleus receives *visual* input from the retina via the optic tract and in turn projects to

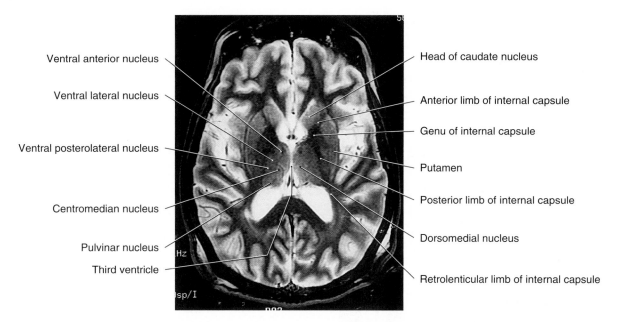

Figure 15-9. T2-weighted MR image of the cerebral hemisphere in the axial plane. Emphasis in labeling is on diencephalic structures. Compare with Figure 15-12.

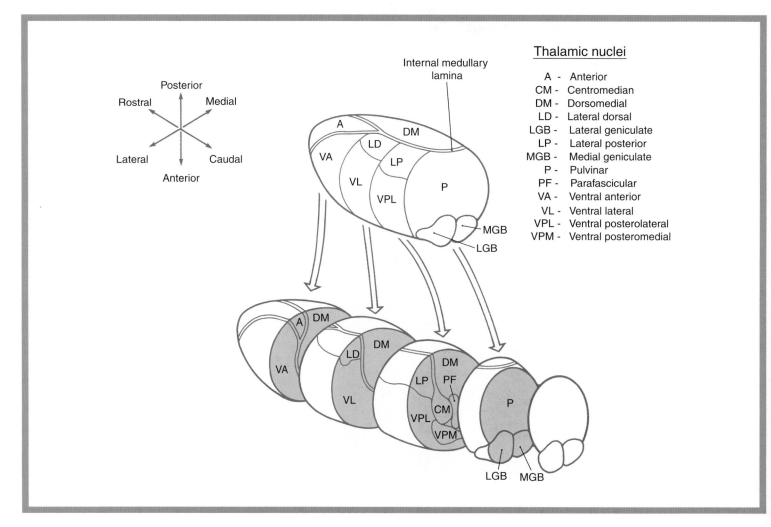

Figure 15-10. Exploded view of the dorsal thalamus illustrating the organization of thalamic nuclei. Compare with Figure 15-6A to D and with Figure 15-8.

the primary visual cortex on the medial surface of the occipital lobe (Fig. 15-11).

Located in the posterior thalamus at about the level of the pulvinar and geniculate nuclei is a cluster of cell groups collectively called the *posterior nuclear complex*. This complex consists of the suprageniculate nucleus, the nucleus limitans, and the posterior nucleus. These nuclei are positioned superior to the medial geniculate and medial to the rostral pulvinar. The posterior nuclear complex receives and sends to the cortex nociceptive cutaneous input that is transmitted over somatosensory pathways.

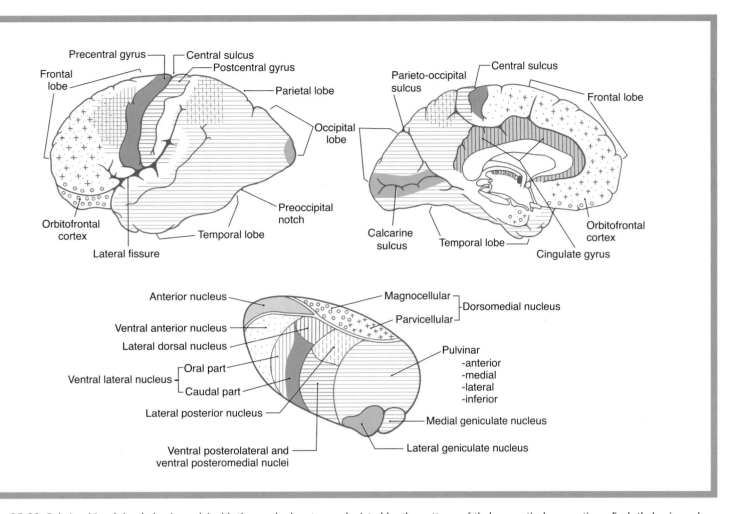

Figure 15-11. Relationship of the thalamic nuclei with the cerebral cortex as depicted by the patterns of thalamocortical connections. Each thalamic nucleus is pattern coded or color coded to match its target area in the cerebral cortex.

Intralaminar Nuclei

Embedded within the internal medullary lamina are the discontinuous groups of neurons that form the *intralaminar nuclei*. These cells are characterized by their projections to the neostriatum and to other thalamic nuclei, along with diffuse projections to the cerebral cortex. Two of the most prominent cell groups are the *centromedian* and *parafascicular nuclei* (Figs. 15-9 and 15-10). The centromedian nucleus projects to the neostriatum and to motor areas of the cerebral cortex, whereas the parafascicular nucleus projects to rostral and lateral areas of the frontal lobe. Other intralaminar nuclei receive input from ascending pain pathways and project to somatosensory and parietal cortex.

Midline Nuclei

The midline nuclei are the least understood components of the thalamus. The largest is the *paratenial nucleus*, which is located just ventral to the rostral portion of the stria medullaris thalami; other cells are associated with the interthalamic adhesion (massa intermedia). Although inputs are poorly defined, efferent fibers reach the amygdaloid complex and the anterior cingulate cortex, suggesting a role in the limbic system.

Thalamic Reticular Nucleus

The cells of this nucleus are situated within the external medullary lamina and between this lamina and the internal capsule (Fig. 15-7B, C). Axons of these cells project medially into the nuclei of the dorsal thalamus or to other parts of the reticular nucleus, but not into the cerebral cortex. Afferents are received

from the cortex and from nuclei of the dorsal thalamus via collaterals of thalamocortical and corticothalamic axons. It appears that thalamic reticular neurons modulate, or gate, the responses of thalamic neurons to incoming cerebral cortical input.

Summary of Thalamic Organization

Each thalamic nucleus (with a few exceptions) gives rise to efferent projections (thalamocortical axons) that target some portion of the cerebral cortex. That region of cortex then typically provides a reciprocal projection (corticothalamic axons) that returns to the original thalamic nucleus. Figure 15-11 reviews the major thalamocortical relationships.

Some thalamic nuclei are primarily associated with a particular function and, in turn, with a specific gyrus (functional area) of the cerebral cortex. The more important of these relationships are as follows: VL/motor/precentral gyrus and anterior paracentral gyrus; VPL/sensory for the body/postcentral gyrus and posterior paracentral gyrus; VPM/sensory for the face/postcentral gyrus; MGB/auditory/transverse temporal gyrus; LGB/vision/cortex on the calcarine sulcus. The anterior nucleus projects primarily to the cingulate gyrus and functions in the broad area of behavior. Consult Figure 15-11 for these interrelationships.

The nuclei of the thalamus have been classified according to their connections as either *relay nuclei* or *association nuclei*. A *relay nucleus* is one that receives input predominantly from a single source such as a sensory pathway or a cerebellar nucleus, or from the basal nuclei. The incoming neural information is processed and then sent to a localized region of either sensory, motor, or limbic cortex. *Relay nuclei* include the medial and lateral geniculate nuclei, VPL, VPM, VL, VA, and the anterior thalamic nuclei. It is important to note that these nuclei do not *merely* relay neural signals; in fact, considerable neural processing also takes place in these nuclei. However, their position in a modality-specific pathway linking one particular source to one particular destination makes the word "relay" a useful designation. In contrast, an *association nucleus* receives input from a number of different structures or cortical regions and usually sends its output to more than one of the *association areas* of the cerebral cortex (i.e., areas that are neither sensory nor motor cortex; see Chapter 32). *Association nuclei* include DM, LD, LP, and the nuclei of the pulvinar complex.

A thalamic nucleus can also be designated *specific* or *nonspecific* on the basis of thalamocortical signals generated in response to electrical stimulation delivered to a localized site in that thalamic nucleus. Focal electrical stimulation of a *specific* nucleus produces a rapidly conducted, sharply localized evoked response in the ipsilateral cerebral cortex. All relay nuclei and association nuclei are *specific nuclei*. Focal electrical stimulation of a *nonspecific* nucleus produces widespread activity in the cortex of *both* hemispheres, at a significantly longer time delay than with stimulation of a specific nucleus. It is thought that *nonspecific* nuclei play a role in modulating the excitability of large regions of cortex. *Nonspecific* nuclei include the midline nuclear group, the intralaminar nuclear group (such as the CM nucleus), and a portion of the VA. Chapter 32 contains additional information on the connections of thalamic nuclei.

Internal Capsule

Axons pass between the diencephalon, particularly the dorsal thalamus, and the cerebral cortex in a fan-shaped mass of fibers, the *internal capsule*, that courses from the central core of the hemisphere into the brainstem (Figs. 15-7 and 15-12). Even though this structure consists mostly of axons that reciprocally link the thalamus and cerebral cortex, it also contains cortical efferent fibers that project to the brainstem (corticorubral, corticoreticular, corticonuclear/corticobulbar) or spinal cord (corticospinal).

Although the internal capsule is described in detail in Chapter 16, it is summarized here because of its important relationship to the thalamus. As seen in axial section (Fig. 15-12) the internal capsule consists of an *anterior limb, genu,* and *posterior limb.* The genu is located immediately lateral to the anterior thalamic nucleus, at about the same level as the interventricular foramen. The anterior limb extends rostrolateral from the genu and is insinuated between the caudate and lenticular nuclei. The posterior limb extends caudolateral from the genu and consists of a large part separating the thalamus from the globus pallidus

and smaller portions that link temporal and occipital lobes with thalamic nuclei.

Hypothalamus

Unlike the thalamus, which is primarily related to somatic functions, the hypothalamus (Figs. 15-8A, B and 15-9) is mainly involved in *visceromotor, viscerosensory,* and *endocrine* activities. The hypothalamus and related limbic structures receive sensory input regarding the internal environment and, in turn, regulate through four mechanisms the motor systems that modify the internal environment. *First,* the hypothalamus is a principal modulator of autonomic nervous system function. *Second,* it is a viscerosensory transducer, containing neurons with specialized receptors capable of responding to changes in the temperature or osmolality of blood, as well as to specific hormonal levels in the general circulation. *Third,* the hypothalamus regulates the activity of the anterior pituitary through the production of releasing factors (hormone-releasing hormones), and, *fourth,* it performs an endocrine function by producing and releasing oxytocin and vasopressin into the general circulation within the posterior pituitary.

The hypothalamus can be divided into lateral, medial, and periventricular zones (Figs. 15-7A and 15-13). The *lateral zone,* often called the *lateral hypothalamic area,* extends the full rostrocaudal length of the hypothalamus and is separated from the medial zone by a line drawn through the fornix in the sagittal plane (Fig. 15-14C). The *medial zone* is divided from rostral to caudal into three regions: the chiasmatic, the tuberal, and the mammillary regions (Figs. 15-13 and 15-14). The *periventricular zone* includes the neurons that border the ependymal surfaces of the third ventricle.

Lateral Hypothalamic Zone

The *lateral hypothalamic area* (Fig. 15-14) is composed of diffuse clusters of neurons intermingled with longitudinally oriented axon bundles. The latter, which form the *medial forebrain bundle,* are diffusely organized in the human brain. No discrete named nuclei are present in this lateral area, although the supraoptic nucleus (see later on) is considered by some authorities to be part of it. Cells of the lateral hypothalamic area are involved in cardiovascular function and in the regulation of food and water intake.

Medial Hypothalamic Zone

In contrast to the lateral zone, the medial hypothalamus contains discrete groups of neurons whose function and connections are established. Within the *chiasmatic* (anterior) *region* are five nuclei: the *preoptic, supraoptic, paraventricular, anterior,* and

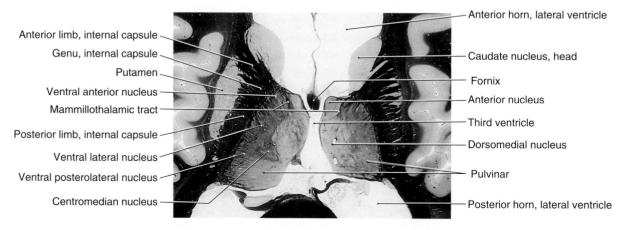

Figure 15-12. Axial view of the forebrain showing the relationship of the thalamus to the limbs of the internal capsule. Weil stain.

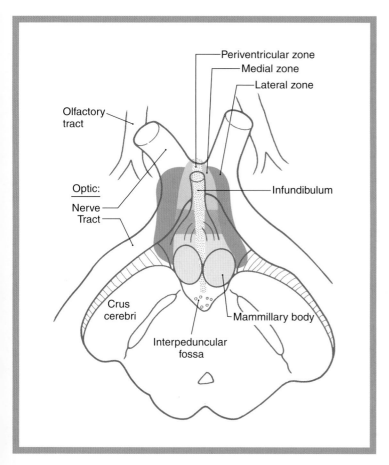

Figure 15-13. Anterior (ventral) view of the diencephalon illustrating the three zones of the hypothalamus as superimposed on external structures. The colors used for medial and lateral zones correlate with those in Figure 15-14.

suprachiasmatic nuclei (Fig. 15-14A, B). Nuclei in the chiasmatic region are generally involved in regulating hormone release (preoptic, supraoptic, periventricular), cardiovascular function (anterior), circadian rhythms (suprachiasmatic), and body temperature and heat loss mechanisms (preoptic). In the *tuberal region* are the *dorsomedial, ventromedial,* and *arcuate nuclei* (Fig. 15-14A, C). The *ventromedial nucleus* is regarded as the food intake (satiety) center. Bilateral lesions of this hypothalamic region produce *hyperphagia,* a greatly increased food intake with resultant obesity. Cells of the *arcuate nucleus* deliver peptides to the portal vessels and, through these channels, to the anterior pituitary. Some of these peptides are *releasing factors,* which cause an increase in the secretion of specific hormones by the anterior pituitary, and some are *inhibiting factors,* which inhibit the secretion of specific hormones by the anterior pituitary.

At caudal levels, the *mammillary region* is composed of the *posterior nucleus* and the *mammillary nuclei* (Fig. 15-14A, D). In humans, the mammillary nuclei consist of a large medial and a small lateral nucleus. Although both of these nuclei receive input via the fornix, only the medial nucleus projects to the anterior thalamic nucleus through the mammillothalamic tract. This latter bundle traverses the internal medullary lamina as it enters the anterior nucleus (Figs. 15-7A and 15-12). The neurons of the posterior nucleus are involved in activities that include elevation of blood pressure, pupillary dilation, and shivering or body heat conservation. The mammillary nuclei are involved in the control of various reflexes associated with feeding, as well as mechanisms relating to memory formation.

Afferent Fiber Systems

Although many axonal systems extend into the hypothalamus, only four inputs are mentioned here; the entire group is discussed in Chapter 30. The fornix and the stria terminalis are

two major afferent fiber bundles that reach the hypothalamus (Fig. 15-7). The *fornix* consists of axons that largely originate in the hippocampus, and the *stria terminalis* arises from neurons in the amygdaloid complex (see Fig. 16-16). Fibers composing the *ventral amygdalofugal bundle* exit the amygdala and course through the substantia innominata to enter the hypothalamus and thalamus (see Fig. 16-16). As mentioned earlier, the *medial forebrain bundle* passes bidirectionally through the lateral hypothalamic region. This composite fiber bundle consists of ascending axons that originate in areas throughout the neuraxis and terminate in the hypothalamus and other axons that exit the hypothalamus to reach forebrain and brainstem targets.

Efferent Fibers

The hypothalamus is the source of a diverse array of efferent fibers (see Chapter 30). Several nuclei give rise to descending fibers that contribute to the dorsal longitudinal fasciculus and the medial forebrain bundle and to diffuse projections that pass into the tegmentum. These fiber systems project directly to numerous brainstem nuclei, as well as to preganglionic sympathetic and parasympathetic neurons in the spinal cord. Other projections reach the thalamus and frontal cortex, and still others extend to the posterior pituitary or to the tuberohypophysial portal system for delivery of substances to the anterior pituitary.

Ventral Thalamus (Subthalamus)

The *ventral thalamus* (also called *subthalamus*) includes the large *subthalamic nucleus,* the medially adjacent *prerubral area (field H of Forel),* and, posteriorly, the *zona incerta* (Figs. 15-4 and 15-7B). As the term *ventral thalamus* (or subthalamus) implies, these cell groups are located ventral (anterior) to the large expanse of the dorsal thalamus. The *subthalamic nucleus* is a lens-shaped cell group situated rostral and posterior to the substantia nigra and immediately inferior to a distinct myelinated fiber bundle, the *lenticular fasciculus* (Fig. 15-7B; see Chapter 26 for more information). The cells of the subthalamic nucleus receive input from motor areas of the cerebral cortex, project to the substantia nigra, and are reciprocally connected with the globus pallidus. The subthalamic nucleus can be affected by vascular lesions involving posteromedial branches of the posterior cerebral or posterior communicating arteries, which results in a characteristic clinical condition known as *hemiballismus.* Patients with this involuntary movement disorder exhibit rapid and forceful flailing movements, which usually involve the contralateral upper extremity. These movements can be very debilitating because the patient has no control over their initiation or duration.

The *zona incerta* is located superior to the subthalamic nucleus and is separated from it by the *lenticular fasciculus* (Fig. 15-7B). Superior to the zona incerta are the myelinated axons of the thalamic fasciculus. The zona incerta contains output neurons that project to a variety of locations, including the cerebral cortex, the superior colliculus, the pretectal region, and the basilar pons. Afferent projections arise from the motor cortex and as collaterals from the medial lemniscus.

The *prerubral area (Forel's field H)* is located just rostral to the red nucleus and medial to the subthalamic nucleus (Fig. 15-7B). There are scattered neurons in this region, and traversing the prerubral area are fibers from the *lenticular fasciculus* (Forel's field H_2) that enter the *thalamic fasciculus* (Forel's field H_1).

Epithalamus

The *pineal gland, habenular nuclei,* and *stria medullaris thalami* are the principal components of the epithalamus (Figs. 15-2, 15-4, and 15-15). The pineal gland consists of richly vascularized

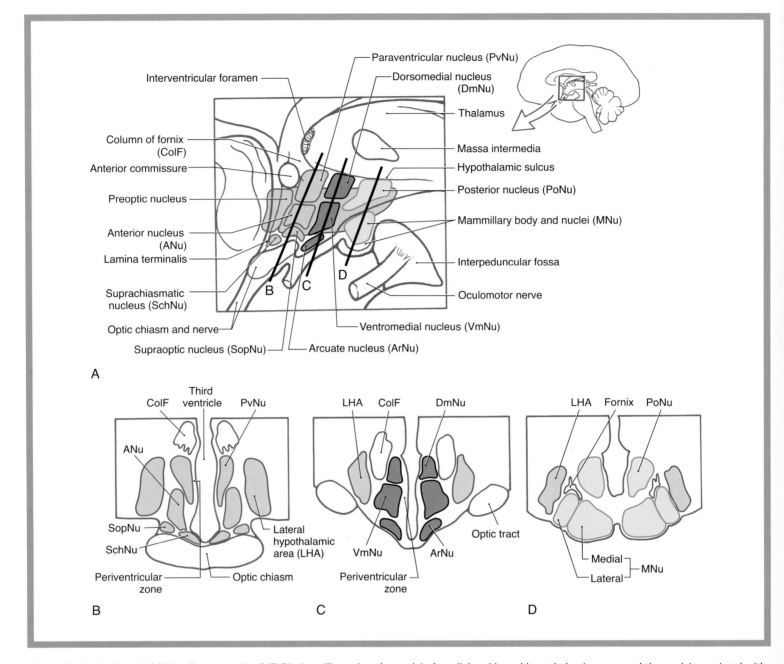

Figure 15-14. Midsagittal (**A**) and cross-sectional (**B-D**) views illustrating the nuclei of medial and lateral hypothalamic zones and the nuclei associated with chiasmatic (**B**), tuberal (**C**), and mammillary (**D**) regions. The colors used here correlate with those in Figure 15-12. (A adapted from Haymaker W, Anderson E, Nauta WJH: The Hypothalamus. Springfield, IL, Charles C Thomas, 1969, with permission.)

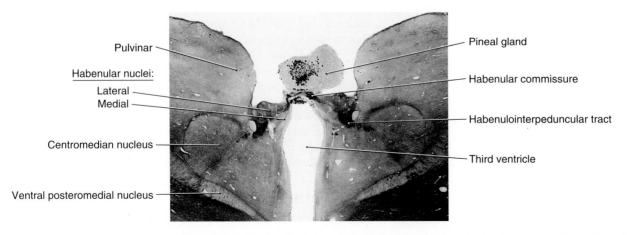

Figure 15-15. Caudal level of the diencephalon showing the habenular nuclei, pineal gland, and related structures. The stria medullaris thalami has disappeared at this level because its fibers have dispersed to end in the habenular nuclei.

connective tissue containing glial cells and pinealocytes but no true neurons. Mammalian pinealocytes are related to the photoreceptor elements found in this gland in lower forms, such as amphibians. In humans, however, they remain only indirectly light sensitive and receive information concerning photic stimuli through a multisynaptic neural circuit.

Pinealocytes have club-like processes that are apposed to blood vessels but do not have direct synaptic contacts with central nervous system neurons. These cells synthesize melatonin from serotonin via enzymes that are sensitive to diurnal fluctuations in light. Levels of serotonin *N*-acetyltransferase increase during the night (in the absence of photic stimulation), and the synthesis of melatonin is enhanced. Exposure to light turns off the enzymatic activity, and melatonin production is diminished. Thus, the production of melatonin by pinealocytes is rhythmic and calibrated to the 24-hour cycle of photic input to the retina. This is called a *circadian rhythm*.

Photic stimulation of pinealocytes occurs through an indirect route. Retinal ganglion cells project to the suprachiasmatic nucleus of the hypothalamus, which in turn influences neurons of the intermediolateral cell column in the spinal cord through descending connections. These preganglionic sympathetic neurons project to the superior cervical ganglion, which in turn innervates the pineal gland via postganglionic fibers that travel on branches of the internal carotid artery.

Pinealocytes also produce serotonin, norepinephrine, and neuroactive peptides, such as thyrotropin-releasing hormone (TRH), which are normally associated with the hypothalamus. These secretory products are released into the general circulation or the cerebrospinal fluid.

Pinealomas (tumors with large numbers of pinealocytes) are accompanied by depression of gonadal function and delayed puberty, whereas lesions that lead to the *loss* of pineal cells are associated with precocious puberty. This indicates that pineal secretory products exert an inhibitory influence on gonadal formation.

The habenular nuclei are located just anterior to the pineal gland and consist of a large lateral nucleus and a small medial nucleus (Figs. 15-2 and 15-15). Both nuclei contribute axons to the *habenulointerpeduncular tract* (fasciculus retroflexus), which terminates in the midbrain interpeduncular nucleus. The *stria medullaris thalami*, which arches over the medial aspect of the dorsal thalamus near the midline, conveys input to both habenular nuclei. The *habenular commissure*, a small bundle of fibers riding on the upper edge of the posterior commissure, connects the habenular regions of the two sides.

Vasculature of the Diencephalon

The diencephalon is supplied by smaller vessels that branch from the various arteries making up the cerebral *arterial circle* (circle of Willis) and by larger arteries that originate from the proximal parts of the posterior cerebral artery (Figs. 15-16 and 15-17A, B). The hypothalamus and subthalamus are supplied by *central (perforating or ganglionic) branches* of the circle. Anterior parts of the hypothalamus are served by central branches *(anteromedial group)* arising from the anterior communicating artery and the A_1 segment of the anterior cerebral artery and from branches of the proximal part of the posterior communicating artery. Caudal hypothalamic regions and the ventral thalamus are supplied by branches of the *posteromedial group;* these branches arise from the posterior communicating artery and the P_1 segment of the posterior cerebral artery. The specific relationships of the anteromedial and posteromedial groups originating from the cerebral arterial circle can be reviewed in Chapter 8, Figure 8-16.

Some of the branches of the *posteromedial group* that arise from the P_1 segment near the basilar bifurcation are called the *thalamoperforating arteries*. These vessels (of which there may be more than one on each side) penetrate deeply to supply rostral areas of the thalamus (Figs. 15-16 and 15-17A, B). If these vessels are occluded during surgery in this region, as can occur, for example, when an aneurysm of the basilar bifurcation is clipped, the patient can be rendered permanently comatose. Slightly more distal branches, which usually arise from the P_2 segment, are the *posterior choroidal* and *thalamogeniculate* arteries. These arteries also supply portions of the diencephalon (Figs. 15-16 and 15-17A, B). A narrow portion of the caudal and medial thalamus bordering on the third ventricle is supplied by the *medial posterior choroidal artery*, whereas the thalamogeniculate branches irrigate the caudal thalamus, including the pulvinar and the geniculate nuclei (Figs. 15-16 and 15-17B). In addition, branches of the medial posterior choroidal artery also serve the choroid plexus of the third ventricle.

The *anterior choroidal artery* originates from the cerebral portion of the internal carotid artery and courses caudolaterally along the trajectory of the optic tract (Fig. 15-18A, B). This vessel serves important structures in this general area. It sends

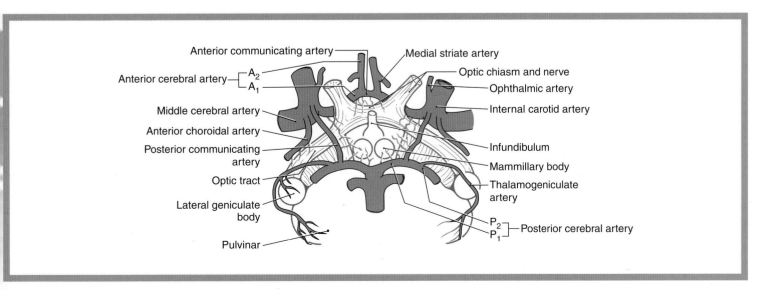

Figure 15-16. Anterior (ventral) view of the diencephalic region showing the arterial circle of Willis and the distribution of central branches to hypothalamic structures.

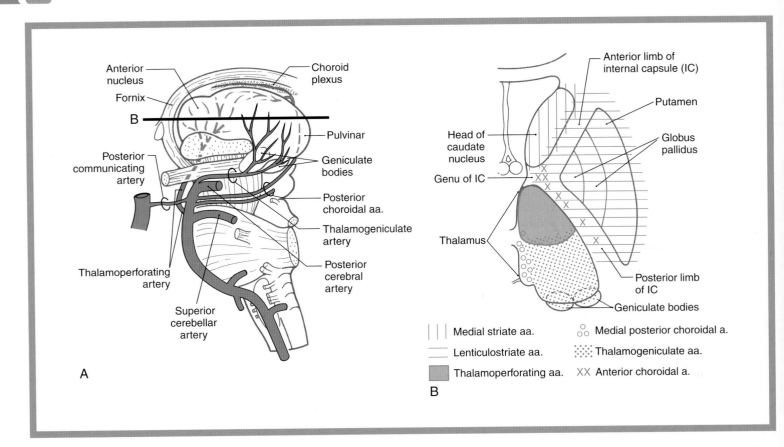

Figure 15-17. Blood supply to the dorsal thalamus. The lateral aspect (**A**) shows the general distribution of the main arteries. A view in the axial plane (**B**) through the hemisphere shows the internal territories served. The distribution of the main striate arteries, especially to the internal capsule, is also shown.

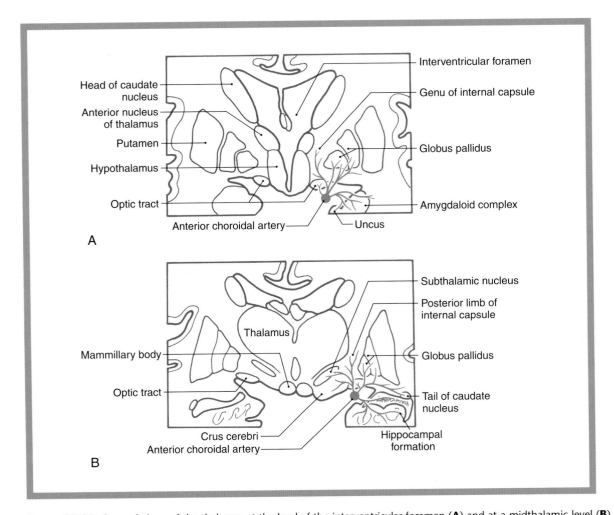

Figure 15-18. Coronal views of the thalamus at the level of the interventricular foramen (**A**) and at a midthalamic level (**B**), both showing the territory served by the anterior choroidal artery at these respective levels.

penetrating branches into the *genu* of the internal capsule and into the more inferior aspect of the *posterior limb* of the internal capsule (Fig. 15-18A, B). In addition it serves the optic tract, inferior portions of the lenticular nucleus, the choroid plexus of the inferior horn of the lateral ventricle, and large parts of the hippocampal formation. An occlusion of this vessel, an *anterior choroidal artery syndrome*, results in characteristic visual and motor deficits that reflect damage to the optic tract and the inferior portion of the posterior limb of the internal capsule (see Chapters 24 and 25 for additional information).

Although the thalamus receives a blood supply largely separate from that of the internal capsule (Fig. 15-17B), vascular lesions in the thalamus may extend into the internal capsule or vice versa. Ischemic or hemorrhagic strokes in the hemisphere may result in *contralateral hemiparesis* in combination with *hemianesthesia*. These losses correlate with damage to corticospinal and thalamocortical fibers in the internal capsule. On the other hand, strokes involving the larger thalamic arteries, such as the thalamogeniculate artery, may result in total or dissociated sensory losses. These patients may subsequently experience persistent, intense pain *(thalamic pain, Dejerine-Roussy syndrome)*.

Synopsis of Clinical Points

- A craniopharyngioma (or Rathke pouch tumor) is a developmental defect related to the diencephalon (p. 231).
- Rathke pouch tumors mimic pituitary tumors (p. 231).
- A T2-weighted magnetic resonance image that does not contain a massa intermedia is normal (p. 231).
- Lesions of the ventral posterolateral nucleus will most directly affect the relay of somatosensory information from the body to the primary somatosensory cortex (p. 234).
- Damage to the ventral lateral nucleus will most specifically affect the efficacy of motor activity (p. 233).
- A small vascular lesion that damages the ventral posteromedial nucleus will interrupt the transmission of somatosensory information from the face to the somatosensory cortex (p. 234).
- Lesions of the lateral geniculate nucleus will result in a partial loss of vision (p. 235).
- Damage to the hypothalamus will result in a variety of visceromotor dysfunctions (p. 238).
- Hypothalamic lesions may affect sleep-wake cycles, eating behavior, the ability of the patient to maintain body temperature, the activity of a variety of releasing hormones, and other visceral activities (p. 238).
- Lesions of the subthalamic nucleus may result in hemiballismus (p. 239).
- Pinealomas may have an effect on gonadal function (p. 241).
- Occlusion of the anterior choroidal artery (ACA syndrome) results in visual and motor deficits (p. 243).

Sources and Additional Reading

Alexander GE, Crutcher MD, DeLong MR: Basal ganglia-thalamocortical circuits: Parallel substrates for motor, oculomotor, "prefrontal" and "limbic" functions. In Uylings HBM, Van Eden CG, DeBruin JPC, Corner MA, Feenstra MGP (eds): Progress in Brain Research, Vol 85, The Prefrontal Cortex: Its Structure, Function, and Pathology. Amsterdam, Elsevier Biomedical Press, 1990.

Burt AM: Textbook of Neuroanatomy. Philadelphia, WB Saunders, 1993.

Hirai T, Jones EG: A new parcellation of the human thalamus on the basis of histochemical staining. Brain Res Rev 14:1-34, 1989.

Jones EG: The Thalamus. New York, Plenum Press, 1986.

Nieuwenhuys R, Voogd J, van Huijzen C: The Central Nervous System, A Synopsis and Atlas, 3rd ed. Berlin, Springer-Verlag, 1988.

Parent A: Carpenter's Human Neuroanatomy, 9th ed. Baltimore, Williams & Wilkins, 1996.

Schell GR, Strick PL: The origin of thalamic inputs to the arcuate premotor and supplementary motor areas. J Neurosci 4:539-560, 1984.

Ungerleider LG, Galkin TW, Mishkin M: Visuotopic organization of projections from striate cortex to inferior and lateral pulvinar in rhesus monkey. J Comp Neurol 217:137-157, 1983.

Walker AE: The Primate Thalamus. Chicago, University of Chicago Press, 1938.

The Telencephalon

D. E. Haines and G. A. Mihailoff

The telencephalon is the largest part of the human brain, constituting about 85% of total brain weight, and is that portion in which all modalities are represented. Various sensory inputs (such as vision and hearing) are localized in some areas, whereas motor functions are represented in other regions and are modulated by subcortical nuclei. The telencephalon contains circuits that interrelate regions that have specific functions, such as motor or visual, with other regions called *association areas*. Seeing a familiar image may precipitate a cascade of neural events having olfactory, emotional, sensory, and motor components. Damage to association areas results in complex neurologic deficits. The patient may not be blind or paralyzed but may be unable to recognize sensory input *(agnosia)*, express ideas or thoughts *(aphasia)*, or perform complex goal-directed movements *(apraxia)*.

Overview

The telencephalon consists of two large *hemispheres* separated from each other by a deep *longitudinal cerebral fissure*. Each hemisphere has an outer surface, the *cerebral cortex*, which is composed of layers of cells. The cortex is thrown into elevations called *gyri* (singular, *gyrus*) that are separated by grooves called *sulci* (singular, *sulcus*). Internal to the cortex are large amounts of *subcortical white matter*, along with aggregates of gray matter that form the *basal nuclei (ganglia)* and the *amygdala*. Although not parts of either the telencephalon or the basal nuclei, the *subthalamic nucleus* (of the diencephalon) and the *substantia nigra* (of the mesencephalon) have important connections that functionally link them with the basal nuclei.

Information passing into or out of the cerebral cortex must traverse the subcortical white matter. The myelinated fibers forming the white matter are organized into (1) association bundles that connect adjacent or distant gyri in one hemisphere; (2) commissural bundles that connect the two hemispheres, the largest of these being the *corpus callosum;* and (3) the *internal capsule*. The internal capsule contains axons projecting to numerous downstream nuclei *(corticofugal fibers)* and axons conveying information to the cerebral cortex *(corticopetal fibers)*. The terms *corticofugal* and *corticopetal* are umbrella terms that include all *efferent* and all *afferent* fibers, respectively, of the cerebral cortex. In later chapters, specific populations of cortical efferent fibers (such as *corticospinal* or *corticostriatal fibers*) and of cortical afferent fibers (such as *thalamocortical fibers*) are discussed.

The *hippocampal complex* and the *amygdala* are located in the walls of the temporal horn of the lateral ventricle. The axons of cells in these structures coalesce to form the *fornix* and *stria terminalis*, respectively.

Development

Enlargements of the prosencephalon, the *telencephalic (cerebral) vesicles*, appear at about 5 weeks of gestation. As the cerebral vesicles enlarge in all directions, they pull along portions of the neural canal that will form the cavities of the telencephalon, the *lateral ventricles* (Fig. 16-1A, B). The primitive lateral ventricles extend into frontal, parietal, temporal, and occipital areas as they develop and form that portion of the ventricle found in each of these lobes in the adult. The *interventricular foramina*, which

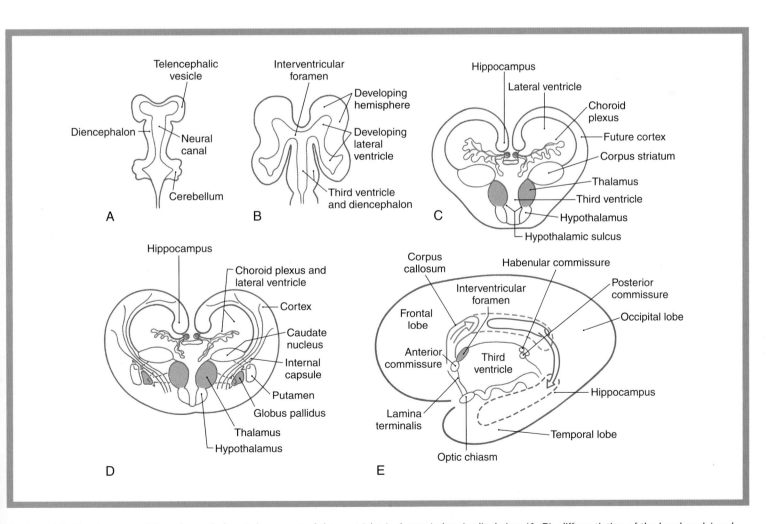

Figure 16-1. Development of the telencephalon. Enlargement of the ventricles is shown in longitudinal view (**A, B**), differentiation of the basal nuclei and internal capsule in cross section (**C, D**), and growth of the corpus callosum (in *red*) and hippocampus (in *green*) in the sagittal plane (**E**).

connect each lateral ventricle to the midline *third ventricle* (cavity of the diencephalon), are initially large but become smaller as development progresses. In the adult brain, each interventricular foramen is bordered rostromedially by the column of the fornix and caudolaterally by the anterior tubercle of the dorsal thalamus (see Fig. 15-12).

Cells forming the *corpus striatum* appear in the floor of the developing lateral ventricle at the time when primordial cell groups in the wall of the third ventricle are giving rise to diencephalic structures (Fig. 16-1C, D). As development progresses, the corpus striatum is bisected by axons growing to and from the cerebral cortex. These axons form the *internal capsule* of the adult and divide the corpus striatum into a medially located *caudate nucleus* and a laterally located *putamen*. As the diencephalon enlarges, it gives rise to the thalamus and hypothalamus *and to cells that migrate across the developing internal capsule to assume a position medial to the putamen* (Fig. 16-1D). These cells become the *globus pallidus* of the adult and, in combination with the putamen, form the *lenticular nucleus*.

The initial development of the major commissural bundles and of the hippocampus takes place along the medial aspect of the hemisphere (Fig. 16-1C-E). In the adult brain there are three major interhemispheric commissures: the *anterior commissure*, the *hippocampal commissure*, and the *corpus callosum*. The first of these to appear, the *anterior commissure*, arises within the lamina terminalis. The latter is a membrane-like structure that extends from the anterior commissure anteriorly (ventrally) to the rostral edge of the optic chiasm (see Fig. 15-4). The second to form, the *hippocampal commissure*, develops along with the hippocampal primordium. As growth occurs, the hippocampus, which originates in the posteromedial part of the hemisphere, is displaced into the temporal lobe, where it assumes a position characteristic of the adult (Fig. 16-1E). In the process, fibers from one side cross to the other side, as the *hippocampal commissure*, just anterior (ventral) to the area that will be occupied by the corpus callosum. The third commissure to develop, the *corpus callosum*, originates from the area of the lamina terminalis as a structure initially composed of astrocytic processes. Axons from developing neurons in each hemisphere traverse this glial structure to access the contralateral side. As this takes place, the corpus callosum enlarges in a caudal direction to form the prominent structure found in the adult (Figs. 16-1E and 16-2A).

Developmental Defects

There are numerous developmental events that may cause defects in the configuration of the telencephalon; many of these are described in Chapter 5 and will be only briefly mentioned here. One of the developmental failures that will result in aberrant development of the telencephalon is the improper migration of maturing neurons on *radial glia*. This failure results in structural, and in some cases corresponding functional, defects in the arrangement of the cerebral cortex. Some examples include *lissencephaly* (a lack of gyri and sulci, a smooth brain), *pachygyria* (abnormally large gyri that are few in number), and *microgyria* (abnormally small gyri that are greater in number).

Holoprosencephaly is a pre-neurulation defect that is represented by three general forms. *Alobar holoprosencephaly*, the most severe form, consists of a midline ventricle, no hemispheres or corpus callosum, and severe retardation. *Semilobar holoprosencephaly* consists of a partial formation of lobes with the ventricles formed; the frontal lobes may be fused, and the occipital lobes may be separated by an incomplete longitudinal fissure. Although the ventricles are formed, midline structures such as the septum pellucidum are missing. In *lobar holoprosencephaly*, the least severe form, the longitudinal fissure is largely complete, hemispheres exist, generally normal patterns

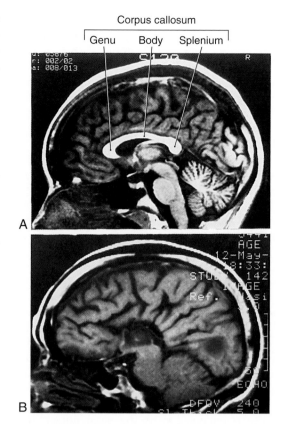

Figure 16-2. MR image in the sagittal plane of a normal adult (**A**) and of another adult with agenesis of the corpus callosum (**B**). A comparison of **B** with **A** reveals an absence of the corpus callosum, aberrant gyri on the medial surface of the hemisphere, and other structural defects.

of sulci and gyri are seen, but there is a fusion of the hemispheres at the frontal pole or at the orbital surface of the frontal lobe.

Anencephaly is a severe developmental failure in which the telencephalon and the surrounding skull are largely absent. This defect is catastrophic and not compatible with life. Anencephaly is generally associated with a failure of the anterior neuropore to close. The lamina terminalis represents the adult position of the anterior neuropore.

Failure of the corpus callosum to develop *(agenesis of the corpus callosum)* may be accompanied by an absence of the anterior and hippocampal commissures (Fig. 16-2A, B). Although some patients with this condition may experience focal seizures and have mental retardation, others live for many years with few or no obvious neurologic deficits. These individuals frequently have developmental abnormalities in other parts of the nervous system.

Lobes of the Cerebral Cortex

On the basis of the arrangement of major sulci, the cerebral cortex is divided into six lobes, five of which are exposed on the surface of the cerebral hemisphere and one (the insular lobe) located internal to the lateral sulcus. Four of these lobes are named according to the overlying bones of the skull.

On the lateral surface of the hemisphere the major sulci are the *central sulcus*, the *lateral (sylvian) sulcus*, and a small lateral end of the *parieto-occipital sulcus* (Fig. 16-3; see also Fig. 16-5). The *preoccipital notch* is a small but distinct indentation along the lateral margin of the hemisphere. An imaginary line connecting the terminus of the parieto-occipital sulcus with the *preoccipital notch* intersects with another line drawn caudally from the lateral sulcus. These lines, along with the central and lateral sulci, divide the lateral surface into *frontal*, *parietal*, *temporal*, and *occipital lobes* (Fig. 16-3).

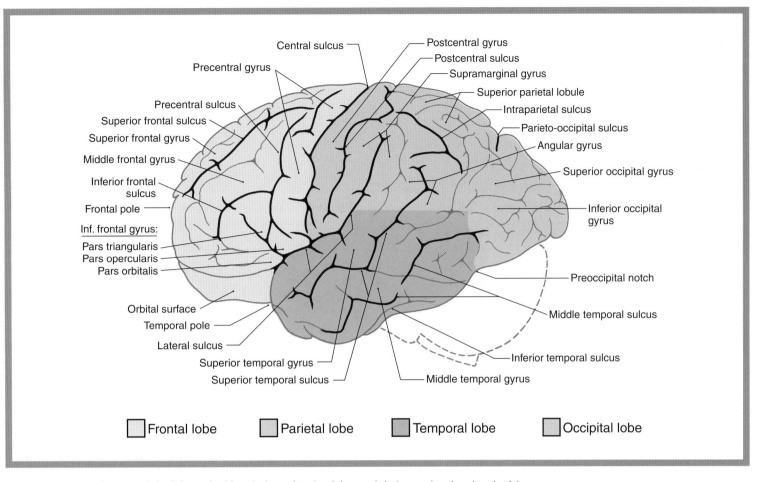

Figure 16-3. Lateral aspect of the left cerebral hemisphere showing lobes and their associated gyri and sulci.

On the medial surface of the hemisphere, the major sulci separating lobes are the *cingulate, parieto-occipital,* and *collateral* (Figs. 16-4 and 16-5). Two imaginary lines also separate lobes on the medial surface. One connects the medial end of the central sulcus with the cingulate sulcus; the other joins the parieto-occipital sulcus with the preoccipital notch. This combination of sulci and lines separates the four lobes noted previously, plus the *limbic lobe,* on the medial surface of the hemisphere (Fig. 16-4).

Deep to the lateral (sylvian) sulcus is an infolded region of cortex called the *insula* (Fig. 16-10). This region is separated from the opercula of the frontal, parietal, and temporal lobes by the *circular sulcus of the insula.* Consequently, this region satisfies the definition of a subdivision of the cerebral cortex in that it is separated from the adjoining cortical structures by a named sulcus and thus defines the *insular lobe.*

Frontal Lobe

The lateral surface of the frontal lobe is divided by *inferior* and *superior frontal sulci* into *inferior, middle,* and *superior frontal gyri* (Fig. 16-3), the latter folding onto the medial aspect of the hemisphere (Figs. 16-4 and 16-5B). The inferior frontal gyrus is divided into a *pars opercularis, pars triangularis,* and *pars orbitalis* (Fig. 16-5A). The anterior (orbital) surface of the frontal lobe is composed of the *gyrus rectus,* the *olfactory sulcus,* and a series of *orbital gyri* (Fig. 16-6). The most rostral point of this lobe is the *frontal pole* of the brain.

The *olfactory bulb* and *tract,* which relay sensory information, lie on the anterior surface of the frontal lobe in the olfactory sulcus (Fig. 16-6). At the point where the olfactory tract attaches to the hemisphere, it bifurcates into *medial* and *lateral striae* (Fig. 16-7). The triangle formed by this bifurcation is called the *olfactory trigone.* Immediately caudal to this trigone, the surface

of the hemisphere is characterized by numerous small holes formed by vessels (lenticulostriate arteries) as they enter the brain; this is the *anterior perforated substance* (Fig. 16-7). The olfactory tract and striae and the cell groups associated with the anterior perforated substance are functionally related to the limbic system.

The *precentral gyrus* is continuous on the medial surface of the hemisphere with the *anterior paracentral gyrus;* the latter is separated from the superior frontal gyrus by the *paracentral sulcus* (Fig. 16-4). These two gyri collectively form the *primary somatomotor cortex.*

Specific functions are associated with some of the gyri of the frontal lobe, and lesions of these areas result in characteristic deficits. The body is somatotopically represented in the precentral and anterior paracentral gyri; these gyri collectively form the *primary somatomotor cortex* (Brodmann area 4). Beginning at the lateral sulcus (Fig. 16-8) the face is represented in about the lateral one third of the precentral gyrus, the hand and upper extremity in about the middle third (emphasis on the hand area), and the trunk in about the medial third of the precentral gyrus. The hip is represented at about the point where the precentral gyrus turns over the edge of the hemisphere to become the anterior paracentral gyrus, and the lower extremity and foot are represented in the anterior paracentral gyrus (Fig. 16-8). Lesions of these areas of the motor cortex may result in weakness or paralysis of the corresponding part of the body on the contralateral side (details are discussed in Chapters 24 to 27).

The *frontal eye field* in humans is located in the depths of the precentral sulcus and in the cortex forming the rostral bank of the precentral sulcus (Fig. 16-9). This cortical area is largely coextensive with Brodmann area 6 and extends to the transitional area between areas 6 and 8 in the most caudal portion of

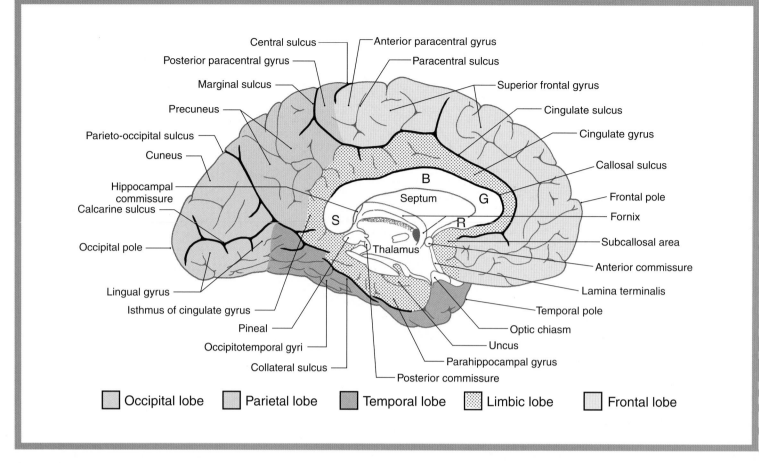

Figure 16-4. Medial aspect of the left cerebral hemisphere showing lobes and their associated gyri and sulci. The parts of the corpus callosum are R, rostrum; G, genu; B, body (or trunk); and S, splenium.

the middle frontal gyrus (Fig. 16-9). The current best evidence in humans supports the view that the frontal eye field is primarily in area 6. This cortical area projects to nuclei in the midbrain and pons that, in turn, project to the oculomotor, trochlear, and abducens nuclei that control eye movement. *Irritative* cortical lesions of the frontal eye field result in conjugate deviation of the eyes away from the side of the lesion, whereas *destructive* lesions result in conjugate deviation of the eyes toward the side of the lesion. An easy way to remember this is "the patient looks away from the irritation but toward the destruction."

The inferior frontal gyrus in the left (dominant) hemisphere is sometimes called the *Broca convolution* because lesions in this area (especially in the pars opercularis, Brodmann area 44, and extending into the pars triangularis) result in *Broca aphasia*. These patients do not have paralysis of the speech apparatus but have great difficulty translating thoughts/concepts into coherent sentences. Broca aphasia is also called *expressive aphasia*.

Parietal Lobe

The parietal lobe consists of the *postcentral gyrus*, located between the *central* and *postcentral sulci*, and the *superior* and *inferior parietal lobules*, which are separated by the *intraparietal sulcus* (Fig. 16-3). Gyri forming the superior parietal lobule extend onto the medial surface of the hemisphere as the *precuneus*, whereas the inferior parietal lobule is made up of the *angular* and *supramarginal gyri*. The latter is a crescent-shaped ridge of cortex around the caudal terminus of the lateral sulcus.

As the *postcentral gyrus* extends onto the medial surface of the hemisphere, it is continuous with the *posterior paracentral gyrus* (Figs. 16-4 and 16-5). This cortical area is bordered rostrally by an imaginary line that connects the central sulcus to the cingulate sulcus and caudally by the *marginal ramus of*

the cingulate sulcus. The latter is frequently called the *marginal sulcus*. Taken together, the postcentral gyrus and posterior paracentral lobule constitute the *primary somatosensory cortex*.

Specific functional areas in the parietal lobe include the *primary somatosensory cortex* (Brodmann areas 3, 1, 2) and the gyri that are part the *Wernicke area* (supramarginal gyrus—Brodmann area 40, and the angular gyrus—Brodmann area 39). Clinically the *Wernicke area* is regarded as extending into the temporal lobe and encompasses portions of Brodmann areas 22 and some of 21. The body is somatopically laid out in the post-central and posterior paracentral gyri in a pattern generally quite similar to that seen in the precentral gyrus (Fig. 16-8). Within the postcentral gyrus the face is represented in about the lateral third, the upper extremity (with emphasis on the fingers) in about the middle third, and the trunk, hip, and thigh in about the medial third; the leg, foot, and genitalia are represented in the posterior paracentral lobule. Damage to the primary somato-sensory cortex results in an alteration of sensory (pain, thermal, and proprioception) perception.

The *angular gyrus* (Brodmann area 39) and the *supramarginal gyrus* (Brodmann area 40) collectively form a portion of the Wernicke area; these two gyri also represent the inferior parietal lobule. Lesions of the Wernicke area result in a constellation of deficits that are called *Wernicke aphasia* (or *receptive aphasia*). These patients cannot understand what they hear, cannot read or write, and speak in a jumble of words that makes no sense. Theirs is a receptive problem; information comes in but it cannot be understood or used to express coherent thought.

Temporal Lobe

The gyri that form the temporal lobe are found on lateral and inferior aspects of the hemisphere between the *lateral sulcus* and the *collateral sulcus* (Figs. 16-3 to 16-6). These gyri are,

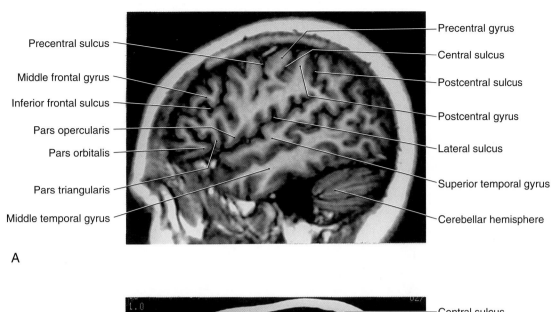

Precentral sulcus
Middle frontal gyrus
Inferior frontal sulcus
Pars opercularis
Pars orbitalis
Pars triangularis
Middle temporal gyrus

Precentral gyrus
Central sulcus
Postcentral sulcus
Postcentral gyrus
Lateral sulcus
Superior temporal gyrus
Cerebellar hemisphere

A

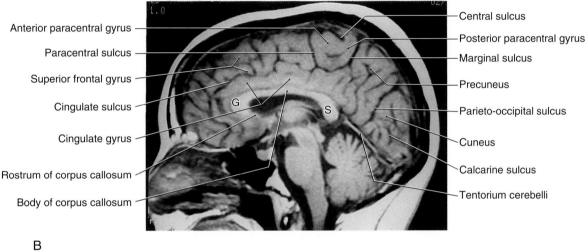

Anterior paracentral gyrus
Paracentral sulcus
Superior frontal gyrus
Cingulate sulcus
Cingulate gyrus
Rostrum of corpus callosum
Body of corpus callosum

Central sulcus
Posterior paracentral gyrus
Marginal sulcus
Precuneus
Parieto-occipital sulcus
Cuneus
Calcarine sulcus
Tentorium cerebelli

G   S

B

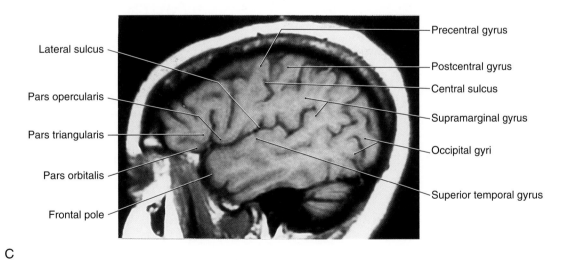

Lateral sulcus
Pars opercularis
Pars triangularis
Pars orbitalis
Frontal pole

Precentral gyrus
Postcentral gyrus
Central sulcus
Supramarginal gyrus
Occipital gyri
Superior temporal gyrus

C

Figure 16-5. T1-weighted MR images in the sagittal plane at about the midline (**B**), at the lateralmost aspect of the cerebral hemisphere (**C**), and through approximately the lateral two thirds of the hemisphere (**A**). Gyri and sulci of the cerebral cortex are labeled. G, genu of corpus callosum; S, splenium of corpus callosum. (From Haines DE: Neuroanatomy: An Atlas of Structures, Sections, and Systems, 5th ed. Philadelphia, Lippincott Williams & Wilkins, 2000.)

beginning at the lateral sulcus, the *superior, middle,* and *inferior temporal gyri* and a broad area of cortex, the *occipitotemporal gyri,* extending from the *temporal pole* to the occipital lobe. The *superior temporal sulcus* ends in the loop of cortex forming the angular gyrus of the inferior parietal lobule. An *inferior temporal sulcus* may be found between the inferior temporal and occipitotemporal gyri, or it may be absent, in which case these gyri blend around the inferior margin of the hemisphere.

On the upper edge of the temporal lobe, and extending into the depths of the lateral fissure, are the *transverse temporal gyri* (of Heschl). These gyri (Fig. 16-10) form the *primary auditory cortex.* Lesions of the auditory cortex may result in difficulty in interpreting a sound, or localizing a sound in space, but do not result in deafness in one ear. In the case of cortical lesions, these somewhat subtle auditory deficits may be masked by other more obvious signs or symptoms.

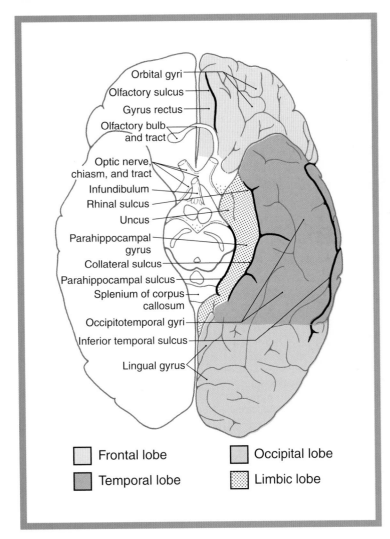

Figure 16-6. Anterior (ventral) aspect of the left cerebral hemisphere showing lobes and their associated gyri and sulci.

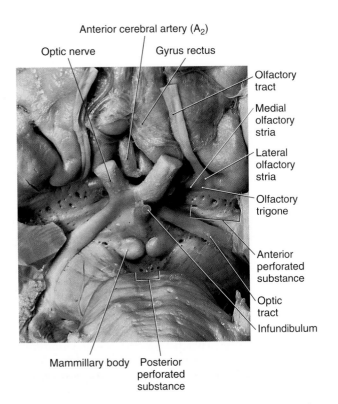

Figure 16-7. Anterior (ventral) aspect of the hemisphere in the area of the anterior perforated substance.

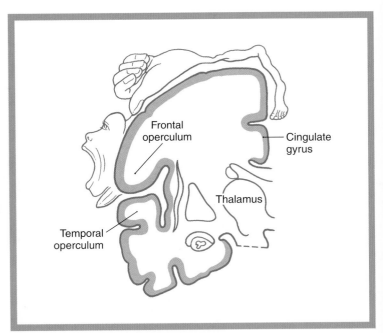

Figure 16-8. Coronal representation showing the somatotopy of the body in the primary motor cortex, which is located in the precentral and anterior paracentral gyri. (Adapted from Penfield and Rasmussen, 1968, with permission.)

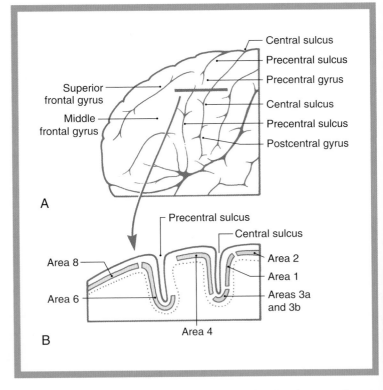

Figure 16-9. Lateral (**A**) view of the hemisphere showing the general area of the frontal eye field, and a cross-sectional representation (**B**) showing the location of area 6 and its general relationship to other adjacent cortical areas.

Insular Lobe

The oval region of cortex located deep inside the lateral fissure is the *insular lobe* (Figs. 16-5C and 16-10). This area is characterized by a set of long gyri in its caudal part (the *gyri longi*) and a set of short gyri in its rostral part (the *gyri breves*). These are separated from each other by the *central sulcus of the insula*. The insular cortex is continuous, at the circular sulcus of the insula, with that of the adjacent frontal, parietal, and temporal

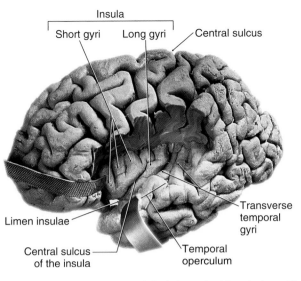

Figure 16-10. Lateral view of the left cerebral hemisphere. The frontal and parietal opercula are removed, and the temporal operculum is retracted to expose the insula and transverse temporal gyri.

lobes. This continuity forms lips on each lobe that overlie the insula to form the *frontal, parietal,* and *temporal opercula* (Figs. 16-10 and 16-12). The *limen insulae* (threshold to the insula) is the area in which the inferior surface of the hemisphere is continuous with the insular cortex (Fig. 16-10). Although the function of the insula is still somewhat unclear, it is known that the insular cortex receives *nociceptive* and *viscerosensory input.*

Occipital Lobe

The occipital lobe forms the caudal portion of the hemisphere; its caudal extreme is the *occipital pole* of the brain (Figs. 16-3 to 16-5B). The irregular collection of gyri on the lateral surface of the occipital lobe constitutes the *occipital gyri.* On the medial surface of the hemisphere the *parieto-occipital sulcus* separates the cuneus, an occipital lobe structure, from the precuneus, a parietal lobe structure.

An important landmark on the medial aspect of the occipital lobe is the *calcarine sulcus.* This sulcus separates the *cuneus,* which is superior to it, from the *lingual gyrus,* which is inferiorly located. The *primary visual cortex* (Brodmann area 17) is located in the portions of these gyri that border directly on the calcarine sulcus. A lesion of the primary visual cortex of one occipital lobe results in a loss of visual input from the contralateral one half of the visual field of each eye. This is called *homonymous hemianopia* and it may be further designated *right* or *left* depending on whether the deficit involves the right or left half of each visual field.

Limbic Lobe

The *limbic lobe* is part of a more complex entity commonly called the *limbic system.* As discussed in Chapter 31, the limbic system includes this lobe plus its afferent and efferent connections with other telencephalic, diencephalic, and brainstem nuclei.

The limbic lobe is a ring of cortex that makes up the most medial rim of the hemisphere. Although not specified as a separate lobe in some texts, it is designated here as such because of its unique functional characteristics. Beginning anteriorly (and just ventral to the rostrum of the corpus callosum) this ring of cortex consists of the *subcallosal area, cingulate gyrus, isthmus of the cingulate gyrus, parahippocampal gyrus,* and *uncus* (Figs. 16-4 and 16-6). The limbic cortex is separated from adjacent cortical areas by the *cingulate sulcus* and the *collateral sulcus* and from the *corpus callosum* by the *callosal sulcus.* On the

inferior surface of the temporal lobe, the *rhinal sulcus* is located between the rostral extreme of the parahippocampal gyrus and the laterally adjacent occipitotemporal gyri (Fig. 16-6).

The function of the limbic lobe is complex and cannot be designated as, for example, primarily sensory or motor. Rather, it is linked to circuits that influence complex functions such as memory, learning, and behavior.

Vasculature of the Cerebral Cortex

The lobes composing the cerebral cortex receive their blood supply via terminal branches of the *anterior, middle,* and *posterior cerebral arteries.* Details of individual branches are given in Chapter 8; only general points are reviewed here.

The *anterior cerebral artery,* the smaller of the terminal branches of the internal carotid artery, passes rostromedially and is joined to its counterpart by the *anterior communicating artery.* The anterior cerebral artery distal to the anterior communicating artery arches superiorly around the genu of the corpus callosum and courses caudally to serve the medial surface of the hemisphere to about the level of the parieto-occipital sulcus (Fig. 16-11). The part of the anterior cerebral artery between the internal carotid and the anterior communicator is the A_1 segment. Branches of A_1 serve structures in the immediate vicinity, including the optic chiasm and anterior parts of the hypothalamus. The branches of the anterior cerebral distal to the anterior communicator collectively form segments A_2 to A_5 (see Chapter 8 for details). These serve the medial surface of the frontal and parietal lobes, including the *anterior* (lower extremity part of motor cortex) and *posterior* (lower extremity part of somatosensory cortex) *paracentral gyri.*

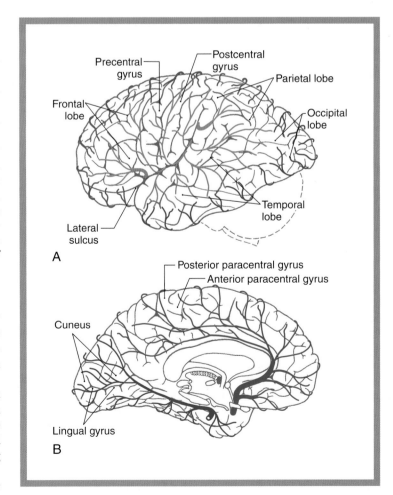

Figure 16-11. Lateral (**A**) and medial (**B**) views of the left cerebral hemisphere showing the distribution of the anterior (in *green*), middle (in *red*), and posterior (in *blue*) cerebral arteries.

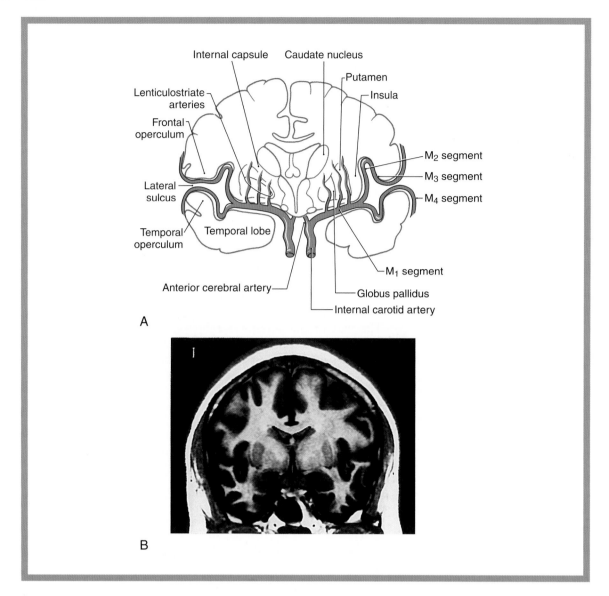

Figure 16-12. Cross section of the cerebral hemisphere showing the main branches of the middle cerebral artery (**A**) and an MR image (**B**) in the coronal plane at a comparable level. (**B** from Haines DE: Neuroanatomy: An Atlas of Structures, Sections, and Systems, 6th ed. Philadelphia, Lippincott Williams & Wilkins, 2004.)

The *middle cerebral artery*, the larger of the terminal branches of the internal carotid artery, passes laterally to the *limen insula*, where it generally branches into *superior* and *inferior trunks* (Figs. 16-11 and 16-12). This initial part of the middle cerebral, the M_1 segment, gives rise to the *lenticulostriate (lateral striate) arteries*. The superior and inferior trunks and their distal branches collectively form the M_2, M_3, and M_4 segments. The insular lobe itself is served by branches of M_2. As the distal branches of the superior and inferior trunks pass onto the inner surface of the opercula they become the M_3 segment, and upon exiting the lateral sulcus they become the M_4 segment (Fig. 16-12A; see also Chapter 8). Important cortical regions served by the M_4 segment include the trunk, upper extremity, and head areas of the motor cortex *(precentral gyrus)*, somatosensory cortex *(postcentral gyrus)*, auditory cortex *(transverse temporal gyri)*, parietal association cortex *(parietal lobules)*, and large parts of the superior and lateral surface of the frontal lobe.

The *posterior cerebral artery* begins at the basilar bifurcation (Fig. 16-11). The first and second parts of this vessel (P_1 and P_2 segments) are located, respectively, between the *basilar bifurcation* and the *posterior communicating artery* and just distal to the latter vessel. Midbrain and diencephalic structures are the main targets of branches of P_1 and P_2 segments. The P_3 segment of the posterior cerebral artery is the part from which

the *temporal branches* originate, and P_4 is the segment that gives rise to *parieto-occipital* and *calcarine arteries*. The calcarine artery is the source of blood to the *primary visual cortex*, which borders on the calcarine sulcus. Other important telencephalic structures in the domains of P_3 and P_4 include the *parahippocampal gyrus* and the *precuneus*.

White Matter of the Cerebral Hemisphere

All information entering or leaving the cerebral cortex or connecting one part of the cortex with another must pass through the subcortical white matter. In general, the white matter core of the hemisphere contains *association fibers*, *commissural fibers*, and *projection fibers*.

Association Fibers

The *association fibers* interconnect various areas of cortex within the same hemisphere. These may be *short association fibers* that connect the cortices of adjacent gyri or *long association fibers* that interconnect more distant areas of cortex (Fig. 16-13). Important examples of the latter are the *cingulum* located internal to the cingulate gyrus and continuing into the parahippocampal

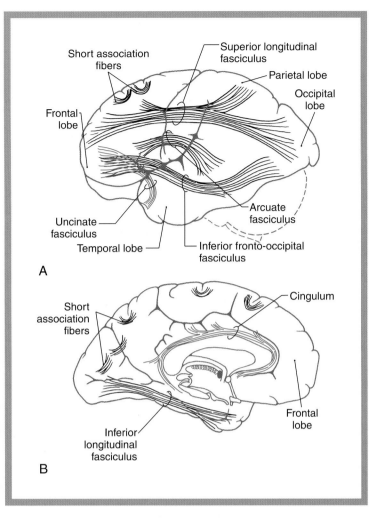

Smaller commissural bundles include the *anterior commissure* and the *hippocampal commissure* (Fig. 16-4). In sagittal views, the anterior commissure is located caudal to the rostrum of the corpus callosum but rostral to the main part of the fornix. This bundle interconnects various parts of the frontal and temporal lobes. The *hippocampal commissure* is formed by fibers that originate in the hippocampal formations and cross the midline as a thin layer inferior to the splenium of the corpus callosum.

The *posterior commissure* and the *habenular commissure* are small fiber bundles traversing the midline that connect caudal parts of the diencephalon (Figs. 16-1 and 16-4). The former crosses the midline at the base of the pineal gland and just posterior (dorsal) to the cerebral aqueduct. The latter is a small fascicle running along the upper aspect of the posterior commissure and interconnecting the habenular nuclei.

Projection Fibers: The Internal Capsule

The projection fibers of the hemispheres include both the axons that originate outside the telencephalon and project to the cerebral cortex *(corticopetal)* and the axons that arise from cerebral cortical cells and project to downstream targets *(corticofugal)*. A prime example of the former are projections from the thalamus to the cerebral cortex *(thalamocortical fibers)*; examples of the latter are *corticospinal*, *corticopontine*, and *corticothalamic fibers*. Projection fibers are organized into a large, compact bundle called the *internal capsule* (Fig. 16-14), which has intimate structural associations with the diencephalon and basal nuclei. Consequently, to divide the internal capsule into its constituent parts, reference must be made to these adjacent cell groups.

In an axial plane through the hemisphere, the internal capsule appears as a prominent "V"-shaped structure with the "V" pointing medially (Figs. 16-14 and 16-15). It is divided into three parts: (1) an *anterior limb* insinuated between the head of the caudate nucleus and the lenticular nucleus, (2) a *posterior limb* located between the dorsal thalamus and the lenticular nucleus, and (3) a *genu* located at the intersection of the anterior and posterior limbs, which is located approximately at the level of the interventricular foramen (Fig. 16-14).

The *anterior limb of the internal capsule* contains *thalamocortical/corticothalamic fibers* (collectively called the *anterior thalamic radiations*) that interconnect the dorsomedial and anterior thalamic nuclei with areas of the frontal lobe and the cingulate gyrus. *Frontopontine fibers*, especially those from the prefrontal areas, also pass through this structure.

The *genu of the internal capsule* contains *corticonuclear (corticobulbar) fibers* that arise in the frontal cortex just rostral to the precentral sulcus and from the precentral gyrus (primary motor cortex) and project to the motor nuclei of cranial nerves. Lesions of these fibers give rise to motor deficits of cranial nerves, most notably deficits related to the facial and hypoglossal nerves.

The *posterior limb of the internal capsule* is larger and more complex (Fig. 16-14). It is sometimes divided into a *thalamolenticular part* (located between the thalamus and the lenticular nucleus), a *sublenticular part* (fibers passing ventral to the lenticular nucleus), and a *retrolenticular part* (fibers located caudal to the lenticular nucleus). However, contemporary terminology and common usage refer to the "thalamolenticular part" as the *posterior limb*, the "sublenticular part" as the *sublenticular limb*, and the "retrolenticular part" as the *retrolenticular limb*. This latter terminology is considerably less cumbersome and much easier to remember and is the convention followed here (Figs. 16-14 and 16-15). By this scheme the internal capsule consists of five parts: an *anterior limb, genu, posterior limb, sublenticular limb,* and *retrolenticular limb*.

The major fiber populations passing through the posterior, sublenticular, and retrolenticular limbs of the internal capsule

Figure 16-13. Main association bundles as visualized from lateral (**A**) and medial (**B**) aspects of the left hemisphere.

gyrus, the *inferior longitudinal fasciculus* (temporal-occipital interconnections), and the *uncinate fasciculus* (frontal-temporal interconnections). The *superior longitudinal fasciculus*, located in the core of the hemisphere, interconnects frontal, parietal, and occipital cortices, whereas the *arcuate fasciculus* interconnects frontal and temporal lobes (Fig. 16-13). In the white matter of the temporal lobe, fibers passing between the frontal and occipital areas make up the *inferior fronto-occipital fasciculus*.

The *claustrum*, a thin layer of neuron cell bodies located internal to the insular cortex, is sandwiched between two small association bundles (Fig. 16-12). The *external capsule* is insinuated between the claustrum and putamen, and the *extreme capsule* is located between the claustrum and the insular cortex.

Commissural Fibers: The Corpus Callosum

In general, commissural fibers interconnect corresponding structures on either side of the neuraxis. The largest bundle of commissural fibers is the *corpus callosum* (Figs. 16-2 and 16-4). This huge bundle is located superior to the diencephalon and forms the roof of much of the lateral ventricles. The corpus callosum consists of, from rostral to caudal, a *rostrum, genu, body* (also called *trunk*), and *splenium* (Figs. 16-4 and 16-5B). Many of the fibers passing through the genu arch rostrally to interconnect the frontal lobes; these form the *minor* (or *frontal*) *forceps*. The fibers interconnecting the occipital lobes loop through the splenium of the corpus callosum, forming the *major* (or *occipital*) *forceps*. The *tapetum*, which is located in the lateral wall of the atrium and posterior horn of the lateral ventricle, is also composed of fiber bundles that cross in the splenium.

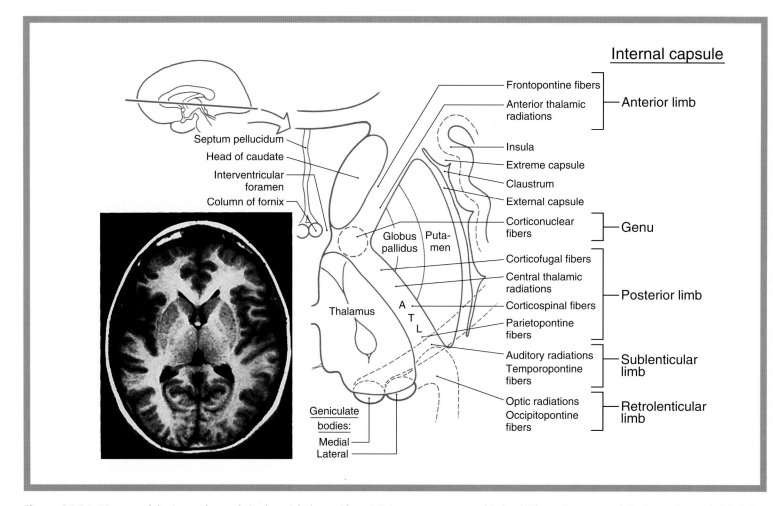

Internal capsule

Figure 16-14. Diagram of the internal capsule in the axial plane with an MR image at a comparable level. The various parts of the internal capsule labeled in the drawing can be identified. *Corticofugal* is an umbrella term under which specific populations of descending fibers, such as corticoreticular, corticorubral, and corticotectal, are included. Although not labeled here, specific types of corticofugal fibers are also present in the sublenticular and retrolenticular limbs of the internal capsule. A, upper extremity; T, thoracic; L, lower extremity. (From Haines DE: Neuroanatomy: An Atlas of Structures, Sections, and Systems, 6th ed. Philadelphia, Lippincott Williams & Wilkins, 2004.)

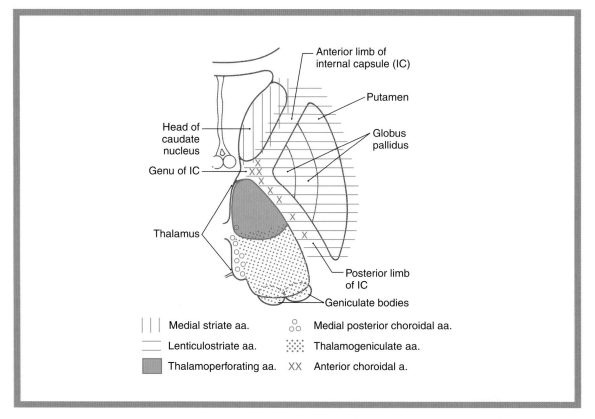

Figure 16-15. Blood supply to the basal nuclei, internal capsule, and thalamus shown in the axial plane.

are summarized in Figure 16-14. Included in the posterior limb are *corticospinal fibers* arising from the motor cortex and projecting to the contralateral spinal cord and *thalamocortical/corticothalamic fibers* (as part of the *central thalamic radiations*) that interconnect nuclei of the dorsal thalamus with the overlying cortex. Studies in humans have revealed that corticospinal fibers are somatotopically arranged in about the caudal half of the posterior limb. *Geniculotemporal radiations (auditory radiations)* convey auditory information from the medial geniculate nucleus to the transverse temporal gyri through the sublenticular limb. Visual input from the lateral geniculate body to the occipital cortex is conveyed via *geniculocalcarine radiations (optic radiations)* through the retrolenticular limb (Fig. 16-14). Optic radiations form a distinct lamina of fibers immediately lateral to the tapetum as they course caudally into the occipital lobe.

Fibers of the internal capsule flare out into the hemisphere as they pass distal to the caudate and putamen. This abrupt divergence of internal capsule fibers forms the *corona radiata* ("radiating crown"), which contains *converging corticofugal fibers*, as well as *diverging corticopetal fibers* (Fig. 16-20).

Vasculature of the Internal Capsule
The blood supply to the genu and most of the posterior limb of the internal capsule is via the *lenticulostriate arteries;* these are branches of the M$_1$ segment (Figs. 16-12 and 16-15; see also Fig. 15-18). Branches of the *anterior choroidal artery* supply the inferior region of the posterior limb, the optic tract, and the immediately adjacent retrolenticular limb. An occlusion of this vessel gives rise to a constellation of deficits, called the *anterior choroidal artery syndrome*, reflecting damage to these structures.

The anterior limb receives somewhat of a dual blood supply, in that lenticulostriate arteries and branches of the *medial striate artery* (usually a branch of A$_2$) serve this area.

While a variety of clinical events may damage the fibers of the internal capsule, the vast majority (about 95%) that produce rapid onset deficits are vascular related. *Hemorrhagic stroke* (about 15% of cases: rupture of, or bleeding from, a vessel serving the capsule) or *occlusive stroke* (about 85% of cases: occlusion of a vessel serving the capsule) are the most common causes. Lesions of the posterior limb may result in a combination of motor (*corticospinal tract* involvement) and sensory (*thalamocortical fiber* involvement) deficits that are seen on the side of the body contralateral to the lesion. Indeed, a characteristic feature of hemisphere lesions is the appearance of motor and sensory deficits on the same side of the body. Lesions of the retrolenticular

limb result in visual deficits (*optic radiation fiber* involvement) that may, depending on the extent of the damage, involve the contralateral hemifield (one half of each visual field, a *hemianopia*) or a contralateral quadrant (about one fourth of each visual field, a *quadrantanopia*) of the visual field of each eye.

Basal Nuclei (Ganglia)
The term *basal ganglia* is somewhat of a misnomer. The cells forming these structures are not "ganglia"—a term usually reserved to describe aggregations of neuronal somata in the peripheral nervous system—but are "nuclei" in the central nervous system. In addition, the definition of what cell groups make up the basal nuclei has been revised over the years, with contemporary views focusing on the functional characteristics of these nuclei. In this respect, *the basal nuclei consist of (1) the caudate and lenticular nuclei (together forming the dorsal basal nuclei), (2) the nucleus accumbens plus parts of the adjacent olfactory tubercle (the ventral striatum), and (3) the substantia innominata (ventral pallidum)* (Fig. 16-16). As described previously, the *subthalamic nucleus* and the *substantia nigra* are not components of the basal nuclei, but they are included in this discussion because of their important structural and functional relationship with the caudate and lenticular nuclei.

The basal nuclei function primarily in the motor sphere. Damage to these nuclei, as in vascular lesions, degenerative genetic disorders, or problems of unknown etiology, results in a variety of motor deficits, some of which are recognized as characteristic involuntary movements.

Caudate and Lenticular Nuclei
Collectively, the caudate and lenticular nuclei form the *corpus striatum*. The corpus striatum, in turn, is divided into the *neostriatum*, consisting of the *caudate nucleus* and the *putamen*, and the *paleostriatum*, or *globus pallidus* (Fig. 16-16). Collectively, the globus pallidus and putamen form the *lenticular nucleus*.

The caudate nucleus is characteristically located in the lateral wall of the lateral ventricle and consists of three parts; a *head, body,* and *tail* (Figs. 16-17 and 16-18). The *head of the caudate nucleus* forms a prominent bulge in the anterior horn of the lateral ventricle. In *Huntington disease* (also called *Huntington chorea*), an inherited neurodegenerative disease, the head of the caudate nucleus is characteristically absent in magnetic resonance imaging or computed tomography. At about the level of the interventricular foramen, the caudate diminishes in size but continues caudally as the *body of the caudate nucleus* in the

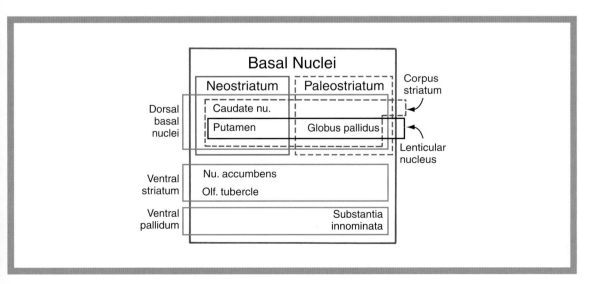

Figure 16-16. A series of stacked boxes showing which nuclei form the various parts of the basal nuclei and the terms used to describe them.

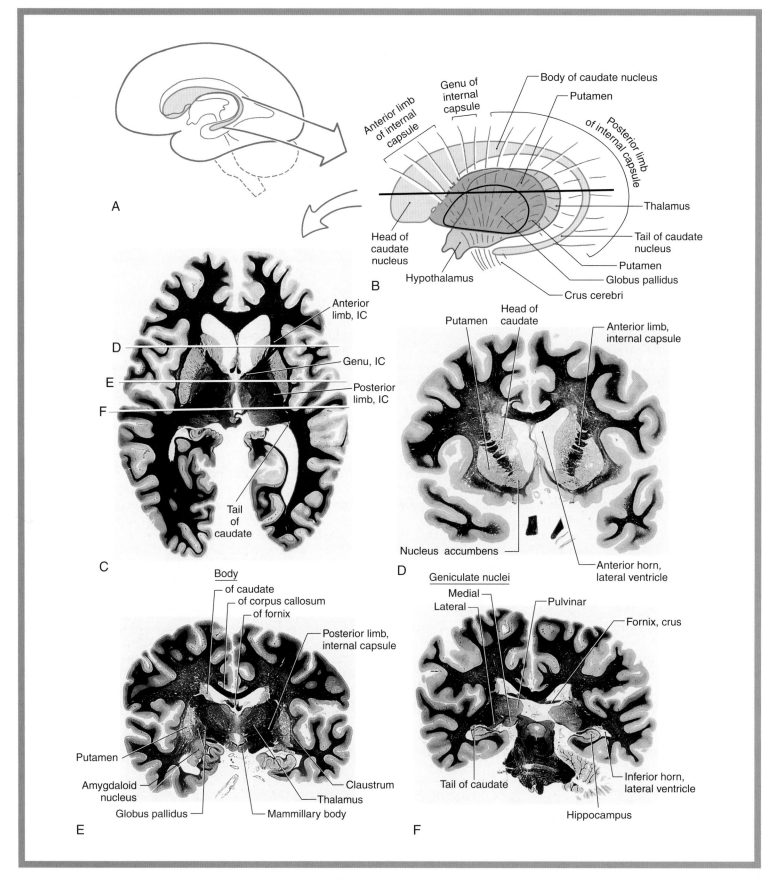

Figure 16-17. Three-dimensional drawings (**A**, **B**) of the relationships of the internal capsule (IC), basal nuclei, and thalamus. The axial section (**C**) represents the approximate plane shown in **B**; the coronal sections (**D-F**) are taken from the three levels indicated in **C**. **C-F**, Weil stains.

lateral wall of the body of the lateral ventricle. In the lateral wall of the atrium of the lateral ventricle, the body of the caudate nucleus turns inferiorly and rostrally to continue as the *tail of the caudate nucleus* in the posterolateral (dorsolateral) wall of the temporal horn of the lateral ventricle. Thus, the "C" shape of the caudate nucleus faithfully follows the "C" shape of the

lateral ventricle (excluding the posterior horn) (Figs. 16-17A, B and 16-18A, B and E-H).

The *lenticular nucleus* is located within the base of the hemisphere and is surrounded by white matter (Figs. 16-17 and 16-18). The internal capsule borders the lenticular nucleus medially, and the external capsule separates it from the claustrum laterally.

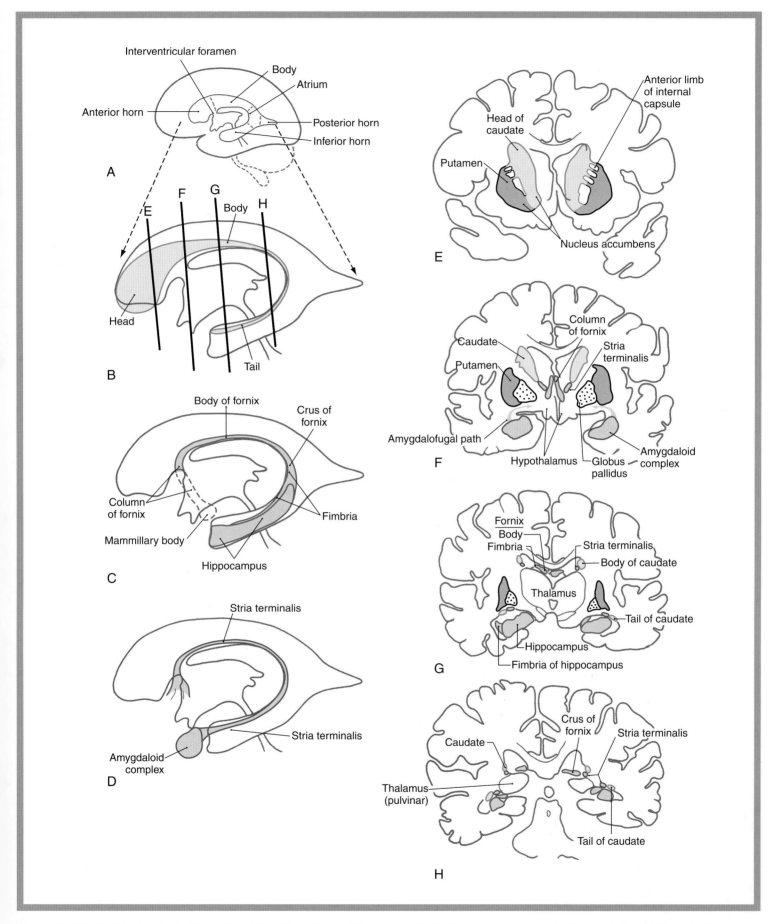

Figure 16-18. The lateral ventricle (**A**) and its relationship to the caudate nucleus (**B**), the hippocampus and fornix (**C**), and the amygdala and stria terminalis (**D**). The coronal levels in **E** through **H** correlate with the planes indicated in **B** and are color coded to match the corresponding structure in **B**, **C**, or **D**.

The lenticular nucleus consists of a larger lateral part, the *putamen,* and a small medial portion, the *globus pallidus* (or *pallidum*). The putamen extends more superior, more rostral, and more caudal when compared with the globus pallidus and is clearly the larger part of the lenticular nucleus when viewed in axial or coronal planes (Fig. 16-17B-E). The *globus pallidus* is located internal to the putamen and is smaller in all dimensions (Figs. 16-17 and 16-18). It is divided into *medial (internal)* and *lateral (external) parts* by thin sheets of vertically oriented white matter. The globus pallidus is also separated from the putamen by a thin lamina of white matter.

Nucleus Accumbens and Substantia Innominata

The *nucleus accumbens* is located rostrally in the hemisphere where the putamen is continuous with the head of the caudate nucleus (Fig. 16-19). This cell group is also closely apposed to the septal nuclei and the nucleus of the diagonal band, both of which extend into the base of the septum pellucidum. At a slightly more caudal level, the *substantia innominata* (basal nucleus of Meynert) is located internal to the anterior perforated substance in the area inferior to the anterior commissure (Fig. 16-19). Although many areas of the nervous system are affected in Alzheimer disease, there is an especially noticeable loss of larger neurons in the substantia innominata.

Subthalamic Nucleus and Substantia Nigra

Although not a part of the telencephalon either developmentally or geographically, the subthalamic nucleus and the substantia nigra are intimately allied with the basal nuclei based on their connections (Fig. 16-20). The *subthalamic nucleus,* a component of the diencephalon, is a flattened, lens-shaped cell group located rostral to the substantia nigra. It is medial to the internal capsule and is capped by a thin sheet of fibers called the *lenticular fasciculus.* Lesions of the subthalamic nucleus, which are com-

monly hemorrhagic in origin, result in a characteristic motor deficit of the contralateral extremities (primarily the upper) called *hemiballismus.*

The *substantia nigra,* a part of the midbrain, is found internal to the crus cerebri and immediately caudal to the subthalamic nucleus. It is divided into a reticulated part *(pars reticulata)* and a compact part *(pars compacta);* the latter is characterized by numerous melanin-containing neuron cell bodies. These melanin-containing cells of the pars compacta utilize dopamine as their neurotransmitter. The progressive loss of these cells, due largely to unknown causes, gives rise to the characteristic motor deficits seen in *Parkinson disease.*

Major Connections of the Basal Nuclei

The connections of the basal nuclei are discussed in their entirety in Chapter 26. It is appropriate, however, to briefly review these relationships here, with particular emphasis on the major fiber bundles of the basal nuclei (Fig. 16-20).

The two largest bundles of efferent fibers exiting the basal nuclei are the *lenticular fasciculus* and the *ansa lenticularis.* The former leaves the globus pallidus, passes through the posterior limb of the internal capsule at right angles to most fibers in the posterior limb, and forms a thin sheet of fibers insinuated between the subthalamic nucleus and the zona incerta. These fibers loop around the medial aspect of the zona incerta and pass laterally (and superiorly) as the *thalamic fasciculus* (Fig. 16-20). The fibers of the *ansa lenticularis* originate at a slightly more rostral level, arch around the inferomedial aspect of the internal capsule, and pass caudally to join with the fibers of the lenticular fasciculus as they enter the thalamic fasciculus (Fig. 16-20).

Two smaller but equally important bundles are the *subthalamic fasciculus* and *connections between the substantia nigra and neostriatum* (Fig. 16-20). The subthalamic fasciculus is composed of bidirectional connections between the globus pallidus and

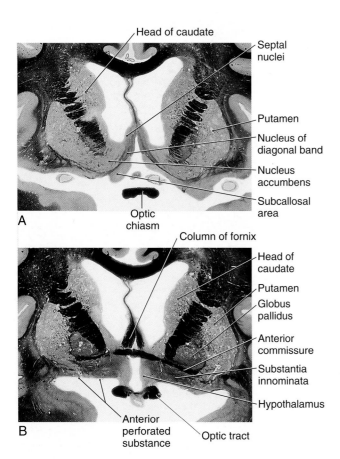

Figure 16-19. Cross sections of the telencephalon at rostral levels showing the nucleus accumbens (**A**) and the substantia innominata (**B**) and adjacent structures. Weil stain.

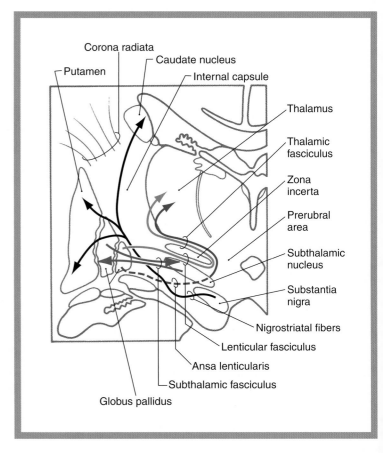

Figure 16-20. Major fiber bundles associated with the basal nuclei and with the subthalamic nucleus and substantia nigra.

the subthalamic nucleus; these fibers also traverse the posterior limb of the internal capsule similar to those of the lenticular fasciculus. The connections between the substantia nigra and the neostriatum are named according to the origin and termination of the fiber. Axons that project from nigral cells to the neostriatum are *nigrostriatal* projections, and fibers that project from striatal cells to the substantia nigra are *striatonigral* fibers. These bidirectional connections between the neostriatum and the substantia nigra course through the lateral aspect of the midbrain-diencephalic junction at the interface between the crus cerebri and the substantia nigra (Fig. 16-20).

Vasculature of the Basal Nuclei and Related Structures

The blood supply to the caudate and putamen is provided by branches of the *medial striate artery, lenticulostriate branches* of the M_1 segment, and the *anterior choroidal artery* (Figs. 16-12 and 16-15). The medial striate artery, usually a branch of A_2, serves much of the head of the caudate nucleus. Most of the lenticular nucleus and the surrounding internal and external capsules are supplied by the lenticulostriate branches of M_1. Inferior (ventral) and medial portions of the head of the caudate, as well as the body of the caudate, are also served by these arteries. The tail of the caudate, adjacent portions of the lenticular nucleus, and adjacent temporal lobe structures (hippocampus, choroid plexus) receive their blood supply via the anterior choroidal artery, a branch of the internal carotid artery. It is important to remember that the anterior choroidal artery also serves the optic tract and inferior regions of the posterior limb of the internal capsule.

The blood supply to the subthalamic nucleus and the substantia nigra arises from the *posteromedial branches* of the P_1 segment and branches of the posterior communicating artery. These vessels penetrate the brain at the midbrain-diencephalon junction through the posterior perforated substance.

Hippocampus and Amygdala

The *hippocampal formation* and the *amygdaloid complex* are located in the temporal lobe. The former lies in the inferomedial floor of the temporal horn of the lateral ventricle and the latter in the rostral end of this space. Through a variety of pathways (see Chapter 31), these structures interconnect with numerous telencephalic and diencephalic centers.

Developmentally, the hippocampus is formed by an invagination of primitive cortex to form the curved, multilayered structure characteristic of the adult brain (Fig. 16-17F). The hippocampal formation is found internal to the parahippocampal gyrus and is composed of the *subiculum*, the *hippocampus proper* (also called *Ammon horn*), and the *dentate gyrus*. The cortex of the parahippocampal gyrus is continuous with the subiculum, which, in turn, is continuous with the hippocampus proper. The dentate gyrus forms a reverse loop adjacent to the hippocampus and, in doing so, presents a serrated surface that is medially exposed to the subarachnoid space. Details of the internal structure of the hippocampal formation are discussed in Chapter 31 and summarized in Figure 31-4.

Axons of hippocampal neurons converge to form a prominent bundle that arches around caudal, superior, and rostral aspects of the thalamus. This bundle, the *fornix*, is a major efferent path of the hippocampal formation (Fig. 16-18A-C and F-H). It is composed of a flattened caudal part, the *crus*; a compact superior portion, the *body*; and a part that arches around the rostral part of the thalamus and passes through the hypothalamus to terminate in the mammillary body—this is the *column of the fornix*. Located along the edge of the dentate gyrus and continuing on the lateral edge of the crus and body of the fornix is a thin fringe of fibers called the *fimbria*.

The *amygdaloid nuclear complex* (commonly called the *amygdala*) is located internal to the cortex of the uncus (Figs. 16-4 and 16-18D-F). It is composed of several cell groups including caudomedial, basolateral, and central subdivisions. Two major efferent bundles are related to the amygdala. First, the *stria terminalis* follows a looping trajectory that shadows, in a reverse direction, the orientation of the caudate nucleus (Fig. 16-18D). In the temporal horn, the stria terminalis is located just medial to the tail of the caudate nucleus. As the stria terminalis arches superiorly and rostrally, it assumes a position in the shallow groove between the caudate nucleus and the dorsal thalamus (Fig. 16-18G, H), where it is accompanied by the terminal vein (superior thalamostriate vein). At about the level of the interventricular foramen, the fibers of the stria terminalis fan out to enter and terminate in the hypothalamus, the septal area, and the neostriatum.

The second major efferent bundle of the amygdala is the diffusely arranged *ventral amygdalofugal pathway*. These fibers leave the amygdaloid complex, pass medially through the *substantia innominata*, and continue medially to enter hypothalamic and septal nuclei, or turn caudally and distribute to the brainstem (Fig. 16-18F).

Cell groups located internal to the subcallosal area collectively form the *septal nuclei* (Fig. 16-19). Consequently, the subcallosal area together with a small strip of cortex located adjacent to the lamina terminalis, the *paraterminal gyrus*, is commonly called the *septal area*. The septal nuclei are medially adjacent to the nucleus accumbens and continuous with sheets of neuronal cell bodies that extend into the *septum pellucidum*. The latter structure extends, in general, from the fornix to the inner surface of the corpus callosum. It forms the medial wall of the anterior horns and a small part of the bodies of the lateral ventricles (Figs. 16-14 and 16-17). In general, the septal nuclei have complex interconnections with hippocampal, amygdaloid, and other limbic structures.

Temporal Lobe Lesions

Injury to the temporal lobe, especially bilateral damage, almost always involves the hippocampus and amygdala. Deficits most directly linked to trauma to these structures include profound changes in eating and sexual behavior, a decrease in aggression levels, and deficits in memory function. Regarding memory deficits, the patient may demonstrate a loss of recent memory or show an inability to acquire new memory (learn new tasks) while memory of events that took place in the distant past remains intact.

Vasculature of the Hippocampus and Amygdala

The blood supply to the hippocampal formation and amygdaloid complex is primarily via the *anterior choroidal artery*. This vessel arises from the internal carotid, passes along the medial edge of the temporal horn, and sends branches into the hippocampus and amygdala. It also serves the tail of the caudate, the choroid plexus of the temporal horn, and inferior regions of the lenticular nucleus. The cortex of the uncus and that of the parahippocampal gyrus are served by superficial branches of the *middle cerebral* and *posterior cerebral arteries*, respectively.

Synopsis of Clinical Points

■ A failure of maturing neurons to properly migrate on radial glia may result in altered patterns of gyri in the cerebral cortex (p. 246).

■ A lack of gyri resulting in a smooth cerebral cortex is lissencephaly (p. 246).

■ Abnormally large gyri that are few in number are known as pachygyria (p. 246).

■ Abnormally small gyri that are numerous are known as microgyria (p. 246).

■ Anencephaly is a catastrophic developmental defect that is incompatible with life (p. 246).

■ Cortical lesions located in the pars opercularis and the adjacent pars triangularis of the dominant hemisphere result in an expressive (Broca) aphasia (p. 248).

■ Damage to the frontal eye field results in conjugate deviation of the eyes (p. 248).

■ A lesion centered mainly in the inferior parietal lobule (supramarginal and angular gyri) of the dominant hemisphere results in a receptive (Wernicke) aphasia (p. 248).

■ The body is somatotopically arranged in the primary somatomotor and somatosensory cortices (pp. 247–248).

■ Damage to the auditory cortex may result in an altered perception of sound, but not deafness, in one ear (p. 249).

■ A lesion of the primary visual cortex results in a homonymous hemianopia (p. 251).

■ The major conduit in and out of the cerebral cortex is the internal capsule (p. 253).

■ A small lesion in the genu of the internal capsule results in motor deficits related primarily to cranial nerves VII, XI, and XII (p. 253).

■ The anterior choroidal artery syndrome includes deficits reflecting damage to the internal capsule and optic tract (p. 255).

■ Lesions of the posterior limb of the internal capsule result in motor and sensory deficits on the same side of the body (pp. 253, 255).

■ The retrolenticular limb of the internal capsule contains optic radiations; lesions of these fibers result in visual deficits on the contralateral side (pp. 253, 255).

■ Huntington chorea is a neurodegenerative disease characterized by loss of the head of the caudate nucleus on magnetic resonance imaging (p. 255).

■ A lesion of the subthalamic nucleus results in a contralateral motor deficit called hemiballismus (p. 258).

■ A loss of the dopamine containing cells in the substantia nigra, the pars compacta, results in the motor defects seen in Parkinson disease (p. 258).

■ Temporal lobe lesions may result in changes in sexual behavior and in memory deficits (p. 259).

Sources and Additional Reading

Bailey P, von Bonin G: The Isocortex of Man. Urbana, IL, University of Illinois Press, 1951.

Crosby EC, Humphrey T, Lauer EW: Correlative Anatomy of the Nervous System. New York, Macmillan, 1962.

Kretschmann H-J, Weinrich W: Cranial Neuroimaging and Clinical Neuroanatomy, Magnetic Resonance Imaging and Computed Tomography, 2nd ed. New York, Thieme Medical Publishers, 1992.

Kuhlenbeck H: The Central Nervous System of Vertebrates: A General Survey of Its Comparative Anatomy with an Introduction to the Pertinent Fundamental Biologic and Logical Concepts, vol 5, part I: Derivatives of the Prosencephalon: Diencephalon and Telencephalon. Basel, S. Karger, 1977.

Kuhlenbeck H: The Central Nervous System of Vertebrates: A General Survey of Its Comparative Anatomy with an Introduction to the Pertinent Fundamental Biologic and Logical Concepts, vol 5, part II: Mammalian Telencephalon: Surface Morphology and Cerebral Cortex. Basel, S. Karger, 1978.

Nieuwenhuys R, Voogd J, van Huijzen C: The Human Central Nervous System, A Synopsis and Atlas, 3rd ed. Berlin, Springer-Verlag, 1988.

Parent A: Carpenter's Human Neuroanatomy, 9th ed. Baltimore, Williams & Wilkins, 1996.

Paxinos G (ed): The Human Nervous System. San Diego, Academic Press, 1990, pp 439-755.

Penfield W, Rasmussen T: The Cerebral Cortex of Man, A Clinical Study of Localization of Function. New York, Hafner Reprint of 1950 Macmillan Edition, 1968.

Rosano C, Sweeney JA, Melchitzky DS, Lewis DA: The human precentral sulcus: Chemoarchitecture of a region corresponding to the frontal eye fields. Brain Res 972:16-30, 2003.

Varnavas GG, Grand W: The insular cortex: Morphological and vascular anatomic characteristics. Neurosurgery 44:127-138, 1999.

Zola-Morgan S, Squire LR: Neuroanatomy of memory. Annu Rev Neurosci 16:547-563, 1993.

Section 3

Systems Neurobiology

Chapters

17–33

Chapter 17

The Somatosensory System I: Tactile Discrimination and Position Sense

S. Warren, N. F. Capra, and R. P. Yezierski

If you reach into your pocket to determine the types of coins present, you are gathering information through the activation of specialized receptors of the *somatosensory system*. Specifically, the size of a coin is determined by noting the joint angles when the coin is held between the forefinger and thumb. "Heads and tails" may be identified using *slowly adapting* receptors sensitive to stimuli that indent the skin. Dimes can be distinguished from pennies by stroking their edges with the fingertips and activating *rapidly adapting* receptors. This information is transmitted to the cerebral cortex by a multisynaptic pathway called the *posterior column–medial lemniscal* system. At the same time, much of this information, along with information concerning muscle tension and length, is also transmitted to the cerebellar cortex, where it is used to regulate muscle activity that allows manipulation of the coins. The *spinocerebellar pathways* are among those that subserve these nonconscious somatosensory functions.

Overview

In general, the somatosensory system transmits and analyzes *touch* or *tactile* information from external and internal locations on the body and head. The result of these processes leads to the appreciation of somatic sensations, which can be subdivided into the submodalities *discriminative touch, flutter-vibration, proprioception (position sense), crude (nondiscriminative) touch, thermal (hot and cold) sensation, and nociception (pain)*. The following anatomically and functionally discrete pathways transmit these signals: (1) the *posterior column–medial lemniscal* pathway, (2) the *trigeminothalamic* pathways, (3) the *spinocerebellar* pathways, and (4) the *anterolateral system*.

This chapter describes pathways that transmit discriminative touch, flutter-vibration, and proprioceptive information. These pathways are the *posterior column–medial lemniscal* pathway, portions of the trigeminothalamic pathways originating in the *principal trigeminal sensory nucleus*, and the *spinocerebellar* pathways. The pathways subserving the submodalities of pain, thermal sense, and crude touch, itch, and tickle compose the anterolateral system. These and portions of the trigeminothalamic pathways are described in Chapter 18.

Posterior Column–Medial Lemniscal System (PCMLS)

The posterior column–medial lemniscal pathway, shown in Figures 17-7 and 17-8, is involved with the perception and appreciation of mechanical stimuli. It underlies the capacity for fine form and texture discrimination, form recognition of three-dimensional shape *(stereognosis)*, and motion detection. This pathway is also involved in transmitting information related to conscious awareness of body position *(proprioception)* and limb movement *(kinesthesia)* in space.

Characteristic features of the PCMLS include transmission in general somatic afferent (GSA) fibers that have fast conduction velocities, a limited number of synaptic relays in which processing of the signal occurs, and a precise somatotopic organization. These features provide the basis for the accurate localization of the body region touched. There is only limited convergence along the pathway; consequently, the signal is transmitted with high fidelity and a high degree of spatial and temporal resolution. This pathway signals somatic sensations using *frequency* and *population codes*. *In frequency coding, a cell's firing rate signals stimulus intensity or temporal aspects of the tactile stimulus. In population coding, the distribution in time and space of activated cells in the central nervous system signals location of the stimulus, as well as its motion or direction if any.*

The high degree of resolution in the PCMLS is the result of inhibitory mechanisms such as *lateral (surround) inhibition*. This mechanism is a feature found initially within the posterior column nuclei and is present through all the relays of the PCML pathway. It sharpens and enhances the discrimination between separate points on the skin and is critical for *two-point discrimination*. The ability to discriminate between two points simultaneously applied varies widely over different parts of the body.

Peripheral Mechanoreceptors

The first step in evoking somatic sensations is the activation of peripheral mechanoreceptors. Mechanical pressure, such as skin deformation, is *transduced* into an electrical signal in the peripheral process of a primary afferent neuron (see Chapter 3). This leads to a depolarizing *graded membrane potential* across the membrane of the neuron. If this potential depolarizes the *trigger zone*, located at the first myelin segment of the axon, to *threshold*, an *action potential* is produced (see Chapter 3). In most receptors, transduction occurs between the mechanoreceptor and subjacent primary afferent membrane. In contrast, Merkel cells may influence their associated primary afferent axon by vesicular release of a transmitter substance.

Each morphologic type of receptor responds to different tactile stimuli. *Cutaneous tactile receptors* (Table 17-1; Fig. 17-1) are located in the basal epidermis and dermis of *glabrous* (palms, soles, lips) and *hairy* skin. These low-threshold mechanoreceptors may be encapsulated, such as *Meissner, pacinian, and Ruffini*

Table 17-1. Cutaneous Mechanoreceptors and Their Associated Fiber Types and Sensations

Receptor Type (Adaptation Rate)	Sensation Produced by Microstimulation	Fiber Type (Group)	Receptive Field Size (Average)	Number per cm^2	
				Fingertip	Palm
Meissner corpuscle (RA)	Tap, flutter 5–40 Hz	II	Small (54.9 ± 8.6 mm^2)	>100	40
Hair follicle receptors (RA, SA)	Motion, direction	II	N/A	N/A	N/A
Pacinian corpuscle (RA)	Vibration 60–300 Hz	II	Large	20	10
Merkel cell (SA)	Touch—pressure	II	Small (44.7 mm^2)	70	30
Ruffini complex (SA)	Unknown	II	Large	50	15

RA, rapidly adapting; SA, slowly adapting.

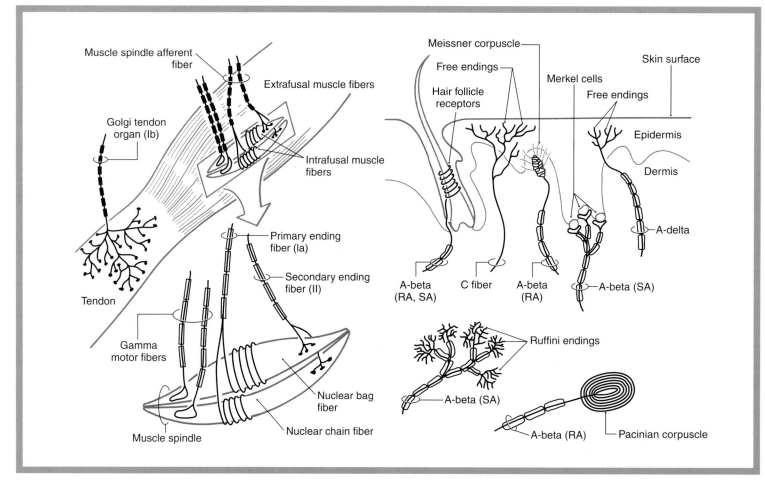

Figure 17-1. Proprioceptive receptors and cutaneous mechanoreceptors and their afferent fibers. Cutaneous receptors are either rapidly adapting (RA) or slowly adapting (SA).

corpuscles, or unencapsulated, such as *Merkel cell neurite complexes* and *hair follicle receptors*. Meissner corpuscles, some hair follicle receptors, and pacinian corpuscles respond to transient, phasic, or vibratory stimuli. These receptors respond to each initial application or removal of a stimulus but fail to respond during maintained stimulation. Consequently, they are *rapidly adapting* (RA) *receptors* (Fig. 17-2A). Hair follicle receptors are also capable of signaling motion, its direction or orientation, and its velocity.

Merkel cells, Ruffini corpuscles, and some hair follicle receptors signal tonic events such as discrete small indentations in the skin. They provide input related to both the displacement and velocity of a stimulus. They are also capable of encoding stimulus intensity or duration because they are *slowly adapting* (SA) and

are active so long as the stimulus is present (Fig. 17-2A). For example, Merkel cell complexes are crucial to reading Braille.

Deep tactile mechanoreceptors are found within the dermis of the skin and in the fascia surrounding muscles and bone and in the peridontium. These receptors include *pacinian corpuscles*, *Ruffini corpuscles*, and other encapsulated nerve endings located in the periosteum, the deep fascia, and the mesenteries. The receptors of this group respond to pressure, vibration (Fig. 17-2B and Table 17-1), or skin stretch and distention or tooth displacement.

Proprioceptive receptors (Table 17-2; see also Fig. 17-1) are located in muscles, tendons, and joint capsules. These receptors include the nuclear bag and nuclear chain intrafusal muscle fibers of *muscle spindles* and their associated nerve fibers. The *Golgi*

Table 17-2. Muscle and Joint Proprioceptors and Their Associated Fiber Types and Sensations

Receptor Type (Adaptation Rate)	Sensation	Function/Signal	Fiber Type (Group)
Nuclear bag fiber (SA—primary annulospiral endings)	High dynamic sensitivity	Length and rate of change; length and velocity	Ia
Nuclear chain fiber (SA—secondary flower spray ending)	Low dynamic sensitivity	Length; tension	II
Golgi tendon organ (SA)	Tension	Muscle force; tension	Ib
Ruffini endings (SA)	Limb position	Joint movement and pressure	I
SA, slowly adapting.			

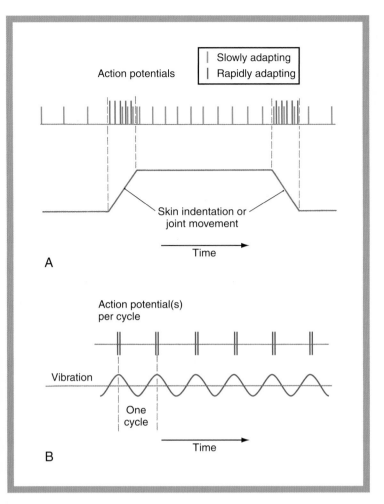

Figure 17-2. Diagrammatic action potentials (*top trace,* **A**) evoked by skin indentation and removal of a cutaneous stimulus or of joint movement (*bottom trace,* **A**) in primary afferent fibers innervating slowly adapting (SA: *red*) and rapidly adapting (RA: *green*) cutaneous mechanoreceptors. Diagrammatic action potentials (*blue,* **B**) evoked in a Pacinian corpuscle afferent fiber by sinusoidal stimulation of the skin surface (*bottom trace,* **B**).

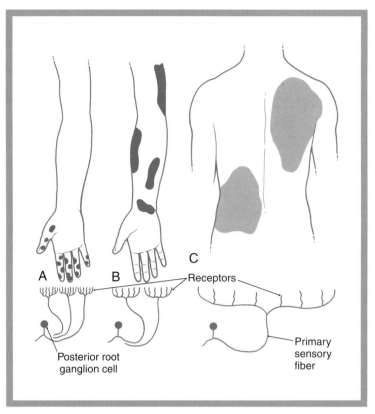

Figure 17-3. A to **C,** Variation in the size of receptive fields as a function of peripheral innervation density. The greater the density of receptors, the smaller the receptive fields of individual afferent fibers.

tendon organs and their group Ib fibers and the encapsulated Ruffini-type joint receptors also function in this capacity. They respond to static limb and joint position or to the dynamic movement of the limb *(kinesthesia)* and are important sources of information for balance, posture, and limb movement.

The accuracy with which a tactile stimulus is detected depends on the density of receptors and the size of receptive fields (Fig. 17-3). The greatest density of cutaneous tactile receptors is found on the tips of the glabrous digits and in the perioral region. Other regions, like the back, have much lower density, thus creating a receptor density gradient between various body parts. The *receptive field* is the area of skin innervated by branches of a GSA fiber, the stimulation of which activates its receptors (Fig. 17-3). *Small receptive fields* are found in areas, such as the fingertips, where receptor density is high and each receptor serves an extremely small area of skin. In such regions the individual is able to discriminate small variations in a variety of sensory inputs. In other regions, receptor density is low and each receptor serves an expansive area of skin, creating *large receptive fields* with resultant reduction in discriminative ability.

At all levels of the tactile pathway, densely innervated body parts are represented by greater numbers of neurons and take up a disproportionately large part of the somatosensory system's body representation. In this respect there is an inverse relationship between the size of the receptive field and the representation of that body part in the somatosensory cortex. For example, the trunk, with its large receptive fields, has a small representation

in the somatosensory cortex, while the fingers, with their small receptive fields, have a large representation in the somatosensory cortex (compare Figure 17-3 with 17-12). As a result, the fingertips and lips provide the central nervous system with the most specific and detailed information about a tactile stimulus.

Primary Afferent Fibers

As initially described in Chapter 9, primary afferent GSA fibers consist of (1) *a peripheral process* extending from the posterior root ganglion to either contact peripheral mechanoreceptors or end as free nerve endings, (2) *a central process* extending from the posterior root ganglion into the central nervous system, and (3) *a pseudounipolar cell body* in the posterior root ganglion. The peripheral distribution of the afferent nerves associated with each spinal level delineates the segmental pattern of *dermatomes.* In clinical testing, these ribbon-like strips of skin are associated primarily with fibers and pathways that convey pain and thermal information; they are considered in Chapter 18.

Peripheral nerves are classified by two schemes. One is based on their contribution to a compound action potential (A, B, and C waves) recorded from an entire mixed peripheral nerve (e.g., sciatic nerve) after electrical stimulation of that nerve. The other scheme specific to cutaneous fibers (e.g., lateral antebrachial cutaneous nerve, sural nerve) is based on fiber diameter, myelin thickness, and conduction velocity (classes I, II, III, and IV) (Table 17-3; Fig. 17-4). The two schemes are related because conduction velocity determines a fiber's contribution to the compound action potential. Discriminative touch, vibratory sense, and position sense are transmitted by group Ia, Ib, and II fibers (Tables 17-1 and 17-2).

Spinal Cord and Brainstem

On the basis of cell and fiber diameter, primary sensory fibers are categorized as *large* and *small.* Large-diameter fibers subserve discriminative touch, flutter-vibration, and proprioception

Table 17-3. Peripheral Sensory and Motor Fibers: Groups, Diameters, and Conduction Velocities

Electrophysiologic Classification of Peripheral Nerves	Classification of Afferent Fibers ONLY (Class/Group)	Fiber Diameter (μm)	Conduction Velocity (m/s)	Receptor Supplied
Sensory Fiber Type				
Aα	Ia and Ib	13–20	80–120	Primary muscle spindles, Golgi tendon organ
Aβ	II	6–12	35–75	Secondary muscle spindles, skin mechanoreceptors
Aδ	III	1–5	5–30	Skin mechanoreceptors, thermal receptors, and nociceptors
C	IV	0.2–1.5	0.5–2	Skin mechanoreceptors, thermal receptors, and nociceptors
Motor Fiber Type				
Aα	N/A	12–20	72–120	Extrafusal skeletal muscle fibers
Aγ	N/A	2–8	12–48	Intrafusal muscle fibers
B	N/A	1–3	6–18	Preganglionic autonomic fibers
C	N/A	0.2–2	0.5–2	Postganglionic autonomic fibers

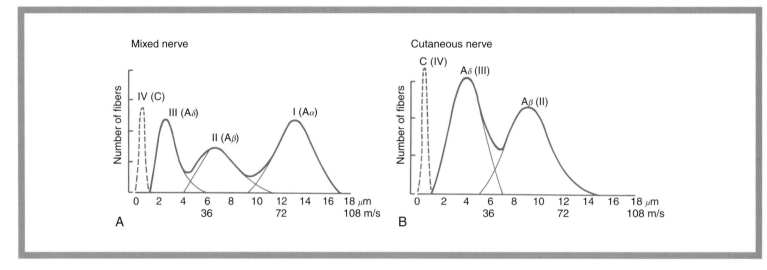

Figure 17-4. Compound action potential evoked in a mixed nerve (**A**) and a cutaneous nerve (**B**) in response to electrical stimulation. Note the increase in the number of small-diameter fibers and the absence of the Aα fibers in the cutaneous nerve (**B**).

(groups Ia, Ib, II, and Aβ; Tables 17-1 and 17-2). They enter the spinal cord via the *medial division of the posterior root* (see Chapter 9) and then branch (Fig. 17-5). One set of branches terminates on second-order neurons in the spinal cord gray matter at, above, and below the level of entry. These branches contribute to a variety of spinal reflexes and to ascending projections such as *postsynaptic posterior column fibers*. The largest set of branches ascends cranially and contributes to the formation of the *gracile* and *cuneate fasciculi*. These fiber bundles are collectively termed the *posterior columns*, owing to their position in the spinal cord (Figs. 17-5 to 17-7).

Within the posterior columns, fibers from different dermatomes are organized topographically. Sacral level fibers assume a medial position, and fibers from progressively more rostral levels (up to thoracic level T6) are added laterally to form the *gracile fasciculus* (Figs. 17-5 and 17-6). Thoracic fibers from above T6 and cervical fibers form the laterally placed *cuneate fasciculus* in the same manner. Thus, the lower extremity is represented medially and the upper extremity is represented laterally within the posterior columns (Figs. 17-5 and 17-6). Compromise of blood flow in the posterior spinal artery, which supplies the posterior funiculus, or mechanical injury to the posterior columns (as in *Brown-Séquard syndrome*) results in an *ipsilateral*

reduction or loss of discriminative, positional, and vibratory tactile sensations at and below the segmental level of the injury. Symptoms indicative of damage to fibers of the posterior columns are also seen in *tabes dorsalis (progressive locomotor ataxia)*. This disease is caused by infection with *Treponema pallidum* and is associated with neurosyphilis. The fibers of the posterior columns degenerate, and the patient has ataxia (related to the lack of sensory input), a loss of muscle stretch (tendon) reflexes, and proprioceptive losses from the extremities.

The *posterior column nuclei*, the *gracile* and *cuneate nuclei*, are found in the posterior medulla at the rostral end of their respective fasciculi. They are supplied by the posterior spinal artery (Fig. 17-7). The cell bodies of the gracile and cuneate nuclei are the *second-order neurons* in the PCMLS. They receive input from *first-order neurons*, having cell bodies in the ipsilateral posterior root ganglia (Figs 17-7 and 17-8). The gracile nucleus receives input from sacral, lumbar, and lower thoracic levels via the *gracile fasciculus;* the cuneate nucleus receives input from upper thoracic and cervical levels through the *cuneate fasciculus.*

In addition to the somatotopic organization of projections to the posterior column nuclei, there is a submodality segregation of tactile inputs within these nuclei. The relay neurons that receive excitatory input from primary afferent fibers form

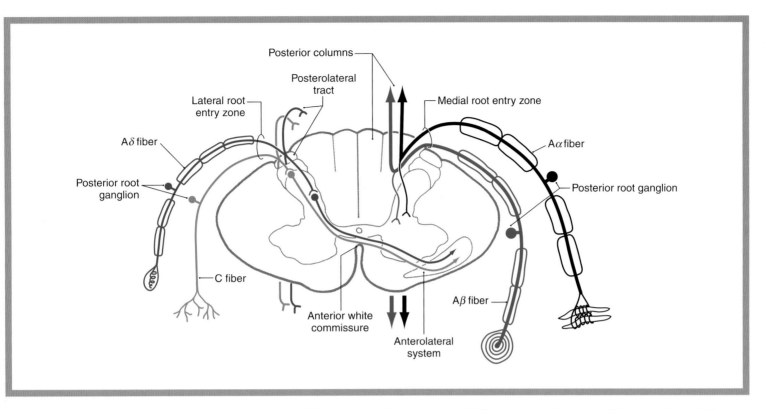

Figure 17-5. A representative section of the cervical spinal cord showing large-diameter Aα and Aβ fibers on the right and small-diameter Aδ and C fibers on the left.

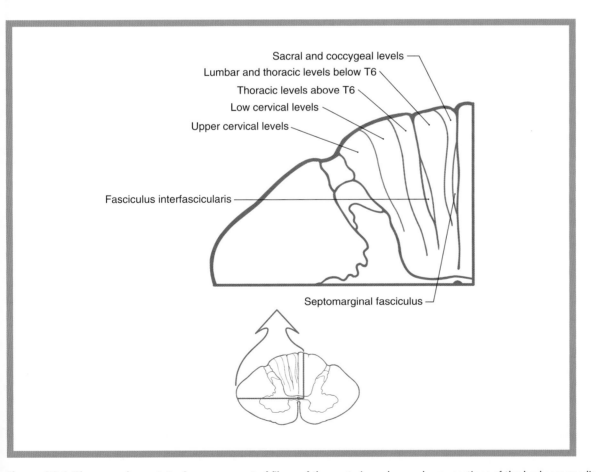

Figure 17-6. The general somatotopic arrangement of fibers of the posterior columns; lower portions of the body are medial and progressively more rostral portions are more lateral within the posterior funiculus. The septomarginal fasciculus is composed of descending collaterals of primary afferent fibers from sacral, lumbar, and low thoracic levels while the fasciculus interfascicularis is composed of descending collaterals from upper thoracic and cervical levels. These fibers are involved in reflexes mediated by posterior column afferents.

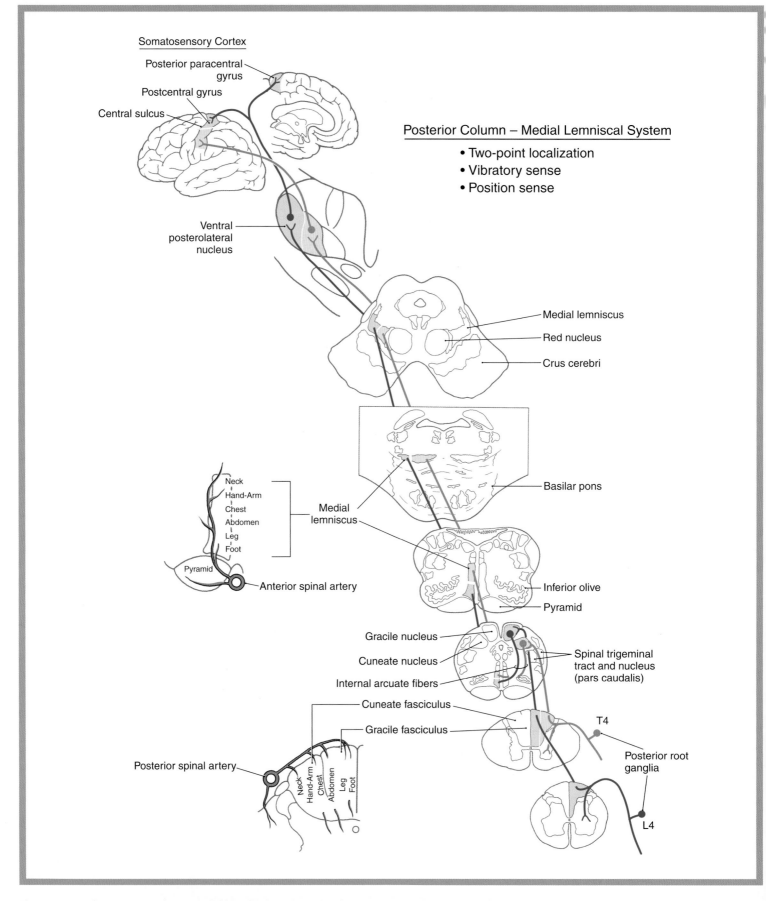

Figure 17-7. The posterior column-medial lemniscal system. Note the somatotopic arrangement of body parts at each level of this pathway.

submodality-specific rostrocaudal bands (Fig. 17-9). *Rapidly adapting* inputs terminate centrally and caudally within the nuclei. *Slowly adapting* cutaneous input and muscle spindle and joint inputs project to the rostral pole of the cuneate and gracile nuclei and to the rostrally adjacent *nucleus z*. The posterior column

nuclei also receive descending axons from the contralateral primary somatosensory cortex and from the medullary reticular formation (nucleus reticularis gigantocellularis) (Fig. 17-9).

The posterior column nuclei have an "inner core" region of large projection neurons surrounded by a diffuse "shell" of small

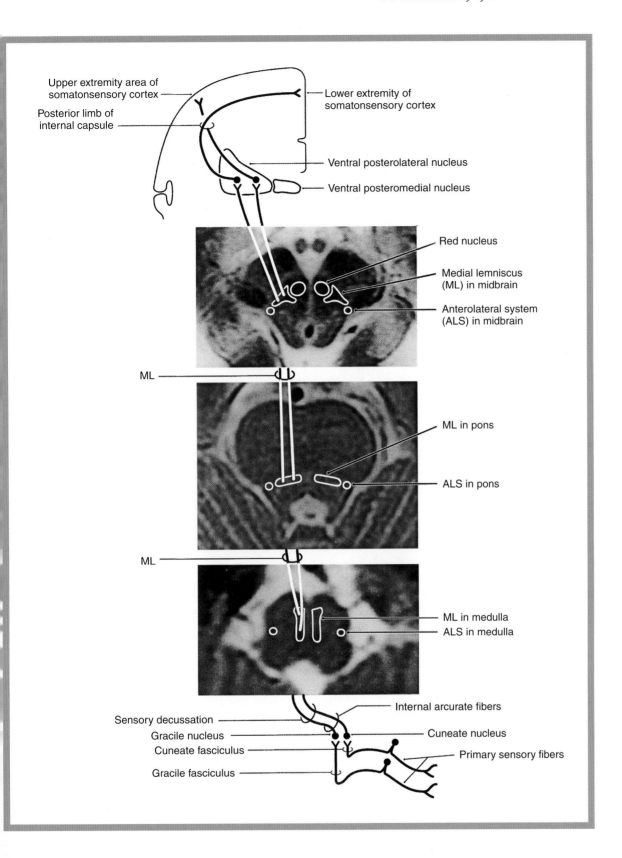

Upper extremity area of somatonsensory cortex

Posterior limb of internal capsule

Lower extremity of somatonsensory cortex

Ventral posterolateral nucleus

Ventral posteromedial nucleus

Red nucleus

Medial lemniscus (ML) in midbrain

Anterolateral system (ALS) in midbrain

ML

ML in pons

ALS in pons

ML

ML in medulla
ALS in medulla

Internal arcurate fibers

Sensory decussation

Gracile nucleus

Cuneate fasciculus

Gracile fasciculus

Cuneate nucleus

Primary sensory fibers

Figure 17-8. The location of posterior column-medial lemniscus (PCML) fibers in MR images at representative levels of the medulla, pons, and midbrain. This illustrates the location of PCML fibers when viewed in images routinely used in the clinical setting.

fusiform and radiating cells (Fig. 17-9). The shell area contains interneurons responsible for feedback inhibition in the posterior column nuclei. This feedback alters activity of projection neurons of the inner core. In addition, the presence of non–posterior column inputs to these projection cells suggests that information received by the posterior column nuclei is not simply relayed but undergoes signal processing.

The *second-order cells* in the core regions of the posterior column nuclei send their axons to the contralateral thalamus

(Figs. 17-7 and 17-8). In the medulla, the *internal arcuate fibers*, axons of cells in the posterior column nuclei, arc anteromedially toward the midline, decussate, and ascend as the *medial lemniscus* on the opposite side. Fibers in the medial lemniscus that arise in the cuneate nucleus are located posterior to those that originate from the gracile nucleus (Figs. 17-7 and 17-8). The anterior spinal artery supplies the medial lemniscus in the medulla, and penetrating branches of the basilar artery supply it in the pons. Vascular damage at these brainstem levels leads to deficits

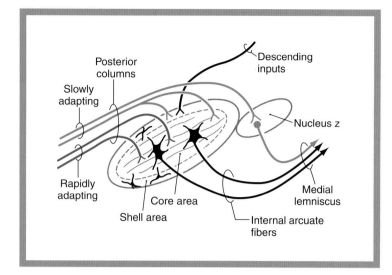

Figure 17-9. Schematic representation of the posterior column nuclei and nucleus z. Slowly adapting inputs, including those from joint and muscle receptors, terminate preferentially in the shell region. Rapidly adapting inputs, including Meissner corpuscles and some hair follicle receptors, project to the core region. The output of the posterior column nuclei is influenced by descending inputs arising in other brainstem and cortical areas.

in discriminative touch, vibratory, and positional sensibilities over the contralateral body. As the medial lemniscus moves rostrally through the brainstem, it rotates laterally so that the upper extremity representation comes to lie medially and the lower extremity laterally (Figs. 17-7 and 17-8). This somatotopic organization is maintained as the lemniscus ascends through the brainstem and terminates on cells in the *ventral posterolateral nucleus* (VPL) of the thalamus.

The *postsynaptic posterior column pathway*, a small supplemental pathway in humans that relays nondiscriminative tactile signals to supraspinal levels, consists of non–primary afferent axons carrying tactile signals in the posterior columns (Fig. 17-10). The cells of origin of this pathway are located in laminae III and IV of the posterior horn. Axons of these second-order *postsynaptic posterior column fibers* travel in the posterior columns and, together with other tactile primary afferent fibers, terminate in the posterior column nuclei. Cells of these nuclei relay this postsynaptic posterior column input to the contralateral thalamus via the medial lemniscus. Although this pathway is small, it may provide the morphologic basis for the return of some tactile sensation after vascular lesions involving the PCML system (Fig. 17-10).

Ventral Posterolateral Nuclei

The *ventral posterior nucleus*, sometimes called the *ventrobasal complex*, is a wedge-shaped cell group located caudally in the thalamus. Its lateral border abuts the internal capsule, and ventrally it borders on the external medullary lamina. The ventral posterior nucleus is composed of the laterally located *ventral posterolateral nucleus* (VPL) and the medially located *ventral posteromedial nucleus* (VPM). Although these nuclei have also been termed the ventralis caudalis externus and ventralis caudalis internus in humans, the more widely used, and recognized, terms VPL and VPM are used in this book. The VPL is separated from the VPM by fibers of the *arcuate lamina*. The ventral posterior nucleus (VPM and VPL) is supplied by thalamogeniculate branches of the posterior cerebral artery, and compromise of these vessels can result in loss of all tactile sensation over the contralateral body and head (Fig. 17-11).

The VPL receives ascending input from the medial lemniscus, and input to the VPM is from the trigeminothalamic tracts.

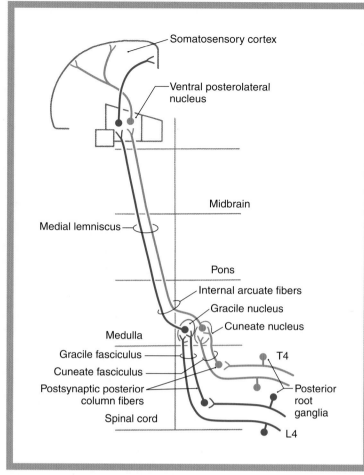

Figure 17-10. Summary of the postsynaptic posterior column pathway.

Within VPL, medial lemniscal fibers from the contralateral cuneate nucleus terminate medial to those from the gracile nucleus. As a result, the representation of the lower extremity is lateral and that of the upper extremity is medial in the VPL (Fig. 17-11). The representation of an individual body part is organized as a "C"-shaped lamina. Tactile signals are also represented in other thalamic nuclei receiving lemniscal input, including the ventral posterior inferior nucleus and the pulvinar and lateral posterior group.

In addition to their somatotopic organization, the medial lemniscal fibers that terminate in the ventral posterior nucleus are segregated on the basis of their functional properties. Rapidly and slowly adapting inputs terminate on different cell groups within the "core" region of VPL. Pacinian inputs and inputs arising from joints and muscles are confined to a "shell" region on the posterior, rostral, and anterior edges of the nucleus. Individual lemniscal axons arborize in the sagittal plane to terminate on longitudinal cell clusters, called *rods*, in the VPL. This arrangement of inputs and target cells creates isorepresentations consisting of neurons with similar receptive fields and submodalities arranged along a rostrocaudal axis.

The VPL, for the trunk and extremities (and VPM for the head), contains two populations of identified neurons. The first consists of large-diameter multipolar cells that give rise to axons that traverse the posterior limb of the internal capsule and terminate mainly in the primary (SI) and secondary (SII) somatosensory cortices. These *thalamocortical cells* and *fibers* are the *third-order neurons* in the PCMLS that provide excitatory (glutaminergic) input to the cortex. The second population consists of inhibitory (GABAergic) *local circuit interneurons*, which receive excitatory corticothalamic inputs and influence the firing rates of thalamocortical cells. In addition, these thalamocortical

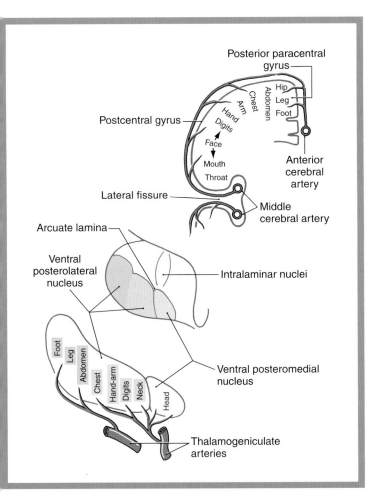

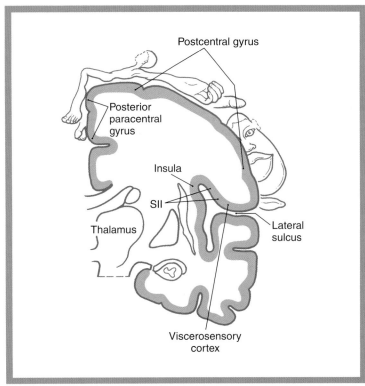

Figure 17-12. The homunculus (body representation) of the primary somatosensory (SI) cortex. (Adapted from Penfield W, Rasmussen T: The Cerebral Cortex of Man: A Clinical Study of Localization of Function. New York, Hafner Publishing, 1968, with permission.)

Figure 17-11. Blood supply and somatotopic organization of the body in the ventral posterolateral and posteromedial nuclei and in the primary somatosensory (SI) cortex.

cells are also influenced by GABAergic input from the thalamic reticular nucleus and by excitatory (glutaminergic) corticothalamic fibers that arise in layer VI of the primary and secondary somatosensory cortices.

Primary Somatosensory Cortex (SI)

Axons from third-order thalamic neurons terminate in the *primary somatosensory cortex* (SI) (Figs. 17-7, 17-11, and 17-12). This cortical region is bordered anteriorly by the central sulcus and posteriorly by the postcentral sulcus and comprises the postcentral gyrus and the posterior paracentral gyrus (Fig. 17-13). The cortex contains a somatotopic representation of the body surface (a *homunculus*, or "little man"), which is laid out in a "foot-to-tongue" pattern along the medial-to-lateral axis (Fig. 17-12). Body regions, such as the hand and the lips, with a high density of receptors have a disproportionately large amount of cortical tissue dedicated to their central representation. In contrast, regions, such as the back, with low receptor density have small cortical representations (Figs. 17-3 and 17-12). Blood supply to the SI cortical areas is provided by the anterior and middle cerebral arteries. Vascular lesions involving the middle cerebral artery produce tactile loss over the contralateral upper body and face, and those involving the anterior cerebral artery affect the contralateral lower limb (Fig. 17-9).

Histologically, the primary somatosensory cortex is subdivided into four distinct areas; from anterior to posterior, these are *Brodmann areas 3a, 3b, 1,* and *2* (Fig. 17-13). Area 3a is located in the depths of the central sulcus and abuts area 4 (primary motor cortex). Areas 3b and 1 extend up the bank of the sulcus onto the shoulder of the postcentral gyrus, whereas area 2 lies

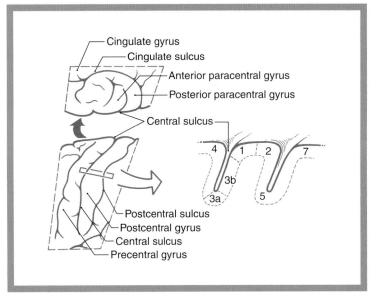

Figure 17-13. The primary somatosensory cortex (SI) of the parietal lobe. The views on the left show the location of SI in the postcentral gyrus (lateral view, *bottom*) and as it extends medially into the posterior paracentral gyrus (top view). See Figure 17-12 for an overview of the entire hemisphere. The cross section at right shows the subdivisions of the SI cortex into the four cytoarchitecturally distinct areas 3a, 3b, 1, and 2. Rostral to these is motor cortex (area 4), and caudal to them are association areas 5 and 7.

on the gyral surface and abuts area 5 (somatosensory association cortex).

Each of these four cytoarchitectural areas of the SI cortex receives submodality-specific inputs. Areas 3a and 2 are primarily targeted by neurons in the "shell" region of VPL. They receive proprioceptive inputs arising from muscle spindle afferents (mainly area 3a), Golgi tendon organs, and joint afferents (mainly area 2). These two areas are capable of processing kinesthetic information related to muscle length and tension, as well as static and transient joint position. Areas 3b and 1 are mainly targeted by neurons in the "core" region of the VPL. They receive cutaneous afferents from receptors such as Meissner corpuscles (RA) and Merkel cells (SA). In addition to receiving input that originates from cutaneous touch receptors such as Meissner and Merkel endings, areas 3b and 1 also receive input from cutaneous receptors that transmit information concerned with pain and thermal sensations. The anterolateral system, the pain pathway, is described in Chapter 18.

Small lesions in various parts of the somatosensory cortex may result in characteristic types of sensory losses. Lesions involving area 1 produce a deficit in texture discrimination, whereas damage to area 2 results in loss of size and shape discrimination *(astereognosis)*. Injury to area 3b has a more profound effect than that from damage to either area 1 or 2 alone, producing deficits in both texture and size and shape discrimination. This difference suggests that there is hierarchical processing of tactile information in SI cortex, with area 3b performing the initial processing and distributing the information to areas 1 and 2. However, it is important to remember that lesions involving the somatosensory cortex usually include larger areas and frequently result in more global deficits, such as a loss of proprioception, position sense, vibratory sense, and pain and thermal sensations on the contralateral side of the body.

Additional Cortical Somatosensory Regions
The secondary somatosensory cortex (SII) lies deep in the inner face of the upper bank of the lateral sulcus (Fig. 17-12). It, too, contains a somatotopically organized representation of the body surface. Inputs to SII cortex arise from the ipsilateral SI cortex, as well as from the ventral posterior inferior nucleus (VPI) of the thalamus, a triangle-shaped nucleus lying anterior (ventral) to VPL and VPM. This cortical area is also supplied primarily by the middle cerebral artery, so it cannot substitute functionally for SI following vascular compromise of this artery (Fig. 17-11).

Posterior to area 2, additional parietal cortical regions also receive tactile inputs. These regions include area 5 and lateral portions of area 7 (7b). The anterior pulvinar and lateral posterior group, which receive some medial lemniscal input, project to areas 5 and 7 (Fig. 17-13). In addition, they also receive input from primary somatosensory cortex. Lesions in the parietal association area can produce *agnosia*, in which contralateral body parts are lost from the personal body map. Sensation is not radically altered, but the limb is not dressed and is not recognized as part of the patient's own body.

Trigeminal System

Most of the somatosensory information from craniofacial structures, including the oral and nasal cavities, is transmitted to the brainstem over the trigeminal nerve. The relay and central processing of input from trigeminal primary afferent neurons occur in a column of brainstem neurons that begins rostrally in the middle pons and extends caudally to overlap with the posterior horn of the upper cervical spinal cord. The primary afferent neurons of the trigeminal nerve, the brainstem nuclei, and pathways described in the following discussion are referred to as the trigeminal system. Like spinal cord somatosensory pathways, trigeminal pathways can be subdivided into those for tactile discrimination, flutter-vibration, and proprioception (as described in this chapter), and those for pain and thermal sensations (as described in Chapter 18).

Trigeminal Nerve
As its name implies, the trigeminal nerve has three peripheral divisions: *ophthalmic* (V_1), *maxillary* (V_2), and *mandibular* (V_3).

A few nerve fibers in the *facial* (cranial nerve VII), the *glossopharyngeal* (cranial nerve IX), and the *vagus* (cranial nerve X) nerves transmit GSA innervation from a small cutaneous area around the ear. The peripheral distribution of these nerves delineates the facial "dermatomes" (see Chapter 18).

The cell bodies of trigeminal primary afferent neurons are located in the *trigeminal (gasserian or semilunar) ganglion* (Figs. 17-14 and 17-15) and in the mesencephalic trigeminal nucleus. The central processes of trigeminal ganglion cells form the large *sensory root (portio major)* of the trigeminal nerve as they enter the lateral aspect of the pons. Within the brainstem, central processes of most trigeminal ganglion cells bifurcate into ascending and descending branches before terminating on *second-order neurons* in the brainstem trigeminal sensory nuclei. The ascending branches terminate in the *principal sensory nucleus*, located in the pons, and the descending branches coalesce to form the *spinal (descending) tract of the trigeminal nerve*. The axons of this tract terminate throughout the rostrocaudal extent of the *spinal nucleus of the trigeminal nerve*, which lies just medial to the tract. Discussion in this chapter focuses on the more rostral components of the trigeminal system, including the *principal sensory nucleus* and the *trigeminal mesencephalic nucleus*. These nuclei and their connections are primarily involved in tactile discrimination, proprioception, and kinesthesia from the head. The role of more caudal components of the trigeminal system, which serve a primary role in pain and thermal sensations, is considered in Chapter 18.

Anterior and Posterior Trigeminothalamic Tracts

Peripheral Receptors
Tactile sensations originating in the head are transduced into nerve impulses by the same types of nerve terminals and specialized sensory receptor organs found in other parts of the body (Fig. 17-1). However, owing to their association with structures unique to this region, some of these sensory endings serve specialized functions. For example, receptors in the periodontal ligament (the primarily collagenous connective tissue surrounding each tooth) are exquisitely sensitive to tooth displacement and bite force. A large number of encapsulated receptors, particularly Meissner corpuscles, are found beneath the surface of the lips and perioral skin. The precision of two-point tactile discrimination on the lips and perioral regions is comparable with that on the fingertips. Most of the primary afferent neurons concerned with perception of discriminative sensation from the face and oral cavity have large-diameter (e.g., Aβ) axons. Some of these ascend without branching, whereas others bifurcate before terminating in the *principal sensory nucleus*.

The *principal (chief) sensory nucleus* is situated in the middle pons at the rostral pole of the spinal trigeminal nucleus (Figs. 17-14 and 17-15). The principal sensory nucleus can be divided into dorsomedial and ventrolateral regions. The *dorsomedial division* receives most of its primary afferent input from the oral cavity, and the *ventrolateral division* receives input from all three components of the trigeminal nerve. Thus, the somatotopic representation within the principal sensory nucleus is inverted, with V_1 (the ophthalmic division) being anterior, V_3 (the mandibular division) being posterior, and V_2 (the maxillary division) sandwiched in between (Fig. 17-14). This certainly is the case when the brain is viewed in the anatomic orientation, anterior/ventral is down and posterior/dorsal is up. However, when the brain is viewed in the clinical orientation, as in magnetic resonance imaging or computed tomography, the somatotopic representation of the face is upright. This point is discussed further, and illustrated, in Chapter 18.

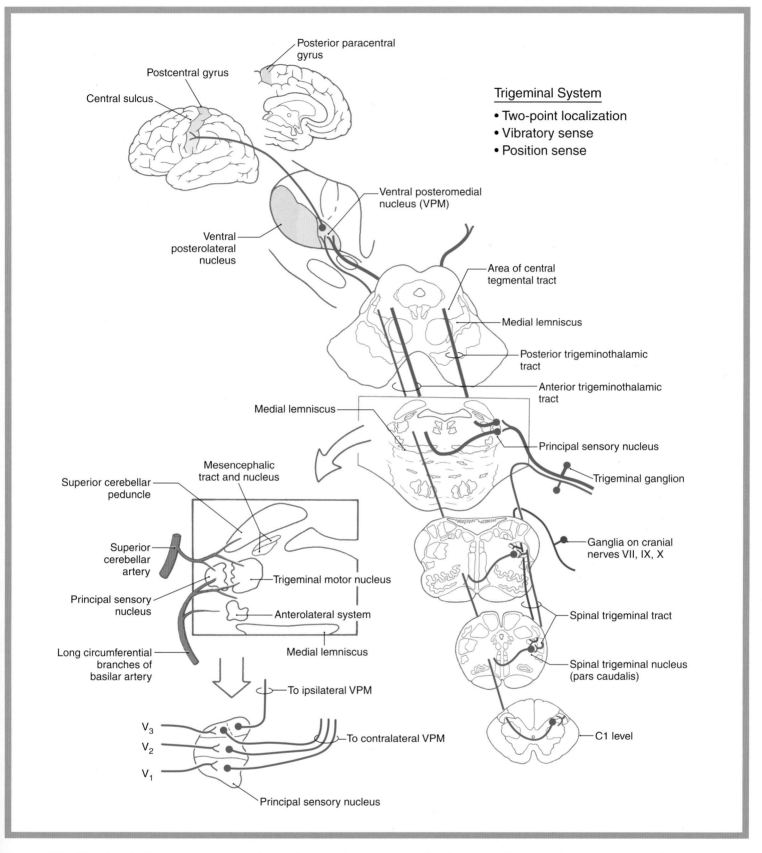

Figure 17-14. The trigeminal pathways carry two-point localization, vibratory sense, and position sense. Thick *green* lines represent large-diameter primary afferent fibers, and thin *green* lines represent smaller-diameter fibers conveying primarily thermal and nociceptive information. Note the inverted pattern of primary afferent fibers in the principal sensory nucleus.

Second-order neurons in the principal sensory nucleus have relatively small receptive fields. In addition, they are subject to the same types of intranuclear modulations as are cells in the posterior column nuclei (e.g., lateral inhibition and descending modulation from the SI cortex), which serves to sharpen the contrast between adjacent receptive fields. Neurons in the principal sensory nucleus relay discriminative tactile information from the head to the *ventral posteromedial nucleus* (VPM). Neurons in the ventrolateral part of the principal sensory nucleus give rise to axons that project to the contralateral VPM along with fibers that originate in the more caudally located spinal trigeminal nucleus. This combined ascending projection forms the *trigeminal lemniscus*, or *anterior (ventral) trigeminothalamic tract* (Figs. 17-14 and 17-15), which courses in close proximity

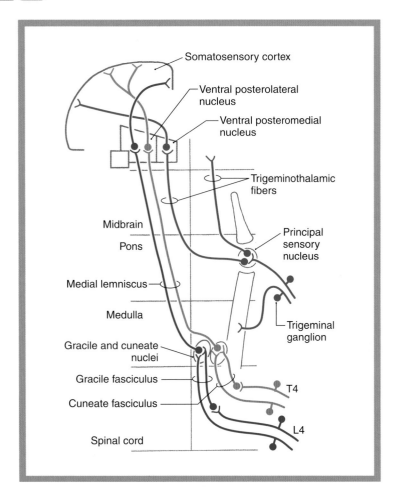

Figure 17-15. Summary of posterior column-medial lemniscal and trigeminothalamic pathways carrying discriminative touch, flutter-vibration, and position sense to the contralateral primary somatosensory cortex.

to the medial lemniscus. Neurons in the dorsomedial division of the principal sensory nucleus project to the ipsilateral VPM by way of the *posterior (dorsal) trigeminothalamic tract* (Fig. 17-14). This pathway ascends in the pontine tegmentum lateral to the periaqueductal gray in close association with the central tegmental tract. The afferent projections from the principal sensory nucleus terminate somatotopically within the VPM so that the oral cavity is represented medially and the external facial structures are represented more laterally (Figs. 17-11 and 17-14). Third-order thalamocortical neurons in the VPM project via the posterior limb of the internal capsule to the laterally placed face area of SI in the postcentral gyrus (Figs. 17-11 and 17-12). Perioral regions have the highest peripheral innervation density, and consequently the largest representation, along the postcentral gyrus (Fig. 17-12).

Proprioceptive endings (muscle spindles) in jaw muscles and some periodontal ligament receptors (modified Ruffini endings and free nerve endings) are innervated by primary afferent neurons located in the *trigeminal mesencephalic nucleus*. This brainstem nucleus consists of a slender column of pseudounipolar cells of neural crest origin that remain within the neural tube during development. Cells of the mesencephalic nucleus extend from the rostral pons to upper midbrain levels, where they form a thin band of neurons along the lateral edge of the periaqueductal gray. An important difference between the cell bodies of the mesencephalic nucleus and typical ganglion cells is that the former receive synaptic inputs from peptidergic and mono-aminergic neurons in the brainstem. This synaptic influence on the neurons of the trigeminal mesencephalic nucleus provides a unique form of presynaptic modulation before central relay of the primary afferent information.

The processes of cells in the trigeminal *mesencephalic nucleus form the mesencephalic tract of the trigeminal nerve*. This tract is located directly adjacent to the mesencephalic nucleus (Figs. 17-14 and 17-18), and also extends rostrally, where it borders the midbrain aqueductal gray. The central processes of the trigeminal mesencephalic neurons generally branch in the area posterior (dorsal) to the trigeminal motor nucleus to inner-vate cells of the motor nucleus. This input to the motor nucleus forms the afferent limb of the *myotatic jaw jerk reflex*. This clinically useful reflex consists of the processes of trigeminal mesencephalic nucleus neurons that innervate muscle spindles in jaw closing muscles and terminate monosynaptically on trigeminal motor neurons. In turn, the axons of trigeminal motor neurons innervate muscles (i.e., temporalis) that elevate the jaw. A gentle tap on the jaw activates the afferent fibers of this reflex and initiates a contraction of the homonymous muscle (e.g., temporalis) as well as its synergists (e.g., masseter). Trigeminal mesencephalic afferents from the periodontal ligament provide feedback to jaw muscle motor neurons during mastication to regulate bite force, although this input is not monosynaptic. In addition to providing collaterals to the trigeminal motor nucleus, a bundle of descending branches of mesencephalic tract fibers (called the Probst tract) distributes to the reticular formation, the spinal trigeminal nucleus, and the cerebellum. The central connections of the trigeminal mesencephalic nucleus are con-sistent with their broad participation in the coordination of oral motility patterns, including mastication, swallowing, and speech.

Proprioceptive input from the mesencephalic nucleus is also provided to the principal sensory nucleus and the spinal trigeminal nucleus. Some proprioceptive receptors are innervated by trigeminal ganglion cells, such as those with receptors in the temporomandibular joint, the extraocular muscles, and some periodontal ligaments. Because most trigeminal ganglion axons bifurcate when they enter the brainstem, both the principal sensory and the spinal trigeminal nucleus receive proprioceptive input. Proprioceptive input to the spinal trigeminal nucleus is relayed to the cerebellum, the spinal cord, and the thalamus. However, the principal sensory nucleus receives a dispropor-tionate share of large-diameter, heavily myelinated fibers and may be considered the trigeminal homologue of the posterior column nuclei. These pathways provide the substrate for cortical processing that permits the full hedonic appreciation of foods with different textural properties (oral stereognosis).

Receptive Field Properties of Cortical Neurons

Neurons located in cortical areas representing the body and head are organized into functional units called *cortical columns* (see Fig. 32-9). These are distributed from the pial surface to the cortical white matter. Each column contains neurons responsive to one submodality, and the cells in a column all have similar peripheral receptive field loci. Thalamocortical inputs terminate on stellate cells in layer IV and lower parts of layer III of the SI cortex. Axons of the stellate cells distribute information vertically to the pyramidal cells within individual columns.

The receptive field properties of cortical neurons are more complex than those at subcortical levels. Cortical neurons respond to a specific stimulus orientation (edges) and to specific textures. They are also capable of coding the velocity, speed, and direction of moving stimuli. At least three distinct populations of neurons receive proprioceptive inputs. The first consists of simple neurons that receive input from a single joint or muscle group. These rapidly adapting cells signal movement. The second group consists of postural neurons that signal the final position of a joint once the movement is completed. The third is made of neurons that receive inputs from several joints and muscle groups (multijoint) and signal complex joint-muscle interactions.

The functional properties of cortical neurons reflect the processing and integration of sensory information as it ascends from the posterior column and ventral posterior nuclei to the final processing station in the cortical columns. This sensory signal processing can include (1) convergence of afferent input, which increases receptive field size while decreasing resolution; (2) divergence of output signal, which allows relay cells to amplify the sensory signal and supply it to multiple targets; (3) facilitation; and (4) inhibition. These processes act in concert to enhance the signal-noise ratio in terms of both space and time.

In general, cortical neurons display larger receptive fields and more complex inhibitory surrounds than displayed by their sub-cortical inputs. For example, a tactile stimulus in the center of a receptive field results in amplification of the sensory signal and increased activity in a restricted population of cortical cells. Conversely, stimulation at the edge of the receptive field suppresses the activity in these neurons. This mechanism provides the circuits active in two-point discrimination.

Neuroimaging and Functional Localization

Neuroimaging techniques including functional magnetic resonance imaging (fMRI), regional cerebral blood flow (rCBF) studies, positron emission tomography (PET), and magneto-encephalography (MEG) have been used in recent clinical studies of the somatosensory pathway in humans. These techniques have elegantly demonstrated the functional organization of somatosensory areas activated by application of various tactile stimuli. For example, PET studies have identified cortical areas 3b and 1 as participating in the discrimination of moving stimuli, whereas cortical area 2 is activated when subjects palpate objects focusing on shape and curvature. Functional MRI studies have identified two areas of increased blood flow, suggesting a concomitant increase in cerebral cortical activity in response to air puff stimulation applied to various loci on the upper limb. One cortical area, located in the depth of the central sulcus, corresponds to area 3b. The other cortical locus of increased activity identified in these studies is posterior and lateral and corresponds to area 1. PET studies have also provided evidence that a tactile stimulus activates both primary (SI) and secondary somatosensory (SII) cortices.

Plasticity and Reorganization in the Primary Somatosensory Cortex

Brain injury, whether resulting from birth or other trauma, tumors, or stroke, can affect anyone and can be devastating. However, on closer examination, some individuals appear to "recover" lost functions, whereas others remain relatively unchanged. In general, the younger the person suffering the trauma, the more "recovery" is noted.

To understand possible mechanisms for this apparent recovery we must first look at brain development. The brain of a child is quite malleable or plastic. It forms multiple, redundant neural connections linking various brain areas. Many of these connections will be retained, through usage and experience, whereas others will be "pruned" by programmed cell death (apoptosis) and other cellular mechanisms. These processes will continue for a finite period of time (a critical period), thus giving many brain regions the potential to function in a variety of ways. Children suffering brain trauma due to a birth injury may appear to be quite normal with respect to sensory, motor, and cognitive abilities. It is only after inspection of a brain scan (e.g., from MRI) that the abnormal brain anatomy resulting from the injury is appreciated. The developing brain possesses the ability to reassign brain functions to other brain regions. This is commonly referred to as plasticity.

In contrast to that in children, the nervous system in the adult has passed beyond the critical periods of brain development and has become relatively nonmalleable. It has been a common view that most neural connections in the adult are stable and have lost much of their capacity to form new synapses. Evidence suggests, however, that the somatosensory cortex can undergo reorganization. An example of this phenomenon is the changes in the cortical map following limb or digit amputation. Normally (Fig. 17-16A), each digit has a sequential representation in the somatosensory cortex. When digits are amputated, there is a loss of input to the corresponding area(s) of the somatosensory cortex from the missing digits. There appears to be an expansion of cortical representation of body parts flanking the amputated digits into those cortical regions that previously had the map of the now-missing body parts (Fig. 17-16B). The cortical neurons or areas representing the missing body part now respond when skin regions adjacent to the amputated body part are stimulated. Although many of these cortical changes are subtle, one study suggests that the time course of this reorganization can be quite rapid, beginning within 10 days after amputation. Thus, it appears that the adult brain can exhibit plastic changes and undergo reorganization in response to specific peripheral perturbations. Similar phenomena have been described by molecular biologic methods within hours after experimental induction by appropriate stimuli.

A similar mechanism is also probably at work in older patients who suffer a stroke. In these patients there may initially be a complete loss, followed by a partial recovery that may extend over many months. In contrast to young patients, who may experience a complete (or almost complete) recovery, older patients may experience less than full recovery. In other words, the older the brain, the less plasticity it seems to have.

Nonconscious Proprioception: Spinocerebellar Pathways

Four spinocerebellar pathways transmit proprioceptive information and limited exteroceptive signals from cutaneous mechanoreceptors to the cerebellum (Fig. 17-17). These sensory signals include information about limb position, joint angles, and muscle tension and length. Input to the cerebellum plays an integral role in guiding cerebellar control of body muscle tone, movement, and posture.

Spinocerebellar tract axons terminate in the cerebellar nuclei and, as mossy fibers, in the vermis and paravermal region of the cerebellum. Sometimes these areas are collectively called the spinocerebellum. This afferent input to the cerebellum forms a pair of somatotopic representations of the body surface in the anterior lobe and the paravermis of the posterior lobe (Fig. 17-17). Degeneration of the major spinocerebellar tracts occurs in diseases such as Friedreich ataxia. The result is cerebellar ataxia—lack of coordination during walking and other movements that occurs because the cerebellum is not receiving the sensory feedback necessary to regulate movement.

Posterior Spinocerebellar Tract

Proprioceptive afferents and a limited number of exteroceptive (cutaneous) afferents from the lower limb and lower trunk travel in the posterior spinocerebellar tract to reach the ipsilateral cerebellar cortex (Fig. 17-17). Posterior root fibers from the trunk and lower limb terminate on cells in the dorsal nucleus of

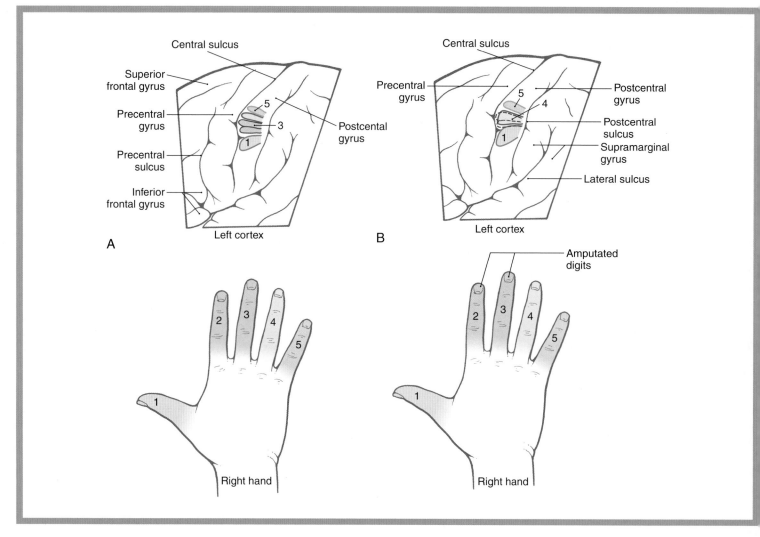

Figure 17-16. A representation of the digit region of the somatosensory cortex (**A**) and how this area is reorganized following amputation of the second and third digits (**B**).

Clarke, which is located in lamina VII of the intermediate zone in spinal segments T1 to L2. Primary afferent fibers from the spinal cord levels caudal to L2 ascend in the posterior funiculus to reach this nucleus.

Group I muscle spindle and Golgi tendon organ afferents monosynaptically activate cells in the Clarke nucleus. The discharge rate of these posterior spinocerebellar tract cells shows a linear relationship to muscle length; therefore, their firing rate can encode muscle length as a frequency code. Group II and group III tactile fibers also terminate on other spinocerebellar cells in the Clarke nucleus. Axons from cells in the dorsal nucleus of Clarke traverse the ipsilateral lateral funiculus and collect on the surface of the spinal cord lateral to the corticospinal tract. These fibers ascend to reach the cerebellum via the restiform body.

Cuneocerebellar Tract

The cuneocerebellar tract is the upper limb equivalent of the posterior spinocerebellar tract (Fig. 17-17). Posterior root fibers in spinal segments C2 to T4 carry muscle spindle and exteroceptive information in the ipsilateral cuneate fasciculus to the cuneate nucleus. In the lower medulla, proprioceptive primary afferent fibers terminate somatotopically in the *lateral cuneate nucleus.* Cells of the lateral cuneate nucleus project as *cuneocerebellar fibers* to the cerebellum via the restiform body. Exteroceptive input arising from the rostral end of the cuneate nucleus also ascends to the cerebellar cortex to terminate in the folia of the anterior lobe in lobule V.

Anterior Spinocerebellar Tract

This pathway relays information from group I afferents arising in the lower limb. The cells of origin of this pathway are located in lumbar segments L3 to L5. They are located in the lateral part of Rexed laminae V to VII, as well as along the anterolateral border of the anterior horn, where they are called *spinal border cells* (Fig. 17-17). The axons of anterior spinocerebellar tract (ASCT) cells immediately *cross the midline* in the anterior white commissure and ascend in the lateral funiculus anterior to the posterior spinocerebellar tract. In the pons, these fibers turn posterolateral to enter the cerebellum via the *superior cerebellar peduncle.* Most fibers *recross* to terminate in the cerebellum ipsilateral to their side of origin. These ASCT fibers are distributed more laterally in the cerebellum than are those of the posterior tract. Cells giving rise to ASCT fibers are strongly influenced by descending projections of the reticulospinal and corticospinal pathways. Reticulospinal input inhibits ASCT cells, and the corticospinal input facilitates ASCT cells. Vestibulospinal and rubrospinal projections also monosynaptically excite ASCT cells.

Rostral Spinocerebellar Tract

This tract, the upper limb equivalent of the ASCT, arises from cell bodies located in lamina VII of the cervical enlargement (C4 to C8) (Fig. 17-17). The efferent projections from these neurons ascend uncrossed in the lateral funiculus of the spinal cord. Although most of these axons enter the cerebellum via the restiform body, some travel in the superior cerebellar peduncle. The rostral spinocerebellar tract from the upper limb and the

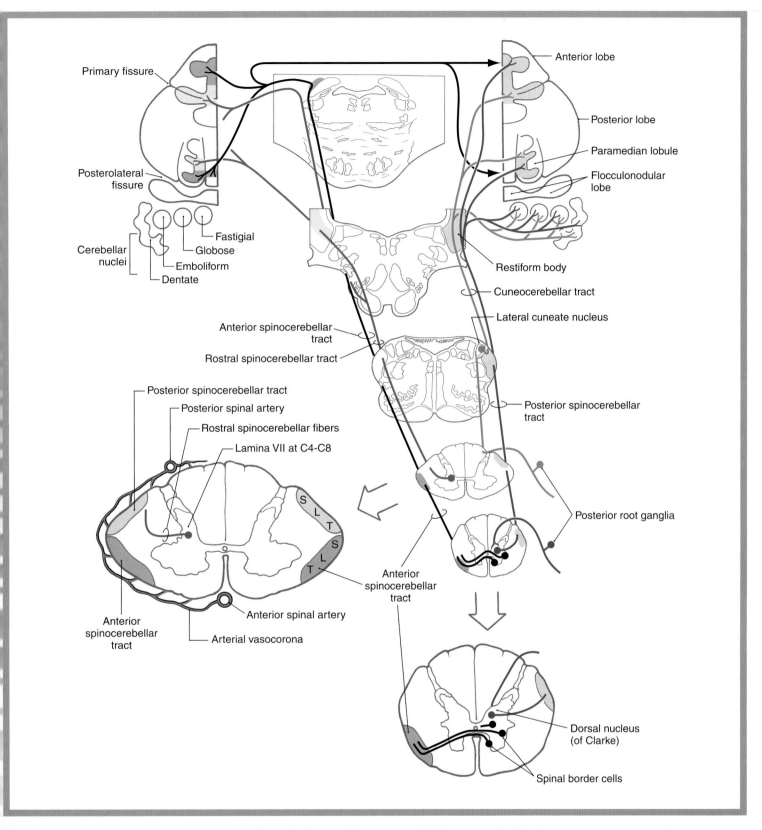

Figure 17-17. Organization of posterior, anterior, and rostral spinocerebellar tracts and of the cuneocerebellar tract.

anterior spinocerebellar tract from the lower limb relay cutaneous tactile information from Meissner, Merkel, and pacinian mechanoreceptors (group II and group III afferents) to the cerebellum.

Trigeminocerebellar Connections

The oral motor system requires continual feedback during mastication. As food is chewed, its texture and consistency are altered, changing the demands on jaw muscles. In addition, adaptation is required for long-range functional changes. For example, there are modifications in jaw motility patterns during the transition from suckling to chewing in the newborn and from natural

dentition to the use of dentures. It is probable that proprioceptive information reaching the cerebellum from jaw muscle spindles, periodontal afferents, and the temporomandibular joint is involved in these processes.

Branches of the central processes of the mesencephalic trigeminal neurons are distributed to the cerebellar hemispheres and nuclei via the superior cerebellar peduncle (Fig. 17-18). Additional proprioceptive signals from the spinal trigeminal nucleus *pars interpolaris* and *pars candalis* enter the cerebellum by way of the restiform body. They contribute a head representation to the two somatotopic maps in the cerebellar cortex.

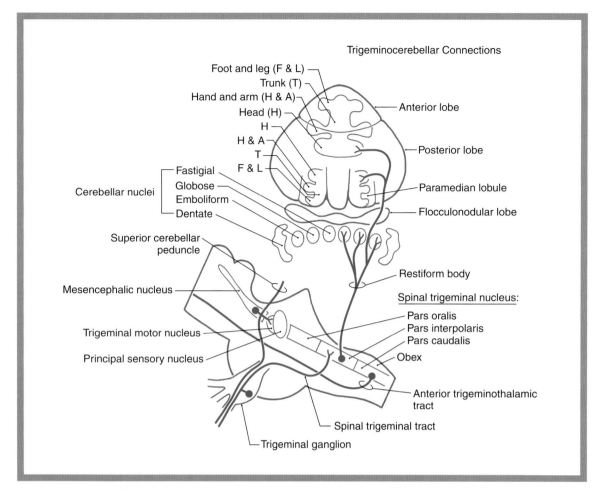

Figure 17-18. Organization of the trigeminocerebellar pathways. Foot and leg refer to the lower extremity, and hand and arm to the upper extremity.

Synopsis of Clinical Points

- Blind patients rely on slowly adapting receptors such as Merkel cell complexes (p. 264).
- The ataxia seen in tabes dorsalis is due to a loss of input via the posterior columns (p. 266).
- The causative agent in tabes dorsalis (progressive locomotor ataxia) is *Treponema pallidum* (p. 266).
- Posterior column deficits may be seen in cases of trauma or vascular compromise (p. 266).
- Lesions of the posterior column–medial lemniscus system caudal to the sensory decussation result in ipsilateral sensory deficits; lesions rostral to this decussation result in contralateral deficits (pp. 269–270).
- Vascular lesions may result in posterior column–medial lemniscus deficits at any level of the neuraxis or cerebral hemisphere (pp. 266, 269–271).
- Bilateral compromise of the posterior columns in the spinal cord result in a loss of discriminative touch, vibratory sense, and position sense bilaterally below the level of the lesion (p. 266).
- Damage to portions of the somatosensory cortex may result in astereognosis (p. 272).
- Lesions in the parietal association cortex may result in agnosia (p. 272).
- In cortical lesions there is characteristically a loss of sensory information (discriminative touch, position sense, vibratory sense, thermal sensation) on the contralateral side (p. 272).
- Damage to the sensory trigeminal root, or the principal sensory nucleus, may result in a loss of tactile discrimination, proprioception, and kinesthesia from the head (p. 272).
- The afferent and efferent limbs of the jaw jerk reflex (myotatic jaw jerk reflex) are carried on the trigeminal nerve (p. 274).
- Predetermined cell loss in the developing nervous system is accomplished through apoptosis (p. 275).
- The ability of the damaged brain, especially in the very young patient, to reassign function is called plasticity (p. 275).
- Amputation of digits, due to a medical condition, will result in remodeling/plasticity in the sensory cortex (p. 275).

Sources and Additional Reading

Bodegard A, Geyer S, Naito E, Zilles K, Roland PE: Somatosensory areas in man activated by moving stimuli: Cytoarchitectural mapping and PET. Neuroreport 11:187-191, 2000.

Bodegard A, Ledberg A, Geyer S, Naito E, Zilles K, Roland PE: Object shape differences reflected by somatosensory cortical activation in human. J Neurosci 20:Rapid Communication 51, 2000.

Brodal A: Neurological Anatomy in Relation to Clinical Medicine, 3rd ed. New York, Oxford University Press, 1981.

Burgess PR, Perl ER: Cutaneous mechanoreceptors and nociceptors. In Iggo A (ed): Handbook of Sensory Physiology, vol 2: Somatosensory System. New York, Springer-Verlag, 1973, pp 30-78.

Frot M, Mauguiere F: Timing and spatial distribution of somatosensory responses recorded in the upper bank of the sylvian fissure (SII area) in humans. Cerebral Cortex 9:854-863, 1999.

Johansson RS, Vallbo AB: Tactile sensory coding in the glabrous skin of the human hand. Trends Neurosci 6:27-32, 1983.

Johnsen-Berg H, Christensen V, Woolrich M, Matthew PM: Attention to touch modulates activity in both primary and second somatosensory areas. Neuroreport 11:1237-1241, 2000.

Jones EG: Cortical and subcortical contributions to activity-dependent plasticity in primate somatosensory cortex. Annu Rev Neurosci 23:1-37, 2000.

Kuwabara S, Mizobuchi K, Toma S, Nakajima Y, Ogawara K, Hattori T: "Tactile" sensory nerve potentials elicited by air-puff stimulation: A microneurographic study. Neurology 54:762-765, 2000.

Lenz FA, Dostrovsky JO, Tasker RR, Yamashiro K, Kwan HC, Murphy JT: Single-unit analysis of human ventral thalamic nuclear group: Somatosensory responses. J Neurophysiol 59:299-316, 1988.

Mountcastle VB: Neural mechanisms in somesthesia. In Mountcastle VB (ed): Medical Physiology, 14th ed, vol I. St. Louis, CV Mosby, 1980, pp 348-390.

Nelson RJ (ed): The Somatosensory System: Deciphering the Brain's Own Body Image. Methods & New Frontiers on Neuroscience Series, CRCPress, Boca Raton, 2002.

Parent A: Carpenter's Human Neuroanatomy, 9th ed. Baltimore, Williams & Wilkins, 1995.

Penfield W, Rasmussen T: The Cerebral Cortex of Man: A Clinical Study of Localization of Function. New York, Hafner Publishing, 1968 (Facsimile of 1950 edition).

Pizella V, Tecchio F, Romani GL, Rossini PM: Functional localization of the sensory hand area with respect to the motor central gyrus knob. Neuroreport 10:3809-3814, 1999.

Servos P, Zacks J, Rumelhart DE, Glover GH: Somatotopy of the human arm using fMRI. Neuroreport 9:605-609, 1998.

Vallbo AB, Olsson KA, Westberg K-G, Clarke FJ: Microstimulation of single tactile afferents from the human hand: Sensory attributes related to unit type and properties of receptive fields. Brain 107:727-749, 1984.

Weiss T, Miltner WHR, Huonker R, Friedel R, Schmidt I, Taub E: Rapid functional plasticity of the somatosensory cortex after finger amputation. Exp Brain Res 134:199-203, 2000.

The Somatosensory System II: Touch, Thermal Sense, and Pain

S. Warren, R. P. Yezierski, and N. F. Capra

One crucial role of the somatosensory system is to supply the brain with information related to insults that could damage tissue. These signals ascend the neuraxis in a fiber bundle called the *anterolateral system* (ALS). Anyone who has used a hammer or hot skillet has had experience with this system. Hit your thumb with a hammer and, if you are lucky, only *high-threshold mechanoreceptors* that signal excess skin deformation will be activated. If you are unlucky, tissue is damaged and the result is pain *(nociception)*. Specifically, *mechanonociceptors* have been stimulated. One common response is to gently rub the damaged area. This activates central nervous system (CNS) pathways that decrease the transmission of nociceptive signals and alter the perception of pain.

After the blow, damaged tissues release chemicals that activate another type of pain receptor, *chemonociceptors*. These receptors may contribute to the mechanism underlying long-term pain and tenderness *(hyperalgesia)*. Similarly, the temperature of a skillet is detected by *thermoreceptors* in the skin and transmitted through the ALS. If a burn is produced, the tissue damage is signaled by high-frequency firing of *thermonociceptors*. ALS activation can lead to a variety of responses, including withdrawal reflexes, the conscious perception of pain, emotional effects such as suffering, and behavioral changes aimed at avoiding the cause of the pain.

Overview

Nondiscriminative (crude or poorly localized) touch, innocuous thermal, and *pain (mechanical, chemical,* and *thermal)* sensations (from the body and back of the head) are conveyed by bundles of fibers that collectively make up the ALS. This system transmits signals originating in peripheral receptors to spinal cord and brainstem neurons (Fig. 18-1). These signals are then forwarded to thalamic nuclei and from there to the trunk and extremity representations in the primary somatosensory cortex. The *anterior trigeminothalamic pathway* (Fig. 18-1; see also Fig. 18-11) carries similar signals that originate from receptors in the face and front of the head. These are relayed through brainstem and thalamic nuclei to the face area of the somatosensory cortex. The touch fibers of the ALS differ from those described for the posterior column–medial lemniscal (PCML) system (see Chapter 17) in several ways: (1) they yield a generalized feeling of being touched but do not give precise localization, (2) their receptive fields are larger, and (3) they are smaller in diameter and more slowly conducting. Disruption of the ALS can produce symptoms ranging from reduced sensibility *(hypesthesia)*, to numbness, tingling, and prickling *(paresthesia)*, to a complete loss of sensibility *(anesthesia)*.

Anterolateral System

The ALS is a composite bundle that includes *spinothalamic, spinomesencephalic, spinoreticular, spinobulbar,* and *spinohypothalamic fibers*. Spinothalamic fibers project directly from the spinal cord to the ventral posterolateral (VPL) nucleus, the posterior nuclear group, and intralaminar nuclei (central lateral and centromedian-parafascicularis nuclei) of the thalamus. Collaterals to the reticular formation arise from some of these axons. Spinomesencephalic axons project to the periaqueductal gray (PAG) and to the tectum; the latter are *spinotectal fibers*. Although spinoreticular fibers project to the reticular formation of the medulla, pons, and midbrain, collaterals may ascend to other targets such as the thalamus. Projections of less relevance to the somatosensory system, such as *spino-olivary fibers*, are grouped under the category of *spinobulbar fibers*. Spinohypothalamic fibers terminate in hypothalamic areas and nuclei, including some that give rise to hypothalamospinal axons.

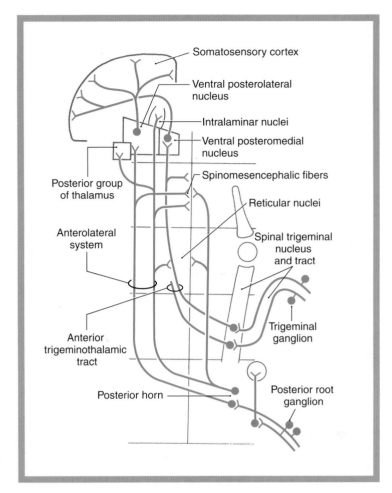

Figure 18-1. Summary of anterolateral system and anterior trigeminothalamic tract fibers conveying nondiscriminative tactile, thermal, and nociceptive inputs to the contralateral somatosensory cortex.

Fibers classically described as composing the lateral spinothalamic tract were considered to carry *only* pain and thermal information, whereas the anterior spinothalamic tract was concerned *only* with nondiscriminative touch. This older view of separate tracts conveying separate types of information is not used in this chapter. Current thinking holds that all parts of the ALS carry all modalities (pain, temperature, and touch) but that there are direct and indirect routes. The former is the *neospinothalamic pathway* (spinal cord → thalamus), whereas the latter is the polysynaptic *paleospinothalamic pathway* (spinal cord → reticular formation → thalamus). Both of these pathways, plus other fibers as defined previously, collectively form the ALS.

Receptors and Primary Neurons

The receptors for nondiscriminative touch, innocuous thermal stimuli, and nociceptive stimuli are distributed in glabrous and hairy skin, as well as in deep tissues including joints and muscles (Table 18-1). Morphologically, these receptors are all *free (naked) nerve endings* (see Fig. 17-1); that is, they lack specialized receptor cells or encapsulations. Because of this lack, the basis for their submodality specificity is unclear. These submodalities are transduced by activation of peripheral branches of either *thinly myelinated Aδ fibers* or *unmyelinated C fibers*. The density of free nerve endings and the corresponding size of receptive fields vary over the body surface in the same way as for other cutaneous receptors (see Fig. 17-3), being highest on the hands and in the perioral area. Regardless of size or location, however, each field is exquisitely sensitive to thermal, chemical, or mechanical stimuli.

Nociceptors (pain receptors) are found in cutaneous as well as in deep structures. Two major classes of cutaneous pain receptors

Table 18-1. Classification of Cutaneous Mechanical, Thermal, and Nociceptive Receptors Using Small-Diameter Fibers and Their Adequate Stimuli

Receptor	Stimulus
Cutaneous Mechanoreceptors	Respond to nondiscriminative tactile
Aδ and C fiber high-threshold	stimuli
mechanoreceptors	Pinch, rub, stretch, squeeze
Cutaneous Thermo- receptors	Respond to transient changes in temperature
Warm and cool thermoreceptors	Innocuous warm and cool stimuli
Cutaneous Nociceptors	Mediate cutaneous pain
Aδ mechanonociceptors	Mechanical tissue damage
C-polymodal nociceptors	Mechanical tissue damage, noxious thermal stimuli, algesic compounds
Other Cutaneous Nociceptors	Mediate cutaneous pain
C fiber mechanonociceptors	Mechanical tissue damage
Aδ, heat thermonociceptors	Noxious thermal stimuli, tissue damage (?)
Aδ, C fiber cold thermonociceptors	Noxious thermal stimuli, tissue damage (?)
C fiber chemonociceptors	Algesic compounds

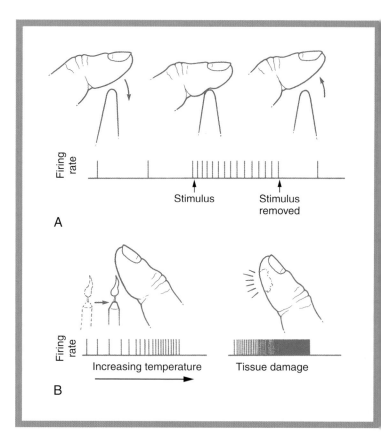

Figure 18-2. Fibers conveying information from high-threshold mechanoreceptors (**A**) respond to the application of a punctate stimulus. Thermoreceptors show a graded response to increases in temperature (**B**, *left*), whereas burns produced by prolonged thermal stimulation evoke high-frequency response in thermonociceptors (**B**, *right*).

have been identified. They are the Aδ (A-delta) *mechanical nociceptors* and the C-*polymodal nociceptors*. These receptors are found at the end of the peripheral processes of thinly myelinated (Aδ) or nonmyelinated (C) fibers (Table 18-1). The cutaneous receptive field of an *Aδ nociceptor* consists of a number of small sensitive spots (2 to 30) scattered over an area of skin. Each spot ranges from 50 to 180 μm in diameter. Aδ mechanical nociceptors respond to mechanical injury accompanied by tissue damage. C-polymodal nociceptors respond to mechanical, thermal, and chemical stimuli. The cutaneous receptive field of a *C-polymodal nociceptor* usually consists of one to two sensitive spots, with each spot covering an area of skin of 1 to 2 mm². For a comparable region of skin, the C-fiber spots are larger but fewer in number than the Aδ spots, which are smaller but more numerous. In addition, other cutaneous receptors that respond to high threshold or noxious stimuli have been identified. They include receptors that respond to temperature changes (thermoreceptors or thermonociceptors) (Table 18-1) and receptors that respond to chemicals, irritants, or algesic compounds (chemonociceptors) (Table 18-1).

Nondiscriminative touch results from the stimulation of free nerve endings that act as non-noxious *high-threshold mechanoreceptors* (Table 18-1). These receptors respond to any rough stimulus, including tapping, squeezing, rubbing, and stretching of the skin, that does not result in tissue damage (Fig. 18-2A). Nerve fibers associated with these receptors generally have no background activity when unstimulated and when stimulated they respond with a sustained discharge that signals stimulus duration (Fig. 18-2A).

Non-nociceptive *thermoreceptors* fall into two classes: those activated by heat (35-45°C) and those activated by cold (17-35°C). They show a graded response to changes in ambient temperature (Fig. 18-2B). With repeated stimulation, these receptors become sensitized and show a decreased threshold and larger response to the application of a stimulus. Levels of heat (>45°C) or cold (<17°C) that burn or freeze the skin produce high-frequency firing in both Aδ and C *thermonociceptors* (Fig. 18-2B).

Tissue damage causes the release of a number of chemical substances that activate a class of free nerve endings called *chemonociceptors* (Table 18-1). Specifically, chemonociceptors are activated by the release of endogenous substances such as

bradykinin, H⁺ ions, and foreign irritants such as insect venoms. These free nerve endings are the peripheral processes of C fibers.

Peripheral Sensitization and Primary Hyperalgesia

Pain receptors, unlike Meissner corpuscles or Merkel cells, demonstrate a unique phenomenon called *sensitization*. Following an insult, these receptors become more sensitive (lower pain threshold) and thus more responsive (increases in firing rate) to noxious stimulation within their receptive fields. Although the mechanisms responsible for receptor sensitization are not completely known, chemicals released by the damaged skin or byproducts from plasma, or both, are thought to contribute to this phenomenon. As a result of this heightened sensitivity, the affected area is exquisitely sensitive to painful stimuli and patients experience a sensory disturbance called *hyperalgesia* (exaggerated response to a painful stimuli). This condition can be differentiated into *primary hyperalgesia* and *secondary hyperalgesia*. *Primary hyperalgesia* occurs in the region of damaged skin and is probably the result of receptor sensitization. *Secondary hyperalgesia* occurs in the skin bordering the damaged tissue. Although receptor sensitization may contribute to secondary hyperalgesia, there is likely to be a central (e.g., spinal) component as well.

Central Sensitization and Secondary Hyperalgesia

Sensitization of peripheral nociceptors causes an increase in spontaneous activity in the Aδ and C fibers. The central processes of these fibers enter the posterior horn of the spinal cord, where they activate posterior horn neurons. Ongoing inputs from these injured peripheral nociceptors evoke a number of changes in the central processing of sensory information by the posterior horn neurons. These changes include a marked increase in the receptive field size of the posterior horn neuron (to include skin areas not involved in the initial injury), an increased response of the cells to the application of suprathreshold stimuli, a decreased threshold to stimulus application in the receptive field, and activation of the cell by novel inputs (e.g., a light breeze). This phenomenon is known as *central sensitization*, and it represents *a potentiated state in which the system has been shifted from one functional level (normal) to another (sensitized) by a change in transcription*. In some persons, an innocuous stimulus, such as a gentle breeze or a light touch, can evoke pain sensation in the skin bordering the damaged tissue. The perception of an innocuous stimulus as painful is referred to as *allodynia* and can be the result of central sensitization.

Pain Receptors in Muscles, Joints, and Viscera

In addition to the cutaneous pain receptors, pain receptors in muscles, joints, and viscera have also been identified (Table 18-2). *Muscle pain* is mediated by receptors of both group III (thinly myelinated) and group IV (nonmyelinated) afferent fibers. Excessive stretch or contraction following strenuous exertion may activate the muscle pain receptors of group III fibers. Receptors of the group IV fibers may be activated in response to the release of algesic compounds after muscle injury or ischemia. *Joint pain*, including arthritis, may be caused by inflammation. This pain is mediated by receptors associated with group III and group IV fibers. *Visceral pain* is often described as being diffuse and difficult to localize and is frequently referred to an overlying somatic body location. In addition, visceral pain usually involves autonomic reflexes. Visceral pain receptors located in the heart, respiratory structures, the gastrointestinal tract, and the urogenital tract are poorly identified (Table 18-2). These receptors can be activated by intense mechanical stimuli

including overdistention or traction, ischemia, and endogenous compounds, including bradykinin, prostaglandins, H⁺ ions, and K⁺ ions. Activation of these receptors produces pain.

Of the two primary afferent fiber types carrying nociceptive sensations, Aδ fibers have a slightly faster conduction velocity (5 to 30 m/s) than that of C fibers. They carry well-localized sensations, which do not evoke an affective component to the sensory experience. A pinprick, used clinically to test ALS function, is one stimulus that activates Aδ fibers. On the other hand, C fibers are smaller and conduct more slowly (0.5 to 2 m/s). They transmit poorly localized sensations that produce a noticeable affective component. For example, the dull, persistent ache that follows a muscle pull results from activation of C fibers. Both Aδ and C fibers are considerably smaller and conduct more slowly than fibers of the PCML system. *Nerve blocks* or *anoxia* preferentially affects large-diameter, heavily myelinated fibers and thus usually results in loss of discriminative tactile, vibratory, and postural sensations to varying degrees. *Local anesthetics*, such as lidocaine or bupivacaine, preferentially affect small-diameter Aδ and C fibers and thus result in loss of nociception *(analgesia)*.

The cell bodies of C and Aδ fibers are generally small compared with other pseudounipolar neurons in the posterior root ganglion. The central processes of these cells enter the spinal cord via the lateral division of the posterior root (see Fig. 17-5). Many smaller fibers contain excitatory amino acids such as glutamate, as well as peptides such as substance P and calcitonin gene-related peptide (CGRP), which may serve as neurotransmitters. The central processes of these fibers also contain surface membrane receptors. They include an adenosine triphosphate (ATP) receptor, a γ-aminobutyric acid (GABA) receptor, a serotonin (5-hydroxytryptophan) receptor, and a mu opioid receptor (MOR). Pharmacologic therapies, as well as descending inhibitory fibers, can act at these *presynaptic sites* and suppress the initiation of the pain signal. In addition to their normal trajectory into the posterior horn, a small number of C fibers enter the spinal cord through the anterior root of a spinal nerve. It is possible that these fibers provide a basis for the return of pain after *posterior rhizotomy*, a procedure in which posterior roots are sectioned in an attempt to alleviate intractable pain.

The strip of skin that is innervated by the peripheral cutaneous branches of a given spinal nerve is called a *dermatome* (Figs. 18-3 and 18-4). The central processes of these nerves that convey cutaneous input terminate in the posterior horn. It is clinically useful to examine dermatomes that have relationships to landmarks on the body: for example, C7 for the index finger, the T4-T5 border at the nipples, T10 at the navel, L1 along

Table 18-2. Classification of Deep and Visceral Nociceptors and Their Adequate Stimuli

Receptor	Adequate Stimulus
Muscle Nociceptors	Mediate muscle pain
Group III afferent fibers	Bradykinin, 5-HT, K⁺ ions, prostaglandin (PGE₂)
Group IV afferent fibers	Bradykinin, 5-HT, K⁺ ions, prostaglandin (PGE₂)
Joint Nociceptors	Mediate joint pain: arthritis (?)
Group III afferent fibers	Inflammation (e.g., K⁺, bradykinin) kaolin, carrageenan
Group IV afferent fibers	Inflammation (e.g., K⁺, bradykinin) kaolin, carrageenan
Visceral Nociceptors	Mediate visceral pain
Heart	
Aδ and C afferent fibers	Prostaglandin (PGE₂), H⁺ ions, bradykinin, K⁺ ions, ischemia
Respiratory System	
Lung irritant receptors (Aδ fibers)	Irritant aerosols and gases, mechanical stimuli
J receptors (C fibers?)	Capsaicin, pulmonary congestion or edema, inhaled irritants
Gastrointestinal Tract	
Rapidly adapting mechanoreceptors, slowly adapting mechanoreceptors, chemoreceptors (Aδ and C fibers?)	Irritation of the mucosa, distention, powerful contraction, torsion, traction, bloat, cramping, appendicitis, impaction
Urogenital Tract	
C-polymodal nociceptors: testis	Intense mechanical stimuli, noxious heat, algesic chemicals

5-HT, 5-hydroxytryptamine.

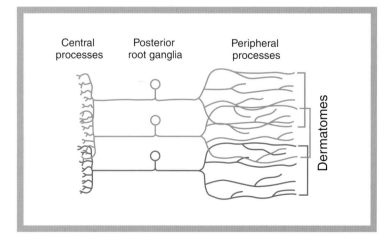

Figure 18-3. The dermatomes formed by the peripheral processes of adjacent spinal nerves overlap on the body surface (see Fig. 18-4). The central processes of these fibers also overlap in their spinal distribution.

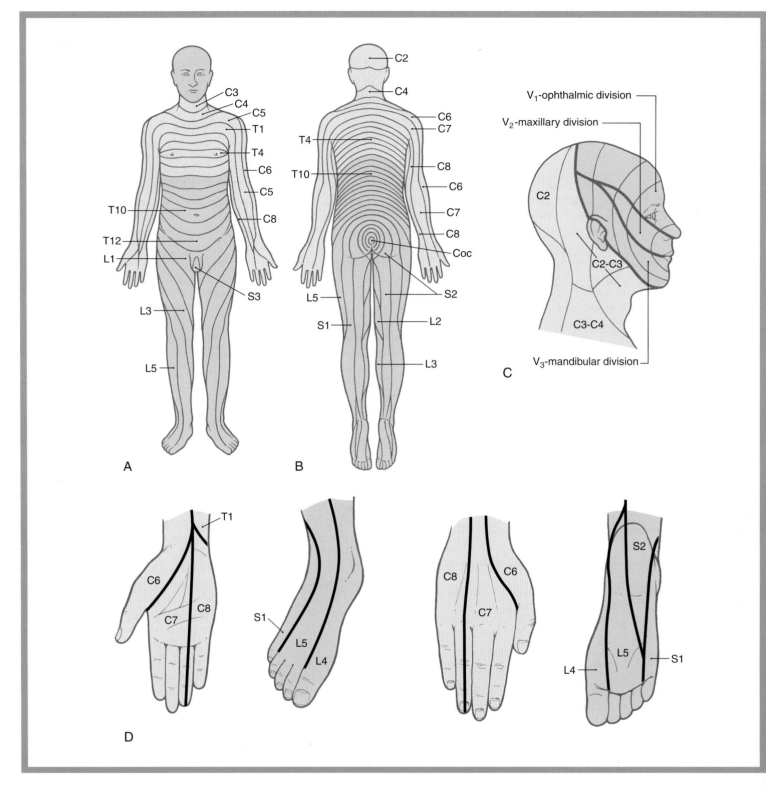

Figure 18-4. A representation of the dermatomal maps on the anterior (**A**) and posterior (**B**) surfaces of the body, on the face (**C**), and on the hands and feet (**D**). The patterns of the body may vary slightly from patient to patient, but the more commonly used landmarks are shown here and include the shoulder (C5-C6), hand (C6-C8), nipple (T4), umbilicus (T10), inguinal region (T12-L1), knee (L3, L4), and the great toe (L4). More can easily be filled in from these landmarks.

the pelvic rim, L5 for the big toe, and S4 and S5 for the genitalia and anus (Fig. 18-4). There is overlap between both the peripheral and central distribution of adjacent spinal nerves and consequently between their dermatomes (Fig. 18-3). This overlap reduces the effects of injury to a single spinal root.

Shingles *(herpes zoster)* is a disease of viral etiology that is noteworthy for its dermatomal distribution (Fig. 18-5). Subsequent to a bout of chickenpox, viral DNA may infect and become latent in trigeminal and posterior root ganglion cells. The virus may reactivate periodically, producing infectious virions that travel down the peripheral processes of the neurons to

produce a painful skin irritation in the dermatomal distribution of the ganglion (Fig. 18-5). When an injury or disease process affects a series of nerve roots, the result is diminished sensibility *(hypesthesia)* over the dermatomes served by those roots. The borders of the hypesthetic region correspond to dermatomal boundaries. However, the most debilitating aspect of this disease is a poorly understood recurrence of pain. Known as *postherpetic neuralgia,* this condition is a neuropathic pain.

Clinically, it is important to test patients for intact ALS and PCML systems function. In testing the ALS, a single pin point applied to the skin should evoke a response *(perception of pain)*

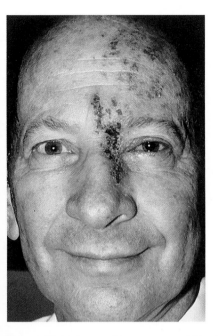

Figure 18-5. A case of herpes zoster (shingles) in a male adult. The ophthalmic division of the trigeminal nerve is involved; note that the lesions do not cross the midline. The border between the ophthalmic and maxillary divisions on the lateral aspect of the nose may very slightly between patients.

from the patient. Function of the intact PCML system is tested by the simultaneous application of two points spaced at measured intervals. As the points are moved closer, the ability to identify them as separate stimuli *(two-point discrimination)* decreases and eventually disappears. The PCML system is also tested by applying a 128-Hz tuning fork (vibratory sense) to a bony prominence or the tip of a finger or toe. The patient perceives this as a buzzing sensation. It is common to test both pain/thermal sense and discriminative touch/vibratory sense on both sides of the face and body to see if there are asymmetries.

Central Pathways

As mentioned previously, Aδ and C fibers enter the spinal cord via the *lateral division* of the *posterior root entry zone*. The fibers enter the posterolateral fasciculus *(Lissauer tract)* and bifurcate into ascending and descending branches (see Fig. 17-5). Some collaterals terminate on interneurons in the spinal gray matter. These connections participate in the circuits that mediate spinal reflexes such as the *flexor withdrawal reflex* (see Chapter 9).

Posterior horn neurons exhibit numerous surface membrane receptors. These include NK1 (the substance P receptor), a GABA receptor, a serotonin receptor, a mu opioid receptor, a receptor for glycine, and an AMPA receptor for glutamate. Descending inhibitory fibers can act on the *postsynaptic sites* and can effectively block forward transmission of the pain signal.

The functional properties of posterior horn neurons reflect the type of primary afferent fiber input received. These neurons are classified as *low-threshold* (non-nociceptive), *nociceptive-specific* (noxious), *wide dynamic range* (non-nociceptive and noxious), or *deep* on the basis of their responses to different stimulus modalities.

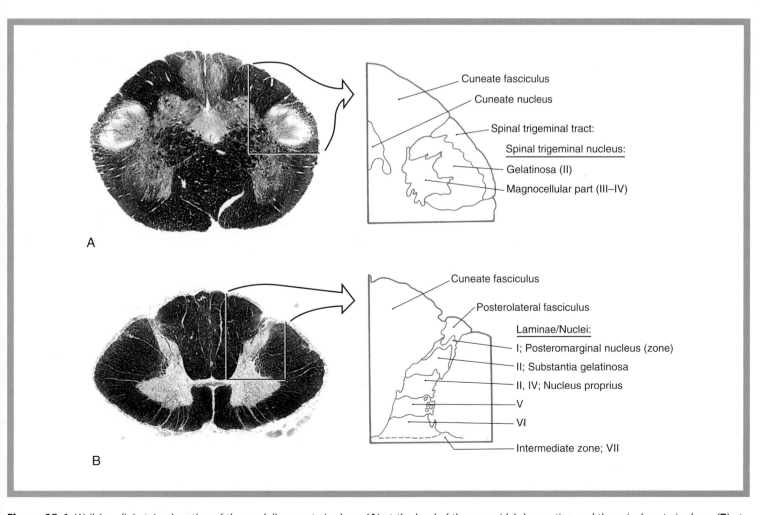

Figure 18-6. Weil (myelin)-stained section of the medullary posterior horn (**A**) at the level of the pyramidal decussation and the spinal posterior horn (**B**) at levels C7 to C8. The spinal laminae that correspond to medullary structures are labeled.

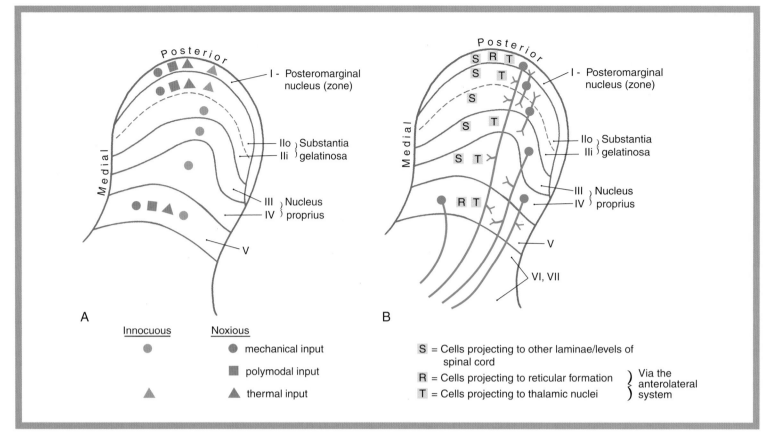

Figure 18-7. Summary of posterior horn laminae and their major sensory inputs (**A**) and major outputs (**B**).

The central target of nociceptive primary afferent fibers includes laminae I, II, and V of the posterior horn (Fig. 18-6). Aδ fibers target laminae I and V. Rexed lamina I, the *posteromarginal nucleus* (or *zone*), receives mainly input from Aδ fibers (Fig. 18-7A). Neurons in this nucleus (or zone) project to other spinal cord laminae, the brainstem reticular formation, and the thalamus (Fig. 18-7B). Lamina II, the *substantia gelatinosa*, is divided into outer (IIo) and inner (IIi) layers. Input to IIo and IIi is derived primarily from C fiber primary afferents, and IIi also receives input from collaterals of non-nociceptive afferent fibers. Lamina II contains excitatory and inhibitory interneurons that project to other laminae of the posterior horn. In addition, some neurons in IIo are involved in relaying sensory information to supraspinal sites, including the thalamus (Fig. 18-7B).

Neurons in laminae III and IV, the *nucleus proprius* (also called the *posterior proper sensory nucleus*), receive non-noxious inputs from the periphery. Cells in these laminae project to deeper laminae of the spinal cord, to the posterior column nuclei, and to other supraspinal relay centers including the midbrain, thalamus, and hypothalamus (Fig. 18-7B).

Lamina V neurons receive both noxious and non-noxious (nociceptive and non-nociceptive) inputs and project to the medullary and mesencephalic reticular formation, thalamus, and hypothalamus (Fig. 18-7B). Neurons in deeper laminae of the spinal gray receive (directly and indirectly) noxious and non-noxious inputs and connect with neurons in other spinal cord levels *(propriospinal connections)*.

As mentioned previously, the fibers of the ALS participate in both direct and indirect spinothalamic pathways (Fig. 18-1). Most Aδ fibers participate in the *direct (neospinothalamic)* pathway, which carries nondiscriminative tactile, innocuous thermal, and nociceptive signals. When these Aδ fibers enter the posterolateral fasciculus and bifurcate, their branches travel rostrocaudally for three to five spinal levels. The descending branches terminate on interneurons within the spinal gray that participate in segmental spinal reflexes. The ascending branches terminate on second-order neurons (tract cells) in lamina I of the posterior horn (Fig. 18-7A). These tract cells, in turn, project to the thalamus. The great majority of their axons cross the midline of the spinal cord obliquely via the anterior (ventral) white commissure and ascend in the contralateral ALS. A few ascend in the *ipsilateral* ALS. The thalamic (third-order) neurons of these pathways are located mainly in the VPL, the posterior nucleus, and the intralaminar nuclei.

The polysynaptic *indirect (paleospinothalamic)* component of the ALS relays noxious and innocuous mechanical and thermal information to the brainstem reticular formation. The input to this pathway originates chiefly from C fibers. Branches of these fibers ascend and descend by one or two levels in the posterolateral fasciculus to synapse on interneurons in laminae II and III (Fig. 18-7B). These interneurons influence tract cells in laminae V to VIII, which send axons that cross obliquely through the anterior white commissure (over a distance of one to three segments) to join the contralateral ALS. These *spinoreticular fibers* terminate in the brainstem reticular formation, which in turn projects to the thalamus.

Fibers in the ALS are arranged *somatotopically* in the spinal cord. Axons from lower levels (coccygeal and sacral) of the body are found posterolaterally, whereas those from more rostral levels of the cord are added in an orderly anteromedial sequence (Figs. 18-8 and 18-9). The deficits seen in patients with certain types of spinal cord lesions reflect this somatopical pattern (Fig. 18-8). For example, an intramedullary tumor that expands laterally results in a loss of pain and thermal sensations that initially begins in cervical levels on the contralateral side and proceeds caudally as the lesion enlarges. On the other hand, an extramedullary tumor that expands medially results in a loss of these same sensations that first begins in lumbosacral levels on the contralateral side and proceeds rostrally as the lesion expands (Fig. 18-8).

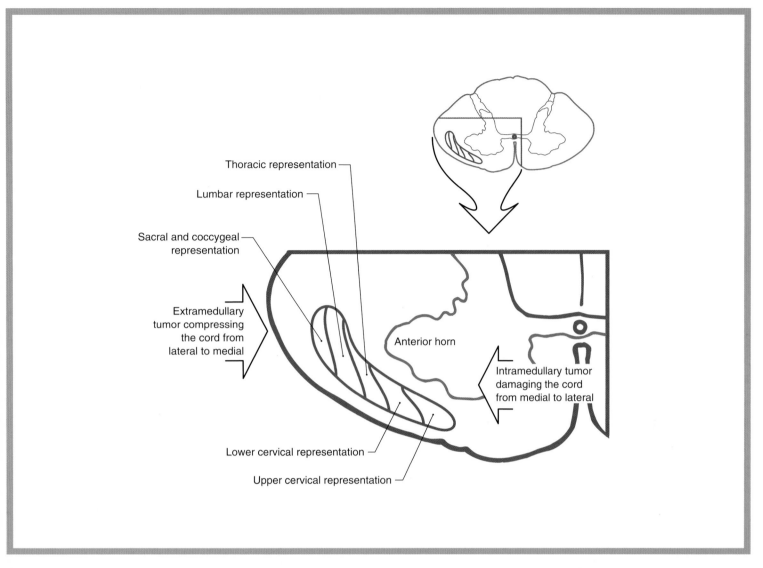

Figure 18-8. The general somatotopic arrangement of the anterolateral system; lower portions of the body are represented more posterolaterally and upper portions are represented anteromedially. Ascending deficits may result from expanding extramedullary lesions, while descending deficits may be seen in patients with expanding intramedullary lesions; all deficits would be experienced on the side contralateral to the lesion.

Because of its location, the ALS does not receive blood supply from a single vessel. Instead, its blood supply originates from the *arterial vasocorona* and via *sulcal branches* of the *anterior spinal artery* (Fig. 18-8). Consequently, occlusion of either of these vessels results in a *patchy loss of nociceptive, thermal*, and *touch sensations over* the contralateral side of the body beginning about two spinal segments below the lesion. In contrast, a *complete loss of these sensations* is seen in patients who have had an *anterolateral cordotomy* for relief of intractable pain.

The ALS may be involved in trauma or diseases of the spinal cord. For example, a hemisection of the spinal cord (as in the *Brown-Séquard syndrome*) results in a combination of sensory and motor losses. Sensory deficits include (1) *contralateral* loss of nociceptive and thermal sensations over the body below the level of the lesion (ALS damage) and (2) *ipsilateral* loss of discriminative tactile, vibratory, and position sense over the body below the level of the lesion (posterior column damage) (Fig. 18-10A). The motor loss is manifested as an ipsilateral paralysis of the leg or leg and arm, depending on the level of the hemisection (see Chapter 24).

Syringomyelia, a condition in which there is cystic cavitation of central regions of the spinal gray matter, may impinge on the anterior white commissure and decussating ALS fibers (Fig. 18-10B). When located at the C4 to C5 levels of the spinal cord, this lesion produces *bilateral loss* of nondiscriminative

tactile, nociceptive, and thermal sensations beginning several segments below the level where the fibers are interrupted. The symptoms present as sensory losses in the configuration of a cape draped over the shoulders and extending down to nipple level.

In the medulla, ALS fibers retain their position near the anterolateral surface. They are located anterior to the spinal trigeminal nucleus and posterolateral to the inferior olive and remain separated from the PCML system as both course through the medulla and pons (Figs. 18-9 and 18-11). Therefore, *vascular lesions or tumors in the lower brainstem can affect discriminative touch and nociception differentially*. For example, a lesion in medial portions of the medulla may result in a contralateral loss of discriminative touch and vibratory sense but not of pain and thermal sensation; this is a *dissociated sensory loss* (one modality absent but not another). At the pontomedullary junction the medial lemniscus begins to rotate to a mediolateral orientation (see Fig. 12-11). By midpontine levels the ALS is adjacent to the lateral extreme of the medial lemniscus (Figs. 18-9 and 18-11); this is the portion of the medial lemniscus containing fibers relaying information from the contralateral lower extremity. Within the midbrain ALS fibers retain their position adjacent to the lateral aspect of the medial lemniscus (Figs 18-9 and 18-11), even though this latter structure has been shifted somewhat laterally by the decussation of the superior cerebellar peduncle and the red nucleus. Thereafter, the PCML and ALS

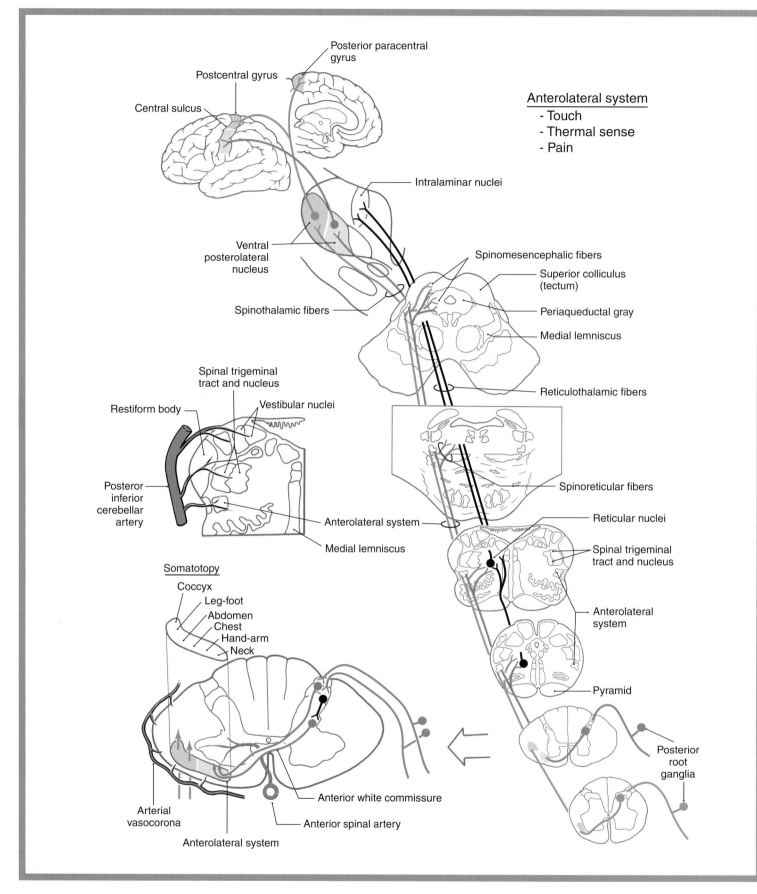

Figure 18-9. The anterolateral system in its entirety and blood supply to these fibers in the spinal cord and medulla.

pathways course together to terminate in the thalamus (Figs. 18-9 and 18-11).

As the ALS ascends through the medulla, it decreases in size because of the departure of the *spinoreticular axons*, which originate in laminae V to VIII and terminate in the reticular formation. The reticular formation also receives *collaterals from*

lamina I spinothalamic axons (Fig. 18-9). Several other pathways ascend in the ALS. For example, spinomesencephalic axons may terminate in the PAG or, as *spinotectal fibers*, in deep layers of the superior colliculus and anterior pretectum. Many tract cells with axons in the ALS project via collaterals to multiple targets as the primary axon ascends through the brainstem.

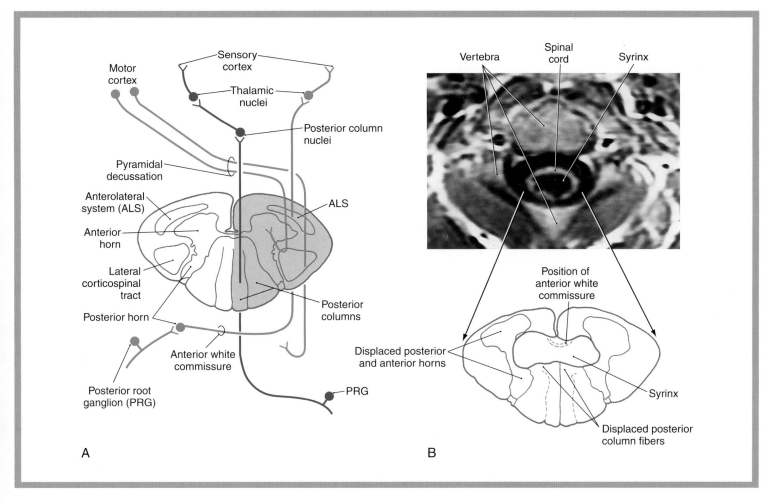

Figure 18-10. Major tracts interrupted in a spinal cord hemisection (**A**, Brown-Séquard syndrome) that account for the characteristic sensory and motor losses. MR image of a cervical syringomyelia (**B**) with resultant expansion of the lesion into fibers of the anterior white commissure. In both **A** and **B**, the cross section of the spinal cord is shown in an orientation identical to that seen in the clinical setting.

In addition to direct spinothalamic fibers, spinal cord neurons also project to brainstem targets that indirectly influence thalamic nuclei. Most notably, the reticular formation, which receives *spinoreticular fibers*, projects via *reticulothalamic fibers* to the intralaminar nuclei and posterior group (Fig. 18-9). The intralaminar nuclei project to the striatum and wide areas of cerebral cortex and subserve the alerting response to painful stimuli. Nuclei of the posterior thalamic group project to the secondary somatosensory (SII) cortex and to the retroinsular cortex. These polysynaptic pathways may underlie the dull, poorly localized, but persistent painful sensations that are perceived with localized thalamic lesions.

Somatosensory information, including nociceptive input from posterior horn cells, also ascends directly to the hypothalamus via the *spinohypothalamic fibers* of the ALS. In addition, spinal input is indirectly conveyed to the hypothalamus by way of synaptic relays in the reticular formation and in the PAG (Fig. 18-19). Through these ascending pathways, nociceptive information is transmitted to brain centers, such as the limbic system, that underlie emotional and autonomic responses to nociceptive stimuli.

Input to the VPL is somatotopically organized such that lower body areas are represented laterally and that upper body regions (exclusive of the head) are represented medially (Figs. 18-10 and 18-12). Within the VPL, fibers of the ALS terminate on clusters of cells located in the periphery of the nucleus. Most of these cells are different from the ones targeted by PCML axons. However, some VPL neurons, called *multinodal cells*, receive input from both ALS and PCML pathways. The functional classes of cells found in VPL reflect the peripheral input received by tract cells of the spinal cord. These classes include, as in the spinal cord, *nociceptive-specific, wide dynamic range, low-threshold non-nociceptive,* and *deep neurons.*

Thalamocortical axons carrying nondiscriminative tactile, nociceptive, and thermal signals project via the posterior limb of the internal capsule to the somatosensory cortices (Figs. 18-9 and 18-11). Fibers originating in the VPL project mainly to SI cortex (areas 3, 1, and 2), whereas those from the posterior nucleus terminate principally in the SII cortex. The somatotopy observed in the VPL is reflected in the cortex. Thalamocortical fibers from lateral areas of the VPL project to the *posterior paracentral gyrus* (thigh, leg, and foot), whereas progressively more medial parts of the VPL project in an orderly manner to sequentially more lateral areas of the *postcentral gyrus* (Figs. 18-9, 18-11, and 18-12). These thalamocortical fibers terminate primarily at the 3b/1 border on specific physiologic classes of SI neurons: *low-threshold non-nociceptive, nociceptive-specific,* and *wide dynamic range cells.* Loss of nociceptive and thermal sensations over the contralateral body and face can result from vascular compromise of either the middle (for trunk, upper extremity, and face) or the anterior (for the lower extremity) cerebral artery (Fig. 18-12). Not only the sensation but also the ability to localize is lost.

Not all nociceptive information reaches the thalamus via the ALS. The *spinocervicothalamic pathway* is a supplemental multimodal pathway that carries discriminative innocuous tactile information as well as nociceptive signals (Fig. 18-13). This pathway begins with afferent fibers that terminate on second-order cells in laminae III and IV of the posterior horn. The axons of these second-order cells travel in the *ipsilateral lateral*

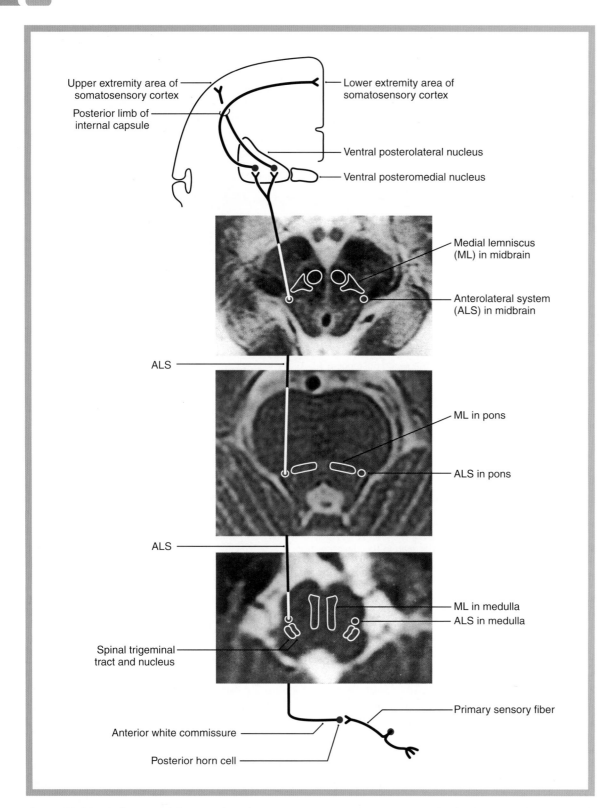

Figure 18-11. The location of the anterolateral system in MR images at representative levels of the medulla, pons, and midbrain. This illustrates the location of fibers comprising the anterolateral system when viewed in images routinely used in the clinical setting.

funiculus to spinal levels C1 and C2, where they terminate on third-order neurons in the *lateral cervical nucleus*. The axons of these cells decussate at the level of the spinomedullary junction and ascend in the medial lemniscus (Fig. 18-13). Like PCML axons, these *cervicothalamic axons* terminate in the VPL nucleus. This pathway is not essential for pain perception and is not especially prominent in humans. However, these fibers and the uncrossed axons in the ALS may be the basis for the retention of some nociceptive function after lesions involving the ALS or for the return of pain perception after *anterolateral cordotomy*.

Spinal Trigeminal Pathway: Anterior Trigeminothalamic Tract

Primary Neurons

Cranial nerves V, VII, IX, and X serve the cutaneous receptors of the face, the oral cavity, and the dorsum of the head except for the area served by the cervical nerves (Figs. 18-14 and 18-15). In addition to cutaneous structures, the trigeminal nerve also innervates deep tissues, including the temporomandibular joint, the meninges, and the peridontium. The primary sensory fibers of these nerves have their cell bodies in the *trigeminal ganglion*,

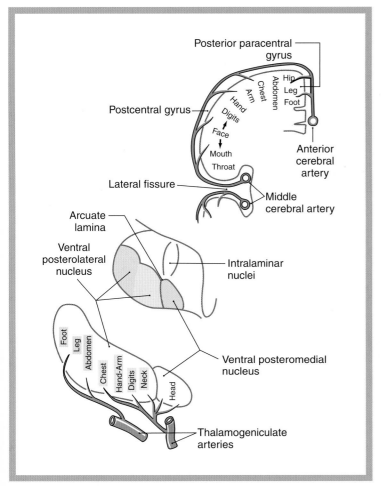

Figure 18-12. Somatotopic organization of, and blood supply to, the ventral posteromedial and posterolateral nuclei and the SI somatosensory cortex.

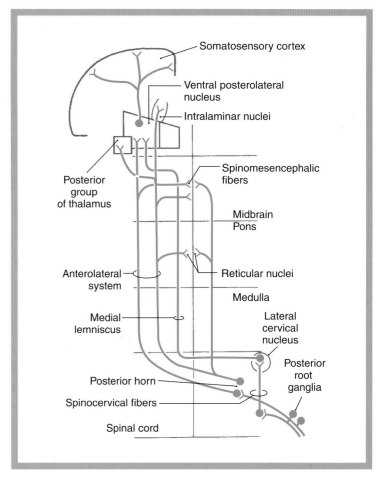

Figure 18-13. Summary of the spinocervicothalamic tract that carries innocuous discriminative tactile, thermal, and nociceptive sensations.

the *geniculate ganglion* of cranial nerve VII, and the *superior ganglia* of cranial nerves IX and X. Aδ and C fiber nociceptors are found throughout the face and oral cavity, and they are particularly prominent in the tooth pulp. Some of these fibers extend into the dentinal tubules, and carious lesions of the tooth expose these and other pulpal nerves to stimuli that result in dental pain. It is probable that the dull aching pain caused by pulp inflammation is the product of C fiber activity. Dental hypersensitivity, often characterized by sharp sensation, represents Aδ fiber activity. The cornea also receives a large number of nociceptive fibers. This corneal innervation forms the afferent limb of the *corneal (blink) reflex*. The meninges are also supplied by fibers of the trigeminal ganglion cells that terminate in the spinal trigeminal nucleus. These fibers are thought to be involved in the pain of migraine headaches.

The central processes of small and large trigeminal ganglion cells are part of the *trigeminal sensory root*, which attaches to the pons (Figs. 18-16 and 18-17). The bifurcating small-diameter axons course posteromedially into the pontine tegmentum, sending an ascending branch to the *principal sensory nucleus*. The descending branch of these fibers joins with numerous other unbranched small-diameter fibers to form a prominent fiber bundle in the posterolateral brainstem, the *spinal trigeminal tract* (Fig. 18-16). Through the caudal pons and the rostral medulla, this tract is internal to the restiform body. However, in the lower medulla caudal to the obex, it forms a superficial landmark lateral to the cuneate tubercle, known as the *trigeminal tubercle (tuberculum cinereum)*. This landmark served as a useful reference point for surgeons, who discovered that sectioning the *spinal tract of the trigeminal nerve* at this level

(tractotomy) provides substantial relief from facial pain on the operated side.

The spinal trigeminal tract extends from the middle pons to the second or third cervical spinal cord segment, where its fibers interdigitate with those of the posterolateral fasciculus (the Lissauer tract) (Figs. 18-6 and 18-16). In addition to the large contributions from the trigeminal nerve, small numbers of fibers conveying general somatic afferent information from the ear on cranial nerves VII, IX, and X also enter the spinal trigeminal tract and terminate in the spinal nucleus. The primary afferent neurons associated with cranial nerves VII, IX, and X have cell bodies in their respective ganglia, enter the medulla, and take a position adjacent to those of the mandibular division in the spinal trigeminal tract.

When the medulla, and the spinal trigeminal tract and nucleus, is viewed in an *anatomic orientation* the face is represented upside down in these structures (Fig. 18-14). In other words, the hemiface representation is inverted from its normal anatomic position (Fig. 18-14). The ophthalmic representation is located inferiorly in the tract/nucleus and the mandibular representation is located superiorly. In this orientation, commonly illustrated in basic and clinical science texts, posterior (i.e., posterior column nuclei, fourth ventricle) is up and anterior (i.e., pyramids) is down in the image of the medulla (Fig. 18-14). It is even more important to emphasize that when viewing the medulla in a *clinical orientation* (as seen in MRI or CT), the face is represented right side up (in its normal anatomic orientation) in the spinal trigeminal tract and nucleus (Fig. 18-15). When the medulla is viewed in the clinical setting, the pyramid is up in the image, the fourth ventricle is down, and within the spinal tract

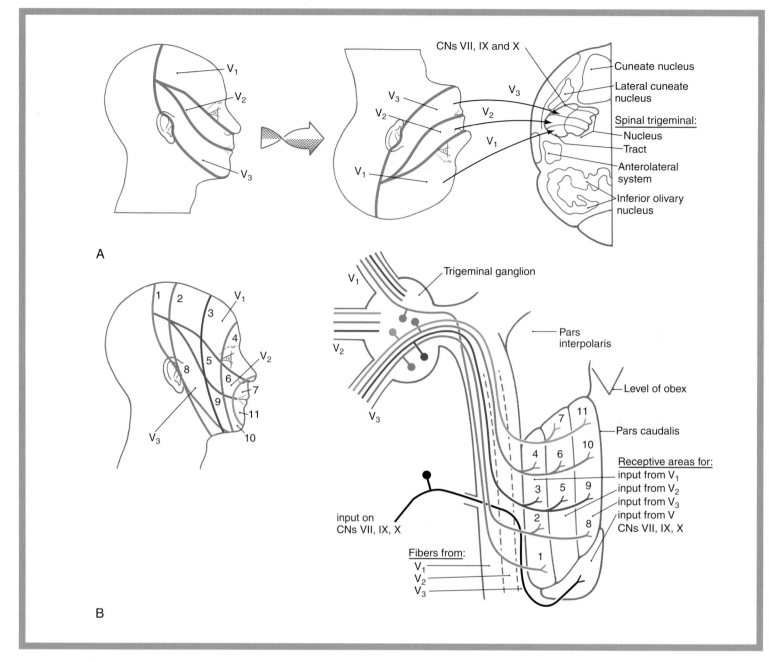

Figure 18-14. Peripheral distribution of the trigeminal nerve and the inverted somatotopic arrangement of the hemiface within the spinal trigeminal nucleus pars caudalis (**A**). Functional onion-skin pattern of facial pain is superimposed along the caudal to rostral axis of the pars caudalis (**B**). CN, cranial nerve. Compare with Figure 8-15.

and nucleus the ophthalmic representation is superior and the mandibular representation is inferior (Fig. 18-15). *Understanding pathways in the clinical orientation is essential when dealing with the neurologically compromised patient.*

The peripheral distribution of the branches of the trigeminal nerve (V_1, V_2, and V_3) delineates the facial dermatomes (Figs. 18-14 and 18-15). Unlike the spinal segmental dermatomes, which partially overlap, the *boundaries between adjacent facial dermatomes are sharply defined.* This segregation of trigeminal branches is maintained by their central processes in the spinal trigeminal tract. An unfortunate clinical condition that illustrates the divisional pattern of the trigeminal system is *herpes zoster,* or *shingles.* Patients with shingles have a characteristic rash that outlines the affected dermatome or spinal cord segment; the ophthalmic or maxillary division is usually affected, and the rash is unilateral (Fig. 18-5).

Injury to trigeminal nerve fibers produces a *paresthesia* restricted to specific regions of the face. The pain of *tic douloureux*

(trigeminal neuralgia) produces episodic "paroxysmal" pain usually restricted to the peripheral distribution of the maxillary or mandibular division on one side. Trigeminal neuralgia is further characterized by the presence of "trigger zones," which, upon the most gentle stimulation (such as a light breeze or a brush with a wisp of cotton), produce stabbing pain on one side of the face. The precise etiology of this condition remains enigmatic, but vascular compression of the trigeminal nerve root and the presence of microneuromas are likely causes.

Central Pathways

The *spinal trigeminal nucleus,* located medial to the spinal tract, is the site of termination for fibers of the spinal trigeminal tract (Figs. 18-16 and 18-17). On the basis of cytoarchitecture, this nucleus is divided into a *pars caudalis,* a *pars interpolaris,* and a *pars oralis.* The caudal subnucleus *(pars caudalis)* (Figs. 18-14 and 18-15) extends from C2 or C3 rostrally to the level of the obex. This part of the spinal nucleus shares many cytoarchitectural

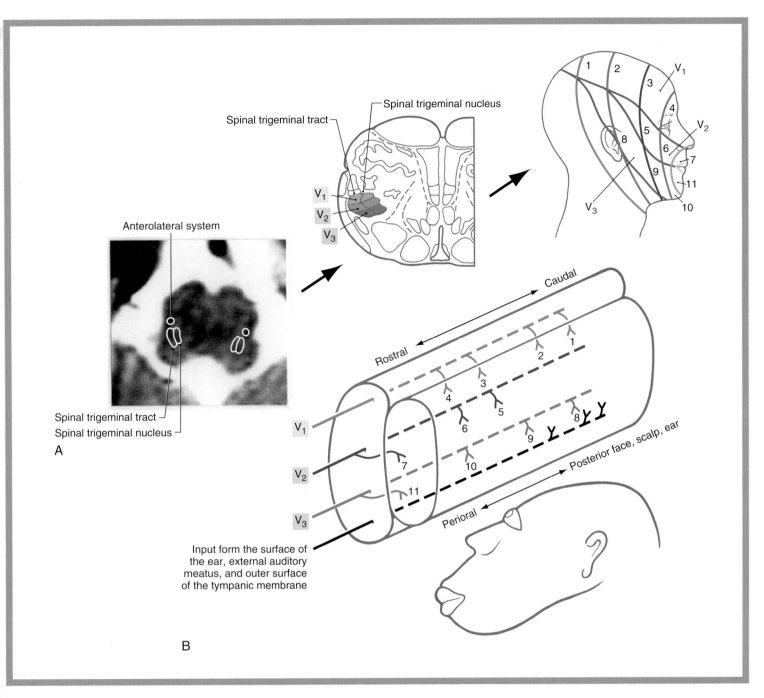

Figure 18-15. The somatotopic organization of the spinal trigeminal tract and nucleus when viewed in a clinical (axial MRI/CT) orientation (**A**); in this orientation the face is represented right-side-up. The posteroanterior arrangement of the facial dermatomes (V₁, V₂, V₃) in the spinal trigeminal tract and nucleus and the respective rostrocaudal termination patterns of spinal trigeminal tract fibers within the spinal trigeminal nucleus in this orientation (**B**). This illustrates, in a three-dimensional view, the anatomic basis for the onion-skin pattern of sensory representation and corresponding deficits. As seen by the numbers, perioral regions of the face are represented rostrally in the pars caudalis and progressively more posterior facial regions in progressively more caudal regions of the pars caudalis and in upper cervical cord levels. Compare with Figure 18-14.

similarities with the posterior horn. For this reason, it has been termed the *medullary posterior horn* and has been divided into layers that correspond to Rexed spinal cord laminae (Fig. 18-6). The *substantia gelatinosa* is largely continuous with lamina II of the spinal cord, and the *magnocellular* region is continuous with laminae III and IV. The pars caudalis and the posterior horn also show homology in the distribution of neurotransmitters. For example, substance P and calcitonin gene-related peptide (CGRP) are localized in nociceptive C fibers that terminate in both of these areas.

The pars caudalis plays an important role in the transmission of nondiscriminative touch, nociceptive, and thermal sensations. This role is reflected by the fact that central processes of Aδ and C fibers terminate somatotopically in this subnucleus. In addition to the somatotopy within the pars caudalis, an *onionskin*

pattern of facial pain representation is oriented along the rostrocaudal axis of the subnucleus (Figs. 18-14B and 18-15). The nociceptive fibers that innervate circumoral and intraoral zones (teeth, gums, and lips) terminate rostrally, close to the obex at the interface of the pars interpolaris with the pars caudalis. Fibers innervating progressively more caudal and lateral regions of the face terminate in progressively more caudal regions of the spinal trigeminal nucleus, pars caudalis (Fig. 18-15). Many second-order neurons in the subnucleus caudalis receive convergent input from small-diameter fibers that innervate cutaneous and deep tissues (jaw muscles and the temporomandibular joint). Convergence of information from different regions is thought to contribute to the referral of pain and may be involved in the manifestation of less well-understood clinical problems such as *temporomandibular disorders* and atypical facial pain.

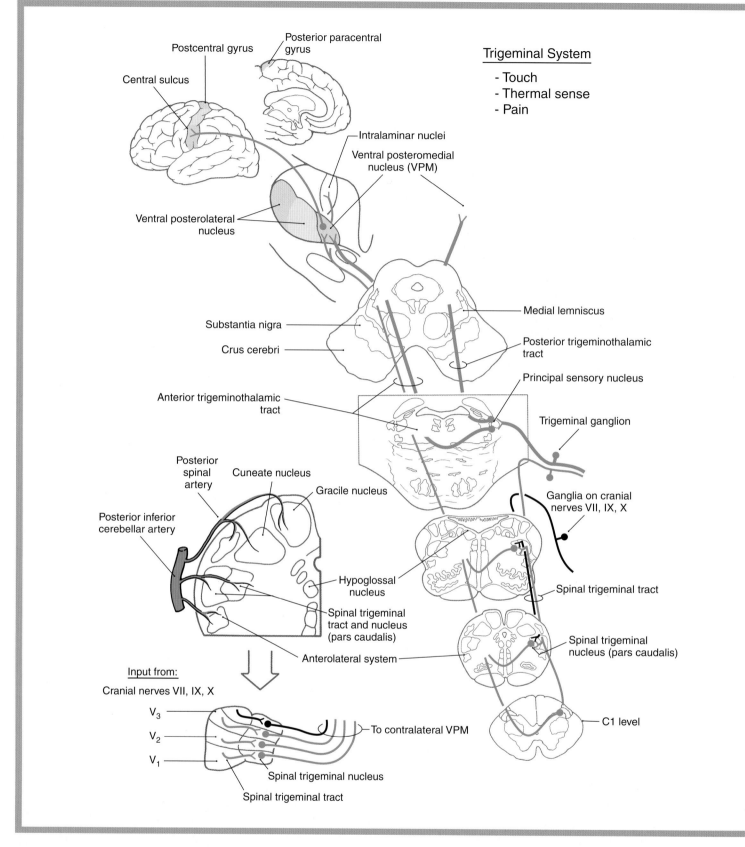

Figure 18-16. The distribution of primary trigeminal fibers, of trigeminothalamic fibers to the ventral posteromedial nucleus (VPM), and of the blood supply to trigeminal structures in the medulla. The large-diameter fibers convey discriminative touch, vibratory, and proprioceptive input, whereas the smaller-diameter fibers constitute the pathway for nondiscriminative tactile, thermal, and nociceptive signals.

At medullary levels, the posterior inferior cerebellar artery supplies the territory of the ALS fibers, as well as the spinal trigeminal nucleus and tract (Figs. 18-9 and 18-16). Vascular lesions involving this vessel produce characteristic sensory symptoms collectively known as the *lateral medullary (Wallenberg) syndrome* or the *posterior inferior cerebellar artery syndrome*. The sensory symptoms of this syndrome may include a

contralateral loss of pain *(hemianalgesia)* and temperature *(hemithermoanesthesia)* sensibility over the body and ipsilateral loss of these modalities over the face. However, the extent of damage following posterior inferior cerebellar artery lesions shows remarkable variation, and the combination of symptoms is representative of the structures served by this artery (Fig. 18-18).

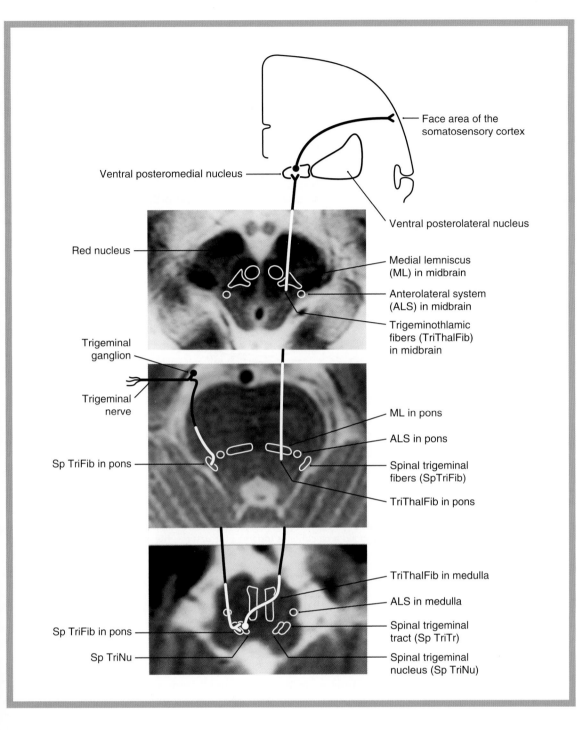

Ventral posteromedial nucleus

Face area of the somatosensory cortex

Ventral posterolateral nucleus

Red nucleus

Medial lemniscus (ML) in midbrain

Anterolateral system (ALS) in midbrain

Trigeminothlamic fibers (TriThalFib) in midbrain

Trigeminal ganglion

Trigeminal nerve

Sp TriFib in pons

ML in pons

ALS in pons

Spinal trigeminal fibers (SpTriFib)

TriThalFib in pons

TriThalFib in medulla

ALS in medulla

Sp TriFib in pons

Sp TriNu

Spinal trigeminal tract (Sp TriTr)

Spinal trigeminal nucleus (Sp TriNu)

Figure 18-17. The location of the spinal trigeminal tract and nucleus and anterior trigeminothalamic fibers in MR images at representative levels of the medulla, pons, and midbrain. This illustrates the location of these fibers when viewed in images routinely used in the clinical setting. It is essential to remember that the face is represented right side up when the spinal trigeminal tract and nucleus is viewed in the clinical orientation. Compare with Figure 18-16.

The interpolar subnucleus *(pars interpolaris)* is located between the level of the obex and the rostral pole of the hypoglossal (XII) nucleus. The most rostral subdivision is the oral subnucleus *(pars oralis)*, which extends from the level of the rostral pole of the hypoglossal nucleus to the caudal end of the trigeminal motor nucleus (Figs. 18-14 and 18-16). Some neurons in the pars interpolaris and the pars oralis contribute to ascending somatosensory pathways, whereas others project to the cerebellum. In addition to projection neurons, the spinal trigeminal nucleus, particularly the subnucleus oralis, contains many local circuit neurons involved in brainstem reflexes.

The axons of *second-order trigeminothalamic neurons* in the spinal trigeminal nucleus decussate, then coalesce to form the *anterior trigeminothalamic tract*, and ascend through the brainstem just posterior to the medial lemniscus (Figs. 18-16 and 18-17). These fibers terminate in the ventral posteromedial (VPM), the posterior, and the intralaminar nuclei of the thalamus. As noted in Chapter 17, this pathway also carries crossed fibers

from the principal trigeminal nucleus. The principal nucleus fibers terminate in the core of VPM, whereas spinal nucleus fibers terminate in its periphery. At the pontomesencephalic junction, anterior trigeminothalamic fibers are adjacent to ALS fibers at the lateral margin of the medial lemniscus (Figs. 18-9 and 18-12). Like ALS fibers, ascending anterior trigeminothalamic axons terminate in, or give rise to collaterals that supply, the reticular formation.

A particularly prominent target of some of these collaterals is the parabrachial nuclear complex. Located adjacent to the superior cerebellar peduncle (brachium conjunctivum), the parabrachial nuclei serve as an important relay for spinal and trigeminal pain fibers, as well as for ascending axons carrying visceral sensory information. In addition to regulating oral and facial reflexes, projections from the reticular formation terminate in the dorsal thalamus in the intralaminar nuclei and the medial region of the posterior nucleus. The intralaminar nuclei project widely to the striatum and cortex, especially the frontal

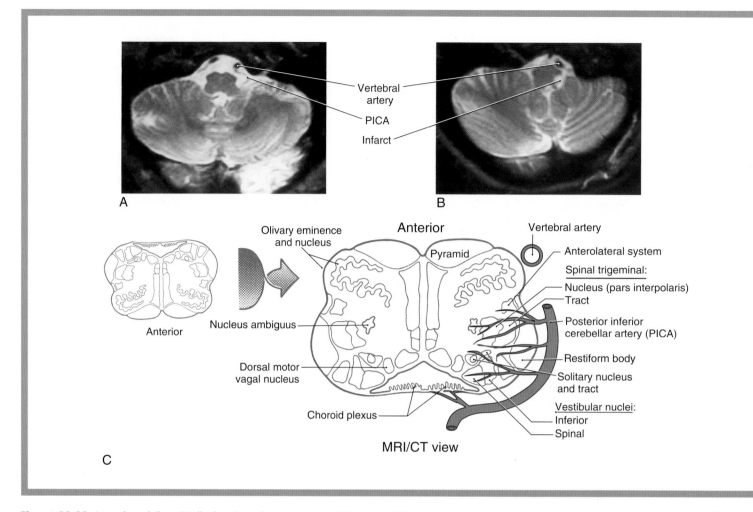

Figure 18-18. Lateral medullary (Wallenberg) syndrome. A normal MR image (**A**) showing vertebral artery and posterior inferior cerebellar artery (PICA). An occlusion of PICA (**B**) resulting in an infarct of the posterolateral medulla. The lesioned area contains trigeminal structures, the anterolateral system, and other important nuclei and tracts (**C**).

and somatosensory cortex. The medial region of the posterior nucleus projects to the head representation in the secondary somatosensory cortex.

Imaging Studies of Pain in the Somatosensory Pathway

Imaging studies including electroencephalography (EEG), positron emission tomography (PET), functional magnetic resonance imaging (fMRI), and magnetoencephalography (MEG) have provided insight into the localization of brain regions responsible for the processing of pain signals. EEG recordings show patterns of increased brain activity following application of painful stimuli. This increased activity is especially prevalent in the somatosensory cortex and the frontal cortex.

When PET is used to identify changes in regional cerebral blood flow, painful stimuli are found to activate SI and SII cortices, as well as the anterior cingulate cortex, the anterior insula, the supplemental motor area of motor cortex, and different thalamic nuclei. The cingulate cortex and the anterior insula are connected with nontraditional somatosensory brain regions, including the limbic cortex. This widespread cortical activation may provide a morphologic basis for integrating the location of painful stimuli with memory and emotion. PET has also been used to study possible gender differences in pain perception to noxious heat stimuli. Similar increases in cortical activation in the posterior insula and anterior cingulate cortex, as well as in the cerebellar vermis, have been described for both sexes.

However, increases in the contralateral prefrontal cortex activity, contralateral insula, and thalamus noted in female subjects suggest that pain perception and processing may be different in males and females.

fMRI techniques reveal increased thalamic and cortical activation in response to application of innocuous (tactile, cool, and warm) and nociceptive (cold and hot) stimuli. Regions of increased activity in response to innocuous stimuli included the contralateral thalamus (VPL), posterior insula, and bilateral SII cortex. Application of innocuous thermal stimuli fail to activate SII. Painful thermal stimuli, however, activate the anterior insular cortex, as well as the contralateral SII cortex.

By using a CO_2 laser to activate Aδ and C nociceptors, MEG revealed that both the contralateral SI and bilateral SII cortices are involved in the processing of pain stimuli. These results support the view that SI provides a mechanism to code spatial, temporal, and intensity qualities of a painful stimulus. These various methods are providing a more complete identification of structures included in pain pathways and responsible for the processing of painful stimuli.

Pain Perception

Vascular compromise of middle or anterior cerebral arteries (Fig. 18-12) produces a loss of sensibility (discriminative, nondiscriminative, thermal, and nociceptive) over contralateral regions of the body. Over time, however, appreciation of sensation may return (partially/totally). Pain sensations are first to return, followed by nondiscriminative tactile and thermal sensations. Discriminative tactile, vibratory, and proprioceptive sensations lag far behind and often fail to return to normal levels. If occlusion of the middle cerebral artery affects most of the postcentral gyrus, sensation begins returning first on the face and oral regions, then on the neck and trunk, and finally on the extremities and the distal parts of the limbs. This return of function indicates that other cortical areas may partially take over the appreciation of somatosensory stimuli, using the input they receive through nonlemniscal, non-ALS pathways.

At least some forms of somatosensory stimuli can be perceived at subcortical levels. In fact, electrical stimulation of the primary somatosensory cortex does not result in a complaint of pain, whereas thalamic stimulation may elicit paresthesia and sensations of dull pain and pressure. Furthermore, painful stimuli can be recognized and produce suffering without the presence of primary and secondary cortices, leading to the concept that *pain is perceived at subcortical levels*. However, damage to specific cortical regions eliminates the ability to precisely localize pain, suggesting that such localization is a function of the somatosensory cortex and its lemniscal inputs (Fig. 18-15A).

A second dissociation can occur in pain pathways. Pain perception and its affective component, suffering, are served by separate brain regions. The neospinothalamic pathway to the primary somatosensory cortex is involved in the localization of painful stimuli (Fig. 18-19A). Paleospinothalamic pathways that access the hypothalamus and limbic system via the reticular formation and PAG are involved in the suffering component of the pain experience (Fig. 18-19B). This dissociation can be regulated pharmacologically, as some drugs eliminate suffering without affecting pain perception. For example, patients taking benzodiazepines report that the pain is still present but that its unpleasant nature is diminished.

Pain Perception in the Somatosensory Thalamus

Results of stereotaxic surgery for treatment of chronic pain or movement disorders have provided tremendous insights into the role of the thalamus in pain perception. Before the performance of such surgical procedures, physiologic identification of the desired target is undertaken in these patients. Single-neuron recording and microstimulation have demonstrated that neurons within the human VPM/VPL (collectively called ventrocaudal [Vc] nuclei by some neurosurgeons) are involved with processing of tactile, thermal, and pain signals. Patients report that microstimulation of Vc evokes sensations of touch, warmth, coolness, tingling, burning, or pain localized to specific body areas. These recordings also reveal that a population of thalamic cells activated by innocuous tactile stimuli are mixed with other neurons activated by mechanical and thermal stimuli in the painful range. Single-neuron recording has demonstrated that microstimulation in VPM/VPL (Vc) evokes the sensation of angina, suggesting that these nuclei play a role in pain localization regardless of its origin, that is, cutaneous or visceral.

The human VPL/VPM (Vc) can undergo changes (i.e., it exhibits plasticity) following *deafferentation*, which can occur directly as a result of damage to ascending pathways or secondarily as a result of removing sensory inputs (e.g., amputation). These changes may contribute to *chronic pain* or *phantom limb pain*. They involve the upregulation and downregulation of neurochemicals within the nucleus, changes in local circuitry, and changes in the functional state of Vc neurons. For example, in patients who have undergone leg amputation, single-neuron recordings reveal that the thalamic region formerly receiving input from the lower leg and foot responded to stimulation of the stump (thigh). These patients also described the presence

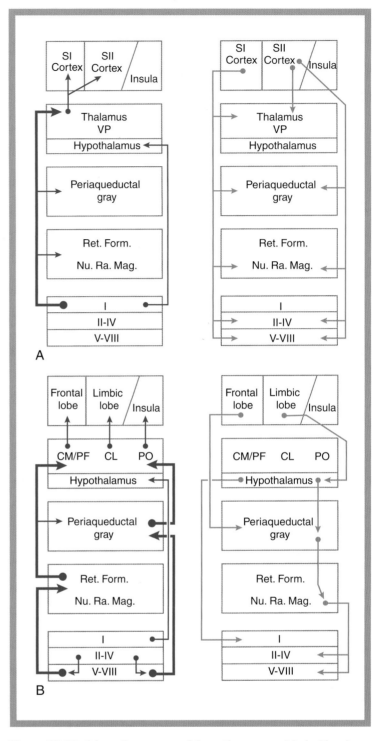

Figure 18-19. Schematic summary of the pathways associated with pain localization (**A**) and the motivational-affect (**B**) components of pain perception. Ascending excitatory connections are shown in *blue;* descending modulatory connections are shown in *red.* The spinothalamic tract *(neospinothalamic tract)* inputs influence specific descending modulatory circuits involved with pain localization (**A**). Spinoreticular and spinomesencephalic tract *(paleospinothalamic tract)* inputs activate specific descending modulatory circuits involved in motivational-affect components of pain perception (**B**). CL, central lateral nucleus; CM/PF, centromedian-parafascicular nucleus; Nu. Ra. Mag., nucleus raphe magnus; PO, posterior group of the thalamus; Ret. Form., reticular formation; SI and SII, primary and secondary somatosensory cortices, respectively; VP, ventral posterior nuclei.

of nonpainful tingling over the stump in response to microstimulation in this same area.

In an attempt to bring about relief for chronic or neuropathic pain, two therapies have been utilized: *thalamic lesioning* and *deep brain stimulation*. Lesions have been centered in either the lateral thalamus or the medial thalamus. Lateral thalamic lesions involve the somatosensory thalamus (VPL/VPM). Although producing some transient relief for pain, these lesions produce unwanted side effects, including loss of cutaneous and position sense in the affected limb, as well as impaired motor function. Lesions in the medial thalamus involve the centromedian-parafascicular (CM-PF) complex as well as the central lateral nucleus (CL) and the medial dorsal nucleus. Medial thalamic lesions produce transient relief from intractable pain but fail to produce loss of pain and thermal sensations. These lesions do not produce the unwanted sensory loss seen with lateral thalamic lesions.

Deep brain electrical stimulation has been used for more than several decades in patients suffering from chronic pain or deafferentation pain. Stimulating electrodes centered in the somatosensory thalamus, the CM-PF complex, or the periventricular gray (PVG)–PAG activate neurons within their vicinity and thus may contribute to stimulus-induced analgesia. Cortical stimulation has also been shown to produce relief of chronic pain of neuropathic origin. An evaluation of different brain regions that may contribute to the stimulus-induced analgesia was carried out using PET. Following thalamic stimulation, increased regional cortical blood flow was noted in the rostral insula, a region activated in studies of experimental pain, neuropathic pain, and warm and cool innocuous stimuli, as well

as in the anterior insular cortex. These results suggest that stimulation of the somatosensory thalamus may activate a pain modulation circuit that involves thalamocortical thermal pathways.

Central or *thalamic pain* is a poorly understood sequela of natural or surgical lesions of structures involved in somatic sensibility. Central pain was originally observed with thalamic lesions, but it can occur with lesions of the ALS below the level of the thalamus.

Central pain syndrome can also result from vascular lesions. Patients surviving the *Wallenberg syndrome* (Fig. 18-18) may ultimately develop central pain, suggesting some sparing of alternate or parallel pain pathways. In *central pain syndrome*, the analgesia that initially results from the lesion is replaced after a period of weeks, months, or years by spontaneous *paresthesia*, *dysesthesia*, or unusual painful responses. *Allodynia*, pain resulting from a stimulus that does not normally evoke pain, and *hyperalgesia*, an increased response to a stimulus that is normally painful, are common neurologic signs associated with the central pain syndrome. Patients often characterize central pain as burning, aching, pricking, or lacerating and as occurring in paroxysms that vary in intensity and are poorly localized.

Central pain may last for years and is intractable to current analgesics. Pharmacologic agents, such as antidepressants and

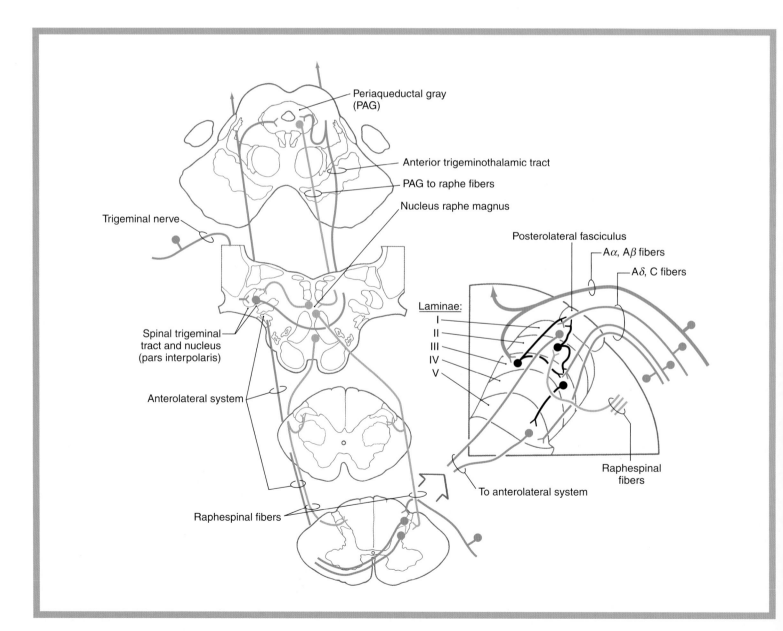

Figure 18-20. Descending brainstem pathways that influence and control pain transmission within the brainstem (for trigeminal pathways) and in the spinal cord (for anterolateral system projections).

antiepileptic drugs, have been used with varying degrees of success to treat central pain. Although the etiology for this condition has not been elucidated, it is possible that this type of pain represents a deafferentation phenomenon, that is, it results from removal of primary afferent influence on central neurons. The time course and symptoms of central pain suggest that it may be due to the sprouting of inappropriate connections of non-nociceptive or nociceptive fibers, to increased excitability of central pain neurons, or to removal of inhibitory influences on pain neurons.

Patients experiencing central pain may obtain temporary relief from *transcutaneous electrical nerve stimulation (TENS)* (electrical stimulation of nerves through the skin), from electrical stimulation of the posterior columns, or from chronic stimulation of the PAG or PVG regions by stereotaxically positioned electrodes *(deep brain stimulation)*. Neuroablative surgical procedures that have been used in the treatment of central pain include anterolateral cordotomy, trigeminal tractotomy, lesions of the posterior root entry zone, thalamotomies, and cortical ablation. Unfortunately none of these procedures is successful in the long term.

Pain Transmission and Control

The relaying of information from the spinal cord to supraspinal centers is an important event in the higher-order processing of nociceptive sensory signals. On the basis of the localization of putative neurotransmitters and secondary messengers in the posterior horn, several candidates, such as *peptides* (calcitonin gene-related peptide, substance P), *glutamate*, and *nitric oxide*, may be involved in this process. These and other chemical agents underlie the central pharmacology of nociceptive transmission and are responsible for the varied qualities associated with central pain pathways. Pain can be classified as acute or chronic, fast or slow, dull or sharp, or burning, throbbing, or aching. Because pain is such a complex sensory experience, reduction or elimination of nociceptive sensations is of obvious clinical importance. Effective clinical approaches that can be used for the purpose of controlling pain include *pharmacologic intervention* and *stimulation-produced analgesia.*

The CNS has neural circuits designed to modulate pain transmission (Figs. 18-19 to 18-21). These systems have components at all levels of the neuraxis. They are capable of controlling nociceptive neuron firing and are sensitive to opiates. Central structures implicated in the *descending control* of nociceptive transmission include (1) the somatosensory cortex, frontal and limbic cortices, (2) the periventricular nucleus of the hypothalamus, (3) the PAG, and (4) raphe nuclei and adjacent medullary reticular formation. Descending pathways originating in these structures are activated by ascending afferent pain signals.

Cortical input may upregulate sites in the brainstem and hypothalamus that modulate the processing of nociceptive information in the brainstem and spinal cord (Figs. 18-19 and 18-20). The PVG of the hypothalamus communicates with the PAG of the midbrain via an enkephalinergic pathway. Descending PAG fibers exert an excitatory influence on *serotoninergic neurons* in the medullary *nucleus raphe magnus*, both directly and through interneurons in the medullary reticular formation (Fig. 18-20). This PAG-to-NRM projection uses *serotonin, neurotensin, somatostatin,* and *glutamate. Raphespinal neurons* project, in turn, to the posterior horn and pars caudalis of the trigeminal nucleus (Figs. 18-20 and 18-21). These raphespinal *serotoninergic axons* terminate on *enkephalinergic interneurons* in laminae II and III, which act presynaptically and postsynaptically to suppress incoming activity in the pain fibers (Figs. 18-20 and 18-21). In addition, the hypothalamus (via *hypothalamospinal fibers*) projects directly to the medullary and spinal cord posterior horns

to act on incoming nociceptive signals (Fig. 18-19). *Cholecystokinin* and substance P are among the putative neurotransmitters used by PAG projection neurons.

Stimulation-produced analgesia (SPA) relies on electrical stimulation of CNS structures to induce the release of endogenous chemicals, such as *enkephalin*, from cells in pain control circuits. As noted previously, endogenous opiates such as enkephalin inhibit pain transmission. Stimulation of PVG, the PAG, or the nucleus raphe magnus results in the release of enkephalin or monoamines producing analgesia. Systemic administration of pharmacologic opiates, such as *morphine*, excites periventricular and periaqueductal neurons, supplementing their natural activity. This increase in activity suppresses neurons in the spinal and medullary posterior horns that transmit painful information, also producing analgesia. The direct delivery of opioids to the spinal cord (*epidural* anesthetic techniques) also is used to produce a powerful analgesia for surgical procedures and deliveries.

Current therapies for the control of pain transmission include transcutaneous electrical nerve stimulation and chronic stimulation of the posterior columns by implanted electrodes. Posterior column stimulation activates large-diameter myelinated fibers. Antidromic activation of these fibers discharges collaterals in the posterior horn (Fig. 18-21). These collaterals stimulate the enkephalinergic interneurons in the posterior horn that inhibit the transmission of pain signals. This stimulation also provides long-term diminution of pain for reasons that are poorly understood. *Acupuncture-like stimulation* also may produce local analgesia by stimulating these fibers.

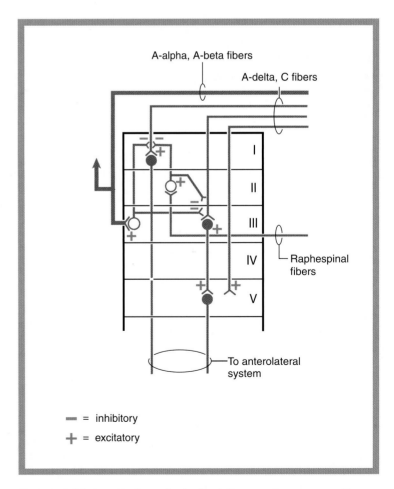

Figure 18-21. Posterior horn circuits that influence primary sensory fibers and ascending tract cells conveying nociceptive inputs. In addition to raphespinal fibers, some reticulospinal fibers also influence pain transmission in the posterior horn.

Synopsis of Clinical Points

- Pain, thermal, and nondiscriminative touch sensations are transmitted via a composite bundle called the anterolateral system (p. 281).
- Aδ and C fibers respond to mechanical stimuli with tissue damage; C fibers respond to noxious stimuli such as thermal or chemical, (p. 282).
- Hyperalgesia (primary or secondary) is a heightened sensitivity to painful stimuli (p. 282).
- Receptor sensitization is the situation whereby pain receptors develop a lower threshold to, and are thereby more sensitive to, noxious stimuli (p. 282).
- Central sensitization may result in allodynia (p. 283).
- Allodynia is a situation in which an innocuous stimulus will result in a perception of pain in the absence of a proper pain stimulus (p. 283).
- Somatic pain can be well localized; visceral pain is difficult to localized and may be referred to an overlying body part/area (referred pain) (p. 283).
- Local anesthetics preferentially block Aδ and C fibers to produce analgesia (p. 283).
- Posterior rhizotomy is a procedure used to alleviate intractable pain (p. 283).
- Shingles is caused by *herpes zoster*, resulting in pain and vesicle eruption in a dermatomal distribution (p. 284).
- Hypesthesia is a sense of diminished sensibility (p. 284).
- Vibratory sense is tested by applying a 128-Hz tuning fork to a bony prominence (p. 285).
- The direct, or neospinothalamic, pathway is concerned with the perception of sharp, immediate pain (p. 286).
- The indirect, or paleospinothalamic, pathway is concerned with the perception of dull, aching pain (p. 286).
- The Brown-Séquard syndrome is a hemisection of the spinal cord (p. 287).
- Syringomyelia is a cavitation of central regions of the spinal cord resulting is a characteristic bilateral sensory loss (p. 287).
- A lesion in the medulla may result in a dissociated sensory loss (p. 287).
- The afferent limb of the corneal (blink) reflex travels on the trigeminal nerve; the efferent limb travels on the facial nerve (p. 291).
- Trigeminal neuralgia (tic douloureux) is an intense idiopathic pain originating from the general area of the cheek or corner of the mouth (p. 292).
- An alternating hemianesthesia (ipsilateral face, contralateral body) is usually characteristic of a lateral medullary syndrome (p. 294).
- Hemianalgesia is a loss of pain perception on one side of the body (p. 294).
- Hemithermoanesthesia is the loss of temperature perception on one side of the body (p. 294).
- Phantom limb pain is the perception of pain from an absent body part (p. 297).
- Thalamic lesions or deep brain stimulation may be used to treat intractable pain (pp. 297–298).
- Central, or thalamic, pain is most commonly seen in lesions of the thalamus (pp. 298–299).
- Paresthesia (burning, prickling, tingling), dysesthesia (impaired, disagreeable, or abnormal sensations), or hyperalgesia (increased sensitivity to stimuli) may be seen in a central pain syndrome (p. 299).
- Transcutaneous electrical nerve stimulation may be used in cases of central pain (p. 299).
- Morphine is an effective anesthetic agent (p. 299).
- The hypothalamospinal pathway is concerned with the suppression of pain transmission in the brainstem and spinal cord (p. 299).

Sources and Additional Reading

Brodal A: Neurological Anatomy in Relation to Clinical Medicine, 3rd ed. New York, Oxford University Press, 1981.

Burgess PR, Perl ER: Cutaneous mechanoreceptors and nociceptors. In Iggo A (ed): Handbook of Sensory Physiology, vol 2. Somatosensory System. New York, Springer-Verlag, 1973, pp 30-78.

Bushnell MC, Duncan GH, Hofbauer RK, Ha B, Chen JL, Carrier B: Pain perception: Is there a role for primary somatosensory cortex? Proc Natl Acad Sci U S A 96:7705-7709, 1999.

Davis KD, Kwan CL, Crawley AP, Mikulis DJ: Functional MRI study of thalamic and cortical activations evoked by cutaneous heat, cold and tactile stimuli. J Neurophysiol 80:1533-1546, 1998.

Dubner R, Bennett GJ: Spinal and trigeminal mechanisms of nociception. Annu Rev Neurosci 6:381-418, 1983.

Dubner R, Sessle B, Storey A: The Neural Basis of Oral and Facial Function. New York, Plenum Press, 1978.

Duncan GH, Bushnell MC, Marchand S: Deep brain stimulation: A review of basic research and clinical studies. Pain 45:49-59, 1991.

Kiss ZHT, Dostrovsky JO, Tasker RR: Plasticity in human somatosensory thalamus as a result of deafferentation. Stereotact Funct Neurosurg 62:153-163, 1994.

Lenz FA, Dougherty PM: Pain processing in the human thalamus. In Steriade M, Jones EG, McCormick DA (eds): Thalamus, vol II. Oxford, Elsevier, 1997, pp. 617-651.

Light A: The Initial Processing of Pain and Its Descending Control: Spinal and Trigeminal Systems, Vol 12, Pain and Headache. New York, Karger, 1992.

Mayer DJ, Liebeskind JC: Pain reduction by focal electrical stimulation of the brain: An anatomical and behavioral analysis. Brain Res 68:73-93, 1974.

Paulson PE, Minoshima S, Morrow TJ, Casey KL: Gender differences in pain perception and patterns of cerebral activation during noxious heat stimulation in humans. Pain 76:223-229, 1998.

Poggio GF, Mountcastle VB: A study of the functional contributions of the lemniscal and spinothalamic systems to somatic sensibility: Central nervous mechanisms in pain. Johns Hopkins Hosp Bull 106:266-316, 1960.

Talbot JD, Marrett S, Evans AC, Meyer E, Bushnell MC, Duncan GH: Multiple representations of pain in the human cerebral cortex. Science 251:1355-1358, 1991.

Wall PD, Melzack R: Textbook of Pain, 4th ed. Edinburgh, Churchill Livingstone, 1999.

Willis WD: The Pain System: The Neural Basis of Nociceptive Transmission in the Mammalian Nervous System, Vol 8, Pain and Headache. New York, Karger, 1985.

Young RF: Effect of trigeminal tractotomy on dental sensation in humans. J Neurosurg 56:812-818, 1982.

Chapter 19

Viscerosensory Pathways

S. G. P. Hardy and J. P. Naftel

The somatosensory system conveys information from sensory receptors in the skin, joints, and skeletal muscles that allows one to perceive and respond to input from the external environment. Functioning in parallel with somatosensory pathways are fibers that convey information from visceral receptors. This input allows the body to make appropriate responses to changes in its internal environment.

Viscerosensory Receptors

Viscerosensory receptors may be categorized as nociceptors or physiologic receptors (Table 19-1). *Nociceptors* in the viscera are the free nerve endings of Aδ and C fibers located in the heart, respiratory structures, gastrointestinal tract, and urogenital tract (Table 19-1). These receptors respond to stimuli that have the potential to damage tissue or to stimuli resulting from the presence of damaged tissue. For example, intense mechanical stimuli (such as overdistention or traction), ischemia, and endogenous compounds (including bradykinin, prostaglandins, and H$^+$ and K$^+$ ions) can activate these receptors and produce pain. These receptors signal changes in visceral structures that result from pathologic processes such as myocardial ischemia or appendicitis or from benign conditions such as gastrointestinal cramping or bloating. *Visceral pain* is often described as being diffuse and difficult to localize and is frequently referred to an overlying somatic body location.

Physiologic receptors are responsive to innocuous stimuli, and they monitor the functions of visceral structures on a continuing basis. These receptors also mediate normal visceral reflexes such as the baroreceptor reflex. Examples of physiologic receptors are (1) rapidly adapting mechanoreceptors, (2) slowly adapting mechanoreceptors, and (3) various types of specialized receptors.

Rapidly adapting mechanoreceptors (Table 19-1) signal the occurrence of dynamic events such as movement or sudden changes in pressure. This type of receptor is present in organs of the thoracic, abdominal, and pelvic cavities. In the thoracic cavity, it is represented by free nerve endings that exist in the epithelia of pulmonary airways. Because these nerve endings are sensitive to the presence of inhaled particles, they have been referred to as "cough receptors." Rapidly adapting mechanoreceptors in the abdominal and pelvic cavities vary greatly in size and location and may be either unencapsulated or encapsulated.

The largest example of a rapidly adapting mechanoreceptor is the pacinian corpuscle.

Slowly adapting mechanoreceptors (Table 19-1) signal the presence of stretch or tension within a visceral structure. These typically unencapsulated receptors are located in the smooth muscle layer of the pulmonary airways and in the smooth muscle layers of hollow abdominal and pelvic viscera. They are essential for the perception of a sense of fullness in certain viscera, such as the stomach or bladder.

Certain *specialized receptors* (Table 19-1) are unique to the viscerosensory system. These include baroreceptors, chemoreceptors, osmoreceptors, and internal thermal receptors. *Baroreceptors* (Fig. 19-1A) are found in the walls of the aortic arch and carotid sinus and respond to rapid increases or decreases in blood pressure. For baroreceptors to effectively perform this task, blood pressure must be in the range of 30 to 150 mm Hg. *Chemoreceptors* (Fig. 19-1B) are found in structures called *carotid bodies* (located at the bifurcation of the common carotid artery) and *aortic bodies* (located in the aortic arch) and are activated by changes in the composition of arterial blood. These changes include alterations in oxygen and carbon dioxide tension and in acidity. The presence of certain drugs such as nicotine or cyanide may also alter arterial blood gases.

In addition, specialized visceroreceptors also exist in the hypothalamus as *chemoreceptors, osmoreceptors,* and *internal thermal receptors.* These viscerosensory receptors are activated by changes in blood chemistry or osmolarity or by changes in the temperature of blood circulating through the hypothalamus. Hypothalamic neurons that respond to these changes by altering their firing rates are considered to be the "receptor" cells.

Viscerosensory Fibers

Sympathetic and parasympathetic divisions of the autonomic (visceral motor) nervous system (see Chapter 29) have traditionally been considered to consist of only visceromotor (general visceral efferent [GVE]) fibers. These fibers travel through sympathetic nerves (such as splanchnic and cardiac nerves) or through parasympathetic nerves (such as vagus and pelvic nerves). However, these *sympathetic and parasympathetic nerves also contain viscerosensory (general visceral afferent [GVA]) fibers* that serve many important functions. In this chapter, *the*

Table 19-1. Classification of Nociceptive Receptors and Physiologic Receptors in the Viscera and Their Adequate Stimuli

Viscerosensory Receptors	Adequate Stimulus(i)
Nociceptors	Mediate visceral pain
Heart	
Aδ and C afferent fibers	Prostaglandin (PGE$_2$), H$^+$ ions, bradykinin, K$^+$ ions, ischemia
Respiratory System	
Lung irritant receptors (Aδ fibers)	Irritant aerosols and gases, mechanical stimuli
J receptors (C fibers?)	Capsaicin, pulmonary congestion/edema, inhaled irritants
Gastrointestinal Tract	
Rapidly adapting mechanoreceptors, slowly adapting mechanoreceptors, chemoreceptors (Aδ and C fibers?)	Irritation of the mucosa, distention, powerful contraction, torsion, or traction, bloating, cramping, appendicitis, impaction
Urogenital Tract	
C-polymodal nociceptors	Intense mechanical stimuli, noxious heat and algesic chemicals
Physiologic Receptors	Monitor physiologic state of viscera; mediate visceral reflexes
Rapidly adapting visceral mechanoreceptors	Movement, sudden change in pressure
Slowly adapting visceral mechanoreceptors	Stretch/tension
Baroreceptors	Increase or decrease in blood pressure
Chemoreceptors	Changes in oxygen, carbon dioxide tension, H$^+$ ions
Osmoreceptors	Changes in blood osmolarity
Internal thermal receptors	Change in circulating blood temperature

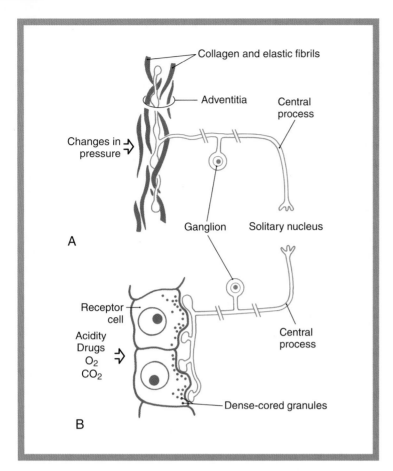

Figure 19-1. Diagrammatic representation of a baroreceptor (**A**) and a chemoreceptor (**B**). The baroreceptor is located in the adventitia in apposition to collagen and elastic fibrils. This receptor alters its firing rate in response to changes in blood pressure. The chemoreceptor is composed of a receptor cell and the numerous afferent endings it contacts. Changes in blood chemistry trigger responses in the receptor cell that result in an action potential in the subjacent afferent ending.

terms *"sympathetic afferent"* and *"parasympathetic afferent"* are used to describe viscerosensory fibers contained in sympathetic and parasympathetic nerves, respectively. In addition to its conciseness, this usage complies with the terminology introduced by Langley, a pioneer in studies on the autonomic nervous system (see Cervero and Foreman, 1990).

Visceral afferents tend to predominate in parasympathetic nerves but are comparatively sparse in sympathetic nerves. For example, more than 80% of the fibers in the vagus nerve (a parasympathetic nerve) are viscerosensory whereas less than 20% of the fibers in the greater splanchnic nerve (a sympathetic nerve) are visceral afferents. Most visceral afferents (90%; both sympathetic and parasympathetic) are either unmyelinated or thinly myelinated and, therefore, are slowly conducting fibers.

Information originating from *nociceptors* is conducted *almost exclusively by sympathetic nerves*. In contrast, input originating from *physiologic receptors* (innocuous input) travels *primarily in parasympathetic nerves*. Thus, there is a division of responsibility between parasympathetic and sympathetic nerves in terms of viscerosensory input.

Ascending Pathway for Sympathetic Afferents

Afferent fibers conveying nociceptive information from thoracic and abdominal viscera travel via the cardiac and splanchnic nerves (Fig. 19-2). For example, primary sensory fibers that originate from the stomach join the greater splanchnic nerve,

enter the sympathetic trunk, and pass through a white ramus to join the spinal nerve. Nociceptive input from pelvic viscera such as the prostate and sigmoid colon is conveyed by viscerosensory fibers traveling through the hypogastric plexus and lumbar splanchnic nerves.

The cell bodies of origin of sympathetic afferent fibers are located in posterior root ganglia at about levels T1 to L2 (Fig. 19-2). The central processes of these fibers enter the spinal cord via the lateral division of the posterior root. They may ascend or descend one or two spinal levels in the posterolateral fasciculus before terminating in laminae I and V and/or laminae VII and VIII. Cells in laminae I and V project mainly to the contralateral side as part of the *anterolateral system*, whereas the neurons in laminae VII and VIII project bilaterally as *spinoreticular fibers*. In addition, some primary viscerosensory fibers terminate on preganglionic sympathetic cell bodies located in the intermediolateral cell column at spinal levels T1 to L2 (Fig. 19-2). The axons of these latter cells, in turn, exit through the anterior root as GVE preganglionic sympathetic fibers.

In general, viscerosensory fibers that enter the spinal cord at a particular level originate from structures that receive GVE input from the same spinal level (Fig. 19-2). For example, visceral afferent fibers from the stomach enter the spinal cord over the posterior roots of T5 to T9 and terminate in the same spinal segments that convey visceral efferent outflow to the stomach.

Projections to Thalamus

Some neurons located in laminae I and V receive nociceptive input from sympathetic afferent fibers and send their axons rostrally via two routes in the anterolateral system (ALS) (Fig. 19-3). Some fibers cross in the anterior white commissure and ascend in the ALS, whereas others ascend in this bundle on the ipsilateral side. These ALS fibers terminate in the ventral posterolateral nucleus (VPL), which, in turn, projects to the inferolateral part of the postcentral gyrus (the parietal operculum) and to the insular cortex (Fig. 19-3). The location from which this visceral nociceptive information originated is encoded in these particular regions of the cerebral cortex. However, visceral pain is poorly localized (lacks detailed point-to-point representation) because receptor density is low and receptive fields correspondingly large and because this input converges in the pathway. Consequently, it is not possible to tell whether pain is coming from the stomach or the duodenum; rather, it can be determined *only* that the pain is coming from the general area of the upper abdomen.

Projections to Reticular Formation

In addition to the direct path to the thalamus and sensory cortex via the ALS and VPL, there are indirect routes via the reticular formation through which visceral nociceptive information can reach the cortex. The reticular formation receives spinoreticular inputs (mainly from laminae VII and VIII) and collaterals from the ALS (Fig. 19-3). In turn, cells of the reticular formation project to progressively higher levels of the neuraxis, thus relaying viscerosensory information in a multisynaptic fashion to progressively higher levels of the brain. Neurons located in the reticular formation and in the periaqueductal gray ultimately project to the hypothalamus and to the intralaminar nuclei of the thalamus (Fig. 19-3). These latter cell groups project to the cortex.

Reticulohypothalamic fibers travel via the *dorsal longitudinal fasciculus*, the *mammillary peduncle*, and the *medial forebrain bundle*. The first originates mainly from the periaqueductal gray, and the latter two originate mainly from the mesencephalic reticular formation. These midbrain centers receive both viscerosensory and somatosensory input and, through their projections, hypothalamic centers may be influenced by either system. For

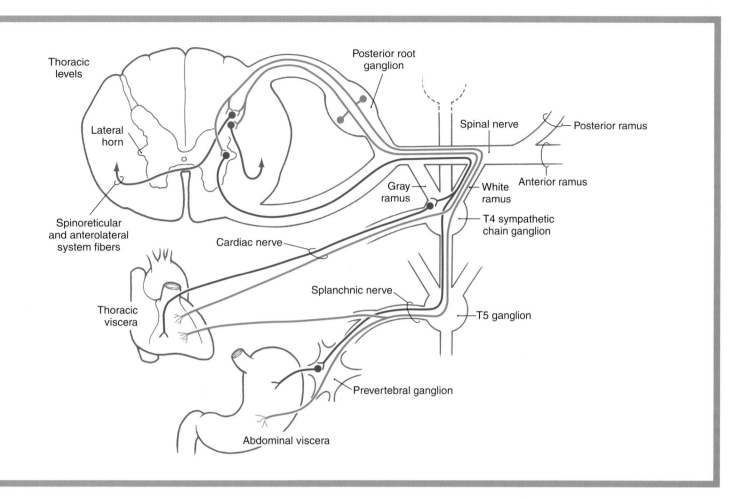

Figure 19-2. Primary sensory sympathetic afferent fibers *(red)* shown in relation to posterior horn tract cells *(green)* conveying visceral information to the thalamus and to general visceral efferent neurons *(blue)*.

example, viscerosensory input resulting from distention of the bowel may result in increased heart rate or cutaneous flushing. On the other hand, somatosensory stimuli such as those associated with coitus or suckling may increase the release of the hypothalamic hormone oxytocin.

Referred Pain

Referred pain is the phenomenon whereby noxious stimuli that originate in a visceral structure, such as the heart or the stomach, are perceived by the patient as pain arising from a somatic portion of the body wall such as the skin, bones, or skeletal muscles (Fig. 19-4). Although such referral of pain may mask the true origin of the information, certain patterns of referred pain are clearly diagnostic of diseases in particular visceral locations. For example, pain in the chest (sometimes perceived as intense pressure) that radiates down the left arm may be indicative of a serious heart problem. A stomach condition may be perceived as pain in the epigastric region. Visceral pain is transmitted by sympathetic sensory fibers and is typically referred to those somatic structures whose afferents enter the cord via the same posterior roots.

The mechanism underlying referred pain is thought to involve a convergence of somatic and visceral afferent information onto pools of posterior horn neurons, the axons of which ascend to higher levels of the neuraxis (Fig. 19-5). Normally, a visceral nociceptive fiber (e.g., from the heart) synapses on a spino-thalamic tract cell whose axon will travel to the VPL, and from there the information is relayed to visceral parts of the sensory cortex. Consequently, this sensory input is perceived as arising from deep within one of the body's cavities (e.g., the thoracic cavity) (Fig. 19-5A). In some situations, however, collaterals of

visceral afferent fibers may synapse on and excite posterior horn tract cells that usually transmit only somatosensory information (Fig. 19-5B). In this case, the tract cell is activated by a visceral afferent collateral but sends information via the VPL to a part of the somatosensory cortex that represents the body wall (Fig. 19-5B). Consequently, the pain is "referred" to (interpreted as coming from) the surface of the body (Fig. 19-4) even though the stimulus actually originated from a visceral structure.

Angina

Referred pain may occur in conjunction with disease affecting any internal organ; however, it is frequently associated with diseases of the heart (Fig. 19-4). The pain resulting from heart disease is termed *angina*. In about 80% of patients, angina is initially perceived as an unpleasant squeezing sensation originating from behind the sternum. This discomfort may also be perceived as pain radiating down the left arm or, more rarely, down both arms. On rare occasions, the pain has been reported to radiate bilaterally into the neck, jaw, and temporomandibular joints. The predilection of the pain for the left side of the chest, or extending down the left arm, reflects the predominance of myocardial disease in the left side of the heart. Consequently, nociception from the left side of the heart is referred to the left side of the body. Because angina is typically perceived as a pain of the chest, including the sternum and pectoral muscles, it is frequently called *angina pectoris*.

The pathways involved in angina are shown in Figure 19-6. Afferent fibers from the heart enter the sympathetic trunk through either the *cervical cardiac* or *thoracic cardiac nerves*. The former join the sympathetic chain at superior, middle, and inferior cervical ganglia, whereas the latter nerves join the

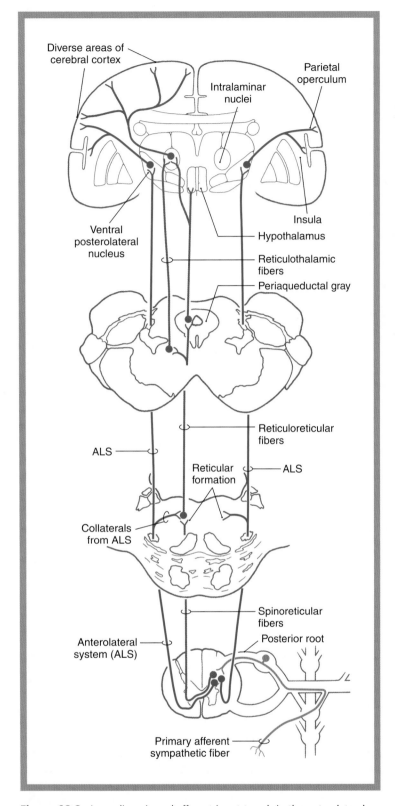

Figure 19-3. Ascending visceral afferent input travels in the anterolateral system *(green)* and through multisynaptic circuits via the reticular formation of the brainstem *(gray)*. These fibers influence specific and diverse areas of the cerebral cortex.

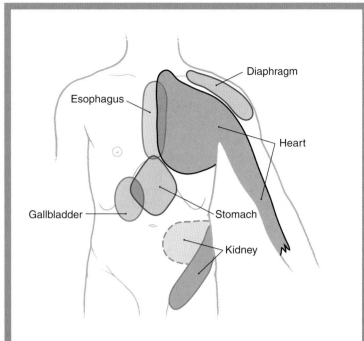

Figure 19-4. Superficial areas to which pain is commonly referred from the corresponding deep structures.

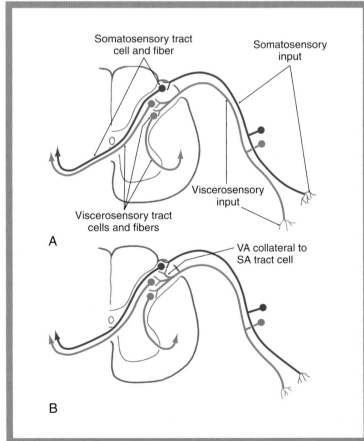

Figure 19-5. The circuits involved in referred pain. Somatic afferent *(blue)* and visceral afferent *(red)* fibers terminate on tract cells that convey their respective types of information to the thalamus (**A**). Collaterals from visceral afferent fibers (VA) may activate tract cells that usually convey somatic afferent (SA) data (**B**). The brain interprets this input as originating from the body wall.

sympathetic ganglia associated with spinal nerves T1 to T5 (Fig. 19-6). These primary viscerosensory fibers enter the spinal cord and terminate in laminae I and V of the posterior horn. These same spinal segments also receive cutaneous somatosensory input from dermatomes of the chest wall and arm (Fig. 19-6). Tract cells in the posterior horn that receive primarily somatosensory input may also be activated, as noted previously, by collaterals of visceral afferent fibers from the heart. Consequently, the cerebral cortex interprets the pain as originating

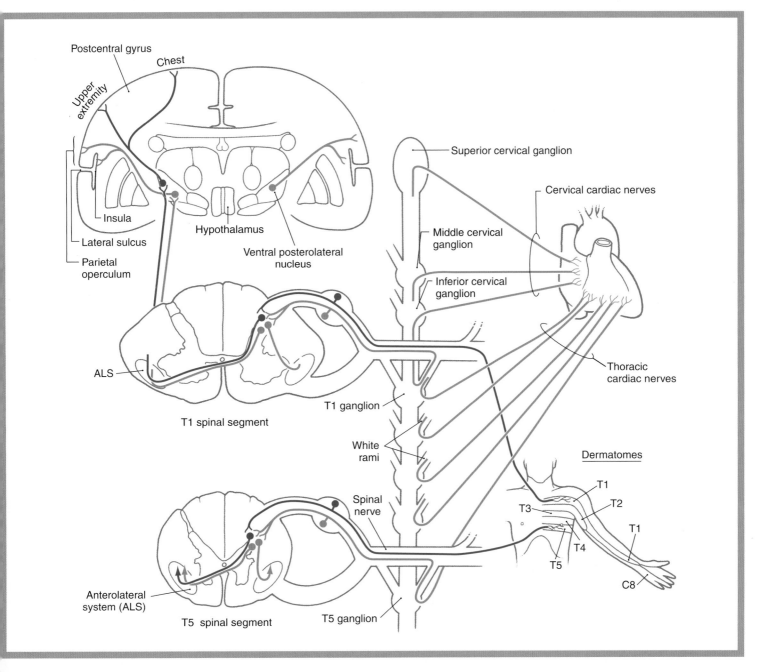

Figure 19-6. The pathways mediating cardiac pain and the circuits through which cardiac pain may be referred to superficial parts of the body wall.

from the surface of the body (over the upper chest and/or arm) when actually the stimulus that has produced the painful input is located in a visceral structure (the heart).

Pathways for Parasympathetic Afferents

Sacral Parasympathetic Afferents

The *pelvic nerves* are parasympathetic and contain viscerosensory fibers passing to cord levels S2 to S4 and GVE preganglionic fibers originating from these levels. These primary sensory parasympathetic fibers pass through the pelvic nerves, enter the spinal nerves, and have their cell bodies in posterior root ganglia of S2 to S4 (Fig. 19-7). Many of the central processes then pass through the posterior root to enter the spinal cord. However, a large number of other central processes, known as *recurrent fibers*, enter the spinal cord by traversing the anterior root (Fig. 19-7).

Once in the cord, these viscerosensory fibers terminate in the posterior horn and in the immediate vicinity of the visceral efferent preganglionic motor neurons. The posterior horn cells relay information on bladder or bowel distention (a sense of "fullness") to the VPL via the ALS and spinoreticular pathways described earlier and then, through this thalamic nucleus, to the insular and parietal opercular cortices (Figs. 19-3 and 19-6). In this way, a full bladder is perceived and interpreted as such. In addition, ascending input from the pelvic viscera is also shunted into the hypothalamus for the initiation of *supraspinal autonomic reflexes*. Those GVE cell groups in S2 to S4 that receive viscerosensory afferents give rise to parasympathetic preganglionic axons that synapse on postganglionic cells located in pelvic viscera (Fig. 19-7). This relationship between viscerosensory fibers and the GVE cell groups to which they project forms the basis for *spinal autonomic reflexes*.

Cranial Parasympathetic Afferents

Cranial nerves III, VII, IX, and X contain fibers of GVE preganglionic parasympathetic motor neurons. However, only cranial nerves VII, IX, and X have sensory ganglia. Of these, only cranial nerves IX (the *glossopharyngeal*) and X (the *vagus*) have significant numbers of parasympathetic afferent fibers.

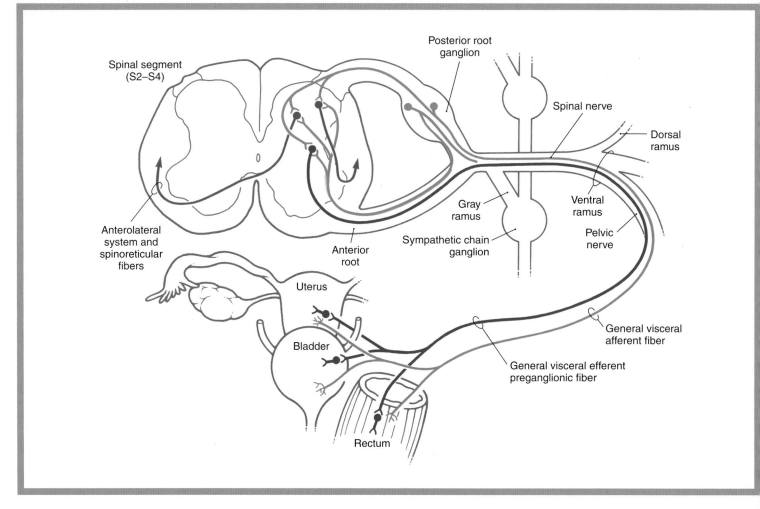

Figure 19-7. Primary sensory parasympathetic fibers *(red)* shown throughout their trajectory in relation to posterior horn tract cells *(green)*, and general visceral efferent neurons *(gray)*.

Visceral afferent fibers traveling in the glossopharyngeal nerve originate primarily from *chemoreceptors* of the carotid body and *baroreceptors* of the carotid sinus wall (Fig. 19-8). In addition, nociceptive and tactile input from the oropharynx (the general area of the palatine tonsil) is also conveyed on the ninth cranial nerve. These sensory fibers form the afferent limb of the gag reflex.

The *carotid body* is composed of specialized neural elements, *chemoreceptors*, and is innervated by viscerosensory branches of the glossopharyngeal nerve. Within the carotid body, these chemoreceptors are located in close proximity to a fenestrated capillary network. As a result, they are responsive to changes in arterial oxygen and carbon dioxide tension, to the acidity of the blood, and to drugs. Carotid *baroreceptors* are located in the carotid sinus wall and respond to rapid changes in arterial blood pressure (Fig. 19-8). The *aortic arch* also contains chemoreceptors and baroreceptors that are similar in structure and function to those found in the carotid body and sinus. These specialized receptors, however, are innervated by aortic or cardiac branches of the vagus nerve.

Fibers of the vagus nerve transmit a wide variety of physiologic information from thoracic viscera and from all viscera of the abdominal cavity above the level of the splenic flexure of the large colon. These vagal fibers convey information regarding the functional status of these structures but are not responsible for conveying information on pain.

The peripheral viscerosensory fibers, traveling in the glossopharyngeal and vagus nerves, enter the skull through the jugular foramen. Within this foramen there is a superior and an inferior ganglion on each nerve (Fig. 19-8). Cell bodies of primary viscerosensory neurons (GVA) are found within the inferior ganglion, whereas the superior ganglion contains the cell bodies of primary somatosensory neurons (general somatic afferent [GSA]).

The central processes of primary visceral fibers in cranial nerves IX and X enter the medulla, form the *solitary tract*, and synapse with neurons of the adjacent *solitary nucleus* (Fig. 19-8). Some of these fibers use substance P and cholecystokinin as their transmitters. Second-order neurons in the solitary nucleus project to and influence a variety of neurons in the brainstem and hypothalamus. These targets include the dorsal vagal nucleus, the nucleus ambiguus, rostral areas of the anterolateral medulla, and the parabrachial nuclei. The *dorsal vagal nucleus* is the primary source of preganglionic parasympathetic neurons that project to thoracic and abdominal viscera. In addition, the *nucleus ambiguus* also contains some parasympathetic visceromotor cells (GVE, autonomic) that innervate cardiac ganglia. However, the targets of most nucleus ambiguus cells (these are special visceral efferent [SVE] motor neurons) are muscles of the larynx, pharynx, and esophagus.

Visceral efferent (GVE) motor neurons of the nucleus ambiguus and the dorsal vagal nucleus receive input from the solitary nucleus and project, via the vagus nerve, to parasympathetic ganglia of the heart. Activation of this pathway causes a decrease in heart rate and a corresponding decrease in blood pressure, a "vasodepressor" response (Fig. 19-9). Conversely, neurons located in rostral parts of the anterolateral medulla receive solitary input and project to the spinal cord, where they influence the activity of preganglionic sympathetic motor

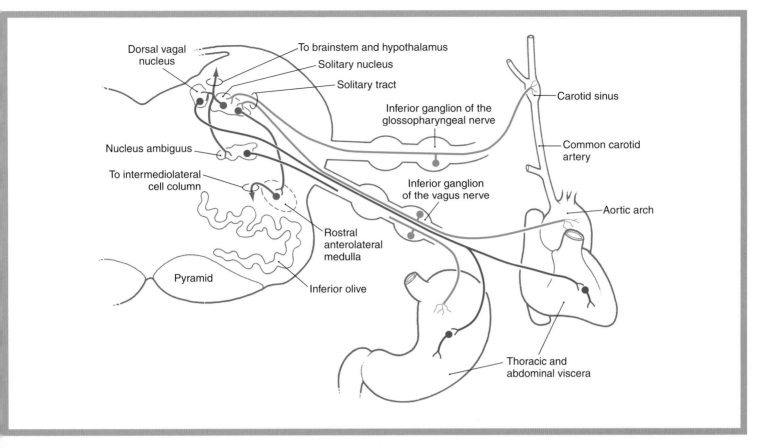

Figure 19-8. The nucleus of the solitary tract receives viscerosensory fibers via the glossopharyngeal (IX) and vagus (X) nerves and projects to a variety of other nuclei.

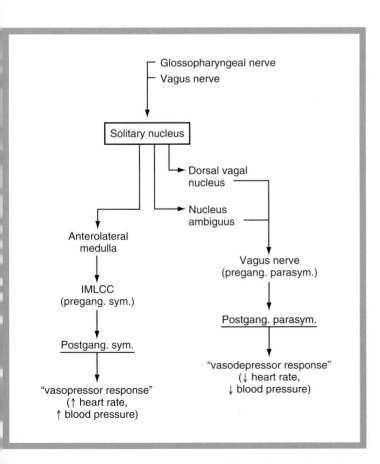

Figure 19-9. A diagrammatic representation of the pathways that mediate the "vasodepressor" and "vasopressor" responses. Compare these circuits with Figure 19-8.

neurons in the intermediolateral cell column. In doing so, this medullary center causes an increase in blood pressure and thereby serves a "vasopressor" function (Fig. 19-9).

Baroreceptor Reflex

Projections from the solitary nucleus to the dorsal vagal nucleus, to cells associated with the nucleus ambiguus, and to rostral parts of the anterolateral medulla are essential to the normal operation of the *baroreceptor reflex* (Fig. 19-8). In this reflex, afferent input from carotid and aortic baroreceptors enters the medulla on cranial nerves IX and X and terminates in the solitary nucleus. Increases in blood pressure cause the baroreceptors to increase their discharge frequency, whereas decreases in blood pressure result in a lower rate of baroreceptor discharge. In this manner, blood pressure is continuously monitored and the resulting information is forwarded to the solitary nucleus. Within this nucleus, neurons projecting to the dorsal vagal nucleus and the nucleus ambiguus respond in a manner opposite to those neurons projecting to the rostral parts of the anterolateral medulla. For example, during a period of acute *hypertension*, solitary neurons excite "vasodepressor" cells of the dorsal vagal nucleus and nucleus ambiguus and inhibit "vasopressor" neurons of the rostral anterolateral medulla (Figs. 19-8 and 19-9). The inhibitory solitary neurons may be GABAergic, whereas the excitatory neurons presumably use one of the excitatory amino acids. As a result of this dual influence from solitary neurons, blood pressure is lowered and the hypertension is diminished. Conversely, during a period of acute *hypotension*, projections from the solitary nucleus inhibit "vasodepressor" cells and excite "vasopressor" neurons, leading to an elevation of blood pressure. Consequently, blood pressure is elevated and the hypotension relieved.

In addition to projections from the solitary nucleus to ambiguus, dorsal vagal, and medullary nuclei, solitary neurons also project into the reticular formation. Consequently, visceral afferent information entering the medulla on the vagal and glossopharyngeal nerves may also influence the hypothalamus and diverse areas of the cerebral cortex. The solitary nucleus does not relay any appreciable amount of general visceral sensation to the dorsal thalamus. Consequently, most of the GVA afferent information conveyed by the glossopharyngeal and vagal nerves does not reach a level of consciousness. On the other hand, the solitary nucleus does relay taste information to the cerebral cortex via the ventral posteromedial nucleus.

Visceral Input to the Reticular Activating System

The reticular formation of the brainstem receives a wide range of inputs and projects to, among other targets, the intralaminar nuclei of the thalamus. These cell groups, in turn, send their axons to broad areas of the cerebral cortex, with the largest number terminating in the frontal lobe. These reticulothalamic and thalamocortical pathways "alert" or "activate" the cerebral cortex as a whole and constitute one important part of the *ascending reticular activating* system (ARAS) (see also Chapters 18 and 32).

As discussed previously, the reticular formation receives viscerosensory input via spinoreticular fibers and collaterals from the ALS. Some of these ascending fibers to the reticular formation convey nociceptive visceral afferent information originating from the gut on sympathetic afferent fibers. Other ascending fibers convey a sense of bladder (or bowel) fullness originating from pelvic viscera on parasympathetic afferents. Both types of viscerosensory input feed into the reticular formation and participate in the "arousal" of the cerebral cortex through the ARAS. For example, either sudden pain from the stomach or small intestine or the stimulus of a full bladder will excite the reticulothalamocortical circuit and wake a person from a deep sleep. The initial sensation is not one of specific information (full bladder, stomach pain) but rather the sense of just being awakened. However, once the cortex has been "alerted," the conscious/perceptive part of the brain takes over (recognizes the source of the arousal) and addresses the problem.

Synopsis of Clinical Points

- Pain from the gut is mediated by visceral nociceptors that are activated by tissue damage, ischemia, mechanical stimuli (distention), or endogenous substances (p. 303).
- Disease processes that alter blood chemistry, osmolarity, or body temperature will activate visceral receptors (p. 303).
- Visceral pain is poorly localized and may be referred (p. 303).
- Visceral pain is transmitted primarily via sympathetic nerves (p. 304).
- Referred pain is the phenomenon whereby pain from a visceral structure is perceived as coming from an overlying portion of the body (p. 305).
- Referred pain may be indicative of a disease process of a visceral structure (p. 305).
- Angina, or angina pectoris, is referred pain usually to the chest and left arm indicative of cardiac disease (p. 305).
- Rapid changes in blood pressure activate baroreceptors in the carotid sinus (p. 308).
- Hypertension is abnormally elevated blood pressure; it is a major health issue and has a variety of causes (p. 309).
- Hypotension is abnormally low blood pressure (p. 309).
- Damage to the reticular activating system may result in a comatose patient due to a failure of cortical arousal (p. 310).

Sources and Additional Reading

Ammons WS: Cardiopulmonary sympathetic afferent excitation of lower thoracic spinoreticular and spinothalamic neurons. J Neurophysiol 64:1907-1916, 1990.

Bieger D, Hopkins DA: Viscerotopic representation of the upper alimentary tract in the medulla oblongata in the rat: The nucleus ambiguus. J Comp Neurol 262:546-562, 1987.

Brody MJ: Central nervous system mechanisms of arterial pressure regulation. Fed Proc 45:2700-2706, 1986.

Cechetto DF, Saper CB: Evidence for a viscerotopic sensory representation in the cortex and thalamus in the rat. J Comp Neurol 262:27-45, 1987.

Cervero F, Foreman RD: Sensory innervation of the viscera. In Loewy AD, Spyer KM (eds): Central Regulation of Autonomic Functions. New York, Oxford University Press, 1990, pp 104-125.

Coggeshall RE, Applebaum ML, Frazen M, Stubbs TB III, Sykes MT: Unmyelinated axons in human ventral roots, a possible explanation for the failure of dorsal rhizotomy to relieve pain. Brain 98:157-166, 1975.

Garrison DW, Chandler MJ, Foreman RD: Viscerosomatic convergence onto feline spinal neurons from esophagus, heart and somatic fields: Effects of inflammation. Pain 49:373-382, 1992.

Procacci P, Zoppi M, Maresca M: Heart, vascular and haemopathic pain. In Wall PD, Melzack R (eds): Textbook of Pain, 4th ed. Edinburgh, Churchill Livingstone, 1999, pp 621-639.

Reis DJ, Granata AR, Joh TH, Ross CA, Ruggiero DA, Park DH: Brain stem catecholamine mechanisms in tonic and reflex control of blood pressure. Hypertension 6(Suppl II):7-15, 1984.

Willis W: Visceral pain. In Brooks FP, Evers PW (eds): Nerves and the Gut. Thorofare, NJ, Charles B. Slack, 1977, pp 350-364.

Chapter 20

The Visual System

J. C. Lynch, J. J. Corbett, and J. B. Hutchins

Vision is the sensory modality that perhaps captures the imagination more than any other. Phrases such as "He is the apple of my eye," or "Her eyes flashed with anger," or "I see what you mean," are common in the language and literature of most cultures and date back thousands of years. Furthermore, because of the way the nervous system converts optical images into neural signals and eventually visual experiences, the visual system is technically easier to study than other sensory systems. The visual system has consequently been studied in greater depth, both in its anatomy and its physiology, than other sensory systems, and the neural mechanisms by which physical energy in the environment is translated into psychological perceptions are better understood in the visual system than in any other sensory system. It turns out that many of the basic anatomic features and physiologic properties of the visual system, especially at the level of the cerebral cortex, are shared with other sensory systems. In this chapter, we present the visual system both as a sensory system important in its own right, particularly its importance in neurologic diagnosis, and also as a convenient example of some basic principles of neural processing that are found in many neural systems, including sensory, motor, and associational systems.

Overview

Like other sensory systems, the visual system creates a location-coded (visuotopic) "map" of its sensory field (the visual world) that is preserved at all levels. Light information is received by the retinal photoreceptors, and the initial processing of the visual signal occurs in the retina. Although the retina projects to several diencephalon and midbrain structures, most retinal axons terminate in a thalamic relay nucleus, the lateral geniculate nucleus, which in turn innervates primary visual cortex, a region in the occipital lobe. From there, visual information is sent to a number of *visual association areas* in the occipital, temporal, and parietal lobes.

Anatomy of the Eye

The human eye forms an optical image of an individual's surroundings and focuses that image on an array of approximately 125 million photoreceptors (rods and cones) that are located in the neural retina. The image is inverted and reversed by the lens. The anatomy of the eye is briefly summarized here.

Cornea

The *cornea* provides a transparent protective coating for the optical structures of the eye (Fig. 20-1). Its lateral margin is continuous with the *conjunctiva*, a specialized epithelium covering the "white" *(sclera)* of the eye. Although the conjunctiva and sclera have a blood supply (most evident when the eyes are irritated), the central cornea is normally not vascularized.

There are a variety of conditions that may affect the cornea and, by disturbing the transmission of light through the cornea, degrade the quality of the visual image. Damage to the cornea may occur in chronic infections of herpesvirus, of *Chlamydia trachomatis*, or of the bacteria that causes conjunctivitis. Trauma may, of course, cause permanent damage to the cornea. In addition, various metabolic diseases may result in crystal deposits, or other opacities, in the cornea.

Chambers of the Eye

Just behind the cornea is the fluid-filled *anterior chamber,* which is bound posteriorly by the *iris* and the opening of the *pupil* (Fig. 20-1). A second fluid-filled space, the *posterior chamber,* is bound anteriorly by the iris and posteriorly by the lens and its encircling suspensory ligament (zonule fibers). Fluid is continuously produced by the epithelium over the *ciliary body* around the rim of the posterior chamber and flows through the pupillary opening into the anterior chamber. It then drains into a set of modified veins, the *canals of Schlemm,* that are located around the rim of the anterior chamber in the *angle* where the iris meets the cornea. Because the suspensory ligament encircling the lens

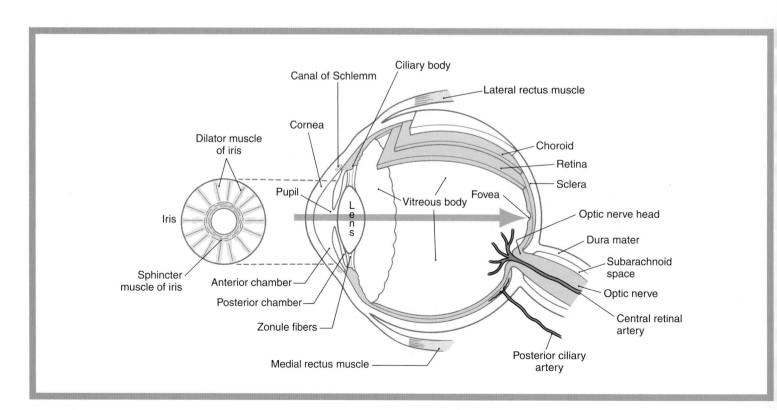

Figure 20-1. Cross section of the human eye. The *gray arrow* shows the path of light through the optical apparatus.

consists of discrete strands, the fluid in the posterior chamber is in contact with the *vitreous body*, the gelatinous mass that fills the main space of the eyeball between the lens and the retina.

Any condition that obstructs the outflow of fluid via the canals of Schlemm can lead to *glaucoma*, a buildup of fluid, and hence pressure, in the entire eyeball with resultant damage to the retina and optic nerve and eventual blindness. Patients with glaucoma often comment that their vision is blurred but not dimmed. A normal amount of light reaches the retina, but the progressive loss of photoreceptors causes blurring of the visual image. Damage proceeds from the periphery of the retina toward the central region where the *fovea* is located. In most cases of glaucoma (about 90%), the angle between the iris and cornea is normal *(open-angle glaucoma)* and the cause of the increase of pressure is unknown. In about 5% of patients, the angle between cornea and iris is abnormally acute *(closed-angle glaucoma)* and blocks the normal flow of fluid. In the remaining cases, the canals of Schlemm are blocked by debris from infection, complications of diabetes, or hemorrhage into the anterior chamber. When the intraocular pressure (IOP) is above 20 mm Hg, optic nerve damage is a concern. The resulting visual loss proceeds from partial (in the periphery first) to total.

Iris

The *iris* is a pigmented structure lying directly anterior to the lens (Fig. 20-1). The connective tissue, or *stroma*, of the iris contains melanocytes that reflect or absorb light to give the iris its characteristic color. Also embedded in the stroma are the circumferentially organized *sphincter muscle* of the iris and the radially arranged *dilator muscle* (Fig. 20-1).

The innervation of the *iris sphincter*, which closes the pupil, is parasympathetic. This pathway begins with preganglionic neurons whose cell bodies lie in the *Edinger-Westphal nucleus* and whose axons terminate in the *ciliary ganglion*. Axons of postganglionic ciliary ganglion neurons, in turn, end as neuromuscular synapses on the sphincter muscle and release acetylcholine. When activated, this pathway results in a reduction in pupil diameter, or *miosis*.

The innervation of the *iris dilator*, which opens the pupil, is sympathetic. The pathway begins with preganglionic neurons whose cell bodies lie in the *intermediolateral cell column* of the spinal cord at upper thoracic levels and whose axons terminate in the *superior cervical ganglion*. Axons of postganglionic superior cervical ganglion neurons, in turn, end as neuromuscular synapses on the dilator muscle and release norepinephrine. When activated, this pathway results in an increase in pupil diameter, or *mydriasis*. This phenomenon is a measure of the general state of the sympathetic tone. Anger, pain, or fear may result in an enlargement of the pupil in the absence of a change in lighting conditions. The *pupillary light reflex*, a contraction of the pupil in response to light, is used to assess the function of the nervous system at midbrain levels (see Chapter 28).

The circumference of the pupillary margin changes by a factor of 6. This proportional change in muscle length is greater than any other in the human body. To accomplish this change, acetylcholine is released onto *both* the sphincter and dilator muscles. The effect is to activate muscarinic receptors that *depolarize* sphincter muscle cells and cause contraction. Additionally, acetylcholine released by collaterals onto the dilator muscle mediates presynaptic inhibition of norepinephrine release and *blocks* dilator contraction. Thus, as the sphincter contracts, the dilator relaxes, strengthening the pupillary response to light.

Lens

The *lens* is a clear structure that focuses light on the *retina* (Fig. 20-1). The lens of the eye is a simple convex lens that inverts and reverses the image on the retina. Mechanisms that change the curvature of the lens are discussed in detail in Chapter 28.

Beginning at about age 40, the lens begins to lose its elasticity, so that the shape it adopts when relaxed is more flattened than earlier in life. This change reduces the affected person's ability to focus on near objects, a condition called *presbyopia*. Reading or bifocal corrective lenses are prescribed to aid the patient in performing tasks requiring close, detailed vision.

Cataract

Opacities in the lens, known as *cataracts*, are relatively common and can be seen as a cloudiness of the lens. Cataracts may be caused by *congenital defects* (e.g., secondary to maternal infection with *rubella*), persistent exposure to *ultraviolet light*, diabetes, high doses of some medications, radiation therapy, or poorly understood mechanisms that occur in aging. Current therapy consists of replacement of the lens with an inert plastic prosthesis, restoring sight but with a concomitant loss of accommodation.

Uvea

The iris, ciliary body, and choroid make up the *vascular tunic* of the eye, also called the *uvea*. The *choroid* is a highly vascularized, pigmented tissue layer lying between the *retinal pigment epithelium* and the *sclera*, the tough outer coating of the eye. *Uveitis* is an inflammation of these structures, often secondary to eye injury.

The Neural Retina and Pigment Epithelium

The inner surface of the posterior aspect of the eye is covered by the *retina*, which is composed of the *neural retina* and the *retinal pigment epithelium* (Fig. 20-2). In describing the layers and cells of the retina, it is common to use the terms *inner* and *outer*. *Inner* refers to structures located toward the vitreous (i.e., the center of the eyeball), whereas *outer* is used in reference to structures located toward the pigment epithelium and choroid.

The *retinal pigment epithelium* is a continuous sheet of pigmented cuboidal cells bound together by tight junctions that block the flow of plasma or ions. Its functions are as follows: (1) it supplies the neural retina with nutrition in the form of glucose and essential ions; (2) it protects retinal photoreceptors from potentially damaging levels of light; and (3) it plays a key role in the maintenance of photoreceptor anatomy via phagocytosis.

The *neural retina* contains the photoreceptors and associated neurons of the eye and is specialized for sensing light and processing the resultant information. The *photoreceptors* absorb quanta of light (photons) and convert this input to an electrical signal. The signal is then processed by retinal neurons as discussed further on. Finally, the retinal neurons called *ganglion cells* send the processed signal to the brain via axons that collectively form the optic nerve.

The contact between the neural retina and the pigment epithelium is the adult remnant of the ventricular space of the developing eye cup. As such, it is mechanically unstable. This instability is demonstrated in a *retinal detachment*, in which the neural retina tears away from the pigment epithelium. Because photoreceptors are metabolically dependent on their contact with pigment epithelial cells, a detached retina must be repaired to avoid further damage. The detached part of the neural retina is reattached to the pigment epithelium using surgical procedures. The degree of functional recovery in the reattached part of the retina depends upon its location. It also depends on how soon the reattachment is performed after the injury.

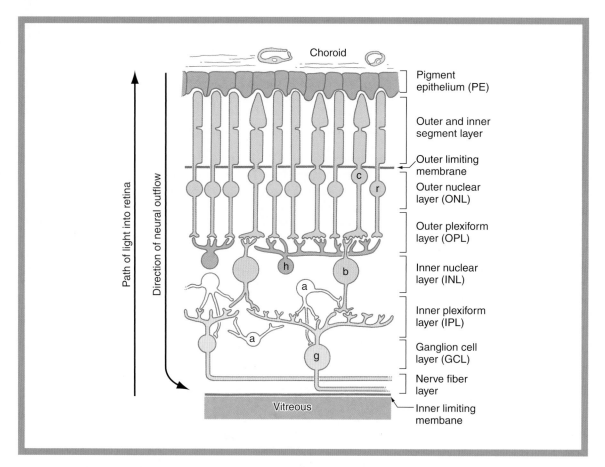

Figure 20-2. Cells and layers of the retina. Photoreceptors (rods, r, and cones, c) are shown in *green*. Horizontal cells (h, *gray*) and bipolar cells (b, *blue*) receive input from photoreceptors; the bipolar cells, in turn, synapse onto amacrine cells (a, *white*) and ganglion cells (g, *red*).

The neural retina has seven characteristic layers (Fig. 20-2). From outer to inner they are (1) a layer containing the *photoreceptor cell outer and inner segments;* (2) an *outer nuclear layer* consisting of the nuclei of photoreceptor cells; (3) the *outer plexiform layer,* consisting of the synaptic connections of photoreceptors with second-order retinal cells; (4) the *inner nuclear layer,* containing somata of second-order and some third-order retinal cells; (5) the *inner plexiform layer,* another area of synaptic contact; (6) the *ganglion cell layer,* containing the cell bodies of the *ganglion cells;* and (7) the *nerve fiber layer* (or *optic fiber layer*), composed of the axons of the ganglion cells. These axons converge at the *optic disc* to form the *optic nerve.* Layers 2 through 7 are flanked by a pair of *limiting membranes,* which consist of glial cell processes joined by tight junctions. The *outer limiting membrane* is located between layers 1 and 2, and the *inner limiting membrane* is located between the nerve fiber layer and the vitreous.

The *photoreceptor outer segments* interdigitate with the melanin-filled processes of pigment epithelial cells (Fig. 20-2). These processes are mobile, and they elongate into the pigmented layer when the light is bright (*photopic* conditions) and retract when the light is dim (*scotopic* conditions). This mechanism combines with contractions of the iris to protect the retina from light conditions that would otherwise damage the photoreceptors. The iris, pigment epithelium, and circuitry of the retina all contribute to the eye's ability to resolve the visual world over a wide range of light conditions.

The blood supply of the neural retina arises from branches of the *ophthalmic artery:* the *central artery of the retina* and the *ciliary arteries.* The central artery branches out from the optic nerve head to serve inner portions of the neural retina. The ciliary arteries penetrate the sclera around the exit of the optic

nerve and feed the *choriocapillaris* (a portion of the choroid), which, in turn, provides nutrients to the outer portions of the neural retina.

Photoreceptor Cells

The rods and cones of the retina are responsible for *photoreception,* the process by which photons are detected and the information is transduced into an electrochemical signal. There are two basic types of photoreceptors: *rods* and *cones* (Figs. 20-3 and 20-4). Both types have the same overall design. Light is detected and transduced in an *outer segment* that points toward the pigment epithelium. A narrow stalk, the *cilium,* connects the outer segment to a second expanded region called the *inner segment,* which contains mitochondria and produces the energy that maintains the cell. The cilium contains nine pairs of microtubules emanating from a basal body located in the inner segment. The nucleus and perikaryon of the cell are found in the outer nuclear layer; finally, the cell terminates in the outer plexiform layer in an expansion that makes synaptic contacts with neurons. This synaptic expansion is called the *spherule* in rod cells and the *pedicle* in cone cells. Both rod and cone synaptic terminals contain a characteristic dark sheet of protein called the *synaptic ribbon.* This structure may act as a "conveyor belt," organizing vesicular release of transmitter.

Rods

Rod cells are named for the shape of their outer segment, which is a membrane-bound cylinder containing hundreds of tightly stacked membranous discs (Fig. 20-3). The rod outer segment is a site of *transduction.* Photons travel through cells of the neural retina before striking the membranous discs of the rod outer

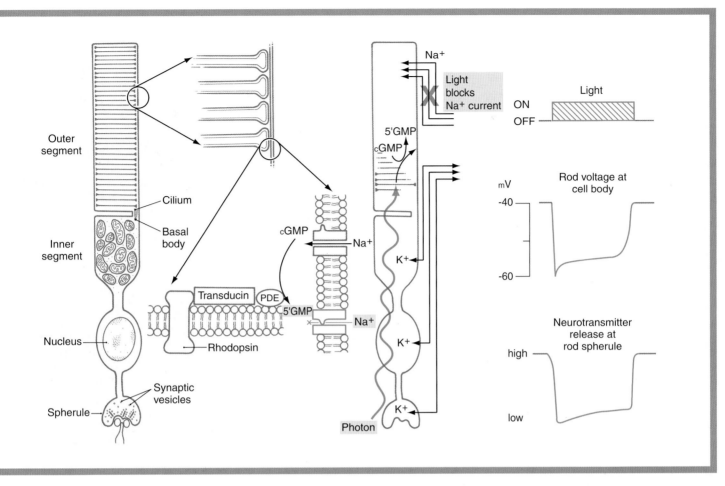

Figure 20-3. The rod photoreceptor and the physiologic and chemical changes that occur in response to light. Events associated with light are shown in *red.* cGMP, cyclic guanosine monophosphate; 5'GMP, 5'-guanosine monophosphate; PDE, phosphodiesterase.

segment. Molecules of *rhodopsin* within these membranes undergo a conformational change and along with transducin and phosphodiesterase (PDE) induce biochemical changes in the rod outer segment, which reduce levels of cyclic guanosine monophosphate (cGMP). In the dark, cGMP levels in the rod outer segment are high. This cGMP mediates a *standing sodium current.* At rest, in the dark, sodium ions flow into the rod outer segment. This high resting level of sodium permeability results in a relatively high resting potential for rod cells, about –40 mV. These sodium channels of the outer segment membrane, which are normally open, close in response to increased calcium or a reduction in cGMP. This drives the membrane potential away from the sodium equilibrium potential and toward the potassium equilibrium potential, and the rod cell is *hyperpolarized* in response to a light stimulus (Fig. 20-3). Note that photoreceptors are the only sensory neurons that hyperpolarize in response to the relevant stimulus.

The hyperpolarization of the rod outer segment propagates passively (i.e., without firing an action potential) through the perikaryon to the rod spherule. In the absence of light, the photoreceptor terminals constantly release the transmitter *glutamate* at these synapses. The arrival of a light-induced wave of hyperpolarization causes a transient *reduction* in this tonic release of glutamate. As explained further on, this event can *depolarize* some of the cells that receive synapses from photoreceptor terminals while *hyperpolarizing* others.

Rhodopsin molecules are capable of a huge but finite number of photoisomerization events. Rather than replace individual rhodopsin molecules, every morning the distal one tenth of the outer segment is broken off and phagocytosed by the pigment epithelium. Through this process of *rod shedding,* the outer segment is constantly renewed. New discs are formed at the base of the outer segment and move outward so that the shed discs are replaced. In this way, the rod remains a constant length and the outer segment is renewed about every 10 days.

Cones

Like rod outer segments, *cone outer segments* also consist of a membranous stack (Fig. 20-4). Unlike in rods, however, these stacks of cone membranes are of constantly decreasing diameter (from cilium to tip), giving the cell its characteristic shape. Also, they are not enclosed within a second membrane but are open to the extracellular space adjacent to the pigment epithelium (Fig. 20-4).

The process of transduction in cones is generally similar to that in rods. *Cone opsin* absorbs photons and undergoes a con-formational change, resulting in a hyperpolarization of the cell membrane (Fig. 20-4). This hyperpolarization propagates passively to the cone's synaptic ending, the *cone pedicle,* in the outer plexiform layer. Cone pedicles and rod spherules both contain synaptic ribbons surrounded by vesicles, but cone pedicles are larger (Fig. 20-4). Serial-section electron microscopy has shown that the synaptic ribbons are actually a single extensive sheet of protein. Like rods, cones release the neurotransmitter *glutamate* tonically in the dark and respond to light with a decrease in glutamate release.

There are three types of cones, each tuned to a different light wavelength (Fig. 20-5). *L-cones* (red cones) are sensitive to long wavelengths, *M-cones* (green cones) to medium wavelengths, and *S-cones* (blue cones) to short wavelengths. Because any pure

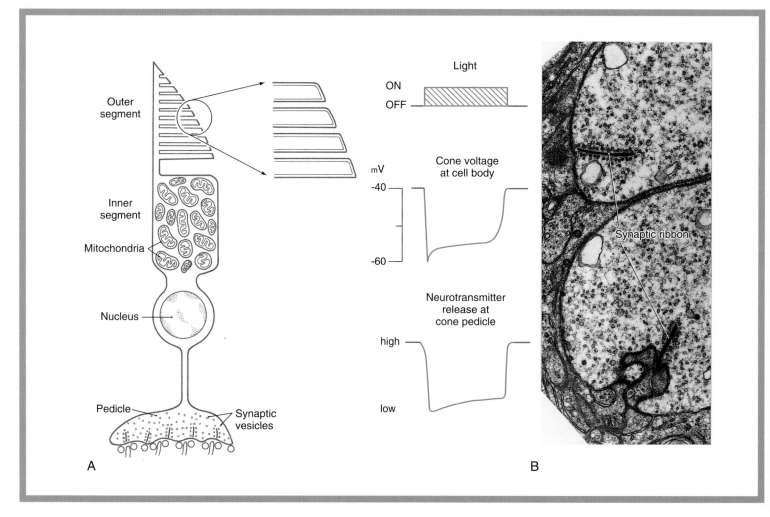

Figure 20-4. The cone photoreceptor (**A**). Cones, like rods, reduce their levels of neurotransmitter release when stimulated by photons. Cones and rods are also distinguished by prominent electron-dense *synaptic ribbons* in their terminals (**B**).

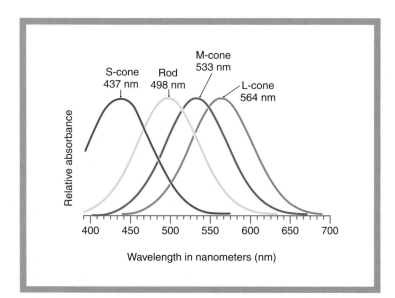

Figure 20-5. Absorption spectra of rods and the three types of cones. Because the three cone spectra are different but overlapping, any wavelength of light in the visual spectrum *(bottom scale)* will elicit a set of response intensities in the three types of cones that is different from the set elicited by any other wavelength. Therefore, any color in the visual spectrum can be uniquely encoded. The rod spectrum is shown for comparison even though rod input is not used in color recognition. Dim red light can be used to adapt humans to maximum rod sensitivity because red light (620 to 700 nm) is not absorbed by rods to any significant extent.

color represents a particular wavelength of light, each color will be represented by a unique combination of responses in the L-, M-, and S-cones.

If one of these cone types is absent because of a genetic defect in the corresponding opsin, the affected person will confuse certain colors that look different to visually normal people and is said to be "*color blind*." It is better, however, to think of this condition as "color confusion" because the patient can still see all colors of the visible spectrum; it is the ability to *distinguish* certain colors that has been lost. Because the genes for the L-cone (red-absorbing) and M-cone (green-absorbing) opsins are located on the X chromosome, color blindness is more common in men. Alteration of the gene for the S-cone (blue-sensitive) pigment, which is located on an autosome, is much rarer. The inability to detect a pure red is known as *protanopia*, and inability to detect green is known as *deuteranopia*.

Macula and Fovea
At the posterior pole of the eye is a yellowish spot, the *macula lutea*, the center of which is a depression called the *fovea centralis* (Fig. 20-6). Near the fovea, the inner retinal layers become thinner and eventually disappear so that, at the bottom of the foveal pit, only the outer nuclear layer and photoreceptor outer segments remain. This allows a maximum amount of light to reach the photoreceptors with optimal fidelity.

Most of the visual input that reaches the brain comes from the fovea. Cones, which are responsible for color vision, are the only type of photoreceptor present in the fovea. In contrast, rods, which are most sensitive at low levels of illumination, are

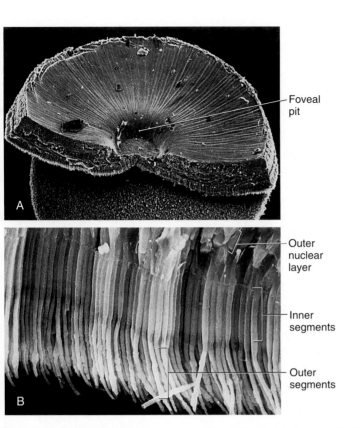

Figure 20-6. Scanning electron micrographs of the primate fovea centralis (**A**) and of inner and outer segments of photoreceptors (**B**), mostly rods, in more peripheral areas of the retina. Only cones are present in the foveal pit. The surface striations (**A**) are ganglion cell axons en route to the optic nerve head. (Photographs courtesy of Dr. Bessie Borwein. From Borwein B: Scanning electron microscopy of monkey foveal photoreceptors. Anat Rec 205:363-373, 1983, with permission of Wiley-Liss, Inc.)

the predominant photoreceptors in the periphery of the retina. The visual world is a composite formed from a succession of foveal images carrying form and color information supplemented with input from the peripheral retina carrying motion information.

Receptive Fields

The *receptive field* of a visually responsive neuron is defined as that region of the visual world in which a stimulus of the proper characteristics will influence the activity of the neuron. The influence may be either excitatory or inhibitory. Some neurons will exhibit an excitatory influence when the stimulus is in one location and an inhibitory influence when the stimulus is in a nearby location. The *receptive field* of a neuron is the sum of the areas in which the stimulus affects the activity of that neuron.

In the early stages of visual information processing, receptive fields have a characteristic *concentric center-surround* organization. The receptive field is roughly circular (Fig. 20-7). Stimuli in the center of this circle tend to evoke one type of response (e.g., depolarization), whereas stimuli in the doughnut-shaped outer rim evoke the opposite response (e.g., hyperpolarization). In later stages of visual processing, in the visual cortex, receptive field properties are more complicated.

Processing of Visual Input in the Retina

Among retinal cells, only retinal ganglion cells have *voltage-gated sodium c*hannels on their axonal membranes. As a result, only ganglion cells use action potentials to carry information.

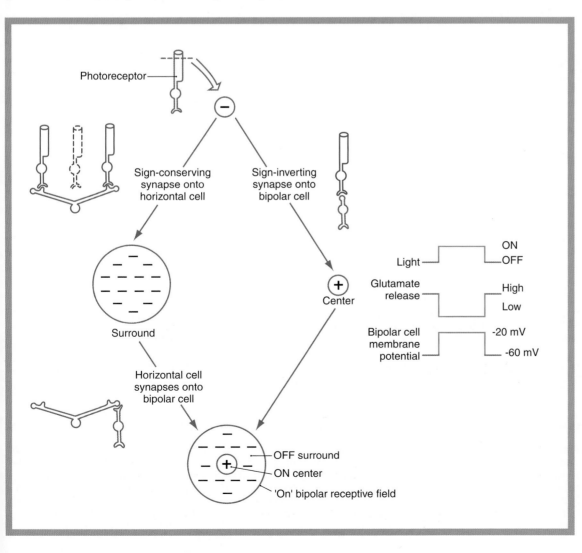

Figure 20-7. How center-surround receptive fields are built in the visual system. Inputs from both receptors and horizontal cells contribute to the characteristic center-surround receptive fields of bipolar cells. A "sign-conserving" synapse is one in which hyperpolarization in the presynaptic cell promotes hyperpolarization in the postsynaptic cell. A "sign-inverting" synapse is one in which hyperpolarization in the presynaptic cell promotes depolarization in the postsynaptic cell. The example illustrated is of an "on" bipolar cell.

So-called *calcium spikes* resulting from an increase in calcium permeability are seen in amacrine cells. All other retinal cells use only *graded potentials* to process information.

The receptive field properties of each retinal cell depend on the processing of information passing through the neurons between the photoreceptor and the retinal cell in question. For example, a bipolar cell's response is directly related to the activity of photoreceptors and horizontal cells (Figs. 20-7 and 20-8). As with all sensory systems, the structural, electrical, and synaptic properties of the cell are reflected in receptive field properties.

Outer and Inner Plexiform Layers

Synaptic contacts in the retina are concentrated into the *outer* and *inner plexiform layers* (Fig. 20-2). The *outer plexiform layer* contains synapses among and between retinal photoreceptors, horizontal cells, and bipolar cells. Contacts between a single cone pedicle or rod spherule, a centrally placed postsynaptic bipolar cell process, and two laterally placed horizontal cell processes form a *triad*.

The *inner plexiform layer* contains synaptic contacts among and between bipolar, amacrine, and ganglion cells. In this layer "off" and "on" bipolar cells terminate, making synaptic contact with the corresponding type ganglion cell. Amacrine cells also synapse with ganglion cells, other amacrine cells, and bipolar cells.

Horizontal Cells

Horizontal cells consist of a cell body and its associated dendrites and an axon that courses parallel to the plane of the retina to nearby and distant photoreceptors (Fig. 20-2). These cells receive glutaminergic input from photoreceptors, and, in turn, form GABAergic synaptic contacts on adjacent rods and cones. This arrangement allows horizontal cells to sharpen the edge of a receptive field by inhibiting surrounding photoreceptor cells.

Bipolar Cells

In their position between photoreceptor cells and ganglion cells, *bipolar cells* help to form a straight-through pathway for

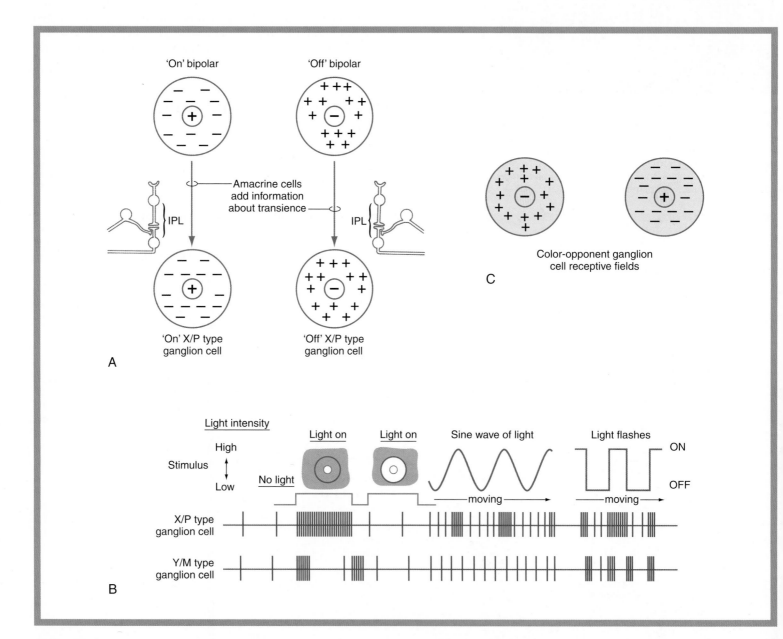

Figure 20-8. How ganglion cell receptive fields are built in the visual system. Both "on" and "off" bipolar cells contribute to the formation of receptive fields (**A**) in ganglion cells. Amacrine cells add information about transience (i.e., how long since the light has changed from on to off). X- or P-type ganglion cells respond linearly to the sine wave grating; the frequency of action potentials rises and falls in synchronization with the sine wave of light intensity used to stimulate them (**B**). When light strikes both center and surround, there is no net change in ganglion cell activity in either cell type. On the other hand, Y- or M-type ganglion cells respond best to the changes between light onset and offset. X- or P-type ganglion cells are also responsive to color (**C**). Two examples are shown, called R⁻G⁺ (for red inhibitory center and green excitatory surround) and R⁺G⁻. There are also G and G cells and blue-yellow combinations. IPL, inner plexiform layer.

visual input (Fig. 20-2). *Cone bipolar cells* and *rod bipolar cells* are differentiated based on their principal synaptic inputs.

Bipolar cells are the comparators, or edge detectors, of the retina. With the horizontal cells, they compare the activity in each region of the visual field with that in a nearby location. They are the first visual cells to exhibit the *center-surround receptive field* organization. In terms of physiologic response, there are two basic types of bipolar cells. "On," or *depolarizing*, cells respond to a light stimulus in the receptive field center by depolarizing, whereas "off," or *hyperpolarizing*, bipolar cells have the opposite center response (Figs. 20-7 and 20-8).

Imagine a series of photons striking a photoreceptor outer segment. Recall that the photoreceptor is *hyperpolarized* in response to light input, so that release of its neurotransmitter, glutamate, is *decreased* in the presence of light.

In an "on" bipolar cell, glutamate must act through receptors to hyperpolarize the bipolar cell. Then, when the glutamate that is released constantly in the dark is removed by the presence of light, the "on" bipolar cell depolarizes. This effect can be confusing, because we are used to thinking of most glutamate receptors as excitatory, or "sign conserving." These receptors must be of a different type from that found elsewhere, namely, inhibitory, or "sign inverting" (Table 20-1).

In an "off" bipolar cell, the opposite type of glutamate receptor must be present on the postsynaptic membrane. In the dark, glutamate released tonically by the photoreceptor depolarizes the "off" bipolar cell. Then, when photons activate the photoreceptor, it hyperpolarizes and reduces its release of glutamate. The decrease in the amount of neurotransmitter causes a hyperpolarization of the postsynaptic "off" bipolar cell membrane. This effect could take place using the "conventional" type of glutamate receptor, which is "excitatory" or "sign conserving."

Thus, the designation "sign conserving" means that the electrical responses of the photoreceptor and bipolar cell are the same (hyperpolarization in one leads to hyperpolarization in the other; depolarization in one leads to depolarization in the other), and "sign inverting" means that the electrical response is inverted (hyperpolarization in one leads to depolarization in the other, and vice versa). The terms "excitation" and "inhibition" lead to confusion in this context and therefore are avoided.

Amacrine Cells

These cells have a small soma, no obvious axon, and dendrites that are few but highly branched (Fig. 20-2). Their cell bodies are usually found in the inner nuclear layer but may be displaced into the ganglion cell layer. Amacrine cells may contain two different transmitters, for example, γ-aminobutyric acid (GABA) and acetylcholine or glycine and a neuropeptide.

Like horizontal cells, amacrine cells also have dendrites that extend over long distances, sampling and modifying bipolar cell output. Whereas horizontal cells sense change, amacrine cells *sense change in change*. For example, a fan blade rotating at constant speed alters the activity of horizontal cells as the dark and light areas of the fan blade stimulate them but the amacrine cell network will not change its activity. However, if the fan is speeding up or slowing down, the amacrine cell network is maximally stimulated.

Ganglion Cells

Ganglion cells are the output cells of the retina (Fig. 20-2). Their somata form the ganglion cell layer, and their axons converge on the *optic disc* and form the *optic nerve*. Ganglion cells are grouped in two ways: by size and by physiologic role. These classifications largely coincide. Like bipolar cells, ganglion cells have center-surround types of receptive fields.

The largest ganglion cells, called *alpha cells*, predominate in the peripheral retina and receive input mainly from rods. They have more extensive dendritic trees and thicker axons than those of other ganglion cell types. Physiologically, alpha cells correspond to the cell type called "Y" cells. They participate little in color perception, in line with their largely rod input, and they show the "on" or "off" center-surround patterns of the bipolar cells with which they connect. These cells are also called "M" cells because in humans and other primates, they consistently connect to other large cells in the *magnocellular* layers in the lateral geniculate nucleus (Fig. 20-17). Medium-sized ganglion cells, *beta cells*, are found predominantly in the central retina and receive input mainly from cones. They correspond to the physiologic class of "X" cells. In keeping with their central location and small dendritic arbors, they have small receptive fields. They are responsive to color stimuli, and this fact gives the center-surround organization a new twist. The center responds to one color, and the surround responds maximally to the color opposite it on a color wheel (Fig. 20-8C). For example, an "X" cell may have a yellow-responsive center and a blue-responsive surround. Still, the "*on-center*" and "*off-center*" categories remain. These cells are also called "P" cells because in humans and other primates they consistently connect to other, smaller cells in the *parvocellular* layers in the lateral geniculate nucleus.

All ganglion cells left out of the preceding two categories are classified anatomically as *gamma*, *delta*, and *epsilon cells* and physiologically as "W" cells. These cells tend to have smaller cell bodies and axons, and they show a variety of receptive field sizes and physiologic responses.

Retinal Projections

Retinal ganglion cells send axons to a variety of locations in the diencephalon and midbrain. Among the targets are the *suprachiasmatic nucleus*, a hypothalamic region that controls diurnal rhythms (see Chapter 30); the *accessory optic* and *olivary pretectal nuclei*, which subserve the pupillary light reflex (see Chapter 28); and the *superior colliculus*, which helps to control eye movements (see Chapter 28) and mediates so-called visual reflexes. The superior colliculus, in turn, projects to the *pulvinar*, the largest nucleus of the thalamus. The pulvinar receives input from the superior colliculus, pretectum, and visual cortex (see below) and sends information to *visual association areas*. This brief overview illustrates the point that the visual system influences a wide range of areas of the brain.

Retinogeniculate Projections

Most retinal ganglion cells send their axons to the *lateral geniculate nucleus* by way of the optic nerve, chiasm, and tract. This connection is called the *retinogeniculate projection* (Fig. 20-9). In this pathway, an orderly map of visual space must

Table 20-1. Responses of Bipolar Cells to Stimuli

Condition	Bipolar Cell Response in Receptive Field Center	
	ON	OFF
Light	Depolarized	Hyperpolarized
No light	Hyperpolarized	Depolarized
Photoreceptor depolarization	Hyperpolarized	Depolarized
Photoreceptor hyperpolarization	Depolarized	Hyperpolarized
Increased transmitter release	Hyperpolarized	Depolarized
Decreased transmitter release	Depolarized	Hyperpolarized

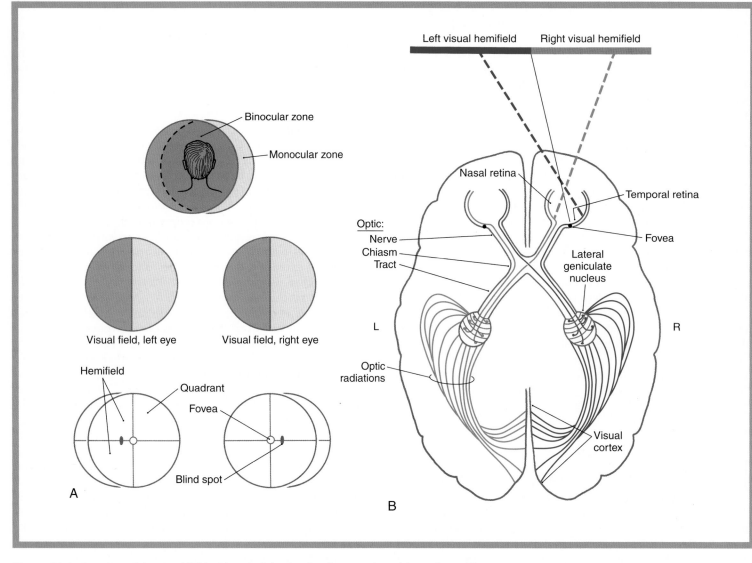

Figure 20-9. Overview of the visual fields (**A**) and of the visual pathway as viewed from above (**B**).

be maintained. The receptive fields of photoreceptors (and of the ganglion cells to which they are connected) lie in a precise arrangement on the retinal surface. Adjacent points in the visual world are perceived by adjacent ganglion cells. This orderly representation of the visual world on the retina is called a *retinotopic map*.

The *visual field* is the part of the world seen by the patient with both eyes open and looking straight ahead (Fig. 20-9A). It consists of a *binocular zone*—a broad central region seen by both eyes—and right and left *monocular zones* (or *monocular crescents*) seen only by the corresponding eye. In the clinical setting, it is common to test the visual function of the two eyes separately by covering first one eye and then the other (see Chapter 33). Consequently, visual field deficits are commonly illustrated as losses from the visual field of each eye (see, for example, Figs. 20-14 and 20-15). Each *visual field* is divided into nasal and temporal halves *(hemifields)*, and each of these halves is divided into upper and lower parts (resulting in *quadrants*) (Fig. 20-9A).

A stream of photons can be thought of as a ray of light that enters the eye. The light ray is bent *(refracted)* by the cornea and lens so that the image is focused on the retina. The image is inverted and reversed by the lens, as described earlier. Light from the inferior visual world strikes the superior retina. Light from the right visual world (in the binocular zone) strikes the temporal retina of the left eye and the nasal retina of the right eye (Fig. 20-9). These patterns are essential to understanding

normal vision and the defects in visual fields seen in patients with lesions in the visual pathways. The *retinotopic map* is maintained throughout the visual system.

Optic Nerve, Chiasm, and Tract

Axons of retinal ganglion cells conveying input from all areas of the retina converge at the *optic disc*, where they penetrate the choroid and sclera to form the *optic nerve*. Within the *nerve fiber layer* of the retina, ganglion cell axons are unmyelinated. However, as they pass through the sclera, they become ensheathed with myelin formed by oligodendrocytes. Because there are no photoreceptor cells in the optic disc (only ganglion cell axons), light striking this area is not perceived. Consequently, this part of the retina is commonly called the *blind spot* (Fig. 20-10A, B). Visual acuity is greatest at the fovea, but the peripheral retina has little form vision: fine details cannot be perceived in the peripheral retina because the "pixel density" (density of rod photoreceptors) is much lower.

The *optic nerve* extends from the caudal aspect of the eye to the *optic chiasm* (Fig. 20-9). This nerve is enclosed in a sleeve of dura and arachnoid mater that is continuous with the same layers around the brain. Thus, the subarachnoid space extends along the optic nerve, which is bathed in cerebrospinal fluid. For this reason, increases in intracranial pressure may be transmitted along the optic nerve(s) and can cause blockage of axoplasmic flow at the optic nerve head. This axoplasmic stasis results in swelling of the optic nerve head *(papilledema)* (Fig. 20-10D).

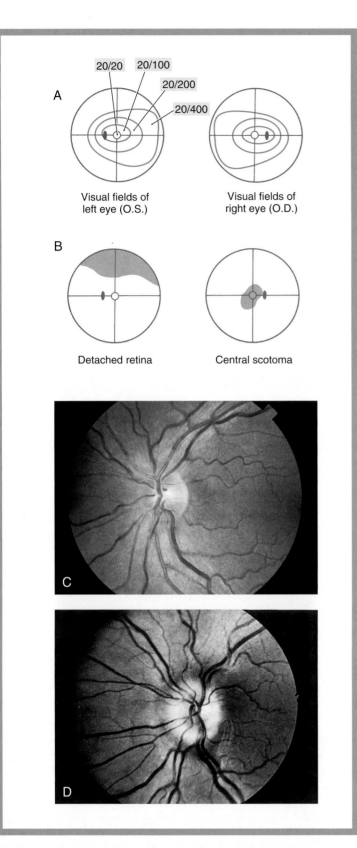

The resulting damage to the optic nerve may result in partial or complete loss of vision in that eye (similar to Fig. 20-14).

Terminal branches of the *central retinal artery*, a branch of the *ophthalmic artery*, issue from the optic disc and radiate over the retina. Examination of these vessels through an *ophthalmoscope* can help assess the health of the eye and the central nervous system (Fig. 20-10C, D). Changes in the configuration of the retinal vessels or in the size or shape of the optic disc may indicate diseases of the retina, the vascular system, or the central nervous system.

Just rostral to the pituitary stalk, the optic nerves come together to form the *optic chiasm*, from which the *optic tracts* diverge as they pass caudally. In the chiasm, the fibers from the *nasal* half of each retina (corresponding to the temporal hemifields) cross to enter the contralateral optic tract, whereas the fibers from the *temporal* half of each retina (corresponding to the nasal hemifields) remain on the same side and enter the ipsilateral optic tract. In this way, each half of the brain receives the fibers corresponding to the contralateral half of the visual world (Figs. 20-9, 20-11, and 20-12).

Although many clinical events can affect the optic chiasm, this structure is especially susceptible to tumors of the pituitary gland. Enlarging pituitary tumors that damage the crossing fibers in the midline of the chiasm will interrupt visual input from the temporal halves of both visual fields, resulting in a *bitemporal hemianopia* (Figs. 20-11, 20-12D-F). A lesion that damages the lateral part of the chiasm may interrupt only fibers conveying information from the nasal visual field on the same side, although in practice this situation is quite rare. This deficit is called an *ipsilateral* (either *right* or *left*) *nasal hemianopia*.

Extending caudolaterally from the chiasm, the axons of retinal ganglion cells continue as a compact bundle, the *optic tract*. This structure courses over the surface of the crus cerebri at its junction with the hemisphere and ends in the lateral geniculate nucleus of the diencephalon (see Fig. 15-5). Because the optic tract contains fibers conveying visual input from the ipsilateral nasal hemifield and the contralateral temporal hemifield, lesions of the optic tract result in a *contralateral (right or left) homonymous hemianopia* (Fig. 20-11; see also Fig. 20-16).

The optic chiasm receives blood from the small *anteromedial branches* of the anterior communicating artery and A_1 segment of the anterior cerebral artery. The optic nerve receives its blood supply from small branches of the ophthalmic artery traveling parallel to the nerve. As noted previously, the optic nerve head and retina are supplied by the central artery of the retina. The optic tract receives its main blood supply from the *anterior choroidal artery* (see Figs. 15-16 and 15-18), whereas the lateral geniculate nucleus is in the domain of the *thalamogeniculate artery*, a branch of the posterior cerebral artery.

Visual Fields Correlated With Visual Structures as Seen in Magnetic Resonance Imaging

The convention for describing and illustrating *visual fields* was established long before the advent of magnetic resonance imaging (MRI) or computed tomography (CT) and continues long after this imaging technology has become commonplace. This convention dictates that visual fields are shown as the *patient would see the environment* (Fig. 20-13). This is also as the examiner sees his/her environment. In this format the visual field of the patient's right eye (*oculus dexter*, OD) is on the right and the visual field of the patient's left eye (*oculus sinister*, OS) is on the left.

Early in the development of MRI and CT technology, it became the standard to view *axial images* as if the observer

Figure 20-10. Contour diagram of visual acuity on the retinal surface (**A**). The contour lines are isopters, lines of equal retinal sensitivity. Visual acuity is sharpest in the fovea (20/20) and drops precipitously in the outer parts of the retina (to 20/600). This drop correlates with a lower density of photoreceptors and ganglion cells in the peripheral regions of the retina. The standard abbreviations O.S. and O.D. stand for left eye (*oculus sinister*) and right eye (*oculus dexter*), respectively. Diagrams showing location of defects in the visual field (**B**). A detached retina in the lower part of the eye results in an irregular defect in the upper visual field (**B**, *left*), whereas an irregular lesion of the macula or compression of the optic nerve produces a central scotoma (area of reduced vision) in the center of the visual field (**B**, *right*). Ophthalmoscopic view of the fundus of a normal right eye (**C**). Increased intracranial pressure may produce a "choked disc" (papilledema), which is swelling of the optic nerve head visible through an ophthalmoscope (**D**). Blood vessels emerge from the optic disc, the light area in the center of the photograph.

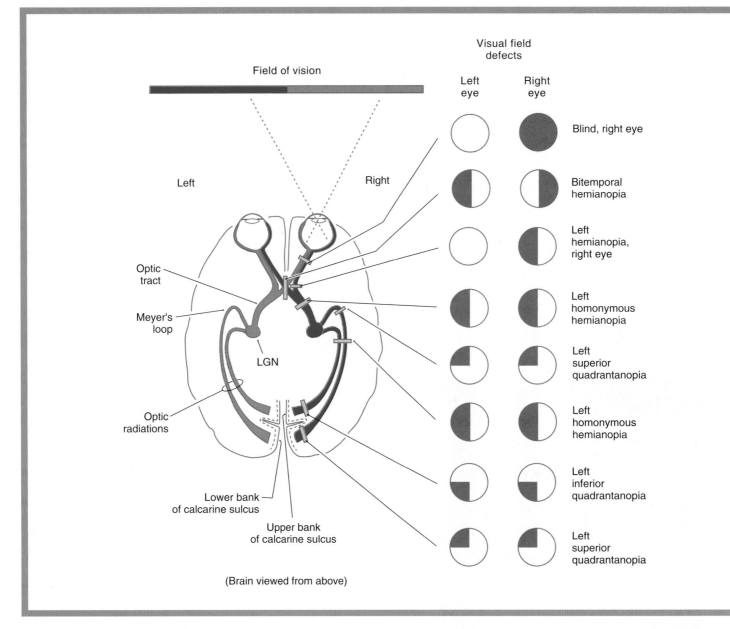

Field of vision

Visual field
defects

Left   Right

Left
eye

Right
eye

Blind, right eye

Bitemporal
hemianopia

Left
hemianopia,
right eye

Left
homonymous
hemianopia

Left
superior
quadrantanopia

Left
homonymous
hemianopia

Left
inferior
quadrantanopia

Left
superior
quadrantanopia

Optic
tract

Meyer's
loop

LGN

Optic
radiations

Lower bank
of calcarine sulcus

Upper bank
of calcarine sulcus

(Brain viewed from above)

Figure 20-11. Visual field defects produced by lesions at different places in the visual pathway. Visual fields are diagrammed as described in Figure 20-9. Regions of normal vision are indicated in *white;* regions of loss of vision are indicated in *black.*

were standing at the patient's feet looking toward the head and *coronal images* as if standing in front of the patient looking at his/her face (Fig. 20-14; see also Chapter 1). *In both axial and coronal images, the left side of the patient is on the observer's right and the right side of the patient is on the observer's left* (Fig. 20-14). Understanding this relationship between the observer (the physician) and the patient is absolutely essential to the successful diagnosis and treatment of the neurologically compromised patient. This applies to all aspects of the clinical neurosciences, not only to just the visual system.

With this in mind, it is not difficult to make the correlation between a visual field deficit and the location of a central lesion as seen in MRI or CT. Just remember, when looking at a representation of the patient's visual field "*you see what the patient sees*"; the patient's right visual field is on the physician's right and the patient's left visual field on the physician's left (Fig. 20-13). When looking at a lesion of a visual structure in MRI the physician is "*looking at the patient's face or feet*"; the patient's right is on the physician's left and the patient's left is on the physician's right (Fig. 20-14). As we will see later in this chapter, this correlates with the deficits seen following lesions at

various points in the visual pathway. For example, a lesion of the right optic nerve (the left side of the MR image as the physician looks at the image) will result in a complete loss of vision in the right eye (Figs. 20-11 and 20-15). On the other hand, a lesion of the left optic tract, which is caudal to the partial crossing of optic fibers in the optic chiasm, will result in a loss of vision in the right half of the visual field in *each eye*—a hemianopia (Figs. 20-11 and 20-16). The patterns of deficits following lesions at representative points in the visual pathway are explored in the following sections of this chapter.

Lateral Geniculate Nucleus

The *lateral geniculate nucleus* is located internal to an elevation on the caudoventral aspect of the diencephalon, the *lateral geniculate body* (Fig. 20-17). The human lateral geniculate nucleus consists of six cellular layers with thin sheets of myelinated fibers sandwiched between them. The ventral base of this nucleus is formed by the incoming *optic tract* fibers, whereas its dorsal and lateral borders are formed by the outgoing *optic radiations*. The cell layers are numbered 1 through 6 from ventral to dorsal. As

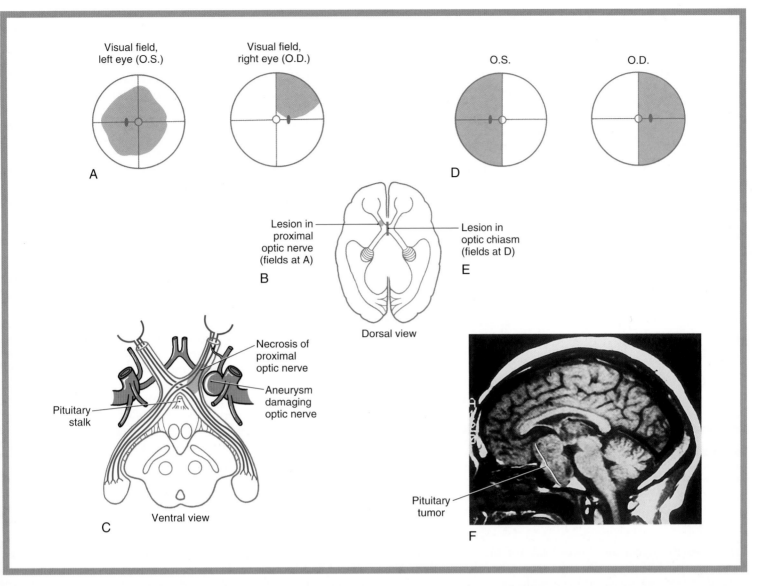

Figure 20-12. Visual field deficits (**A**) resulting from a lesion of the left optic nerve (**B** and **C**) at its junction with the optic chiasm *(junctional lesion)*. This combination of field defects is caused by destruction of fibers of the left optic nerve plus some of the crossed fibers from the lower nasal hemiretina on the right, producing an upper temporal field deficit in the right eye. Visual field deficits (**D**, *bitemporal hemianopia*) resulting from damage to the crossing fibers in the optic chiasm (**E**). Pituitary tumors, such as the one shown in the magnetic resonance image (**F**), are a common cause of such deficits.

explained in the next two sections, the layers can be grouped by both the type of ganglion cell input they receive and the side of the retina from which the input originates.

Magnocellular and Parvocellular Layers

Layers 1 and 2 of the lateral geniculate contain cells with large somata and are called the *magnocellular* (M) layers. Layers 3 through 6 contain small cells and are therefore termed the *parvocellular* (P) layers (Fig. 20-17C, D). The subdivision of the lateral geniculate into magnocellular and parvocellular layers correlates with the subdivision of the retinal ganglion cells into "Y" and "X" classes. The "Y" (or "M") fibers terminate in the magnocellular layers (layers 1 and 2), whereas the "X" (or "P") fibers terminate in the parvocellular layers (layers 3 through 6). Recall that the "Y" ("M") ganglion cells receive their input mainly from rods, have larger receptive fields and thick, rapidly conducting axons, and are particularly sensitive to moving stimuli. The "X" ("P") ganglion cells receive input mainly from cones, have small receptive fields and slower-conducting axons, and are tonically responsive to stationary stimuli; they arise mainly in the central retina and are responsible for high-acuity color vision. The ganglion cells of the remaining, mixed "W" class terminate on small cells scattered between the main layers.

Ipsilateral and Contralateral Layers

The ganglion cell axons that arise in the *temporal* retina remain uncrossed as they pass through the chiasm and terminate in layers 2, 3, and 5 of the *ipsilateral* lateral geniculate nucleus. On the other hand, the axons that arise in the *nasal* retina cross in the chiasm and terminate in layers 1, 4, and 6 of the *contralateral* lateral geniculate (Fig. 20-9).

Ganglion cell axon terminals and relay cells on which they synapse are arranged so that the same point in visual space is represented six times, once for each layer of the lateral geniculate nucleus, and at the same medial-lateral point in each layer. The map progresses from the midline to the periphery in visual space as the layer runs from medial to lateral in the lateral geniculate nucleus. Layers also run rostral to caudal, representing the inferior-superior axis.

Optic Radiations

Relay cells forming the layers of the lateral geniculate nucleus receive input from ganglion cells (as *retinogeniculate fibers*) and send their axons to the ipsilateral primary visual cortex as a large bundle of myelinated fibers, the *optic radiations* (Figs. 20-9, 20-18, and 20-19). The primary visual cortex (striate cortex) is

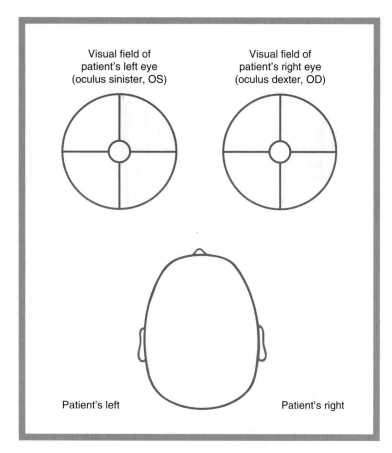

Figure 20-13. Relationship of visual field diagrams to patient being examined. The observer draws the diagrams as if they were on the wall the patient is looking at.

located on the upper and lower banks of the *calcarine sulcus*. Consequently, the optic radiations are also called the *geniculostriate* or *geniculocalcarine pathway*.

The optic radiations can be divided into two main bundles, one serving the lower and one the upper quadrant of the contralateral hemifields (Figs. 20-18 and 20-19). The fibers that carry visual information from the lower quadrant of the contralateral hemifields originate from the dorsomedial portion of the lateral geniculate nucleus, arch directly caudally to pass through the retrolenticular limb of the internal capsule, and synapse in the cortex of the superior bank of the calcarine sulcus, on the cuneus. Consequently, a lesion in the upper portion of the optic radiations results in a loss of vision in the contralateral inferior visual field, termed *contralateral (right or left) inferior quadrantanopia* (Fig. 20-11).

The fibers corresponding to the upper quadrant of the contralateral hemifields originate from the ventrolateral portion of the lateral geniculate nucleus. These fibers do not pass directly caudal to the visual cortex. Instead they arch rostrally, passing into the white matter of the temporal lobe, to form a broad U-turn *(loop of Meyer or Archambault)* before passing caudally to synapse in the inferior bank of the calcarine sulcus, on the lingual gyrus (Figs. 20-11, 20-18, and 20-19). Damage to the Meyer loop in the temporal lobe, or to these fibers en route to the calcarine sulcus, results in a *contralateral (right or left) superior quadrantanopia* (Fig. 20-19). Geniculostriate fibers conveying information from the macula (and fovea) originate from central regions of the lateral geniculate nucleus and pass to caudal portions of the visual cortex.

Lesions of the optic radiations may result in a *quadrantanopia* or may involve only a portion of a quadrant of the visual field

(Fig. 20-19). Lesions in the optic tracts and optic radiations are described as *congruous* or *incongruous*. A deficit is called *congruous* when the visual field loss of one eye can be superimposed on that of the other eye. The closer a lesion is to the visual cortex, the more congruous it is likely to be. Conversely, the more anterior a lesion is in the optic tract or radiations, the more likely it is that it will be *incongruous*.

The blood supply to the optic radiations is via branches of the *middle* and *posterior cerebral arteries* that penetrate deep into the white matter. In general, the more laterally located fibers of the optic radiations and the fibers of the loop of Meyer are served by branches of the middle cerebral artery. The more medially located fibers and the visual cortex receive their blood supply predominantly from the posterior cerebral artery.

Primary Visual Cortex

Primary visual cortex (striate cortex, area 17, V1) receives most of the axons from the lateral geniculate nuclei. It lies on either bank of the calcarine sulcus in the occipital lobe. The superior bank of the calcarine sulcus, on the *cuneus*, receives input from the inferior part of the contralateral hemifields, whereas the inferior bank of the sulcus, on the *lingual gyrus*, receives input from the superior part of the hemifields (Fig. 20-12). The *central part* of the visual field (i.e., the macula and fovea) is represented in the portion of the primary visual cortex closest to the occipital pole, and the more peripheral regions of the visual field are represented more rostrally on the cuneus and lingual gyrus (Fig. 20-12). The central 10 degrees of the visual field occupies about one half of the visual cortex.

The six-layered neocortex of area 17 is characterized by a wide layer IV. This layer contains an extra band of myelinated fibers, the *stria of Gennari* (Fig. 20-20). This structure is visible to the naked eye in the freshly cut brain and accounts for the name *striate cortex*. It is indicative of the large geniculocalcarine input to this layer. Layer VI is also prominent in striate cortex. It is the source of a cortical feedback projection to the lateral geniculate nucleus. The neurons of the visual cortex are organized into an elaborate array of *cortical columns* (see below), which extend perpendicularly from the pial surface to the white matter.

A large lesion of the visual cortex on one side (e.g., from occlusion of the calcarine artery) will result in a *contralateral (right or left) hemianopia*. *Macular sparing* may result because caudal parts of the visual cortex can also be served by collateral branches of the middle cerebral artery.

Functional Organization of Visual Cortex

The functional organization of the visual cortex has for decades been the subject of intense anatomic and physiologic investigation. Much is now known about the receptive field properties and the neural connections of neurons in the visual cortex, and about the neurotransmitters they employ. Although most of the information was initially gained from animal research, recent experiments using functional MRI have confirmed that the physiologic and anatomic organization of the visual system in humans is extremely similar to that in nonhuman primates. Consequently, the general principles of organization described here are directly applicable to the human visual system.

In a typical study of the receptive field properties of neurons in visual cortex, an anesthetized primate is placed in front of a projection screen (Fig. 20-21), with its eyes directed toward and focused on a fixation point in the center of the screen. The neural activity of a single cortical neuron is isolated using a microelectrode, amplifier, and oscilloscope. A movable projector projects a small circular spot of light or a long, narrow bar of light onto the screen, and it is moved around the screen until a

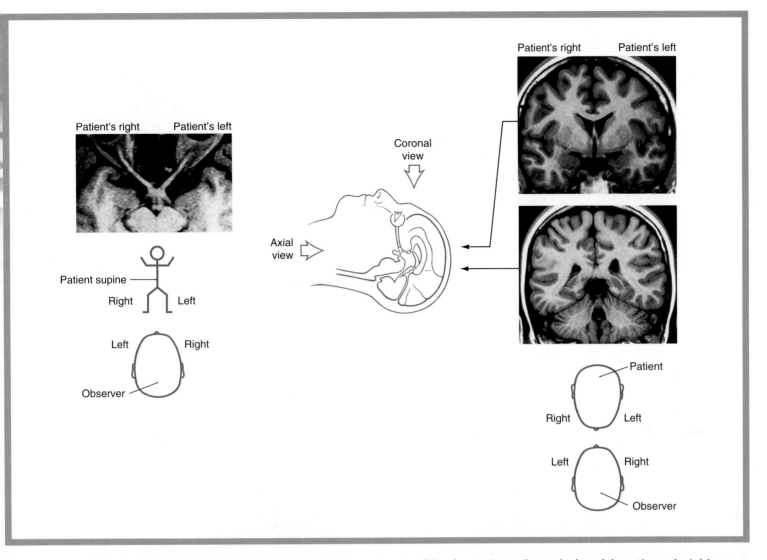

Figure 20-14. Relationship of MR images to observer. Axial images *(left)* are viewed as if the observer is standing at the feet of the patient, who is lying on his back. Coronal images *(right)* are viewed as if the observer is looking into the face of the patient.

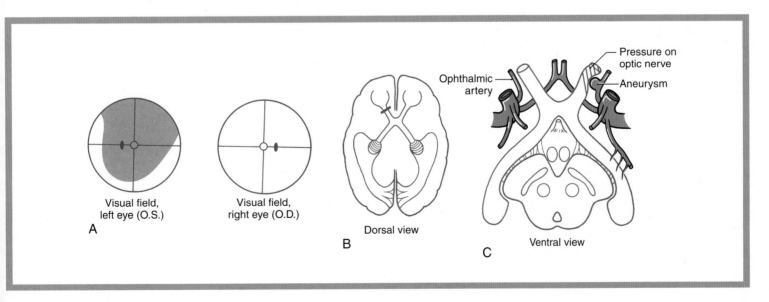

Figure 20-15. A visual field deficit, such as blindness in the left eye (**A**), may result from a lesion of the left optic nerve (**B**, *seen from above*). An aneurysm of the ophthalmic artery (**C**, *seen from below*) may cause damage to the optic nerve on that side.

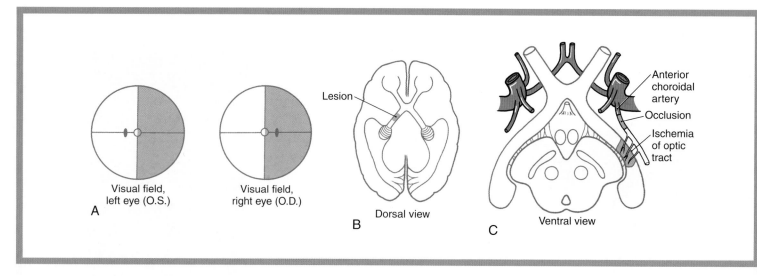

Figure 20-16. Visual field deficits (**A**, right homonymous hemianopia) resulting from a lesion of the left optic tract (**B**, *seen from above*). Interruption in the blood supply to the optic tract (**C**, *seen from below*) may produce such deficits.

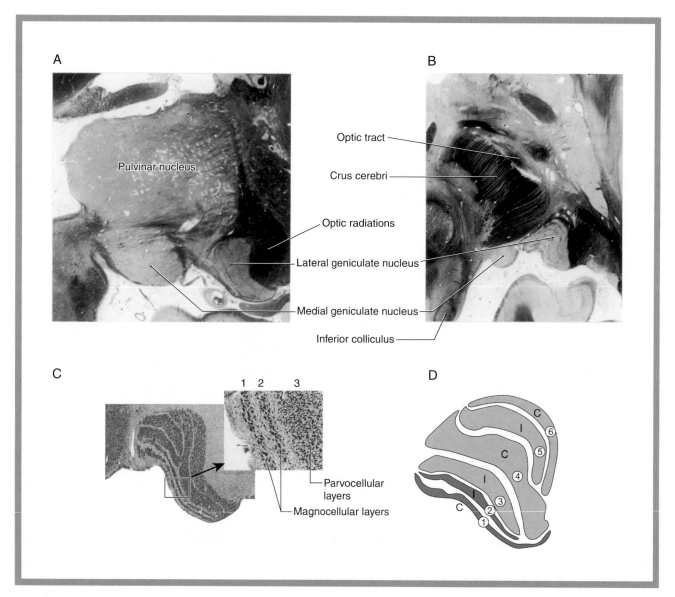

Figure 20-17. The lateral geniculate nucleus (LGN). The LGN has a characteristic layered structure in either cell or myelin stains (**A**, coronal; **B**, axial). **C**, Coronal section through the posterior third of the left LGN. At this level, six layers are obvious in the medial portion of the nucleus, but layers 3 and 5 merge into one layer laterally, as do layers 4 and 6. *Inset* shows the large cell bodies in the magnocellular layers and the small, densely packed cell bodies in one parvocellular layer. (Section courtesy of Joseph Malpeli.) **D**, Drawing of a coronal section through the middle third of the LGN. Layers 1 and 2 are magnocellular layers; 4 to 6 are parvocellular layers. C indicates layers that receive retinal input from the contralateral eye; I indicates retinal input from the ipsilateral eye.

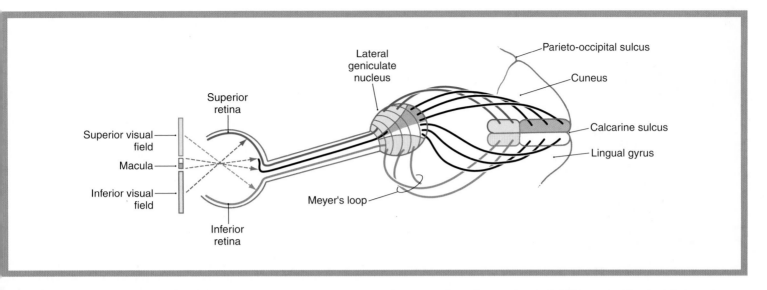

Figure 20-18. The retinogeniculate and geniculostriate pathways in the sagittal plane. Input from the *superior visual field* is received by the inferior retina and is relayed to the lower bank of the calcarine cortex. Similarly, input from the *inferior visual field* reaches the upper bank of the calcarine sulcus. Note the disproportionately large representation of the macula; the central 10 degrees of visual field space occupies about one half of the visual cortex.

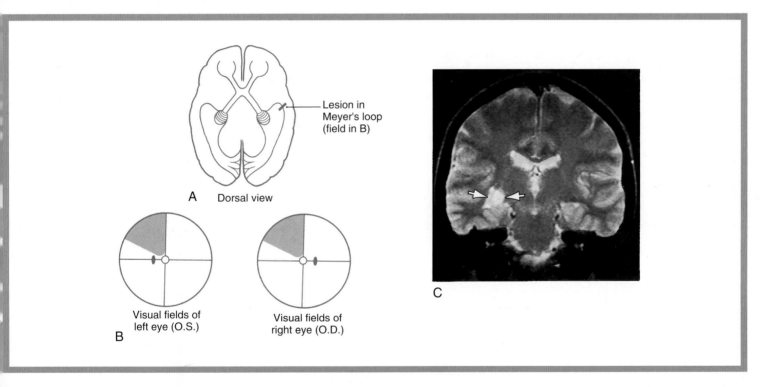

Figure 20-19. Visual field deficits (**B**, left superior homonymous quadrantanopia) resulting from lesions in the lower part of the optic radiations (**A**). Such a defect can be produced by lesions in the right Meyer loop, as shown in the magnetic resonance image (**C**).

location is found at which the light causes action potentials to occur in the neuron under study.

Receptive Field Properties of Cortical Neurons

The receptive field of a neuron is defined as that region of the visual field in which the correct stimulus will have an effect on the activity of the neuron (either excitatory or inhibitory). Depending on exactly where within the receptive field of the neuron the light is projected, the neuron may give an "on" response, when a burst of action potentials occurs when the light is turned on (Fig. 20-21), or an "off" response, when background activity in the neuron is inhibited when the light is turned on but a burst of action potentials occurs when the light is then turned off (rebound excitation) (Fig. 20-21).

The most common receptive field arrangements in primary visual cortex are illustrated in Figure 20-22. Some cortical neurons have concentric receptive fields, similar to the receptive fields of retinal ganglion cells and lateral geniculate cells (Fig. 20-22A). Cortical neurons with concentric receptive fields are almost all in layer IV of the cortex and are probably stellate neurons that receive synaptic contacts from lateral geniculate nucleus neuron axons. A small spot of light within the center region of the receptive field will produce a small "on" response in the neuron being studied; a larger spot of light that completely fills the center of the receptive field will produce a stronger "on" response. In contrast, a small spot of light in the surround region of the receptive field will produce an "off" response and a "doughnut" of light that completely fills the surround region will

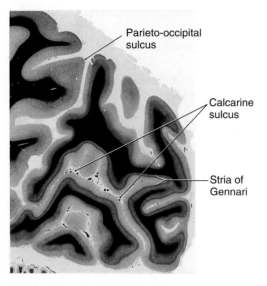

Parieto-occipital sulcus

Calcarine sulcus

Stria of Gennari

Figure 20-20. The characteristic appearance of the stria of Gennari in the primary visual cortex bordering on the calcarine sulcus.

produce the maximal "off" response. As in the retina and lateral geniculate nucleus, about half of the cortical concentric neurons have receptive fields with "on" centers and "off" surrounds; the other half have "off" centers and "on" surrounds. A large spot of light that fills both the center and the surround regions of the receptive field produces no response at all, as the excitatory and inhibitory influences on the neuron cancel each other out.

In layers II, III, V, and VI of the visual cortex, the receptive fields of neurons are organized quite differently. Instead of circular receptive fields, virtually all other cortical neurons have elongated receptive fields and respond best to long, narrow bars of light. One class of neurons, those with simple receptive fields, give a small "on" response when a small spot of light is presented anywhere in the excitatory region of the receptive field (*pluses*, Fig. 20-22A, B) and a small "off" response when the spot of light is presented somewhere in the inhibitory region of the receptive field (*triangles*, Fig. 20-22A, B). However, the maximal response is produced by a bar of light that completely fills either the excitatory or inhibitory region of the field. To produce a maximal "on" response, the light bar must be positioned exactly within the excitatory zone of the receptive field, and its angle with respect to the horizontal must match the angle of the excitatory zone (*pluses*, Fig. 20-22B). Thus a neuron with simple receptive field characteristics is sensitive to both the position and the angle (or orientation) of the stimulus. Different simple cells have

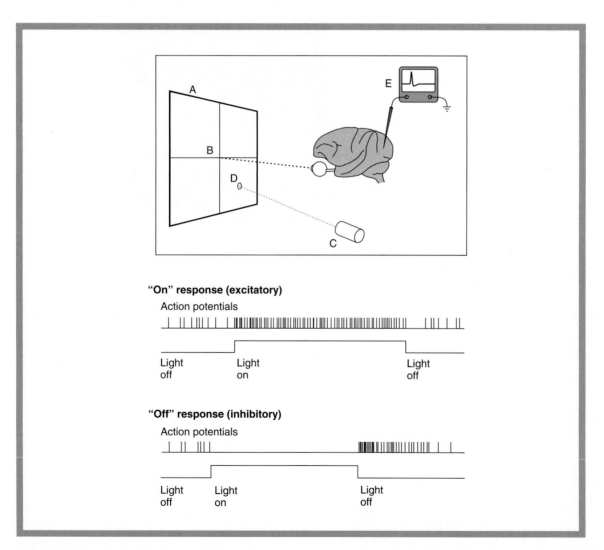

"On" response (excitatory)

Action potentials

Light off   Light on   Light off

"Off" response (inhibitory)

Action potentials

Light off   Light on   Light off

Figure 20-21. Experimental setup in which the activity of a single neuron in primary visual cortex of a monkey is analyzed. A projection screen is placed a few feet in front of the animal (A); the animal's eyes are focused on the center of the screen (B); a movable projector (C) creates a spot or bar of light (D) anywhere on the screen. The activity of a single, electrically isolated neuron is recorded via microelectrode, amplifier, and oscilloscope (E). Activity in representative neurons is illustrated in the traces below the diagram. Some neurons give a high-frequency burst of action potentials when a properly positioned stimulus is turned on ("on" response). Other neurons have their background rate of activity reduced when the stimulus is turned on and give a small burst of action potentials when the light is turned off ("off" response).

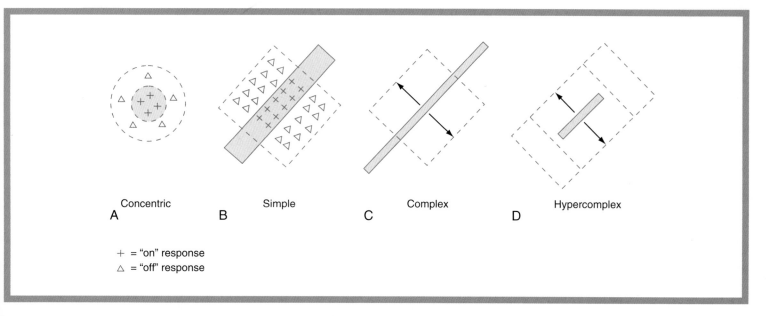

Concentric
A

Simple
B

Complex
C

Hypercomplex
D

+ = "on" response
△ = "off" response

Figure 20-22. A to **D**, Representative receptive field organization of neurons in primary visual cortex.

different preferred stimulus orientations throughout the entire range of 360 degrees.

A second class of visual neurons, which are also found throughout layers II, III, V, and VI, intermixed with simple cells, are cells with complex receptive field properties (Fig. 20-22C). A complex neuron responds best to a bar of light in a certain orientation, just as simple cells do. However, a complex cell will respond maximally to a stimulus of the correct orientation anywhere within its receptive field. Additional types of receptive fields have been described, including hypercomplex receptive fields, which are similar to complex receptive fields except that now the length of the stimulus is also critical to producing the maximal "on" response (Fig. 20-22D). If the stimulus is too long, it extends into inhibitory zones adjacent to the excitatory zone and diminishes the neuron's response.

The variety of receptive field types that are observed in V1 are the result of progressive convergence of neural connections. Figure 20-23A illustrates how several stellate neurons (1) in layer IV, each having a concentric receptive field, converge upon a pyramidal neuron (2) in layer II, III, V, or VI, to produce a simple receptive field. A small spot of light in the center of the receptive field of any one of the stellate cells produces an "on" response in that cell, which in turn produces enough excitation in the pyramidal cell to generate a modest "on" response in it. A maximal "on" response in the pyramidal cell is generated when a long narrow bar of light is in the proper position and angle to activate the center of all of the concentric receptive fields simultaneously. If the light stimulus is moved laterally, so that it illuminates only the inhibitory surrounds of the concentric fields, then the simple cell gives an "off" response. Similarly, several simple cortical cells (2, Fig. 20-23B) might converge on another neuron to produce a complex receptive field (3, Fig. 20-23B). In this case, a properly oriented bar of light that illuminates any of the simple receptive fields would produce enough excitation to generate activity in the complex cell.

Orientation Columns

Another general property of neural organization in the visual cortex is the *columnar organization* of the neurons. This is a general property of cerebral cortex and was first described in primary somatosensory cortex (see also Columnar Organization in Chapter 32). In the visual cortex, there are two types of cortical columns. The first are referred to as *orientation columns*

(Fig. 20-24). If a microelectrode is introduced into the visual cortex at a right angle with respect to the cortical surface, and is advanced slowly through the cortex recording the receptive field properties of each neuron that is encountered, it will be observed that neurons with simple, complex, and hypercomplex receptive field properties are more or less randomly intermixed but *every* neuron encountered, regardless of its type, will have the same optimal stimulus orientation. The exception would be that the neurons in layer IV, which receive direct input from lateral geniculate neurons, would have predominantly concentric receptive fields.

If another electrode penetration is made a few hundred microns away from the first, every neuron will again have the same preferred stimulus orientation but in this case the preferred stimulus orientation will be slightly different from that in the first column of neurons. If a microelectrode were to traverse the cortex parallel to the surface, it would encounter neurons with regularly changing preferred stimulus orientations. Over a distance of about 800 microns, the preferred stimulus orientation would rotate through 180 degrees. The visual cortex is therefore divided into many small regions, or columns, that extend from the pial surface to the white matter and code the various angles that a linear stimulus might take. This columnar organization is repeated for each point on the retina, as it is mapped onto the visual cortex.

Ocular Dominance Columns

Superimposed upon the orientation column organization is a second system of columns, the *ocular dominance columns* (Fig. 20-24; see also Chapter 32). These columns are critical to *stereopsis*, one of the ways in which depth is perceived in the visual world. Each eye receives a slightly different image in an individual's surroundings. This can be verified by pointing your finger at an object in your immediate environment and closing first one eye and then the other. These two images are kept separate in the alternating layers of the lateral geniculate nucleus (Figs. 20-17 and 20-24) and in the projection of each lateral geniculate layer to primary visual cortex (Fig. 20-24). In one cortical ocular dominance column, all simple, complex, and hypercomplex cells have a stronger response when the optimal stimulus is presented to one eye (e.g., contralateral) and a lesser response when the same stimulus is presented to the other eye (e.g., ipsilateral). In the adjacent ocular dominance column,

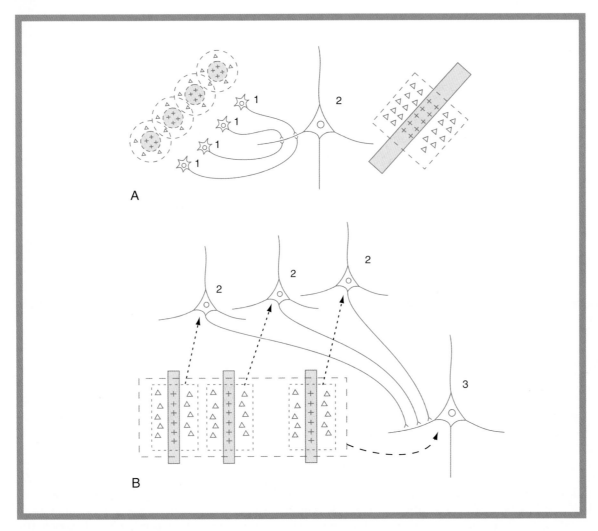

A

B

Figure 20-23. A, Diagram of how four stellate cells in layer IV with *concentric* receptive fields (1, *on left*) could converge onto a pyramidal cell (2) to produce *simple* receptive field characteristics (2, *on right*). **B,** Diagram of how several neurons, each having a *simple* receptive field (2), could converge on another neuron (3) to produce a *complex* receptive field.

the reverse relationship is observed. The relationship between ocular dominance columns and orientation columns is normally depicted as if they were arranged at right angles to each other, although their exact relationship is probably not so simple. Ocular dominance columns are about 400 microns wide. A collection of orientation columns in which the preferred stimulus orientation rotates through 180 degrees occupies about 800 microns. A combination of one contralateral-dominant column (*blue*, C_I, Fig. 20-24) and one ipsilateral-dominant column (*white*, I_C, Fig. 20-24), which includes a complete 180 degree shift in stimulus orientation, is referred to as a *hypercolumn* and occupies a region of cortex about 800 microns on a side.

The establishment of the neural connections in ocular dominance columns occurs after birth and requires proper visual stimulation in both eyes to develop normally. If disorders of vision such as strabismus, amblyopia, or congenital cataracts prevent the formation of simultaneous, superimposed, sharply focused images in both eyes during the early years of life, the neural connections that form the basis of the ocular dominance columns do not develop normally and the individual will not be able to experience stereopsis, although other aspects of vision may be normal or near-normal.

Using the neural mechanisms described previously, the visual system assembles progressively more complex representations of the visual world, beginning with tiny dots in the retina that are translated into lines and areas of light and dark in primary visual cortex and then into more and more sophisticated representations in visual association cortex (see next). For additional

information on the processing of neural signals in the visual system, see the list of suggested readings.

Abnormal Development of Visual Cortex

During development of the visual system, the axons of visually responsive cells in the lateral geniculate nucleus compete for synaptic space on cortical cells. If both eyes receive the same detailed visual information, in focus and exactly superimposed in the two retinae, this competition results in the devotion of equal numbers of layer IV visual cortical cells to inputs from the right and the left eyes (Fig. 20-24). However, if the visual input from one eye is disrupted (e.g., by congenital cataracts, strabismus, or amblyopia), the lateral geniculate axons from that eye do not compete successfully and most of the layer IV stellate cells eventually receive synaptic contacts primarily from the normal eye. Stereopsis is then lost. This competition is limited to a *critical period* during postnatal development. At some point, the synaptic connections made during the competition phase become permanent, the lateral geniculate neurons that lost the competition are permanently shut out, and binocular vision cannot be regained. This critical period is believed to last several years in humans. Once the neural connections are established successfully, later disruption of visual input does not have a marked effect on the synaptic efficiency of the input to the visual cortex.

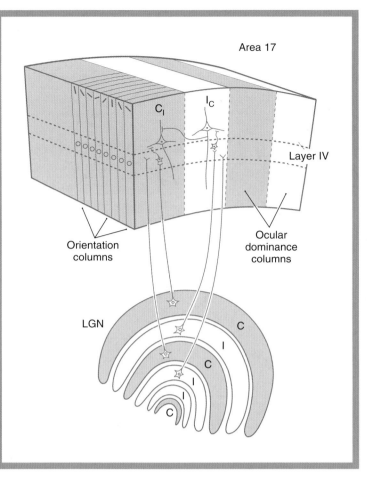

Area 17

C_I

I_C

Layer IV

Ocular
dominance
columns

Orientation
columns

LGN

C
I
C
I
I
C

Figure 20-24. Ocular dominance columns and orientation columns in the cortex, and their relationship to the layers of the lateral geniculate nucleus (LGN).

Other Visual Cortical Areas

The primary visual cortex, which we have been discussing up to this point, is responsible for much of the initial cortical processing of neural information relating to vision. However, what happens in primary visual cortex is only a first step in the conversion of an image on the retina into a psychological perception. Many additional regions of the brain, generally termed *visual association cortex* and *multimodal association cortex* (see Chapter 32), participate directly or indirectly in this process. Figure 20-25 depicts a simplified "road map" of some of the most important paths that visual information takes as it is processed by the brain.

One of the surprising features of the visual system is that different aspects of the visual experience are processed by different regions of visual association cortex. Thus, localized damage in one region of visual association cortex can impair a person's ability to perceive the colors of objects without impairing the person's ability to recognize what the object is *(achromatopsia)*. (This is a different defect from color blindness of retinal origin.) Cortical damage in another region can impair a person's ability to accurately perceive the speed and direction of moving objects in the visual field, and damage in yet another region can impair the person's ability to recognize familiar faces, even though standard ophthalmologic tests might reveal normal visual acuity.

One feature of visual processing that contributes to the parcellation of different aspects of the overall perception has already been introduced. The ganglion cells in the retina that project to the parvocellular layers of the lateral geniculate nucleus are most sensitive to small, stationary stimuli and are concentrated in the central region of the retina. These cells are the origin of a

pathway, or a "stream of processing," that is specialized at every level for the processing of the finely detailed, high resolution aspects of vision, the aspects necessary to recognize an object, a word, or a face in the visual environment. This pathway is called the parvocellular ("P") stream of processing, or the "what" pathway (Fig. 20-25C).

A second general stream of processing originates in the retinal ganglion cells that project to the magnocellular layers of the lateral geniculate. These ganglion cells are most sensitive to moving stimuli and to relatively large areas of light and dark and are more common in the peripheral retina. This pathway is specialized for the detection and analysis of movement in the environment and also for the spatial localization of objects in the environment. Curiously, it is possible for damage in this pathway, particularly in parietal association cortex, to render a person unable to judge which of two objects is closer to him, although he has no difficulty in recognizing what the objects are (see Chapter 32). This pathway is called the magnocellular (M) stream of processing, or the "where" pathway (Fig. 20-25C).

Starting in area 18, the "M" and "P" pathways that originate in the respective retinal ganglion cells diverge. Up to this level, both of these pathways, or "streams of processing," have been located in the same general regions: "M" and "P" cells coexist in retina, lateral geniculate nucleus, and area 17, even though they process separate streams of information. This arrangement persists in the *V2 subregion* of area 18, but as the streams emerge from the V2 subregion, they take different routes (Fig. 20-25C). The *"M" stream* proceeds to a subregion of area 18 called *V3* and then to the medial temporal area *(V5 or MT)*, and finally goes to the *posterior parietal area* (area 7). (Remember that the information carried by this stream originates largely in rod cells and in the peripheral portions of the retinas and that the receptive fields involved are large.) Appropriately, this information is used in determining where relevant visual stimuli are located and whether they are moving.

The *"P" stream* proceeds from the V2 subregion to the *V4* subregion of Brodmann area 19 and from there to the *inferior temporal cortex* (area 37). This stream, which originates mainly in cones and in the central area of the retina, codes for form and for color (Fig. 20-19C). In fact, starting in the lateral geniculate nucleus, form and color information are carried by two separate portions of the "P" stream. The portion that subserves form perception makes use of the small receptive fields and consequent high acuity of the "P" ganglion cells. The color-opponent receptive fields of these ganglion cells form the basis for color perception, but these signals are relayed by a different subset of lateral geniculate neurons.

Stroke or trauma to higher-order visual processing areas may produce syndromes that seem odd to the casual observer, some of which are described in the popular book, *The Man Who Mistook His Wife for a Hat*, by Oliver Sacks. For example, the process of perception seems to be anatomically distinct from the process of attaching meaning to what we see. Thus, an *apperceptive agnosia*, in which the patient cannot identify objects because of a perceptual deficit, is a separate entity from an *associative agnosia*, in which the patient can perceive the object, face, or photograph but cannot attach any meaning to it. This latter phenomenon was described by Teuber as "percepts stripped of their meaning."

These *agnosias* arise from lesions of the inferotemporal region in areas 18, 20, and 21, alone or in combination. In most people, the left hemisphere is dominant for speech. Thus, lesions in areas 18, 20, and 21 of the left (dominant) hemisphere typically result in *object agnosia*, in which the patient is unable to recognize (i.e., identify or name) real objects, although they are perceived. Lesions in these areas in the right (nondominant) hemisphere produce agnosia for drawings of objects. Smaller bilateral lesions

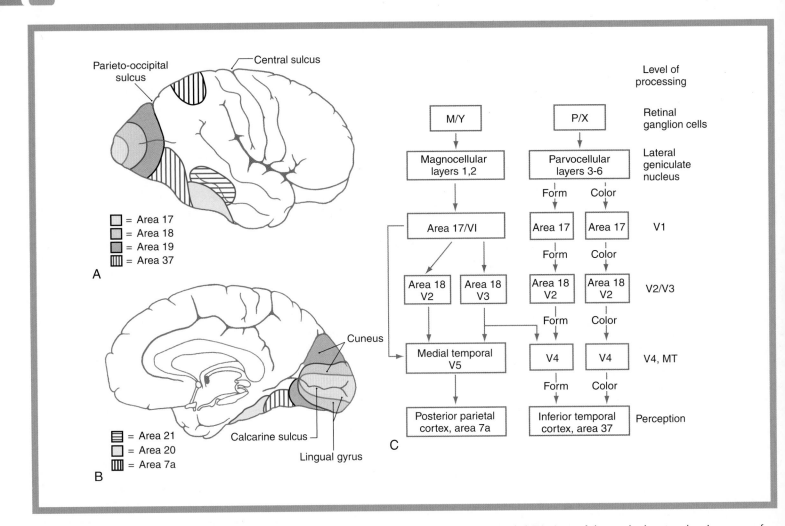

Figure 20-25. Simplified diagram of the cortical processing of visual information. Lateral (**A**) and medial (**B**) views of the cerebral cortex showing some of the cortical areas (using Brodmann's numbers) involved in the processing of visual input. **C,** The paths through which these areas interact to create a perceived image. Area 18 is divided into V2 and V3 subregions on the basis of its cortical connections. V4 represents a physiologically distinct subregion of Brodmann's area 19. The magnocellular pathway *(on the left)* is sometimes termed the *dorsal stream* of processing, or the *where* pathway. The parvocellular pathway *(on the right)* is sometimes termed the *ventral stream* of processing, or the *what* pathway. MT, medial temporal.

in these areas, especially in the fusiform gyrus, may produce *prosopagnosia,* the inability to recognize faces. The patient can see the face and recognize it as a face but cannot distinguish one face from another, even the faces of old friends and family members.

Balint syndrome results from bilateral lesions in the parieto-occipital junction region. It consists of impairment of voluntary eye movements (reflex eye movements are preserved) and optic ataxia (inaccurate eye movements related to visual-motor coordination).

Another dissociation of functions that we normally think of as linked occurs in the phenomenon of *alexia without agraphia.* In this syndrome, affected persons can write but cannot read what they have written (or what anyone else has written). A lesion of the splenium of the corpus callosum, carrying visual information from one visual cortex to another, combined with damage to the adjacent occipital region can produce this syndrome, which usually (but not always) occurs in conjunction with a homonymous hemianopia.

Synopsis of Clinical Points

- Damage to the cornea, as in infections, trauma, or metabolic diseases, degrade the quality (and perception) of an image (p. 312).
- Any obstruction to the egress of fluid into the canals of Schlemm may cause glaucoma (p. 313).
- In most patients the cause of the increased pressure in glaucoma is unknown (p. 313).
- Open-angle glaucoma is much more common than closed-angle glaucoma (p. 313).
- Glaucoma may result from infections, complications of diabetes, or hemorrhage into the anterior chamber (p. 313).
- The relative size of the pupil is a reflection of its innervation (p. 313).
- Mydriasis is increased pupil diameter (pupillary dilation) (p. 313).
- The pupillary light reflex is evaluated as part of the neurologic examination (p. 313).
- A loss of the elasticity of the lens may result in presbyopia (p. 313).
- A cataract is an opacity or cloudiness of the lens; this degrades the quality of the image (p. 313).
- Uveitis is an inflammation of the vascular tunic of the eye (p. 313).
- The initial processing of visual input takes place in the retina (p. 314).
- Rods and cones are the photoreceptors of the retina (p. 314).
- A patient who is color blind is unable to distinguish certain colors (p. 316).
- Protanopia is the loss of red-sensitive cones, resulting in a confusion of red and green (p. 316).
- Deuteranopia is the loss of green-sensitive cones, resulting in a confusion of green and red (p. 316).
- Each layer of the retina participates in the processing of visual information (pp. 317–319).
- Ganglion cells are the output cells of the retina; damage to these cells, or to their axons, may result in various patterns of blindness and potential compromise of the pupillary light reflex (p. 319).
- Increases in intracranial pressure may result in papilledema with a consequent partial or complete loss of vision in that eye (p. 320).
- Lesions of the optic nerve, chiasm, or tract result in visual deficits that characteristically correlate with the level of the lesion (pp. 320–322).
- A loss of vision in one half of the visual field in each eye is a hemianopia (p. 321).
- Visual fields are viewed as the patient sees the environment (pp. 321–322).
- Visual structures in MRI or CT are viewed as if looking at the patient's face (coronal) or feet (axial) (pp. 321–322).
- Damage to fibers comprising the optic radiations result in a quadrantanopia that may be specified by the side (right/left) and elevation (superior/inferior) (p. 324).
- Lesions in the visual cortex may result in macular sparing (p. 324).
- The visual cortex is highly organized in its receipt and processing of visual information (p. 324).
- If visual input from one eye is interrupted during the critical period, stereopsis (a perception of three dimensions in the image—commonly called depth perception) is lost (pp. 329–330).
- Achromatopsia is an inability to perceive the color of an object even though the object itself is recognized (p. 331).
- Lesions of association cortices that process visual information may result in various types of agnosia (pp. 331–332).

Sources and Additional Reading

Borwein B: Scanning electron microscopy of monkey foveal photoreceptors. Anat Rec 205:363-373, 1983.

Choisser B: Face Blind! Bill's Face Blindness (Prosopagnosia) Pages. Available at http://www.choisser.com/faceblind/

Curcio CA, Sloan KR, Kalina RE, Hendrickson AE: Human photoreceptor topography. J Comp Neurol 292:497-523, 1990.

Hubel DH: Eye, Brain and Vision. New York, Henry Holt & Co., 1995.

Hubel DH, Wiesel TN: Functional architecture of the macaque visual cortex (The Ferrier Lecture). Proc R Soc Lond B 198:1-59, 1977.

Koretz JF, Handelman GH: How the human eye focuses. Sci Am 259:92-99, 1988.

LeVay S, Hubel DH, Wiesel TN: The pattern of ocular dominance columns in macaque visual cortex revealed by a reduced silver stain. J Comp Neurol 159:559-576, 1975.

Masland RH: Functional architecture of the retina. Sci Am 255:102-111, 1986.

Rodieck RW: The First Steps in Seeing. Sunderland, MA, Sinauer, 1998.

Stryker MP: Is grandmother an oscillation? Nature 338:297-298, 1989.

Werblin FS: The control of sensitivity in the retina. Sci Am 228:70-79, 1973.

Zeki S: A Vision of the Brain. Boston, Blackwell Scientific Publications, 1993.

The Auditory System

C. K. Henkel

Hearing is one of the most important senses. In combination with vision and the ability to speak, it contributes, in a significant way, to the quality of life. In our daily routine, we unconsciously sort out meaningful sounds from background noise, localize the source of sounds, and react (many times in a reflex mode) to unexpected sounds. About 12% of people in the general population experience a diminution or loss of hearing during their lifetime, which in some cases may represent a significant disability.

Overview

The auditory apparatus is adapted for receiving sound waves at the tympanic membrane and transmitting auditory signals to the central nervous system. Injury to elements of the peripheral apparatus, such as the ear ossicles, may result in *conductive deafness*. Alternatively, damage to the cochlea or the cochlear portion of the eighth cranial nerve may result in *sensorineural (nerve) deafness*. When central auditory pathways are injured, the apparent hearing dysfunction *(central deafness)* is usually combined with other signs and symptoms. Central lesions seldom result in complete deafness in one ear. These three types of hearing losses are considered in more detail when we discuss the external and middle ear, the cochlea and cochlear nerve, and central auditory pathways, respectively. To understand the neurophysiologic and audiologic methods used in assessing peripheral and central auditory disorders, it is essential to understand the structure and function of the cochlea and central auditory pathways.

Properties of Sound Waves and Hearing

Complex sounds are mixtures of pure tones that are either *harmonically related*, thus having *pitch*, or that are *randomly related* and therefore called *noise*. The cochlear apparatus is designed to analyze sounds by separating complex waveforms into their individual frequency components.

The *frequency* of audible sounds is measured in cycles per second, or hertz (Hz). A simple sine wave (Fig. 21-1) depicts the cyclic increase and decrease in the compression of air molecules that constitutes a pure tone. The time interval between two peaks is the *period*, the distance traveled is the *wavelength*, and the number of cycles per second is the *frequency*. The *intensity* is the peak-to-trough amplitude of force at the eardrum.

The normal frequency range for human hearing is 50 to 16,000 Hz. Most human speech takes place in the range of 100 to 8,000 Hz, and the most sensitive part of the range is between 1,000 and 3,000 Hz. Exposure to loud noise can result in selective hearing loss for certain frequencies, and normal aging may reduce the range.

The hearing apparatus is exquisitely sensitive to sound *intensity* over an enormous *dynamic range*. Intensity of sound is related to the perception of loudness and is usually measured in units called *decibels* (dB). Intensity is also related to a measure of *sound pressure level* at the tympanic membrane. A sound that has 10 times the power of a just-audible sound is said to have a 20-dB sound pressure level. Normal conversational levels of sound are about 50 dB. Sounds above 120 to 130 dB elicit pain, and permanent damage to the hearing apparatus is probable for exposure to repeated sounds above 150 dB (e.g., jet engine).

The brain derives the location of a sound by computing differences in the shape, timing, and intensity of the waveforms that reach each ear. The path of the sound is affected by the distance to the ears and by obstacles such as the head (Fig. 21-1). Thus, *interaural time and intensity differences* are related to the angle between the direction in which the head is pointing and

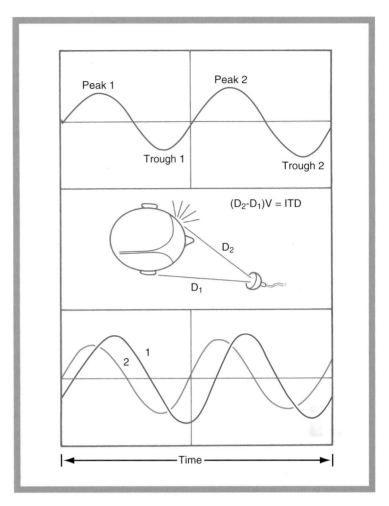

Figure 21-1. *Upper panel* shows the cyclic changes in a simple, pure tone. *Lower panel* shows that the arrival of a tone at right (D_1) ear and left (D_2) ear is affected by the distance traveled and shadowing effect of the head *(center panel)* when the source of the sound is displaced from the midline. The interaural time difference (ITD) is calculated by the equation $(D_2 - D_1)V = ITD$, where V is the speed of sound.

the direction of the sound source. *Interaural time differences are more important for localizing low-frequency sounds, whereas interaural intensity differences are more important for localizing high-frequency sounds.*

Processing of Sound: The Ear

External (Outer) Ear

Sound waves are captured by the *external ear (pinna)* and channeled through the *external auditory meatus* to the *tympanic membrane* (Fig. 21-2A). Resonance features of the pinna and meatus enhance some frequencies more than others in a direction-dependent fashion. For example, sounds coming toward the back of the head are baffled compared with those coming toward the side of the head. *Monaural (single-ear) localization* depends on such cues, and accuracy in localizing sound is impaired by damage to the pinna.

Middle Ear

The *middle ear* or *tympanic cavity* is an air-filled space in the temporal bone that is interposed between the tympanic membrane and the inner ear structures (Fig. 21-2A). Sounds are transmitted across the space from the tympanic membrane to the fluid-filled inner ear by a chain of three bony *ossicles*: the *malleus, incus,* and *stapes*. On one end of this chain, the arm of the malleus is attached to the tympanic membrane, and at the other end the footplate of the stapes fits into the *oval window* of the membranous labyrinth of the inner ear. The three bones act

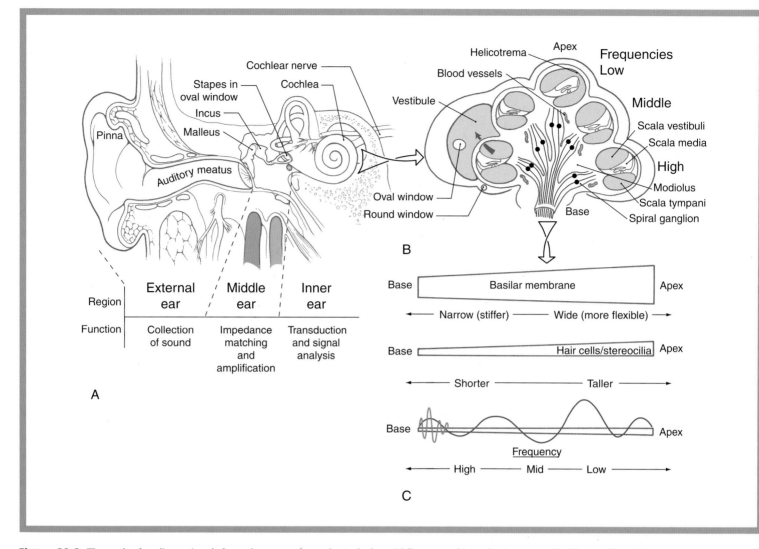

Figure 21-2. The path of auditory signals from the external ear, through the middle ear, and into the inner ear (**A**). The cochlea (**B**) is shown in cross section from apex to base. The basilar membrane (**C**) functions to separate waves of different frequencies within a sound. This membrane is narrow and stiff at its base and becomes wider and more flexible toward the apex, and the hair cell stereocilia increase correspondingly in height. These features "tune" the membrane so that each frequency of sound in the audible range will cause a wave in the basilar membrane that has its peak amplitude at a unique spot (near the base for high frequencies and near the apex for low frequencies). At this spot, the hair cells are excited most intensely, producing a peak in neural output.

as levers to *reduce the magnitude of movements of the tympanic membrane while increasing their force* at the oval window.

The mechanical stiffness of the ossicle chain acts to *compensate for the difference in impedance* between air and fluid environments (a function called *impedance matching*) so that there is optimal transfer of energy between the two media. Diseases such as *otosclerosis* and *otitis media* result in conductive hearing loss by affecting the efficiency of the ossicle movement. *Otosclerosis*, the cause of middle ear conductive hearing loss in about one half of cases, may be an inherited disease and is characterized by tissue overgrowth and resultant fixation of the stapes in the oval window. *Otitis media* is an inflammation of the middle ear and may be accompanied by the accumulation of pus or exudate. In addition, fractures of the temporal bone with direct damage to the ossicles, or indirect damage by bleeding into the middle ear, may result in a conduction deafness. The stiffness of the ossicle chain can also be modified by two muscles of the middle ear, the tensor tympani and stapedius muscles (middle ear reflex).

Conduction Deafness

A *conductive deafness* is a deficit related to an obstructed, or altered, transformation of sound to the tympanic membrane and/or through the ossicle chain of the middle ear. For example, damage to the pinna results in a failure of sound waves to be properly conducted to the auditory meatus. In addition, infection involving the auditory canal (*otitis externa*, sometimes called *swimmer's ear*), inflammation or trauma to the tympanic membrane, or even the excessive accumulation of cerumen (wax) in the auditory canal are other causes of conduction deafness. The deficit experienced by the patient may range from decreased hearing to total deafness in the affected ear. Depending on the cause, conduction deafness may resolve with medication or by removal of the obstruction.

Inner Ear: Structure of the Cochlea

The cochlea is named for its similarity to a conch shell (Fig. 21-2B). The *membranous cochlea*, the coiled portion of the inner ear, is encased in the osseous cochlea and consists of three spiraling chambers. The cochlea makes approximately two and two-thirds turns from base to apex. Uncoiled, it is about 34 mm long. The base of the cochlear spiral is connected to the saccule of the membranous labyrinth by the *ductus reuniens*.

The central chamber of the membranous cochlea is the *cochlear duct*, also called the *scala media* (Fig. 21-2B). Above it, the *scala vestibuli* is positioned to communicate with the vestibule, the portion of the membranous inner ear between the oval window and the cochlea. Below, the *scala tympani* ends at the *round window*, which separates this space from the middle ear cavity. The scala vestibuli is continuous with the scala

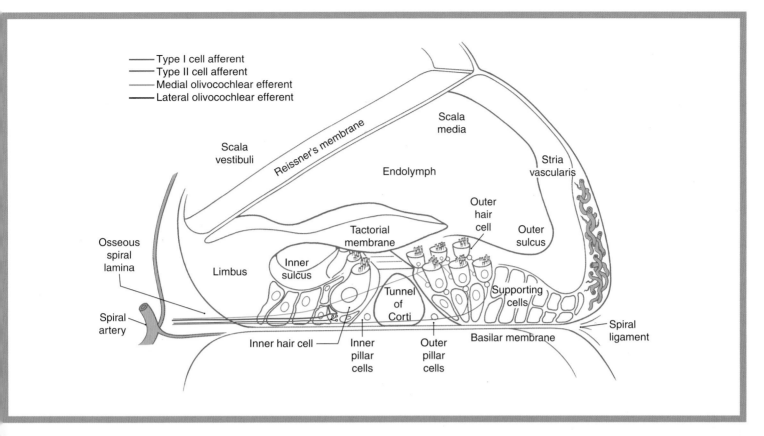

----- Type I cell afferent
----- Type II cell afferent
----- Medial olivocochlear efferent
----- Lateral olivocochlear efferent

Figure 21-3. Cross section through a typical turn of the membranous cochlea.

tympani through an opening at the apex of the cochlea called the *helicotrema* (Fig. 21-2B). In cross section, the scala media is bounded by the *basilar membrane* below, the *vestibular* or *Reissner membrane* above, and the *stria vascularis* externally (Figs. 21-2B and 21-3). The screw-like bony core of the cochlea is the *modiolus*. A spiral osseous lamina extends outward from the modiolus to join the basilar membrane. The basilar membrane, in turn, is continuous laterally with the *spiral ligament*. The scala vestibuli and tympani are filled with *perilymph*. The *endolymph*, which fills the cochlear duct, is elaborated by the cells and rich capillary bed of the *stria vascularis* (Fig. 21-3).

The *organ of Corti* is the specialized sensory epithelium resting on the basilar membrane (Fig. 21-3). It comprises inner and outer hair cells, supporting cells, and the tectorial membrane. The inner hair cells are separated from the outer hair cells by the *tunnel of Corti* (Fig. 21-3). This tunnel is formed by the filamentous arches of the *inner and outer pillar cells* and is filled with fluid.

Inner hair cells form a single line spiraling from base to apex, and the *outer hair cells* form three parallel lines that follow the same course (Fig. 21-4). Once damaged, human hair cells do not regenerate. Research has not yet found a way to augment this. It is uncertain how many of the inner (about 3500) or outer (about 12 000) hair cells must be lost to disease, trauma, or aging before a just-noticeable sensorineural hearing loss ensues. Projecting from the apical surface of each hair cell is a *hair bundle* consisting of 50 to 150 *stereocilia* arranged in curving rows (Fig. 21-4). Each hair bundle is polarized so that the longest stereocilia are on the outer border (Fig. 21-4), and the rows of stereocilia are linked by filamentous material at their tips.

The *tectorial membrane* is a gelatinous arm that extends outward over the sensory epithelium from the limbus of the osseous spiral lamina (Fig. 21-4). The taller stereocilia in each hair bundle are in contact with or embedded in the tectorial membrane. Consequently, movement of the basilar membrane and the organ of Corti will bend the stereocilia against the tectorial membrane and cause a graded depolarization of the hair cells.

The bony modiolus, around which the cochlear duct turns, houses the *spiral ganglion* (Figs. 21-2 and 21-3). At the edge of the osseous spiral lamina, the peripheral processes of the bipolar cells of this ganglion lose their myelin and pass through perforations to the basilar membrane, where they synapse on the base of the inner and outer hair cells (Fig. 21-4). The central processes of the spiral ganglion cells form the *cochlear portion of the vestibulocochlear nerve (cranial nerve VIII)*. *Efferent fibers* to the cochlea either spiral along the inner part of the basilar membrane to synapse on inner hair cells or travel radially across the tunnel of Corti to contact outer hair cells (Fig. 21-4).

Mechanoelectrical Transduction

Inner hair cells are extremely sensitive transducers that convert the mechanical force applied to the hair bundle into an electrical signal (Fig. 21-4). Endolymph, like extracellular fluid, has a high concentration of K^+. In contrast, perilymph, like cerebrospinal fluid, has a high concentration of Na^+. As indicated in Figure 21-4, the potential difference between the endolymph and the perilymph is +80 mV. This endolymphatic potential appears to be due to the selective secretion and absorption of ions by the stria vascularis. At the same time, ion pumps in the hair cell membrane produce a resting intracellular potential of about −70 mV (Fig. 21-4).

As the basilar membrane moves up in response to fluid movement in the scala tympani, the taller stereocilia are displaced against the tectorial membrane. This causes ion channels at the tips of the stereocilia to open, allowing K^+ flow along the electrical gradient to depolarize the cell (Fig. 21-4). The large potential difference between the endolymph and the hair cell interior creates a force of 150 mV that drives K^+ into the cell and that increases the range of the cell's graded electrical response to mechanical displacement. Damage to the stria vascularis results in loss of the endolymphatic potential and failure of mechanoelectrical transduction.

When a hair cell depolarizes, voltage-gated Ca^{2+} channels at the base of the cell open and the resulting influx of Ca^{2+} causes

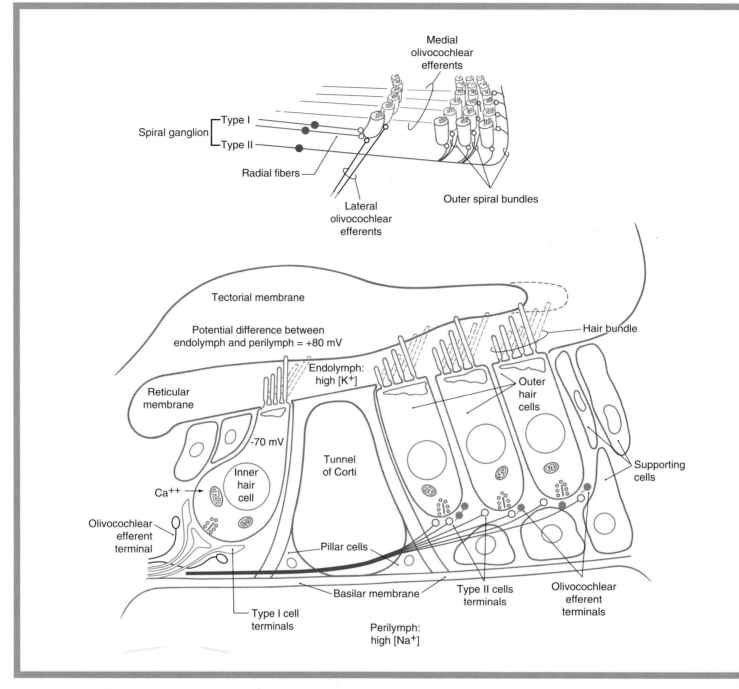

Figure 21-4. The structure and function of the organ of Corti *(lower)* and the relation of type I and type II afferent fibers to the spiraling ranks of inner and outer hair cells *(upper)*. Note that the designation as lateral or medial olivocochlear efferents refers to their origin in the superior olive, not to their target in the organ of Corti.

synaptic vesicles to fuse to the cell membrane and release a neurotransmitter into the synaptic cleft between the hair cell and the cochlear nerve fibers (Fig. 21-4). The transmitter causes depolarization of the afferent fiber, and an action potential is transmitted along the cochlear nerve fiber.

The stimulus-related changes in the electrical potential between the perilymph and the hair cells can be recorded anywhere in the cochlea. The potential varies synchronously with the sound stimulating the ear and is therefore referred to as the *cochlear microphonic*. This electrical record provides a clinically useful monitor of cochlear function.

Tuning of the Cochlea

The cochlea acts as a frequency filter to separate and analyze individual frequencies from complex sounds. These tuning properties result from anatomic and physiologic characteristics of hair cells and the basilar membrane (Figs. 21-2 and 21-3).

The plunger-like motion of the stapes in the oval window compresses the perilymph. In the fluid medium of the cochlea, this pressure variation imparts motion to the basilar membrane, causing a wave to travel along it (Fig. 21-2C). The basilar membrane is stiffest at its base and becomes progressively more flexible toward its tip. Therefore, any given frequency of sound (pure tone) will cause a wave in the basilar membrane that has its maximum displacement at a unique point along the membrane. For high tones, this point is close to the base of the cochlea; and for lower frequencies, it is more distal. The response of hair cells to the tone is strongest at the point of greatest displacement. Therefore, the position from base to apex along the spiral of the basilar membrane and organ of Corti is directly related to the frequency of the tone that will elicit a response. This relationship of frequency and cochlear position is the basis for the *place theory of cochlear tuning*. The *cochleotopic order,* and thus *tonotopic representation,* are highly conserved throughout the auditory pathways.

In patients with profound sensorineural hearing loss, some audible sensation may be regained with *cochlear implants* having a number of fine wire electrodes. Each wire is tuned to a broad frequency band from an electrical receiver, and the wires are implanted so that each stimulates nerve terminals at the appropriate tonotopic point along the cochlear spiral.

Primary Afferent Innervation and Function

The spiral ganglion is made up of two types of bipolar sensory neurons. *Type I cells* make up 90% to 95% of the cells in the spiral ganglion and have radial branches that synapse with only one or two inner hair cells (Fig. 21-4). As many as 20 or more type I radial fibers converge on each inner hair cell. As a result, type I cochlear nerve fibers respond to a narrow frequency range. In contrast, *type II ganglion cells* have widely distributed peripheral processes, which traverse the tunnel of Corti and synapse with over 10 outer hair cells (Fig. 21-4). Thus, type II cochlear fibers are more sensitive to low-intensity sounds than are type I cells, but they may be less precisely tuned to frequency.

Frequency is coded in the cochlear nerve by the position of afferent fibers along the cochlear spiral. For loud sounds, each afferent fiber responds over a range of frequencies. As the intensity of the sound drops to near threshold, the frequency response range narrows. A *tuning curve* can be constructed that plots the threshold intensity for each frequency that will elicit a response (Fig. 21-5A). The *characteristic frequency* is the frequency at which the fiber has the lowest threshold. The discharge pattern of primary afferents over time to pure tone bursts is shown with post-stimulus histograms of the number of action potentials summed over many presentations (Fig. 21-5B). Stimulus onset produces an initial high-frequency discharge followed by a lower sustained discharge level that is related to stimulus intensity. When the tone ends, the fiber drops back to a low, spontaneous discharge rate. For low-frequency fibers, the timing of each impulse is *phase locked* with the stimulus cycle, so that the fiber output preserves the timing information of the signal.

The enormous dynamic range of the human ear to intensity cannot be coded in the response of single nerve fibers. Intensity is coded both by the discharge rate of cochlear nerve fibers and by recruitment of activity in additional afferents as stimulus intensity increases. The discharge rate for the cochlear nerve fibers increases proportionally with intensity over a range of about 40-dB sound pressure level and then plateaus (Fig. 21-5C). At higher stimulus intensities, additional cochlear nerve fibers having sequentially greater thresholds are recruited.

Sensorineural Deafness

Sensorineural deafness (this may sometimes be called *nerve deafness*) results from damage to the cochlea or to the cochlear root of the vestibulocochlear nerve. The causes of sensorineural deafness are varied and may include repeated exposure to loud noises, treatment with certain antibiotics, infections such as rubella, mumps, or bacterial meningitis, and tumors at different levels of the neuraxis. When the cause is infectious or inflammatory, it is called *labyrinthitis* or *otitis interna*. As is the case with the middle ear, trauma in the form of skull fracture may also result in sensorineural deafness. The deficits experienced by the patient are deafness in the ear on the affected side, varying degrees of *tinnitus*, a perception of ringing in the ears if the cochlea is damaged, and additional signs and symptoms indicative of damage to the adjacent vestibular root.

The Weber and Rinne Tests

As described earlier, conduction deafness and sensorineural deafness may have different causes and, therefore, different tests may be used to diagnose these deficits. These tests take advan-

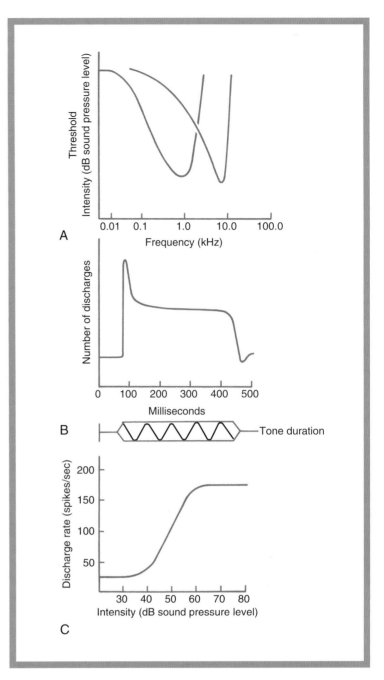

Figure 21-5. Typical response characteristics of type I cochlear afferent fibers. Frequency-tuning curves (**A**), post-stimulus time histogram of discharges through the duration of a tone burst at the characteristic frequency of a primary afferent fiber (**B**), and rate-intensity curve illustrating how a limited range of intensity can be coded in the response of primary afferent fibers to increasing intensity of a tone at its characteristic frequency (**C**).

tage of the difference between *conduction of sound through air* versus *conduction of sound through bone*. To test air conduction, a vibrating tuning fork, usually with a 512-Hz frequency, is held about 1 inch (2.5 cm) from the opening of the auditory canal. Hearing this sound means that *the sound waves generated are passing through the external and middle ears; disease or damage in these areas would result in decreased or lost hearing in this ear*. To test bone conduction, a vibrating tuning fork is placed directly on the skull. Perceiving these vibrations as sounds means that *the sound (vibration) is transmitted directly to the cochlea of the inner ear and bypasses the external ear and the middle ear*.

Both the *Rinne test* and the *Weber test* use these principles to differentiate conduction deafness from sensorineural deafness. For the *Rinne test* (bone + air conduction) the tuning fork is placed against the mastoid process. The normal patient perceives the sound in the ear on that side, and after the sound is no longer perceived by bone conduction the tuning fork is immediately moved to the auditory canal and the sound is again heard (air conduction). If the patient has middle ear disease/deafness, the sound is perceived by bone conduction but not by air conduction; this is a *negative Rinne test*. If the patient has sensorineural deafness (cochlea or cochlear nerve damage), the sound is not perceived by bone conduction but is perceived by air conduction; this is a *positive Rinne test*.

For the *Weber test* the tuning fork is placed on the midline of the skull or forehead. In a patient with normal hearing the sound (vibration) is perceived about equally in both ears. A patient with sensorineural deafness (e.g., cochlear damage) would perceive the sound of the tuning fork in the normal (opposite) ear, whereas a patient with conduction deafness (canal middle ear obstruction) would perceive the sound of the tuning fork in the ear on the side of the damage.

An Overview of Central Auditory Pathways

In the major ascending auditory connections from cochlea to cortex, *the place code of the cochlea is, as a rule, strictly maintained* (Fig. 21-6). Within this tonotopic framework, projections connect similar frequency regions of successive nuclei. Information processing is, therefore, hierarchical with increasing complexity of feature extraction.

All fibers in the cochlear nerve synapse in the *cochlear nuclei*. As cochlear information ascends to the auditory cortex, information is distributed through multiple parallel pathways that ultimately converge in the inferior colliculus. The hierarchy of auditory nuclei involved in these parallel pathways includes the *cochlear nuclei, nuclei of the superior olive and trapezoid body, nuclei of the lateral lemniscus,* and *inferior colliculus*. Specific fiber bundles that convey this information from one level to the next are the *trapezoid body, acoustic stria,* and *lateral lemniscus*. From the midbrain, auditory information is conveyed from the inferior colliculus by its *brachium* to the *medial geniculate nucleus* of the thalamus and then through the *sublenticular limb of the internal capsule to the auditory cortex*. The hierarchy of auditory regions and the fiber bundles that connect one level to the next are summarized in Figures 21-6 and 21-10.

Although fibers conveying auditory input decussate at several levels, this information is routed in one of two orderly ways: (1) *monaural information* (information about sounds at a single ear) *is routed to the contralateral side* and (2) *binaural information* (information about differences between sounds at both ears) *is handled by central pathways that receive, compare, and transmit this input*. Binaural pathways perform the neural computation needed to localize brief sounds.

Unilateral damage to the cochlear nerve or cochlear nucleus results in monaural deafness. In contrast, unilateral damage at or above the superior olivary complex leaves intact routes from either

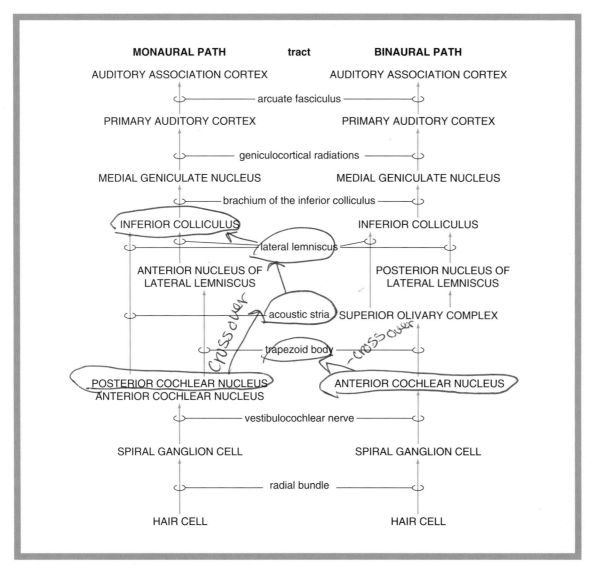

Figure 21-6. Hierarchical order of central auditory pathways.

ear that are conveyed through binaural pathways, so monaural deafness does not occur. The auditory decussations, particularly the trapezoid body, are functionally similar to the optic chiasm in the visual system and have been collectively referred to as a *functional acoustic chiasm*. Thus, central hearing dysfunction may result in inattention to stimuli on the contralateral side.

Vascular Supply of the Auditory Brainstem and Cortex

The blood supply to the cochlea and the auditory nuclei of the pons and medulla originates from the *basilar artery*. The *internal auditory (labyrinthine) artery*, usually a branch of the *anterior inferior cerebellar artery* (AICA), supplies the inner ear and the cochlear nuclei. Occlusion of the AICA will result in a monaural hearing loss. This lesion may also damage the emerging fibers of the facial nerve and the pontine gaze center, resulting in monaural deafness combined with ipsilateral facial paralysis and an inability to look toward the side of the lesion.

Vascular lesions higher in the ascending auditory system necessarily interrupt pathways conveying information from both ears. The superior olivary complex and lateral lemniscus are mainly supplied by *short circumferential branches of the basilar artery*. The *superior cerebellar* and *quadrigeminal arteries* supply the inferior colliculus, and the medial geniculate bodies lie in the vascular territory of the *thalamogeniculate arteries*. The blood supply to the primary auditory and association cortices is via branches of the M_2 segment of the *middle cerebral artery*.

When damage occurs to neural tissue from vascular insults, tumors, or demyelinating diseases such as multiple sclerosis, the effect on conduction time and activity levels in the auditory system can be utilized in clinical neurophysiology to assist in localization of the pathologic process. Brainstem auditory evoked responses are average scalp potentials elicited by a train of clicks and recorded much as for an electroencephalogram. A pattern of seven waves occurs in the auditory evoked response, with peaks at regular latencies after the clicks that are correlated with activity levels of the ascending auditory system. The activity from one or more auditory structures may be correlated with a specific wave, as summarized in Figure 21-7; and shifts in latency and amplitude of specific waves may be used to localize the lesion, assess hearing, or indicate swelling in response to neurosurgical procedures.

Brainstem Auditory Nuclei and Pathways

Cochlear Nuclei

The *posterior cochlear nucleus (dorsal cochlear nucleus)* and the *anterior cochlear nucleus (ventral cochlear nucleus)* are located lateral and posterior to the restiform body and are partially on the surface of the brainstem at the pontomedullary junction (Fig. 21-8A). The posterior cochlear nucleus drapes over the restiform body just inferior to the pontomedullary junction. At this level the posterior part of the anterior cochlear nucleus is small in proportion to the posterior cochlear nucleus (Fig. 21-8A, B). The anterior cochlear nucleus extends rostral to the posterior cochlear nucleus (Fig. 21-8C), where it may be covered by the flocculus and by caudal fascicles of the middle cerebellar peduncle.

All cochlear nerve fibers end in the cochlear nuclei on the ipsilateral side (Fig. 21-9). As these fibers enter the brainstem at the cerebellopontine angle, they divide into ascending and descending bundles. Fibers in the ascending bundle synapse in the anterior part of the anterior cochlear nucleus, whereas fibers in the descending bundle synapse in the posterior part of the anterior cochlear nucleus and in the posterior cochlear nucleus.

In the cochlear nuclei, each afferent nerve fiber makes specialized synaptic contacts with several different cell types. Individual fibers and their synaptic contacts distribute along orderly rows so that the resulting order produces distinct tonotopic maps in each division (Fig. 21-9C). The frequency-related lines are organized so that low frequencies are represented laterally and high frequencies medially (Fig. 21-9C).

Specific cell types of the cochlear nuclei, in turn, give rise to parallel but separate ascending pathways in the auditory system that analyze and code different sound features while preserving

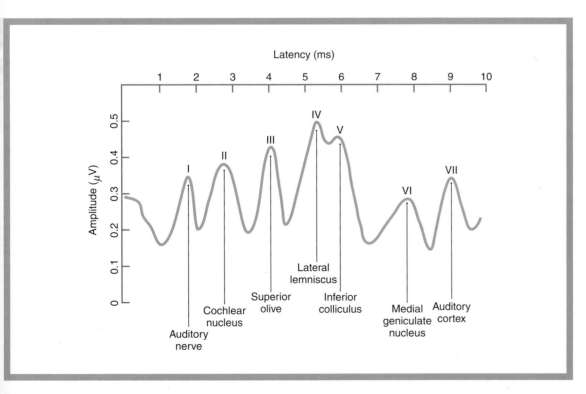

Figure 21-7. Stylized example of an auditory brainstem response recording. Waves I to VII are labeled above, while below the sequence of auditory structures in which activity may be correlated with each wave is indicated. The *vertical lines* indicate the approximate correlation of wave and auditory structure, although more than one structure is likely to contribute to various waves. Levels and latency may vary in actual recordings.

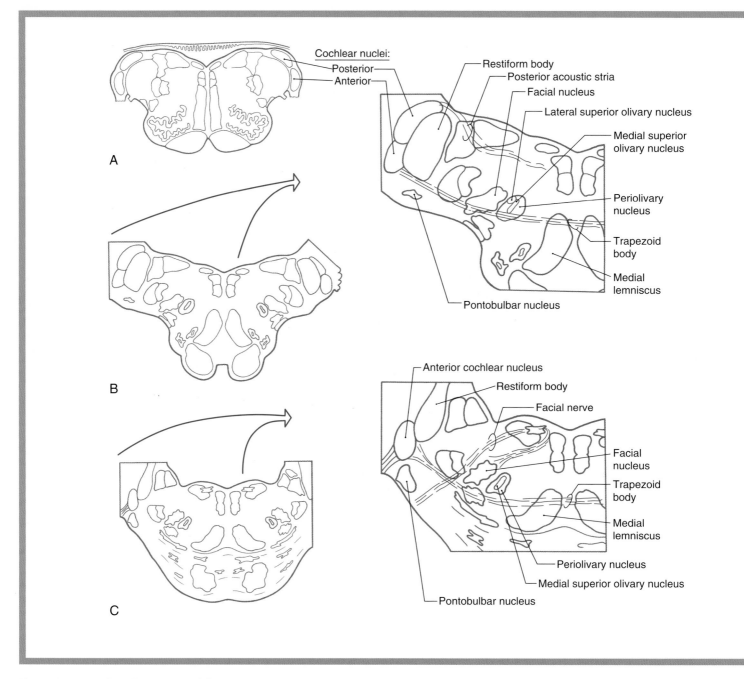

Figure 21-8. Levels of the rostral medulla (**A**, **B**) and caudal pons (**C**) illustrating the relation of the cochlear nuclei and superior olivary complex.

frequency information. These projections are subdivided into pathways conveying monaural information to the inferior colliculus and those providing input to the superior olivary complex for binaural processing. Most fibers from the anterior cochlear nucleus course anterior to the restiform body part of the inferior cerebellar peduncle to form the *trapezoid body* (Fig. 21-8B, C). Projections from the posterior cochlear nucleus and some from the anterior cochlear nucleus course posteriorly over the restiform body as the *posterior acoustic stria* and decussate in the pontine tegmentum before joining the lateral lemniscus.

Many of the cells in the posterior cochlear nucleus contribute to complex local circuits and are not easily correlated with distinct ascending channels. *Pyramidal cells* have fusiform cell bodies with apical and basal dendrites. A major output of the posterior cochlear nucleus is via a direct pyramidal cell projection to the contralateral inferior colliculus (Fig. 21-10).

The anterior cochlear nucleus is distinguished by the presence of anatomically and physiologically distinct output cell types (Fig. 21-9). The anterior part of the anterior cochlear nucleus contains mainly *spherical* and *globular bushy cells*. There is almost a one-to-one relation between the synaptic endings of a cochlear nerve fiber and each bushy cell. Consequently, the temporal pattern of activity in bushy cells is remarkably similar to that of the primary afferents, and these cells show sustained responses to short tones that convey information about the timing and phase of the tone. Axons of bushy cells travel in the trapezoid body. They are the central origin of ascending channels that process *binaural information*, which is useful for sound localization (Figs. 21-6 and 21-10).

Multipolar cells in the anterior cochlear nucleus are sensitive to changes in sound pressure level. Accordingly, they convey information in a *direct monaural pathway*, primarily to the contralateral inferior colliculus (Fig. 21-10) about the intensity of the sound.

Also in the posterior part of the anterior cochlear nucleus are *octopus cells*, which have long, relatively unbranched dendrites and integrate inputs from a wider array of cochlear afferents. Axons of octopus cells synapse mainly in the contralateral anterior nucleus of the lateral lemniscus, which, in turn, projects to the inferior colliculus. This *indirect monaural pathway* conveys

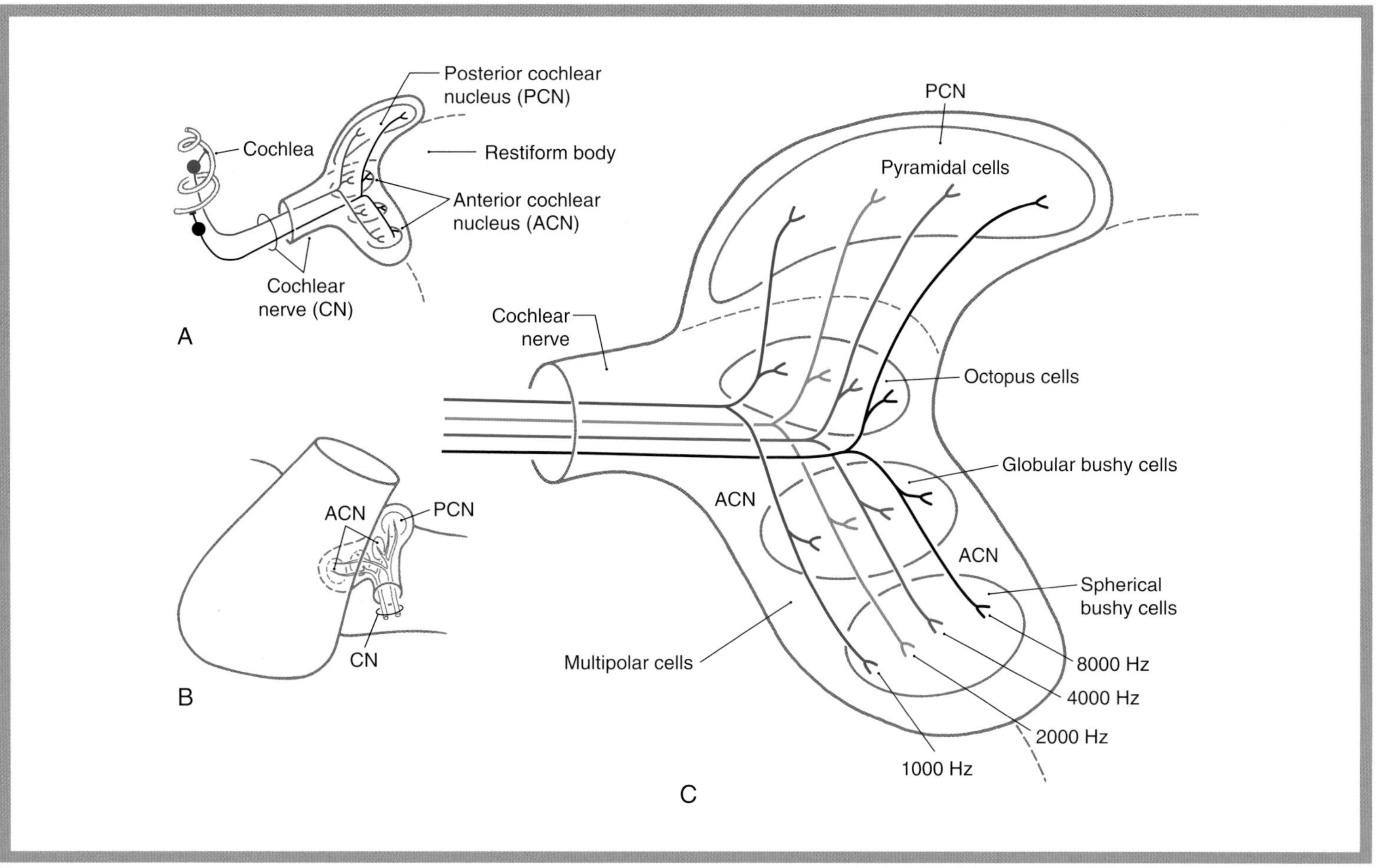

Figure 21-9. The posterior and anterior cochlear nuclei in cross section (**A**, **C**) and as viewed from the lateral aspect on the left (**B**). The anterior cochlear nucleus extends rostral to the posterior nucleus (**B**). The course, tonotopic organization of cochlear afferent fibers, and the locations of main cell groups are also indicated (**C**).

information that is useful in analyzing brief components of speech sounds.

Superior Olivary Complex

The superior olivary complex is located near the facial motor nucleus in the caudal pons (Figs. 21-8B, C and 21-10). It is the first site in the brainstem where information from both ears converges. This binaural processing is essential for accurate sound localization and the formation of a neural map of the contralateral auditory hemifield.

The *medial superior olivary nucleus* (MSO), which forms a distinct vertical bar within a diffuse group of *periolivary nuclei*, is the principal nucleus in the human superior olivary complex (Figs. 21-8B, C and 21-10). The *lateral superior olivary nucleus* (LSO), located lateral to the MSO, is not distinct and contains fewer cells.

The *trapezoid body* is a bundle of myelinated fibers passing anterior to the superior olivary complex and intermingling with fibers of the medial lemniscus as it crosses the midline (Figs. 21-8B and 21-10). Decussating fibers of the trapezoid body end in the contralateral superior olivary complex or ascend in the contralateral lateral lemniscus. The medial nucleus of the trapezoid body lies medial to the MSO. It receives projections from globular bushy cells in the contralateral anterior cochlear nucleus and gives rise to important local inhibitory circuits within the superior olive.

The topographic organization of the afferents to the MSO and the LSO conserves the orderly representation of the cochlea (Fig. 21-10). In the MSO, cells with low characteristic frequencies are found posteriorly, and those with higher characteristic frequencies are found more anteriorly. These are bipolar cells with medially and laterally directed dendrites (Fig. 21-10). Axons in the trapezoid body arising from ipsilateral spherical bushy cells make excitatory synapses with the laterally directed dendrites. Axons from the contralateral spherical bushy cells decussating in the trapezoid body make excitatory synapses with the medially directed dendrites. The excitatory neurotransmitter is probably *glutamate* or *aspartate*. Local inhibitory circuits in the superior olivary complex use *glycine* as a neurotransmitter.

The pathways to the MSO from spherical bushy cells in the anterior cochlear nucleus are anatomically arranged so that signals from the contralateral ear arrive close enough in time to those from the ipsilateral ear to summate at each cell only for a sound from a specific point in the contralateral hemifield of space. This mechanism, referred to as *coincidence detection*, accounts for computation by the MSO of interaural time differences that constitute the basis for sound localization (Fig. 21-11). Coincidence of the signals occurs when the shorter neural conduction time in the path from the ipsilateral cochlear nucleus compensates for the shorter delay of the sound path to the contralateral ear (Figs. 21-10 and 21-11).

Ascending projections from the MSO travel largely in the ipsilateral side in the lateral lemniscus and synapse in the *central nucleus* of the inferior colliculus (Fig. 21-10). These fibers synapse in corresponding frequency regions (low to low, and so on) of the inferior colliculus (Fig. 21-10). The LSO also contributes in a small way in humans to both of these pathways. Branches of these projections always end in the posterior nucleus of the lateral lemniscus (dorsal nucleus of the lateral lemniscus). This nucleus, in turn, projects to the contralateral inferior colliculus and constitutes an indirect binaural pathway from the superior olive to the inferior colliculus (Fig. 21-10).

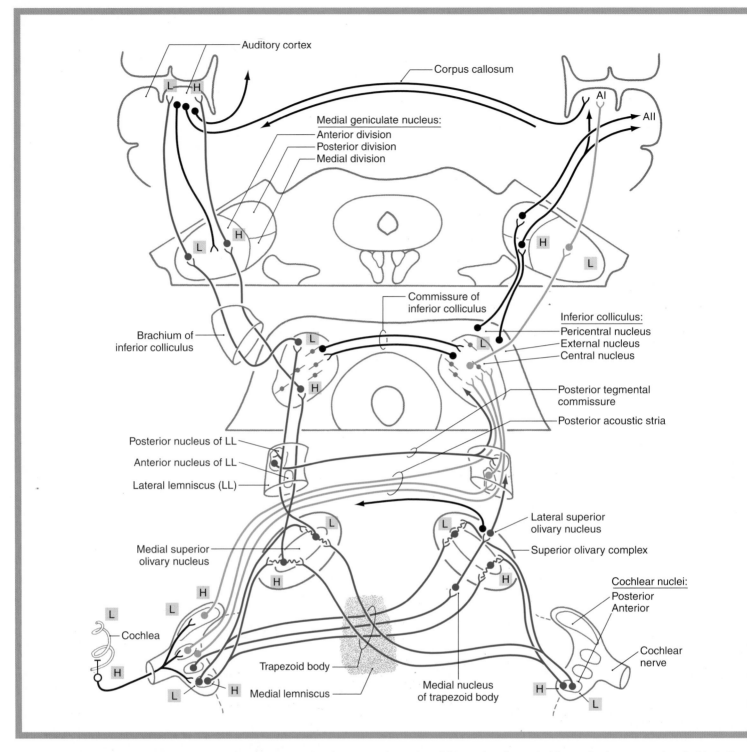

Figure 21-10. Ascending central auditory pathways. Monaural pathways are shown in *red,* binaural pathways in *blue,* and other connections in *black.* AI and AII, primary and secondary auditory cortices; H, high frequencies; L, low frequencies.

Detection of interaural intensity differences, which provide spatial cues for high-frequency stimuli caused by shadowing of sounds by the path from the contralateral side of the head, is also accomplished by summation of excitatory and inhibitory inputs to LSO neurons. Humans are capable of detecting small sound differences between the two ears for high-frequency signals, which serve as cues to the source of the auditory signal.

Lateral Lemniscus and Its Nuclei

The lateral lemniscus contains axons from second-order neurons in the cochlear nuclei, third-order neurons in the superior olive, and fourth-order neurons in the adjacent nuclei of the lateral lemniscus (Fig. 21-10). *It is precisely this heterogeneous collection that prevents a simple correlation of nuclei or tracts with specific wave components of the auditory evoked responses that are widely*

used to assess clinically the level of brainstem function. The interposition of synaptic delays in each of these components of the lateral lemniscus imparts temporal differences that contribute to at least the second, third, and fourth wave components of the evoked responses.

The larger *anterior nucleus of the lateral lemniscus (ventral nucleus of the lateral lemniscus)* consists of cells scattered among the ascending fibers of the lateral lemniscus (Fig. 21-10). It extends from the rostral limit of the superior olive to just below the inferior colliculus. These cells project to the inferior colliculus, completing an *indirect monaural pathway* (Fig. 21-10).

The smaller *posterior nucleus of the lateral lemniscus (dorsal nucleus of the lateral lemniscus)* is intercalated in the ascending fiber bundles of the lateral lemniscus just caudal to the inferior colliculus (Fig. 21-10). This nucleus receives input mainly from

The central nucleus integrates information from multiple hindbrain auditory sources and, in turn, projects to the anterior division of the medial geniculate nucleus (Fig. 21-10). The central nucleus consists of parallel layers of cells with disc-shaped dendritic fields. Afferents from the lateral lemniscus course parallel to these dendritic fields, forming a series of *fibrodendritic laminae*. Ascending projections diverge and converge in a point-to-plane order in the central nucleus. As a result, each point along the cochlear spiral is represented in an *isofrequency lamina*. Functionally, cells in the central nucleus are narrowly tuned, with the lowest frequencies represented posterolaterally and higher frequencies anteromedially (Fig. 21-10).

Many cells in the inferior colliculus respond to input from either ear. Among cells with low characteristic frequencies, many are sensitive to interaural time delays, and those with high characteristic frequencies are sensitive to interaural intensity differences. Thus, binaural responses of inferior collicular neurons resemble those of the superior olivary neurons, from which they receive a dominant binaural input. These responses are probably further modified by indirect binaural pathways from the posterior nucleus of the lateral lemniscus and by intrinsic circuits in the fibrodendritic laminae. Other cells in the fibrodendritic laminae of the central nucleus are monaural and are mainly excited only by the contralateral ear. Their responses resemble those of cells in the contralateral cochlear nucleus.

Cells in the *paracentral nuclei* are broadly tuned to frequency, and they habituate rapidly to repetitive stimuli. They receive input from the central nucleus and the cerebral cortex and nonauditory input from the spinal cord, posterior column nuclei, and superior colliculus. These nuclei project to the medial geniculate nucleus (Fig. 21-10), superior colliculus, reticular formation, and precerebellar nuclei. Thus, the paracentral nuclei are probably involved in functions related to attention, multisensory integration, and auditory-motor reflexes (Fig. 21-15).

Medial Geniculate Nucleus

The medial geniculate nucleus forms a small protuberance on the lower caudal surface of the thalamus between the lateral geniculate body and the pulvinar (Fig. 21-10; see also Fig. 15-10). The *anterior division* of the medial geniculate nucleus receives afferents from the central nucleus of the inferior colliculus and projects to the primary auditory cortex. Isofrequency contours in the anterior division are arranged so that low frequencies are represented laterally and higher frequencies are represented medially (Fig. 21-10). As a result of collicular and thalamic integration, however, most cells are not reliably excited by simple tones and are probably involved in complex feature detection.

The *posterior division* receives input from the pericentral nucleus of the inferior colliculus and projects to secondary auditory cortex (Fig. 21-10). These projections are also tonotopically arranged. More broadly tuned and sensitive to habituation, this pathway may convey information about moving or novel stimuli that direct auditory attention.

The *medial (magnocellular)* division receives afferents from the external nucleus of the inferior colliculus and projects to association areas of auditory cortex. It contains cells that are broadly tuned to auditory and other sensory stimuli, including vestibular and somesthetic inputs. The medial division projects to temporal and parietal association areas and to the amygdala, putamen, and pallidum. In view of the multisensory convergence that occurs in this pathway, it may be a part of the reticular activating system.

Central Deafness

Central deafness results from damage to the cochlear nuclei and/or the central pathways that relay auditory information to the auditory cortex. Damage to the cochlear nuclei may cause

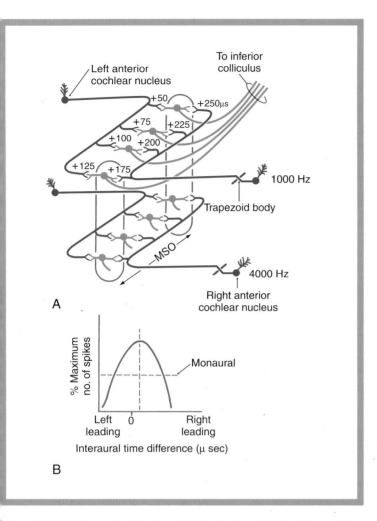

Figure 21-11. The mechanism by which the brain calculates interaural time differences. Diagrammatic representation of how time delay lines are established in connections between spherical bushy cells in anterior cochlear nucleus and two medial superior olivary nucleus (MSO) isofrequency columns (**A**). Transmission times in microseconds for the neural signals are shown in the delay line that maps interaural time delay along the rostral-caudal axis of MSO. When the interaural delay is precisely the reciprocal of this delay (that is, when the arrival at the right ear precedes the arrival at the left ear by the same increment as the signal on the left precedes the signal on the right), then summation occurs as shown in the delay-response curve (**B**). The *dotted horizontal line* indicates the response level to a monaural stimulus.

the superior olivary complex. Ascending projections from the posterior nucleus of the lateral lemniscus decussate in the *posterior tegmental commissure*. These fibers terminate in the contralateral inferior colliculus and, to a lesser degree, in the contralateral posterior nucleus of the lateral lemniscus (Fig. 21-10). This pathway is largely inhibitory, using γ-aminobutyric acid (GABA) as the neurotransmitter. It conveys binaural information and inhibits activity from the opposite hemifield.

Inferior Colliculus

Virtually all ascending auditory pathways terminate in the inferior colliculus (Fig. 21-10). The egg-shaped core of the inferior colliculus, the prominent *central nucleus*, is nested in a base of afferent fibers formed by fibers of the lateral lemniscus. These fibers are the major source of input to the inferior colliculus. In a shell around the central nucleus, other cells form the smaller *paracentral nuclei* (Fig. 21-10). These are the *pericentral nucleus*, which lies posterior and is traversed by fibers from the commissure of the inferior colliculus, and the *external (lateral) nucleus*, which lies lateral and is intersected by fibers that form the *brachium of the inferior colliculus*.

deafness in the ear on the affected side. On the other hand, central lesions within the brainstem, diencephalon, or auditory cortices may alter the perception of sound but infrequently result in deafness in one ear. In some cases pontine lesions may result in *pontine auditory hallucinosis*, such as an orchestra out of tune, buzzing insects, or strands of music. These perceived auditory events are accompanied by more typical symptoms of pontine lesions, such as cranial nerve deficits and/or long tract signs. A perception of noise or sounds may also be experienced by patients with temporal lobe seizures or a temporal lobe lesion that damages auditory cortices.

Auditory and Related Association Cortices

The *primary auditory cortex* (AI) is located in the *transverse gyri of Heschl* (Fig. 21-12; see also Fig. 21-10). Two transverse temporal gyri are buried in the lateral sylvian sulcus, covered by parts of the frontal and parietal opercula, and continuous with the superior temporal gyrus. Caudal to the transverse temporal gyri is a smooth area, the *planum temporale*, which is usually larger on the left side than on the right.

The primary auditory cortex (AI, Brodmann area 41) is located in the first (anterior) transverse temporal gyrus but may extend into the second (posterior) gyrus (Fig. 21-12A). Cyto-architecturally, area 41 encompasses the *granular cortex*, with its well-developed layer IV containing small granule cells and densely packed small pyramidal cells in layer VI (Fig. 21-12B). Adjacent to the granular cortex in the second transverse gyrus and planum temporale is area 42, which constitutes the *secondary auditory* cortex (AII) (Fig. 21-12A).

Area 41 is reciprocally connected with the anterior division, and area 42 with the posterior division, of the medial geniculate body (Fig. 21-13). Through the corpus callosum, each auditory cortical area is connected with the reciprocal areas in the other cerebral hemisphere. The tonotopic organization of constituent cells of the cortical layers and incoming afferent fibers form a series of orderly isofrequency columns that extend through the primary auditory cortex as long stripes (Fig. 21-12). High frequencies are represented medially and low frequencies laterally. The series of stripes so formed have one subcomponent composed of cells excited by stimulation of both ears (EE) alternating with a subcomponent composed of cells excited by the contralateral ear and inhibited by the ipsilateral ear (EI).

The *auditory association cortex* surrounds the primary auditory area and is located mainly in the posterior portion of the superior temporal gyrus (Fig. 21-12A). It is connected to the primary auditory cortex by the *arcuate fasciculus* (Fig. 21-12A). Area 22 includes a part of the planum temporale and the posterior portion of the superior temporal gyrus. It receives connections from the primary auditory cortex, as well as visual and somesthetic information. This speech receptive area, known as the *Wernicke area*, may be as much as seven times larger on the left side than on the right. When this area is damaged by occlusion of branches of the middle cerebral artery, an *auditory aphasia (Wernicke aphasia)* results. In such cases, comprehension of speech sounds is impaired but discrimination of nonverbal sounds is largely unaffected.

The higher association areas of auditory cortex also extend into the inferior parietal lobule (Fig. 21-12A). This lobule is made up of the angular gyrus (area 39) and supramarginal gyrus (area 40). These two areas are important in aspects of language such as reading and writing and are sometimes included in the Wernicke area.

Brodmann areas 44 and 45 are known as the *Broca area* for expressive speech and language. They are located in the *pars opercularis* and *pars triangularis* of the *inferior frontal gyrus* (Fig. 21-12A). The major pathway connecting these areas with the primary and association auditory cortex is the *arcuate fasciculus* (Fig. 21-12). If areas 44 and 45 are damaged along

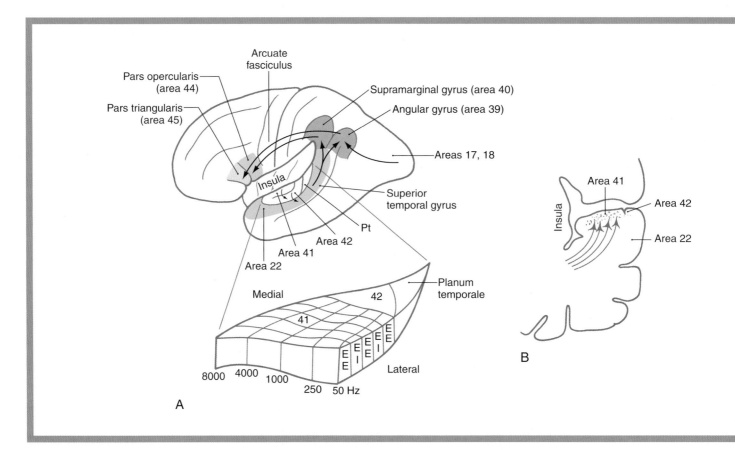

Figure 21-12. The organization of auditory cortical areas. Location and interconnections of auditory cortical areas (**A**) and of the granular cortex in area 41 (**B**), and the orthogonal isofrequency and binaural response columns in the primary auditory cortex (*detail* from **A**).

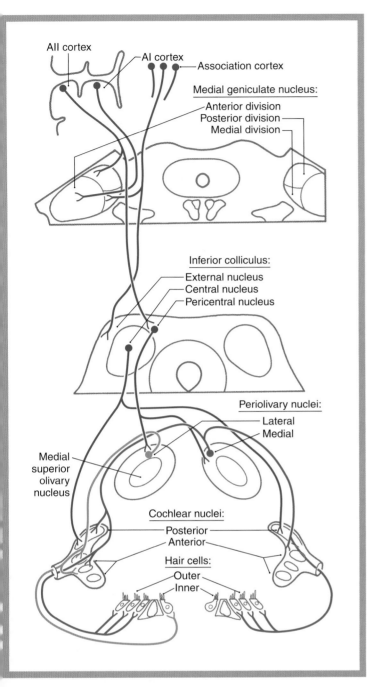

Figure 21-13. Descending auditory pathways that modulate sensory processing at central and peripheral auditory sites. The lateral olivocochlear efferents are shown in *red* and the medial olivocochlear efferents in *green.* AI and AII, primary and secondary auditory (cortices).

with other motor cortices on the left side by a stroke involving branches of the middle cerebral artery, the result is *Broca aphasia.* In this disorder, speech is nonfluent, but comprehension of verbal and nonverbal sounds is largely unimpaired.

Descending Auditory Pathways

Descending projections make reciprocal connections throughout the auditory pathway. They form feedback loops that provide circuits to modulate information processing from the peripheral level to the cortex (Fig. 21-13). For example, the auditory cortex projects to the medial geniculate nucleus and nuclei of the inferior colliculus. The inferior colliculus projects to the periolivary nuclei, which, in turn, send olivocochlear efferents to the cochlea. There are also descending projections from the periolivary nuclei to the cochlear nuclei.

The Olivocochlear Bundle

The *olivocochlear efferent system* arises from groups of cells in the periolivary nuclei of the superior olivary complex (Fig. 21-13). These efferent systems travel as the *olivocochlear bundle* in the vestibular part of the vestibulocochlear nerve. *Lateral olivocochlear efferent* cells project to the ipsilateral inner hair cells, where they make axoaxonic synapses with type I spiral ganglion afferent fibers (Figs. 21-4 and 21-13). *Medial olivocochlear efferent* cells have bilateral projections that terminate directly on outer hair cells (Figs. 21-4 and 21-13).

Direct efferent feedback to outer hair cells, in particular, may influence cochlear mechanics and, consequently, the sensitivity and frequency selectivity of the cochlea. Efferent-induced changes in outer hair cell membrane potentials result in changes in the height of the cells and the stiffness of their stereocilia. These changes modulate basilar membrane motion and thereby influence cochlear function. The tight coupling of the basilar membrane to the tectorial membrane by the outer hair cells enables this efferent mechanism to feed energy back to the cochlea to amplify responses to specific tones. The cochlear amplifier effect is important in selectively tuning the cochlea to important sounds.

Middle Ear Reflex

The small striated muscles of the middle ear affect the mechanical impedance of the ossicular chain. These muscles are activated by the *middle ear reflex* (Fig. 21-14).

The *stapedius muscle* is innervated by *facial motor neurons,* and the *tensor tympani muscle* is innervated by *trigeminal motor neurons.* These motor neurons are intimately associated with the caudal end of the superior olivary complex, in the case of the stapedius muscle, and with the rostral end of the superior olivary complex, in the case of the tensor tympani muscle. In these

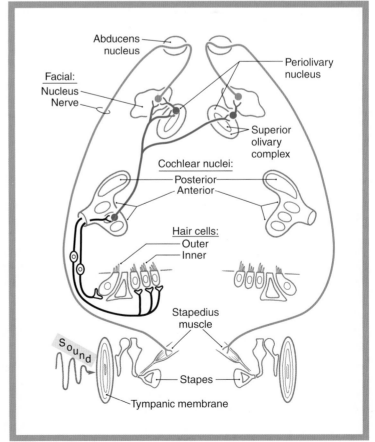

Figure 21-14. The pathway of the middle ear reflex arc. For simplicity, only the stapedius reflex is shown.

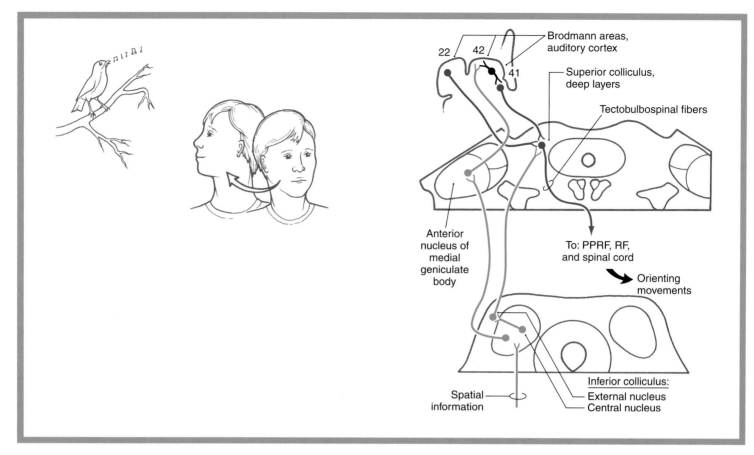

Figure 21-15. The pathways that subserve auditory-motor integration involved in simple orientation to a novel auditory stimulus. RF, reticular formation; PPRF, paramedian pontine reticular formation.

positions, auditory input via axons of neurons in the cochlear nuclei or the superior olivary complex provides the sensory limb of the reflex. The sensory pathways are bilateral, so that stimuli may be presented by earphones to one ear while the device to measure impedance is placed in the ear canal on the other side.

Acoustic Startle Reflex, Orientation, and Attention

Reflexive and learned responses to sound require sensory-motor integration. In addition to corticocortical interconnections for the dissemination of auditory information, there is also integration of auditory sensory input with motor pathways in the brainstem. Reticulospinal neurons in the region of the lateral lemniscus have dendrites that sample lemniscal activity and are involved in rapid *acoustic startle reflex* pathways. In addition, the *deep layers of the superior colliculus* receive auditory information from the inferior colliculus and auditory cortical areas (Fig. 21-15). The deep layers of the superior colliculus integrate auditory, visual, and somesthetic information and project to brainstem and cervical spinal cord nuclei via tectobulbospinal fibers, which are involved in controlling orientation of the head, eyes, and body to sound (Fig. 21-15).

Synopsis of Clinical Points

- Obstruction of the ear canal or damage to the ossicles may result in conduction deafness (pp. 335, 336).
- Sensorineural deafness results from damage to the cochlea or cochlear portion of the eighth nerve (pp. 339, 335).
- Lesions within the brain may result in central deafness; these patients rarely perceive deafness in one ear (pp. 335, 340, 346).
- Otosclerosis results in conductive hearing loss (p. 336).
- Patients with otitis media may have an accumulation of pus or exudate in the middle ear (p. 336).
- Otitis externa may cause conduction deafness (p. 336).
- Any alternation of the transmission of sound waves through the middle ear may produce a conduction deafness (p. 336).
- Patient's with profound hearing loss may benefit from a cochlear implant (pp. 338–339).
- Sensorineural hearing loss results from damage to the cochlea or cochlear nerve (pp. 335, 339).
- Inflammation of the inner ear is otitis interna or labyrinthitis (p. 339).
- Tinnitus may result from damage to the cochlea (p. 339).
- Sensorineural hearing loss may result from a variety of causes such as mumps, infections, or tumors (p. 339).

Synopsis of Clinical Points   *(Continued)*

- The Weber and Rinne tests differentiate bone from air conduction (pp. 339–340).
- Middle ear disease will result in the negative Rinne test (p. 340).
- A tuning fork, usually with a 512-Hz frequency, is used in the Weber and Rinne tests (p. 339).
- Auditory brainstem responses are electrical potentials that measure neural conduction in peripheral and central parts of the auditory pathway and they are a clinically important tool (pp. 341, 344).
- Brainstem lesions rarely produce hearing loss in one ear (pp. 340, 346).
- A perception of sound may be experienced by patients with temporal lobe lesions or seizure (p. 346).
- Pontine auditory hallucinosis may occur in brainstem lesions (p. 346).
- Cortical lesions that involve temporoparietal areas may result in auditory aphasia (p. 346).
- Auditory aphasia is a component of Wernicke aphasia (p. 346).
- Speech patterns are altered in Broca aphasia (p. 347).
- The middle ear reflex activates the small striated muscles of the middle ear that affect the mechanical impedance of the ossicular chain (p. 347).
- Clinically, parameters of acoustic startle can be used to evaluate attentional states modulated through connections of the lateral lemniscus and reticular formation (p. 348).

Sources and Additional Reading

Interesting web links related to the auditory system:

Promenade 'round the Cochlea. Available at http://www.iurc.montp.inserm.fr/cric/audition/english/start.htm

The Cochlea—graphic tour of the inner ear's machinery. Available at http://www.vimm.it/cochlea/index.htm

Altschuler RA, Bobbin RP, Hoffman DW: Neurobiology of Hearing: The Cochlea. New York, Raven Press, 1986.

Altschuler RA, Bobbin RP, Clopton BM, Hoffman DW: Neurobiology of Hearing: The Central Auditory System. New York, Raven Press, 1991.

Gelfand SA: Hearing: An Introduction to Psychological and Physiological Acoustics. New York, Marcel Dekker, 1990.

Pickles JO: An Introduction to the Physiology of Hearing, 2nd ed. London, Academic Press, 1988.

Webster D, Fay RR, Popper AN: Springer Handbook of Auditory Research, vol I. The Auditory Pathway: Neuroanatomy. New York, Springer-Verlag, 1992.

Yost WA: Fundamentals of Hearing: An Introduction. San Diego, Academic Press, 1994.

The Vestibular System

J. D. Dickman

Humans have the ability to control posture and movements of the body and eyes relative to the external environment. The *vestibular system* mediates these motor activities through a network of receptors and neural elements. This system integrates peripheral sensory information from vestibular, somatosensory, visceromotor, and visual receptors, as well as motor information from the cerebellum and cerebral cortex. Central processing of these inputs occurs rapidly, with the output of the vestibular system providing an appropriate signal to coordinate relevant movement reflexes. Although the vestibular system is considered to be a special sense, most vestibular activity is conducted at a subconscious level. However, in situations producing unusual or novel vestibular stimulation, such as rough air in a plane flight or wave motion on ships, vestibular perception becomes acute, with dizziness, vertigo, or nausea often resulting.

Overview

The vestibular system is an essential component in the production of motor responses that are crucial for daily function and survival. Throughout evolution, the highly conserved nature of the vestibular system is revealed through striking similarities in the anatomic organization of receptors and neuronal connections in fish, reptiles, birds, and mammals.

For the present discussion, the vestibular system can be divided into five components:

1. The *peripheral receptor apparatus* resides in the inner ear and is responsible for transducing head motion and position into neural information.
2. The *central vestibular nuclei* comprise a set of neurons in the brainstem that are responsible for receiving, integrating, and distributing information that controls motor activities such as eye and head movements, postural reflexes, and gravity-dependent autonomic reflexes and spatial orientation.

3. The *vestibulo-ocular network* arises from the vestibular nuclei and is involved in the control of eye movements.
4. The *vestibulospinal network* coordinates head movements, axial musculature, and postural reflexes.
5. The *vestibulo-thalamo-cortical network* is responsible for the conscious perception of movement and spatial orientation.

Peripheral Vestibular Labyrinth

The vestibular labyrinth contains specialized sensory receptors and is located lateral and posterior to the cochlea in the inner ear (Fig. 22-1). The vestibular labyrinth consists of five separate receptor structures, *three semicircular canals* and *two otolith organs*, which are contained in the petrous portion of the temporal bone. The labyrinth is actually composed of two distinct components. The *bony labyrinth* is a surrounding shell that contains and protects the sensitive underlying vestibular sensory structures (Fig. 22-1). In humans, the bony labyrinth can be visualized only on excision of the mastoid process. Inside the bony labyrinth is a closed, fluid-filled system, the *membranous labyrinth*, which consists of connecting tubes and prominences (Fig. 22-2). Vestibular receptors are located in specialized regions of the membranous labyrinth.

Between the membranous and bony labyrinth is a space containing fluid called *perilymph*, which is similar to cerebrospinal fluid. Perilymph has a high sodium content (150 mM) and a low potassium content (7 mM), and it bathes the vestibular portion of the eighth cranial nerve.

The membranous labyrinth is filled with a different type of fluid, called *endolymph*, which covers the specialized sensory receptors of both the vestibular and the auditory systems. Endolymph has a high concentration of potassium (150 mM) and a low concentration of sodium (16 mM). It is important to note the differences in these two fluids because both are involved in the normal functioning of the vestibular system. Disturbances

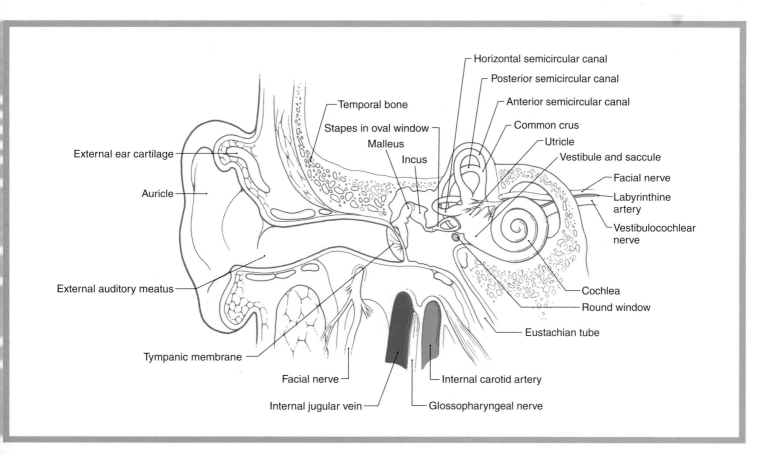

Figure 22-1. A cross section of the outer, middle, and inner ear.

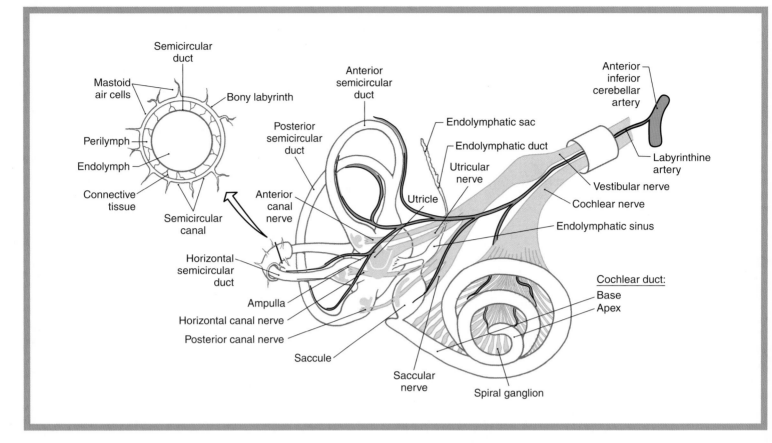

Figure 22-2. The membranous labyrinth and associated vessels and nerves. The approximate configuration of the receptor sites in the ampullae, utricle, and saccule are shown in *green*. The detail shows the relationship between bony and membranous labyrinths.

in the distribution or ionic content of endolymph often lead to vestibular pathology.

Vestibular Receptor Organs

The five vestibular receptor organs in the inner ear complement each other in function. The semicircular canals (horizontal, anterior, and posterior) transduce rotational head movements (angular accelerations). The otolith organs (utricle and saccule) respond to translational head movements (linear accelerations) or to the orientation of the head relative to gravity. Each semicircular canal and otolith organ is spatially aligned to be most sensitive to movements in specific planes in three-dimensional space.

In humans, the horizontal semicircular canal and the utricle both lie in a plane that is slightly tilted anterodorsally relative to the naso-occipital plane (Fig. 22-3). When a person walks or runs, the head is normally declined (pitched downward) by approximately 30 degrees, so that the line of sight is directed a few meters in front of the feet. This orientation causes the plane of the horizontal canal and utricle to be parallel with the earth and perpendicular to gravity. The anterior and posterior semicircular canals and the saccule are arranged vertically in the head, orthogonal to the horizontal semicircular canal and utricle (Fig. 22-3). The two vertical canals in each ear are positioned orthogonal to each other, whereas the plane of the anterior canal on one side of the head is coplanar with the plane of the contralateral posterior canal (Fig. 22-3).

The receptor cells in each vestibular organ are innervated by primary afferent fibers that join with those from the cochlea to comprise the *vestibulocochlear (eighth) cranial nerve*. The cell bodies of these bipolar vestibular afferent neurons are in the vestibular ganglion (Scarpa ganglion), which lies in the internal acoustic meatus (Fig. 22-4). The central processes of these bipolar cells enter the brainstem and terminate in the ipsilateral vestibular nuclei and cerebellum.

The blood supply to the labyrinth is primarily via the *labyrinthine artery*, usually a branch of the anterior inferior cerebellar artery. This vessel enters the temporal bone through the internal auditory meatus. Although not as important as the labyrinthine artery, the *stylomastoid artery* also provides branches to the labyrinth, mainly to the semicircular canals. An interruption of blood supply to the labyrinth will compromise vestibular (and cochlear) function, resulting in labyrinth-associated symptoms such as vertigo or oscillopsia, and clinical signs such nystagmus or unstable gait.

Membranous Labyrinth

The membranous labyrinth is supported inside the bony labyrinth by connective tissue. The three *ducts of the semicircular canals* connect to the utricle, and each duct ends with a single prominent enlargement, the *ampulla* (Fig. 22-2). Sensory receptors for the semicircular canals reside in a neuroepithelium at the base of each ampulla. The receptors in the utricle are oriented longitudinally along its base, and in the saccule they are oriented vertically along the medial wall (Fig. 22-2). Endolymph in the labyrinth is drained into the endolymphatic sinus via small ducts. In turn, this sinus communicates through the *endolymphatic duct* with the *endolymphatic sac*, which is located adjacent to the dura mater (Fig. 22-2). The saccule is also connected to the cochlea by the *ductus reuniens*.

Ménière Disease

The balance between the ionic contents of endolymph and perilymph is maintained by specialized secretory cells in the membranous labyrinth and the endolymphatic sac. In cases of advanced *Ménière disease*, there is disruption of normal

---

endolymph volume resulting in *endolymphatic hydrops* (an abnormal distention of the membranous labyrinth). Symptoms of Ménière disease include severe vertigo (a sense of spinning in space), positional nystagmus, and nausea. Affected persons often suffer unpredictable attacks of auditory and vestibular symptoms, including vomiting, tinnitus (ringing in the ears), and a complete inability to make head movements or even stand passively. For patients with frequent debilitating attacks, the first course of treatment is often administration of a diuretic (e.g., hydrochlorothiazide) and a salt-restricted diet to reduce the hydrops. If persistent symptoms of Ménière disease continue, second treatment options include either the implantation of a small shunt into the abnormally swollen endolymphatic sac or the delivery of a vestibulotoxic agent such as gentamicin into the perilymph.

Semicircular Canal Dehiscence

Occasionally, a condition may develop in which a portion of the temporal bone overlying either the anterior or the posterior semicircular canal thins so much that an opening (dehiscence) is created next to the dura (Fig. 22-5). In affected patients, the canal dehiscence exposes the normally closed bony labyrinth to the extradural space. Symptoms can include vertigo and oscillopsia (a sense that objects are moving to and fro, oscillating, in the visual fields) in response to loud sounds (the Tullio phenomenon) or in response to maneuvers that change middle ear or intracranial pressure. The eye movements evoked by these stimuli (nystagmus) align with the plane of the dehiscent superior canal. Surgical closure of the defect by bone replacement is often performed.

Vestibular Sensory Receptors

Hair Cell Morphology

The sensory receptor cells in the vestibular system, like those in the auditory system, are called *hair cells*, owing to the *stereocilia* that project from the apical surface of the cell (Fig. 22-6A). Each hair cell contains 60 to 100 hexagonally arranged stereocilia and a single longer *kinocilium*. The stereocilia are oriented in rows of ascending height, with the tallest lying next to the lone kinocilium. The stereocilia arise from a region of dense actin, the *cuticular plate*, located at the apical end of the hair cell. The cuticular plate acts as an elastic spring to return the stereocilia to the normal upright position after bending. Each stereocilium is connected to its neighbor by small filaments.

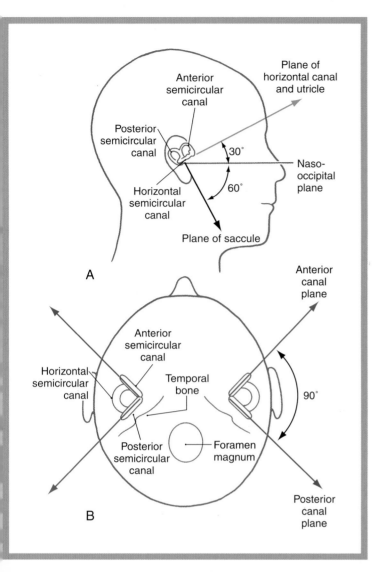

Figure 22-3. Orientation of the vestibular receptors. In the lateral view (**A**), the horizontal semicircular canal and the utricle lie in a plane that is tilted relative to the naso-occipital plane. In the axial view (**B**), the vertical semicircular canals lie at right angles to each other.

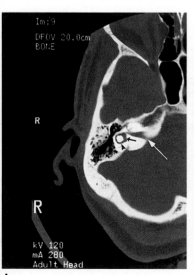
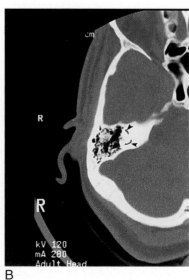

Figure 22-4. CT scans of the human temporal bone. The horizontal (**A**, *arrowhead*) and anterior and posterior (**B**, *arrowheads*) semicircular canals, utricle (**A**, *small arrow*), and internal acoustic canal (**A**, *large arrow*) are visible.

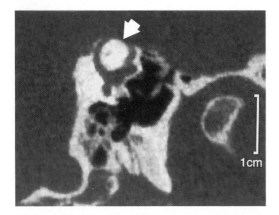

Figure 22-5. CT scan of the temporal bone projected into the plane of the left superior canal in a patient with superior canal dehiscence syndrome. The patient developed vertigo, oscillopsia, and eye movements in the plane of the left superior canal in response to loud noises and pressure in the left ear. A dehiscence is noted overlying the left superior canal *(arrowhead)*.

There are two types of hair cells, and they differ in their pattern of innervation by fibers of the eighth cranial nerve (Fig. 22-6A). Type I hair cells are chalice shaped and typically are surrounded by an afferent terminal that forms a *nerve calyx*. Type II hair cells are cylindrical and are innervated by simple synaptic boutons. Excitatory amino acids such as aspartate and glutamate are the neurotransmitters at the receptor cell–afferent fiber synapses. Both types of hair cells, or their afferents, receive synapses from *vestibular efferent fibers* that control the sensitivity of the receptor. These efferent fibers contain acetylcholine and calcitonin gene–related peptide (CGRP) as neurotransmitters. Efferent cell bodies are located in the brainstem just rostral to the vestibular nuclei and lateral to the abducens nucleus. They are activated by behaviorally arousing stimuli or by trigeminal stimulation.

Within each ampulla, the hair cells and their supporting cells lie embedded in a saddle-shaped neuroepithelial ridge, the *crista*, which extends across the base of the ampulla (Fig. 22-6B). Type I hair cells are concentrated in central regions of the crista, and type II hair cells are more numerous in peripheral areas. Arising from the crista and completely enveloping the stereocilia of the hair cells is a gelatinous structure, the *cupula*. The cupula attaches to the roof and walls of the ampulla, forming a fluid-tight partition that has the same specific density as that of endolymph. Rotational head movements produce angular accelerations that cause the endolymph in the membranous ducts to be displaced, so that the cupula is pushed to one side or the other like the skin of a drum. These cupular movements displace the stereocilia (and kinocilium) of the hair cells in the same direction.

For the otolith organs, a structure analogous to the crista, the *macula*, contains the receptor hair cells (Fig. 22-6C). The hair cell stereocilia of otolith organs extend into a gelatinous coating called the *otolith membrane*, which is covered by calcium carbonate crystals called *otoconia* (from the Greek, meaning "ear stones"). Otoconia are about three times as dense as the surrounding endolymph, and they are not displaced by normal endolymph movements. Instead, changes in head position relative to gravity, or linear accelerations (forward-backward, upward-downward), produce displacements of the otoconia, resulting in bending of the underlying hair cell stereocilia.

Hair Cell Transduction

The response of hair cells to deflection of their stereocilia is highly polarized (Figs. 22-7 and 22-8A). Movements of the stereocilia *toward the kinocilium* cause the hair cell membranes to *depolarize*, which results in an increased rate of firing in the

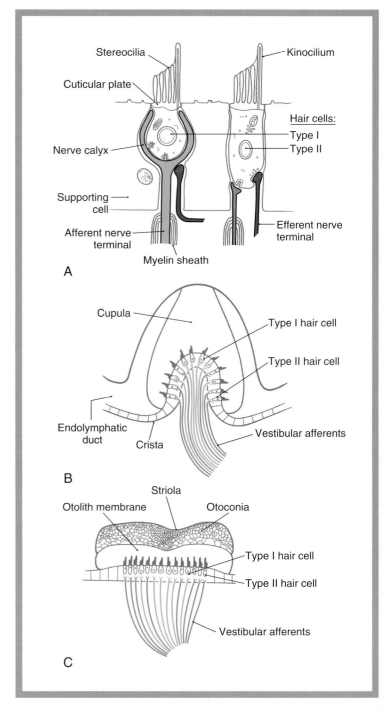

Figure 22-6. The receptor cells (**A**, type I and type II hair cells) of the vestibular system. The relation of these cells to the crista and cupula (**B**) in the ampullae and to the macula and otolith membrane (**C**) of the otolith organs is shown.

vestibular afferent fibers. If the stereocilia are *deflected away from the kinocilium*, however, the hair cell is *hyperpolarized* and the afferent firing rate decreases.

The mechanisms underlying the depolarization and hyperpolarization of vestibular hair cells depend, respectively, on the potassium-rich character of endolymph and the potassium-poor character of the perilymph that bathes the basal and lateral portions of the hair cells. Deflection of the stereocilia *toward* the kinocilium causes potassium channels in the apical portions of the stereocilia to open. K^+ flows into the cell from the endolymph, depolarizing the cell membrane (Fig. 22-7). This depolarization in turn causes voltage-gated calcium channels at the base of the hair cells to open, allowing Ca^{2+} to enter the cell. The influx of Ca^{2+} causes synaptic vesicles to release their transmitter (aspartate or glutamate) into the synaptic clefts,

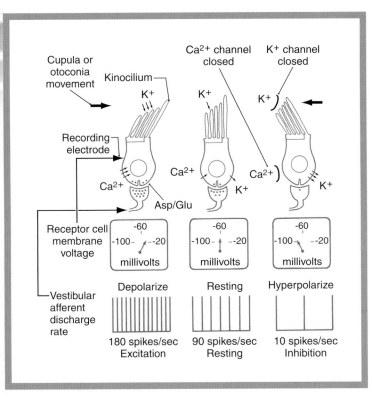

Figure 22-7. Physiologic responses of vestibular hair cells and their vestibular afferent fibers. Asp, aspartate; Glu, glutamate.

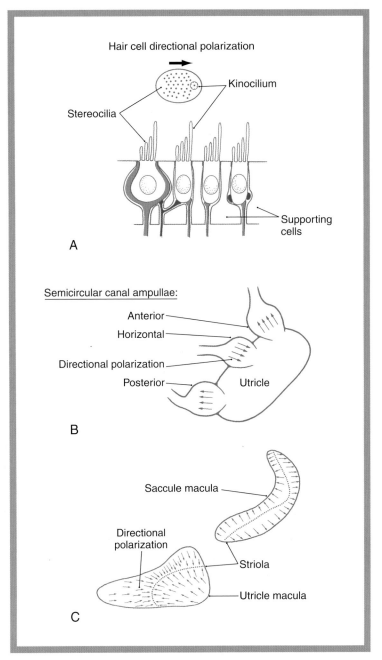

Figure 22-8. Morphologic polarization of vestibular receptor cells showing polarity of stereocilia and kinocilia (**A**), and the orientation of receptors in the ampullae (**B**) and maculae (**C**).

and the afferent fibers respond by undergoing depolarization and increasing their rate of firing. When the stimulus subsides, the stereocilia and kinocilium return to their resting position, allowing most calcium channels to close and voltage-gated potassium channels at the base of the cell to open. K⁺ efflux returns the hair cell membrane to its resting potential (Fig. 22-7).

Deflection of the stereocilia *away* from the kinocilium causes potassium channels in the basolateral portions of the hair cell to open, allowing K⁺ to flow out from the cell into the interstitial space. The resulting hyperpolarization of the cell membrane decreases the rate at which the neurotransmitter is released by the hair cells and, consequently, decreases the firing rate of afferent fibers.

Almost all vestibular primary afferent fibers have a moderate spontaneous firing rate at rest (approximately 90 spikes per second). Therefore, it is likely that some hair cell calcium channels are open at all times, causing a slow, constant release of neurotransmitter. The ototoxic effects of some aminoglycoside antibiotics (e.g., streptomycin, gentamicin) may be due to direct reduction of the transduction currents of hair cells.

Morphologic Polarization of Hair Cells

Given that deflections of the stereocilia toward and away from the kinocilium cause opposing physiologic responses, it is clear that the directional orientation of the hair cells in the vestibular organs will play an essential role in signaling the direction of movement. On the cristae of the horizontal semicircular canal, the hair cells are all arranged with their kinocilium on the side closer to the utricle (Fig. 22-8B). Thus, *movement of endolymph toward the ampulla in the horizontal canal* causes the stereocilia to be deflected toward the kinocilium, resulting in depolarization of the hair cell. In the vertical semicircular canals, the hair cells are arranged with their kinocilia on the side farther from the utricle (closest to the endolymphatic duct). Thus the *hair cells of the vertical canals are hyperpolarized by movement of endolymph toward the ampulla* (ampullipetal movement) and are depolarized by movement away from the ampulla (ampullifugal movement).

In both the utricle and the saccule, the otolith membrane overlying the hair cells contains a small, curving depression, the *striola*, that roughly bisects the underlying macula (Fig. 22-8C). Hair cells on the utricular macula are polarized so that the kinocilium is always on the side toward the striola (Figs. 22-6C and 22-8C), which effectively splits the receptors into two morphologically opposed groups. In contrast, the kinocilia of saccular hair cells are oriented on the side away from the striola. Because the striola curves through the macula, otolith hair cells are polarized in *many different directions* (Fig. 22-8C). In this way, utricular and saccular hair cells are directionally sensitive to a wide variety of head positions and linear movements.

Semicircular Canals and Otolith Organs

As stated previously, the vestibular receptors transduce *movement and position* stimuli into neural signals that are sent to the brain. The *semicircular canals are responsive to rotational acceleration* resulting from turns of the head or body. The *otolith organs are responsive to linear accelerations.* The most prominent linear acceleration on earth is the constant force of gravity. Linear motion, such as experienced during swinging on a swing or flying in an airplane through turbulence, couples with gravity to change the direction and amplitude of the resultant *gravitoinertial acceleration* (GIA). The GIA is sensed by the otolith organs and can be greatly reduced during space flight. Linear accelerations also occur in situations such as up-and-down motion during running or acceleration of an automobile. The otolith organs are also responsive to tilting of the head relative to gravity (pitch and roll movements). Forward and backward tilting is called *pitch;* side-to-side tilting is called *roll.*

Function of Semicircular Canals

The membranous semicircular duct can be thought of as a fluid-filled tube with a partition (the cupula) in the middle (Fig. 22-6B). Because the utricles are located medially, as compared with the horizontal canals, on each side of the head, the hair cells of the complementary left and right semicircular canals are *oppositely polarized.* An example is seen in rotational head movements made in the horizontal plane (Fig. 22-9). When the head is stationary (no angular acceleration), the endolymph and the cupula remain still and the afferents from the two horizontal semicircular canals fire at the same (resting) rate (Fig. 22-9A). When the head turns to the right or left, however, the horizontal semicircular ducts turn with it, but the endolymph lags owing to inertial forces and the viscous drag between the fluid and the duct wall. The lagging endolymph deflects the cupula, which in turn deflects the stereocilia of the hair cells. As Figure 22-9B shows, a leftward turn of the head causes the stereocilia in the left horizontal canal ampulla to be deflected toward their kinocilia, resulting in an increase in the discharge rate of the eighth nerve afferents on the left side. Simultaneously, the hair cells in the right horizontal canal ampulla are hyperpolarized, so their afferents show a decreased rate of firing. A rightward head turn produces the opposite pair of responses (Fig. 22-9C).

The left and right semicircular canals of each functional pair (such as the left and right horizontal canals) *always* respond oppositely to any head movement that affects them. This fact leads to the "push-pull" concept of vestibular function, which states *that directional sensitivity to head movement is coded by opposing receptor signals.* Because of commissural connections, neurons in the vestibular nuclei receive information from receptors on both sides of the head. These neurons act as *comparator units* that interpret head rotation on the basis of the relative

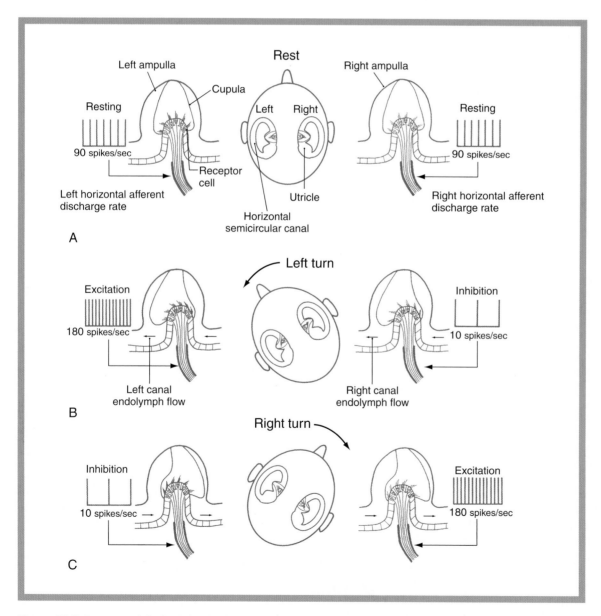

Figure 22-9. Response of the horizontal semicircular canals to head rotations in the horizontal plane. At rest (**A**), the firing rates of horizontal canal afferents are equivalent on both sides. With a leftward head turn (**B**) or a rightward head turn (**C**), there is receptor depolarization and afferent fiber excitation toward the side of the turn and corresponding inhibition on the opposite side.

discharge rates of left and right canal afferents. This pattern of connections also increases the sensitivity of the system, so that even small differences in the discharge rates of afferents from corresponding canal pairs (such as in slow head movements) can be perceived. During a leftward head turn, the comparator units receive impulses at a higher frequency from the left horizontal canal than from the right horizontal canal; the difference is interpreted as a left head turn. Similar conditions exist when the head is pitched or rolled so that the vertical semicircular canals are stimulated by rotational accelerations in their respective planes. However, in the case of the vertical canals, the opposing push-pull responses occur between the anterior semicircular canal in one ear and the posterior semicircular canal of the opposite ear (Fig. 22-3).

Head trauma or disease can change the normal resting activity in eighth nerve afferent fibers. This change may be interpreted by the brain as turning, even though the head is stationary. For example, a lesion of the eighth nerve, such as that produced by a glomus tumor or vestibular schwannoma (Fig. 22-10), may reduce the frequency of impulses in the ipsilateral afferent fibers or block their impulse transmission entirely. The comparator units of the vestibular nuclei will then consistently receive a higher impulse frequency from the intact side, which will be interpreted as a head turn away from the side of the lesion.

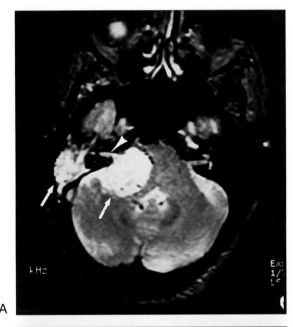

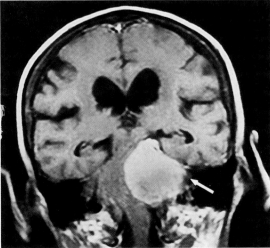

Figure 22-10. MR image of a glomus tumor (**A**, *arrows*) and a vestibular schwannoma (**B**, *arrow*) involving the vestibular nerve *(arrowhead)*. Both patients complained of dizziness, nausea, and spatial disorientation.

Function of Otolith Organs

The receptor hair cells in the maculae do not respond to head rotation but are sensitive to linear acceleration and tilt of the head (Fig. 22-11). When the head is moved with respect to gravity *(rolled or pitched)*, the otoconia crystals are displaced because of their density with respect to the surrounding endolymph. This displacement shifts the underlying gelatinous coating on the maculae and produces stereocilia deflection in the hair cells. As in the responses of semicircular canal hair cells, otolith organ hair cells are either depolarized or hyperpolarized with stereocilia deflection toward or away from the kinocilium, respectively. However, hair cells on the maculae are oriented according to their position relative to the striola (Fig. 22-8). Hair cells on one side of the striola will be depolarized, and hair cells on the other side of the striola will be hyperpolarized (Fig. 22-11). Because the striola is curved, only certain groups of cells will be affected by a specific direction of head tilt or linear acceleration. Thus, movement is encoded by a macular map of directional space. The eighth nerve fibers maintain the directional signal because each afferent only innervates hair cells from a small region on the macular neuroepithelium.

Vestibular Nuclei

Neural information carried on vestibular afferent fibers is transmitted to the four vestibular nuclei, which lie in the rostral medulla and caudal pons (Fig. 22-12). The *superior vestibular nucleus* lies superolaterally in the central pons and is bordered by the restiform body and the fourth ventricle (Fig. 22-12B). The *medial vestibular nucleus* lies in the lateral floor of the fourth ventricle throughout most of its rostrocaudal extent (Fig. 22-12B-E). The *lateral vestibular nucleus* lies lateral to the medial vestibular nucleus (Fig. 22-12B, C) and contains some large neurons known as Deiters' cells. Located lateral to the medial vestibular nucleus, the *inferior* (or *descending*) vestibular nucleus extends through much of the medulla (Fig. 22-12D-F).

The processing of positional and movement information for control of visual and postural reflexes largely takes place in the vestibular nuclei. Consequently, the major targets for efferents of the vestibular nuclei include the oculomotor nuclei, the vestibulocerebellum, the contralateral vestibular nuclei, the spinal cord, the reticular formation, and the thalamus. Each vestibular nucleus differs in its cytoarchitecture and its afferent and efferent connections.

Vestibular Afferent Inputs

Vestibular primary afferent fibers enter the brainstem at the pontomedullary junction. These fibers traverse the restiform body and then bifurcate into ascending and descending branches. Afferent fibers from the semicircular canals project primarily to the superior and medial vestibular nuclei, although lesser inputs also reach the lateral and inferior vestibular nuclei (Fig. 22-13). The otolith organs project primarily to the lateral, medial, and inferior vestibular nuclei. Saccular afferents also project to cell group Y, which, in turn, excites neurons in the contralateral oculomotor nucleus and influences vertical eye movements.

The termination of vestibular afferent fibers on neurons of the vestibular nuclei is highly ordered. Individual central neurons in the superior and medial vestibular nuclei appear to receive information from otolith receptors and from one semicircular canal pair (either horizontal or vertical). Vestibular neurons in the lateral and inferior nuclei mostly receive information from several canal pairs and otolith receptors. As a result of their inputs, neurons in the vestibular nuclei show directional selectivity for particular head movements and can encode both the angular and linear components of head movements. These cells distribute information about both the direction and speed of

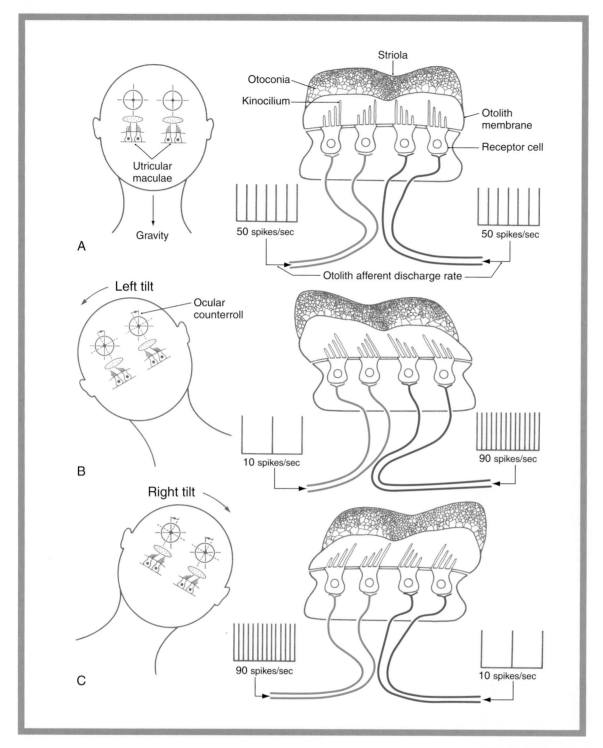

Figure 22-11. Responses of the utricular maculae to tilts of the head. When the head is upright (**A**), the afferent fibers have equivalent firing rates on both sides of the striola *(red and green lines)*. With leftward tilt (**B**) or rightward tilt (**C**), hair cells and their innervating afferents are either excited or inhibited, depending on their position relative to the striola; the weight of the otoconia causes the stereocilia to be deflected. Hair cells on the "upslope" side of the striola increase their firing rate, and those on the "downslope" side decrease their firing rate.

the head movement, as well as the position of the head with respect to gravity, to many different regions of the brain.

Cerebellar Connections
The vestibular labyrinth is the only sensory organ in the body that sends direct primary afferent projections to the cerebellar cortex and nuclei (Fig. 22-13). These *primary vestibulocerebellar* fibers course through the *juxtarestiform body*, the smaller medial part of the inferior cerebellar peduncle. Primary vestibulo-cerebellar fibers send collaterals to the dentate nucleus and terminate as mossy fibers in the nodulus, the uvula, and perhaps the flocculus. Neurons in all four vestibular nuclei also send axons to the cerebellum as *secondary vestibulocerebellar* projections.

These axons end in the flocculonodular lobe, uvula, immediately adjacent portions of the paraflocculus, and the fastigial and dentate nuclei of the cerebellum.

The cerebellum forms reciprocal connections with the vestibular nuclei. This cerebellovestibular projection includes Purkinje cell axons *(cerebellar corticovestibular fibers)* from the nodulus, uvula, flocculus, and other areas of the cerebellar vermis. In addition, projections from the fastigial nucleus *(fastigio-vestibular fibers)* also innervate the vestibular nuclei. Purkinje cells are GABAergic (γ-aminobutyric acid) and therefore inhibitory, whereas the fastigiovestibular fibers use glutamate or aspartate and are excitatory. These *vestibulocerebellar* and *cerebellovestibular* fibers all pass through the juxtarestiform body.

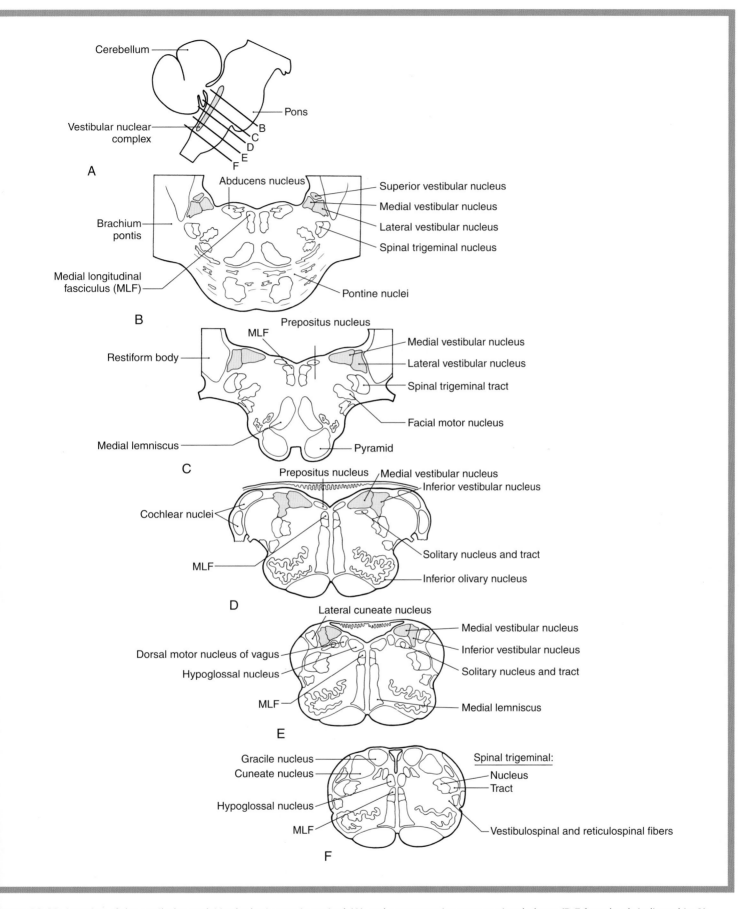

Figure 22-12. Location of the vestibular nuclei in the brainstem in sagittal (**A**) and representative cross-sectional planes (**B-F** from levels indicated in **A**).

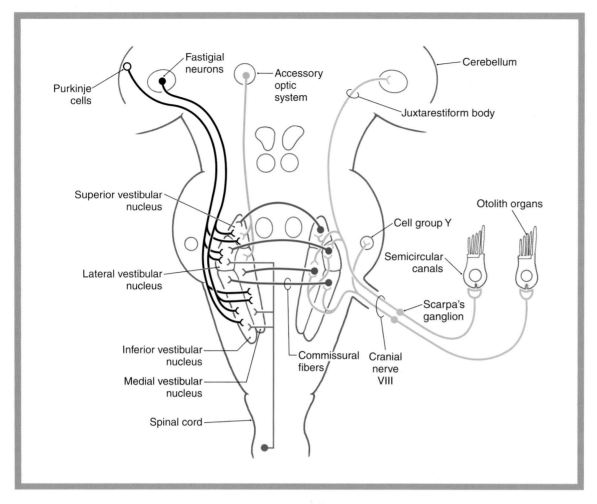

Figure 22-13. Afferents to the vestibular nuclei. Open cell bodies represent inhibitory projections.

The reciprocal connections between the cerebellum and the vestibular nuclei constitute important regulatory mechanisms for the control of eye movements, head movements, and posture.

Commissural Connections
Commissural *vestibulovestibular fibers* arise from all vestibular nuclei, but they appear to be most prominent from the superior and medial nuclei. Many of these fibers form reciprocal connections with the analogous contralateral nucleus. Most vestibulovestibular cells contain the inhibitory neurotransmitter GABA or glycine, although some may use the excitatory amino acids. These commissural fibers provide the pathways by which information from pairs of corresponding semicircular canals and otolith organs can be compared. Commissural fibers also play a major role in *vestibular compensation*, a process by which reflexes and postural control that are impaired as a result of unilateral loss of vestibular receptor function (through trauma or disease) are restored gradually by means of central adjustment.

Other Afferent Connections
Spinovestibular fibers arise from all levels of the spinal cord and provide proprioceptive input primarily to the medial and lateral vestibular nuclei. Information concerning the movement of the head through the visual world also reaches vestibular nuclei neurons through the *accessory optic system* (see Chapter 28). Finally, vestibular nuclear neurons receive input from the reticular formation, primarily from cells relaying information regarding proprioception.

Other Efferent Connections
Vestibular neurons also send efferent projections to the reticular formation, posterior (dorsal) pontine nuclei, and nucleus of the tractus solitarius, or solitary tract. The function of some of these efferent projections remains unknown. However, axons arising from the cells of the medial and inferior vestibular nuclei project to the solitary tract, where it is believed that the vestibular function–mediated changes in breathing and circulation, which occur with changes in posture, are controlled. These compensatory vestibular visceromotor responses serve to stabilize respiration and blood pressure during normal body position changes relative to gravity and during locomotion. They may also be important for induction of motion sickness and emesis.

Vestibulo-ocular Network

It is often necessary to keep one's gaze fixed on an object of interest while the head is moving—as in reading a sign on a building while walking down the street. The vestibular system provides this capability by eliciting compensatory eye movements through a network of neural connections. These stabilizing eye movements, collectively known as the *vestibulo-ocular reflex*, are said to be *compensatory* because they are equal in magnitude and opposite in direction to the head movement perceived by the vestibular system. The vestibulo-ocular reflex occurs for any direction or speed of head movement, whether the movement is rotational, linear, or a combination of both. The reflex can also be suppressed at will if, for example, one wishes to focus on a moving target while turning the head in the same direction (as when watching an airplane or baseball move across the sky).

Rotational Vestibulo-ocular Reflex
There are three types of rotationally induced eye movements: *horizontal*, *vertical*, and *torsional*. Each of the six pairs of eye

muscles (see Chapter 28) must be controlled in unison to produce the appropriate response. Thus, the vertical semicircular canals and the saccule are responsible for controlling vertical eye movements, whereas the horizontal canals and the utricle control horizontal eye movements. Torsional eye movements are controlled by the vertical semicircular canals and the utricle.

For purposes of example, only the horizontal vestibulo-ocular reflex is described here (Fig. 22-14). Primary afferents from the horizontal semicircular canals project to specific neurons in the medial and lateral vestibular nuclei. Most of these cells send excitatory signals through the *medial longitudinal fasciculus* to the *contralateral abducens nucleus.* Abducens motor neurons send impulses via the sixth cranial nerve to excite the *ipsilateral lateral rectus muscle.* At the same time, abducens interneurons send excitatory signals to motor neurons in the *contralateral oculomotor nucleus,* which innervates the *medial rectus muscle.* A second population of vestibular neurons sends excitatory signals to the medial rectus subdivision of the ipsilateral oculomotor nucleus. A third group of vestibular neurons carry inhibitory signals to the ipsilateral abducens nucleus.

During a *leftward head turn,* excitatory signals from the left horizontal semicircular canal afferents increase the firing rate of neurons in the left vestibular nuclei neurons (Fig. 22-14). At the same time, inhibitory signals from the right vestibular nuclei are decreased via commissural neurons. Neurons in the left vestibular nuclei then excite both the contralateral abducens motor neurons and interneurons, which, in turn, produce contraction in the right lateral rectus and the left medial rectus muscle (Fig. 22-14). The resulting *rightward eye movement* keeps the object of interest on the fovea. Through matching bilateral connections, the left lateral rectus and right medial rectus eye muscles are inhibited.

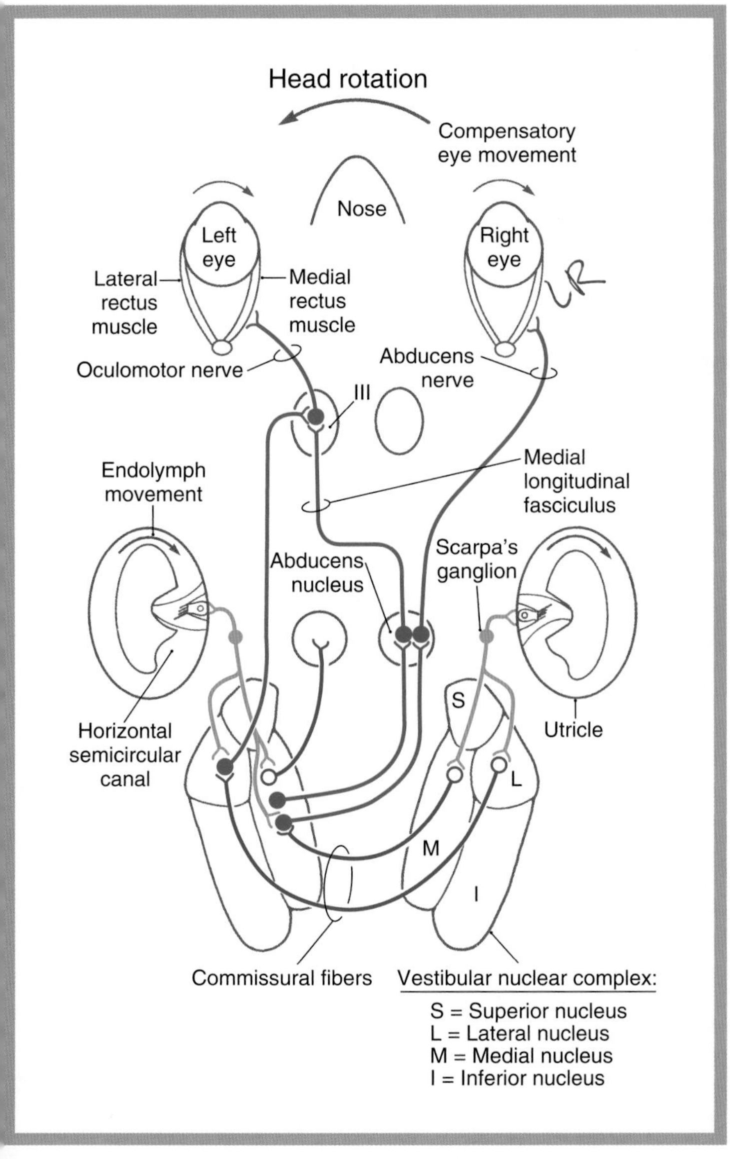

A similar pattern of connections links the vertical semicircular canals with the motor neurons in the trochlear and oculomotor nuclei to control vertical and torsional responses (see also Chapter 28). The vertical vestibulo-ocular reflex originates primarily from neurons in the superior vestibular nucleus, although some medial vestibular nucleus neurons also participate.

Linear Vestibulo-ocular Reflex

During linear movements that do not involve head rotation, an appropriate vestibulo-ocular reflex also occurs. These reflexes depend on input from the otolith organ receptors and involve connections to the extraocular motor neuron pools that are similar to those described previously for the rotational vestibulo-ocular reflex. For example, side-to-side head movements result in a horizontal eye movement in a direction opposite to the head movement. Vertical displacements of the body, such as occur during walking or running, elicit oppositely directed vertical eye movements to stabilize gaze. During roll tilts of the head, the compensatory eye movement is termed a *counter roll* and is actually a torsional eye movement (Fig. 22-11).

Nystagmus

With large head rotations, such as with a 360-degree body turn, compensatory eye movements take another form (Fig. 22-15). Initially, the vestibulo-ocular reflex directs the eyes slowly in the direction opposite to the head motion. This movement is called the *slow phase.* When the eye reaches the limit of how far it can turn in the orbit, it springs back rapidly to a central

Figure 22-14. The connections subserving the horizontal vestibulo-ocular reflex. Open cell bodies represent inhibitory projections. III, oculomotor nucleus.

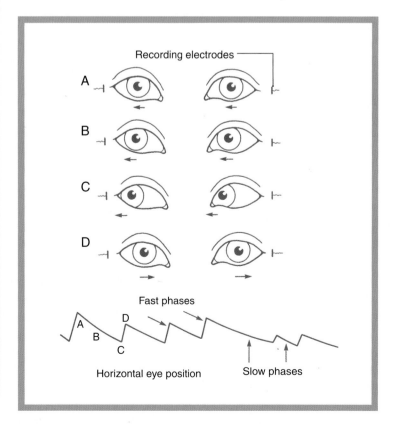

Figure 22-15. Vestibular nystagmus in the horizontal plane showing slow phase (**A-C**) and fast phase (**D**) eye movements.

position, moving in the same direction as that of the head, also known as the *fast phase*. Another slow phase then begins. This combination of slow compensatory phases punctuated by fast return phases is called *nystagmus*. Nystagmus movements are named for the direction of the fast return phase, for example, as leftward-beating nystagmus or downward-beating nystagmus. Nystagmus takes many forms and is often observed clinically (see also Chapter 28). In cases of head injury with acute temporal bone fracture, the semicircular canals can be affected, producing rapid spontaneous nystagmus that can persist for hours or days.

Nystagmus can be used as a diagnostic indicator of vestibular system integrity. Typically, in patients complaining of dizziness or vertigo, the function of the vestibular labyrinth is assessed by administering a *caloric test*. Either warm (40°C) or cold (30°C) water is introduced into the external auditory canal. In normal persons, warm water induces nystagmus that beats toward the ear into which the water has been introduced, whereas cold water induces nystagmus that beats away from the ear into which the water has been introduced. (This relationship is encapsulated in the mnemonic COWS: Cold water produces nystagmus beating to the Opposite side; Warm water produces nystagmus beating to the Same side.) In normal persons, the two ears give equal responses. If there is a unilateral lesion in the vestibular pathway, however, nystagmus will be reduced or absent on the side of the lesion.

Vestibulospinal Network

The vestibular system influences muscle tone and produces reflexive postural adjustments of the head and body through two major descending pathways to the spinal cord, the *lateral vestibulospinal tract* and the *medial vestibulospinal tract* (Fig. 22-16). There is also a *reticulospinal pathway* that receives input from the vestibular system.

Lateral Vestibulospinal Tract

The lateral vestibulospinal tract (LVST) arises primarily from neurons in the lateral and inferior vestibular nuclei and projects to all levels of the ipsilateral spinal cord. This projection is topographically organized. Cells in anterorostral areas of the lateral nucleus project to the cervical cord, while cells in posterocaudal regions project to the lumbosacral cord. These vestibulospinal neurons receive substantial input from orthogonal semicircular canal pairs, the otolith organs, the vestibulocerebellum, and the fastigial nucleus, as well as proprioceptive inputs from the spinal cord.

Fibers of the LVST course through the lateral medulla dorsal to the inferior olivary complex, and then through the anterior funiculus of the cord (Fig. 22-16) to terminate directly on alpha and gamma motor neurons and on interneurons in lamina VII to IX. Axons of many LVST neurons give off collaterals in different

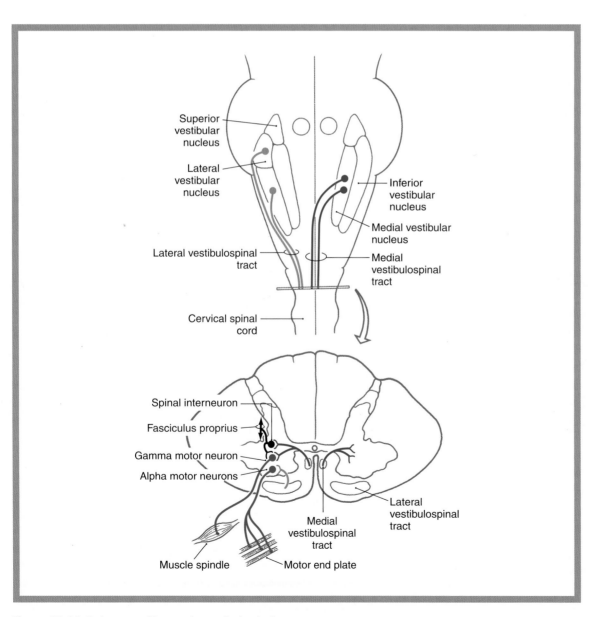

Figure 22-16. Pathways making up the vestibulospinal system.

segments of the cord, thus ensuring that different muscle groups will be coordinated during postural control. The LVST neurons contain either acetylcholine or glutamate as a neurotransmitter and exert an excitatory influence on extensor muscle motor neurons. The coordinated actions of neurons that make up the LVST and provide postural stabilization are not completely understood. However, if a person begins tilting to the right, ipsilateral LVST fibers elicit extension of the left axial and limb musculature. Concurrently, right extensor muscles are inhibited. These actions stabilize the body's center of gravity and preserve upright posture.

Medial Vestibulospinal Tract

The action of vestibular stimulation on neck muscles arises primarily through neurons in the medial vestibulospinal tract (MVST). These fibers originate primarily from the medial vestibular nucleus, although lesser projections arise from the inferior and lateral vestibular nuclei. Similar to LVST neurons, cells of the MVST receive input from vestibular receptors and the cerebellum, as well as somatosensory information from the spinal cord. Fibers of the MVST descend bilaterally through the medial longitudinal fasciculus to terminate in laminae VII to IX of the cervical spinal cord (Fig. 22-16). These MVST fibers carry both excitatory and inhibitory signals, and they terminate on neck flexor and extensor motor neurons, as well as on propriospinal neurons.

The effects of vestibular function–induced responses can be seen in the *vestibulocolic* reflex, which is actually a series of responses that stabilize the head in space. If, for example, a person falls forward, MVST neurons will receive signals on downward linear acceleration from the saccule, signals on the changing head position relative to gravity from both the utricle and the saccule, and signals on forward rotational acceleration from the vertical semicircular canals. The MVST neurons process this information and transmit excitatory signals to the dorsal neck flexor muscles (splenius, biventer cervicis, and complexus muscles). At the same time, inhibitory signals are sent to the anterior neck extensor muscles. The result is a neck movement upward, opposite to the falling motion, to protect the head from impact.

Vestibulo-Thalamo-Cortical Network

Vestibular Thalamus

The cognitive perceptions of motion and spatial orientation arise through the convergence of information from the vestibular, visual, and somatosensory systems at the thalamocortical level. Neurons in the superior, lateral, and inferior vestibular nuclei project bilaterally to two thalamic areas (Fig. 22-17). The first is located in the *ventral posterolateral (VPL) nucleus and includes adjacent cells in the ventral posteroinferior (VPI) nucleus*. The second is the *posterior nuclear group*, located near the medial geniculate body. In humans, electrical stimulation of these areas produces sensations of movement and dizziness. Thalamic VPL and posterior nucleus neurons constitute separate, parallel pathways transmitting vestibular information from the brainstem to the cortex, because their connections with cortical areas are distinct. In addition, vestibular signals indirectly project to the *anterior thalamic nuclei*, where cells respond only when facing a preferred heading direction. These neurons are thought to be involved in spatial navigation and loose their directional selectivity with vestibular ablation.

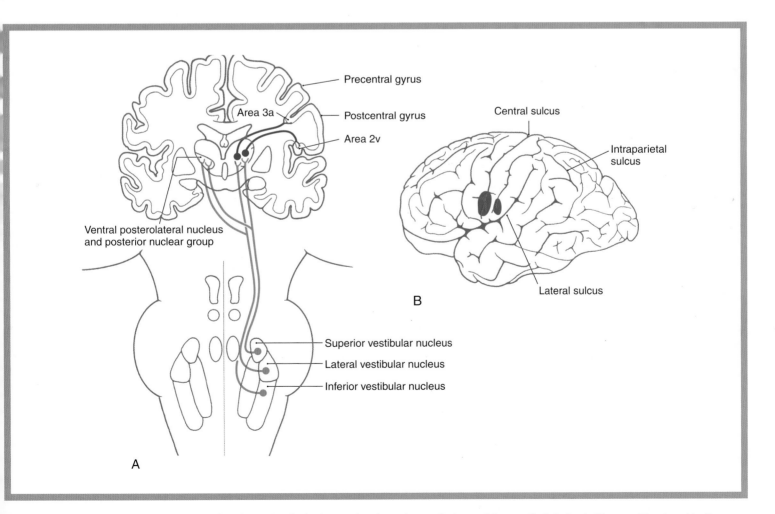

Figure 22-17. The vestibulo-thalamo-cortical pathway. Vestibular input arises from the vestibular nuclei as vestibulothalamic fibers and is relayed to the cortex as thalamocortical fibers (**A**). Areas 3a and 2v (**B**) are the main cortical regions that receive this input.

Vestibular Cortex

Two cortical areas respond to vestibular stimulation (Fig. 22-17). One region, *area 2v*, lies at the base of the intraparietal sulcus just posterior to the hand and mouth representations in the postcentral gyrus. Electrical stimulation of this area in humans produces sensations of moving, spinning, or dizziness. Area 2v neurons respond to head movements and receive projections from the posterior thalamic nucleus. These 2v cells also receive visual and proprioceptive inputs. Area 2v is probably involved with motion perception and spatial orientation, because it has reciprocal connections with other parietal regions involved in similar functions (e.g., areas 5 and 7). Lesions of parietal cortical areas result in confusions in spatial awareness.

The second cortical area responding to vestibular stimulation, *area 3a*, lies at the base of the central sulcus, adjacent to the motor cortex (Fig. 22-17) and receives input from VPL or VPI thalamic nuclear neurons. In addition, area 3a cells receive inputs from the somatosensory system. Because these cells project to area 4 of the motor cortex, it is believed that one of their functions is to integrate motor control of the head and body.

Dizziness and Vertigo

Dizziness is a *nonspecific* term that generally means a spatial disorientation that may or may not involve feelings of movement. Dizziness may be accompanied by nausea or postural instability. A large number of factors may produce a dizzy sensation, and many are not exclusively vestibular in origin.

Vertigo is a *specific* perception of body motion, often spinning or turning, experienced when no real motion is taking place. As children, we all learn to produce vertigo by whirling in place as fast as possible and then abruptly stopping. For a few moments, the world seems to be spinning in the opposite direction.

Examination of the eyes during this phase will reveal a nystagmus that beats in the direction opposite to the original direction of rotation. Vertigo can also be elicited optokinetically if the visual surroundings are revolved while the body remains stationary. Many modern amusement games take advantage of this phenomenon to produce the sensation of motion.

Benign Paroxysmal Positional Vertigo

One of the most common vestibular disorders observed clinically is *benign paroxysmal positional vertigo*. This condition is characterized by brief episodes of vertigo that coincide with particular changes in body position. Typically, episodes may be triggered by turning over in bed, getting up in the morning, bending over, or rising from a bent position. The pathophysiology of benign positional vertigo is not clearly understood, but posterior canal abnormalities are implicated. One possible explanation is that otoconial crystals from the utricle separate from the otolith membrane and become lodged in the cupula of the posterior canal (a condition called *cupulolithiasis*). The resulting increased density of the cupula produces abnormal cupula deflections when the head changes position relative to gravity.

Vestibular Neuritis

Often patients present with severe vertigo, nausea, and vomiting, yet have no accompanying hearing loss or other central nervous system abnormalities. In many of these cases, *vestibular neuritis* is diagnosed and is thought to involve edema of the vestibular nerve (or ganglion). The edema is most commonly believed to be produced through an acute viral infection, such as herpes simplex virus. In fact, some patients report a recent history of upper respiratory tract infection, cold, or flu. Treatment options include antiemetics, vestibular suppressants, corticosteroids to reduce inflammation, and antiviral agents.

Synopsis of Clinical Points

- Damage to the petrous portion of the temporal bone may result in vestibular deficits (pp. 351–353).
- Disturbances in the ionic content of endolymph may result in symptoms indicating vestibular dysfunction (p. 357).
- Occlusion of the labyrinthine artery may result in vertigo, oscillopsia, nystagmus, or unstable gait (p. 352).
- Changes in the volume of endolymph may result in Ménière disease (p. 352).
- A patient with Ménière disease may experience vertigo, nausea, nystagmus, vomiting, tinnitus, difficulty maintaining balance, or various combinations of these signs/symptoms (pp. 352, 353).
- Head trauma may result in symptoms indicating damage to the vestibulocochlear nerve and/or the vestibular structures in the petrous bone (pp. 351–353).
- Vestibulocochlear deficits, and deficits indicative of potential damage to the facial nerve, may be seen in a patient with a vestibular schwannoma (p. 357).
- The cerebellum has significant interconnections with vestibular structures; cerebellar lesions may result in signs/symptoms indicating damage to these pathways (p. 358).
- Nystagmus is an indicator of vestibular system dysfunction (p. 361).
- Nystagmus is named according to the direction of fast return phase (p. 362).
- The caloric test is used to determine the integrity of the vestibular system (p. 362).
- The vestibular system influences posture and muscle tone via vestibulospinal fibers (p. 362).
- Dizziness is a perception of spatial disorientation that may be accompanied by nausea and ataxia (p. 364).
- Vertigo is a perception of spinning or turning when no actual movement is taking place (p. 364).
- Benign paroxysmal positional vertigo is an intermittent, or brief, episode of vertigo that may result from a change in body position (p. 364).
- A patient with severe vertigo, nausea, and vomiting but with no hearing loss or other central nervous system lesions may be suffering vestibular neuritis (p. 364).
- Vestibular neuritis may result from an acute viral infection (p. 364).

Sources and Additional Readings

Angelaki DE, Shaikh AG, Green AM, Dickman JD: Neurons compute internal models of the physical laws of motion. Nature 430:560-564, 2004.

Baloh RW, Halmagyi GM: Disorders of the Vestibular System. New York, Oxford University Press, 1996.

Baloh RW, Honrubia V: Clinical Neurophysiology of the Vestibular System. Philadelphia, FA Davis, 1990.

Beitz AJ, Anderson JH: Neurochemistry of the Vestibular System. New York, CRC Press, 2000.

Dickman JD, Byer M, Hess BJ: Three-dimensional organization of vestibular related eye movements to rotational motion in pigeons. Vision Res 40:2831-2844, 2000.

Goldberg JM: The vestibular end organs: Morphological and physiological diversity of afferents. Curr Opin Neurobiol 1:229-235, 1991.

Highstein SM, Cohen B, Buttner-Ennever JA: New directions in vestibular research. Ann NY Acad Sci 781:1-739, 1996.

Highstein SM, McCrea RA: The anatomy of the vestibular nuclei. In Buttner-Ennever JA (ed): Reviews of Oculomotor Research, Vol 2, Neuroanatomy of the Oculomotor System. Amsterdam, Elsevier, 1988.

Hudspeth AJ: How the ear's works work. Nature 341:397-404, 1989.

Minor LB, Solomon D, Zinreich JS, Zee DS: Sound- and/or pressure-induced vertigo due to bone dehiscence of the superior semicircular canal. Arch Otolaryngol Head Neck Surg 124:249-258, 1998.

Wilson VJ, McIvill Jones G: Mammalian Vestibular Physiology. New York, Plenum Press, 1979.

Yates BJ, Miller AD: Vestibular Autonomic Regulation. New York, CRC Press, 1996.

Olfaction and Taste

K. L. Simpson and R. D. Sweazey

The olfactory and taste systems sample the rich chemical environment that surrounds us. Information provided by these systems is intimately associated with the enjoyment of foods and beverages. When we refer to the taste of food, what we mean is a complex sensory experience correctly called *flavor*. Flavor perception results from a combination of the olfactory, taste, and somatosensory cues present in foods and beverages. *Olfaction* is the sensation of odors that results from the detection of odorous substances aerosolized in the environment. In contrast, taste *(gustation)* is the sensation evoked by stimulation of taste receptors located in the oropharyngeal cavity. The somatosensory system contributes to the experience of flavor by detecting irritating components in smells like ammonia or the "hot" in spicy food like peppers. In general, this is made possible by the activation of somatosensory endings by strong "aversive" chemical substances. Somatosensory cues include thermal, tactile, and the common chemical sense, and this information is relayed to the brain by branches of the trigeminal nerve that innervate oral and nasal mucosa.

Overview

For many mammals, smell is the principal means by which information about the environment is received. *Macrosmatic* animals have a well-developed sense of smell on which they rely for recognizing food, detecting predators and prey, and locating potential mates. In animals such as humans that are less dependent on smell *(microsmatic* animals), the olfactory system is less well developed. However, humans are still able to distinguish thousands of odors, many at extremely low concentrations. Through connections with cortical and limbic structures, the olfactory system plays a role in the pleasures associated with eating and with the many scents that make up our world.

In contrast to olfaction, the taste system exhibits a limited range of sensations. Traditionally, taste sensations have been divided into *sweet, salty, sour,* and *bitter*. In addition to these four basic tastes, a taste sensation termed *umami*, best exemplified by the taste of monosodium glutamate, may be important for identification of amino acids. Furthermore, recent evidence suggests that taste mechanisms for fats may also exist. Combinations of these different taste qualities account for much of our taste experience. Taste input, which originates from receptors in the oropharyngeal cavity, is important for determining the acceptance or rejection of foods. This information is relayed by neural pathways that underlie various ingestive and digestive functions.

Disorders of olfaction or taste may adversely affect the individual's quality of life. The intimate association between the chemical senses and ingestion means that chemosensory disorders impair the patient's ability to enjoy eating. In addition, these disorders can render the patient unable to detect hazards such as gas leaks or spoiled foods.

Olfactory Receptors

The olfactory bulb lies on the *cribriform plate* of the *ethmoid bone*. In this location it is inferior to medial aspects of the frontal lobe (Fig. 23-1), at the rostral end of the olfactory sulcus (Fig. 23-7), and in the rostral portions of the anterior cranial fossa. Olfactory structures are especially vulnerable to facial trauma, particularly that involving the nasal bones, frontal bone, or concha of the nose.

The receptors responsible for transduction of odor molecules are found in the *olfactory mucosa*. This portion of nasal mucosa is 1 to 2 cm^2 in size and is located in the roof of the nasal cavity on the inferior surface of the cribriform plate and along the nasal septum and medial wall of the superior turbinate (Fig. 23-2).

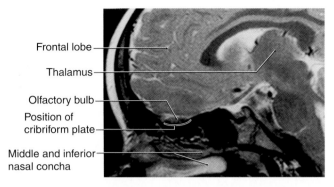

Frontal lobe
Thalamus
Olfactory bulb
Position of cribriform plate
Middle and inferior nasal concha

Figure 23-1. Sagittal MR image of the hemisphere and nasal structures showing the general relationships of the olfactory bulb.

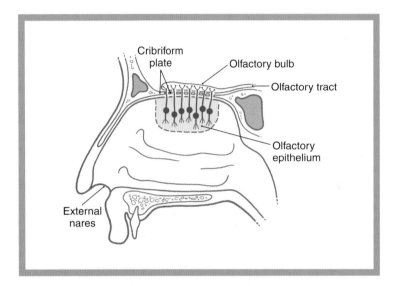

Cribriform plate
Olfactory bulb
Olfactory tract
Olfactory epithelium
External nares

Figure 23-2. Sagittal section through the human nasal cavity showing the relationship of the olfactory epithelium and bulb to the cribriform plate.

The olfactory mucosa is composed of a superficial acellular layer of *mucus* that covers the *olfactory epithelium* and underlying *lamina propria*. The olfactory epithelium is differentiated from the adjacent pinkish respiratory epithelium by its faint yellowish color and greater thickness. In humans the transition between olfactory and respiratory epithelia is gradual.

The olfactory epithelium is pseudostratified and contains three main cell types: *olfactory receptor neurons, supporting cells (sustentacular cells),* and *basal cells* (Fig. 23-3A, B). The small (5 μm) somata of bipolar olfactory receptor neurons are found in the basal two thirds of the epithelium. Each has a single thin apical dendrite and a basally located unmyelinated axon. The apical dendrite extends to the surface of the epithelium, where it terminates in a knob-like *olfactory vesicle* from which 10 to 30 nonmotile *cilia* arise and protrude into the overlying mucus layer (Fig. 23-3C, D). These olfactory cilia contain receptors for odorant molecules.

The unmyelinated axon of an olfactory receptor neuron is about 0.2 μm in diameter, making it one of the smallest in the nervous system. These axons pass through the lamina propria and group together into bundles called *olfactory fila*, which collectively make up the *olfactory nerve* (cranial nerve I) (Fig. 23-3A). The olfactory fila pass through the cribriform plate to terminate in the olfactory bulb.

Olfactory receptor cells are true neurons because they originate embryologically from the central nervous system. Olfactory receptor cells undergo continuous turnover, with an average life span between 30 and 60 days. They are replaced by receptors arising from undifferentiated basal cells by mitotic division

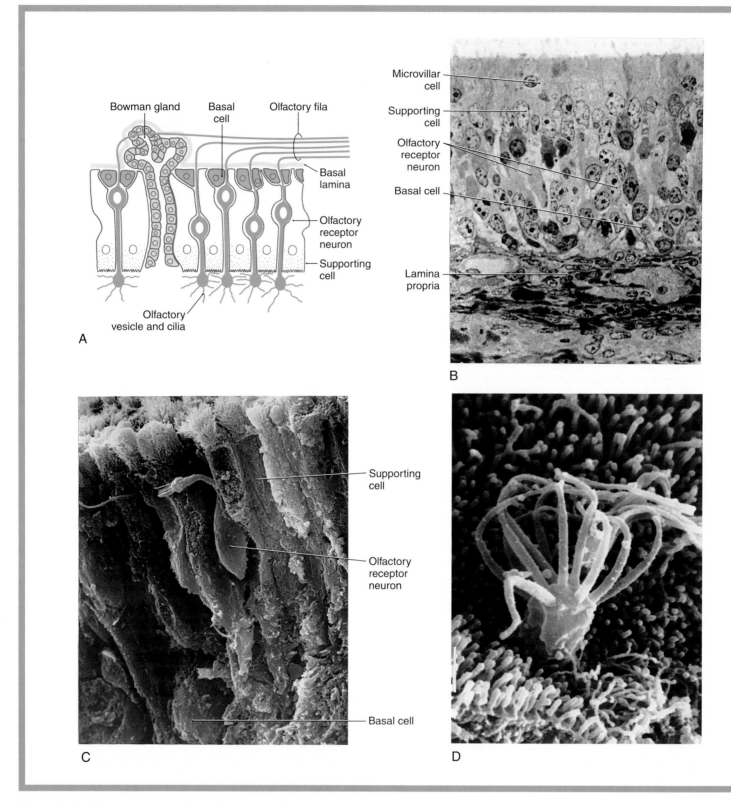

Figure 23-3. Schematic drawing of the olfactory epithelium (**A**). Light micrograph of the human olfactory epithelium and the underlying lamina propria (**B**). Scanning electron micrographs of the human olfactory epithelium showing its characteristic cell types (**C**) and the dendritic knob and cilia of a receptor neuron (**D**). (Photomicrographs courtesy of Dr. Richard M. Costanzo, Virginia Commonwealth University.)

(Fig. 23-3A, C). Thus, basal cells are stem cells that give rise to the receptor cells.

The supporting cells are columnar and extend from the lamina propria to the surface of the epithelium, where they end in short microvilli that extend into the overlying mucus (Fig. 23-3A, C, D). Nuclei of the sustentacular cells are found near the surface of the epithelium. These cells provide mechanical support for the olfactory receptor cells (Fig. 23-3B). In addition, they contribute secretions to the overlying mucus that may play a role in the binding or inactivation of odorant molecules.

A fourth and minor cell type, the *microvillar cell*, is found in the human olfactory epithelium (Fig. 23-3B). These cells have an apical process that projects into the mucus and a basal process that extends to the lamina propria. Although their function is unknown, they may be a second type of receptor neuron.

The lamina propria contains bundles of olfactory axons, blood vessels, fibrous tissue, and numerous *Bowman glands* (Fig. 23-3A). The serous secretions of the Bowman glands, combined with the secretions of the sustentacular cells, provide the mucus covering of the olfactory mucosa.

Olfactory Transduction

Olfactory perception begins when volatile odor molecules are inhaled and contact the mucus layer that bathes the olfactory epithelium. This mucus is an aqueous solution of proteins and electrolytes. Odorants, particularly hydrophobic ones such as musk, cross the mucus by interacting with small, water-soluble proteins called *odorant-binding proteins*. These proteins are ubiquitous in the mucus layer.

After crossing the mucus, odor molecules bind to odorant receptors on the cilia of the olfactory receptor neurons, where transduction occurs (Fig. 23-4). The *odorant receptors* are membrane proteins belonging to a superfamily of G protein–coupled receptors. Binding of the odorant to one of as many as 1000 different types of odorant receptors leads to activation of a second-messenger pathway involving an *olfactory-specific G protein*, which, in turn, activates adenyl cyclase to produce cyclic adenosine monophosphate (cAMP). The transient rise in ciliary cAMP opens a cyclic nucleotide–gated cation channel in the ciliary membrane, allowing cations to flow into the cell (Fig. 23-4). The flow of cations into the cell results in a gradual depolarization (*generator potential*) that travels down the dendrite to the soma of the olfactory receptor neuron. A sufficiently large depolarization initiates an action potential that travels along the axon to the olfactory bulb.

There is also evidence for another intracellular second-messenger pathway in olfactory transduction. This pathway, involving inositol 1,4,5-trisphosphate (IP_3), is thought to act either separately or with the cAMP pathway. In this pathway, binding of odorant to the receptor activates a G protein that, in turn, activates phospholipase C to produce IP_3. The IP_3 opens a channel in the ciliary membrane that permits Ca^{2+} to enter the cell (Fig. 23-4). Current research further supports a role for cyclic guanosine monophosphate and carbon monoxide in olfactory signal transduction.

Studies suggest that olfactory discrimination begins in the olfactory epithelium and that a "receptor map" is utilized to encode complex qualities of a given odor. Receptors, which are tuned to specific structural features of a stimulus, appear not only to be selectively expressed within subsets of the olfactory neuron population but also to exhibit spatial organization. In fact, findings indicate that individual olfactory neurons express only one type of odorant receptor and that specific subtypes of odorant receptors preferentially distribute within one of four bilaterally symmetric zones of the olfactory epithelium. Such specificity permits olfactory information to be patterned for additional processing in the olfactory bulb.

Central Olfactory Pathways

Olfactory Bulb

The olfactory bulb, a forebrain structure, is located on the ventral surface of the frontal lobe in the olfactory sulcus and is attached to the rest of the brain by the *olfactory tract*. The olfactory tract is an inclusive structure that contains fibers of the *lateral olfactory tract*, cells of the *anterior olfactory nucleus*, and fibers of the *anterior limb of the anterior commissure*. The latter part of the olfactory tract is the route through which many centrifugal fibers reach the olfactory bulb (Fig. 23-7).

The olfactory bulb consists of five well-defined layers of cells and fibers, which give it a laminated appearance. From superficial to deep these are the *olfactory nerve layer, glomerular layer, external plexiform layer, mitral cell layer,* and *granule cell layer* (Fig. 23-5).

The afferent projections from the olfactory epithelium form the *olfactory nerve layer* on the surface of the olfactory bulb. These axons terminate exclusively in structures called *olfactory glomeruli*, which are found in the glomerular layer of the bulb (Figs. 23-5 and 23-6). The axon of each olfactory sensory neuron synapses in only one glomerulus. Interestingly, the terminations of these axons are arranged such that neurons expressing the same receptor subtype target the same few glomeruli. This suggests that each glomerulus receives input from only one type of receptor.

Glomeruli are the most prominent feature of the olfactory bulb. The core of an olfactory glomerulus is made up of the axons of olfactory receptor neurons, which branch and synapse on the bushy endings of the *primary dendrites* (apical dendrites) of *mitral* and *tufted* cells (Fig. 23-5). These two cells are functionally similar and together constitute the efferent neurons of the olfactory bulb. Adjacent to the glomerulus are small interneurons (juxtaglomerular cells), of which *periglomerular cells* are the principal type. This cell has short bushy dendrites that arborize extensively within a glomerulus and a short axon that distributes within a radius of about five glomeruli.

There is significant neural convergence at the level of the olfactory glomerulus; thousands of olfactory receptor neurons form excitatory (*glutaminergic, carnosine*) axodendritic synapses on mitral, tufted, and periglomerular cells (Fig. 23-6). The other major synaptic connections within the glomerulus are reciprocal and serial dendrodendritic synapses between mitral or tufted

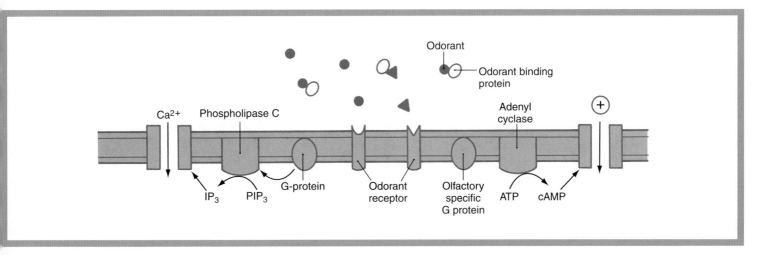

Figure 23-4. Pathways of olfaction transduction. Odorants are transported through the mucus by odorant-binding proteins. Binding of odorants to receptors on the olfactory cilia activates a second-messenger pathway involving either cyclic AMP (cAMP) or inositol 1,4,5-trisphosphate (IP_3). Both pathways lead to the opening of membrane cation channels and depolarization of the olfactory receptor neuron. PIP_3, phosphatidylinositol 4,5-bisphosphate.

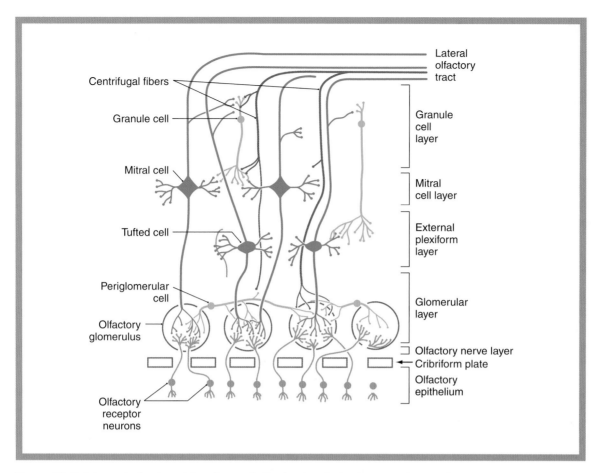

Figure 23-5. Schematic drawing of the olfactory bulb, showing the laminar organization, the major cell types, and the basic neuronal circuitry. Receptor neurons are shown in *blue*, interneurons in *red*, the efferent neurons of the bulb in *green*, and centrifugal fibers in *black*.

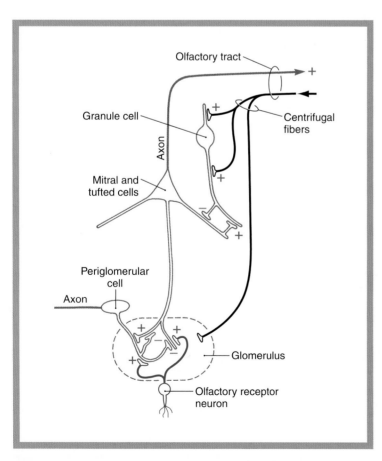

Figure 23-6. Synaptic interaction between the principal cell types of the olfactory epithelium and bulb. Excitatory synapses (+) are shown in *green* and inhibitory ones (−) in *red*. The action of centrifugal axons in the glomerulus is not clearly established.

cells and periglomerular cells. It appears that the synapses of mitral and tufted cells onto periglomerular cells are excitatory (*glutaminergic*), whereas those of periglomerular cells onto mitral and tufted cells are inhibitory (*GABAergic*; GABA, for γ-aminobutyric acid).

The glomerular layer also receives input from other central nervous system areas via *centrifugal afferents* that use a wide variety of neurotransmitters and neuromodulators (Figs. 23-5 and 23-6). *Noradrenergic* centrifugal afferents from the *locus ceruleus* and *serotonergic* fibers from the *raphe nuclei* of the midbrain and rostral pons terminate in the glomeruli. Centrifugal fibers from the ipsilateral *anterior olfactory nucleus* and the *diagonal band* terminate in the periglomerular spaces, primarily on periglomerular cells. Excitatory amino acids, such as *glutamate*, are present in centrifugal fibers that arise in cortical structures.

The *external plexiform layer* is composed of the somata of tufted cells, along with the *primary* and *secondary dendrites* (basal dendrites) of tufted and mitral cells and the apical dendrites of *granule cells* (Fig. 23-5). Within this layer, the apical dendrites of granule cells form reciprocal dendrodendritic GABAergic synapses with the secondary dendrites of tufted and mitral cells. These synapses modulate tufted and mitral cell output through lateral and feedback inhibition. Mitral and tufted cells, in turn, form excitatory (*glutaminergic*) synapses with granule cell dendrites (Fig. 23-6).

The *mitral cell layer* is a thin layer containing the large somata of mitral cells. In addition, the axons of tufted cells, granule cell processes, and centrifugal fibers traverse this layer (Fig. 23-5).

Internal to the mitral cell layer, the *granular cell layer* contains the cell bodies of *granule cells*, the principal interneuron of the olfactory bulb. This layer also contains primary and collateral axons of mitral and tufted cells and centrifugal afferents from the anterior olfactory nucleus, olfactory cortex, cells of the iagonal band, locus ceruleus, and raphe nucleus (Fig. 23-5). Granule cells lack axons, their only output being via dendro-endritic GABAergic synapses with mitral and tufted cells. In addition, granule cells receive numerous synaptic inputs from oth mitral and tufted cell axon collaterals and centrifugal fferent fibers. Granule cells presumably modulate olfactory ulb activity via an inhibitory feedback loop that shuts down the ctivity of the mitral and tufted neurons.

Olfactory Bulb Projections

Axons of mitral and tufted cells emerge from the caudal portion of the olfactory bulb to form the *lateral olfactory tract*. Although *glutamate* is the major neurotransmitter of these efferent fibers, *aspartate*, *dopamine*, and *substance P* also are used. These fibers course caudally to terminate in areas on the ventral surface of the telencephalon, which are broadly defined as the *olfactory cortex* (Fig. 23-7). The principal areas making up the olfactory cortex are the *anterior olfactory nucleus, olfactory tubercle, piriform cortex, anterior cortical amygdaloid nucleus, periamygdaloid*

cortex, and *lateral entorhinal cortex*. The olfactory cortex is an example of *paleocortex*, a phylogenetically older type of cortex that is less complex than the neocortex. Throughout most of its extent, the olfactory cortex has three cell layers, as opposed to the six layers characteristic of neocortex. A unique aspect of the olfactory system is that the olfactory bulb projects directly to the cortex. In other sensory systems, information reaches the cortex after a relay in the thalamus.

Lateral olfactory tract axons send collaterals to the anterior olfactory nucleus, to other areas of olfactory cortex, and to subcortical limbic structures. The major targets of the anterior olfactory nucleus are the olfactory bulbs bilaterally and the contralateral anterior olfactory nucleus (Figs. 23-7 and 23-8). The large numbers of interbulbar connections, via the anterior olfactory nucleus, suggest that interhemispheric processing of odors plays an important role in olfactory functions.

Axons of the lateral olfactory tract course caudally in the form of the *lateral olfactory stria* to terminate in the *olfactory tubercle* and the *piriform cortex* (Fig. 23-7). The piriform cortex is a

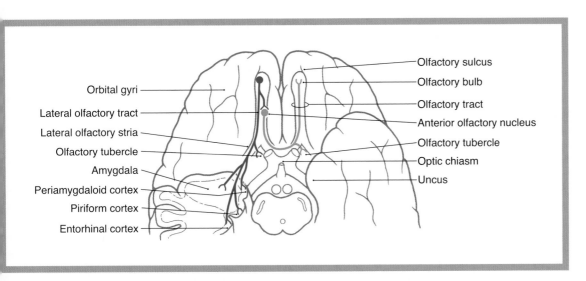

Figure 23-7. Major efferent projections of the olfactory bulb. Direct projections from the olfactory bulb are shown in *blue* and indirect interbulbar connections via the anterior olfactory nucleus are depicted in *red*.

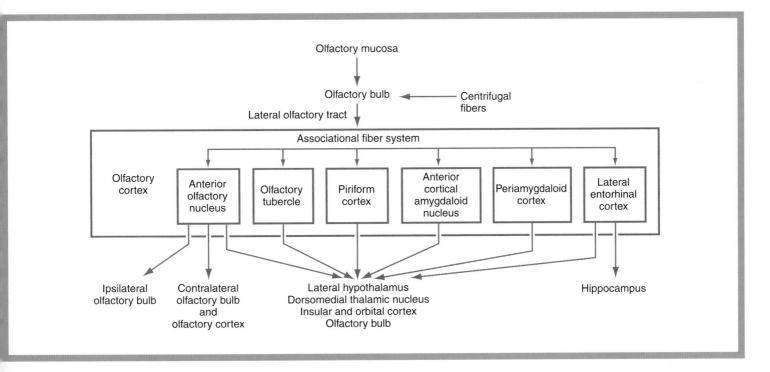

Figure 23-8. Major projections of the olfactory cortex.

major component of the olfactory cortex. Fibers of the lateral olfactory tract also continue posteriorly to terminate in the *anterior cortical amygdaloid nucleus*, the *periamygdaloid cortex* (a part of the piriform cortex overlying the amygdala), and the *lateral entorhinal cortex*.

There is little evidence of a topographic projection from the olfactory bulb onto the various structures constituting the olfactory cortex. Mitral cells project to all areas of the olfactory cortex, whereas tufted cells terminate primarily in its anterior parts. However, each region of olfactory cortex is regarded as receiving input from all areas of the olfactory bulb.

Olfactory Cortex Projections

Cells of the olfactory cortex have reciprocal connections with other regions of the olfactory cortex *(intrinsic or associational connections)* and connections with regions outside the olfactory cortex *(extrinsic connections)* (Fig. 23-8). Most intrinsic connections arise from the anterior olfactory nucleus, piriform cortex, and lateral entorhinal cortex. As a group, these associational fibers distribute to all areas of the olfactory cortex (Fig. 23-8).

Extrinsic connections include extensive projections back to the olfactory bulb. These centrifugal fibers originate from most parts of the olfactory cortex, with the exception of the olfactory tubercle. As in other sensory systems, olfactory information is also relayed to the neocortex. This connection occurs through a direct projection from olfactory cortex to *orbitofrontal* and *ventral agranular insular cortices* or via a relay in the thalamus. The latter pathway originates from cells in the olfactory cortex that project to the *dorsomedial nucleus of the thalamus* (Fig. 23-8). This neocortical representation of olfaction is important for discrimination and identification of odors, and lesions in this area, particularly the orbitofrontal cortex, result in the loss of these capabilities. Another noteworthy point is that the insular and orbitofrontal cortex also receive taste input. The medial orbitofrontal cortex appears to play an especially important role in integrating olfactory, taste, and other food-related cues that produce the experience of flavor.

In addition to neocortical projections, the olfactory cortex also sends fibers directly to the lateral hypothalamus and hippocampus. Those to the lateral hypothalamus arise primarily from the piriform cortex and anterior olfactory nucleus and are probably important for feeding behavior. The projection to the hippocampus arises from the entorhinal cortex and links olfactory input to centers concerned with learning and behavior.

Disorders of the Olfactory System

Disorders of smell are normally classified according to the type of loss experienced by the patient. The loss of smell *(anosmia)* or decreased sensitivity to odorants *(hyposmia* or *olfactory hypesthesia)* is frequently associated with upper respiratory tract infections, sinus disease, and trauma. Nasal and paranasal diseases *(rhinitis, sinusitis)* may block the access of odorants to the olfactory epithelium, but blockage is not the sole cause because even when blockage is absent, olfactory dysfunction may be present. Frequently, treatment with systemic anti-inflammatory drugs results in rapid attenuation of symptoms, suggesting that edema of the olfactory epithelium may be partly responsible for the olfactory dysfunction. In addition, the viruses associated with upper respiratory tract infections may permanently damage the olfactory epithelium. Although the process is not completely understood, it is thought that viral infection of an olfactory receptor cell may lead to cell death.

Head trauma can produce olfactory deficits by damaging central olfactory pathways or olfactory receptor axons as they pass through the cribriform plate. Boxers, for instance, may sustain damage to their olfactory senses as a result of blows to the head

that produce shearing movements of the olfactory bulb relative to the cribriform plate. Transection of the thin axons comprising the olfactory fila may result in a partial or total loss of smell that may persist as a temporary or permanent condition. Fractures along the anterior base of the skull are also commonly observed after head trauma. Dural lacerations may cause drainage of cerebrospinal fluid into the paranasal sinuses and through the nose *(rhinorrhea)*. Involvement of the anterior venous sinuses can further lead to the pooling of blood in the periorbital tissue and produce a characteristic "raccoon" or "panda" bear appearance. The notable lack of subconjunctival hemorrhage can be used to rule out the prospect of direct ocular trauma. In cases of anterior skull base fracture, there is always the threat of olfactory nerve damage as well as the possible complication of meningitis. To reduce the chance of bacterial infection, patients may receive treatment with antibiotics or undergo surgical measures to repair a severe meningeal breach.

Neuroblastomas (malignant) and meningiomas (typically benign) may also compromise olfactory function. Neuroblastoma, a type of primitive neuroectodermal tumor (PNET) deriving from primitive progenitor cells, is rare, occurs in children, and is most frequently localized to the frontoparietal lobe. The olfactory neuroblastoma *(esthesioneuroblastoma)* is believed to originate from olfactory neuroepithelial cells in the nasal cavity and to contribute to nasal obstruction and *epistaxis* (nosebleed) in affected individuals. Olfactory groove meningiomas, however, arise from arachnoid cells along the cribriform plate (see Fig. 7-10). Like medial sphenoid wing and other parasellar meningiomas, these neoplasms may elicit multiple sensory and motor disturbances. In addition to deficits in smell, visual abnormalities may be detected as the tumor compresses the optic nerve and causes blindness, optic atrophy, as well as contralateral papilledema (Foster Kennedy syndrome). Extension of the mass into the cavernous sinus may further produce extraocular palsies and facial numbness.

Olfactory losses are also the result of excessive smoking and prolonged use of cocaine. However, reports also indicate instances whereby healthy individuals with otherwise normal olfactory acuity are unable to perceive the odor of a particular compound or class of compounds. This phenomenon, termed *specific anosmia*, is a condition that may be inherited as an autosomal recessive trait and is likely explained by the absence of a specific odorant receptor. Conversely, increased olfactory acuity *(hyperosmia* or *olfactory hyperesthesia)* has been described in conjunction with migraine and hysteria. Occurrences of hyperosmia have also been found in certain psychotic states and with certain types of substance abuse.

The chief complaint of most patients with chemosensory disturbances is the loss or alteration of taste. However, clinical studies reveal that in all but a small number of patients the dysfunction actually resides in the olfactory system. The reason for this discrepancy is that most people confuse taste with flavor. It is important to remember that when evaluating a patient with a potential olfactory lesion to note whether deficits exist in the individual's ability to perceive, or the ability to recognize a smell. The detection of an odorous substance indicates the integrity of the peripheral nerve and its pathway. Identification of the odor reveals intact cortical function. If the patient is aware of a smell, but he or she cannot recall the name of the scent *(olfactory agnosia)*, the disorder is likely to reside at higher levels of the sensory system. A second relevant point pertains to the fact that olfactory losses may be manifested unilaterally or bilaterally. Unilateral deficiencies are typically observed subsequent to nasal cavity disease or following tumor-associated compression injury of one olfactory bulb/tract. Bilateral anosmia is usually sustained in response to head injury or the common old. However, the absence of smell from either nostril has been noted in advanced cases of olfactory groove meningioma.

Aged-related declines in olfactory function are quite common even in healthy persons. Typically, the loss occurs gradually and the patient often fails to notice these changes. These gradual changes can affect the palatability of foods in the elderly. Olfactory dysfunction is also encountered in neurodegenerative diseases such as Alzheimer and Parkinson disease, or in Huntington chorea. These neurodegenerative diseases involve central olfactory pathways and produce marked reduction in the affected person's olfactory capabilities. Most notably, these olfactory deficits appear very early in the course of the disease and may be among its first manifestations.

Disorders of olfaction are also associated with epilepsy and various depressive and psychiatric disorders such as schizophrenia and Korsakoff psychosis. The patients frequently experience *parosmia (dysosmia)*, a distortion in a smell experience or the perception of a smell when no odor is present *(olfactory hallucination or phantosmia)*. Such episodes, resulting presumably from abnormal sequences of neuronal activity, can be elicited by an irritative lesion of the anterior medial temporal lobe, hippocampus, amygdala, or medial dorsal thalamic nucleus. In the case of epilepsy, focal (partial) seizure activity in the uncal region of the temporal lobe has been found to correlate with the formation of repugnant or disagreeable olfactory auras *(cacosmia)*. This type of attack, known as an uncinate fit, may occur in people who are genetically predisposed to seizure-like discharge, or in individuals who demonstrate tumor growth, a vascular disorder, head trauma, infection, drug usage, or substance withdrawal.

Taste Receptors

The taste experiences of sweet, salty, sour, bitter, and umami result from an interaction between gustatory stimuli and receptor cells located in sensory organs called *taste buds*. Although found throughout the oropharyngeal cavity, taste buds are most obvious on the tongue, where they are ovoid structures with a constriction at their apical end.

Each taste bud contains 40 to 60 *taste receptor cells* that extend from a basal lamina to the surface of the epithelium. The apical ends of these receptor cells are covered with microvilli of variable lengths that extend into a *taste pore*. The pore forms a pocket to permit contact between the microvilli of the taste receptor cells and the external milieu (Figs. 23-9 and 23-10). Numerous junctional complexes located between the apices of receptor cells restrict access of stimuli to the microvilli where taste transduction occurs. The taste pore is filled with a protein-rich substance through which substances must pass to reach the receptor cell microvilli. Taste receptor cells undergo a continuous process of turnover, having a life span of 10 to 14 days. New taste cells are thought to arise from polygonal *basal cells* located in basolateral areas of the taste bud. These cells are not involved in taste transduction.

Afferent fibers penetrate the basement membrane and then branch within the base of the taste bud (Fig. 23-9). Each taste bud is typically innervated by more than one afferent fiber, and an individual fiber may innervate multiple taste buds. The taste afferent fibers form the postsynaptic element of a chemical synapse near the base of the taste receptor cell.

Distribution of Taste Receptors

Lingual Taste Buds

Taste buds are found, in variable numbers, on the human tongue, palate, pharynx, and larynx. On the tongue, taste buds are located exclusively in specialized structures called *papillae*, of

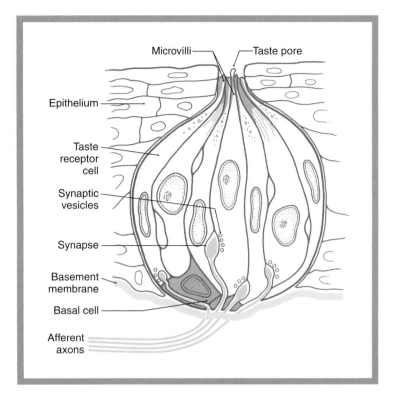

Figure 23-9. The mammalian taste bud and associated structures. (Adapted from Mistretta CM: Anatomy and neurophysiology of the taste system in aged animals. In Murphy C, Cain WS, Hegsted DM [eds]: Nutrition and the Chemical Senses in Aging: Recurrent Advances and Current Research Needs. Ann NY Acad Sci 561:277-290, 1989, with permission.)

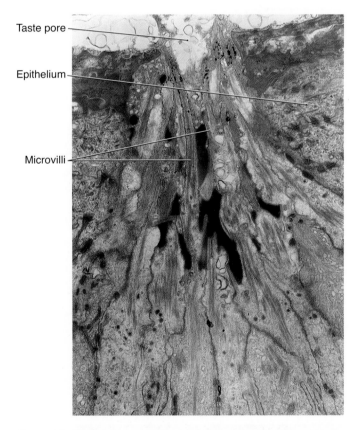

Figure 23-10. Electron micrograph of the pore region of a mouse taste bud in the circumvallate papilla. (Courtesy of Drs. F. Kinnamon and H. Linnen, University of Denver.)

which there are three types (Fig. 23-11A). Taste buds on the anterior two thirds of the tongue reside in mushroom-shaped *fungiform papillae* (Fig. 23-11B). These structures are scattered among the more numerous nongustatory *filiform papillae* distributed over the surface of the tongue. The size, shape, and number of fungiform papillae vary widely, and usually 2 to 4 taste buds are found in the dorsal epithelium of each. The *vallate (circumvallate) papillae* are located on the dorsal surface of the tongue at the junction of the oral and pharyngeal cavities (Fig. 23-11A). There are from 8 to 12 vallate papillae, each of which is composed of a central papilla surrounded by a cleft containing taste buds in its epithelium (Fig. 23-11C). A single

foliate papilla on each side of the tongue appears as a series of clefts along the lateral margin of the tongue (Fig. 23-11A). Each is composed of two to nine clefts, with five being the most common number. Taste buds in foliate papillae are also located in the epithelium that lines the clefts (Fig. 23-11D).

Associated with both the vallate and foliate papillae are the *von Ebner* lingual salivary glands. These glands drain into the base of the clefts and influence their microenvironment. Taste stimulation of vallate and foliate papillae influences the secretions of the von Ebner glands via circuits located in the brainstem.

It was once believed that different regions of the tongue were specialized for the detection of particular taste qualities. It is

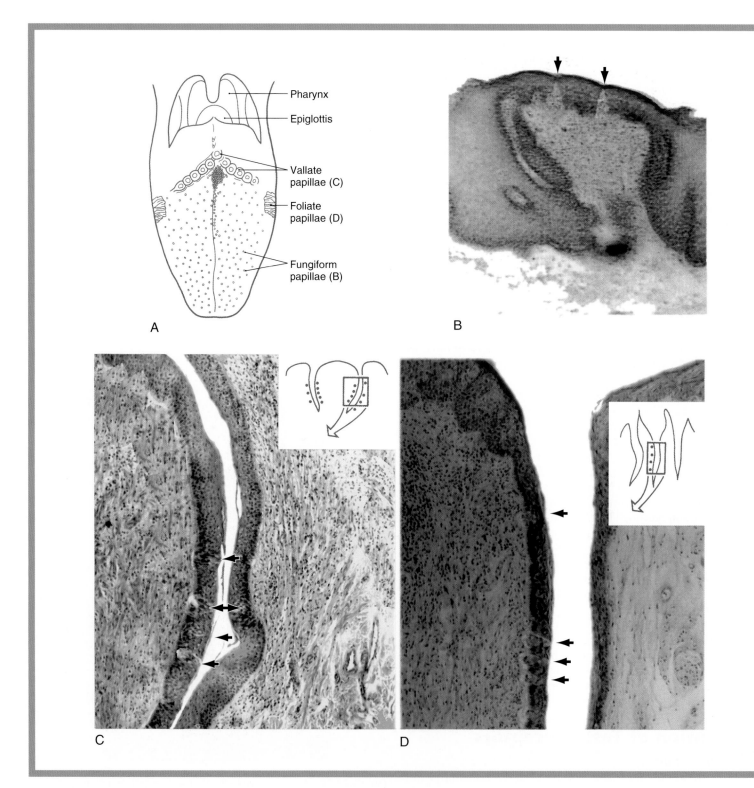

Figure 23-11. Distribution of papillae (**A**), and their associated taste buds, on the human tongue. Light micrographs of transverse sections through human fungiform (**B**), vallate (**C**), and foliate (**D**) papilla. Examples of taste buds are shown at the *arrows*. (Photomicrographs courtesy of Dr. I. J. Miller, Bowman Gray School of Medicine.)

ow known that all taste qualities are detected in all regions of he tongue, although sensitivity to the different taste qualities nd taste transduction mechanisms may vary by tongue region.

Extralingual Taste Buds

Additional taste buds are located on the human soft palate, oral nd laryngeal pharynx, larynx, and upper esophagus. Extralingual aste buds are not located in papillae but rather are situated n the epithelium. Palatal taste buds are located at the juncture of the hard and soft palates and on the soft palate. Laryngeal aste buds are found on the laryngeal surface of the epiglottis nd adjacent aryepiglottic folds. The number of extralingual aste buds is substantial, and they may contribute to the taste xperience. Stimulation of some extralingual taste buds, particularly those near the larynx, elicits brainstem-mediated reflexes hat prevent accidental aspiration of ingested materials.

Taste Transduction

As research has begun to clarify the mechanisms underlying taste ransduction, it has become clear that individual taste qualities or even individual taste compounds utilize several transduction mechanisms. In general, taste transduction is initiated when oluble chemicals diffuse through the contents of the taste pore and interact with receptors located on the exposed apical microvilli of the receptor cells. Several different receptor types have recently been cloned, including a novel variant of the metabotropic glutamate receptor that functions as an umami aste receptor and G protein–coupled receptors that function as bitter receptors. The interaction of the chemical stimulus with the taste cell receptor results in either depolarization or hyperpolarization of the receptor cell microvilli. It is now generally accepted that depolarizing potentials of sufficient magnitude result in action potential generation within the taste receptor cells, which in turn produce an increase in intracellular Ca^{2+}, either by the release of Ca^{2+} from internal stores or by the activation of voltage-gated calcium channels located in the basolateral membrane of the taste receptor cells (Fig. 23-12). This Ca^{2+} release results in a release of chemical transmitters at the afferent synapse, which, in turn, leads to an action potential in the afferent fiber. Although several neurotransmitter candidates have been put forward, the transmitter at the synapses between taste receptor cells and primary afferent fibers remains unknown.

Transduction of stimuli leading to salty and perhaps some sour and bitter tastes appears to be the result of a direct interaction of these tastants with specific ion channels located in the apical membrane of the taste receptor cells. One mechanism for the transduction of sodium salts such as sodium chloride involves movement of Na^+ into the taste receptor cell through apically located amiloride-sensitive cation channels. Similar mechanisms have been proposed for K^+ salts (Fig. 23-12). One pathway responsible for transduction of some sour and bitter stimuli is blockage of apical voltage-sensitive potassium channels. At the resting potential, there is a small outward K^+ current through the apical membranes of taste receptor cells. Protons provided by sour stimuli such as hydrochloric acid block this outward current, causing the cell to depolarize.

At least some sweet, sour, and bitter-tasting compounds are transduced by receptors that activate intracellular G protein–

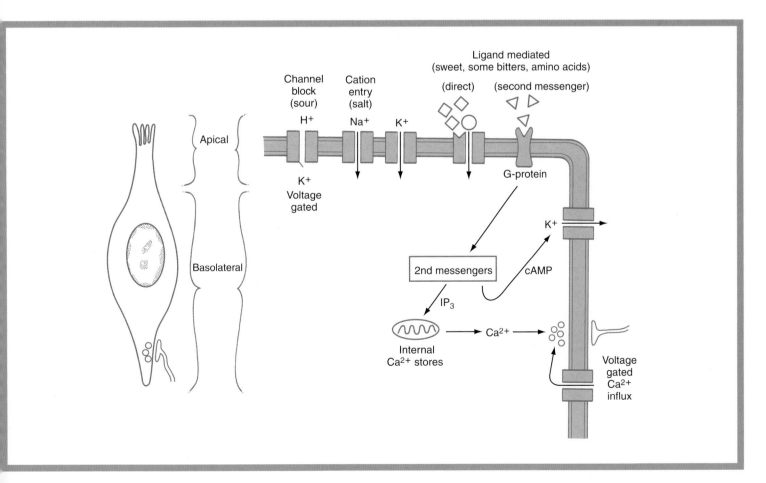

Figure 23-12. Some pathways of transduction in taste receptors. Some sour and bitter substances are transduced by the closing of apical voltage-sensitive potassium channels. The transduction of salts such as sodium chloride, involves the movement of ions (such as Na^+ and K^+) through amiloride-sensitive cation channels in the apical membrane. Sweet and some bitter compounds are thought to activate intracellular second-messenger pathways (cyclic AMP [cAMP], inositol 1,4,5-trisphosphate [IP_3]), which leads to activation of membrane channels in the basolateral membrane of the taste cell. (Adapted from Kinnamon SC: Taste transduction: A diversity of mechanisms. Trends Neurosci 11:491-496, 1988, with permission.)

mediated second-messenger pathways (Fig. 23-12). Binding of sweet-tasting compounds such as sucrose to apically located receptors stimulates an adenylyl cyclase–cAMP second-messenger pathway that closes basolateral potassium channels, leading to depolarization of the taste receptor cell. Additional mechanisms for sweet transduction have been proposed, and there is good evidence for multiple sweet receptor types. One of these mechanisms has also been implicated in the detection of bitter and may potentially be involved in the conduction of umami, the taste sensation conveyed by a glutamate receptor. This particular signaling cascade activates a G protein that stimulates phosphodiesterase, causing a reduction in intracellular cAMP and subsequent changes in receptor cell activity. A different second-messenger pathway (IP$_3$) that releases Ca^{2+} from intracellular stores has been shown in conjunction with some bitter compounds but may also play a role in the perception of sweet. Alkaloids, glucosides, and some amino acids are known to convey a bitter taste.

Evidence exists for several possible transduction pathways for amino acids. One pathway involves binding of amino acids by receptors that are directly coupled to cation channels having properties similar to those of the nicotinic acetylcholine receptor. Another receptor activates a G protein–dependent increase in the second messengers cAMP and IP$_3$.

Peripheral Taste Pathways

The afferent fibers of first-order taste neurons (special visceral afferent [SVA]) innervating oropharyngeal taste buds travel in the *facial* (VII), *glossopharyngeal* (IX), and *vagus* (X) nerves (Fig. 23-13). The *chorda tympani* branch of the facial nerve innervates taste buds in the fungiform papillae on the anterior two thirds of the tongue and in the most anterior clefts of the foliate papillae. The *greater superficial petrosal nerve*, also a branch of the facial nerve, innervates taste buds on the soft palate. The cell bodies of facial nerve fibers subserving taste are located in the *geniculate ganglion*, and their central processes enter the brainstem at the pontomedullary junction in the *intermediate nerve*, which is actually a part of the facial nerve. These primary afferent taste fibers enter the *solitary tract*, travel caudally, and terminate on cells of the surrounding *solitary nucleus* (Fig. 23-13).

Taste buds located in the vallate papillae and posterior clefts of the foliate papillae are innervated by the *lingual-tonsillar branch* of the glossopharyngeal nerve (cranial nerve IX). Those located on the epiglottis and esophagus are innervated by the *superior*

laryngeal nerve, a branch of the vagus nerve (cranial nerve X) (Fig. 23-13). Taste fibers in cranial nerves IX and X have their cell bodies of origin in the *inferior ganglia* (*petrosal* and *nodose* respectively) of these cranial nerves (Fig. 23-13). The central processes of these fibers, like those of the facial nerve, enter the medulla, descend in the solitary tract, and terminate on neurons in the adjacent solitary nucleus (Fig. 23-13).

Central Taste Pathways

The solitary nucleus is the principal visceral afferent nucleus of the brainstem. On the basis of functional characteristics, it is divided into a *rostral* (gustatory) *nucleus* and a *caudal (visceral or cardiorespiratory) nucleus*. Taste fibers traveling in cranial nerves VII, IX, and X terminate primarily in the rostral portions of the solitary nucleus because this region contains most of the second-order neurons in the taste pathway (Fig. 23-13). Although there is considerable overlap in the distribution of the terminals of the primary taste cranial afferents from these three nerves in the gustatory nucleus, information derived from different areas of the tongue is spatially segregated. General visceral afferent fibers of the vagus, and those that travel in the glossopharyngeal nerve, terminate in the caudal part of the solitary nucleus (Fig. 23-13). These visceral fibers are involved in the central control of respiration, cardiac function, and certain aspects of swallowing.

Axons arising from second-order taste neurons in the gustatory nucleus ascend in association with the ipsilateral *central tegmental tract* and terminate in the *parvicellular division of the ventral posteromedial nucleus* of the thalamus (VPMpc), medial to the head representation (Fig. 23-14). Axons from these neurons in the VPMpc travel through the ipsilateral posterior limb of the internal capsule to terminate in the inner portion of the *frontal operculum* and *anterior insular cortex*, and in the rostral extension of *Brodmann area 3b* on the lateral convexity of the postcentral gyrus (Fig. 23-14). This pathway (solitary nucleus → VPMpc → cortex) is responsible for the discriminative aspects of taste and, in contrast to other sensory pathways, is exclusively ipsilateral.

Physiologic studies in primates indicate that there is an additional region of the cortex that processes taste information. The *lateral posterior orbitofrontal cortex* receives inputs from primary taste cortex and acts as a site of integration for taste, olfactory, and visual cues associated with the ingestion of foods. Recent data suggest that cells in this area are involved in the appreciation

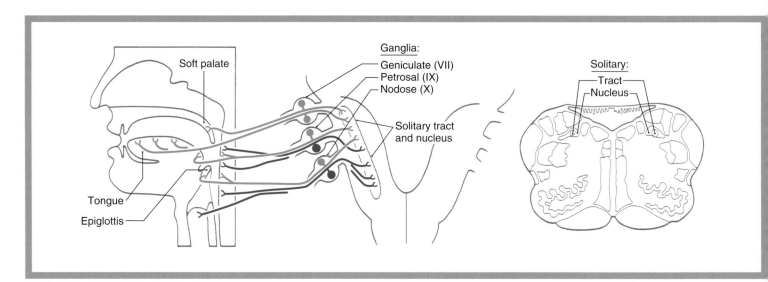

Figure 23-13. Summary of peripheral taste pathways. Special visceral afferent fibers for taste *(in red)* terminate in the rostral (gustatory) areas of the solitary nucleus, whereas general visceral afferent fibers *(in blue)* terminate in the caudal portion of the nucleus.

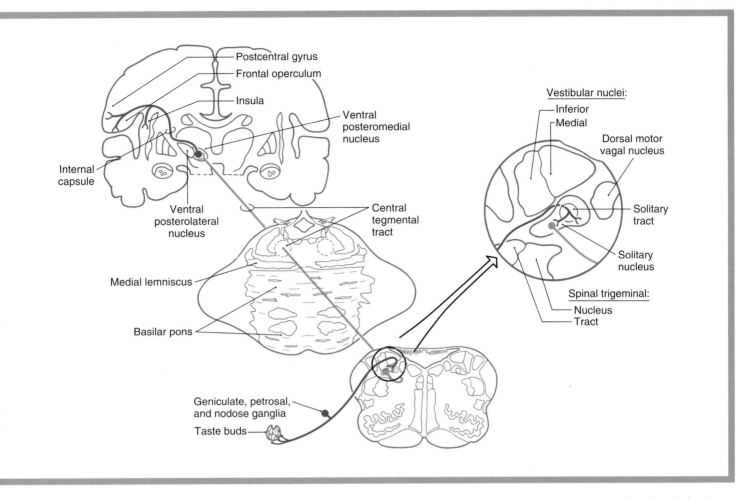

Figure 23-14. The ascending taste pathway to thalamus and cortex. Color coding demonstrates the projections of first *(blue)-*, second *(red)-*, and third *(green)-*order neurons conveying gustatory information.

of flavor, food reward, and the control of feeding. Taste-responsive cells have also been found in the primate amygdala and hypothalamus. These cells do not respond exclusively to taste, and their connecting pathways and role in taste-mediated behavior are not fully understood. Taste information is also relayed from cells in the solitary nucleus into medullary reflex connections that influence salivary secretion, mimetic responses, and swallowing.

Disorders of the Gustatory System

The chorda tympani branch leaves the facial nerve just distal to the geniculate ganglion. Consequently, lesions of the root of the seventh cranial nerve, or tumors in the internal auditory meatus, such as a *vestibular schwannoma*, sometimes called an acoustic neuroma (see Fig. 22-10), will result in loss of taste perception from the anterior two thirds of the tongue on the ipsilateral side. Accompanying this deficit are paralysis of the ipsilateral facial muscles, *hyperacusis* (paralysis of the stapedius muscle), and impaired secretion of the nasal and lacrimal glands and of submandibular and sublingual salivary glands. Damage just distal to the geniculate ganglion may or may not result in taste loss, depending on the origin of chorda tympani branches, but an ipsilateral facial paralysis will be seen (see Fig. 14-14).

The complete loss of taste *(ageusia)* is rarely encountered, in part because of the large numbers of nerves that relay taste information to the central nervous system. Rarely does a patient suffer from bilateral injury to all the nerves innervating the oropharyngeal region. More frequently a patient suffers from *hypogeusia*, decreased taste sensitivity, or *parageusia (dysgeusia)*, distortions in the perception of a taste. One of the most frequent

causes of taste disturbances is drug usage. A wide array of medications can affect taste function, the most frequent complaint being *dysgeusia*. Like olfactory disorders, taste disorders are associated with head trauma, viral infections, and various psychiatric disorders. Notable impairments of taste have been documented in Bell palsy (see Chapter 25). It has been suggested that herpes simplex virus may be a causative factor of this disease and that administration of prednisone may reduce potential damage from nerve swelling in the facial canal. Taste changes have also been documented in the elderly as numbers of taste buds decrease and taste transduction mechanisms become less effective. These changes are often accompanied by alterations in eating habits. For example, a person may use more sugar in his or her coffee to compensate for reduced acuity of sweet stimuli. Taste disturbances are similarly known to occur in cancer patients who receive radiation therapy and chemotherapy and in diabetics where losses are progressive. Another consideration is saliva, an important medium for the relay of chemical information to taste receptors. Diseases that affect the production of saliva may impact on taste quality. Individuals with cystic fibrosis, for instance, have been reported to experience increases in taste sensitivity that may be related to the hyperviscosity of their saliva. Other factors contributing to altered taste sensation include oropharyngeal tumors, which can compromise the function of the chorda tympani or lingual nerves, and foci of seizure activity in central taste processing areas, which can trigger unpleasant taste sensations *(cacogeusia)*. Although experienced less frequently than olfactory auras, gustatory hallucinations have been elicited by electrical stimulation of the frontal and parietal opercula, as well as the hippocampus and amygdala.

Synopsis of Clinical Points

- Anosmia is the loss of the sense of smell (p. 372).
- Olfactory hypesthesia, or hyposmia, is a decreased sensitivity to odorants (decreased ability to perceive odors) (p. 372).
- Rhinitis or sinusitis may decrease the patient's ability to perceive odors (p. 372).
- The sense of smell may be damaged, or lost, as the result of trauma (p. 372).
- Basal skull fractures, especially those extending into the anterior cranial fossa, may cause a loss of smell (p. 372).
- Tumors related to olfactory structures, such as neuroblastomas or meningiomas of the olfactory groove, may alter the ability of the patient to detect odors (p. 372).
- Olfactory groove meningiomas may extend into the cavernous sinus and produce deficits related to damage of the nerves traversing this sinus (p. 372).
- Specific anosmia is the inability to detect a specific odor (p. 372).
- Olfactory hyperesthesia, or hyperosmia, is a increased sensitivity to odors (p. 372).
- Olfactory agnosia is the situation in which the patient is aware of an odor but is not able to specifically identify it (p. 372).
- An olfactory hallucination is the case of the patient sensing an odor when none is present; this may occur in certain types of temporal lobe lesions (p. 373).
- Cacosmia is the perception of a disagreeable disorder; this may be seen in seizure patients (p. 373).
- Parosmia, or dysosmia, is the perception of an unpleasant odor when a pleasant odor is present (p. 373).
- Loss of taste may be seen in a patient with vestibular schwannoma (p. 377).
- Hypogeusia is a decreased sense of taste (p. 377).
- Parageusia, or dysgeusia, is the unpleasant perception of taste when the substance would normally taste good (p. 377).
- A variety of disease processes may affect a patient's perception of taste (p. 377).
- Cacogeusia is the perception of an unpleasant taste sensation (p. 377).

Sources and Additional Reading

Anholt RRH: Molecular neurobiology of olfaction. Crit Rev Neurobiol 7:1-22, 1993.

Buck LB: Smell and Taste: The Chemical Senses. In Kandel ER, Schwartz JH, Jessel TM (eds): Principles of Neural Science, 4th ed. New York, McGraw-Hill, Health Professions Division, 2000, pp 625-647.

Cowart BJ, Young IM, Feldman RS, Lowry LD: Clinical disorders of smell and taste. Occup Med 12:465-483, 1997.

Getchell TV, Doty RL, Bartoshuk LM, Snow JB (eds): Smell and Taste in Health and Disease. New York, Raven Press, New York, 1991.

Gold GH: Controversial issues in vertebrate olfactory transduction. Annu Rev Physiol 61:857-871, 1999.

Haerer AF: The Olfactory Nerve. In DeJong's The Neurologic Examination, 5th ed. Philadelphia, JB Lippincott, 1992, pp 87-92.

Herness MS, Gilbertson TA: Cellular mechanisms of taste transduction. Annu Rev Physiol 61:873-900, 1999.

Kinnamon SC: Taste transduction: A diversity of mechanisms. Trends Neurosci 10:491-496, 1988.

Kinnamon SC: A plethora of taste receptors. Neuron 25:507-510, 2000.

Lewcock JW, Reed RR: ORs rule the roost in the olfactory system. Science 302:2078-2079, 2003.

Mistretta CM: Anatomy and neurophysiology of the taste system in aged animals. In Murphy C, Cain WS, Hegsted DM (eds): Nutrition and the chemical senses in aging: Recent advances and current research needs. Ann NY Acad Sci 561:277-290, 1989.

Mori K: Membrane and synaptic properties of identified neurons in the olfactory bulb. Prog Neurobiol 29:275-320, 1987.

Mori K, Nagao H, Yoshihara Y: The olfactory bulb: Coding and processing of odor molecule information. Science 286:711-715, 1999.

Morrison EE, Costanzo RM: Morphology of the human olfactory epithelium. J Comp Neurol 297:1-13, 1990.

Netter FM: CIBA Collection of Medical Illustrations, Vol. I, Nervous System, Part II Neurologic and Neuromuscular Disorders, CIBA, 1986.

Norgren R: Gustatory System. In Paxinos G (ed): The Human Nervous System. San Diego, Academic Press, 1990, pp 845-861.

Scott JW, Wellis DP, Riggott MJ, Buonviso N: Functional organization of the main olfactory bulb. Microsc Res Tech 24:142-156, 1993.

Speielman AI: Chemosensory function and dysfunction. Crit Rev Oral Biol Med 9:267-291, 1998.

Victor M, Ropper AH: Adams and Victor's Principles of Neurology, 7th ed. New York, McGraw-Hill, 2001.

Wong TW, Gannon KS, Margolskee RF: Transduction of bitter and sweet taste by gustducin. Nature 381:796-800, 1996.

Zald DH, Pardo JV: Functional neuroimaging of the olfactory system in humans. Int J Psychophysiol 36:165-181, 2000.

Chapter 24

Motor System I: Peripheral Sensory, Brainstem, and Spinal Influence on Anterior Horn Neurons

G. A. Mihailoff and D. E. Haines

Spinal anterior horn motor neurons whose axons innervate skeletal muscles are called *lower motor neurons*. These cells stimulate muscles to produce characteristic movements of a body part. The activity of these motor neurons is influenced from two sources. First, *peripheral sensory input* arrives via posterior roots and is transmitted to anterior horn motor neurons and interneurons. Second, extensive descending projections from the cerebral cortex and brainstem, called *supraspinal systems*, terminate at all levels of the spinal cord and are responsible for a mixture of excitatory and inhibitory effects on anterior horn motor neurons. This chapter focuses on the peripheral sensory and brainstem systems that influence anterior horn neurons.

Overview

The *lower motor neurons* of the spinal cord anterior horn form neuromuscular junctions (synapses) with skeletal muscles and are topographically arranged according to the muscle groups they innervate. This is particularly evident in the cervical and lumbosacral enlargements, the levels of the spinal cord that innervate the musculature of the upper and lower limbs, respectively. Motor neurons that supply flexor muscles generally are more posteriorly located in the anterior horn than are extensor motor neurons. In addition, motor neurons that innervate paravertebral and proximal limb muscles are most medial, whereas those that innervate distal musculature are most lateral (Fig. 24-1). The anterior horn motor neurons receive sensory feedback from the muscles they control, as well as from synergist and antagonist muscles. The linkage of peripheral sensory input and anterior horn neurons forms the substrate for a number of spinal reflexes (see Figs. 9-9 to 9-11).

In addition to sensory feedback, the activity of lower motor neurons in the spinal cord is greatly influenced by descending projections from cells in the brainstem and cerebral cortex. These brainstem and cortical neurons are referred to as *upper motor neurons*, and, unlike lower motor neurons, they have no direct synaptic link with muscles. Because of their origin, these descending projections are also called *supraspinal systems*.

Anterior horn motor neurons represent the only direct link (the *final common path*) between the nervous system and skeletal muscle. As such, these neurons play a central role in the production of movement. The regulation of motor neuron activity by peripheral sensory input and descending brainstem influences is crucial to the performance of normal movement.

Anterior Horn Motor Neurons

Types and Distribution

There are two varieties of anterior horn motor neurons, alpha and gamma, which are intermingled within the anterior horn. *Alpha motor neurons* innervate the ordinary, working fibers of skeletal muscles called *extrafusal fibers*, and *gamma motor neurons* innervate a special type of skeletal muscle fiber, the *intrafusal fibers*, which are found only within *muscle spindles*. Recall that the anterior horn also contains small *interneurons* whose axons distribute locally within the spinal gray. Interneurons are numerous in the intermediate zone and anterior horn and are functionally quite essential in the regulation of alpha and gamma motor neurons. Their action on motor neurons may either be excitatory or inhibitory.

The axons of both types of anterior horn motor neurons exit the spinal cord via the anterior roots and course distally in peripheral nerves. These fibers represent the *final common path* that links the nervous system and skeletal muscles. As the axon of an alpha motor neuron reaches the muscle it innervates, it loses its myelin sheath and forms a series of flattened boutons that indent the surface of a group of muscle fibers. This specialized type of synapse is called a *neuromuscular junction* or *motor end plate* (Fig. 24-2).

Neuromuscular Junction

Like synapses in the central nervous system, the junction between a motor axon and skeletal muscle fibers consists of presynaptic and postsynaptic components (Fig. 24-2). The *presynaptic element*, the axon terminal, contains round, clear synaptic vesicles (filled with the neurotransmitter *acetylcholine*), mitochondria, and small patches of dense material around which the vesicles aggregate at the active site. The presynaptic element is separated from the postsynaptic element by an extracellular space called the *synaptic cleft*. The *postsynaptic membrane*, the specialized portion of the muscle cell plasma membrane subjacent to the axon terminal, exhibits a large number of folds that effectively increase the surface area of the muscle cell in contact with the axon terminal (Fig. 24-2). These irregularities, called *subjunctional folds*, contain *nicotinic acetylcholine receptors* on their summit facing into the synaptic cleft (Fig. 24-2). These *nicotinic acetylcholine receptors* are integral membrane proteins with an extracellular domain that actually binds the acetylcholine molecule and a membrane-spanning domain that forms an ion

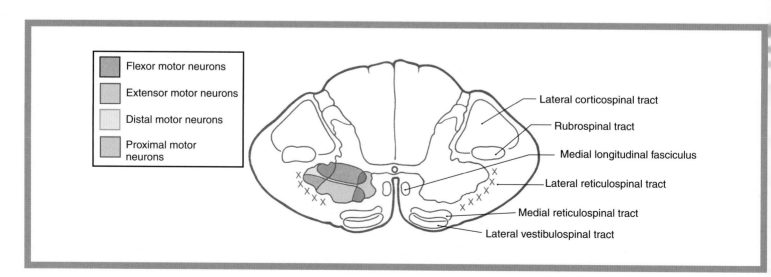

Figure 24-1. The locations of vestibulospinal and reticulospinal tracts at a representative cervical level of the spinal cord. Medial vestibulospinal fibers are located in the medial longitudinal fasciculus. The general positions of motor neuron pools are shown on the *left.*

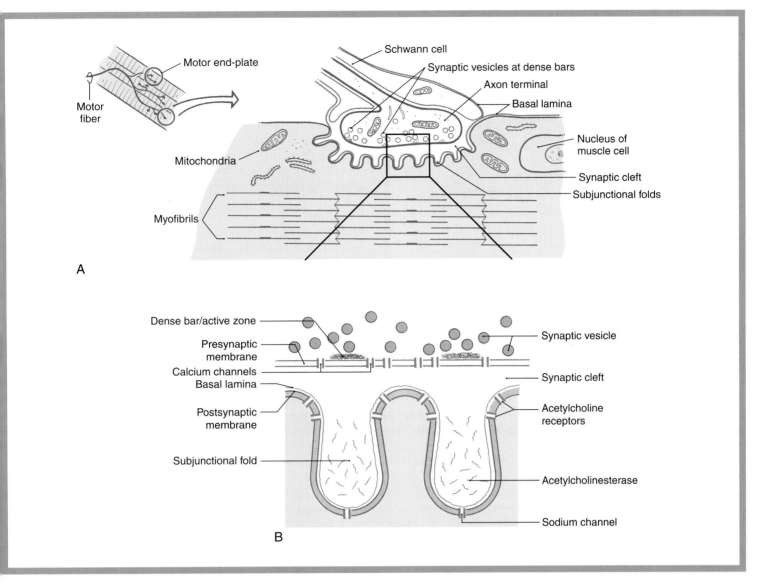

Figure 24-2. The structural elements related to the axon terminal at the neuromuscular junction (**A**) and the details of the synaptic cleft, its receptors, and related elements that enhance transmission and then hydrolyze the transmitter into acetate and choline (**B**).

channel (Fig. 24-2B). Such receptors are called *inotropic receptors* because binding of the neurotransmitter molecule to the extracellular domain typically opens the ion channel and allows the passage of sodium and potassium ions. Thus the receptor and its associated ion channel mediate the ion flux that underlies the transmission of electrical signals from nerve to muscle. Surrounding the exterior surface of the muscle is a *basal lamina* that extends into the synaptic cleft where it becomes continuous with a basal lamina formed by the Schwann cell process that encloses the axon terminal (Fig. 24-2).

When an action potential depolarizes the presynaptic element, there is an influx of calcium through voltage-gated membrane channels. Synaptic vesicles fuse with the presynaptic membrane at the active sites (which are marked by structures called *dense bars*) and release *acetylcholine* into the synaptic cleft. The transmitter binds to receptors on the postsynaptic membrane and opens ion channels. Ion flux then occurs, and a depolarizing potential called an *end plate potential* spreads over the surface of the muscle fiber. This potential triggers the release of Ca^{2+} (from the sarcoplasmic reticulum), which elicits the movement of actin and myosin filaments, resulting in muscle contraction. Synaptic transmission is terminated by an enzyme called *acetylcholinesterase*, which is located in the matrix of the basal lamina in the depths of the postjunctional folds. This enzyme inactivates

acetylcholine by detaching it from its receptor and hydrolyzing it to acetate and choline.

Motor Units

Each muscle fiber receives only one motor end plate, but the number of muscle fibers innervated by a single alpha motor neuron axon varies from a few to many. The aggregate of a motor neuron axon and *all* the muscle fibers it innervates is called a *motor unit* (Fig. 24-3). In general, as the need for fine control of a muscle increases, the size or innervation ratio of its motor unit decreases. That is, the number of muscle fibers innervated by a single axon decreases. The size of a motor unit is also related to the mass of the muscle and its speed of contraction. Small muscles that generate low levels of force typically have *small motor units* (10 to 100 muscle fibers per motor axon), whereas large, powerful muscles that generate high levels of force are usually innervated by *large motor units* (600 to 1000 muscle fibers per motor neuron axon).

Motor units can be divided into two categories *(slow twitch* and *fast twitch)* based on the metabolic and physiologic properties of the muscle fibers and their innervation. *Type I* units are composed of "red" (dark) muscle fibers referred to as *slow-twitch* (S) fibers. These muscles are rich in mitochondria and contain a (red) heme protein that helps bind and store oxygen.

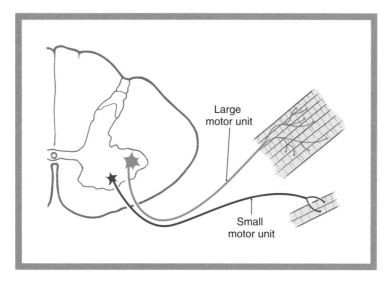

Figure 24-3. Large and small motor units.

Because of their ability to utilize glucose and oxygen from the bloodstream, these fibers can generate abundant adenosine triphosphate (aerobic metabolism) and fuel the contractile apparatus for long periods of contraction time, making these motor units resistant to fatigue. The trade-off, however, is that these muscle fibers can generate only relatively small levels of force or tension. The postural muscles (deep back muscles) are composed predominately of this fiber type; these muscles may contract at a low level of tension but for exceedingly long periods of time.

In contrast, the *type II* or *fast-twitch* units (white or pale muscles) generate much higher levels of force but for comparatively brief periods of time. Muscles used during strenuous exercise are examples of type II fibers: they contract with greater force than postural muscles but for shorter time periods. The fast-twitch fibers actually come in two varieties. The fast-fatigable type (type IIB or FF) contains large stores of glycogen that provide the energy necessary to phosphorylate adenosine diphosphate (glycogen converted to lactic acid) and produce relatively greater amounts of force compared with slow-twitch fibers. However, the rapid depletion of glycogen coupled with the accumulation of lactic acid (anaerobic catabolism) contributes to the relatively brief contraction time. A second fast-twitch unit (type IIA) is actually intermediate between the type I slow-twitch and type II fast-twitch units because it exhibits sufficient aerobic capacity to resist fatigue yet is able to generate nearly as much force as the type IIB units. These units are referred to as fast fatigue-resistant fibers (FFR).

Muscles generally contain a mixture of motor units, and the proportions vary according to the demands placed on the muscle. For example, the soleus muscle is a slow-twitch postural muscle containing mainly S-type units. The relatively slow conduction time of the small-diameter alpha axons serving these motor units is adequate for the demands of this muscle. By contrast, the gastrocnemius muscle is a dynamic, powerful muscle used in running and jumping. It is considered to be a fast-twitch muscle synd contains mainly FF motor units innervated by large-diameter, rapidly conducting axons.

Size Principle

The nervous system uses the size and functional properties of motor units as a means of grading the force of muscle contraction. When an excitatory input reaches a group of motor neurons in the anterior horn, that input will produce a larger change in the membrane potential of the smaller motor neurons than in the larger motor neurons. This is because the firing threshold of a neuron is determined by its total electrical resistance, which is *inversely proportional to its surface area*. Therefore, a given synaptic input to a pool of motor neurons will first recruit the smaller neurons (linked to small motor units) followed in sequence by progressively larger cells (and larger motor units). This is known as the *size principle of motor neuron recruitment*. Thus in a fine movement that requires sustained output with little force, the smaller cells and the small motor units (slow-twitch) are activated first. As the need for a more forceful rapid movement increases, progressively larger cells and larger motor units (fast-twitch) are activated and the movement transitions smoothly from low force to high force with strong bursts of contraction. The force of contraction is also influenced by the firing rate of the participating motor neurons. As the requirement for greater force and speed of contraction increases, the synaptic input increases and recruits more of the larger neurons. The firing rate of the activated larger motor neurons also increases and enhances the speed and force of the movement.

Peripheral Sensory Input to the Anterior (Ventral) Horn

Muscle Spindles

Signals that transmit information from skeletal muscles into the nervous system enter the spinal cord via the posterior roots. For the most part, these signals are generated in specialized structures in muscles called *neuromuscular spindles (muscle spindles)*. The output of the muscle spindle signals a change in muscle length and the rate of change in muscle length.

A muscle spindle (Fig. 24-4) is a long, thin encapsulated structure that typically contains about seven skeletal striated *intrafusal muscle fibers*. Spindles range in length from 4 to 10 mm.

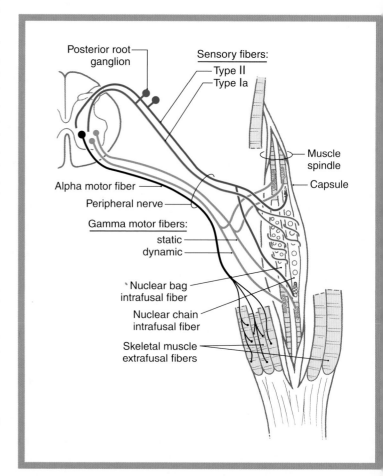

Figure 24-4. Structure of a muscle spindle and the relation of afferent and efferent nerve fibers to intrafusal and extrafusal muscle fibers.

Table 24-1. The Muscle Spindle

Intrafusal Fiber	Ending/Fiber Type/Velocity (Diameter)	Function (Measures)	Nuclei
Nuclear bag fiber			
Dynamic bag	Primary*/Ia/80-120 msec (12-20 μm)	Rate of length change in muscle	Central cluster
Static bag	Primary*/Ia/80-120 m/s (12-20 μm)	Only change in length, not rate of change	Central cluster
Nuclear chain fiber	Secondary†/II/35-70 m/s (6-8 μm)	Change in length, not rate of change	Central row

*Annulospiral ending.
†Flower-spray ending.

The capsule of the spindle (along with its intrafusal muscle fibers) is attached to, and oriented in parallel with, the *extrafusal fibers* that constitute the bulk of the muscle.

There are two basic types of intrafusal fibers: *nuclear bag fibers* and *nuclear chain fibers* (Fig. 24-4 and Table 24-1). Like other skeletal muscle cells, intrafusal fibers are multinucleated, and the arrangement of the nuclei is the most obvious structural feature distinguishing the two types. In both types, the nuclei occupy the central *(equatorial)* region of the cell. In *nuclear bag fibers*, the nuclei are clustered centrally, and give the equatorial region a swollen appearance. In *nuclear chain fibers*, the nuclei are arranged in a linear row, and the equatorial region is not obviously expanded. The contractile elements of both types of cells are located entirely in the two distal (polar) regions of the cell. Because the two ends of the cell are anchored, contraction of the intrafusal fibers causes the equatorial region to be stretched between the two polar regions.

The two types of intrafusal fibers perform different sensory functions. The nuclear bag fibers are actually subdivided into two different categories that have different elastic properties and, correspondingly, different functions (Table 24-1). One type, the *dynamic nuclear bag fiber*, is sensitive mainly to the rate of change in muscle length. The other, the *static nuclear bag fiber*, signals only a change in muscle length but not the rate of that change. Nuclear chain fibers, like static bag fibers, are mainly sensitive to changes in muscle length (Table 24-1).

Intrafusal muscle fibers are associated with two types of sensory fibers, the terminals or receptive ends of which are concentrated at the equatorial (noncontractile) region of intrafusal fibers. The *type Ia fiber* is heavily myelinated, has a conduction velocity of 80 to 120 m/s and is typically associated with dynamic and static nuclear bag fibers (Table 24-1). The distal end of this sensory fiber is wrapped around the central (noncontractile) region of the intrafusal muscle fibers. Because of this relationship, the type *Ia* afferent terminations are called *annulospiral endings*. These endings are, in effect, mechanoreceptors. Stretching of the central region of the intrafusal fiber will also stretch the sensory fiber and mechanically open ion channels that will enable Na$^+$ and K$^+$ ion flux through the membrane. If the induced ion flux raises the membrane potential above threshold, an action potential is initiated in the sensory fiber. The firing frequency is directly proportional to the degree to which the spindle is stretched.

The other type of muscle spindle sensory fiber, the *type II fiber*, is principally associated with nuclear chain fibers (Fig. 24-4 and Table 24-1). Its connection with the equatorial region of the target intrafusal fiber has the form of a cluster of thin, radiating branches and is called a *secondary ending* or *flower-spray ending*. This sensory fiber is also activated by mechanical stretch, but it codes only *the change in muscle length not the rate* of the stretch.

Each type of intrafusal fiber is also innervated by a gamma motor neuron. Dynamic nuclear bag fibers are associated with *dynamic gamma motor neurons*, whereas static nuclear bag fibers and nuclear chain fibers are innervated by *static gamma motor neurons*. When the gamma motor neuron is active, contractile elements at both poles of the intrafusal muscle fiber are activated, resulting in increased stretch on its central region. This increases the frequency of action potentials generated in the *Ia* sensory fibers. As explained further on, dynamic and static gamma motor neurons function to maintain spindle sensitivity and length, respectively.

Gamma Loop

Muscle spindles play an essential role in movement and in the maintenance of muscle tone. Consider two situations: one in which a muscle—for example, the biceps brachii—is passively stretched and another in which it contracts and shortens actively against a load.

A passive stretching of the biceps muscle, produced, for example, by tapping on its tendon, will elongate the muscle spindles. The stretching of the equatorial region of the nuclear bag fibers results in an increase in the firing rate of the Ia fibers (Fig. 24-6A). These sensory fibers enter the cervical spinal cord and form monosynaptic excitatory synapses with alpha motor neurons that innervate the biceps brachii (Figs. 24-5 and 24-6). This is the circuit that forms the basis of the muscle stretch reflex explained in Chapter 9 (see Fig. 9-9).

The connection between the Ia sensory fibers and the alpha motor neurons of a muscle also functions in a more complex mechanism called the *gamma loop*, which is crucial to the maintenance of stretch reflexes and muscle tone. In this mechanism, extrafusal muscle contraction is indirectly produced by supraspinal activation of *gamma* motor neurons (Fig. 24-5 and Table 24-2). Like alpha neurons, gamma motor neurons receive supraspinal input from the cerebral cortex and brainstem. In the gamma loop, this supraspinal input activates the gamma motor neurons so that the intrafusal muscle fibers contract. Because the contraction of an intrafusal fiber has the effect of stretching the equatorial region between its two polar regions, it results in increased Ia fiber activity. In the spinal cord, this increase in Ia fiber discharge activates alpha motor neurons, which then activate extrafusal muscle fibers, resulting in muscle contraction (Fig. 24-5). This circuit involving gamma motor neurons, Ia primary afferent fibers, alpha motor neurons, and extrafusal muscle fibers is called the *gamma loop* (Table 24-2).

Now, consider the situation in which a muscle is contracting actively against a load. Because a muscle spindle is attached parallel to the adjacent extrafusal fibers, one might infer that overall spindle length is determined by the length of the surrounding extrafusal muscle fibers; when the muscle contracts, the spindle shortens. This is not so; if the intrafusal fibers remained passive during extrafusal muscle fiber contraction, the shortening of the spindle would relax the equatorial region of the intrafusal fibers, and the Ia fibers would cease firing (Fig. 24-6B).

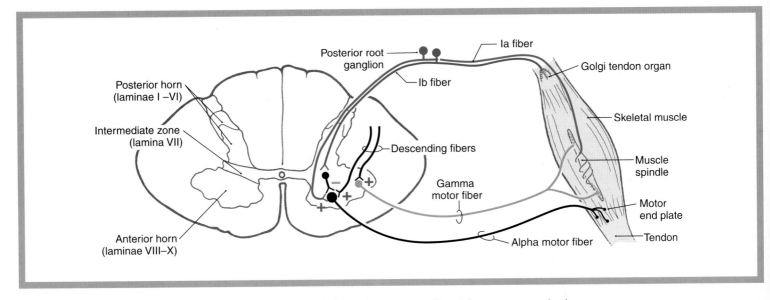

Figure 24-5. Circuits related to input and output mediated by Golgi tendon organs and to alpha-gamma coactivation.

This slack, inactive spindle would be useless for reporting muscle length. In reality, the spindle retains its sensitivity (Fig. 24-6C) and the Ia sensory fibers continue to fire during voluntary muscle contraction, because when *the brain signals the alpha motor neurons to initiate muscle contraction, it sends parallel impulses to the gamma neurons to cause the intrafusal fibers to contract.* Therefore, when the extrafusal muscle fibers shorten, the intrafusal fibers also shorten because their gamma motor neurons are activated at the same time. As a result the equatorial regions of the intrafusal fibers remain under nearly constant tension and thus retain their ability to signal changes in muscle length as movement (muscle contraction) occurs. This phenomenon is called *alpha-gamma coactivation* (Fig. 24-5 and Table 24-3).

Golgi Tendon Organ

Sensory feedback to the spinal anterior horn is also derived from the Golgi tendon organ. These structures are located in tendons near their junctions with muscle fibers and consist of networks of thin nerve fibers intertwined with the collagen fibers of the tendon (Fig. 24-5 and Table 24-4). These nerve fibers, like the sensory fibers of muscle spindles, are mechanoreceptors. However, unlike muscle spindles, the sensory fibers of tendon organs are connected in *series* between the tendon and the extrafusal muscle fibers. When force is applied to the tendon, the sensory fibers are stretched, which opens ion channels in the nerve fiber membrane. The fibers that lead from the tendon organs to the spinal cord are *type Ib* fibers. These fibers are large in diameter and heavily myelinated, with a conduction velocity of 70 to 110 m/s (Table 24-4). After entering the spinal cord, the type Ib fibers traverse the intermediate zone to reach the anterior horn, where they form *excitatory* synapses with interneurons. These interneurons in turn *inhibit* alpha motor neurons that innervate the muscle associated with the activated Golgi tendon organ. This action of the Golgi tendon organ is exactly opposite that of the muscle spindle; activation of the latter leads to excitation of the muscle associated with the activated spindle, whereas

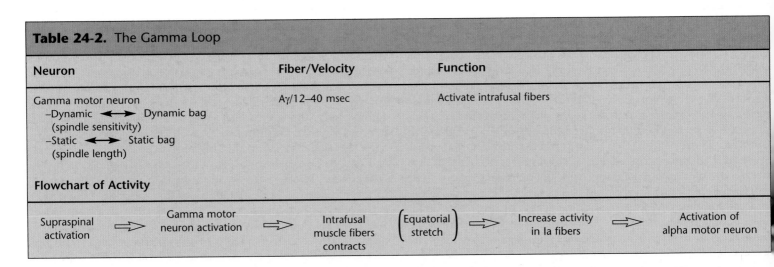

Neuron	Fiber/Velocity	Function

Gamma motor neuron
  –Dynamic ◄──► Dynamic bag
   (spindle sensitivity)
  –Static ◄──► Static bag
   (spindle length)
	Aγ/12–40 msec	Activate intrafusal fibers

Table 24-2. The Gamma Loop

Flowchart of Activity

| Supraspinal activation | ⟹ | Gamma motor neuron activation | ⟹ | Intrafusal muscle fibers contracts | (Equatorial stretch) | ⟹ | Increase activity in Ia fibers | ⟹ | Activation of alpha motor neuron |

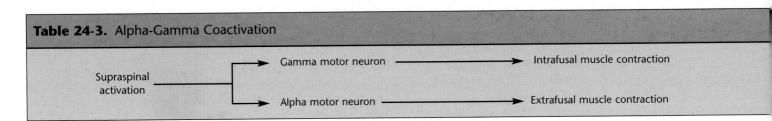

Table 24-3. Alpha-Gamma Coactivation

Supraspinal activation ──┬──► Gamma motor neuron ──────► Intrafusal muscle contraction
               └──► Alpha motor neuron ──────► Extrafusal muscle contraction

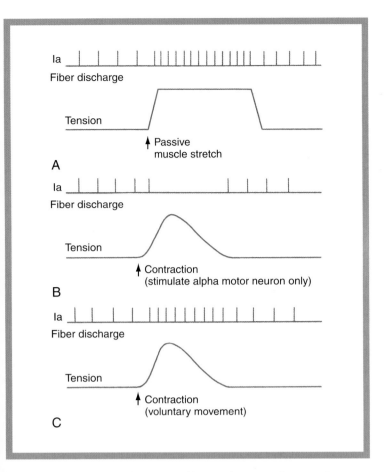

Figure 24-6. Responses shown by Ia fibers in three situations: passive stretching of the muscle (**A**), experimentally induced contraction of the muscle in which only the alpha motor neurons are stimulated (**B**), and a voluntary contraction of the muscle in which gamma and alpha motor neurons are coactivated (**C**). When only alpha neurons are activated (**B**), the intrafusal fibers stay relaxed while the surrounding muscle contracts and the Ia discharge ceases. In a normal contraction (**C**), the shortening of the spindle caused by extrafusal fiber contraction is coupled with the contraction of intrafusal fibers and the Ia discharge persists.

activation of the tendon organ leads to inhibition of neurons innervating the muscle from which the afferent input originated (Table 24-4).

Reflex Circuits

Afferent fibers from muscle spindles and Golgi tendon organs take part in a variety of reflex circuits that directly or indirectly influence the activity of anterior horn motor neurons. Several of the more prominent of these circuits are described in Chapter 9 (see Figs. 9-9 to 9-11); they are summarized only briefly here. As mentioned earlier, many type *Ia* spindle afferents form monosynaptic excitatory connections with alpha motor neurons that innervate the muscle from which the afferents originated. This circuitry is the basis for the *muscle stretch reflex* (see Fig. 9-9). At the same time, these *Ia* fibers activate *Ia inter-neurons* that inhibit motor neurons innervating *antagonist* muscles;

this is called *reciprocal inhibition* (see Fig. 9-9). Incoming muscle afferents can also activate interneurons that project to the contralateral side of the spinal cord, as well as to propriospinal neurons that link the spinal segment at which the spindle afferents entered to more rostral or caudal spinal cord levels. Circuits of the first type, which convey cutaneous somatic inputs, form the basis for the *crossed extensor reflex* (see Fig. 9-11).

In general, the various local spinal reflex pathways primarily target alpha motor neurons or spinal interneurons. For the most part, the activity of these basic spinal reflexes occurs in the background and is not under direct volitional control. However, certain so-called long loop reflexes transmit muscle sensory information through ascending pathways that reach the cerebral cortex by way of a thalamic relay. The cortex can then increase or decrease the gain of spinal reflexes via descending supraspinal pathways.

Brainstem-Spinal Systems: Anatomy and Function

Of the several pathways that project to the spinal cord from the brainstem or cerebral cortex, four are particularly relevant to voluntary movement. Three of the four originate from cell groups in the brainstem. Two of them, the *vestibulospinal* and *reticulospinal systems*, travel in the ventral funiculus of the spinal cord. The other two, the *rubrospinal* and *lateral corticospinal tracts*, travel in the lateral funiculus. The following sections focus on the three systems that originate in the brainstem, the vestibulospinal, reticulospinal, and rubrospinal tracts.

Vestibulospinal Tracts

The vestibulospinal system comprises medial and lateral vestibulospinal tracts (Figs. 24-1 and 24-7). The *medial vestibulospinal tract* is made up of axons that originate in the medial and inferior vestibular nuclei and *descend bilaterally* into the spinal cord as part of the medial longitudinal fasciculus. The *lateral vestibulospinal tract* is formed by axons that originate in cells of the lateral vestibular nucleus and *descend ipsilaterally* through the anterior portion of the brainstem to course in the anterior funiculus of the spinal cord.

The medial vestibulospinal tract projects only as far as cervical or upper thoracic spinal cord levels and influences motor neurons controlling neck musculature. The lateral vestibulospinal tract, in contrast, extends throughout the length of the cord. Cells in rostral portions of the lateral vestibular nucleus project to the cervical cord, cells in the middle portion project to the thoracic cord, and cells in the caudal part terminate in lumbosacral levels. The fibers of this tract terminate in the medial portions of laminae VII and VIII and *excite motor neurons that innervate paravertebral extensors and proximal limb extensors* (Fig. 24-7). These muscles function to counteract the force of gravity and, therefore, are commonly called *antigravity muscles*. Through their effects on these extensor muscles, lateral vestibulospinal fibers function in the control of posture and balance. Evidence from experimental studies suggests that some vestibulospinal

Table 24-4. The Golgi Tendon Organ		
Tendon Organ	**Fiber Type/Velocity (Diameter)**	**Function***
Capsule, collagen fiber bundles interlaced by nerve fiber terminals	Ib/75-110 msec (12-15 μm)	Signal small changes in muscle tension
*While some tendon organs may discharge at high rates under conditions of high force (and may serve a protective function), it is well known that the discharge of many tendon organs forms a continuum from low (rate/force) to high (rate/force).		

Vestibulospinal fibers

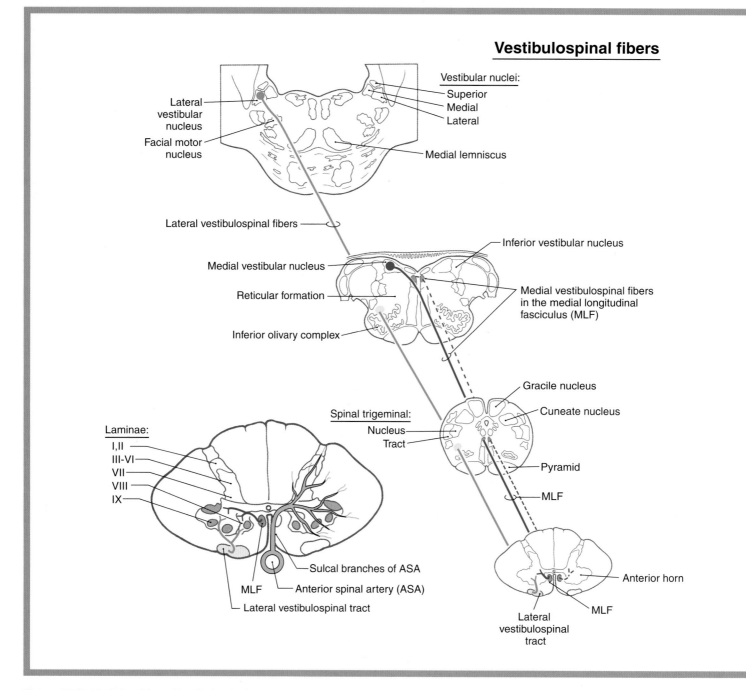

Figure 24-7. Medial and lateral vestibulospinal tracts.

axons synapse directly on alpha motor neurons but that most exert their influence through spinal interneurons.

Activity in the lateral vestibulospinal tract is driven primarily by three ipsilateral inputs—two excitatory and one inhibitory (Fig. 24-8). The two sources of excitatory input are the vestibular sensory apparatus and the cerebellar nuclei, mainly the fastigial nucleus. The inhibitory input consists of Purkinje cell axons from the cerebellar cortex.

The lateral vestibulospinal tract is the path by which input from the vestibular sensory apparatus is used to coordinate orientation of the head and body in space. Maintenance of body and limb posture is also influenced by extensive cerebello-vestibular projections, which can be either excitatory or inhibitory. The cerebral cortex essentially has no direct projections to the vestibular nuclei; consequently, the vestibulospinal tract is not directly influenced by cortical mechanisms.

Reticulospinal Tracts
Cells at many levels of the reticular formation contribute to the reticulospinal system, and these fibers can be found in the lateral and anterior funiculi throughout the spinal cord. Reticulospinal fibers participate in a wide variety of functions ranging from pain modulation to visceromotor activity. Most of the fibers involved in somatomotor function originate either from the oral and caudal pontine nuclei or from the gigantocellular reticular nucleus (Fig. 24-9). The fibers from the *oral* and *caudal pontine reticular nuclei* descend bilaterally, but with an ipsilateral predominance, in the anterior funiculus. They constitute the *medial reticulospinal (or pontine reticulospinal) tract*, which runs the full length of the spinal cord. The fibers from the *gigantocellular reticular nucleus* originate at medullary levels. Most of these *medullary reticulospinal fibers* remain ipsilateral and descend in the anterior funiculus, although a few decussate (Fig. 24-9). Most take up a new position somewhat lateral and anterior to the anterior horn, where they are called the *lateral reticulospinal tract*.

Like the vestibulospinal fibers, reticulospinal fibers terminate in the anteromedial portion of laminae VII and VIII, where they influence *motor neurons supplying paravertebral and limb extensor musculature*. However, in contrast to the vestibulospinal tract, individual reticulospinal fibers commonly terminate at multiple

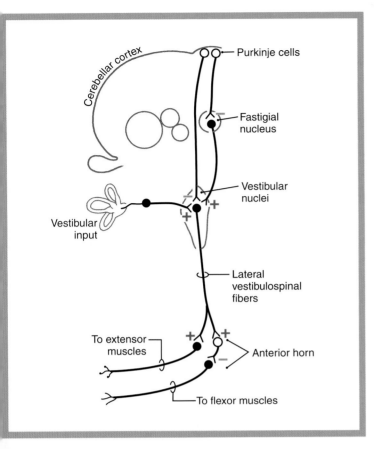

Figure 24-8. Summary of vestibular and cerebellar inputs to vestibular nuclei and the subsequent action of lateral vestibulospinal fibers on spinal motor neurons. Inhibitory neurons have open cell bodies.

spinal levels by means of collateral branches, and there is little evidence for monosynaptic contact with alpha motor neurons.

The reticulospinal system is activated by ipsilateral descending cortical projections *(corticoreticular fibers)* as well as ascending somatosensory systems *(spinoreticular fibers)*, mainly those conveying nociceptive signals. Through its influence on gamma motor neurons, the reticulospinal system is involved in the maintenance of posture and in the modulation of muscle tone. Pontine reticulospinal fibers tend to mediate excitatory effects, and medullary reticulospinal fibers usually produce inhibitory effects.

Rubrospinal Tract

In the midbrain, neurons in the red nucleus give rise to axons that cross the midline in the *anterior (ventral) tegmental decussation* (Fig. 24-9). These fibers descend through the brainstem contralateral to their origin and enter the spinal cord anteriorly adjacent to the lateral corticospinal tract. The red nucleus consists of magnocellular and parvocellular subdivisions. In mammals that have been investigated, and probably also in humans, *the magnocellular part gives rise to most rubrospinal fibers and the parvocellular part gives rise to rubro-olivary fibers.* Each rubrospinal fiber terminates in a restricted area of the spinal cord; they do not innervate multiple cord levels by means of collaterals, as do reticulospinal fibers. In the spinal gray, rubrospinal fibers terminate in laminae V, VI, and VII. For the most part, they provide *excitatory influence to motor neurons innervating proximal limb flexors* (Fig. 24-9).

The magnocellular portion of the red nucleus is relatively smaller in humans than in other mammals, and the rubrospinal tract is correspondingly small. In addition, relatively few rubrospinal axons appear to extend caudal to the cervical enlargement in humans, suggesting that this system is primarily involved with the upper extremity. Clinical findings in patients are consistent with this conclusion, indicating that the rubrospinal system exerts its control mainly over the upper extremity and has little influence over the lower extremity.

The rubrospinal system is influenced by the cerebral cortex and the cerebellar nuclei via *corticorubral* (uncrossed projection) and *cerebellorubral* (crossed projection) fibers, respectively. Precentral and premotor cortices project to the ipsilateral red nucleus, and the supplementary motor area contributes contralateral input. The latter pathways provide a route through which the cortex might influence flexor motor neurons and thus serve as a supplement to the corticospinal system. Connections that link the cerebellar nuclei, inferior olive, red nucleus, and rubrospinal tract may represent circuitry important for modifying motor performance or acquiring new motor skills.

Functional Role of Brainstem-Spinal Interactions

Insight into the functional role of the brainstem and spinal systems has come from animal studies in which lesions have been created in specific locations above or within the brainstem. The resulting deficits mimic those of humans known to have, or suspected of having, damage in the same structures.

Decerebration

The premise in this experiment was to remove the influence of the cortex and other higher centers *on* brainstem-spinal systems with the idea that whatever functions remained were controlled predominantly *by* the brainstem-spinal systems. In the basic experiment, under deep anesthesia, the brainstem was completely transected bilaterally between the superior and the inferior colliculi (Figs. 24-10A and 24-11A). This procedure results in a constellation of deficits that closely resemble those seen in humans with *supratentorial* lesions that cause herniation of the midbrain downward through the *tentorial notch*; this is *central herniation*, also called *transtentorial herniation* (Fig. 24-12). The experimental lesion in animal models, and the comparable lesion in humans, results in unopposed hyperactivity in extensor musculature in all four extremities, a condition called *decerebrate rigidity* (Fig. 24-13).

In this experiment all descending cortical systems are interrupted. These systems include the corticospinal tract, as well as the corticorubral and corticoreticular projections. In addition, the rubrospinal tract is transected, but the excitatory and inhibitory components of the reticular formation are intact. Also unaffected is the ascending somatosensory input to the reticular formation via the anterolateral system, most of which is directed to the excitatory elements of the reticulospinal system. Consequently, when a decerebrate patient receives a painful stimulus to the hands or feet, their rigidity is momentarily exacerbated.

Central (or *transtentorial*) *herniation* in humans may be seen in patients with large tumors in the hemisphere or following a large hemorrhage in the hemisphere (Figs. 24-12 and 24-13). In the diencephalic stage (before herniation through the tentorial notch) the patient may have a decreased level of consciousness, lethargy, small but poorly reactive pupils, and eye movement disorders. In addition, the *withdrawal reflex* to noxious stimuli is intact, reflexes are hyperactive, and there is a bilateral Babinski response. The extremities may be weak, and the patient may become decorticate (Fig. 24-15); first on the ipsilateral side then contralaterally. Once the herniation occurs there is a rapid decline. The patient is *decerebrate* (Fig. 24-13), comatose, pupils are dilated and fixed (do not react to light), and eye movement is absent. As the damage extends downward through the midbrain, respiration is compromised (Cheyne-Stokes, *tachypnea*, followed by shallow rapid rates), and survival is highly unlikely.

Rubrospinal and Reticulospinal tracts

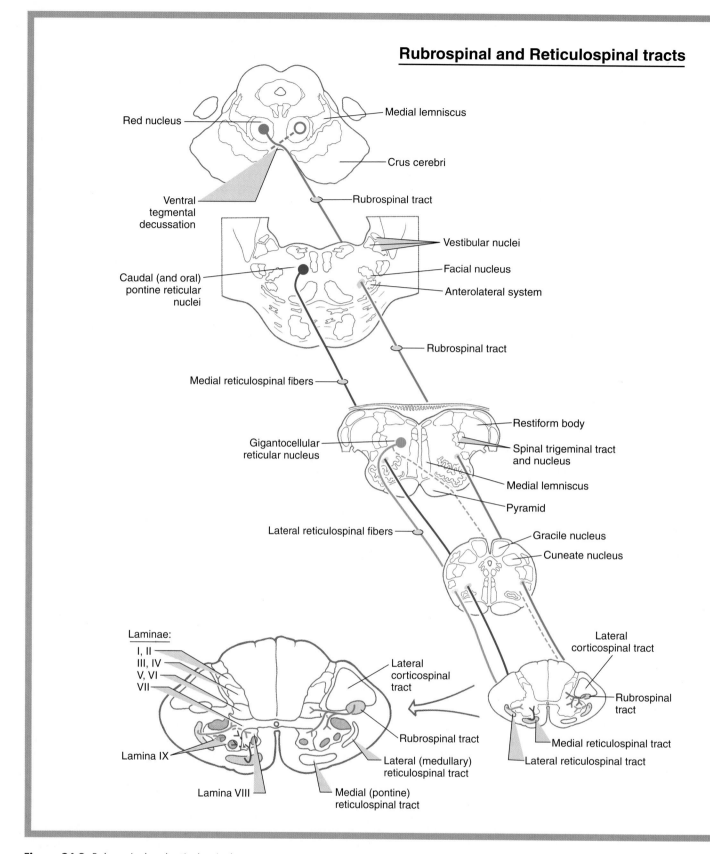

Figure 24-9. Rubrospinal and reticulospinal tracts.

Posterior (Dorsal) Root Section

An important question that arose in relation to the decerebration experiment was whether the extensor hypertonus was due to excessive activation of alpha or of gamma extensor motor neurons. To answer this question, the posterior root input from one extremity was interrupted in a decerebrate animal (Figs. 24-10B, 24-11B, and 24-14). Immediately, the extensor hypertonus in that limb collapsed. What does this result indicate? Remember that supraspinal input can produce muscle

contraction by two routes: by direct activation of alpha motor neurons or indirectly via the *gamma loop*. In the latter, the supraspinal input activates gamma motor neurons, leading to contraction of intrafusal fibers, and the resulting increase in Ia sensory input activates alpha motor neurons, which activates extrafusal fibers and leads to muscle contraction.

In the decerebrate condition, flexor muscles are inactive due to the loss of descending corticospinal and corticorubrospinal input to flexor motor neurons. Conversely, extensor motor neurons

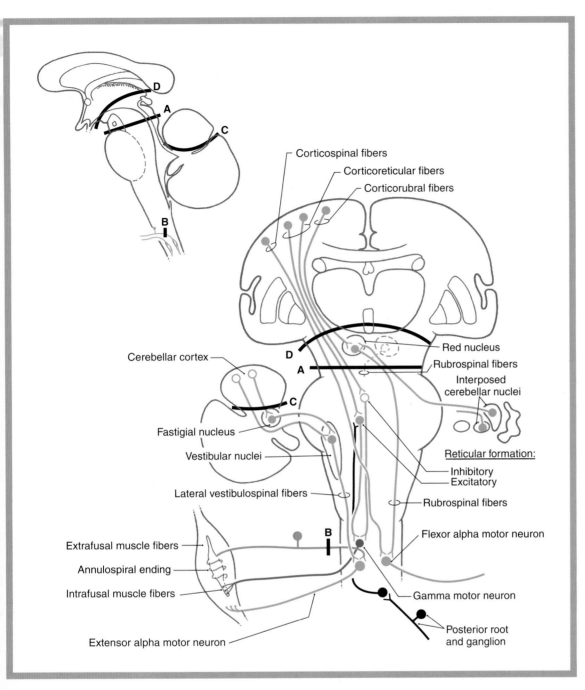

Corticospinal fibers
Corticoreticular fibers
Corticorubral fibers

Red nucleus
Rubrospinal fibers
Interposed cerebellar nuclei

Cerebellar cortex

Reticular formation:
Inhibitory
Excitatory
Rubrospinal fibers

Fastigial nucleus
Vestibular nuclei

Lateral vestibulospinal fibers

Flexor alpha motor neuron

Extrafusal muscle fibers
Annulospiral ending
Intrafusal muscle fibers

Gamma motor neuron

Posterior root and ganglion

Extensor alpha motor neuron

Figure 24-10. Locations of lesions and circuits on a diagrammatic representation of the nervous system that are involved in decerebrate rigidity (A), posterior root section in a decerebrate preparation (B), decerebellate rigidity (C), and decorticate posturing (D). Inhibitory neurons have open cell bodies. Ascending fibers in the anterolateral system *(black fibers)* are an excitatory input to excitatory cells of the reticular formation. This illustration provides a clear appreciation of the relative rostrocaudal positions of the brain areas that are involved in these clinical conditions.

are unaffected by the loss of descending cortical fibers because they are activated by descending reticulospinal and vestibulospinal inputs that are not involved by the decerebration lesion; consequently, these tracts remain intact. While the vestibulospinal system receives no significant descending input from the cortex, the reticular formation is clearly influenced by descending cortical fibers and this influence would be eliminated by the decerebrate lesion. However, the ascending somatosensory input to the reticular formation remains intact and this input primarily reaches the excitatory components of the reticular formation (Figs. 24-10 and 24-11). Since the extensor hypertonus collapses when the posterior roots are sectioned, it can be suggested that the descending reticulospinal influence on extensor motor neurons is focused primarily on *gamma* rather than on *alpha* extensor motor neurons (Fig. 24-14). The posterior root lesion interrupts the gamma loop and eliminates the circuit that would be used by the gamma motor neuron to produce

indirect activation of extensor alpha motor neurons (via activation of Ia sensory fibers) and subsequently, the stimulation of extensor extrafusal muscle fibers (Fig. 24-14). Therefore, decerebrate rigidity has come to be known also as *gamma rigidity*. To support the conclusion that the basic decerebrate paradigm involves a disruption in the balance of excitatory and inhibitory control of extensor gamma motor neurons, another experiment was initiated to determine if the influence of the vestibulospinal system might be focused on extensor *alpha* motor neurons.

Cerebellar Anterior Lobe Section
Assuming that extensor gamma motor neurons receive preferential input from the reticulospinal system, it is reasonable to ask if extensor *alpha* motor neurons are preferentially driven by vestibulospinal fibers. To investigate this point, the cerebellar anterior lobe was removed in a decerebrate animal (by midcollicular transection) (Figs. 24-10C and 24-11C). Under these

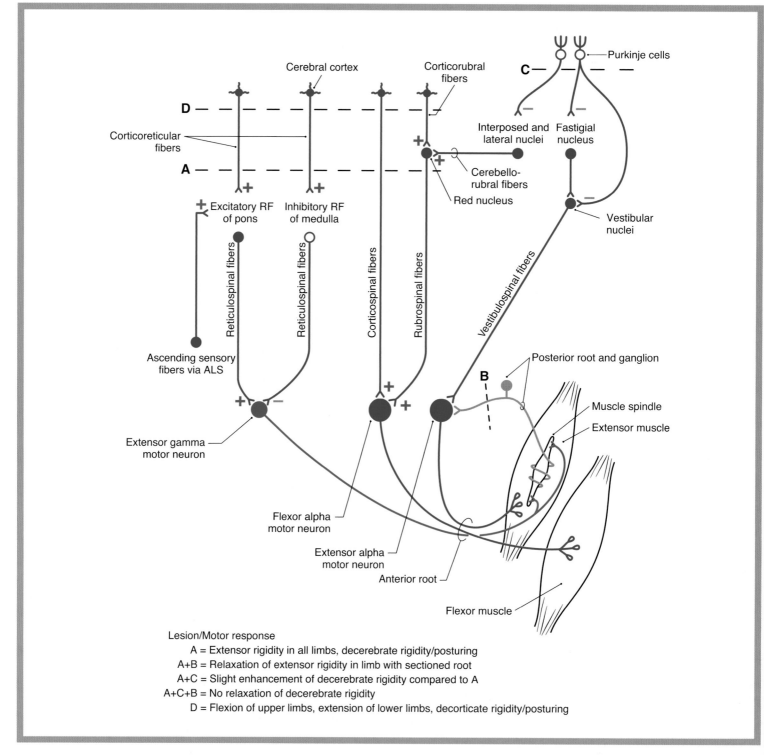

Figure 24-11. A circuit drawing representing the lesions produced in experimental animals to replicate the decerebrate and decorticate lesions/deficits seen in humans. Bilateral transection lesions are indicated by dashed lines A, B, C, and D. The decerebration lesion is at a midcolicular level (A), the decortication lesion is rostral to the superior colliculus (D), the posterior roots sectioned for one extremity (B), and removal of the anterior lobe of the cerebellum (C). The objective was to identify the anatomic substrate responsible for the decerebrate or decorticate rigidity/posturing seen in humans suffering lesions that either isolate the forebrain from the brainstem or separate the rostral brainstem from the caudal brainstem and spinal cord. Compare with Figure 24-10.

conditions the extensor hypertonus actually proved to be enhanced compared with that seen with decerebration alone, and the condition was called *decerebellate rigidity.* Subsequently, section of the posterior roots from one extremity in such an animal produced only a slight decline in extensor rigidity of the limb. Removal of the cerebellar anterior lobe cortex has two effects (Figs. 24-10C and 24-11C). First, *it eliminates direct Purkinje cell inhibition of the vestibular nuclei,* resulting in enhanced output from the vestibular nuclei over the vestibulospinal tract. Second, Purkinje cell *inhibition of fastigial neurons is eliminated.* This increases the fastigial excitatory output to the vestibular

nuclei and further augments the activity in the vestibulospinal tract. Therefore, the overall effect of cerebellar cortex removal is to substantially increase activity in the vestibulospinal system. When cerebellar anterior lobe removal was followed by posterior root section in one limb, the extensor hypertonus persisted in that limb. This suggests that the hypertonus in that limb is not due to enhanced excitatory input to gamma motor neurons from the gamma loop, but instead there is enhanced direct input to extensor *alpha* motor neurons resulting from increased excitatory activity in the vestibulospinal system. Consequently, *decerebellate extensor rigidity* is referred to as *alpha rigidity.*

Bilateral hemorrhage
into the diencephalon

Hemorrhage extending
into the midbrain

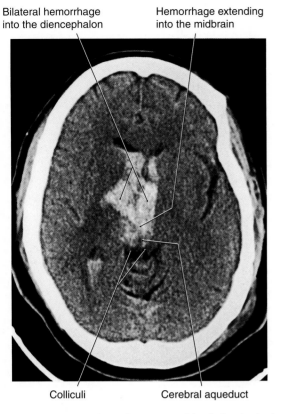

Colliculi   Cerebral aqueduct

Figure 24-12. Axial CT of a patient with a lesion in the forebrain that has herniated through the tentorial notch, into the midbrain, and resulted in decerebrate rigidity (compare with Figure 24-13).

Decortication

An extension of these experiments was undertaken to explain the neural substrate for the phenomenon called *decorticate posturing* or *decorticate rigidity* observed in humans (Fig. 24-15). In the clinic, the patient presents with flexion of the upper extremities at the elbow combined with extensor hypertonus in the lower extremities.

In experimental animals, this posture can be mimicked by transecting the brainstem at a level just *rostral to the superior colliculus* (Figs. 24-10D and 24-11D). This lesion leaves the rubrospinal tract intact while eliminating the cortical input to the red nucleus. The rubrospinal system can still be activated because excitatory projections to the red nucleus from the cerebellar nuclei are unaffected by the lesion. The rubrospinal tract influences primarily *flexor muscles*, and most of this activity, in humans, is limited to the upper extremity. The upper extremities do not exhibit extensor hypertonus but instead show an increase in flexor tone due to the intact rubrospinal system. In contrast, the lower extremities exhibit extensor hypertonus for the same reasons as in decerebration. This characteristic type of posturing is called *decorticate rigidity* (Fig. 24-15).

These two conditions, *decerebration* and *decortication*, are frequently seen (Figs. 24-13 and 24-15), and knowledge of these symptoms and the underlying brain pathology is important in the diagnosis and clinical management of these patients. In some cases, the patient may be comatose and initially exhibit decorticate posturing that subsequently converts to decerebrate posturing. This is an ominous sign, as it suggests that the lesion has continued to progress and now involves more caudal portions of the brainstem. The patient's cardiovascular and respiratory control centers in the medulla may soon be compromised, necessitating prompt intervention.

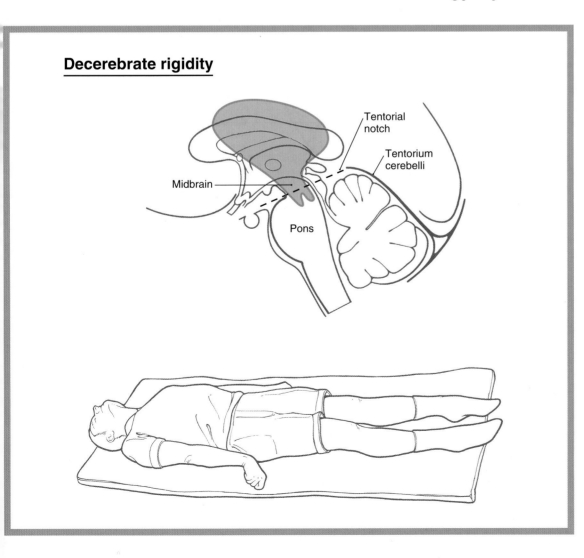

Decerebrate rigidity

Tentorial notch

Tentorium cerebelli

Midbrain

Pons

Figure 24-13. Decerebrate rigidity. A supratentorial lesion has extended through the tentorial notch. The patient's lower extremities are extended, with the toes pointed inward; the upper extremity is extended, with the fingers flexed and the forearms pronated; and the neck and head are extended. The rigidity may be so extreme that the patient's back is arched up off the bed. A patient may become decerebrate after a period of decorticate posturing (see Fig. 24-12).

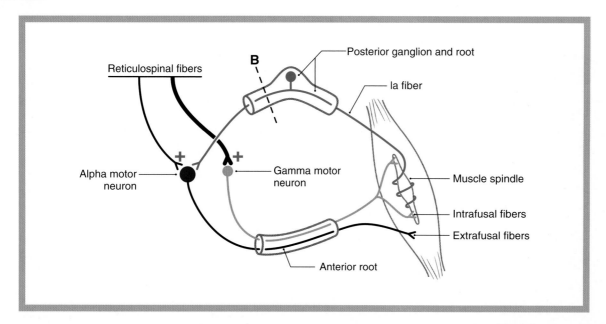

Figure 24-14. The gamma loop is formed by (1) gamma motor neurons that innervate intrafusal muscle fibers, (2) intrafusal muscle fibers that contract, stretching the sensory terminal encircling the central region of the spindle with consequent activation of the Ia fiber, (3) Ia fibers entering the posterior root and activating alpha motor neurons in the anterior horn, and (4) increased Ia activity causing increased alpha motor neuron activity with consequent extrafusal muscle contraction. Sectioning of the posterior root *(broken line, B)* removes the Ia fiber, gamma motor neurons no longer "indirectly" produce contraction of extrafusal muscle fibers; the gamma loop is interrupted.

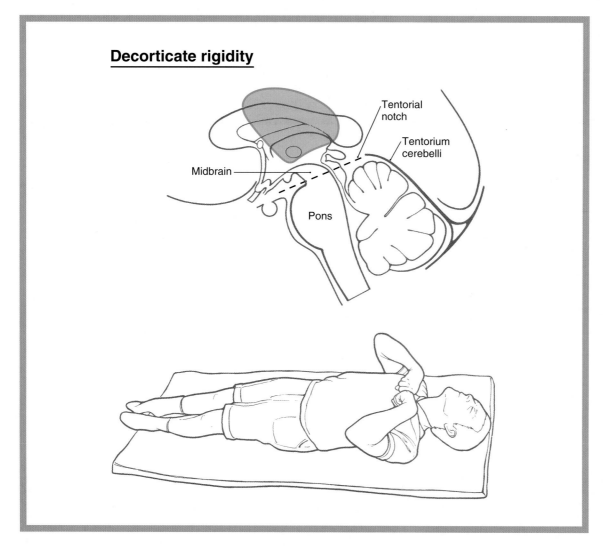

Figure 24-15. Decorticate rigidity. The lesion is in a supratentorial location. The lower extremities are extended, with the toes pointed slightly inward, and the upper extremities are flexed against the chest. The head is extended. A lesion in the supratentorial location may produce decorticate rigidity or posturing that may proceed to decerebrate rigidity or posturing as the lesion expands inferiorly (caudally) through the tentorial notch.

Synopsis of Clinical Points

- A lesion of alpha motor neurons will result in a flaccid paralysis of the muscles enervated (pp. 380–381).
- Tapping the tendon of a patient's muscle activates the muscle spindle and results in a muscle stretch reflex (p. 383).
- Type Ia fibers are heavily myelinated and rapidly conducting (p. 383).
- The muscle spindle is a mechanoreceptor essential to testing the integrity of muscle stretch reflexes (p. 383).
- One function of the Golgi tendon organ (a mechanoreceptor) is to mediate the amount of tension in a skeletal muscle (pp. 384–385).
- Lesions that damage vestibulospinal fibers/tracts will affect the activity of motor neurons innervating paravertebral and proximal limb extensor muscles (p. 385).
- Reticulospinal fibers influence the activity of motor neurons innervating paravertebral and limb extensor muscles (p. 386).
- Rapidly expanding supratentorial lesions may result is transtentorial (central) herniation (p. 387).
- The decerebrate patient presents with a constellation of deficits and progressive deterioration as the damage extends into the brainstem (p. 387).
- In general, the motor appearance of the decerebrate patient is one of rigidity (decerebrate rigidity) of all extremities (p. 387).
- Decerebrate rigidity is sometimes also known as gamma rigidity (p. 389).
- Decerebellate rigidity is sometimes referred to as alpha rigidity (p. 390).
- Decerebrate posturing is an ominous sign (p. 391).
- In general, a patient with decorticate posturing, or decorticate rigidity, has extension of the lower extremities and flexion of the upper extremities (p. 391).

Sources and Additional Reading

Boyd IA: The isolated mammalian muscle spindle. Trends Neurosci 3:258-265, 1980.

Brodal A: Neurological Anatomy in Relation to Clinical Medicine, 3rd Ed. New York, Oxford University Press, 1981, pp 148-211, 264-282.

Brooks VB (ed): Handbook of Physiology, section 1: The Nervous System, vol II. Motor Control, Part 1. Bethesda, MD, American Physiological Society, 1981.

Desmedt JE (ed): Spinal and Supraspinal Mechanisms of Voluntary Motor Control and Locomotion, vol 8. In Progress in Clinical Neurophysiology. Basel, Karger, 1980.

Mathews PBC: Evolving views on the internal operation and functional role of the muscle spindle. J Physiol (Lond) 320:1-30, 1981.

Shepherd GM: Neurobiology. New York, Oxford University Press, 1994.

Sherrington CS: Decerebrate rigidity and reflex coordination of movements. J Physiol (Lond) 22:319-332, 1898.

Taylor A, Prochazka A (eds): Muscle Receptors and Movement. London, Macmillan, 1981.

Chapter 25

Motor System II: Corticofugal Systems and the Control of Movement

G. A. Mihailoff and D. E. Haines

Brushing our teeth seems like a simple voluntary movement. The neural basis for this action is, in fact, richly complex. For example, muscles in the upper limb are used cooperatively with jaw muscles while neck and back muscles provide postural support. Sensory feedback from the teeth and gums is linked to muscle afferents conveying tension and proprioceptive signals from the forearm and hand. Even other, less obvious aspects, such as visual system input and memory of prior experience, are involved. The focus of this chapter is on elements of voluntary movement that are regulated by the cerebral cortex.

Overview

Control of the voluntary movements just described is a complex, multifaceted process that involves many areas of the brain. Several of the principal control sites are located in the cerebral cortex, specifically the *primary motor, premotor,* and *supplementary motor cortices* in the frontal lobe, along with portions of the parietal lobe. Although the frontal and parietal lobes have direct projections to the spinal cord, they also work cooperatively through the *primary motor cortex (upper motor neurons)* and the *corticospinal* and *corticonuclear (corticobulbar) systems* to influence the activity of ventral horn and cranial nerve motor neurons *(lower motor neurons)*. The latter cells and their axons represent the *final common path* that links the central nervous system with skeletal muscles. Lesions that damage the descending cortical systems or lower motor neurons produce signs and symptoms of *upper* or *lower motor neuron disease*, respectively. These signs are among the most useful in diagnosing neurologic deficits related to the control of movement.

General Features of Motor Deficits

Lower Motor Neuron Signs

Lower motor neurons are those cells whose axons synapse directly on skeletal muscle. When these neurons or their axons are damaged, the innervated muscles will show some combination of the following signs: (1) *flaccid paralysis* followed eventually by *atrophy*, (2) *fibrillations* or *fasciculations* (involuntary contractions of one motor unit or a group of motor units), (3) *hypotonia* (decreased muscle tone), and (4) weakening or absence of tendon (stretch) reflexes *(hyporeflexia, areflexia)*.

Upper Motor Neuron Signs

The term *upper motor neuron* is commonly used in reference to corticospinal or corticonuclear cell bodies and their axons. Other neurons, such as rubrospinal or reticulospinal neurons, can also be included under the strict definition of this term. Corticospinal neurons are also called *pyramidal neurons* because their axons pass through the medullary pyramid. Therefore, the terms *upper motor neuron signs* and *pyramidal tract signs* are often used synonymously. However, as described later in this chapter, these characteristic signs of "pyramidal tract damage" are in fact the result of injury to other descending motor systems in *combination* with damage to the pyramidal tract. For example, ischemic lesions of the internal capsule can potentially involve corticostriatal, corticothalamic, and corticoreticular fibers in addition to corticospinal axons.

Damage to upper motor neurons results in muscles that (1) are *initially weak* and *flaccid* but (2) eventually become *spastic*, (3) exhibit increased muscle tone *(hypertonia)*, seen as an increase in resistance to passive movement of an extremity, and (4) show an increase in deep tendon reflexes *(hyperreflexia)*, as may be seen in *clonus*. Upper motor neuron lesions usually *affect groups of muscles*, and certain pathologic reflexes and signs often appear. One of the most common is the *inverted plantar reflex*, also known as the *Babinski sign*. This involves dorsiflexion

of the great toe in response to firm stroking of the lateral aspect of the sole of the foot with a blunt instrument. The response in the normal adult is plantar flexion of the great toe.

Spasticity

Muscles that are no longer under the influence of upper motor neurons exhibit spasticity. That is, when tested by the examiner, the affected muscles offer an *increased resistance to passive movement or manipulation*. These effects are most pronounced in the antigravity muscles, which in humans include the proximal flexors in the upper extremity and extensors in the lower extremity. Also, the increased resistance to passive movement is velocity dependent: *the more rapidly the examiner moves the affected extremity, the greater the resistance*. However, after a relatively brief period of applied force, the increased resistance totally collapses; this response is known as the *clasp-knife effect*.

Several hypotheses have been advanced to explain spasticity. One suggests that spasticity, with its associated hypertonia and hyperreflexia, is the result of a release of *dynamic gamma motor neurons* from descending inhibitory control. This leads to increased gamma motor neuron firing and increased activity transmitted over type Ia muscle spindle afferents, resulting in increased excitatory tonic drive on the associated alpha motor neurons. Another suggestion is that spasticity may represent a *generalized failure of the descending cortical activation of spinal cord inhibitory interneurons*. For example, supraspinal fibers activate *type Ia* inhibitory interneurons that contact extensor motor neurons (Fig. 25-1A). If the upper motor neuron input to inhibitory interneurons were removed, the extensor motor neurons would be *released from inhibitory control*, and the result would be hypertonia and spasticity.

Descending cortical fibers also activate a type of inhibitory (glycinergic) interneuron called a *Renshaw cell* (Fig. 25-1B). The Renshaw cell receives excitatory input from a lower motor neuron via an axon collateral (and in turn it inhibits the same) and potentially from adjacent lower motor neurons. It is also known, for example, that cortical fibers activating ankle flexors also contact Renshaw cells (as well as type Ia inhibitory interneurons) that inhibit the antagonistic ankle extensors (Fig. 25-1B). This circuitry serves to prevent reflex stimulation of the extensors when flexors are active. Therefore, when the cortical fibers are lost (upper motor neuron lesion), the inhibition of antagonists is absent. The result is repetitive, sequential contraction of ankle flexors and extensors. Such a phenomenon is referred to as *clonus* and is often present in combination with spasticity and hyperreflexia.

Corticospinal System

Before the specifics of corticospinal projections are considered, a general point about laterality should be made. The fibers that form the core of the corticospinal system cross the midline in the pyramidal decussation; this structure is commonly called the *motor decussation* because it is where corticospinal fibers cross. Corticospinal fibers arising in the left motor cortex therefore influence muscles on the right side of the body, and vice versa. Consequently, *lesions of corticospinal fibers rostral to the pyramidal (motor) decussation result in contralateral motor deficits, whereas lesions of the corticospinal tract in the spinal cord result in ipsilateral deficits*. An understanding of this concept of laterality is essential in the diagnosis of the neurologically impaired patient.

Origin

Neurons that give rise to *corticospinal* axons are located in deep portions of layer V of the cerebral cortex (Fig. 25-2A). A small number of these pyramidal neurons are especially large, with

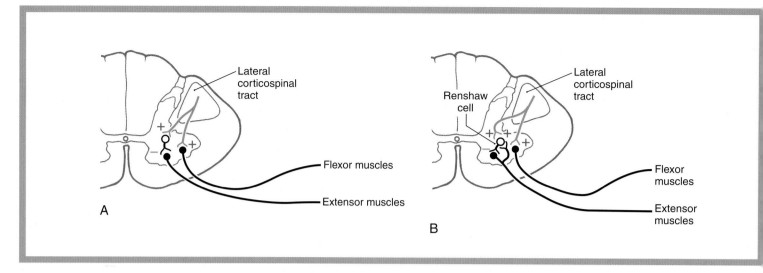

Figure 25-1. Connections by which descending fibers influence lower motor neurons. Direct influence and influence via an inhibitory interneuron (**A**) and influence via a Renshaw cell, which participates in a recurrent inhibition circuit (**B**).

somata that may reach 100 μm or more in diameter. These neurons are called *Betz cells*, and at one time it was believed that they were the sole source of corticospinal axons. Now it is known that they account for only 1% to 2% of this fiber bundle.

Corticospinal neurons are found primarily in six cortical locations (Fig. 25-2B). The single largest concentration (about 31%) is in *Brodmann area 4*, which occupies the posterior portion of the *precentral gyrus* bordering on and extending into the depth of the *central sulcus*. This region is also called *MI*, the *primary motor cortex*. The *premotor* and *supplementary motor cortices*, which are located in *area 6*, give rise to about 29% of corticospinal axons. Thus about 60% of all corticospinal axons arise from neurons in the *frontal lobe*, with more than one half of this group coming from the *precentral* and *anterior paracentral gyri* (Fig. 25-2B). The remaining approximately 40% arise from the *parietal lobe* and a few other regions. Included are cells in the *postcentral gyrus* (areas 3, 1, and 2), the *superior parietal lobule* (areas 5 and 7), and portions of the *cingulate gyrus*.

Within MI, corticospinal neurons are somatotopically organized in patterns that reflect their influence over specific muscle groups. The caricature thus created is called the *motor homunculus* (Fig. 25-3A). Neurons in medial MI, the anterior paracentral gyrus, project to lumbosacral cord levels to influence motor neurons that innervate muscles of the foot, leg, and thigh. Thoracic and cervical cord levels, which contain motor neurons innervating the trunk and upper extremity, receive input from neurons in the medial two thirds of the precentral gyrus. The musculature of the head, face, and oral cavity is influenced by neurons in the lateral one third of the precentral gyrus (Fig. 25-3A). These cells contribute to the *corticonuclear (corticobulbar) tract* that projects to cranial nerve motor nuclei. The disproportion in body part size in the *homunculus* reflects the density and distribution of corticospinal neurons devoted to the control of musculature in each particular region of the body (Fig. 25-3A). Complete, but less precise, body representations are also found in other motor cortical regions. Thus, a single muscle or muscle group can be influenced from multiple locations in the cerebral cortex.

The blood supply to MI arises from branches of the anterior and middle cerebral arteries (Fig. 25-3B). The lower extremity area of MI is served by terminal branches of the A_2 segment of the anterior cerebral artery. Specifically, these branches arise from the *callosomarginal artery*. The trunk, upper extremity, and head areas of the motor cortex are supplied by branches of

the M_4 segment of the middle cerebral artery, mainly its *rolandic* and *prerolandic branches*.

Lesions that involve only areas of motor cortex outside the MI usually do not result in paralysis, and the effects may dissipate over time. For example, vascular infarcts of the premotor or supplementary cortex may produce an *apraxia*. This disorder involves difficulty in using the affected part of the body to perform voluntary actions, such as grasping a pencil, even though there is no obvious spasticity, paralysis, or altered tone in the muscles. For example, a premotor lesion may result in the inability to perform voluntary actions with the contralateral hand, although the strength and tone of the hand muscles are normal. Similarly, unilateral lesions in the supplementary motor cortex affect the ability to coordinate actions on the two sides of the body. The muscles, again, are normal. In contrast, lesions that affect both the primary motor cortex in combination with another motor cortical region usually result in spastic paralysis and hyperreflexia, signs characteristic of upper motor neuron lesions.

Course

The largest axons in the corticospinal tract are myelinated, range from 12 to 15 μm in diameter, and have conduction velocities up to 70 m/s, but they make up less than 10% of the total corticospinal population. The remainder are less than 5 μm in diameter, and many are lightly myelinated or unmyelinated with proportionally slower conduction velocities.

Corticospinal fibers pass through the corona radiata and converge to enter the *posterior limb of the internal capsule* (Fig. 25-4A). Here the fibers are somatotopically organized in about the caudal half of the posterior limb such that the axons that terminate at the highest cord levels are located most rostrally and the axons that terminate at progressively lower levels are located more caudally (Fig. 25-4B).

Unlike lesions of the cortical gray matter, interruption of axons in the posterior limb of the internal capsule often results in catastrophic motor deficits. A common cause of lesions in this area is hemorrhage from *lenticulostriate branches* of the M_1 segment of the middle cerebral artery (Fig. 25-4A). Motor symptoms of capsular infarcts appear in the contralateral upper and lower extremities and consist of weakness and transient flaccid paralysis of variable duration, which is followed by spastic paralysis (upper motor neuron signs) that typically never resolves. Apparently these symptoms appear because not only

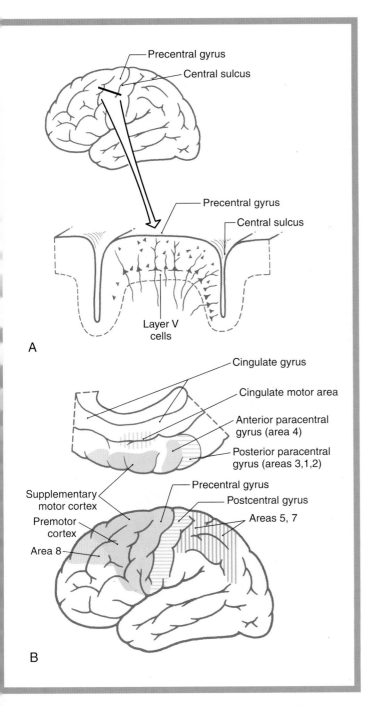

Figure 25-2. The motor-related areas of the cortex. A cross section through the precentral gyrus, showing pyramidal cells in layer V (**A**). The main areas of the cortex that give rise to corticospinal axons (**B**).

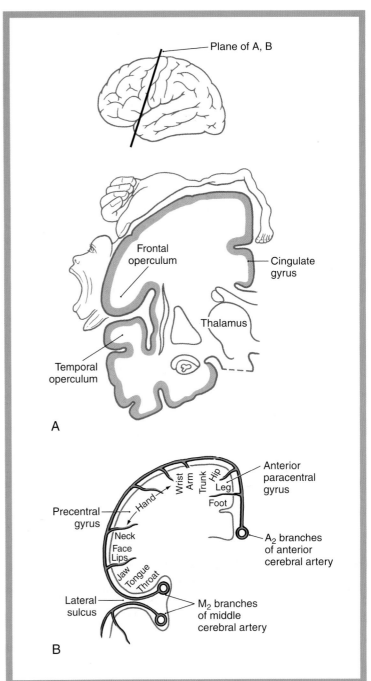

Figure 25-3. Coronal views of the cerebral hemisphere showing the somatotopy of the primary motor cortex (**A**, **B**) and the blood supply of the anterior paracentral lobule and the precentral gyrus (**B**).
(**A** is adapted from Penfield W, Rasmussen T: The Cerebral Cortex of Man: A Clinical Study of Localization of Function. New York, Hafner Publishing, 1968, with permission.)

corticospinal fibers but also many other types of cortical axons are interrupted. Included are axons projecting to the neostriatum, thalamus, and brainstem, as well as thalamocortical axons involved in somatic sensation and vision. Damage to thalamocortical axons explains why *hemisensory loss or homonymous hemianopia may accompany the motor deficit.* It is important to note that deficits such as *spasticity, hypertonia,* and *hyperreflexia,* although commonly associated with pyramidal tract lesions, are in fact due to damage of other descending systems in *combination* with damage to corticospinal fibers.

As they pass caudally from the internal capsule, corticospinal fibers traverse the various divisions of the brainstem. In the midbrain they coalesce to form the middle third of the crus cerebri (Figs. 25-5A, 25-6, and 25-7). Within this part of the crus, fibers from forearm/hand areas of MI are located medially whereas those from leg/foot areas are located laterally.

Fibers in the medial two thirds of the crus cerebri (frontopontine, corticonuclear [corticobulbar], and corticospinal) and the exiting rootlets of the oculomotor nerve fibers are served by *paramedian branches of P_1* and branches from the adjacent *posterior communicating artery* (Fig. 25-6). Hemorrhage of these vessels will damage these groups of fibers, resulting in (1) *contralateral hemiparesis* of the arm and leg with spasticity and (2) *deviation of the ipsilateral eye* down and laterally, owing to the unopposed action of the superior oblique and lateral rectus muscles. *Direct* and *consensual light reflexes* and *accommodation* may also be lost in the eye on the side of the lesion. This condition is known as *superior alternating hemiplegia* because cranial nerve signs are seen on one side and corticospinal signs on the

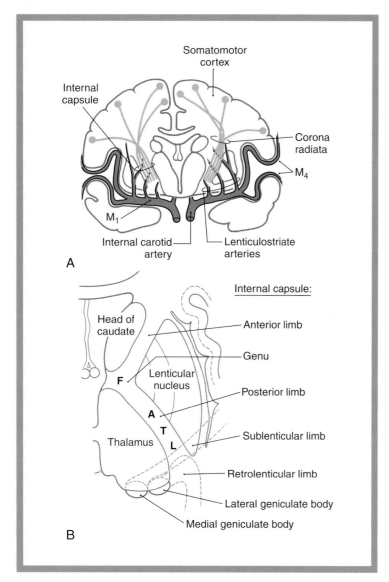

Figure 25-4. Descending fibers of the corticospinal and corticonuclear (corticobulbar) systems in the internal capsule in coronal (**A**) and axial (**B**) planes. The positions of fibers from face (F), arm-upper extremity (A), trunk (T), and leg-lower extremity (L) areas are shown in the internal capsule in the axial plane (**B**).

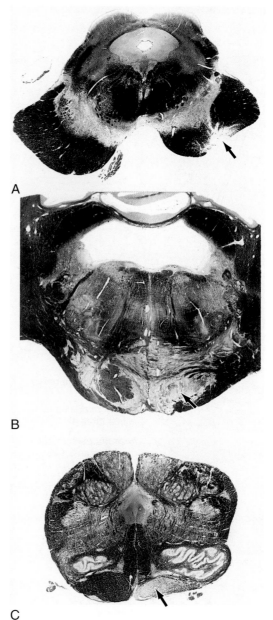

Figure 25-5. Degeneration of corticospinal fibers caused by an infarction in the posterior limb of the internal capsule. The degeneration serves as a marker to show the position of these fibers (at *arrows*) in the middle third of the crus cerebri (**A**), the basilar pons (**B**), and the pyramid of the medulla (**C**).

"alternate" side; also called a *crossed deficit*. In clinical parlance this combination of deficits is known as a *Weber syndrome* (Fig. 25-8 and Table 25-1).

From the midbrain, corticospinal fibers continue into the basilar pons, where they make their way longitudinally between the masses of neurons forming the basilar pontine nuclei (Figs. 25-5B, 25-6, and 25-7). As corticospinal axons pass through the pontine gray, they give rise to collaterals that synapse on these neurons.

Corticospinal fibers in the basilar pons and the exiting fibers of the abducens nerve in the caudal pons are within the domain of the *paramedian branches of the basilar artery*. Occlusion or rupture of these vessels results in *hemiplegia* and *upper motor neuron* signs in the contralateral extremities. The lesion may also involve *intra-axial* abducens fibers, resulting in *lower motor neuron paralysis of the ipsilateral lateral rectus muscle* (Fig. 25-9). This combination of deficits (ipsilateral abducens paralysis and contralateral hemiplegia) is (1) a characteristic of brainstem lesions—that is, a *crossed deficit*, (2) called a *middle alternating hemiplegia*, and (3) one of the variations of the *Foville syndrome* (Table 25-1). The paramedian branches of the basilar artery may penetrate deep into the pons and also serve the medial lemniscus (Fig. 25-9). In such cases, damage to these vessels can produce

not only the motor deficits described earlier but also *contralateral loss of vibratory sense and two-point tactile discrimination*.

In the medulla, corticospinal fibers aggregate on the anterior surface of the brainstem, where they course within the medullary pyramids (Figs. 25-5C, 25-6, and 25-7). Within the pyramid fibers that terminate at cervical levels tend to be located medially whereas those projecting to lumbar and sacral levels are more lateral. Collaterals of these axons innervate the inferior olivary complex, posterior column nuclei, and various medullary reticular nuclei.

The pyramid, the laterally adjacent exiting fibers of the hypoglossal nerve, and the medial lemniscus receive their blood supply through penetrating branches of the *anterior spinal artery* (Fig. 25-6). Occlusion of these branches results in a *contralateral hemiparesis of the extremities* (with spasticity) and an *ipsilateral flaccid paralysis of the tongue*. When protruded, the tongue deviates toward the side of the lesion (the weak or flaccid side). This combination of symptoms is called *inferior alternating hemiplegia*. Because branches of the anterior spinal artery also

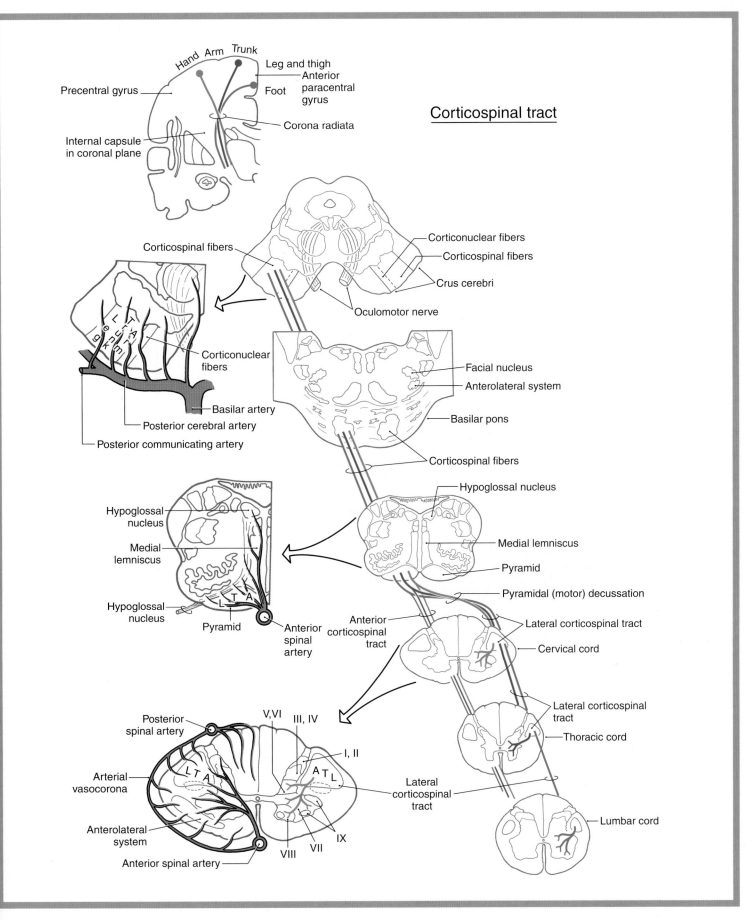

Corticospinal tract

Figure 25-6. The corticospinal system with details showing the blood supply to these fibers in the midbrain, medulla, and spinal cord.

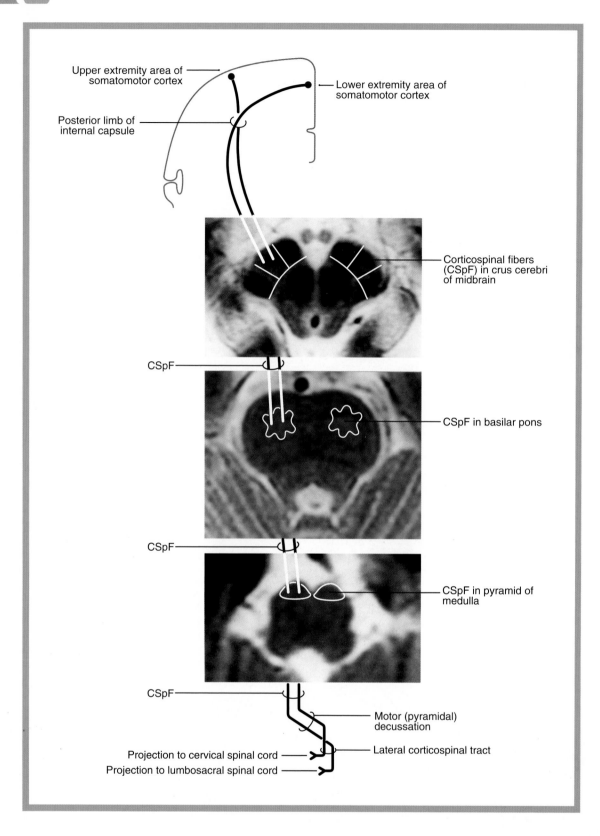

Upper extremity area of somatomotor cortex

Lower extremity area of somatomotor cortex

Posterior limb of internal capsule

Corticospinal fibers (CSpF) in crus cerebri of midbrain

CSpF

CSpF in basilar pons

CSpF

CSpF in pyramid of medulla

CSpF

Motor (pyramidal) decussation

Projection to cervical spinal cord

Projection to lumbosacral spinal cord

Lateral corticospinal tract

Figure 25-7. The location of corticospinal fibers in MR images representative levels of the midbrain, pons, and medulla. This illustrates the location of corticospinal fibers when viewed i images routinely used in the clinical setting.

serve the medial lemniscus, an inferior alternating hemiplegia is typically accompanied by a *contralateral loss of two-point discrimination and vibration sense.* Lesions of the medial medulla characterized by *crossed* (or alternating) *deficits,* as described earlier for other brainstem levels, are also known as the *Dejerine syndrome* (Table 25-1). Additional brainstem syndromes that may involve cranial nerves and corticospinal fibers in various combinations are summarized in Table 25-1.

At the medullospinal junction, 85% to 90% of the corticospinal fibers cross the midline as the *(motor pyramidal) decussation* (Fig. 25-6). Fibers that cross in the rostral and caudal portions of the pyramidal decussation originate, respectively, from the upper and lower extremity areas of MI cortex. This arrangement

explains why small vascular lesions in the decussation (which i also served by branches of the *anterior spinal artery*) may resul in bilateral weakness or paralysis of either the upper or lowe extremities. The decussating fibers extend into the lateral funic ulus to form the *lateral corticospinal tract.* The corticospina axons that do not cross in the decussation continue into the ipsilateral anterior funiculus of the spinal cord as the *anterio corticospinal tract* (Fig. 25-6). Damage to this tract is of littl clinical significance. This is because most of the fibers in thi tract cross in the spinal cord prior to termination.

The crossing of corticospinal fibers at the *motor decussatio* is the anatomic basis for the contralateral deficits seen in . patient with a lesion where these fibers are rostral to (above) thi

Table 25-1. Synopsis of Brainstem Syndromes Involving Corticospinal Fibers and Cranial Nerves*

Syndrome	Structure(s) Involved	Corresponding Deficit
Benedikt syndrome (Weber + Claude)	Corticospinal fibers in crus Oculomotor nerve fibers Red nucleus Cerebellothalamic fibers (Medial lemniscus)	Contralateral hemiplegia Ipsilateral oculomotor palsy, dilated pupil, diplopia Contralateral tremor, hyperkinesias Contralateral ataxia (Contralateral loss of vibratory sense, position sense, discriminative touch)
Claude syndrome[†]	Oculomotor nerve fibers Red nucleus Cerebellothalamic fibers (Trochlear nucleus)	Ipsilateral oculomotor palsy, dilated pupil, diplopia Contralateral tremor, hyperkinesias Contralateral ataxia (Weakness of contralateral superior oblique muscle)
Dejerine syndrome (medial medullary)	Corticospinal fibers in pyramid Hypoglossal nerve fibers/nucleus Medial lemniscus	Contralateral hemiplegia Ipsilateral deviation of tongue on protrusion Contralateral loss of vibratory sense, position sense, discriminative touch
Foville syndrome[‡]	Corticospinal fibers in basilar pons Abducens nerve fibers Middle cerebellar peduncle	Contralateral hemiplegia Ipsilateral abducens (lateral rectus) palsy, diplopia Ataxia
Gubler or Millard-Gubler syndrome[§]	Corticospinal fibers in basilar pons Facial nerve fibers or nucleus (Anterolateral system) (Trigeminal nerve fibers)	Contralateral hemiplegia Ipsilateral weakness of facial muscles (Impaired pain and thermal sense on contralateral side of body) (Impaired pain and thermal sense on ipsilateral side of face)
Midpontine base syndrome	Corticospinal fibers in basilar pons Trigeminal nerve fibers Middle cerebellar peduncle	Contralateral hemiplegia Ipsilateral paralysis of masticatory muscles; ipsilateral loss of pain and thermal sensations on face Ataxia
Raymond syndrome	Corticospinal fibers in basilar pons Abducens fibers in basilar pons	Contralateral hemiplegia Ipsilateral abducens (lateral rectus) palsy, diplopia
Wallenberg syndrome (lateral medullary, PICA)	Spinal trigeminal tract Anterolateral system Vestibular nuclei Nucleus ambiguus Restiform body	Ipsilateral loss of pain and thermal sense on face Contralateral loss of pain and thermal sense on the body Vertigo, nystagmus, nausea, vomiting Hoarseness, dysphagia, deviation of the uvula to opposite side on phonation Ataxia
Weber syndrome	Corticospinal fibers in crus Oculomotor nerve fibers Corticonuclear fibers in crus Substantia nigra	Contralateral hemiplegia Ipsilateral oculomotor palsy, dilated pupil, diplopia Contralateral weakness of facial muscles on lower half of face; deviation of the tongue to contralateral side on protrusion; ipsilateral weakness of trapezius and sternocleidomastoid muscles Contralateral Parkinson-like tremor, akinesia

*Syndromes are listed in alphabetical order.
[†]Although this syndrome does not include corticospinal fibers it is included here for completeness.
[‡]This syndrome is described, in some sources, as including the facial nerve/nucleus, anterolateral system fibers, paramedian pontine reticular formation (lateral gaze center), and the medial lemniscus, each with their corresponding deficits.
[§]Some sources also include the fibers of the abducens nerve as being involved in this syndrome.
Note: Those structures/deficits listed in parentheses are inconsistently seen in these respective syndromes.
Lesions in the lateral areas of the brainstem interrupt descending hypothalamospinal fibers to the interomediolateral cell column (GVE preganglionic sympathetic cells) of the spinal cord. An ipsilateral *Horner syndrome* (*ptosis*, a drooping eyelid; *miosis*, constricted pupil; *anhidrosis*, lack of facial sweating) is commonly seen in these patients.

lecussation. For example, a patient with a capsular lesion *on the right side will have hemiparesis of the upper and lower extremities n the left* (Fig. 25-10). This patient may also exhibit additional leficits related to damage of corticonuclear fibers in the genu of he internal capsule, such as drooping of the face and weakness of the sternocleidomastoid muscle; these deficits are discussed ater in the section on the corticonuclear system.

Termination

Fibers of the lateral corticospinal tract are topographically organized (Figs. 25-6 and 25-7). Axons terminating in cervical cord evels are most medial in this tract, whereas those distributing to

lumbosacral levels are most lateral. This pattern means that, as the medially located fibers enter and terminate in the spinal gray, the adjacent, more lateral fascicles shift medially.

Corticospinal fibers that arise from the frontal lobe terminate primarily in the intermediate zone and anterior horn (laminae VII to IX), whereas fibers arising from the parietal lobe terminate in the base of the posterior horn (laminae IV to VI). As might be expected, most fibers terminate in the spinal cord enlargements that serve the extremities; about 55% terminate in the cervical enlargement, and about 25% terminate in the lumbosacral enlargement. The remaining fibers terminate at thoracic levels. As mentioned earlier, some corticospinal fibers terminate, via

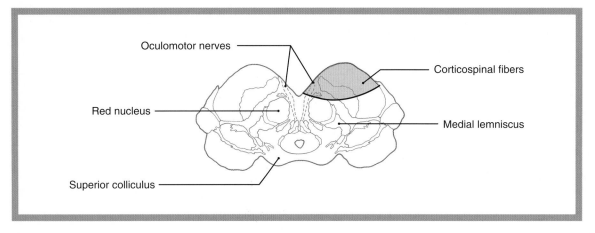

Figure 25-8. The location of a lesion that results in deficits seen in a Weber syndrome. This illustration is in a clinical orientation (as seen in MRI or CT); consequently, the observer's right is the patient's left and the observer's left is the patient's right.

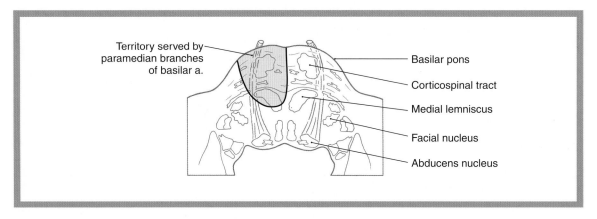

Figure 25-9. A lesion of the pons representing occlusion of the paramedian branches of the basilar artery. This illustration is in a clinical orientation (as seen in MRI or CT); consequently, the observer's right is the patient's left and the observer's left is the patient's right.

their collateral branches, at multiple levels. However, the influence exerted by any single axon or its collaterals depends on the *number* of synapses it forms and the locus of the synaptic contacts on the postsynaptic neuron. Thus, a given corticospinal axon may have a powerful action on some spinal cord neurons and only a weak influence on others.

At their level of termination, particularly in the cord enlargements, corticospinal fibers synapse primarily on *interneurons* in laminae V to VII. In animals capable of dexterous finger movements, such as monkeys and humans, some corticospinal fibers terminate among clusters of lamina IX alpha motor neurons, which innervate distal flexor muscles. However, most corticospinal fibers, at least in nonhuman primates, synapse with excitatory and inhibitory interneurons, which, in turn, influence flexor and extensor motor neurons, respectively.

Interruption of lateral corticospinal axons in the *upper cervical cord* (C1, C2) results in spastic hemiplegia involving the ipsilateral upper and lower extremities (Fig. 25-11). Common upper motor neuron signs such as *hypertonia*, *hyperreflexia*, and the *Babinski sign* will be present ipsilateral to the lesion. If the lesion is sufficiently large, the innervation of the diaphragm (from C3 to C5 via the phrenic nerve) may be disrupted, necessitating the use of a respirator.

A lesion of the *cervical enlargement* results in a different pattern of motor deficits (Fig. 25-11). If the damage involves only the lateral funiculus, then the ipsilateral upper and lower extremities will exhibit typical upper motor neuron signs. If, however, the C6 to C8 anterior horn gray matter and the lateral funiculus white matter are both included in the lesion, then *lower motor neuron signs will appear in the upper extremity*

ipsilaterally, whereas upper motor neuron signs will be seen in the ipsilateral lower extremity. When anterior horn motor neurons or their axons are damaged, the affected muscles exhibit lower motor neuron signs, despite the fact that supraspinal axons providing input to these cells may also have been interrupted.

At *lumbosacral levels*, injury to the spinal cord frequently affects motor neurons in the anterior horn as well as descending supraspinal fibers (Fig. 25-11). Characteristically, affected patients exhibit lower motor neuron signs in the ipsilateral lower extremity if both the corticospinal fibers and anterior horn motor neurons are damaged.

The blood supply to the lateral corticospinal tract is derived from *penetrating branches of the arterial vasocorona* and *sulcal branches of the anterior spinal artery* (Fig. 25-6). The former serve fibers in lateral parts of the tract, and the latter serve the medially located fibers. Hyperextension of the neck may result in injury to the cord or in occlusion of the sulcal arteries *(central cord syndrome)*; either can result in bilateral hemiparesis of the upper extremities secondary to vascular infarcts involving medial regions of both lateral corticospinal tracts. In addition, affected patients may also exhibit both urinary retention and a bilateral patchy loss of pain and temperature sensations below the lesion.

A functional hemisection of the spinal cord, such as may be caused by a tumor or by trauma, results in a characteristic set of deficits known as the *Brown-Séquard syndrome* (Fig. 25-12; also see Fig. 18-9). These deficits begin about two levels below the lesion and consist of (1) *ipsilateral* loss of two-point discrimination and vibration (from damage to the dorsal columns), (2) *contralateral* loss of pain and thermal sensation (from damage to the anterolateral system), and (3) an *ipsilateral* paresis or

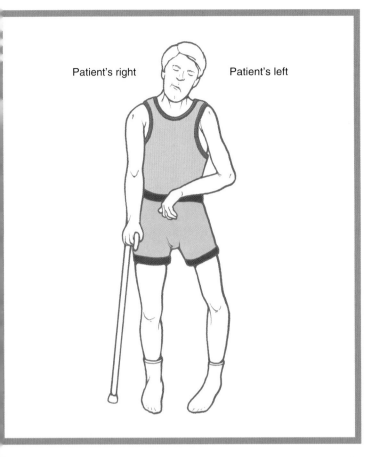

Figure 25-10. Patient with a lesion of the internal capsule on the right side. This man exhibits a left hemiparesis, drooping of the lower part of the face on the left, and slight turning of the head to the right (weak right sternocleidomastoid muscle).

paralysis (from damage to the corticospinal tract). The paralysis involves the upper and lower extremities or only the lower, depending on the level of the injury. Also, if the lesion is large enough that it involves several spinal cord levels, damage to a sufficient number of primary afferent fibers entering the cord may result in a narrow band of complete anesthesia on the side ipsilateral to the lesion in dermatomes corresponding to the damaged cord segments.

Corticonuclear (Corticobulbar) System

Origin

Organized in parallel with the corticospinal system is the *corticonuclear (corticobulbar) system* (Fig. 25-13). As defined here, the corticonuclear system consists of the cortical neurons that influence the movements of striated muscles innervated by the motor nuclei of cranial nerves V, VII, and XII, by the nucleus ambiguus (cranial nerves IX and X), and by the accessory nucleus.

The term "corticobulbar" was historically used to describe all cortical projections to cranial nerve nuclei of the brainstem. The suffix "bulbar" comes from "bulb," an obsolete term for the medulla oblongata. The international committee (see Preface) charged with establishing anatomic terminology studied the inherent problems with this term; for example, how can there be "corticobulbar" projections to cranial nerve nuclei that are not in the "bulb"? After detailed consideration by the committee, and with the publication of the new terminology in 1998, the term "corticobulbar" was replaced with terms that accurately

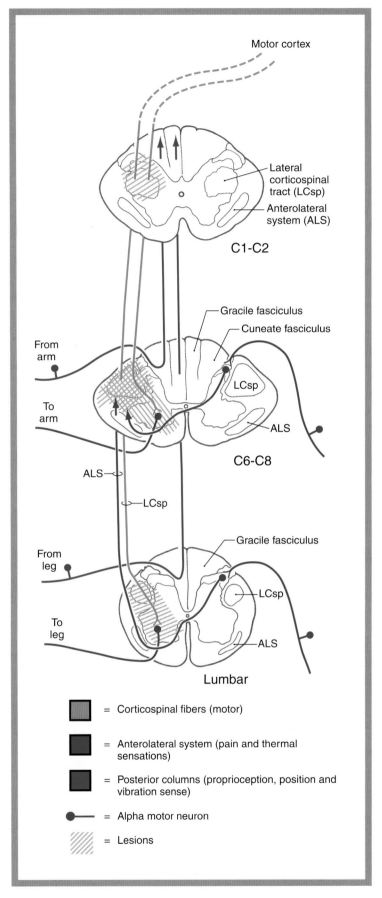

Figure 25-11. Examples of spinal cord lesions at C1 to C2 (involving only corticospinal fibers), at C6 to C8 (involving corticospinal fibers only, or these plus the anterior horn), and at lumbar levels (involving corticospinal fibers and the anterior horn). Arm, upper extremity; leg, lower extremity.

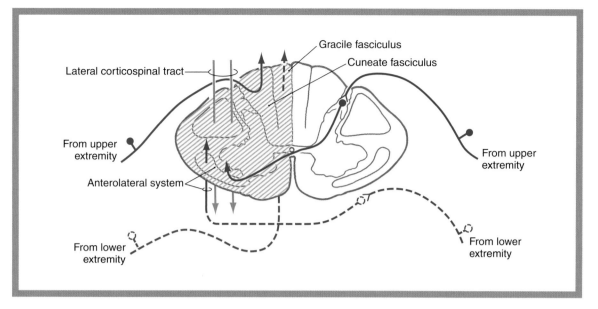

Figure 25-12. Hemisection of the spinal cord (Brown-Séquard syndrome).

describe these connections. These terms are as follows: *fibrae corticonucleares bulbi* for cortical projections to cranial nerve nuclei in the bulb/medulla (medullary corticonuclear fibers), *fibrae corticonucleares pontis* for cortical projections to cranial nerve nuclei of the pons (pontine corticonuclear fibers), and *fibrae corticonucleares mesencephali* for similar projections to the midbrain (mesencephalic corticonuclear fibers). Here these terms are shortened to simply *corticonuclear*, and this new and preferred term is used synonymously with the replaced term "corticobulbar."

Some corticonuclear axons project directly to cranial motor neurons, but most terminate on reticular formation interneurons immediately adjacent to the cranial nerve nuclei. The corticonuclear system originates for the most part from the face and head area of the precentral gyrus (Fig. 25-13). Because most of the musculature innervated by cranial nerves is located in the facial region, this area of MI is typically called *face motor cortex*.

The oculomotor, trochlear, and abducens nuclei do not receive direct input from the face motor cortex. Instead, voluntary control of eye movement is mediated via cortical projections from *frontal* and *parietal motor eye fields* to eye movement (gaze) control centers in the midbrain and pons. These centers in the *midbrain reticular formation* and the *paramedian pontine reticular formation*, in turn, relay input from the cortical eye fields to somatic motor neurons in the nuclei of cranial nerves III, IV, and VI (see Chapter 28 for details). Although the cortex of each hemisphere influences these nuclei bilaterally, the resulting eye movements are conjugate and are toward the side contralateral to the cortex from which the input originated. Because these cortical axons are often several synapses removed from the actual cranial nerve motor neurons, they are not considered part of the corticonuclear system as defined in this text.

Course

Corticonuclear axons that originate from cells in layer V of the face motor cortex funnel into the *genu of the internal capsule* (Fig. 25-4). Corticonuclear fibers continue into the crus cerebri, where they are located medial to corticospinal fibers traveling to cervical cord levels (Figs. 25-6 and 25-13). From here, these axons descend into the pons and medulla in association with corticospinal fibers. Corticonuclear fibers in the genu and in the crus cerebri receive their blood supply from lenticulostrate arteries and from the paramedian branches of the basilar bifurcation, respectively.

Termination

As corticonuclear fibers pass through the basilar pons, branche arch superiorly into the pontine tegmentum to terminate bilaterally in the areas of the trigeminal and facial motor nucle (Fig. 25-13). The fibers to the trigeminal motor nuclei terminate on interneurons adjacent to the nuclei. The corticonuclear system sends nearly equal numbers of fibers to the left and right trigeminal motor nuclei.

Likewise, nearly equal numbers of fibers are sent to the left and right facial motor nuclei. Whereas the muscles of facial expression in the upper half of the face are controlled about equally from both hemispheres, *muscles in the lower half of the face are influenced primarily from the contralateral hemisphere* Consequently, a lesion of corticonuclear fibers rostral to the facial motor nucleus results in drooping of muscles at the corne of the mouth and on the lower portion of the face *on the side opposite the lesion* (Figs. 25-10 and 25-14A). This deficit is called a *central facial paralysis (central seven)*. In contrast, a lesion of the root of the facial nerve will result in a flaccid paralysis of facial muscles of *upper and lower portions of the face on the ipsilateral side* (Fig. 25-14B); this deficit is called a *Bell (facial) palsy*.

At midmedullary levels, corticonuclear fibers pass superiorly to reach the ambiguus and hypoglossal nuclei (Fig. 25-13) Projections to nucleus ambiguus motor neurons are generally bilateral. However, the motor neurons that innervate muscular parts of the soft palate and uvula receive mainly a contralateral input. Consequently, a lesion of corticonuclear fibers to the nucleus ambiguus may produce a weakness in the affected muscles and *result in failure of the soft palate to elevate on the contralateral side and in deviation of the uvula (especially on attempted phonation) toward the side of the lesion* (Fig. 25-15).

In the case of the hypoglossal nuclei, although corticonuclear fibers in general distribute bilaterally, those *motor neurons that innervate the genioglossus muscles receive primarily contralateral corticonuclear input*. Each genioglossus muscle pulls its half of the tongue anteriorly and slightly medially. When the two muscles function together and symmetrically, the tongue protrudes straight out of the mouth. However, a lesion of corticonuclear fibers to the hypoglossal nucleus will cause the tongue to *deviate toward the weak (contralateral to the lesion) side when protruded* because of the unopposed pull of the intact muscle (Fig. 25-15) In this example of a lesion of corticonuclear fibers (upper motor neurons) the tongue will deviate (on protrusion) *toward the side*

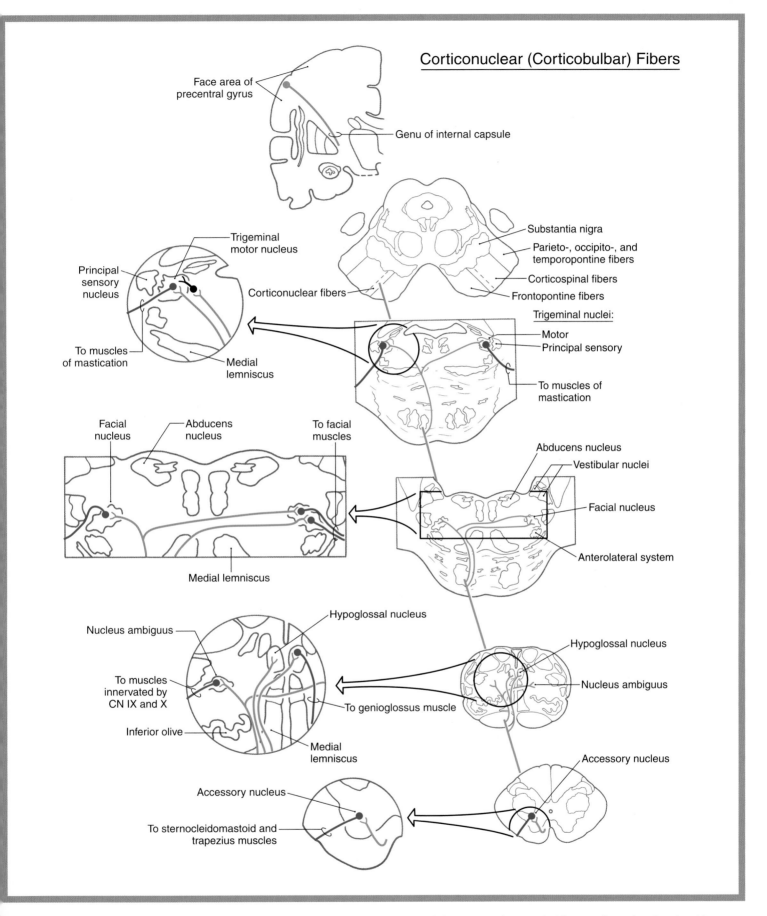

Corticonuclear (Corticobulbar) Fibers

Face area of precentral gyrus

Genu of internal capsule

Trigeminal motor nucleus

Principal sensory nucleus

Corticonuclear fibers

To muscles of mastication

Medial lemniscus

Substantia nigra

Parieto-, occipito-, and temporopontine fibers

Corticospinal fibers

Frontopontine fibers

Trigeminal nuclei:
Motor
Principal sensory

To muscles of mastication

Facial nucleus

Abducens nucleus

To facial muscles

Abducens nucleus

Vestibular nuclei

Facial nucleus

Anterolateral system

Medial lemniscus

Nucleus ambiguus

Hypoglossal nucleus

Hypoglossal nucleus

To muscles innervated by CN IX and X

Nucleus ambiguus

Inferior olive

To genioglossus muscle

Medial lemniscus

Accessory nucleus

Accessory nucleus

To sternocleidomastoid and trapezius muscles

Figure 25-13. The corticonuclear (corticobulbar) system with details shown at the levels of the trigeminal motor, facial motor, hypoglossal and ambiguus, and accessory nuclei. CN, cranial nerve.

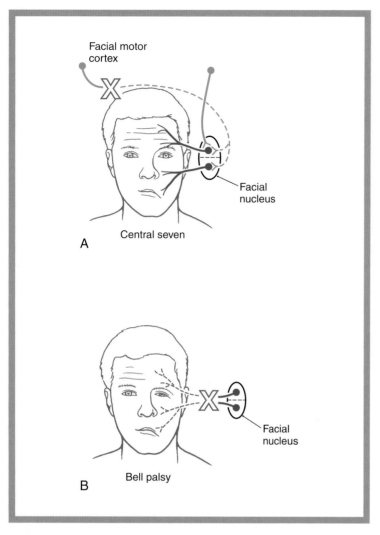

Figure 25-14. Appearance of the face following a lesion of corticonuclear (corticobulbar) fibers to the facial nucleus (**A**) versus a lesion of the root of the facial nerve (**B**). The large "X" indicates the location of the lesion.

opposite the lesion (Fig. 25-15), and the patient may have other symptoms characteristic of a lesion of the genu of the internal capsule, such as a central seven or a deviation of the uvula. In contrast, an injury to the hypoglossal nerve (lower motor neurons) will result in *deviation of the tongue toward the side of the lesion* (weak side) on protrusion (Fig. 25-16) and ultimately lead to the appearance of lower motor neuron signs in the tongue, such as muscle atrophy and a flaccid paralysis. If, however, the lesion is in the medial medulla and involves the root of the hypoglossal nerve, pyramid, and medial lemniscus, the patient may experience an ipsilateral deviation of the tongue along with a contralateral hemiparesis (corticospinal fiber involvement) and a contralateral loss of posterior column modalities (medial lemniscus involvement). This combination of deficits is an *inferior alternating hemiplegia* (*medial medullary* or *Dejerine syndrome*; Table 25-1). Hypoglossal root fibers, corticospinal fibers, and the medial lemniscus have a common blood supply, in the medulla, from the anterior spinal artery.

The final contingent of corticonuclear (corticobulbar) fibers innervates the spinal portion of cranial nerve XI *(accessory nucleus)* (Fig. 25-13). These fibers continue into the upper cervical spinal cord along with corticospinal fibers. Clinical observations in patients with cortical or internal capsule lesions reveal that the sternocleidomastoid and trapezius muscles (targets of accessory motor neurons) are affected mainly on the side ipsilateral to the lesion. The patient is unable to shrug or elevate that shoulder (especially against resistance) or to turn the head away from the side of the lesion (Fig. 25-10). This finding suggests that *corticonuclear fibers distribute primarily to the ipsilateral accessory nucleus.*

Because the corticospinal and corticonuclear systems course adjacent to each other, it is common for lesions of the internal capsule or midbrain to affect both fiber bundles. For example, lenticulostriate arteries serve portions of the genu and most of the posterior limb of the internal capsule (Fig. 25-4A). Consequently, hemorrhage of these vessels on the *right side* results in (1) a *left spastic hemiparesis* of the extremities (corticospinal damage), (2) a *central facial paralysis* on the left, (3) a *deviation*

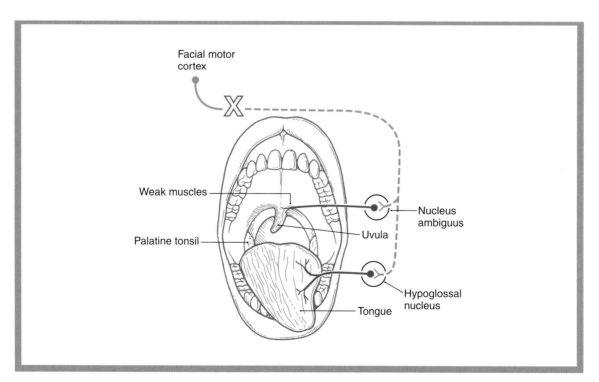

Figure 25-15. Deviation of the uvula and of the tongue following a lesion of corticonuclear (corticobulbar) fibers to the nucleus ambiguus and hypoglossal nucleus, respectively. The large "X" indicates the side of the lesion. Note that the tongue deviates to the side opposite the lesion, whereas the uvula deviates toward the side of the lesion. Compare the deviation of the tongue with that in Figure 25-13.

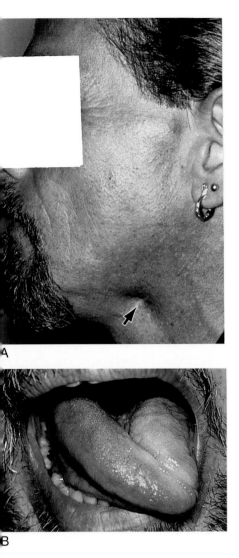

A

B

Figure 25-16. Paralysis of the tongue on the left side. Removal of a lymph node from the left side of the neck (**A**, *arrow*) inadvertently resulted in damage to peripheral fibers of the hypoglossal nerve on that side. The tongue deviates to the left (side of the lesion) on protrusion (**B**).

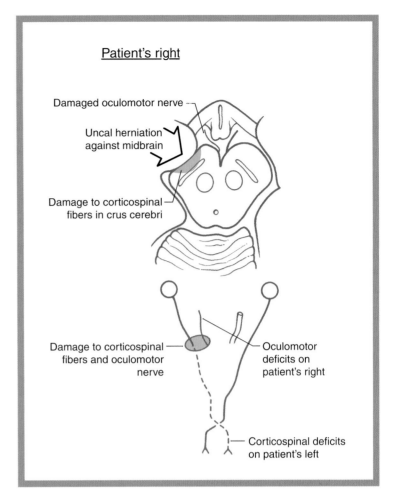

Figure 25-17. Uncal herniation on the patient's right damaging the oculomotor nerve and corticospinal fibers in the crus cerebri, both on the side of the herniation. The result is alternating oculomotor and corticospinal deficits.

of the uvula to the right on phonation, and (4) a *deviation of the tongue to the left* when protruded. The latter three deficits are the result of damage to corticonuclear fibers. Effects on the trapezius and sternocleidomastoid muscles are variable but if present will usually involve the muscles ipsilateral to the lesion of corticonuclear fibers (Figs. 25-10 and 25-14 to 25-16).

Lesions that impinge on, or are located within, any level of the brainstem may produce corticospinal and corticonuclear signs in various combinations depending on the level of the brainstem involved and what cranial nerve root is damaged along with the corticospinal fibers. One example is the case of herniation of the uncus through the tentorial notch (Fig. 25-17). Increased intracranial pressure in a supratentorial compartment forces the uncus over the edge of the tentorium and into the midbrain, damaging the oculomotor nerve and the crus cerebri *on that side*. The deficits experienced by the patient are an ipsilateral paralysis of most eye movement, *diplopia*, and a dilated pupil (oculomotor damage) and a contralateral *hemiplegia* (damage to corticospinal fibers in the crus) (Fig. 25-17). This is an example of one lesion that results in a Weber syndrome (Table 25-1). In patients with corticospinal signs accompanied by cranial nerve signs on the opposite side of the body, two important facts come to mind. *First*, these *alternating* or *crossed* deficits are a *hallmark of brainstem lesions*. *Second*, the cranial nerve deficit is the best *localizing sign* since it provides, in combination with a long-tract

deficit (corticospinal in this example), the most precise location/level of the lesion.

Having made this distinction, concerning the localizing sign, it is important to realize that there are examples of what are called *false localizing signs*. These are cases in which the signs are counter to what one would expect. One example of this is the *Kernohan syndrome* (also called the *Kernohan notch phenomenon*). This is a variation on uncal herniation against the midbrain (Fig. 25-18). In a Kernohan lesion the herniating uncus displaces the midbrain (and crus cerebri) against the edge of the tentorium cerebelli on the side contralateral to the herniation (Fig. 25-18). This may result in an oculomotor nerve palsy and a hemiplegia of the extremities, *both on the side of the herniation* (Fig. 25-18). The former indicates damage to the oculomotor nerve root (by avulsion of the root or by compression of its blood vessels with resultant necrosis of the root) on the side of the herniation and the latter results from the crus cerebri being forced against the edge of the tentorium on the contralateral side with subsequent damage to the corticospinal fibers on that side (Fig. 25-18). In this example (ipsilateral oculomotor paralysis + ipsilateral hemiplegia) the hemiplegia is the false localizing sign. The combination of oculomotor and corticospinal deficits in some combination suggests that uncal herniation may be the underlying cause of these symptoms.

The Kernohan syndrome illustrates an important general concept concerning posterior fossa lesions that may affect the brainstem. This being that *lesions at any brainstem level (midbrain, pons, medulla) may displace the stem to one side, damage ipsilateral cranial nerve roots at that level (for example,*

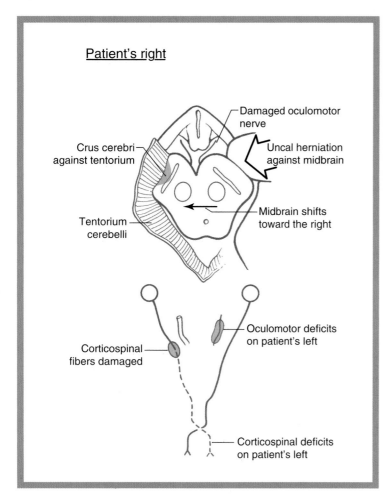

Patient's right

Crus cerebri against tentorium

Damaged oculomotor nerve

Uncal herniation against midbrain

Tentorium cerebelli

Midbrain shifts toward the right

Oculomotor deficits on patient's left

Corticospinal fibers damaged

Corticospinal deficits on patient's left

Figure 25-18. Uncal herniation on the patient's left side. The midbrain shifts toward the right, pressing the crus cerebri against the edge of the tentorium cerebelli on the right and, at the same time, stretching/damaging the oculomotor nerve on the left. The result is oculomotor and corticospinal deficits on the same side of the body; this is characteristic of Kernohan syndrome.

oculomotor, trigeminal, facial, hypoglossal), and damage long tracts on the contralateral side by compression of the stem against bony or meningeal structures. The result is a patient with cranial nerve and long tract signs *on the same side of the body.*

Other Corticofugal Systems

Corticorubral System
Cortical projections to the red nucleus arise primarily from areas 4 and 6, and to a lesser extent from areas 5 and 7. Both large and small neurons in the red nucleus receive ipsilateral corticorubral input. Although pyramidal tract neurons provide some collaterals to the red nucleus, many corticorubral axons are not collaterals of pyramidal tract fibers. In general, the corticorubral-rubrospinal projection is topographically organized. For example, the upper extremity region of the MI cortex projects to cells of the red nucleus that, in turn, send their axons to contralateral cervical levels of the spinal cord (see Fig. 24-13). Because the rubrospinal system primarily influences flexor musculature, this pathway may supplement the function of the corticospinal tract. It is known from experimental studies that section of corticospinal fibers in the medullary pyramid leaves the animal still able to walk, climb, and pick up food but unable to perform fine, dexterous movements with its digits. This finding suggests that the *corticorubrospinal system may partially compensate for the loss of the corticospinal tract.*

The red nucleus also receives input from the contralateral interposed and lateral nuclei of the cerebellum (see Chapter 27).

Consequently, this relatively small population of brainstem upper motor neurons is capable of integrating signals from motor-related areas of the cerebral cortex and from the cerebellum. Input from the interposed nuclei is excitatory, and this projection may be part of a circuit specialized for rapid control or adjustment of movements based on sensory processing by the cerebellum.

Corticoreticular System
The pontine and medullary nuclei that give rise to the reticulospinal tracts receive cortical input from the premotor cortex and, to a lesser extent, from the supplementary motor cortex. Because reticulospinal systems primarily influence extensor muscles, including the paravertebral extensors as well as those of the limbs, the *corticoreticulospinal system* may provide the cortex with the means to influence extensor musculature in parallel with its regulation of flexors (see Figs. 24-9 to 24-11). It should also be noted that the cerebellar nuclei project to the motor-related areas of the reticular formation, thus providing for a cerebellar influence on extensor musculature.

Corticopontine System
Axons from nearly all regions of the cerebral cortex contribute to the corticopontine projection, and this pathway is particularly well developed in the human brain. Although most of these fibers originate from motor-related areas and the somatosensory cortex, nonmotor regions in the frontal lobe and in parietal, temporal, and occipital association cortices also contribute fibers. Corticopontine axons descend through the internal capsule and continue into medial and lateral parts of the crus cerebri. Frontopontine fibers are located medially, and parieto-, occipito-, and temporopontine fibers are laterally placed. These corticopontine projections synapse in the ipsilateral basilar pontine nuclei. Although most neurons in the pontine nuclei send their axons into the contralateral cerebellum via the middle cerebellar peduncle, there is a notable ipsilateral pontocerebellar projection.

Although little is known about the function of this vast corticopontocerebellar system, it certainly must be involved in aspects of motor control. However, recent studies in humans have shown that the cerebellum is also active during mental problem solving and internal (nonvocal) language functions. This finding, in conjunction with animal experiments showing the presence of basilar pontine local-circuit interneurons, implies that the corticopontine system is an important route of communication between the cerebral cortex and the cerebellum, structures that have no direct connections in the mature brain.

Motor Cortex and the Control of Movement

The classic view of voluntary movement control is that the various motor-related areas of the cerebral cortex function hierarchically. At one time, the primary motor cortex was thought to form the apex of this hierarchy, the output of the other cortical areas being funneled through it. Recent findings suggest that the motor-related cortical areas outside MI and their respective descending projections carry out the tasks involved in planning and executing a movement *in parallel* with MI and its descending projections.

Primary Motor Cortex
Recall that the primary motor cortex (MI) is organized into a detailed somatotopic map of the body (Fig. 25-2) and that many corticospinal fibers originate from the pyramidal neurons in its layer V. What is this area's contribution to the control of movement?

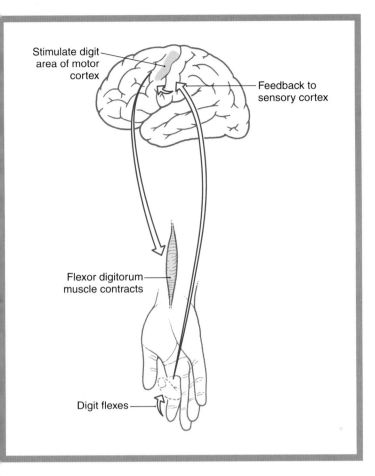

Figure 25-19. Schematic representation of a long-latency reflex.

Like other cortical areas, such as the striate and primary somatosensory cortices, MI is organized into a series of modules or *vertical columns.* Microstimulation in MI can result in discrete movements of individual muscles. For example, stimulation in a vertical column in the hand area of MI may evoke flexion of a digit (Fig. 25-19). Neurons in the same columnar array receive somatosensory feedback from the patch of skin on the volar (glabrous) side of the digit, which is the area that would come in contact with a surface when the digit is flexed, as to grasp an object. These connections are part of *long-latency reflex circuits.* The sensory information reaches MI from the ascending somatosensory systems indirectly via synapses in the thalamus and the primary somatosensory cortex (SI). The inference here is that *motor cortical neurons are informed of the result of their output.*

However, studies have shown that many muscles, particularly distal muscles of the upper extremity, are regulated from more than one cortical location. Conversely, microstimulation at one cortical locus can often activate more than one muscle. Thus, the classic view that a discrete, somatotopically organized projection emanating from area 4 is primarily responsible for the control of individual muscles may be an oversimplification.

The activity of corticospinal neurons in MI can also be modified during a movement. In experiments involving nonhuman primates, microelectrodes placed in layer V identified single corticospinal neurons by their response to *antidromic stimulation* of a medullary pyramid. These monkeys were trained to make wrist flexion or extension movements in a situation in which the movement was either assisted or impeded by a weight attached to the wrist by a pulley system. Under these conditions, corticospinal neurons were found to be *active slightly in advance of the movement,* and they did not simply code for flexion or extension but rather for *the amount of force required to make the movement.* For example, when the weight was arranged to oppose the movement,

increases in the amount of weight were matched by increases in the activity of corticospinal neurons and vice versa; if the weight assisted the movement, the cortical neurons decreased their firing rates.

Other populations of MI cortical neurons encode *movement direction.* When a monkey is trained to move a handle toward one of several targets arranged concentrically around a central starting location, the activity of individual cortical neurons varies with the direction of the required movement. That is, some neurons fire rapidly for a movement in one direction but are silent for a movement in the opposite direction. This directional tuning is rather broad, however, with most neurons firing with movement in a preferred direction but exhibiting less vigorous activity in relation to movements in other directions.

Supplementary Motor Cortex

The supplementary motor cortex occupies the portion of Brodmann area 6 that lies rostral to MI near the convexity of the hemisphere and extends onto the medial wall of the hemisphere rostral to the paracentral gyri (Fig. 25-2). It contains a map of the body musculature that is complete, although less precisely organized than that of MI. It receives input from the parietal lobe and projects to MI and directly to the reticular formation and spinal cord.

Stimulation of the supplementary cortex can evoke movements. In contrast to the single-muscle movements evoked by MI stimulation, however, these movements involve sequences or groups of muscles and orient the body or limbs in space. In addition, stimuli of higher intensities are required than for MI and bilateral movements of the hands or upper extremities are often produced.

Experiments performed in humans illustrate the functional role of the supplementary motor cortex. By using a device similar to a computed tomography scanner and injecting small amounts of a solution containing radioactive xenon into the vascular system, it is possible to measure small increases in local blood flow (as enhanced radioactivity) in brain regions where neuronal activity is believed to be increased. When a volunteer made a series of random finger movements, an increase in neural activity was observed only over the hand region of MI (Fig. 25-20A). The subject was then asked to make movements with several fingers of the same hand, but in a specific sequence. Activity was increased both in the *supplementary motor cortex* and in the hand region of MI (Fig. 25-20B). Finally, when the subject was asked to mentally rehearse a specific sequence of finger movements without actually moving the fingers, increased activity was restricted to the supplementary cortex and the hand region of MI was silent (Fig. 25-20C). These findings indicate that the supplementary motor cortex is involved in *organizing* or *planning* the sequence of muscle activation required to make a movement whereas the primary motor cortex functions mainly to *execute* the movement.

Premotor Cortex

The premotor cortex occupies the portion of area 6 lying just rostral to the anterolateral part of MI (Fig. 25-2). Like the supplementary motor cortex, this region contains a somatotopic representation of the body musculature that is complete, although less precisely organized than that of MI. The premotor cortex receives considerable input from sensory areas of the parietal cortex and projects to MI, the spinal cord, and the reticular formation. The reticular formation gives rise to reticulospinal fibers, which, in turn, influence spinal motor neurons that innervate paravertebral and proximal limb musculature.

On the basis of these connections, it was suggested that premotor cortex, like the supplementary cortex, is involved in the *preparation to move.* That is, it organizes those postural

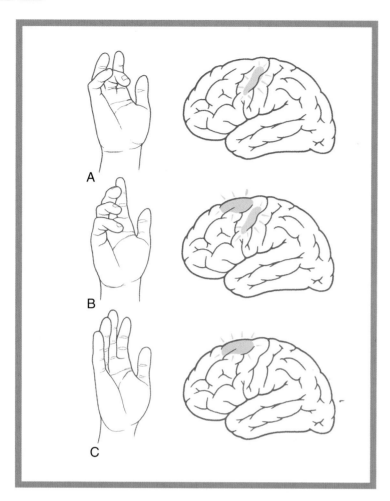

Figure 25-20. Random movements made without prior planning and in no particular order (**A**) result in increased activity in only the hand area of motor cortex. When the movement is planned and executed in a specific sequence (**B**), both motor and supplementary cortices are active. When the movement is mentally planned and rehearsed but never executed (**C**), only the supplementary cortex is activated.

adjustments that are required to make a movement. To test this concept, monkeys were trained to move one hand to a specific target location that differed from trial to trial. The monkey was first given a cue signaling which target to reach for and then a "go" signal to actually make the movement. Recordings of *cell activity* revealed that premotor neurons were active only *during the interval between presentation of the cue and the "go" signal.* The premotor cortex is most active in directing the control of proximal limb muscles that are used to position the arm for movement tasks or, more generally, to orient the body for movement.

Posterior Parietal Cortex

The motor regions of the posterior parietal cortex comprise Brodmann areas 5 and 7, which largely occupy the superior parietal lobule (Fig. 25-2). These areas carry out some of the "background computations" necessary for making movements in space. To organize such a movement, it is necessary to collate input from a variety of sensory systems to create a map of space and to compute a trajectory by which a body part can reach its target. Area 5 receives extensive projections from somatosensory cortex and input from the vestibular system, whereas area 7 processes visual information related to the location of objects in space. Both areas project primarily to supplementary and premotor cortices and have few spinal or brainstem targets.

Experiments in monkeys provide the best insight into the function of areas 5 and 7. In area 5, *arm projection neurons* are active only when the monkey reaches for a specific object of

interest. They are not active when the same arm movement is made but the object is not present, *hand manipulation neurons* fire only when the hand manually explores an object of interest. In area 7, many different types of neurons are present. One type, the *eye-hand coordination neurons,* are vigorously active only when the eyes fixate a target and the hand reaches for that target.

Cingulate Motor Cortex

Two aggregates of corticospinal neurons are associated with the cingulate gyrus (Fig. 25-2). One occupies the inferior bank of the cingulate sulcus, and the other, located slightly more caudally, occupies both the superior and inferior banks of the cingulate sulcus. Each is topographically organized with respect to its spinal cord projections, and each also projects to primary motor cortex. Little is known about the functional role of these areas, other than that stimulation in either area produces motor effects. Because of their proximity to limbic cortex, these motor neurons may be involved in movements that have an intense motivational or emotional component.

Cerebellar and Pallidal Influences

The basal nuclei and cerebellum play essential roles in the control of movement through their interaction with motor-related areas of the cerebral cortex. Although these pathways are detailed in Chapters 26 and 27, their general relationships are summarized here. The cerebellar nuclei and the globus pallidus each project primarily to their own spatially segregated regions in the ventral anterior, ventral lateral, and oral parts of the ventral posterolateral nuclei of the dorsal thalamus. These so-called motor areas of the thalamus give rise to thalamocortical projections to MI and the supplementary motor area. The thalamic areas that receive input from the globus pallidus project mainly to the supplementary motor cortex, and the thalamic areas that receive input from the cerebellum project to MI. The degree to which these two lines of communication are separate is not clear. Therefore, it is important to realize that signals transmitted through the corticospinal and corticonuclear systems can be modified by outputs that reach the cortex from the cerebellum, basal nuclei, and thalamus.

Hierarchical Organization Versus Parallel Distributed Processing in the Motor System

Until recently, it was generally thought that the control of voluntary movement could be satisfactorily described by the hierarchical scheme shown in Figure 25-21. In this plan, lower motor neurons and their associated interneurons are influenced by (1) segmental peripheral sensory feedback circuits, (2) descending brainstem-spinal systems modulated by the cerebral cortex, and (3) the corticospinal system.

Furthermore, the motor areas in the cortex are hierarchically organized such that the output of the corticospinal system is regulated and modulated by higher-order motor cortices. When a voluntary movement is desired, a plan for the movement is organized by the combined efforts of the higher-order motor areas and then transmitted to MI. The primary motor cortex then executes the plan by communicating with the spinal motor apparatus either directly or indirectly via brainstem-spinal systems (Fig. 25-21). However, a re-examination of the origins of the corticospinal tract indicates that more of these fibers than had been previously thought originate from cells located *outside MI.* In addition, circuits linking the basal nuclei, thalamus, and motor cortical regions are segregated to some extent from pathways linking the cerebellum, thalamus, and motor cortical areas.

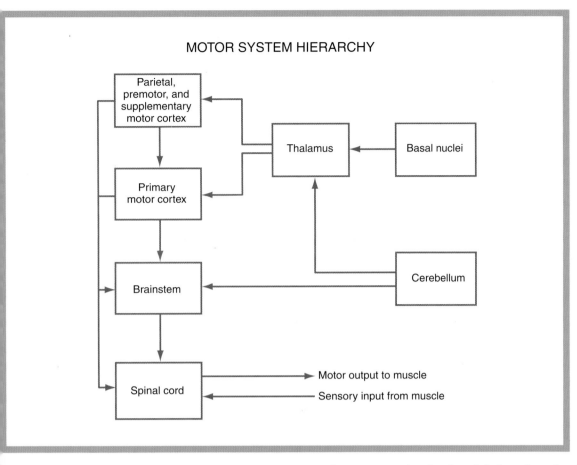

MOTOR SYSTEM HIERARCHY

Figure 25-21. The hierarchical organization of the motor system. Evidence suggests that the direct links from the various brainstem and cortical centers to the spinal cord, which operate as a series of systems, may be more important than was previously thought and that hierarchical organization may be less important.

These observations have led to an evolving hypothesis that motor system control is achieved by a series of *parallel systems* formed by somatotopically organized, descending cortical projections that link the various motor-related areas of cortex more directly with spinal motor circuits. Included here are spinal projections originating from the so-called higher-order motor regions such as the premotor and supplementary motor areas.

The concept is that each descending cortical pathway contributes its own element or series of elements to movement control. This idea is supported by the fact that stimulation in different cortical locations can elicit movements that involve the same muscles or muscle groups, but the characteristics of the movement are different and depend on the site of stimulation. However, additional information is needed before this hypothesis can be validated.

Synopsis of Clinical Points

- Lower motor neuron lesion signs include flaccid muscles with atrophy, fibrillations/fasciculations, hypotonia, and hyporeflexia (p. 395).
- Upper motor neuron lesion signs include muscles that are initially weak but eventually become spastic, hypertonic, and hyperreflexic (p. 395).
- Muscle spasticity refers to the fact that the muscles exhibit an increased resistance to passive movements (p. 395).
- In upper motor neuron lesion spasticity the more rapid the attempted movement of the extremity by the physician, the greater resistance (p. 395).
- The patient with a lesion of the crus cerebri and adjacent midbrain experiences an ipsilateral loss of considerable eye movements, deficits of the pupillary light reflex, and a contralateral hemiparesis (p. 397).
- The Weber syndrome involves a lesion of the midbrain and the oculomotor nerve (p. 398).
- The Foville syndrome involves a lesion of the basilar pons and the abducens nerve (p. 398).
- A middle alternating hemiplegia is a lesion involving the root of the abducens nerve and corticospinal fibers in the pons (p. 398).
- The Dejerine syndrome involves a lesion of the medullary pyramid and the hypoglossal nerve (p. 400).
- A lesion in the territory of the anterior spinal artery may result in an inferior alternating hemiplegia (pp. 398–400).
- Damage to the root of the hypoglossal nerve results in a deviation of the tongue to the ipsilateral side on protrusion (p. 398).

Continued

Synopsis of Clinical Points   *(Continued)*

- Dorsiflexion of the great toe upon aggressive stimulation of the sole of the foot is the Babinski sign (p. 395).
- The Brown-Séquard syndrome involves a hemisection of the spinal cord (p. 402).
- Hemisection of the spinal cord results in ipsilateral paralysis below the lesion and alternating sensory deficits (p. 402).
- A central seven results from a lesion of the genu of the internal capsule or of the crus cerebri (p. 404).
- Damage to the facial root results in a facial (Bell) palsy (p. 404).
- A lesion of corticonuclear fibers results in a deviation of the uvula toward the side of the lesion on attempted phonation (p. 404).
- Damage to the root or nucleus of the hypoglossal nerve will result in weakness of the ipsilateral genioglossus muscle; the tongue deviates to the weak (ipsilateral) side on protrusion (p. 406).
- When long tract and cranial nerve signs are seen resultant to a brainstem lesion, the cranial nerve deficits are usually the best localizing sign (p. 407).
- The Kernohan syndrome, or Kernohan notch phenomenon, results in the appearance of a false localizing sign (p. 407).
- False localizing signs, is present when a patient exhibits corticospinal or other long-tract signs and cranial nerve signs on the same side of the body (p. 407).
- Lesions of the supplemental motor cortex may result in difficulties in planning a movement (p. 409).

Sources and Additional Reading

Asanuma H, Rosen I: Topographical organization of cortical efferent zones projecting to distal forelimb muscles in the monkey. Exp Brain Res 14:243-256, 1972.

Asanuma H: The Motor Cortex. New York, Raven Press, 1988.

Brodal A: Neurological Anatomy in Relation to Clinical Medicine, 3rd ed. New York, Oxford University Press, 1981.

Dum R, Strick PL: The corticospinal system: A structural framework for the central control of movement. In LB Rowell, JT Sheper [eds]: Handbook of Physiology. Section 12, *Exercise: Regulation and Integration of Multiple Systems.* Oxford, Oxford University Press (for the American Physiological Society), 1996.

Evarts EV: Relation of pyramidal tract activity to force exerted during voluntary movement. J Neurophysiol 31:14-27, 1968.

Georgopoulos AP: Higher order motor control. Annu Rev Neurosci 14:361-377, 1991.

Humphrey DR: On the cortical control of visually directed reaching: Contributions by nonprecentral motor areas. In Talbot RE, Humphrey DR (eds): Posture and Movement. New York, Raven Press, 1979, pp 51-112.

Humphrey DR: Representation of movements and muscles within the primate precentral motor cortex: Historical and current perspectives. Fed Proc 45:2687-2699, 1986.

Mihailoff GA, Border BG: Evidence for the presence of pre synaptic dendrites and GABA immunogold labeled synaptic boutons in the monkey basilar pontine nuclei. Brain Res 514:141-146, 1990.

Mihailoff GA, Kosinski RJ, Azizi SA, Border BG, Lee HS: The expanding role of the basilar pontine nuclei as a source of cerebellar afferent information. In Llinas R, Sotelo C (eds) *The Cerebellum Revisited.* New York, Springer-Verlag, 1992.

Penfield W, Rasmussen T: The Cerebral Cortex of Man: A Clinical Study of Localization of Function. New York, Hafner Publishing, 1968 (facsimile of 1950 edition).

Roland PE, Larsen B, Lassen NA, Skinholf E: Supplementary motor area and other cortical areas in organization of voluntary movements in man. J Neurophysiol 43:118-136, 1980.

Terminologia Anatomica: International Anatomical Terminology Federative International Committee on Anatomical Terminology. Stuttgart, Thieme, 1998.

Wolf JK: The Classical Brain Syndromes: Translations of the Original Papers with Notes on the Evolution of Clinical Neuroanatomy. Springfield, IL, Charles C Thomas, 1971.

The Basal Nuclei

T. P. Ma

Voluntary movement is essential to the well-being of living animals. Such behaviors are accomplished by signals that direct the actions of individual muscles. Although these signals originate in the cerebral cortex, they are modulated by a variety of subcortical structures. One such group of structures is the basal nuclei (ganglia) and their functionally associated cell groups. Classically, motor systems have been divided into "pyramidal" and "extrapyramidal" on the basis of whether the pathway is mediated by corticofugal neurons (pyramidal) or by the basal nuclei, cerebellum, or descending brainstem pathways (extrapyramidal). However, this distinction is overly simplistic, if not inaccurate. Consequently, it is not used here. The basal nuclei are involved in a wide variety of motor and affective behaviors, in sensorimotor integration, and in cognitive functions.

Overview

These nuclei are traditionally called the *basal ganglia* rather than the *basal nuclei*, even though "ganglia" is usually reserved for groups of nerve cell bodies in the peripheral nervous system. The official term *basal nuclei* is used throughout this chapter, although the unofficial term *basal ganglia* is also commonly seen in the literature. For practical purposes these terms may be considered interchangeable.

The *basal nuclei* consist of cell groups embedded in the cerebral hemisphere. Although not classified as nuclei of the basal nuclei in a strict sense, the *subthalamic nucleus, substantia nigra,* and *pedunculopontine tegmental nucleus* are integral parts of the pathways passing through these forebrain cell groups. Collectively, the basal nuclei and their associated nuclei function primarily as components in a series of parallel circuits from the

cerebral cortex through the basal nuclei to the thalamus and then back to the cerebral cortex.

Four fundamental concepts are crucial to understanding the basal nuclei. *First,* damage to or disorders of the basal nuclei result in disruption of movements, and may also cause significant deficits in other neural functions such as cognition, perception, and mentation. *Second,* the basal nuclei are anatomically and functionally segregated into parallel circuits that process different types of behaviorally significant information. *Third,* the basal nuclei function primarily through *disinhibition* (release from inhibition). *Fourth,* diseases of the basal nuclei can be described as disruptions of the neurochemical interactions between elements of the basal nuclei. These neurochemical relationships rely not simply on the neurotransmitters involved but also on the characteristics of the transmitter receptors, on the locations of the synapses, and on other inputs received by these cells.

In summary, the basal nuclei integrate and modulate cortical information along multiple independent parallel channels. These channels affect behavior indirectly by feedback to the cerebral cortex and directly by providing information to subcortical centers that influence movements. Disruption of these channels by stroke or disease results in dysfunctions in the motor sphere that are characteristic of the circuits damaged.

Components of the Basal Nuclei

The basal nuclei are typically divided into dorsal and ventral divisions. The dorsal basal nuclei include the *caudate* and *putamen* (together constituting the *neostriatum*) and the *globus pallidus* (constituting the *paleostriatum*) (Fig. 26-1A). Associated with the dorsal basal nuclei, in a functional sense, are the *substantia*

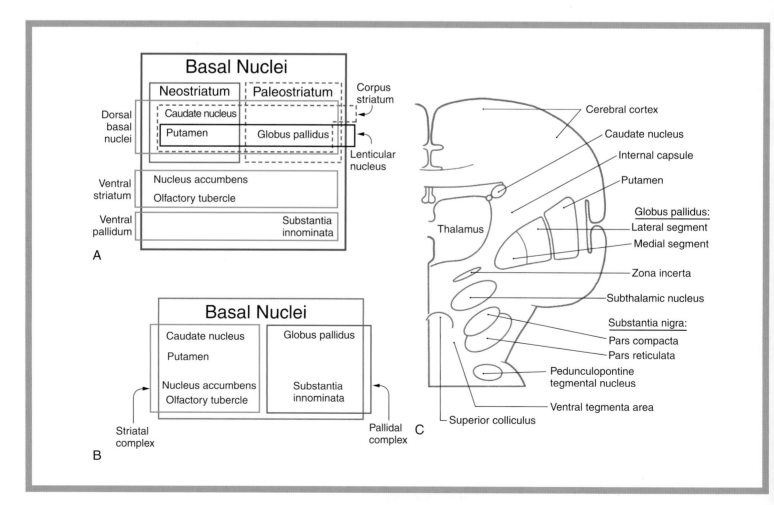

Figure 26-1. A series of stacked boxes (**A**) illustrating which nuclei form the various parts of the basal nuclei and how these groups are used in this chapter (**B**). A standard drawing of the basal nuclei (**C**) used throughout this chapter.

nigra, the *subthalamic nucleus,* and the *parabrachial pontine reticular formation* (containing the *pedunculopontine tegmental nucleus*). The ventral basal nuclei are located inferior to the anterior commissure and include the *substantia innominata, nucleus basalis of Meynert, nucleus accumbens,* and *olfactory tubercle.* This ventral region is intimately associated with portions of the amygdala and ventral tegmental area. For the purposes of this chapter, the basal nuclei are regarded as making up two complexes: the *striatal complex* and the *pallidal complex* (Fig. 26-1B).

The telencephalic regions of the basal nuclei are supplied by the *medial striate artery, lenticulostriate branches* of the M_1 segment of the middle cerebral artery, and the *anterior choroidal artery* (Fig. 26-2). The diencephalic and mesencephalic regions are supplied by the *posteromedial branches* of the P_1 segment of the posterior cerebral artery and branches of the *posterior communicating artery.* Diseases of these vessels may result in various behavioral or motor deficits, depending on which vessel and region is affected.

Striatal Complex

The *striatal complex* is a functional unit composed of the *neostriatum* and *ventral striatum* (Fig. 26-3A, B). The neostriatum consists of the *caudate nucleus* and *putamen.* These two nuclei have the same embryologic origin and similar connections. Although fused rostroventrally, they are separated throughout most of their extents by fibers of the internal capsule. The ventral striatum is composed of the *nucleus accumbens* and the *olfactory tubercle* (Figs. 26-1A, B and 26-3A). The nucleus accumbens is located rostroventrally in the hemisphere, at the point where the putamen is continuous with the head of the caudate (Figs. 26-3A, 26-4). It is internal to part of the anterior perforated substance. Portions of the olfactory tubercle are considered part of the ventral striatum because of functional, cytoarchitectural, and chemoarchitectural similarities. The

olfactory tubercle is unique in that it has striatal characteristics yet receives primary olfactory information.

A defining characteristic of the striatal complex, *striosomes* (also called *patches*) are particularly prominent in the head of the caudate (Fig. 26-4). Striosomes are acetylcholinesterase-poor regions within the striatal complex. They contain large amounts of one or more neuropeptides and one or more types of opiate receptors. The remainder of the striatal complex, called the *matrix,* contains high concentrations of acetylcholinesterase and therefore stains darkly when tissue is histochemically reacted to reveal this enzyme. These regions appear to subserve different components of the basal nuclei pathways.

The largest afferent projections to the striatum are from the cerebral cortex *(corticostriatal fibers)* (Fig. 26-5A). Other afferents are from the thalamus *(thalamostriatal fibers),* substantia nigra *(nigrostriatal fibers),* and parabrachial pontine reticular formation *(pedunculopontostriatal fibers)* (Fig. 26-5A). The efferent projections of the striatum reach primarily the pallidum *(striatopallidal fibers)* and the nigral complex *(striatonigral fibers),* and to a small degree the subthalamic nucleus.

Most of the neurons in the neostriatum are called *medium spiny neurons,* so named because of their medium-sized cell bodies and the large numbers of spines on their dendrites (Fig. 26-6). Most medium spiny cells have dendritic fields that are restricted to the striosomes or matrix compartment in which the cell bodies are located. That is, *medium spiny neurons in striosomes have dendrites that usually ramify within striosomes; medium spiny neurons within the matrix primarily ramify within the matrix.* Both the afferent and efferent connections of neurons within the striosomes and matrix also differ significantly. Adjacent neurons across a striosome-matrix border may receive cortical projections from widely different areas. Axon collaterals of neurons within striosomes remain within striosomes, whereas those from the matrix remain within the matrix. Even when

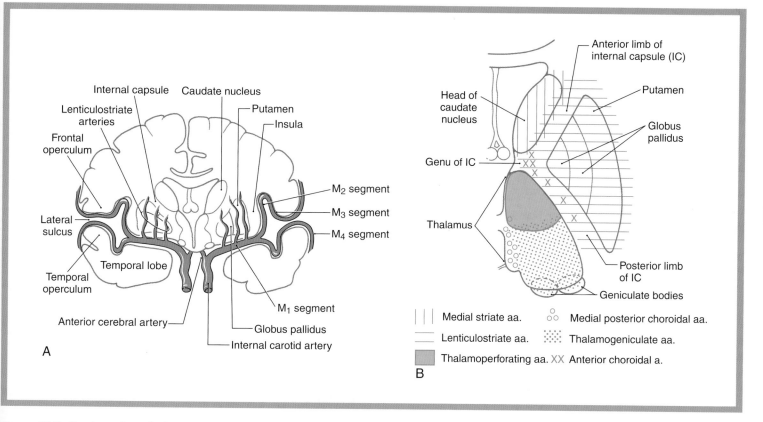

Figure 26-2. Blood supply to the basal nuclei in coronal (**A**) and axial (**B**) planes. The anterior choroidal artery serves the more inferior aspects of the genu and posterior limb; the more superior aspects are served by the lenticulostriate arteries a, artery; aa, arteries.

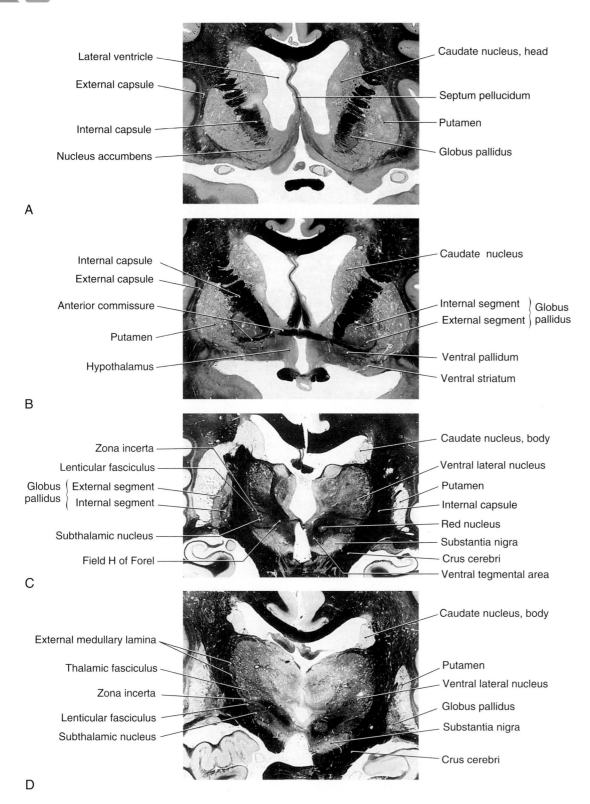

Figure 26-3. Cross sections of the human brain from rostral (**A**) to caudal (**D**) showing the basal nuclei and related structures. Myelin stain. (**A** modified from Haines DE: Neuroanatomy: An Atlas of Structures, Sections, and Systems, 6th ed. Philadelphia, Lippincott Williams & Williams, 2004.)

both compartments project to the same nucleus, they differ in the region to which they project, thus resulting in different functional effects. Medium spiny neurons fire few action potentials spontaneously and thus require activation by their afferent fibers. These cells use the inhibitory neurotransmitter γ-aminobutyric acid (GABA) and may also contain neuroactive peptides such as substance P and enkephalin. Thus, when medium spiny neurons are activated, they subserve both direct inhibitory and neuromodulatory functions at their targets. The axons of medium spiny neurons are the *efferent fibers of the neostriatum*, collectively forming the *striatopallidal fibers*.

Also found in the neostriatum are large, acetylcholine-containing local circuit neurons that modulate local activity within the neostriatum. Huntington disease is characterized by progressive loss of medium spiny neurons and acetylcholine-containing neurons throughout the striatal complex.

Pallidal Complex

The *pallidal complex* is composed of the *globus pallidus* and the *ventral pallidum*. The latter is largely synonymous with the substantia innominata (Fig. 26-3B, C). The pallidal complex contains primarily GABAergic neurons with high rates of

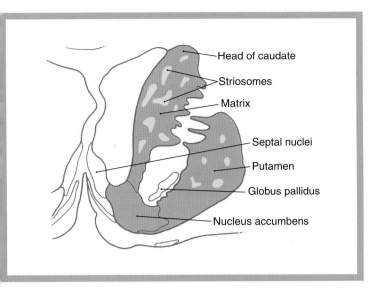

Figure 26-4. Schematic representation of striosomes and matrix in the striatal complex.

spontaneous activity. Consequently, these cells tonically inhibit their targets.

The globus pallidus is divided into *medial (internal)* and *lateral (external) segments* by a sheet of white matter (the medullary lamina) (Fig. 26-3C). The substantia innominata is located inferior to the anterior commissure and internal to the anterior perforated substance. One important cell group in the substantia innominata is the basal nucleus of Meynert. This nucleus has large acetylcholine-containing neurons, which are lost in Alzheimer disease. However, this disease is not considered a basal nuclear disorder because acetylcholine-containing cells in the cerebral cortex, hippocampus, and septum are also lost in Alzheimer disease patients. This disease is further characterized by other biochemical and pathologic features such as senile plaques.

The two divisions of the globus pallidus are reciprocally connected *(pallidopallidal fibers)* (Fig. 26-5B) but subserve different functions. The main afferent input to the pallidum is from the striatal complex. Medium spiny neurons from the striatum that project to the medial segment and substantia nigra use GABA and substance P; those that project to the lateral segment use GABA and enkephalin (Fig. 26-5B).

The medial division is composed of the medial segment of the globus pallidus. It subserves the *direct basal nuclear pathway* (described later) and projects primarily to the thalamus *(pallidothalamic fibers)* (Fig. 26-5B). These fibers exit the globus pallidus as two bundles: the *ansa lenticularis* and the *lenticular fasciculus* (Figs. 26-7 and 26-8). The *ansa lenticularis* originates from lateral portions of the medial segment and loops around the posterior limb of the internal capsule to enter the *prerubral field (field H of Forel)*. The *lenticular fasciculus (field H2 of Forel)*, on the other hand, originates in the posteromedial portion of the medial segment. These fibers traverse the internal capsule as small groups of axons, merge to form the lenticular fasciculus between the zona incerta and subthalamic nucleus, and then enter field H of Forel. In the Forel field, the ansa lenticularis and lenticular fasciculus join the *thalamic fasciculus (field H1 of Forel)*, which courses immediately superior to the zona incerta (Figs. 26-7 and 26-8). These fibers ultimately terminate in ventral anterior, ventral lateral, and centromedian nuclei of the thalamus. The medial division of the pallidal complex is a principal efferent nucleus of the basal nuclei; the axons of these cells comprising the *ansa lenticularis* and the *lenticular fasciculus*.

The lateral division is composed of the external (or lateral) segment of the globus pallidus and the ventral pallidum. This division subserves the *indirect basal nuclear pathway* (see later). These nuclei receive a large input from the striatal complex *(striatopallidal fibers)* and small projections from the subthalamic nucleus *(subthalamopallidal fibers)* and the substantia nigra pars reticulata *(nigropallidal fibers)*. They project strongly to the subthalamic nucleus *(pallidosubthalamic fibers)* and are also connected with the substantia nigra *(pallidonigral fibers)* (Fig. 26-5B).

Subthalamic Nucleus

The subthalamic nucleus is a lens-shaped cell group that makes up the largest part of the ventral thalamus. It is immediately inferior to the zona incerta and rostral to the substantia nigra (Fig. 26-3C, D). It receives projections from the lateral pallidal division *(pallidosubthalamic fibers)*, cerebral cortex *(cortico-subthalamic fibers)*, nigral complex *(nigrosubthalamic fibers)*, and parabrachial pontine reticular formation. The subthalamic nucleus projects to both pallidal divisions *(subthalamopallidal fibers)* and to the substantia nigra *(subthalamonigral fibers)* (Fig. 26-5C). These connections, especially the subthalamopallidal projections to the medial globus pallidus, are an essential part of the indirect pathway underlying basal nuclear function (Fig. 26-8).

Subthalamic neurons use the excitatory neurotransmitter glutamate. Most of the time, subthalamic cells are inactive because of the constant inhibition by cells of the external pallidal segment. However, if this inhibition is removed, subthalamic neurons have a high level of activity resulting in a characteristic motor deficit described later in this chapter. This activity is mediated in part by a large corticosubthalamic projection.

Nigral Complex

The nigral complex is composed of the *substantia nigra* and the *ventral (anterior) tegmental area* (Fig. 26-3C, D). The substantia nigra is divided into a cell-dense portion *(pars compacta)* and a reticulated portion (referred to here as the *pars reticulata*, although it can be divided into a *pars reticulata* and a *pars lateralis*). The pars reticulata is located at and within the medial edge of the descending corticofugal fibers that form the crus cerebri. The pars compacta and the adjacent ventral tegmental area appear to subserve similar functions and to have a similar chemoarchitectural organization. The major afferents to the nigral complex are from the striatal and pallidal complexes. The nigral complex also receives cortical *(corticonigral)*, subthalamic *(subthalamonigral)*, and pedunculopontine fibers (Fig. 26-5D).

The pars compacta includes a large number of neuromelanin-containing cells, whose dark color gives the nucleus its name *(substantia nigra,* "black substance"). Neurons in the pars compacta use the neurotransmitter dopamine and project primarily to the neostriatum as *nigrostriatal fibers*. The dopamine released by these cells may excite or inhibit striatal neurons, depending on the *type of receptor* on the postsynaptic membrane.

The pars reticulata is formed by loose aggregations of medium- to large-sized GABAergic neurons that are indistinguishable from those of the medial pallidum. Neurons in the pars reticulata have axons with an extensive system of collaterals; consequently, they may project to and inhibit one or more target structures. These targets include the neostriatum *(nigrostriatal fibers)*, thalamus *(nigrothalamic fibers)*, superior colliculus *(nigrotectal fibers)*, and the parabrachial pontine reticular formation. These cells have a high rate of discharge and tonically inhibit their targets. Projections of pars reticulata neurons represent an important pathway by which the basal nuclei influence other motor centers.

The pars compacta and the pars reticulata are interconnected. Dendrites of dopaminergic pars compacta neurons extend into the pars reticulata, where they release free dopamine (by a

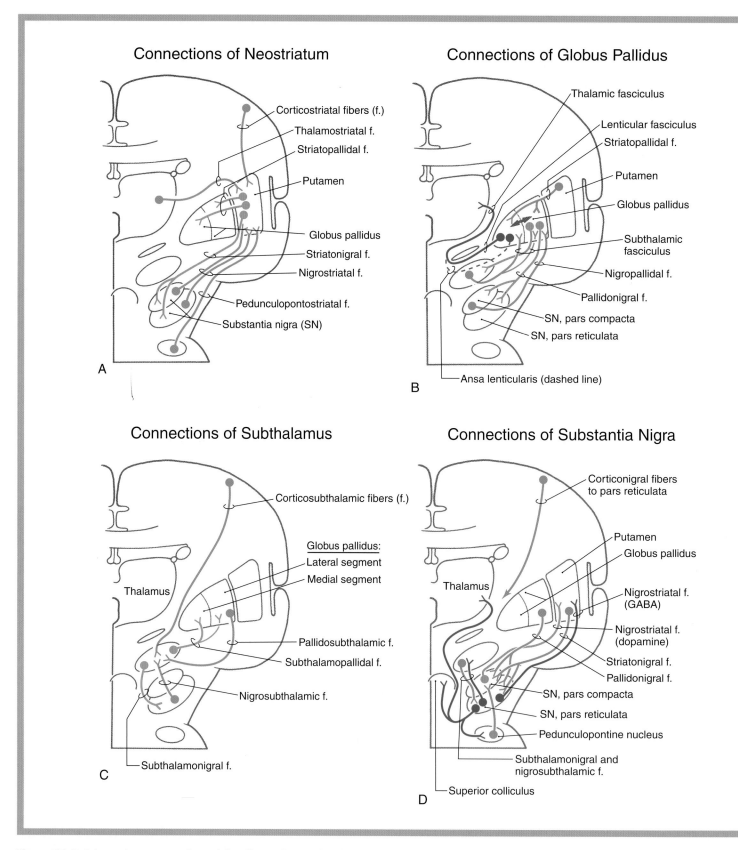

Figure 26-5. Schematic representations of the afferent (in *green*) and efferent (in *red*) connections of the neostriatum (**A**) and subthalamus (**C**) and of the afferent (in *green*) and efferent (in *red and blue*) connections of the globus pallidus (**B**) and substantia nigra (**D**). The *double-headed arrow* in **B** represents pallidopallidal fibers.

nonvesicular mechanism). The level of dopamine modulates the resting membrane potential of pars reticula cells, making them either more or less likely to discharge, depending on the subtype of dopamine receptor they possess. In turn, pars reticulata neurons have axon collaterals that ramify extensively in the pars compacta and form GABAergic synapses. Collectively, these interactions form modulatory loops between neurons of the pars compacta and the pars reticulata.

These modulatory loops are influenced by the segregated output of the striatal striosome-matrix system. Neurons in the striosomes project predominantly onto the cells in the pars compacta, whereas the neurons in the matrix project predominantly onto the cells in the pars reticulata. Thus, the striatonigral projection from the striosomes directly inhibits the dopaminergic nigrostriatal neurons and the projection from the matrix inhibits the GABAergic neurons in the pars reticulata.

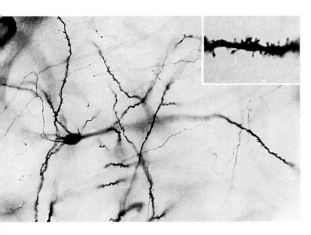

Figure 26-6. Medium spiny neuron from the primate neostriatum. The detail shows the characteristic appearance of dendritic spines on these cells. (Photos courtesy of Dr. José Rafols.)

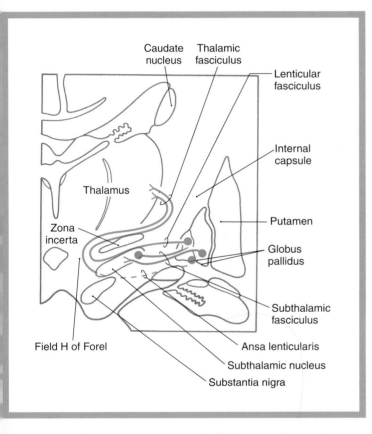

Figure 26-7. Schematic representation of pallidal connections to the thalamus and with the subthalamic nucleus.

Consequently, inhibition of the pars reticulata is reduced and its targets, such as the pars compacta, are released from inhibition and may become more active.

The ventral tegmental area is located medial to the substantia nigra. It contains large numbers of dopaminergic neurons and forms connections with the ventral striatum, the amygdala, and other limbic system structures. Cells of the ventral tegmental area project to, and terminate on, striatal neurons that have postsynaptic D_2 (dopamine) receptors. In schizophrenia there is an increase in number and in sensitivity of these receptors. Neuroleptic drugs help to control schizophrenia by blocking (downregulating) these D_2 receptors.

Parabrachial Pontine Reticular Formation
Nuclei in the region of the parabrachial pontine reticular formation, primarily the pedunculopontine tegmental nucleus,

are intimately connected with all portions of the basal nuclei and their associated nuclei. For example, GABAergic substantia nigra pars reticulata neurons project onto cells of the pedunculopontine tegmental nucleus. In return, acetylcholine-containing pedunculopontine tegmental neurons project to the substantia nigra pars compacta. In addition, the parabrachial pontine nuclei are connected with motor centers in the brainstem, which project to the spinal cord via the descending spinal pathways. Thus, these nuclei serve as an efferent pathway for the basal nuclei. It has been suggested that damage to the connections between the pedunculopontine nucleus and the basal nuclei may partially account for motor deficits, such as tremor or chorea, in some patients.

Ventral Basal Nuclei
The ventral basal nuclear pathways are similar to those of the dorsal basal nuclei. The pathways originate in the allocortex (limbic-related cortical areas) and the orbital and medial prefrontal cortices. The corticostriatal pathway terminates in the ventral striatum (nucleus accumbens and portions of the olfactory tubercle). Striatopallidal neurons then project to the ventral pallidum (substantia innominata). Then the pallidothalamic neurons project to the mediodorsal nucleus of the thalamus, whose neurons then project to the cerebral cortex. As with the dorsal basal nuclei, distinct regions of each nucleus in these pathways are connected with each other. Thus, there is a clear loop through the ventral basal nuclei for information originating from different areas of the cortex, as is discussed later.

Numerous functions are ascribed to the ventral basal nuclei. Generally, they can be grouped as natural or biologic rewards, such as feeding, drinking, sex, exploration, and appetitive learning. Consequently, diseases that can be associated with imbalances of "rewards," such as drug and alcohol abuse, can be related to the ventral basal nuclei. Similarly, other psychiatric disorders such as schizophrenia and certain forms of affective disorders are also linked to the ventral basal nuclei. Thus, it is not surprising that the pharmacologic treatments of many psychiatric disorders have their primary effect in the ventral basal nuclear pathways. Although the most evident symptoms of classic basal nuclear disorders are those of motor disturbances, almost every patient will exhibit psychiatric complications owing to the involvement of the ventral basal nuclei.

Direct and Indirect Pathways of Basal Nuclear Activity

Pathways though the basal nuclei consist of parallel circuits that share certain features. The basic circuit is divided into *direct* and *indirect* pathways that have opposing actions on targets of the basal nuclei (Figs. 26-8 and 26-9). As a general concept, the *direct pathway facilitates* a flow of information through the thalamus and the *indirect pathway inhibits* this flow. These pathways create a balance in the inhibitory outflow of the basal nuclei and function by modulating the extent of this inhibition on target nuclei.

The *direct pathway* (Figs. 26-8, 26-9, and 26-10A) begins as an excitatory, glutamatergic projection from the cerebral cortex to the striatal complex. Striatal neurons inhibit cells in the internal (or medial) segment of the globus pallidus and in the substantia nigra pars reticulata. These *striatopallidal* and *striatonigral fibers* use GABA and substance P. Cells of the internal segment of the globus pallidus (as *pallidothalamic fibers*) and of the substantia nigra pars reticulata (as *nigrothalamic fibers*) project to thalamic neurons. These fibers have a high rate of spontaneous activity and thus tonically inhibit target thalamic neurons. Inhibition of these pallidal and nigral projections by

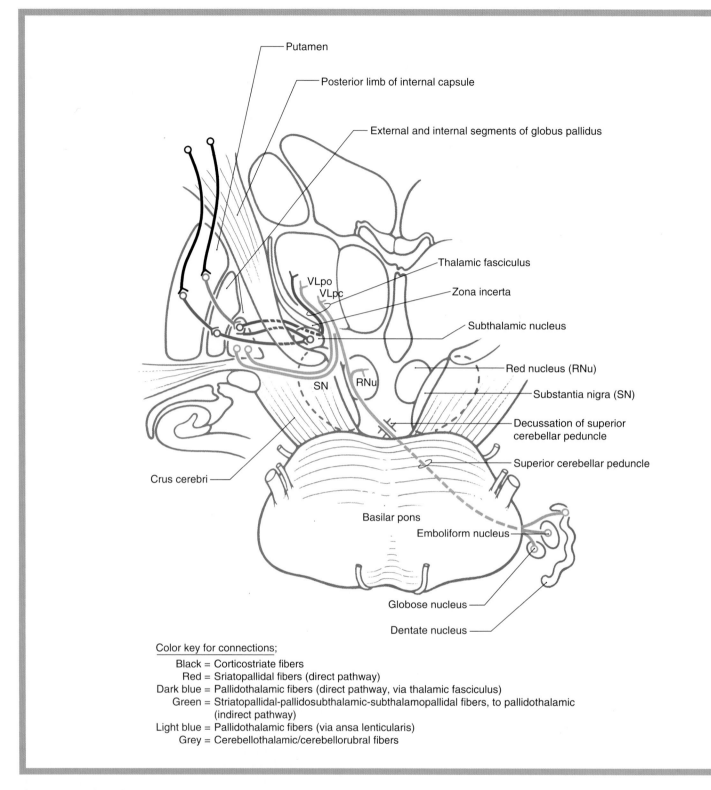

Color key for connections;

    Black = Corticostriate fibers
    Red = Sriatopallidal fibers (direct pathway)
    Dark blue = Pallidothalamic fibers (direct pathway, via thalamic fasciculus)
    Green = Striatopallidal-pallidosubthalamic-subthalamopallidal fibers, to pallidothalamic
           (indirect pathway)
    Light blue = Pallidothalamic fibers (via ansa lenticularis)
    Grey = Cerebellothalamic/cerebellorubral fibers

Figure 26-8. Three-dimensional representation of the connections of the basal nuclei, excluding those with the substantia nigra. Fibers of the thalamic fasciculus *(dark blue)* traverse the internal capsule, pass between the subthalamic nucleus and zona incerta, and then enter the thalamic fasciculus to access the VLpo. Fibers of the ansa lenticularis *(light blue)* arch around the rostromedial edge of the internal capsule and course caudally to enter the thalamic fasciculus en route to the VLpo. Pallidosubthalamic and subthalamopallidal fibers *(both green)* collectively form the subthalamic fasciculus. Cerebellothalamic fibers from the contralateral cerebellar nuclei also use the thalamic fasciculus to get to the VLpc. VLpc, ventral lateral thalamic nucleus, pars caudalis; VLpo, ventral lateral thalamic nucleus, pars oralis. (Modified from Nieuwenhuys, Voogd, and van Huijzen, 1988, with permission.)

striatal cells decreases the inhibitory inputs to thalamocortical neurons *(thalamic disinhibition)*. The *net effect of the direct pathway is to increase the activity of the thalamus and the consequent excitation of the cerebral cortex* (Fig. 26-10B).

The *indirect pathway* includes a loop through the globus pallidus and subthalamic nucleus (Figs. 26-8, 26-9, and 26-10C). *Striatopallidal* neurons involved in this pathway contain

GABA and enkephalin. They project into the lateral pallidal segment, which, in turn, sends *pallidosubthalamic fibers* into the subthalamic nucleus. These pallidosubthalamic fibers are GABAergic, have high spontaneous firing rates, and tonically inhibit subthalamic cells. Inhibition of these fibers by the neostriatum releases these subthalamic cells from their tonically inhibited state *(subthalamic disinhibition)*. These subthalamic

Direct and Indirect Pathways

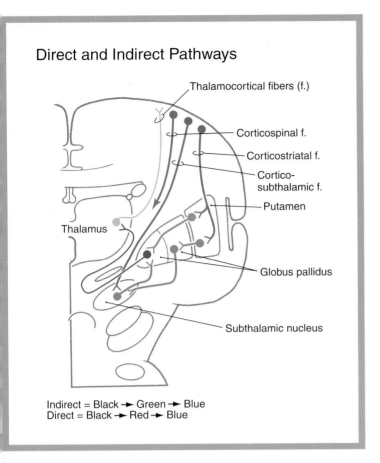

Figure 26-9. Schematic representation of direct and indirect pathways through the basal nuclei.

neurons have spontaneous activity and are also influenced by an excitatory *corticosubthalamic* projection. Together, these inputs increase the firing rates of glutamatergic *subthalamopallidal fibers* to the medial pallidal segment. As a consequence, the firing rate of inhibitory *pallidothalamic fibers* is increased, with a resultant decrease in the activity of thalamocortical neurons. The *net effect of the indirect pathway is to decrease activity of the thalamus and, consequently, decrease activity of the cerebral cortex* (Fig. 26-10D).

Disinhibition as the Primary Mode of Basal Nuclear Function

The function of the direct pathway is to release the thalamus from its pallidal inhibition. This release is accomplished by striatopallidal inhibition of pallidothalamic neurons. In the indirect pathway, the subthalamic nucleus is released from inhibition by the lateral pallidal segment so that it can excite the inhibitory pallidothalamic cells. This mechanism that *releases cells from inhibition* is called *disinhibition*. Balance between *thalamic disinhibition* by the direct pathway and *subthalamic disinhibition* by the indirect pathway results in normal basal nuclear function. Behavioral deficits that accompany basal nuclear disorders can ultimately be traced to imbalances between the direct and indirect pathways.

Although the balance between the direct and indirect pathways determines the net outflow of the basal nuclei, other elements of the basal nuclei are also modulated by disinhibitory mechanisms. For example, in the earlier description of the suggested projections from the striosomes and matrix to the substantia nigra, the striosomal pathway to the pars compacta is a direct inhibitory pathway, whereas the pathway from the matrix, which inhibits the pars reticulata and releases the pars

compacta nigrostriatal neurons, functions to *disinhibit* the pars compacta neurons.

Parallel Circuits of Information Flow Through the Basal Nuclei

Information flow through the basal nuclei is separated into five distinct parallel circuits. They are the *motor loop, oculomotor loop, dorsolateral prefrontal loop, lateral orbitofrontal loop,* and *limbic loop.* The *motor loop* is involved in somatosensory and somatomotor control (Fig. 26-11). The *oculomotor loop* is primarily related to the control of orientation and gaze. The *dorsolateral prefrontal* and *lateral orbitofrontal loops* are related to cognitive processes. The *limbic loop* is concerned with emotional and visceral functions. All of these circuits have both the direct and indirect pathways described previously.

The five circuits originate from functionally distinct regions of the cerebral cortex, pass through distinct regions of each basal nuclear component, modulate different areas of the thalamus, and return to functionally distinct cortical regions (Fig. 26-11). That is, each circuit can be considered an independent channel that processes information from one functional type of cortex by way of its own areas of the basal nuclei and thalamus and returns to the appropriate functionally related part of cortex.

Anatomic studies in nonhuman primates have demonstrated that each loop projects to a restricted portion of each nucleus. Therefore, there is an *anatomic* as well as a *functional* separation of the basal nuclear circuits. This separation is called the *closed component* of the circuitry. However, at every stage of each circuit, the information is modulated and integrated with input from other centers by intrinsic basal nuclear connections. Thus, although the circuits are anatomically and functionally distinct, their activities are modulated by the other modalities of the basal nuclei. This integration is called the *open component* of basal nuclear circuits.

The Motor Loop

Because the most obvious symptoms of basal nuclear disorders are those associated with the motor system, it is important to understand the motor loop. Although this loop contains both direct and indirect pathways, which are associated with specific parts of each nucleus, only the direct path way of the motor loop is described here (Fig. 26-11).

The motor loop originates mainly in supplementary motor area (SMA), primary motor (MC), and premotor (PMC) cortices (Fig. 26-11). These corticostriatal projections terminate in the putamen (Put), which also receives projections from the somatosensory cortex (SC). Efferents from the putamen terminate in specific areas of the internal segment of the globus pallidus (GPi-v) and the substantia nigra pars reticulata (SNr-dl). These two regions project to the oral part of the ventral lateral nucleus (VLo), the ventral anterior nucleus (VA), and the centromedian nucleus (CM) of the thalamus. In turn, the VLo and VA nuclei project to the supplementary motor cortex; the VA nucleus to premotor cortex; and the VLo and CM nuclei to motor cortex. Although the primary projections of the globus pallidus and substantia nigra are to the thalamus, they also project to the superior colliculus and brainstem reticular formation. In this way, this basal nuclear circuit affects both cortical motor efferents and brainstem motor centers.

Comparable circuits also exist in each of the other four loops passing through the basal nuclei. Although the pathways through the other basal nuclear loops are not described here in detail, it is important to note that investigators are giving increasing attention to the deficits resulting from damage to those other

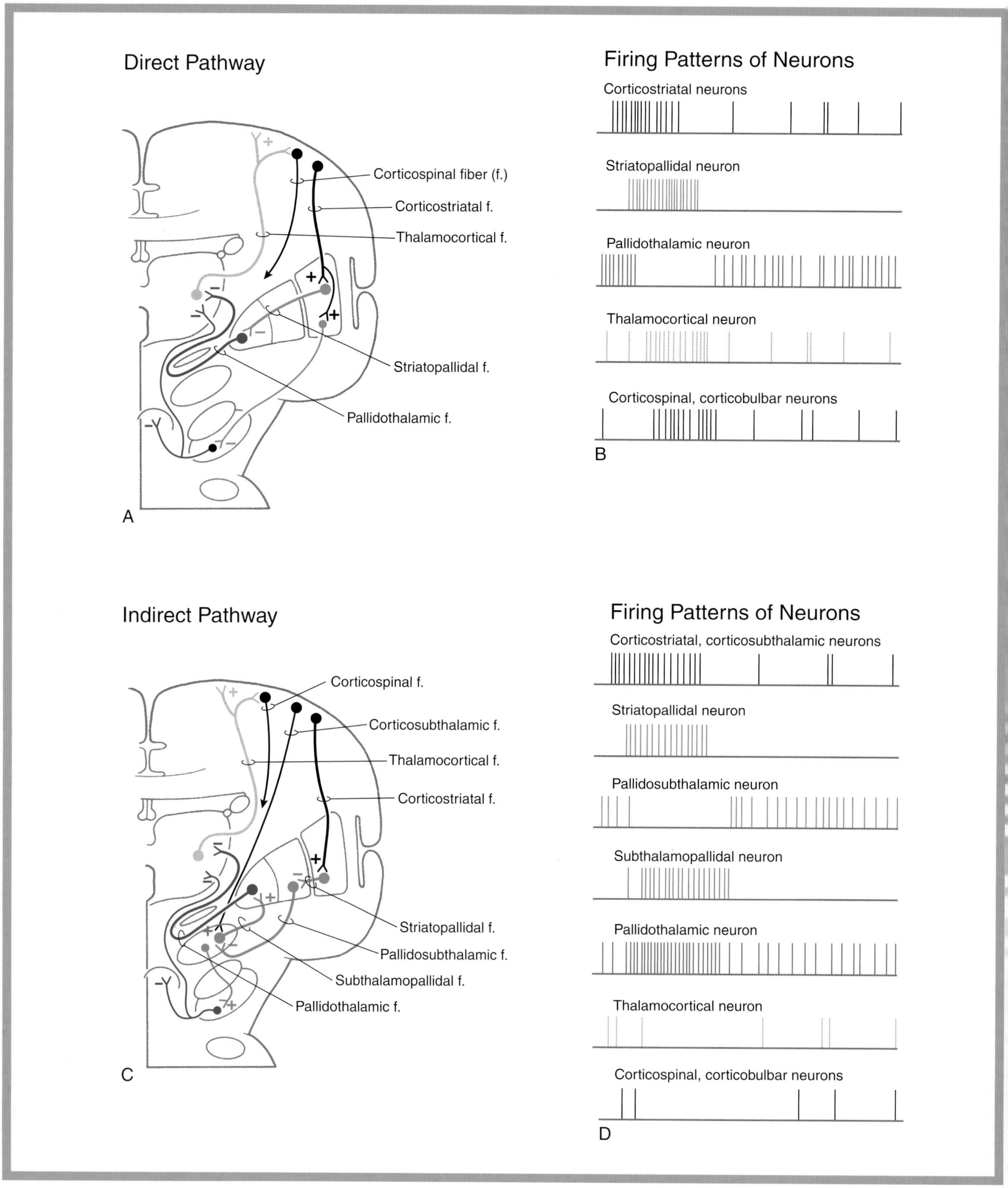

Direct Pathway

- Corticospinal fiber (f.)
- Corticostriatal f.
- Thalamocortical f.
- Striatopallidal f.
- Pallidothalamic f.

A

Firing Patterns of Neurons

Corticostriatal neurons

Striatopallidal neuron

Pallidothalamic neuron

Thalamocortical neuron

Corticospinal, corticobulbar neurons

B

Indirect Pathway

- Corticospinal f.
- Corticosubthalamic f.
- Thalamocortical f.
- Corticostriatal f.
- Striatopallidal f.
- Pallidosubthalamic f.
- Subthalamopallidal f.
- Pallidothalamic f.

C

Firing Patterns of Neurons

Corticostriatal, corticosubthalamic neurons

Striatopallidal neuron

Pallidosubthalamic neuron

Subthalamopallidal neuron

Pallidothalamic neuron

Thalamocortical neuron

Corticospinal, corticobulbar neurons

D

Figure 26-10. The direct and indirect pathways (**A**, **C**) and the corresponding firing patterns of their neurons (**B**, **D**). The color of each fiber correlates with the color of the firing pattern (action potentials) of that neuron (**B** and **D**). The bold fibers in **A** and **C** represent the primary pathway in each example. +, excitatory synapse; –, inhibitory synapse.

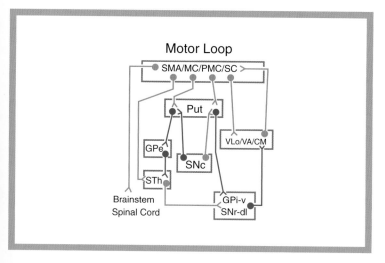

Figure 26-11. Flow diagram of the direct and indirect pathways of the motor loop through the basal nuclei as discussed in the text. CM, centromedian nucleus; GPe, external segments of globus pallidus; GPi-v, internal segment of globus pallidus, ventral portion; MC, motor cortex; PMC, premotor cortex; Put, putamen; SC, somatosensory cortex; SMA, supplementary motor area; SNc, substantia nigra pars compacta; SNr-dl, substantia nigra pars reticulata, dorsolateral portion; STh, subthalamic nucleus; VA, ventral anterior nucleus; VLo, ventral lateral nucleus, oral part.

pathways. These deficits include those related to emotions, cognition, eye movements, and mentation.

Behavioral Functions of the Basal Nuclei

The best-understood functions of the basal nuclei are associated with the motor systems, in particular, the somatomotor (motor loop) and visuomotor (oculomotor loop) systems. Lesions in the basal nuclei resulting from stroke or other disease processes lead to significant changes in the motor behavior of the patient. Examination of the pathways damaged in these cases reveals how disruption of the basal nuclei can lead to seemingly opposite effects in different patients. For example, movements can be either reduced *(hypokinetic disturbances)* or increased *(hyperkinetic disturbances)*.

Hypokinetic Disturbances

The two major types of hypokinetic disturbances seen in patients with basal nuclear disorders are *akinesia* and *bradykinesia* (Fig. 26-16). Akinesia *is an impairment in the initiation of movement;* bradykinesia *is a reduction in velocity and amplitude of movement.* Both disturbances are characteristic in patients with Parkinson disease.

Akinesia, the impaired ability to initiate voluntary movements, may be due to disruption of the ability to plan a movement or to guide a movement to some desired position. Experimental studies in nonhuman primates reveal that many basal nuclear neurons are most active during the *planning phase of a movement* or when the subject is making an *internally guided movement.* The latter is a movement to a location at which no particular stimulus is present. Thus, *patients with akinesia have a generalized disruption of the role of the basal nuclei in planning and generating programmed movements.*

Bradykinesia, the reduction in velocity and amplitude of movements, is due to disruption of the balance between the outflows of the direct and indirect pathways to the thalamus. The result is *an increase in the activation of the antagonist muscles.* Thus, *the observed abnormalities are due to an inappropriate activation*

of the antagonistic muscles, and not necessarily to an overall decrease in muscular activity.

Hypokinetic disorders can be considered as lesions of the neostriatum (Fig. 26-12A, B). These lesions result in the loss of inhibitory connections between the neostriatum and internal segment of the globus pallidus. Thus, tonically active pallidothalamic neurons continuously inhibit their thalamic targets. The thalamus is not disinhibited, so there is a decreased flow of information through the thalamus to the cerebral cortex. This decrease, in turn, causes a decrease in the activity of the appropriate corticospinal and other corticofugal neurons. In addition, most of the connections that subserve the indirect pathway remain intact. Therefore, when those connections are activated, as, for example, by a larger-than-normal burst in cortical neurons, subthalamopallidal cells excite pallidothalamic neurons, which results in increased inhibition of the thalamus. The combination of a *lack of disinhibition of the thalamus* by the direct pathway and an *increased inhibition of the thalamus* by the indirect pathway significantly *decreases the level of appropriate activity in the cerebral cortex and increases the level of inappropriate cortical activity.* Therefore, the patient becomes less able to execute the appropriate movements. Experiments in nonhuman primates have shown that bradykinetic animals have levels of neuronal activity that are consistent with this view.

Hyperkinetic Disturbances

Hyperkinetic disturbances take the form of dyskinesias. The three most common forms are *ballismus, choreiform movements,* and *athetoid movements.*

Ballismus is most typically seen as *hemiballismus* because it usually occurs on one side. It consists of uncontrolled flinging (ballistic) movements of an upper or lower extremity. This motor disorder is most commonly seen in patients with vascular lesions localized to the contralateral subthalamic nucleus (Fig. 26-12C, D).

Choreiform movements, which are present in Huntington disease and sometimes in treated Parkinson disease, are generalized irregular (and brisk) dance-like movements of the limbs. Similar movements may occur in oral and facial musculature. These patients may also have a decrease in muscle tone *(hypotonia).* In Huntington disease, there is an initial selective loss of the medium spiny cells in the striatum, which project to the lateral pallidum, and of acetylcholine-containing neurons in the striatal complex. It is thus likely that the neurons specifically associated with the indirect pathway are lost.

Finally, *athetoid movements (athetosis)* are a continuous writhing of distal portions of the extremity (Fig. 26-13). Athetosis generally presents as slow, sinuous and writhing movements more obvious in the upper extremities and hands (Fig. 26-13) and face, although any muscle group may be affected. However, athetoid movements may also be seen as a range of abnormal movements. When they are more brisk and resemble chorea, the term *choreoathetosis* may be appropriate. When the movements are more intense and sustained, they may resemble dystonia, and the term *athetotic dystonia* may be used.

These hyperkinetic disturbances can most easily be explained by the disruption of the indirect pathway through the motor loop, resulting from the loss of excitatory subthalamopallidal neurons (Fig. 26-12C, D). The balance between excitation of pallidothalamic neurons (by the direct pathway) and their inhibition (by the indirect pathway) is skewed. The result is a decrease in the net amount of inhibition of thalamic cells, which results in more activity in the cerebral cortex.

Integrated Function of the Basal Nuclei

By combining the direct and indirect pathways, it is possible to gain a better appreciation of how the basal nuclei affect

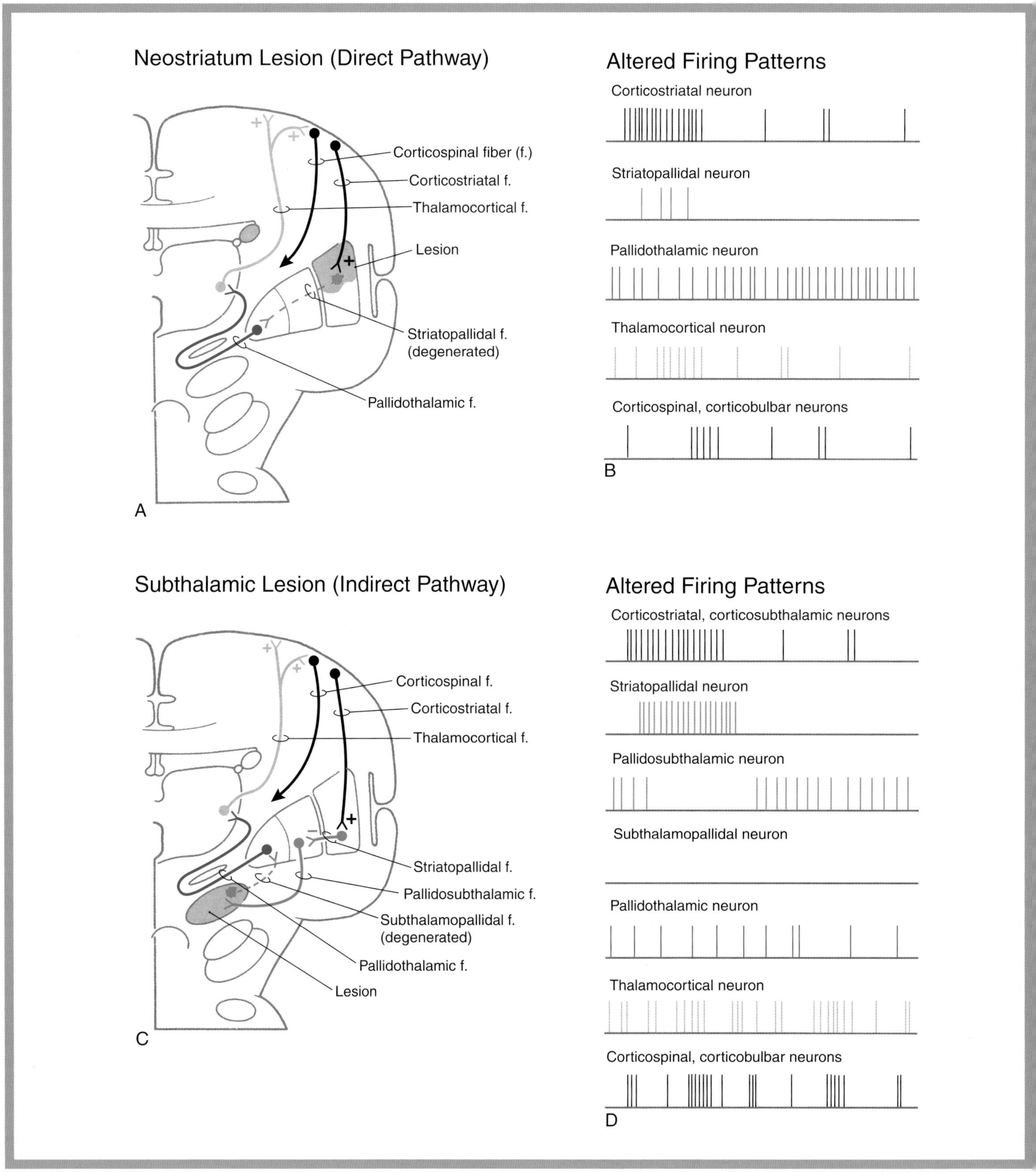

Neostriatum Lesion (Direct Pathway)

- Corticospinal fiber (f.)
- Corticostriatal f.
- Thalamocortical f.
- Lesion
- Striatopallidal f. (degenerated)
- Pallidothalamic f.

A

Altered Firing Patterns

Corticostriatal neuron

Striatopallidal neuron

Pallidothalamic neuron

Thalamocortical neuron

Corticospinal, corticobulbar neurons

B

Subthalamic Lesion (Indirect Pathway)

- Corticospinal f.
- Corticostriatal f.
- Thalamocortical f.
- Striatopallidal f.
- Pallidosubthalamic f.
- Subthalamopallidal f. (degenerated)
- Pallidothalamic f.
- Lesion

C

Altered Firing Patterns

Corticostriatal, corticosubthalamic neurons

Striatopallidal neuron

Pallidosubthalamic neuron

Subthalamopallidal neuron

Pallidothalamic neuron

Thalamocortical neuron

Corticospinal, corticobulbar neurons

D

Figure 26-12. Schematic representation of a lesion in the neostriatum (**A**) and a lesion of the subthalamic nucleus (**C**), and the corresponding alterations of neuronal firing patterns of all fibers involved in each pathway (**B**, **D**). The color of each fiber in **A** and **C** correlates with the colors of the altered firing patterns in **B** and **D**. +, excitatory synapses; –, inhibitory synapse.

their targets through a balance between activation by the direct pathway and inactivation by the indirect pathway, as seen in Figure 26-14A, B. The activity in the cerebral cortex activates the striatopallidal neurons in both the direct *(red)* and indirect *(green)* pathways. Activation of the striatopallidal neurons in the direct pathway will inhibit pallidothalamic neurons *(blue* in Fig. 26-14B1). This pathway may be considered to be the initiator of the pause in pallidothalamic activity. At the same time, activation of the striatopallidal neurons in the indirect pathway inhibits the pallidosubthalamic neurons (Fig. 26-14B2). This inhibition releases the subthalamic neurons, which then excite the pallidothalamic neurons. This excitation by the

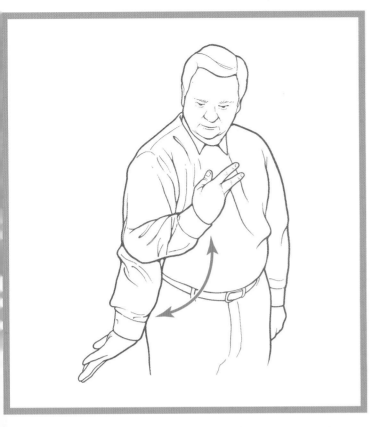

Figure 26-13. Athetoid movements (athetosis) of the upper extremity.

subthalamopallidal neurons is what reactivates the pallidothalamic neurons that were inhibited through the direct pathway. Thus, careful balance of the activity between the two pathways modulates the amount of time during which the thalamocortical neurons are activated.

In addition to the activities of these pathways, the dopaminergic loop from the neostriatum to the substantia nigra and back to the neostriatum is also active. Activity of striatonigral projections originating in the striosomes will inhibit the dopaminergic nigrostriatal pathway (Fig. 26-14B3). Subsequent reactivation of the nigral neurons is due in part to a number of factors, including disinhibition of the pars compacta by means of the striatal projection originating from the matrix. The dopaminergic neurons project back onto striatal neurons. The effect of the dopamine depends on the receptor on the postsynaptic striatal neuron. D_1 receptors are found on striatal neurons in the "direct" pathway. Stimulation of the D_1 receptors causes excitation of the striatopallidal neurons in the direct pathway. This excitation accounts for the slightly longer train of action potentials seen in Figure 26-14B. The neurons belonging to the "indirect" pathway have D_2 receptors. When dopamine binds to the D_2 receptor, the neurons are inhibited. This inhibition accounts for the shorter train of action potentials for indirect striatopallidal neurons in the indirect pathway.

The modulation between the direct and indirect pathways by dopamine is significantly affected if dopamine is absent. For example, in Parkinson disease, the loss of melanin-containing dopaminergic neurons in the nigral complex has the net effect of decreasing thalamocortical neuronal activity (Fig. 26-14C, D). The striatopallidal activity of the direct pathway initiates the pause (Fig. 26-14D1). However, the activity is less sustained owing to the loss of excitation from the substantia nigra. The activity of the striatopallidal neurons in the indirect pathway is not inhibited by the dopamine and thus is of a somewhat longer duration. This longer duration of activity results in a longer-lasting inhibition of the pallidosubthalamic neurons (Fig. 26-14D2), which increases the activity of the subthalamopallidal neurons

and results in increased activation of the pallidothalamic neurons. Consequently, not only is the pause in pallidothalamic activity shortened but the inhibition of the thalamus by these neurons is enhanced. The net result is an increased inhibition of the thalamocortical neurons with decreased activity in the cerebral cortex.

Etiology of Basal Nuclear Related Disorders

The hallmark of basal nuclear disorders is a change in the neurochemical environment within the striatal complex. Careful examination of patients with basal nuclear syndromes reveals that the classic motor signs and symptoms constitute only one characteristic of these disorders and that associative memory and limbic dysfunctions also occur. Recent clinical and basic science studies of the chemistry of basal nuclear disorders have provided significant insight into their etiology and treatment.

Huntington Disease

As originally described, *Huntington disease* is a progressive, untreatable disorder in which patients lose their ability to function and experience increasing dementia; death occurs 10 to 15 years after onset. The initial symptoms indicative of this disease generally begin to appear at 35 to 40 years of age. In the United States, the incidence of Huntington disease is approximately 1 in every 17,000 to 19,000 individuals. In the early stages, this disease is characterized by absentmindedness, irritability, depression, clumsiness, and sudden falls. Gradually, choreiform movements increase until the patient is bedridden. Cognitive functions and speech progressively deteriorate. The later stages of this disease are characterized by severe dementia. One salient feature in the progressive memory loss is a difficulty in integrating newly acquired memory into useful information for planning movements. In addition, a large proportion of these patients develop psychiatric disorders such as major affective disorder, schizophrenia, and other behavioral disturbances.

Postmortem examination reveals decrease in the size of the striatal complex caused by loss of about 90% of all striatal neurons and extensive astrocytosis. In particular, medium spiny cells, which project to the lateral pallidum, and the large acetylcholine-containing local circuit cells are lost. This disease can be demonstrated on magnetic resonance imaging (MRI) as a flattening of the head of the caudate nucleus (Fig. 26-15).

Huntington disease is a genetic disorder inherited in autosomal dominant fashion, and any person who inherits the gene will develop the disease. It is most prevalent among persons of European descent. This disease is known to be due to a mutation on the short arm of chromosome 4. At the molecular level, the mutated gene has dozens of copies of the DNA sequence CAG (cytosine-adenine-guanine), which codes for glutamate. These CAG repeats result in the addition of glutamate residues inside the gene coding for the protein *huntingtin*. Patients with larger numbers of repeats have a more severe illness with an earlier onset. Thus, there are now reliable markers for the disease.

Much effort has been devoted to understanding the mechanism underlying the death of striatal neurons in this disease. In the very earliest stages of the disease, which may be months or years before the onset of clinical features, there is a diminution of glucose metabolism in the neostriatum of some patients. *Glutamate excitotoxicity* is thought to be primarily responsible for this process. Normally, cortical axons release glutamate as their neurotransmitter in the caudate and putamen. Glutamate binds with its receptor on the medium spiny neurons and opens the receptor channel to an influx of ions. This action depolarizes the membrane, resulting in an excitatory postsynaptic potential.

Direct and Indirect Pathways
(Including the Substantia Nigra)

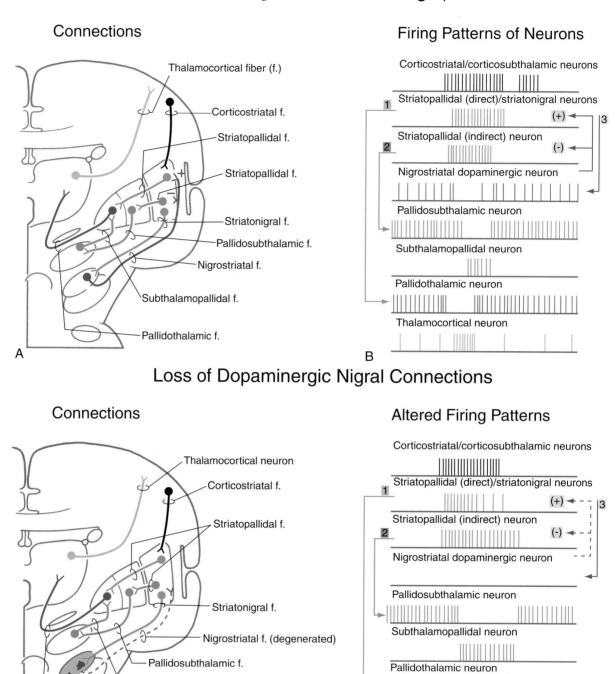

Figure 26-14. The role of the direct and indirect pathways and the influence of dopamine. Fibers and their corresponding firing patterns for the intact pathway are shown in **A** and **B**. The flow of signals through the direct (1), indirect (2), and a striatonigral-nigrostriatal (3) pathways are shown by their respective arrows. Lesions of the pars compacta (**C**), as in Parkinson disease, is characterized by the loss of dopaminergic neurons and results in the altered firing patterns of neurons in the entire pathway (**D**). The colors of the fibers correlate with the colors of the action potentials. +, excitatory synapses; –, inhibitory synapses.

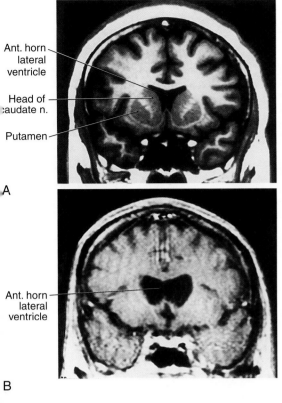

Ant. horn lateral ventricle

Head of caudate n.

Putamen

A

Ant. horn lateral ventricle

B

Figure 26-15. Coronal MR image obtained through the frontal lobe, and head of the caudate nucleus, of a normal person (**A**) and of a patient with Huntington disease (**B**). The head of the caudate normally forms a prominent bulge into the anterior horn of the lateral ventricle (**A**, inversion recovery image). Profound cell loss in the neostriatum in Huntington disease greatly diminishes the size of the caudate and renders the lateral wall of the ventricle flat (**B**, T1-weighted image). The slightly wavy appearance of the image in **B** is the result of movement (tremor) while the scan was being done.

As glutamate dissociates from the receptor, it is cleared from the extracellular space by uptake by astrocytes. In Huntington disease, an unknown mechanism causes glutamate to persist at one type of receptor, the *N*-methyl-D-aspartate (NMDA) receptor, which opens calcium ion channels. The resulting excessive influx of calcium causes an increase in intracellular calcium, which triggers a cascade that leads to cell death. Glutamate excitotoxicity is also thought to be the primary cause of localized neuronal death following acute brain injury, such as stroke (see Chapter 2).

Parkinson Disease

Parkinson disease is also a progressive, debilitating disorder. It affects over 500,000 Americans and there are about 50,000 new cases each year. The vast majority of cases of *adult Parkinson disease* appear initially as signs or symptoms in patients in the age range of 45 to 65 years (mean of 55). These initial signs may include a slight asymmetrical gait and/or vague clumsiness of a hand, less blinking, or a reduction in, or lack, of arm swing when walking. In rare cases, signs or symptoms of Parkinson disease may be seen in patients younger than 20 years of age *(juvenile Parkinson disease)* or in patients in the age range of 20 to 40 years of age *(young-onset Parkinson disease)*. This disease, in these younger patients, is more likely to have a genetic basis. Although equally rare, Parkinson disease may be seen resultant to repeated trauma, such as that experienced by boxers *(pugilistic Parkinson disease)*. Some familial groups with Parkinson disease have been described.

This disorder is characterized by a progressive onset of movement and affective disturbances (Fig. 26-16). The movement disorders include *tremor at rest, cogwheel (gamma) rigidity*

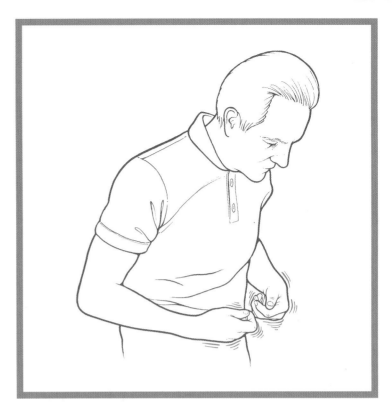

Figure 26-16. Parkinsonian tremor (resting tremor) and characteristic posturing. The patient may have difficulty initiating a movement (akinesia), or once movement is initiated, it may be slow and lack spontaneity (bradykinesia).

(increased muscular tone), *akinesia, bradykinesia, disturbances of eye movements,* and *loss of postural reflexes.* A classic picture of a patient with Parkinson disease is a person sitting or standing with *pill-rolling tremor,* a *blank stare* (reptilian or decreased blink), a *flexed posture,* and a *paucity of movement* (Fig. 26-16). When the patient starts to move there is a shuffling start, as if the feet were stuck in place (also called a *festinating gait*), followed by nearly normal gait.

At autopsy, the nigral complex is found to be devoid of dopaminergic neurons. Although there is degeneration of serotoninergic and noradrenergic pathways, it is this specific loss of dopamine that results in the observed symptoms. The standard treatment aims at replacing the lost dopamine. Because dopamine itself will not cross the blood-brain barrier, patients are given L-3,4-hydroxyphenylalanine (*L-dopa*), which will. This agent is now combined with a second drug, *carbidopa,* which does not cross the blood-brain barrier but has the effect of inhibiting peripheral uptake of L-dopa and thus increasing the amount of L-dopa available to brain tissue. Persons receiving this combination therapy, along with other drugs such as dopamine agonists and monoamine oxidase inhibitors, show significant reductions in signs and symptoms, although progression of the disease is not arrested. Why L-dopa works is not clear. The method by which L-dopa is converted to dopamine in the brain of Parkinson disease patients is not known, as these persons have very little tyrosine hydroxylase, the enzyme that is necessary for this catabolism. Moreover, the dopamine is not localized to specific nerve terminals or to the basal nuclei. Thus, it appears that dopamine simply needs to be in the neural environment of the striatal complex to reduce the signs and symptoms of the patients.

Insight into one possible mechanism of Parkinson disease was inadvertently realized by a group of illicit drug manufacturers whose heroin was contaminated by a compound called 1-methyl-4-phenyl-1,2,3,6-tetrahydropyridine (MPTP). Persons who used this drug developed symptoms exactly like those of patients with Parkinson disease but at an age (early 20s) when this disease is normally never manifested. Autopsy revealed a profound loss of dopaminergic neurons in the substantia nigra pars compacta.

Studies on the mechanism of action of MPTP in animal models showed that MPTP is converted into an active form (MPP$^+$) before it causes a loss of dopaminergic cells. This metabolic pathway requires monoamine oxidase (MAO). Thus, it was hypothesized that the use of MAO inhibitors may affect the progression of Parkinson disease. In fact, clinical trials have now shown that the drug L-deprenyl, an MAO-B inhibitor, slows the progression of Parkinson disease and increases the levels of dopamine in the brain. The increase in dopamine may result both from protection of neurons against toxicity and from blocking of the degradation pathway for dopamine, which requires the MAO enzyme.

In recent years, there has been an increasing number of surgical treatments for Parkinson disease. The most common type of surgical intervention is ablative surgery in which either the ventral intermediate nucleus of the thalamus (thalamotomy) or the posterolateral part of the internal segment of the globus pallidus (pallidotomy) is lesioned. Another surgical approach involves introduction of stimulation electrodes directed at the thalamus, globus pallidus, or subthalamic nuclei. Each of these surgical approaches appears to be effective for treating one set of symptoms. However, none of these approaches completely eliminates the disease or prevents its progression.

A controversial method of treatment for Parkinson disease patients involves the use of human embryonic or autologous transplants. Tissues that produce dopamine, such as substantia nigra (embryonic) and the adrenal cortex (autologous), are obtained and separated into cell suspensions. These are then injected into the lateral ventricles of the patient. The idea is that these cells will adhere to the walls of the ventricle and produce dopamine. The dopamine will then diffuse into the nearby cerebral cortex and basal nuclei. This procedure has now been performed in humans as well as in animals. In the clinical trials to date, only a small number of patients have benefited from this approach.

Wilson Disease

Wilson disease, also known as *hepatolenticular degeneration*, is also related to the basal nuclei. This genetic disorder inherited as an autosomal recessive trait is due to a mutation on the long arm of chromosome 13. Onset of the disorder is typically between 11 and 25 years of age. Wilson disease is a disorder in copper metabolism that results in accumulation of the metal in the liver, resulting in small necrotic lesions leading to cirrhotic nodules and progressive liver damage. Signs of liver damage may precede the onset of neurologic abnormalities by several years. Another metabolic feature, probably due to damage of the tubules in the kidney, is *aminoaciduria*, excessive amounts of amino acids in the urine. In the eye, copper accumulates in the periphery of the cornea; these deposits are responsible for the Kayser-Fleischer ring (Fig. 26-17), which may appear yellow to green to brown. Degeneration of the putamen, often forming small cavities, is the predominant pathoanatomic feature in the brain (Fig. 26-18). However, other regions of the brain, including the frontal lobe of the cerebral cortex, may also show similar changes. This degeneration is due to a loss of neurons, axonal degeneration, and increasing numbers of protoplasmic astrocytes.

As in other basal nuclear disorders, many patients with Wilson disease will develop psychiatric symptoms. However, the motor disturbances are often the most evident signs and include *tremor, dysarthria, diminished dexterity, unsteady gait,* and *rigidity.* The most common form of tremor in this disease is known as *asterixis,* a "wing-beating" tremor. Affected patients do not have a tremor at rest. However, after the arms are extended, a beating

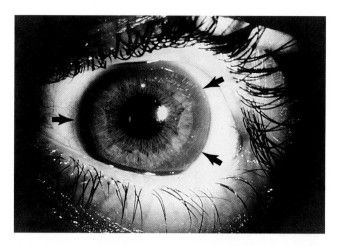

Figure 26-17. Deposition of copper (Kayser-Fleischer ring, *arrows*) in the periphery of the cornea as seen in hepatolenticular degeneration (Wilson disease).

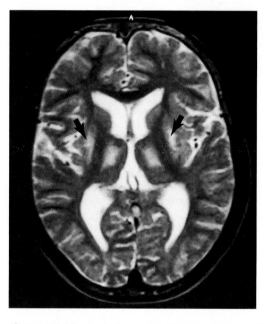

Figure 26-18. Axial T2 weighted MR image of a patient with Wilson disease. Note the bilateral cavitations in the lenticular nuclei *(arrows),* hence the name hepatolenticular degeneration. All Wilson disease patients are somewhat different; this patient also has noticeable signal changes bilaterally in the thalami. Other patients may show similar changes in the dentate nucleus, pons, or midbrain. (Image courtesy of Dr. Madhuri Behari.)

movement develops that can be restricted to the wrists or can result in the arms being thrown up and down in a wide arc. Treatment is essential, and the goal is to decrease the amount of copper within the body, thus limiting its toxic effects. Prognosis for patients who have completed the first few years of treatment is very good, with diminution of neurologic signs within 5 to 6 months from the onset of therapy.

Sydenham Chorea

This is a childhood autoimmune disease that is infrequently seen. This disease typically affects children between the ages of 5 and 15 years. It is a consequence of rheumatic fever, which is caused by infection with group A β-hemolytic streptococci. The disease is self-limited and is rarely fatal; fatalities are usually attributed to consequences of rheumatic fever. The chorea may not appear until 6 months or longer after infection and typically lasts for 3 to 6 weeks. Patients present with rapid, irregular, aimless movements of the limbs, face, and trunk. These movements are more flowing and "restless" than those in Huntington disease.

atients. In addition, patients with Sydenham chorea have some muscular weakness and hypotonia. Other signs and symptoms may include irritability, emotional lability, obsessive-compulsive behaviors, attention deficit, and anxiety. Fortunately, this is a benign disease, and most patients experience complete recovery from the symptoms. However, about one third of patients may have recurrences of signs and symptoms after several months or even years.

Tardive Dyskinesia

Tardive dyskinesia is a basal nuclear disorder that is iatrogenic in nature, that is, caused by medical intervention for another disease. This condition is caused by chronic treatment with neuroleptic medications such as the phenothiazines (e.g., chlorpromazine, thioridazine) and butyrophenones (e.g., haloperidol). The manifestation of this condition is uncontrolled involuntary movements, particularly of the face and tongue, and cogwheel rigidity. These abnormalities may be temporary or permanent. The action of these neuroleptic drugs is to block dopaminergic transmission throughout the brain. The primary target cells are those in the ventral tegmental area that form the mesolimbic dopaminergic pathway. Prolonged treatment with neuroleptic drugs leads to a hypersensitivity at the D_3 dopamine receptor, which causes an imbalance in the nigrostriatal influence on the basal nuclear motor loop and ultimately results in movement disorders.

Synopsis of Clinical Points

- Acetylcholine-containing cells and medium spiny neurons are lost from the striatal complex in Huntington disease (p. 416).
- Acetylcholine-containing cells are lost in a number of areas in the central nervous system in Alzheimer disease (p. 417).
- Loss of the melanin-containing cells in the substantia nigra, pars compacta, is characteristically seen in Parkinson disease (pp. 425, 427).
- When inhibitory neurons are released from inhibition, this is called disinhibition (pp. 414, 421).
- The deficits seen in patients with injury to the basal nuclei are expressed through descending cortical pathways (pp. 414, 423).
- Hypokinetic disturbances are those in which motor activity is reduced (p. 423).
- Hyperkinetic disturbances are those in which motor activity is increased (p. 423).
- Akinesia is impairment in initiating a movement, and bradykinesia is reduced velocity and amplitude of movement; both are seen in Parkinson disease (p. 423).
- Ballism, or hemiballistic movements, is seen in lesions of the subthalamus (p. 423).
- A patient with hemiballistic movements on one side of the body has a lesion in the contralateral subthalamic nucleus (p. 423).
- Choreiform movements are seem in patients with Huntington disease (p. 423).
- Athetosis (or athetoid movements) is one type of hyperkinetic disorder (p. 423).
- Huntington disease is a genetic disorder that results in absentmindedness, depression, memory loss, locomotor deficits, psychiatric disorders, dementia, and death at 10 to 15 years after onset (p. 425).
- Glutamate excitotoxicity is a probable mechanism of cell death in Huntington disease (p. 425).
- Parkinson disease (also called adult Parkinson disease) is characterized by a resting tremor, rigidity, akinesia and bradykinesia, and the loss of postural reflexes (p. 427).
- The symptoms of Parkinson disease may be treated with L-dopa in combination with other drugs (p. 427).
- Wilson disease (hepatolenticular degeneration) is an inherited disease of the teenage years and young adulthood (p. 428).
- Cavitations may be seen in the lenticular nucleus in magnetic resonance images of patients with Wilson disease (p. 428).
- The presence of amino acids in the urine of Wilson disease patients is called aminoaciduria (p. 428).
- A deficit in copper metabolism is the cause of the lesions in Wilson disease; this disease is treatable (p. 428).
- Asterixis, a wing-beating tremor, may be seen in Wilson disease patients (p. 428).
- Sydenham chorea is a childhood autoimmune disease that is usually seen as a consequence to rheumatic fever (p. 428).
- Sydenham chorea is rarely fatal and has characteristic motor deficits, and many patients recover fully (p. 429).
- Tardive dyskinesia is a motor disorder that results in a patient being treated for another disease (p. 429).

Sources and Additional Reading

Alexander GE, DeLong MR, Strick PL: Parallel organization of functionally segregated circuits linking basal ganglia and cortex. Annu Rev Neurosci 9:357-381, 1986.

Brazis PW, Masdeu JC, Biller J: Localization in Clinical Neurology, 4th ed. Philadelphia, Lippincott Williams & Wilkins, 2001.

Caplan LR: Caplan's Stroke: A Clinical Approach, 3rd ed. Boston, Butterworth Heinemann, 2000.

Gerfen CR: The neostriatal mosaic: Multiple levels of compartmental organization in the basal ganglia. Annu Rev Neurosci 15:285-320, 1992.

Goldman-Rakic PS (ed): Basal ganglia research (Special Issue). Trends Neurosci 13:241-308, 1990.

Graybiel AM, Aosaki T, Flaherty AM, Kimura M: The basal ganglia and adaptive motor control. Science 265:1826-1831, 1994.

Haber SN, McFarland NR: The concept of the ventral striatum in nonhuman primates. Ann N Y Acad Sci 877:33-48, 1999.

Hankey GJ, Wardlaw JM: Clinical Neurology. New York, Demos Medical Publishing, 2002.

Middleton FA, Strick PL: Anatomical evidence for cerebellar and basal ganglia involvement in higher cognitive function. Science 266:458-461, 1994.

Nieuwenhuys R, Voogd J, Van Huijzen Chr: The Human Central Nervous System, A Synopsis and Atlas, 3rd ed. Berlin, Springer-Verlag, 1988.

Parent A, Hazrati L-N: Functional anatomy of the basal ganglia: I. The cortico-basal ganglia-thalamo-cortical loop. Brain Res Rev 20:91-127, 1995.

Parent A, Hazrati L-N: Functional anatomy of the basal ganglia: II. The place of the subthalamic nucleus and external pallidum in basal ganglia circuitry. Brain Res Rev 20:128-154, 1995.

Pedro BM, Pilowsky LS, Costa DC, Hemsley DR, Ell PJ, Verhoeff NP, Kerwin RW, Gray NS: Stereotypy, schizophrenia and dopamine D_2 receptor binding in the basal ganglia. Psychol Med 24:423-429, 1994.

Pryse-Phillips W: Companion to Clinical Neurology, 2nd ed. New York, Oxford University Press, 2003.

Rowland LP (ed): Merritt's Neurology, 10th ed. Philadelphia, Lippincott Williams & Wilkins, 2000.

Shultz W: Predictive reward signal of dopamine neurons. J Neurophysiol 80:1-27, 1998.

Chapter 27

The Cerebellum

D. E. Haines, G. A. Mihailoff, and J. R. Bloedel

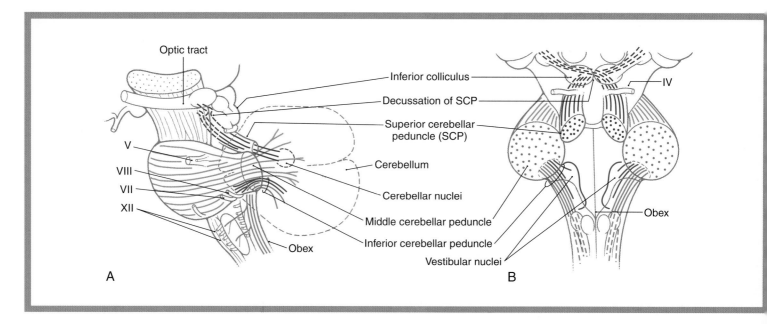

Figure 27-1. Lateral (**A**) and posterior (**B**) views of the brainstem showing the inferior *(dark green + red),* middle *(light green),* and superior *(blue)* cerebellar peduncles. The inferior peduncle is composed of juxtarestiform *(dark green)* and restiform *(red)* bodies. Cranial nerves are identified by Roman numerals.

As indicated by its relative size (about 10% of the weight of the central nervous system), the cerebellum is important in brain function. However, it executes these responsibilities in unique ways. First, it receives extensive sensory input, but it is not involved in sensory discrimination or interpretation. Second, although it profoundly influences motor function, resection of relatively large portions of the cerebellar cortex does not result in lasting paralysis. Large lesions of the cerebellum may result in significant motor deficits (seen as asynergistic movements) but not in paralysis. Third, the cerebellum plays a role in motor learning and higher mental function.

Overview

The cerebellum is composed of a highly convoluted *cerebellar cortex* and a core of white matter containing the *cerebellar nuclei.* This structure is anchored to the brainstem via the *cerebellar peduncles.* The cerebellum is located superior to the brainstem, inferior to the tentorium cerebelli, and internal to the occipital bone. The cerebellum has a *superior surface* apposed to the tentorium and a convex *inferior surface* that abuts the inner surface of the occipital bone.

The cerebellum receives input from many areas of the neuraxis and influences motor performance through connections with the dorsal thalamus and, ultimately, the motor cortices. Lesions of these pathways result in characteristic motor dysfunctions, which may involve either proximal (axial) or distal musculature. These deficits are actually the result of altered activity in the motor cortex and its descending brainstem and spinal projections, which influence lower motor neurons of the spinal cord.

Basic Structural Features

Cerebellar Peduncles

The cerebellum is connected to the brainstem by three pairs of *cerebellar peduncles* (Fig. 27-1). The *inferior cerebellar peduncle* is composed of a *restiform body* and a *juxtarestiform body.* The former is the large ridge on the dorsolateral aspect of the medulla rostral to the level of the obex. This bundle contains mainly fibers that arise in the spinal cord or medulla. The juxtarestiform body is located in the wall of the fourth ventricle.

Its fibers form reciprocal connections between the cerebellum and vestibular structures.

The basilar pons, which is located inferior to the exiting root of the trigeminal nerve, is continuous into the *middle cerebellar peduncle (brachium pontis),* which is located superior to the exiting roots of the fifth cranial nerve (Figs. 27-1 and 27-2). These exiting roots represent the boundary between the basilar pons and the middle cerebellar peduncle. This large peduncle conveys fibers from the nuclei of the basilar pons into the cerebellum.

The *superior cerebellar peduncle (brachium conjunctivum)* sweeps rostrally out of the cerebellum and penetrates into the midbrain just caudal to the exit of the trochlear nerve (Fig. 27-1). This bundle contains predominantly *cerebellar efferent fibers* that originate from neurons of the cerebellar nuclei and distribute to the diencephalon and brainstem.

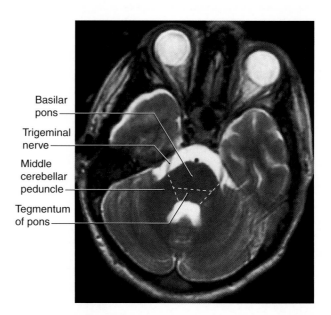

Figure 27-2. Axial MR image of the cerebellum and pons showing the relationship between the root of the trigeminal nerve and the basilar pons (inferior to the root) and the middle cerebellar peduncle (superior to the root). Compare with Figure 27-1.

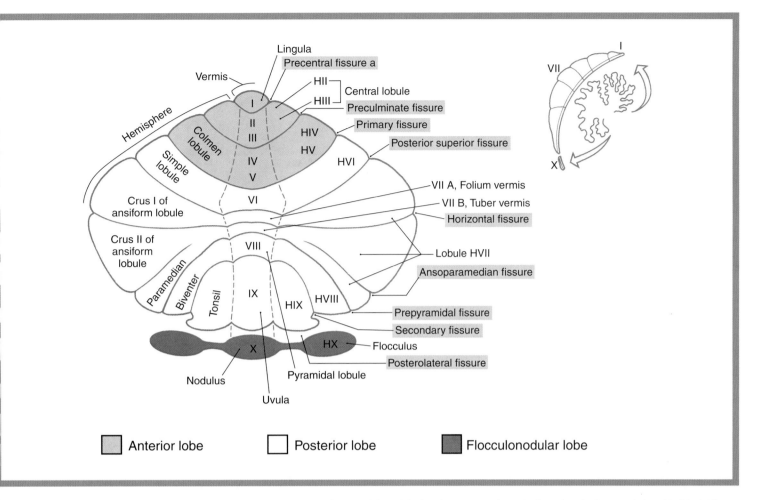

Figure 27-3. Unfolded view (see *upper right*) of the cerebellar cortex showing lobes, lobules *(by name and number),* and main fissures *(printed in blue).* The lobules of the hemisphere are designated by the prefix "H," to show which lobule of the hemisphere (H) is continuous with its corresponding *(designated by the Roman numeral)* vermal lobule.

Cerebellar Lobes, Lobules, and Zones

At the most general level, it is common to divide the cerebellum into a narrow midline *vermis* and expansive lateral *hemispheres* (Figs. 27-3 and 27-4). The cerebellum is further divided into *anterior, posterior,* and *flocculonodular lobes* by the *primary* and *posterolateral fissures,* respectively. The lobes of the cerebellum are composed of yet smaller divisions called *lobules* (Figs. 27-3 and 27-5). The lobules of the vermis are identified by Roman numerals I to X; the corresponding lateral (hemisphere) portion of each vermis lobule is identified by the same Roman numeral but with the prefix "H" (Figs. 27-3 and 27-5). Vermis lobules II to X have hemisphere portions HII to HX (Fig. 27-5); lobule I does not have a hemisphere part in humans. The anterior lobe comprises *lobules I to V and HII to HV,* and the posterior lobe, *lobules VI to IX and HVI to HIX.* The flocculonodular lobe consists of the nodulus (lobule X) and its hemisphere counterpart, the flocculus (lobule HX). In turn, each lobule consists of a series of individual ridges of cortex called *folia* (singular, *folium*).

The individual folia are continuous from one hemisphere to the other, across the midline (Fig. 27-4A). This pattern, obvious on the superior cerebellar surface, is disrupted on the inferior surface by the enlargement of the lateral parts of the cerebellum and consequent infolding of the midline area (Fig. 27-4B).

Superimposed on the lobes and lobules of the cerebellum are rostrocaudally oriented cortical zones that are defined on the basis of their connections. There are three principal zones on each side: the *medial (vermal), intermediate (paravermal),* and *lateral (hemisphere)* zones (Fig. 27-5). On the basis of their connections, these three larger zones can be subdivided further

into nine smaller zones. In general, these zone patterns are the basis for the *modules* discussed later in this chapter. The clinical deficits that result from a cerebellar lesion depend mainly on which of the three principal zones is involved; consequently, the three-zone terminology is used in this chapter.

The *medial (vermal) zone* is a narrow strip of cortex adjacent to the midline that extends throughout anterior and posterior lobes and includes the nodulus (Figs. 27-4A, B and 27-5). This zone is widest in lobule VI and tapers rostrally and caudally. The *intermediate (paravermal) zone* lies adjacent to the medial zone and extends throughout anterior and posterior lobes but has little representation in the flocculonodular lobe (Fig. 27-5). The *lateral (hemisphere) zone* occupies by far the largest part of the cerebellar cortex. It includes large portions of anterior and posterior lobes and the flocculus (Figs. 27-3 and 27-5).

Cerebellar Nuclei

The four pairs of cerebellar nuclei are located within the white matter core of the cerebellum and are accessed easily by fibers traveling to and from the overlying cortex (Figs. 27-5 and 27-6). The *fastigial (medial cerebellar) nucleus* lies immediately adjacent to the midline and is functionally related to the overlying medial zone of the cerebellar cortex. Lateral to the fastigial nucleus are the two interposed nuclei: the *globose (posterior interposed) nucleus* and the *emboliform (anterior interposed) nucleus.* These nuclei are functionally related to the intermediate zone of the cortex. Lateral to the emboliform nucleus is the *dentate (lateral cerebellar) nucleus,* which appears as a large, undulating sheet of cells shaped like a partially crumpled paper bag. Its

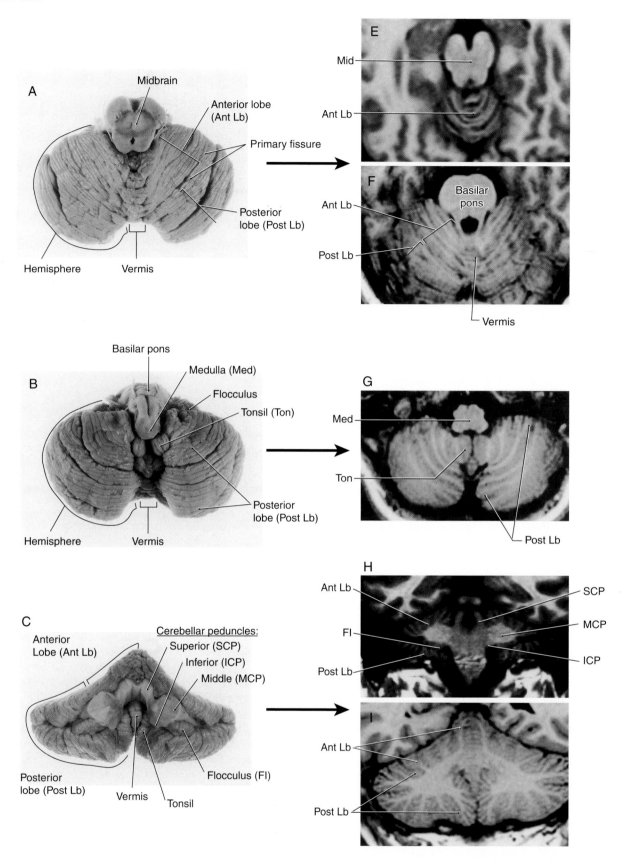

Figure 27-4. Rostral (**A**, superior aspect), caudal (**B**, inferior aspect), anterior or ventral (**C**, with brainstem removed), and a medial sagittal (**D**) views of the cerebellum compared with corresponding views of the cerebellum in MRI (**E-J**). In rostral views (**A + E, J**) the folia of the anterior lobe can characteristically be followed across the midline. The tonsil and its close relationship with the medulla are seen in inferior views (**B + G, H**), while the peduncles and the lobes are clearly evident in anterior/ventral views (**C + H, I**). The medial sagittal views (**D + J**) reveal the relationship of the cerebellum to the fourth ventricle and brainstem.

opening, the *hilus*, is directed anteromedially (Fig. 27-6). This nucleus is functionally related to the lateral zone of the cortex; its large size correlates with the large size of this cortical zone.

Most of the signals that leave the cerebellum do so via axons that arise in the cerebellar nuclei; the remainder travel on fibers that originate in the cerebellar cortex. Collectively, the former constitute *cerebellar efferent projections* (or *fibers*). These axons originate from cells in the cerebellar nuclei and use one of the excitatory neurotransmitters *glutamate* or *aspartate* and thus function to activate their targets. The fastigial nuclei generally project bilaterally to the brainstem through the *juxtarestiform bodies*. Fibers originating in the dentate, emboliform, and globose

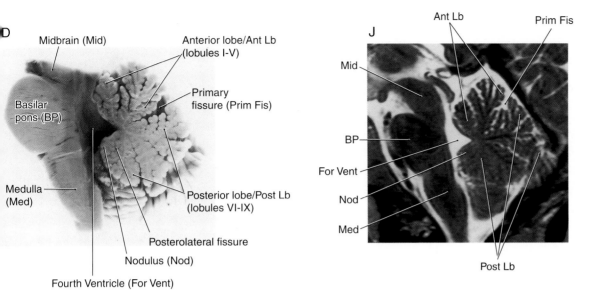

D
Midbrain (Mid)
Anterior lobe/Ant Lb (lobules I-V)
Basilar pons (BP)
Primary fissure (Prim Fis)
Medulla (Med)
Posterior lobe/Post Lb (lobules VI-IX)
Posterolateral fissure
Nodulus (Nod)
Fourth Ventricle (For Vent)

J
Ant Lb
Prim Fis
Mid
BP
For Vent
Nod
Med
Post Lb

Figure 27-4—cont'd.

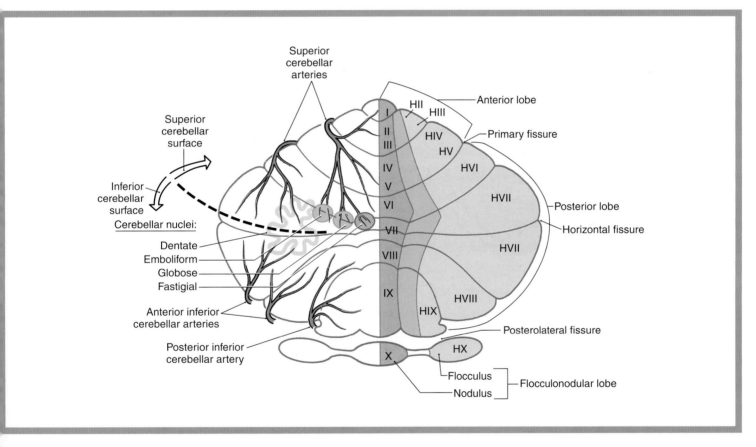

Figure 27-5. An unfolded view of the cerebellum showing medial *(gray)*, intermediate *(green)*, and lateral *(blue)* zones on the right and the nuclei with which each zone is functionally associated on the left in the corresponding color. The general areas of cortex and nuclei served by the cerebellar arteries are also indicated on the *left. Roman numerals* indicate lobules of the vermis; *numerals preceded by H* indicate the corresponding lobules of the hemisphere.

nuclei exit the cerebellum via the *superior cerebellar peduncle* and cross in its decussation.

Some neurons in each cerebellar nucleus send axons or axon collaterals into the overlying cortex, where they terminate in the granular layer as mossy fibers. These axons are called *nucleocortical fibers,* and they exert an excitatory influence on the cerebellar cortex.

Blood Supply to Cerebellar Structures

The blood supply to the cerebellar cortex, nuclei, and peduncles is via the *posterior inferior cerebellar artery* (PICA), *anterior inferior cerebellar artery* (AICA), and *superior cerebellar artery*

(Figs. 27-5 and 27-7). The PICA originates from the vertebral artery and supplies the posterolateral medulla (including the restiform body), the choroid plexus of the fourth ventricle, and caudomedial regions of the inferior cerebellar surface (including the vermis) (Figs. 27-5 and 27-7). Caudal parts of the middle cerebellar peduncle and caudolateral portions of the inferior cerebellar surface are served by the AICA. This vessel may also supply caudal parts of the dentate nucleus (Fig. 27-5). The entire superior surface of the cerebellum, most of the cerebellar nuclei, the rostral parts of the middle cerebellar peduncle, and the superior cerebellar peduncle are served by the superior cerebellar artery (Fig. 27-7).

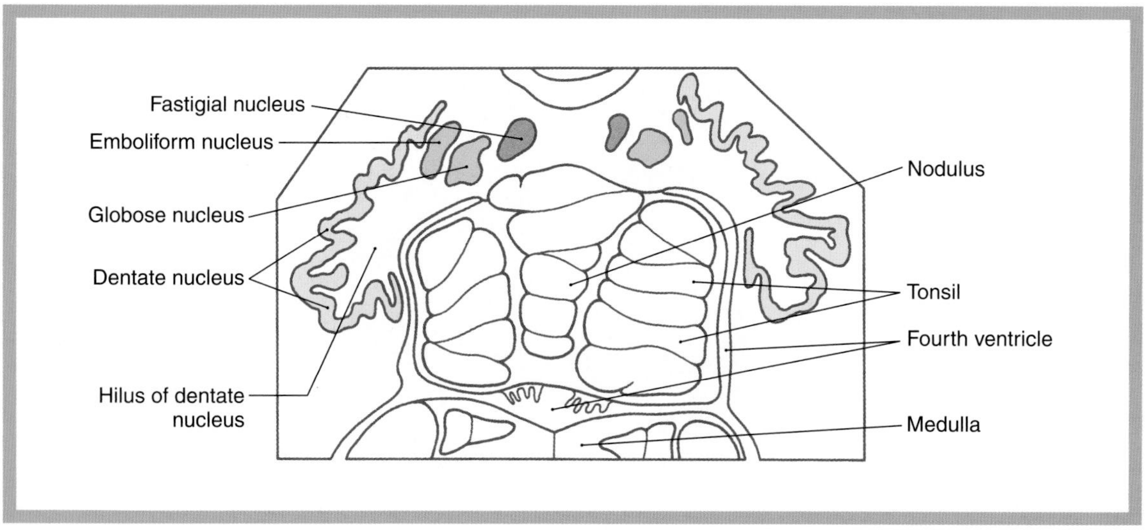

Figure 27-6. The cerebellar nuclei in cross section, drawn from a slide. The color coding of each nucleus corresponds to its appropriate zone in Figure 27-5.

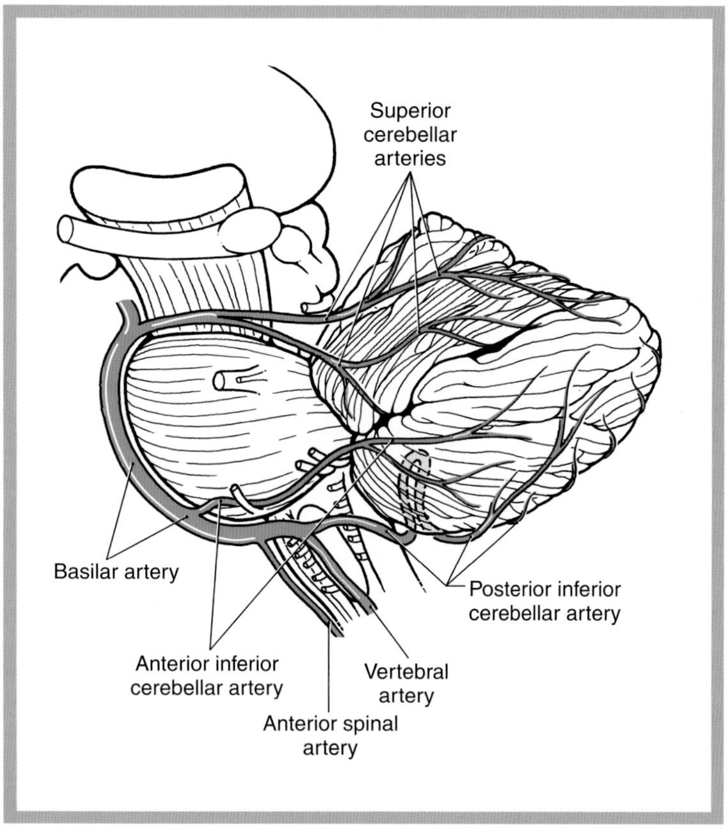

Figure 27-7. Origin and course of arteries serving the cerebellum as seen in lateral aspect.

Cerebellar Cortex

Histologically, each folium of the cerebellum has a superficial cellular layer, the cerebellar cortex, and a core of myelinated fibers traveling to *(afferent)* or from *(efferent)* the overlying cortex. The cortex consists of a *Purkinje cell layer* insinuated between a cell-dense inner region immediately adjacent to the white matter core, the *granule cell layer,* and an outer pale and relatively cell-sparse portion, the *molecular layer* (Figs. 27-8 and 27-9).

Purkinje Cell Layer

The large (40 to 65 μm in diameter) somata of Purkinje cells form a single layer at the interface of the granular and molecular layers (Fig. 27-8). Each Purkinje cell gives rise to an elaborate dendritic tree that radiates into the molecular layer. This dendritic tree is shaped like a fan with its wide flattened aspect oriented perpendicular to the long axis of the folium (Figs. 27-9 and 27-10). The "trunk" of the tree is a single primary dendrite which gives rise to several secondary dendrites, which in turn branch into many tertiary dendrites. Synaptic contacts are formed mainly on short *terminal branchlets* that emerge primarily from the secondary and tertiary dendrites (Figs. 27-9 and 27-10). There are two types of branchlets. *Smooth branchlets* emerge from secondary and tertiary dendrites, whereas *spiny branchlets (gemmules)* arise mainly from tertiary dendrites.

Purkinje cells are the only efferent neurons of the cerebellar cortex. Axons of Purkinje cells arise from the basal aspect of the cell body and may give rise to recurrent collaterals. The former processes traverse the granular layer and the subcortical white matter to eventually terminate in either the cerebellar or the vestibular nuclei. Purkinje cells projecting into the cerebellar nuclei (as *cerebellar corticonuclear fibers*) arise from all areas of the cortex, whereas those projecting into the vestibular nuclei (as *cerebellar corticovestibular fibers*) originate primarily from parts of the vermis and the flocculonodular lobe. Purkinje cells release γ-aminobutyric acid (GABA) at their synaptic terminals and inhibit target neurons in the cerebellar and vestibular nuclei.

Granule Cell Layer

There are three types of neuron cell bodies within the granule layer. These are *granular cells,* which are extraordinarily numerous and found in all areas of the cerebellar cortex, *Golgi cells,* which are larger and also widely distributed, and *unipolar brush cells,* which are small neurons that have a restricted geographic distribution within the cortex.

The most numerous neuron of the granule cell layer is the small (5 to 8 μm in diameter) *granule cell* (Figs. 27-8, 27-9, and 27-10C). The dendrites of these cells form claw-like endings *(dendritic digits)* that ramify in the vicinity of the cell body. Their axons ascend into the molecular layer, where they bifurcate to form *parallel fibers*. As indicated by their name, *parallel fibers run parallel to the long axis of the folium.* Consequently, these fibers pass through the fan-like dendritic trees of the Purkinje cell and, when doing so, make synaptic contacts with spiny branchlets (Figs. 27-9 and 27-10B, F). They also synapse with the cells intrinsic to the molecular layer (discussed later). The distance spanned by the parallel fibers of a granule cell ranges from 0.3 to 5.0 mm, and the number of Purkinje and other cells contacted varies accordingly. Granule cells use *glutamate* (or perhaps *aspartate*) as their neurotransmitter and thus have

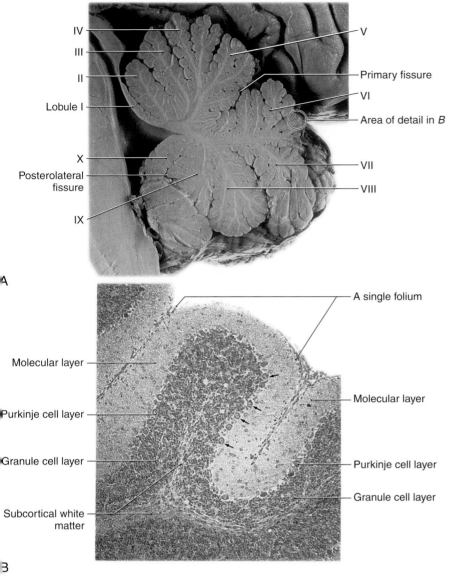

IV

III

II

Lobule I

X

Posterolateral
fissure

IX

V

Primary fissure

VI

Area of detail in *B*

VII

VIII

A

A single folium

Molecular layer

Purkinje cell layer

Granule cell layer

Subcortical white
matter

Molecular layer

Purkinje cell layer

Granule cell layer

B

Figure 27-8. Midsagittal view (**A**) of the cerebellum showing the main fissures and lobules and a detail (**B**) of the cortex showing the cortical layers as seen in a neutral red-stained section. *Arrows* point to representative Purkinje cell bodies.

n excitatory effect on their target cells. In fact, the *granule cells are the primary excitatory neurons of the cerebellar cortex.* The unipolar brush cell, described later, is also excitatory but is found in strikingly fewer numbers and is restricted in its distribution within the cortex. All of the other neurons of the cerebellar cortex, as we shall see, are inhibitory.

The second cell type of the granular layer is the *Golgi cell.* The soma of this neuron is larger (at 18 to 25 μm in diameter) than that of the granule cell and is usually found in the granular layer adjacent to the Purkinje cells (Figs. 27-9 and 27-10D). Dendrites of Golgi cells branch in the granular layer but extend primarily into the molecular layer without regard to plane of orientation. Axons of Golgi neurons branch in the granular layer and form synaptic contacts on granule cell dendrites (Fig. 27-9). The Golgi cell utilizes GABA as a neurotransmitter and is an inhibitory interneuron in the cerebellar cortex.

The third neuronal type found within the granule layer is the *unipolar brush cell.* This neuron has a slightly oval cell body, measuring 9 to 14 μm in diameter at the equator, and a single stout dendritic structure arising from the soma (Fig. 27-11). This dendritic process ends in a brush-like configuration made up of a cluster of *dendrioles.* The axon of the unipolar brush cell arises from the cell body, ramifies within the granular layer, and ends as a series of two to four synaptic structures called *unipolar brush cell rosettes* (Fig. 27-11). In contrast to granule cells, which are distributed throughout the cerebellar cortex, the unipolar brush cells are found primarily in the flocculonodular lobe,

adjacent areas of the paraflocculus, the vermis, and (in very sparse numbers) in hemisphere lobules HVI-HVIII. Mossy fibers arising from primary and secondary vestibulocerebellar fibers and Golgi cell axons contact the dendrioles (Fig. 27-11B). The unipolar brush cell rosette is contacted by granule cell dendrites, dendrioles of the unipolar brush cell, Golgi cells axons, and an occasional Golgi cell dendrite (Fig. 27-11B). Unipolar brush cells use *glutamate* as their neurotransmitter and are, therefore, excitatory to their targets.

The classic *cerebellar glomerulus* is a synaptic complex found throughout all portions of the cerebellar cortex within the neuropil of the granular layer. The glomerulus includes granule cell and Golgi cell dendrites and Golgi cell axons, and a specialized synaptic segment *(the mossy fiber rosette)* of a *mossy fiber,* one type of cerebellar afferent axon (Figs. 27-9 and 27-10C-E). The mossy fiber rosette is centrally located and forms synapses with several granule cell dendrites. Golgi cell axons contact granule cell dendrites in the glomerulus, and the entire complex is encapsulated by glial cell processes.

Some glomeruli within the vermis or flocculonodular lobe are structured as described previously whereas others center on the *unipolar brush cell rosette,* in which case they may be called, in these cortical areas, *unipolar brush cell glomeruli* (Fig. 27-11B). This specific type of glomerulus is composed of the brush cell rosette, small contacts made by granular cell dendrites, larger contacts made by brush cell dendrioles, and small contacts by Golgi cell axons at the periphery of the glomerulus (Fig. 27-11B).

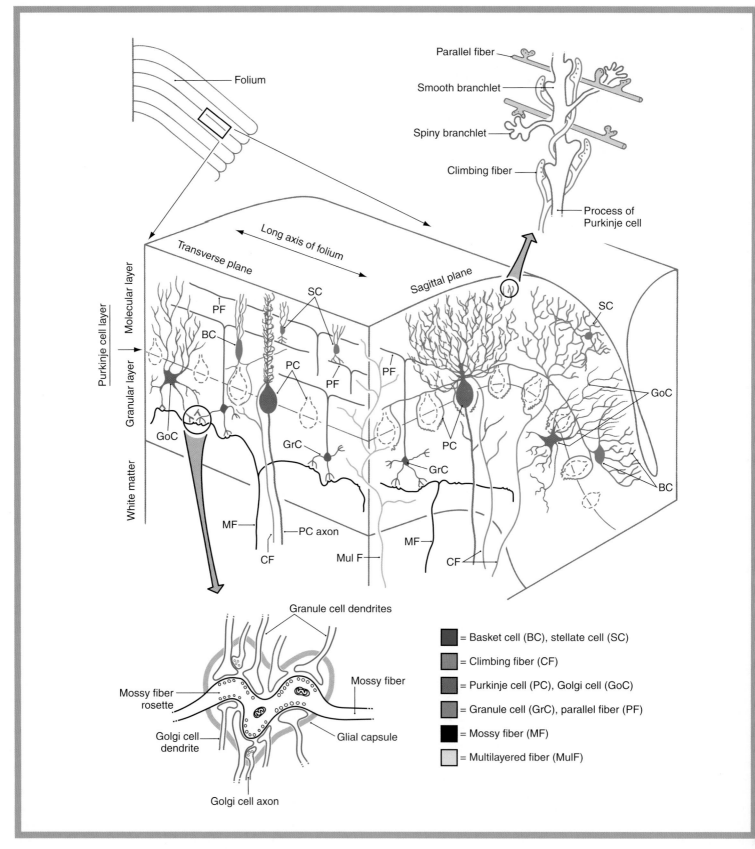

Figure 27-9. Cell types and synaptic relations in the cerebellar cortex in transverse and sagittal planes. Note the structure of the cerebellar glomerulus *(lower left)* and the interaction of parallel and climbing fibers *(upper right)* with the dendritic processes of Purkinje cells. Compare with Figure 27-10. Because of their regional specificity, the unipolar brush cells are not shown (see Fig. 27-11).

Since unipolar brush cells, and their synaptic interactions, are located primarily in the flocculonodular lobe and vermis and since these cells receive vestibular inputs, their function is most likely related to cerebellar (and vestibular) control of eye movements, vestibulo-ocular reflexes, and various postural mechanisms.

Molecular Layer

The molecular layer has considerably fewer cell bodies than the granule cell layer (Fig. 27-8) but has proportionately more cell processes. These processes include *parallel fibers, Purkinje cell dendrites, Golgi cell dendrites, climbing fibers* (see later), and the processes of cells intrinsic to the molecular layer (Fig. 27-9)

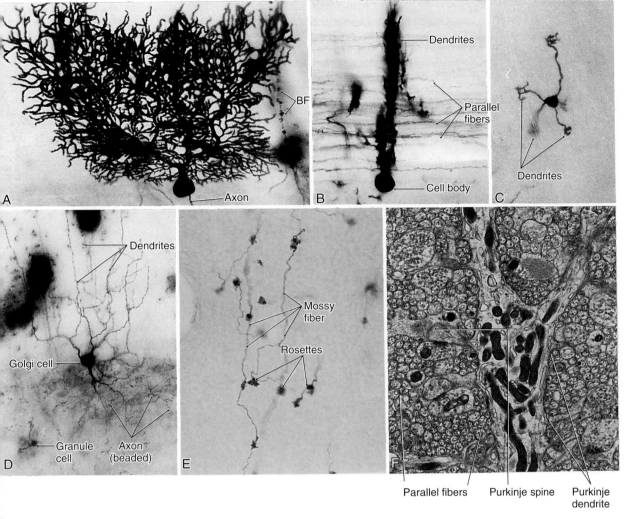

Figure 27-10. Examples of cells of the cerebellar cortex (see Fig. 27-9). The Purkinje cells are shown in sagittal (**A**; note the beaded appearance of the dendrites) and transverse (**B**; note the many parallel fibers) planes. Granule cell (**C**, **D**) dendrites end as a cluster of short, claw-like processes. Dendrites of Golgi cells (**D**) branch into molecular and granular layers, whereas their axons (**D**, beaded structures) ramify in only the granular layer. Mossy fibers (**E**) branch profusely and have many rosettes; synaptic contacts between mossy fibers and granule cell dendrites take place at the rosette in the cerebellar glomerulus (see Fig. 27-9). At the ultrastructural level, the Purkinje cell dendrite is surrounded by the numerous small profiles of parallel fibers. BF, Bergmann fiber, a type of glial cell process. (**A-D**, Courtesy of Dr. José Rafols, Wayne State University.)

The intrinsic cell types of the molecular layer are *stellate cells* and *basket cells* (Fig. 27-9). Stellate cells are usually found in outer regions of the molecular layer and are frequently referred to as *superficial* or *outer stellate cells*. The somata of basket cells are located immediately above the Purkinje cell layer. The *basket cell axon* travels in the sagittal plane and gives rise to descending branches that form elaborate "baskets" around the Purkinje cell body. This cell derives its name from this characteristic feature.

In general, the dendritic and axonal plexuses of basket and stellate cells are *oriented primarily in the sagittal plane*, much like those of Purkinje cell dendrites (Fig. 27-9). Although basket and stellate cells are similar in general shape, the *extent* of the dendritic and axonal fields is much larger in basket cells than in stellate cells. Consequently, basket cells may influence a large number of Purkinje cells, mainly in the sagittal plane, whereas stellate cells influence a much smaller population, but also in the sagittal plane. Stellate and basket cells receive excitatory inputs from parallel fibers.

Basket and stellate cells are GABAergic and inhibit their target neurons. Although these cells influence several targets in the molecular layer, for our purposes the Purkinje cell is the most important. Similarly, Purkinje and Golgi cells are also inhibitory, thus making *the granule cell and the unipolar brush cell the only neurons in the cerebellar cortex whose outputs are excitatory to their targets*. As emphasized earlier, the granule cells are numerous and found in the granular layer throughout all zones and lobules of the cortex; therefore, their excitatory output influences all cortical areas. In contrast, the unipolar brush cells are significantly fewer in number, found primarily in the granular layer of the vermis and flocculonodular lobe; therefore, their excitatory output influences a comparatively restricted area of cortex (and presumably functions in a more specific sphere).

Cerebellar Afferent Fibers

The afferent fibers to the cerebellar cortex are grouped into three types on the basis of the *morphology and connections of their terminals in the cortex*. These three types of cortical terminals arise as *mossy fibers*, *climbing fibers*, and *multilayered (monoaminergic) fibers*.

The cerebellar afferent axons that end as *mossy fibers* originate from cell bodies in the cerebellar nuclei (*nucleocortical fibers*) and from a variety of other nuclei in the spinal cord, medulla, and pons (Table 27-1). En route to the cerebellar cortex, most of these extracerebellar afferent fibers send collaterals into a cerebellar nucleus. In the granular layer, *mossy fibers* branch profusely and their large terminals contact other cells at irregular intervals (the *mossy fiber rosette*). The rosette, which is the central element of the cerebellar glomerulus, gives the fiber a mossy appearance (Figs. 27-9 and 27-10E). Single mossy fibers may form up to 50 rosettes, and each rosette may participate in

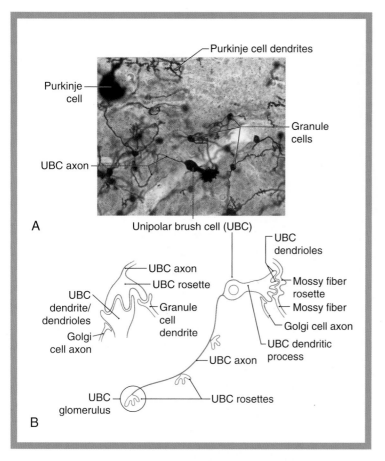

A

B

Figure 27-11. The unipolar brush cell of the granular layer of the cerebellar cortex. This cell has a comparatively small soma when compared with Purkinje and with granule cells (**A**). The cell body, dendrioles, and axon all ramify within the granular layer (**B**) and establish synaptic contact with mossy fibers, granule cells, and Golgi cells. This cell is restricted to vestibulocerebellar structures. (**A**, Courtesy of Dr. Enrico Mugnaini, Northwestern University Institute for Neuroscience).

synaptic contacts with up to 10 to 15 granule cells in a cerebellar glomerulus. In addition, a mossy fiber may branch and distribute to more than one folium. Mossy fibers utilize *glutamate* as their neurotransmitter and are excitatory to granule cell and Golgi cell dendrites in the cerebellar glomerulus and to cerebellar

nuclear neurons on which their collaterals terminate. Mossy fiber rosettes that end in relation to the dendrioles of the unipolar brush cells within the granular layer of the vermis and flocculonodular lobe are also excitatory to this cell type in these cortical regions.

The inferior olivary nuclei are the only source of cerebellar afferent axons that end as *climbing fibers* in the cerebellar cortex (Table 27-1). Olivocerebellar fibers send collaterals to the appropriate cerebellar nucleus. The climbing fibers then terminate in the molecular layer by entwining, ivy like, up the dendritic trees of Purkinje dendrites (Fig. 27-9). Each Purkinje cell is innervated by a single climbing fiber, but olivocerebellar axons may branch to serve several Purkinje cells. Climbing fibers use the neurotransmitter *aspartate*, and they excite Purkinje cells and cerebellar nuclear neurons.

Multilayered fibers (monoaminergic or peptide-containing) originate from cells of the locus ceruleus *(noradrenergic)*, the raphe nuclei *(serotoninergic)*, the hypothalamus (some are *histaminergic)*, and other select locations. These fibers enter the cerebellum via the cerebellar peduncles and, in the case of some hypothalamocerebellar fibers, by passing through the periventricular gray and then into the cerebellum. En route to the cerebellar cortex, many of these fibers send collaterals to the cerebellar nuclei. In the cortex, these axons branch diffusely and terminate in molecular and granular layers, where they may influence all major cell types (Fig. 27-9). In general, these fibers modulate the output of the cerebellar cortex through two mechanisms. First, they decrease the spontaneous discharge rates of Purkinje cells. Second, both directly and via interneurons, multilayered fibers alter the responsiveness of Purkinje cells to excitation by climbing fibers and by the mossy fiber–granule cell projection.

Topographic Localization

The cerebellum receives input from a wide range of sources. Some input that originates in the periphery is conveyed via spinocerebellar and vestibulocerebellar pathways that project *directly* to the cerebellum. Other afferent information is *indirect*, having passed through multiple central pathways before entering the cerebellum. For example, responses can be recorded in selected regions of the cerebellar cortex following stimuli that activate visual, auditory, or sensorimotor areas of the cerebral cortex in primates (Fig. 27-12A). These pathways involve a

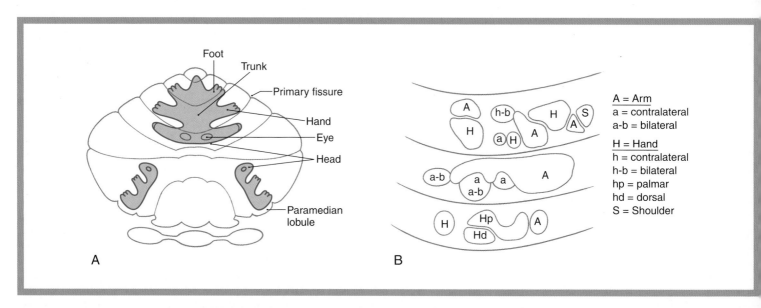

A

B

Figure 27-12. Somatotopy in the cerebellar cortex (**A**) and a summary representation of fractured somatotopy in the paramedian lobule (**B**) of a primate. In the somatotopic map, body areas were originally thought to be continuous (**A**), but more recent studies suggest that discontinuous body parts (or areas) may be represented in immediately adjacent cortical regions (**B**). (**B** is adapted from Welker W, Blair C, Shambes GM: Somatosensory projections to cerebellar granule cell layer of giant bushbaby, *Galago crassicaudatus*. Brain Behav Evol 31:150:150, 1988, with permission.)

Table 27-1. Synopsis of Selected Afferent and Efferent Fibers of the Cerebellum as Contained in, or Associated With, the Cerebellar Peduncles

Cerebellar Peduncles	Laterality	Afferents, Efferents
Inferior Cerebellar Peduncle		
Restiform Body		
Dorsal spinocerebellar fibers	–	Mossy fibers
Cuneocerebellar fibers	–	Mossy fibers
Olivocerebellar fibers	X	Climbing fibers
Reticulocerebellar fibers (from reticulotegmental pontine nucleus)	X,–	Mossy fibers
Reticulocerebellar fibers (from lateral reticular nucleus)	–,(X)	Mossy fibers
Reticulocerebellar fibers (from paramedian reticular nucleus)	–,(X)	Mossy fibers
Trigeminocerebellar fibers	–	Mossy fibers
Raphecerebellar fibers	–,(X)	Multilayered fibers
Fuxtarestiform Body		
Vestibulocerebellar fibers (primary and secondary)	–	Mossy fibers
Cerebellar corticovestibular fibers	–	Vestibular nuclei
Fastigiovestibular fibers	–,X	Vestibular nuclei
Fastigioreticular fibers	–,X	Reticular nuclei
Fastigio-olivary fibers	X	Caudal parts of accessory olivary nuclei
Fastigiospinal fibers	X	Spinal cord
Middle Cerebellar Peduncle		
Pontocerebellar fibers	X,(–)	Mossy fibers
Raphecerebellar fibers	–,(X)	Multilayered fibers
Superior Cerebellar Peduncle		
Ventral spinocerebellar fibers	X,–	Mossy fiber
Rostral spinocerebellar fibers	X,–	Mossy fiber
Ceruleocerebellar fibers	–,X	Multilayered fibers
Hypothalamocerebellar fibers	–,X	Multilayered fibers
Raphecerebellar fibers	–	Multilayered fibers
Cerebellar efferent fibers		
Dentatothalamic	X	Dorsal thalamus
Dentatorubral	X	Red nucleus
Dentatoreticular	X	Reticular nuclei
Dentatopontine	X	Pontine nuclei
Dentato-olivary	X	Principal olivary nucleus
Dentatohypothalamic	X	Hypothalamus
Interpositothalamic	X	Dorsal thalamus
Interpositorubral	X	Red nucleus
Interpositoreticular	X	Reticular nuclei
Interposito-olivary	X	Rostral parts of accessory olivary nuclei
Interpositohypothalamic	X	Hypothalamus
Interpositospinal	X	Spinal cord

–, uncrossed; X, crossed; (–), some uncrossed; (X), some crossed.

cerebropontine-pontocerebellar connection. Visual and auditory cortices project to cells of the basilar pons, which, in turn, provide a mossy fiber input to areas of the cerebellar cortex where the eye and ear are represented (Fig. 27-12A). Similarly, the sensorimotor cortex, also via projections through the basilar pons, influences cerebellar cortical regions containing representations of the body.

At a finer level of resolution, experimental studies in mammals have shown that body parts are not represented continuously over a large area of cerebellar cortex but instead are broken into smaller, discontinuous patches. In this pattern, a small area of cortex that receives sensory input from the arm (via mossy fiber–granule cell connections) may be located adjacent to an area that receives input from a noncontiguous region of the same upper extremity (Fig. 27-12B). In addition, each body part is represented in several locations. This pattern of spatial representation is referred to as *fractured somatotopy*.

Synaptic Interactions in the Cerebellar Cortex

In general, cerebellar function is regulated by modulating the output of the cerebellar nuclei. This modulation results from the excitatory action of the collaterals of cerebellar afferents and the inhibitory action of Purkinje cell axons (corticonuclear fibers) descending from the overlying cortex (Fig. 27-13). These synaptic interactions continuously modify the efferent signals generated by cerebellar nuclear neurons.

Climbing fibers synapse directly on Purkinje cells, whereas mossy fibers act through granule cells. Because a *single climbing fiber* makes numerous synaptic contacts on a *single Purkinje cell*, its influence over that cell is substantial. Consequently, the Purkinje cell response to input from one climbing fiber is represented by a complicated waveform called a complex spike (Fig. 27-14). These spikes are unique and are the result of the combined action of multiple excitatory climbing fiber synapses formed throughout the Purkinje cell dendritic tree. In contrast, each Purkinje cell receives excitatory input from *many granule cells* via their parallel fibers. Summation, both spatial and temporal, of parallel fiber input is responsible for modulating the *simple spike* activity of Purkinje cells (Fig. 27-14). At any given moment in time, there is an ongoing background level of simple spike activity in the cerebellum. This level can be modulated by phasic increases or decreases in afferent inputs to the mossy

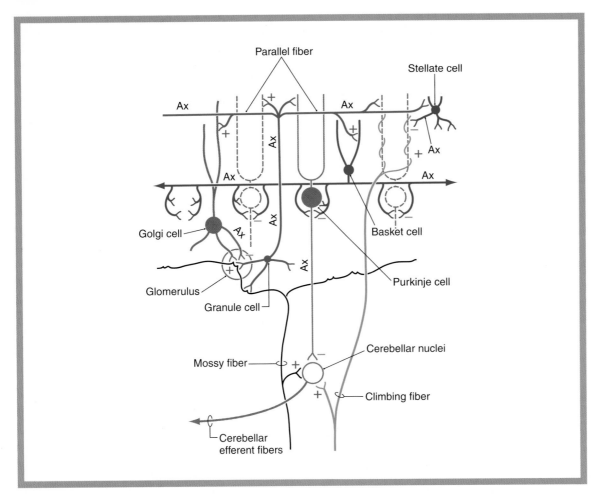

Figure 27-13. A diagrammatic representation of synaptic interactions in the cerebellar cortex. +, excitatory synapses; –, inhibitory synapses; Ax, axon.

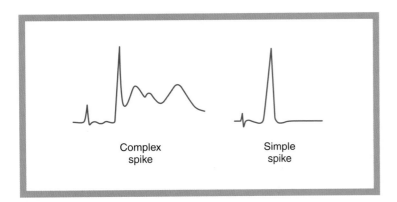

Figure 27-14. Complex and simple spikes of Purkinje cells, as recorded intracellularly following excitation by climbing and mossy fibers, respectively.

fiber–granule cell–parallel fiber system. Collectively, mossy fibers have a powerful influence over Purkinje cells, and this influence may be modulated by climbing fibers through mechanisms not fully understood.

Let us review the mossy fiber–granule cell connection and its effects (Figs. 27-9 and 27-13). In the cerebellar glomerulus, mossy fibers excite granule cell and Golgi cell dendrites. The Golgi cell axon, in turn, synapses on and inhibits granule cell dendrites within the glomerulus. Thus, the Golgi cell provides feedback inhibition to granule cells previously excited by mossy fiber activity. The granule cell axon enters the molecular layer, branches into parallel fibers, and excites Purkinje, stellate, basket, and Golgi cells (Fig. 27-13). At a basic level, mossy fiber input leads to excitation of Purkinje cells via parallel fibers, and the

GABAergic Purkinje cells respond by inhibiting the cerebellar nuclei.

The synaptic interactions within the cerebellar cortex are also described in the following simplified model, which considers the cytoarchitectural and electrophysiologic properties of cerebellar cortical neurons. The inhibitory Purkinje cell outflow is modulated, in part, by the feed-forward inhibition resulting from stellate and basket cell activation (Figs. 27-13 and 27-15). Parallel fibers excite a specific population of Purkinje cells, as well as stellate and basket cells located within their domain (Fig. 27-15). The latter two GABAergic interneurons, in turn, inhibit Purkinje cells located adjacent to (via stellate synapses), or at some distance from (basket synapses), the row of activated parallel fibers. When a narrow bundle of parallel fibers is activated, under certain experimental conditions, basket and stellate cells can define a central row, or beam, of excited Purkinje cells. Within the beam, Purkinje cells are activated by parallel fibers and, in turn, inhibit cells in the cerebellar or vestibular nuclei (Fig. 27-15). Purkinje cells on either side of the activated row are inhibited by stellate and basket axons and, consequently, do not inhibit their target neurons in the cerebellar (or vestibular) nuclei (Fig. 27-15). These target cells are removed from their normal (background) inhibitory influence; that is, they are disinhibited.

Synaptic interactions between cells of the cerebellar cortex contribute to the activity of cerebellar nuclear neurons. The unique structural and functional properties of the cortex provide circuits for the *temporal and spatial processing of information* that contributes substantially to the cerebellar capacity to co-ordinate movement. The exact nature of these interactions has not been fully determined. However, the cytoarchitecture and synaptology within the cerebellum suggest one hypothetical model. According to this model, the *excitatory outflow from each*

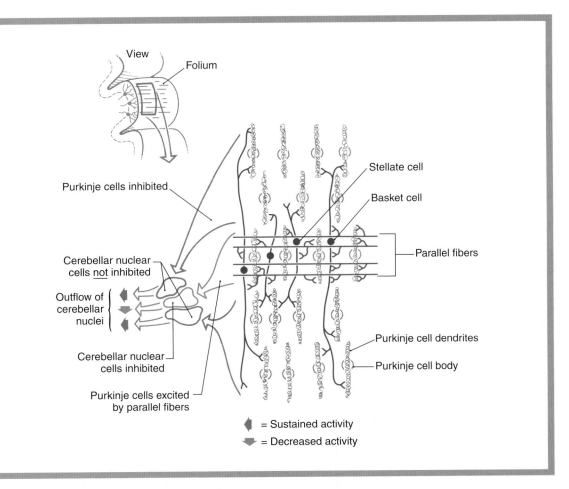

View
Folium

Purkinje cells inhibited

Stellate cell

Basket cell

Parallel fibers

Cerebellar nuclear cells not inhibited

Outflow of cerebellar nuclei

Purkinje cell dendrites

Purkinje cell body

Cerebellar nuclear cells inhibited

Purkinje cells excited by parallel fibers

= Sustained activity

= Decreased activity

Figure 27-15. A diagrammatic representation of a portion of a cerebellar folium as viewed from the surface. Activation of a bundle of parallel fibers *(green)* will lead to activation of a row of Purkinje cells *(red)* located within their domain. Simultaneously, the Purkinje fibers in the flanking zones *(gray)* will be inhibited by the action of basket and stellate cells, which are also activated by parallel fibers. These populations of activated and inhibited Purkinje cells will cause, respectively, inhibition *(red)* and disinhibition *(gray)* of cerebellar nuclear cells via the corticonuclear pathway.

cerebellar nucleus varies dynamically in response to the combined effects of (1) the excitatory input from cerebellar afferent collaterals to cerebellar nuclear neurons and (2) the inhibitory or disinhibitory influence mediated by Purkinje cells through the various circuits of the cerebellar cortex. Temporal processing refers to timing variances that partially depend on the number of synaptic contacts within a given circuit; spatial processing refers to variances in inputs, be they from different body parts or different feedback centers within the brain.

Functional Cerebellar Modules

It is convenient to think of the cerebellum as being arranged into *compartments* or *modules*. Each module consists of (1) an area of cortex (usually a cortical zone), (2) a white matter core that contains afferent and efferent fibers to and from that cortical area, and (3) a nucleus (or nuclei) that is functionally related to the overlying cortical area. A cerebellar cortical zone and its corresponding nucleus (nuclei) and white matter constitute a module.

Vestibulocerebellar Module

The flocculonodular lobe and adjacent portions of vermal lobule IX (the paraflocculus) receive afferents from the ipsilateral vestibular ganglion *(primary vestibulocerebellar fibers)* and vestibular nuclei *(secondary vestibulocerebellar fibers)*. Therefore, these cortical areas are commonly called the *vestibulocerebellum*. Along with the *fastigial nucleus*, they form the *vestibulocerebellar module* (Fig. 27-16). Because this is phylogenetically the oldest part of the cerebellum, the vestibulocerebellum is sometimes

called the archicerebellum (Greek *arche*, "beginning"). However, this latter term is not commonly used and is actually discouraged.

Vestibulocerebellar fibers access the flocculonodular cortex and fastigial nucleus via the juxtarestiform body and convey information concerning the position of the head and body in space, as well as information useful in orienting the eyes during movements. As noted earlier, the unipolar brush cell is largely unique to the granular layer of the vestibulocerebellum and is probably involved in the cerebellar and vestibular regulation of eye movement. This information is supplemented by inputs carried on *olivocerebellar fibers* from the contralateral olivary nuclei and on *pontocerebellar fibers* (only to the flocculus) from the contralateral basilar pons. The latter pathways convey *indirect* inputs from nuclei of the diencephalon and brainstem, which are concerned with a broad spectrum of information regarding visual processing and eye movements (see also Chapter 28).

The outflow of the vestibulocerebellar module consists of *cerebellar corticovestibular fibers* from the flocculonodular lobe, *cerebellar corticonuclear fibers* from the nodulus to the fastigial nucleus, and efferent fibers arising in the *fastigial nucleus* (Fig. 27-16). Purkinje cells in the flocculonodular cortex project, via the juxtarestiform body, directly to the ipsilateral vestibular nuclei *(cerebellar corticovestibular fibers)*. Other Purkinje cells in the nodulus project into caudal regions of the fastigial nucleus as *cerebellar corticonuclear fibers*. Both of these projections are inhibitory (GABAergic) pathways. Fastigial neurons provide bilateral excitatory inputs to the vestibular and reticular nuclei (Fig. 27-16). On the ipsilateral side, these axons pass directly through the juxtarestiform body. Fibers passing to the

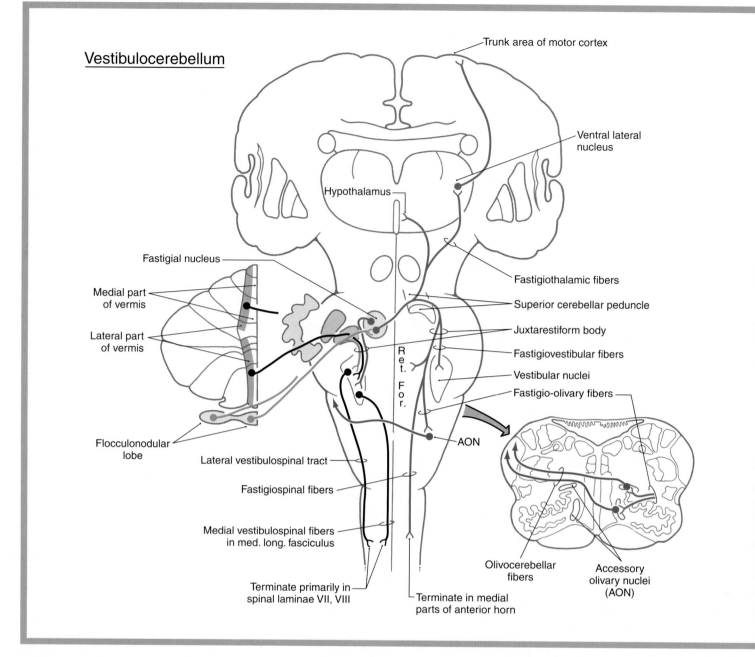

Vestibulocerebellum

Figure 27-16. Projections of the vestibulocerebellum and of the lateral part of the medial zone through the fastigial and vestibular nuclei. med. long., medial longitudinal; Ret. For., reticular formation.

contralateral side cross in the cerebellar white matter and form the *uncinate fasciculus* as they loop over the superior cerebellar peduncle. These crossed fibers enter the vestibular complex via the juxtarestiform body.

The brainstem targets of cerebellar corticovestibular fibers and of fastigial efferent fibers, the vestibular and reticular nuclei, are the sources of vestibulospinal and reticulospinal tracts, respectively. The action of cerebellar corticovestibular fibers on the vestibular nuclei is inhibitory, whereas the action of fastigial efferents on the vestibular and reticular nuclei is excitatory.

Vestibulocerebellar Dysfunction
The vestibulocerebellum influences posture, balance, and equilibrium through vestibulospinal and reticulospinal projections to extensor motor neurons that influence axial and proximal limb muscles. The vestibular nuclei also bilaterally innervate the motor nuclei of cranial nerves III, IV, and VI through fibers that ascend in the medial longitudinal fasciculus (see Chapter 28).

Damage to the flocculonodular lobe, or to midline structures such as the nodulus and fastigial nucleus, will result in an

unsteady lurching gait *(truncal ataxia)* that resembles that seen with drunkenness. This instability is also manifested as exaggerated movements of the legs and a *tendency to fall* to the side, forward, or backward. The patient may stand with feet farther apart than usual *(wide-based stance)* in an effort to maintain balance. Patients with such lesions are *unable to walk in tandem* (heel-to-toe) or to walk on their heels or on their toes. Midline lesions may also result in a tremor of the axial body or head called *titubation*. This tremor can range in amplitude from barely noticeable to so powerful that the patient is unable to sit or stand unsupported. *Nystagmus* is frequently seen, and deficits in pursuit eye movements are also common. In addition, the patient's head may *tilt* or turn to one side, the direction being unrelated to the laterality of the lesion.

Vestibular Connections of the Vermis
In addition to the nodulus (of the flocculonodular lobe), most lobules of the vermal zone also have vestibular connections (Fig. 27-16). For example, lateral portions of the vermal cortex receive secondary vestibulocerebellar fibers and project to

Spinocerebellum - Vermal Zone

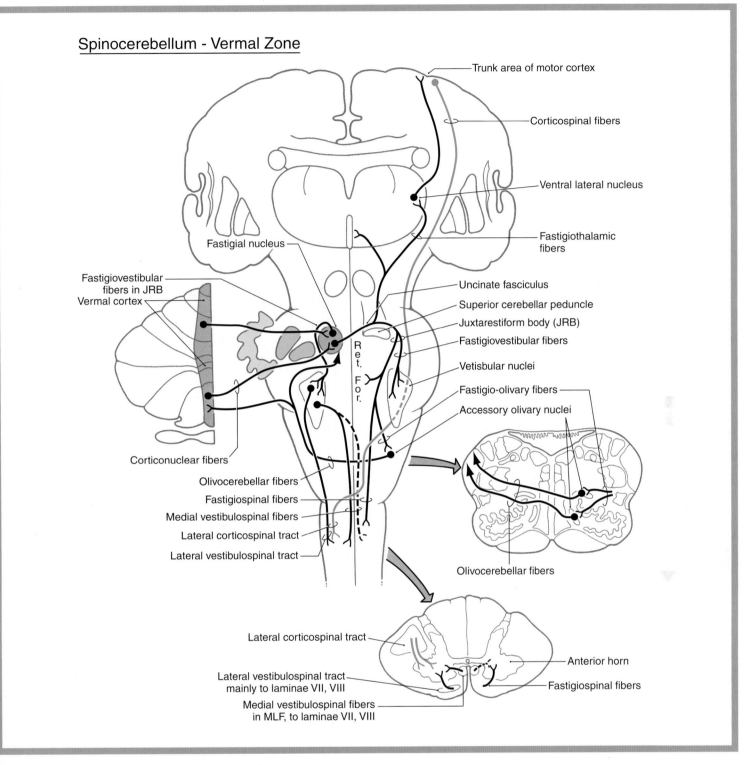

Figure 27-17. Projections of the spinocerebellum (vermal zone) through the fastigial and vestibular nuclei. MLF, medial longitudinal fasciculus; Ret. For., reticular formation.

the ipsilateral vestibular nuclei. Like the nodular cortex of the vestibulocerebellar module, the medial portions of the vermal cortex send cerebellar corticonuclear fibers into the ipsilateral fastigial nucleus (Fig. 27-17). Consequently, the *fastigial nucleus* links vestibulocerebellar cortex *and* portions of the vermal cortex with the vestibular and reticular nuclei of the brainstem. In this respect, the vermal cortex and fastigial nucleus share the task of influencing axial musculature along with vestibulocerebellar and spinocerebellar modules.

Spinocerebellar Module

The vermal and intermediate zones receive input mainly via the *posterior* and *anterior spinocerebellar tracts* and, from the upper extremity, through *cuneocerebellar fibers*. Owing to this predominant input, these zones are collectively called the *spinocerebellum* (sometimes the *paleocerebellum*, although this term is not frequently used) (Figs. 27-17 and 27-18). Posterior spinocerebellar and cuneocerebellar fibers enter the cerebellum via the restiform body, whereas anterior spinocerebellar fibers course into the cerebellum in association with the superior cerebellar peduncle. Fibers that enter the vermal zone send collaterals into the *fastigial nucleus*, and those passing into the intermediate zone send branches into the *emboliform* and *globose nuclei*.

The output of the spinocerebellum is focused primarily on the control of axial musculature through vermal cortex and fastigial efferents, and on the control of limb musculature through efferents

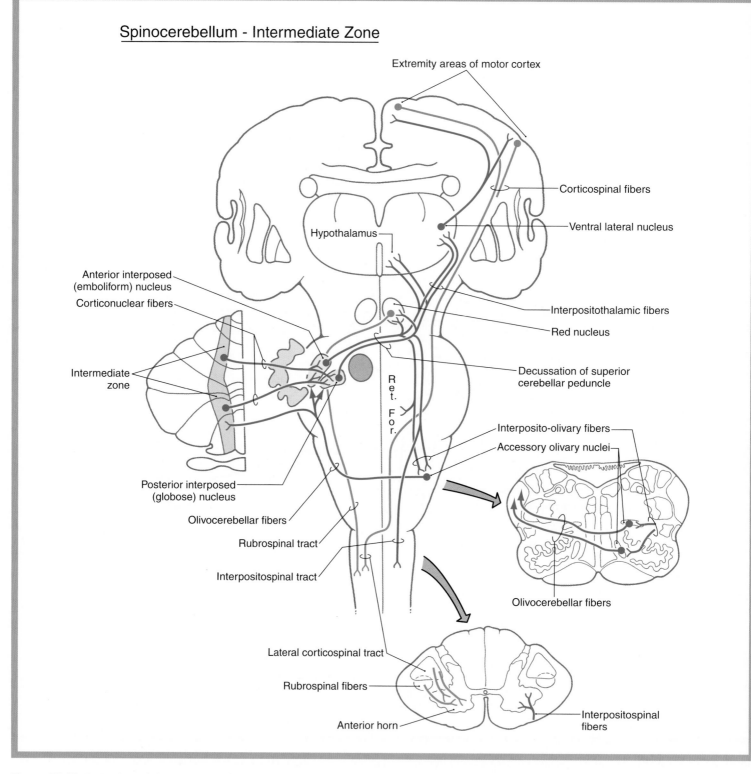

Spinocerebellum - Intermediate Zone

Figure 27-18. Projections of the spinocerebellum (intermediate zone) through the emboliform and globose nuclei. Ret. For., reticular formation.

of the globose and emboliform nuclei. Posterior spinocerebellar and cuneocerebellar fibers inform the cerebellum of limb position and movement. This information is processed in the cerebellum and, through connections with the motor cortex via the neurons of the ventral lateral thalamic nucleus, the pars caudalis (VLpc), influences movements of the extremities and muscle tone. Cells in the spinal cord that give rise to anterior spinocerebellar fibers receive primary sensory inputs and are also under the influence of descending reticulospinal and corticospinal fibers. In this respect, anterior spinocerebellar fibers provide afferent signals and feedback to the cerebellum regarding motor circuits in the spinal cord.

There are additional inputs to the spinocerebellar cortex. These arise in the contralateral accessory olivary nuclei *(olivo-cerebellar fibers)*, the vestibular nuclei *(secondary vestibulo-cerebellar fibers)*, the contralateral pontine nuclei *(pontocerebellar fibers)*, and the reticular nuclei *(reticulocerebellar fibers)*. These afferent axons also send collaterals into the fastigial and interposed nuclei.

The outflow of the spinocerebellar module consists of *cere-bellar corticonuclear fibers* from vermal and intermediate cortex to *fastigial, emboliform,* and *globose nuclei* and of *cerebellar efferent axons* arising in these nuclei (Figs. 27-17 and 27-18). Corticonuclear fibers project in a topographic sequence into heir respective nuclei on the ipsilateral side. For example, fibers rom anterior parts of the vermis enter rostral portions of the astigial nucleus, whereas those of the posterior vermis project nto caudal areas of the same nucleus. In general, this pattern s repeated between the intermediate zone and the emboliform nd globose nuclei.

As indicated previously, the *fastigial nucleus* projects bi-aterally to vestibular and reticular nuclei, which, through their pinal projections, influence axial muscles. The fastigial nucleus ilso projects to (1) the contralateral *medial accessory olivary* nucleus, from which it receives input; (2) the medial areas of the nterior horn in upper levels of the spinal cord as *fastigiospinal ibers,* and (3) the ventral lateral nucleus of the thalamus, which, n turn, projects to trunk regions of the motor cortex (Fig. 27-17).

Axons from the *globose* and *emboliform* nuclei exit the :erebellum via the superior cerebellar peduncle and cross in ts decussation (Fig. 27-18). From this point, some of these :erebellar efferent fibers course rostrally to terminate in the magnocellular part of the red nucleus *(cerebellorubral fibers)* and n the VLpc nucleus of the thalamus *(cerebellothalamic fibers).* These particular thalamic neurons project mainly to areas of the primary motor cortex. The red nucleus, via *rubrospinal fibers,* ind the motor cortex, through *corticospinal fibers,* influence motor neurons in the contralateral spinal cord that control distal limb musculature (Fig. 27-18). Other globose and emboliform efferents travel caudally to terminate in the reticular formation *(cerebelloreticular fibers)* and in the inferior olivary complex *(cerebello-olivary fibers).* Reticular cells influence spinal motor neurons and project back to the spinocerebellum as *reticulo-cerebellar fibers.* The globose and emboliform nuclei also receive olivocerebellar fibers from the accessory olivary nuclei to which they project (Fig. 27-18).

Damage to spinocerebellar structures is frequently the result of extension from more medially or laterally located lesions. Consequently, the clinical picture is dominated by deficits characteristic of these medial or lateral regions. The lateral regions are more frequently affected.

Pontocerebellar Module

The large lateral zone receives significant input from the *basilar pontine nuclei* via a primarily crossed *pontocerebellar fiber* projection. These fibers enter the cerebellum via the middle cerebellar peduncle. Because of this predominant source of afferent fibers, the lateral zone is called the *pontocerebellum* (Fig. 27-18). Because the pontine nuclei receive a major projection from the ipsilateral cerebral cortex (as *corticopontine fibers),* this lateral zone is sometimes called the *cerebrocerebellum* (or *neocerebellum).* However, the term *pontocerebellum* is more appropriate and is in parallel with vestibulocerebellum and spinocerebellum. Afferent fibers that enter the lateral zone also send collaterals into the *dentate nucleus* (Fig. 27-19).

The pontocerebellum functions in the planning and control of precise dexterous movements of the extremities, particularly in the arm, forearm, and hand, and in the timing of these movements. Through its connections to motor cortical areas, the dentate nucleus is capable of modulating activity in cortical neurons that project to the contralateral spinal cord.

Another important source of afferents to the pontocerebellum is the *principal inferior olivary nucleus* (Fig. 27-19). These *olivocerebellar fibers* are exclusively crossed. They enter the cerebellum via the restiform body, send collaterals to the dentate nucleus, and end in the molecular layer as climbing fibers.

The outflow of the pontocerebellar module consists of *cerebellar corticonuclear fibers* from the lateral zone to the dentate nucleus and *cerebellar efferent fibers* originating in the dentate nucleus (Fig. 27-19). As for other cerebellar regions, corticonuclear fibers of the lateral zone are topographically organized; rostral and

caudal areas of the zone project to the corresponding portions of the dentate nucleus.

Neurons of the *dentate nucleus* send their axons out of the cerebellum via the superior cerebellar peduncle and through its decussation (Fig. 27-19). The fibers that pass rostrally project mainly to the parvocellular part of the red nucleus *(dentatorubral fibers)* and to the intralaminar and VLpc nuclei of the thalamus *(dentatothalamic fibers).* Some neurons of the red nucleus project, as part of the central tegmental tract, to the ipsilateral inferior olivary complex *(rubro-olivary fibers).* At the same time, cells of the VLpc nucleus project to wide areas of the motor and premotor cortices. The motor cortex, in turn, projects to the contralateral spinal cord (as *corticospinal fibers)* to influence motor neurons that innervate distal limb musculature (Fig. 27-19). Descending crossed projections from the dentate nucleus pass mainly to the principal olivary nucleus *(dentato-olivary fibers)* and, in limited numbers, to the reticular and basilar pontine nuclei. *Olivocerebellar fibers* arising in the principal nucleus cross the midline and distribute to the cortex of the lateral zone and to the dentate nucleus. There is also feedback to the dentate nucleus via pontocerebellar and reticulocerebellar fibers.

The relationship between the dentate nucleus and movement has been explored in experiments in monkeys. A cooling probe implanted in the cerebellar white matter adjacent to the dentate nucleus halts most of the electrical activity in dentate neurons. This significant reduction in electrical signals temporarily disconnects the dentate nucleus from its targets without permanently destroying the nucleus. Reversing the cooling results in a resumption of normal neuronal activity. After dentate cooling, the *electrical activity of neurons in the primary motor cortex (MI) that signals the initiation of a movement (in response to a visual stimulus) was delayed, as was the execution of the movement itself.* This observation indicates that dentate projections, which reach the cortex via the VLpc nucleus, are *essential for the initial activation of MI corticospinal neurons at the beginning of a movement.*

As a result of the delay of excitatory output from the motor cortex, there are corresponding delays in muscle contraction. For example, the *initial activation* of an agonist muscle (biceps brachii) to a load is slowed and its overall contraction time is longer. Similarly, the activation of the antagonist muscle (triceps brachii) that occurs when the load is removed is also delayed. Furthermore, the reciprocal pattern of activation in agonists and antagonists that accompanies some movements is dramatically disrupted. Thus, cerebellar output is involved in *timing* muscle activation (and inactivation), as well as influencing the duration of muscle contraction.

Pontocerebellar Dysfunction

Before the consequence of lesions affecting the pontocerebellar module is considered, two important points merit emphasis. First, damage that involves *only* the cerebellar cortex rarely results in permanent motor deficits. However, damage to the cortex plus nuclei or to only the nuclei results in a wide range of motor problems. Second, *lesions of the cerebellar hemisphere result in motor deficits on the ipsilateral side of the body because the motor expression of cerebellar injury is mediated primarily through corticospinal and rubrospinal pathways.* In brief, the right lateral and interposed nuclei influence the left motor cortex and red nucleus, which, in turn, project to the right side of the spinal cord. Thus, a lesion in the cerebellum on the right results in deficits on the right side of the body. The exception is a midline lesion, which produces bilateral deficits restricted to axial/truncal parts of the body. Lesions that involve the cerebellar hemisphere frequently affect portions of the lateral and intermediate modules. It is common for these disorders to be

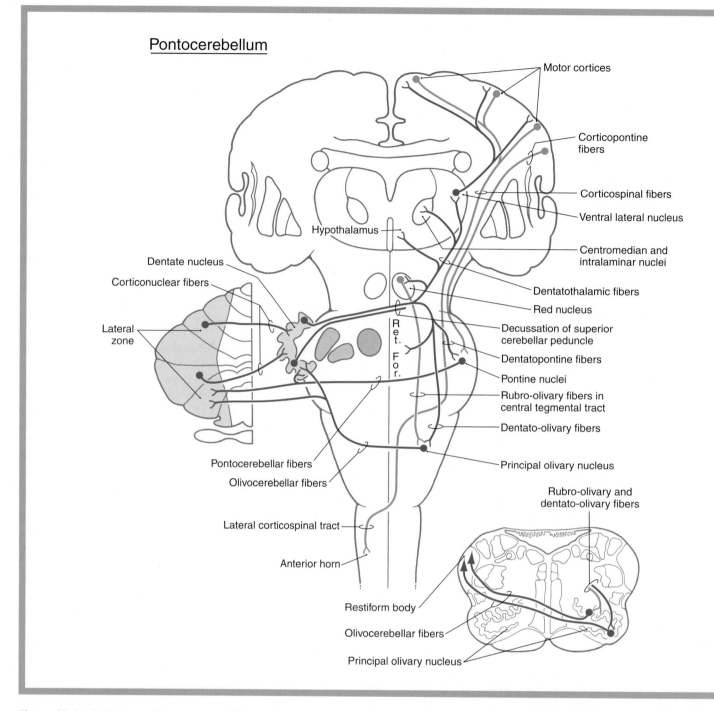

Pontocerebellum

Figure 27-19. Projections of the pontocerebellum (lateral zone) through the dentate nucleus. Ret. For., reticular formation.

categorized as disorders of the *lateral* (or *hemisphere*) *zone* or as *neocerebellar disorders*.

In general, lesions of the lateral cerebellum result in a deterioration of coordinated movement, which is sometimes referred to as a *decomposition of movement* (or *dyssynergia*). This deficit consists of the breakdown of movement into its individual component parts. There may also be a decrease in muscle tone *(hypotonia)* and in deep tendon reflexes. *Ataxia* involving the extremities generally is also seen in patients with lateral cerebellar lesions. Because of ataxia of the lower extremity, these patients may also have an *unsteady gait* and a tendency to lean or fall to the side of the lesion.

Dysmetria (also called *past-pointing*) is apparent in patients when they attempt to point accurately or rapidly to moving or stationary targets. The patient may reach past the target *(hypermetria)* or fall short of the target *(hypometria)*.

Tremor is a consistent finding in patients with lateral cerebellar lesions. A *kinetic tremor*, commonly called an *intention tremor*,

is evident when the patient performs a voluntary movement and is most obvious as the end-point, or target, is approached. This deficit is commonly seen when the patient extends the arm and then attempts to touch the index finger to the nose (Fig. 27-20). At rest there is little or no tremor, but as the finger approaches the nose, the tremor is markedly accentuated. This finding is opposite to that seen in patients with Parkinson disease, whose tremor is evident at rest *(resting tremor)* but largely diminishes during a voluntary movement. Patients with cerebellar lesions may also demonstrate a *static tremor*. This tremor is manifested when the patient stands with the arms extended (muscles contracted against gravity). There is rhythmic movement of the shoulders that also involves the upper extremities.

Awkward performance of rapid alternating movements, such as supinating and pronating the hand against the thigh, is called *dysdiadochokinesia* (Fig. 27-21). The patient may also be unable to perform rhythmic movements. This deficit is demonstrated by asking the patient to rapidly tap the table three times with the

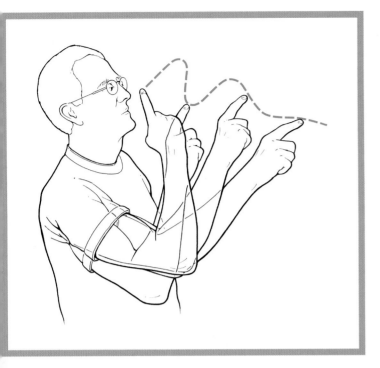

Figure 27-20. Intention tremor. Note that as the patient moves his finger closer to the target (his nose), the tremor becomes worse. In other words, as the patient "intends" to make a precise movement, the tremor gets progressively worse as the target is approached; this sequence of events is an easy way to remember this deficit.

index finger, pause two seconds, tap three times, and so on. For patients with lateral cerebellar lesions, this task will be difficult or impossible.

Other lateral zone deficits include rebound phenomena, dysarthria, and ocular motor dysfunction. The *rebound phenomenon* (or *impaired check*) is an inability of agonist and antagonist muscles to adapt to rapid changes in load. For example, if the patient is asked to push against the physician's hand and the hand is then unexpectedly removed, the patient's arm will overshoot beyond the point where it would normally halt. Tremors or oscillations may also be evident as the arm returns to its starting point. Patients with *dysarthria* have slurred, garbled speech that may also be alternately slow or staccato in nature *(scanning speech)*. This is a motor problem (not an aphasia), because the patient is still able to use words and grammar correctly. Characteristic ocular motor dysfunctions seen in patients with lateral cerebellar lesions are *nystagmus* and abnormalities of target-directed eye movements. Nystagmus most commonly presents as abnormal horizontal eye movements that consist of a slow conjugate movement away from the side of the lesion. This abnormality is opposite to that seen in lesions of the vestibular receptors, primary sensory fibers, and nuclei. In other cases, the velocity of these conjugate movements may be the same in both directions *(pendular nystagmus)*. Abnormal target-directed eye movements may present as an inability to follow a slowly moving target (disturbed pursuit movements) or difficulty in maintaining fixation on a stationary target.

Cerebellar Influence on Visceromotor Functions

The cerebellum receives input from the *solitary* and *dorsal motor vagal nuclei* and from a number of nuclei in the *hypothalamus*. These areas are directly involved in the control and modulation of a variety of visceromotor functions. The hypothalamus, in addition to having direct connections with the cerebellar cortex

and nuclei, also projects to brainstem and spinal nuclei that are involved in the regulation of visceral functions.

Neurons in several hypothalamic areas and nuclei project to the cerebellar cortex and nuclei *(hypothalamocerebellar fibers)*. The cerebellar nuclei, in turn, send a primarily crossed projection to the hypothalamus *(cerebellohypothalamic fibers)* via the superior cerebellar peduncle (Figs. 27-17 and 27-19). Through these reciprocal connections, the cerebellum may receive visceral input and influence neurons that control visceral functions.

Visceral deficits related to cerebellar lesions are rarely reported, for two reasons. First, the somatomotor deficits seen in such cases are overwhelmingly diagnostic and there is no need to look further. Second, cerebellar lesions may cause an increase in intracranial pressure with resultant pressure on the medulla. Consequently, it is difficult to separate visceral deficits that relate to the cerebellar lesion from those that relate to pressure on the medulla.

In some situations, however, visceral deficits can be related directly to the cerebellar lesion. For example, deficits of this type occurred in a patient who had an occlusion of branches of the left superior cerebellar artery with resultant damage to the cerebellar nuclei on that side. There was no indication of increased intracranial pressure. This patient had characteristic somatomotor tremors in the left arm and leg *during attempted movement* on that side and showed two distinct visceral responses *that occurred concurrent with the somatomotor tremor*, but not before or after. First, the patient's pupils dilated *during* the tremor. Second, the skin on the patient's face flushed and felt warm to the touch *during* the tremor. Immediately upon cessation of the attempted movement (and resulting tremor) of the left hand, the patient fanned his face with his right hand and complained, "It's hot in here." In other cases, small lesions restricted to the fastigial nucleus have been noted to result in decreases in heart rate and blood pressure. These observations suggest that the cerebellum is actively involved in the regulation of visceral function concurrent with its classically recognized influence in the somatomotor sphere.

The Cerebellum and Motor Learning

The involvement of the cerebellum in the learning of movements has been an interesting if not controversial topic in part because the cerebellar often affects the performance of the movement being learned. Consequently, it has been difficult to separate the effects of cerebellar dysfunction on motor learning from those related to performance. In addition, these effects are somewhat dependent on the type of behavior being learned. This task-dependent characteristic may reflect the fact that the cerebellum can be involved in different aspects of the learning process (i.e., acquisition, consolidation, and memory storage) when different behaviors are learned. The cerebellum plays a very critical role in the learning of relatively simple reflexive motor behaviors. These movements include the adaptation of the vestibulo-ocular reflex and the classical (pavlovian) conditioning of reflexes evoked by aversive stimuli, such as the eye-blink and withdrawal reflexes.

Because damage to specific regions of the cerebellum will eliminate the classically conditioned eyeblink reflex and impair the adapted vestibule-ocular reflex, this structure is considered to be a possible storage site for the plastic changes established during the acquisition of these behaviors. Some researchers contend that sites outside the cerebellum also may be involved. However, it has been difficult to demonstrate which locations are most important because the cerebellum is so critical to the function of circuits required for the performance of these reflexes. Current studies utilizing methods that do not impair its contribution to performance will likely contribute significantly to resolving this question.

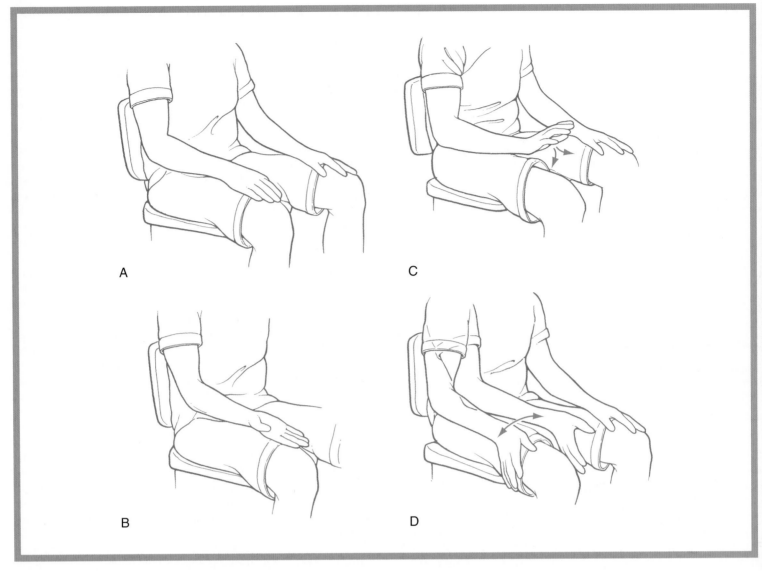

Figure 27-21. Difficulty performing rapid alternating movements: dysdiadochokinesia. Normally the patient can rapidly and precisely pronate (**A**) and supinate (**B**) his hand, but with a cerebellar lesion the patient cannot perform this task. This affected hand flails about the target (**C, D**) and is unable to make the movement smoothly or otherwise. If the patient has a lesion in the right side of the cerebellum, the right hand will be affected.

Although the cerebellum also is believed to be involved in the learning of voluntary, complex motor skills, the extent and nature of its involvement has been more difficult to understand than its role in the learning of certain reflexes. Initial studies demonstrated that normal subjects performed better after practicing a new task than did patients with cerebellar damage. This finding was first ascribed to the presence of a learning deficit in these patients. However, recent experiments that examined the rate at which a new motor skill is acquired revealed that cerebellar patients can learn to perform new movements even though the *quality* of the performance is affected by their deficit. Furthermore, animals can learn volitional limb movements even when the cerebellar nuclei are inactivated. Thus the cerebellum is not as essential for the learning of many volitional movements as it is for the modification of the specific reflexes reviewed previously. However, cerebellar dysfunction does result in a decrease in the quality and consistency of the learned behaviors.

Together these findings suggest that, even though the cerebellum is not essential for learning volitional movements, it is involved in the acquisition process. This argument is supported further by imaging experiments showing that specific regions in the cerebellum are activated *during* the learning of novel movements. In addition, the acquisition of complex behaviors in animals is associated with increased modulation of cells in the cerebellar nuclei when the animal first learns to perform the task correctly and consistently on successive trials.

The cerebellum is not likely a critical storage site for the memory established during the learning of volitional movements. Experiments in animals focused on this issue demonstrated that the patterns of movements required to perform previously learned complex volitional motor tasks could be recalled during the inactivation of the ipsilateral dentate and interposed nuclei. For those learned motor behaviors that may require intracerebellar memory storage sites, the mechanism responsible for establishing the storage and even the location of these changes has not yet been resolved despite extensive experimentation in this area. It has been proposed that the climbing fiber input to the dendrites of Purkinje cells can induce plastic changes that modify the responsiveness of these neurons to specific inputs mediated by parallel fibers. However, the relevance of this mechanism to normal physiologic conditions continues to be debated. There is stronger evidence that the cerebellar nuclei may be a storage site in certain types of motor learning such as the classically conditioned eye-blink reflex through processes such as long-term depression.

In summary, certain reflexes cannot be modified in the absence of the cerebellum and lesions of this structure impair the *performance* of certain previously learned behaviors. This structure plays an important role in the *acquisition of several motor behaviors including skilled volitional movements*, although the nature of its contribution to this process has not been characterized. The cerebellum may be a storage site for the learning of certain reflex behaviors. However, it is not considered to be essential for storing engrams related to complex volitional movements. Current research also has demonstrated that this structure is involved in cognitive processes, some of which may also be related to important aspects of motor learning.

Synopsis of Clinical Points

- Cerebellar lesion may result in motor deficits but not in paralysis (p. 432).
- The exit of the trigeminal nerve is an important landmark indicating the boundary between the basilar pons and the middle cerebellar peduncle (p. 432).
- The superior cerebellar artery supplies the anterior lobe and most of the cerebellar nuclei (pp. 433–436).
- The excitatory neurons of the cerebellar cortex are the granules cell and the unipolar brush cell (p. 437).
- Midline cerebellar lesions result in truncal ataxia (p. 444).
- Patients with medial cerebellar lesions are unable to walk in tandem, on their heels, or on their toes (p. 444).
- Titubation is a tremor of axial portions of the body and/or head (p. 444).
- Lesions of the flocculonodular lobe may result in nystagmus (pp. 443–446).
- The output of the vestibulocerebellum relates to eye movements and axial and proximal limb musculature (pp. 443–446).
- The output of the spinocerebellum relates to the control of axial muscles and limb musculature (pp. 445–446).
- The output of the pontocerebellum relates to the planning, timing, and control of precise upper extremity movements (p. 447).
- Damage to only the cerebellar cortex usually results in transient deficits (p. 447).
- Cerebellar lesions that involve the cerebellar cortex and the nuclei usually result in long-term deficits (p. 447).
- Damage to the cerebellar cortex + nuclei result in motor deficits on the side of the body ipsilateral to the lesion (p. 447).
- Lesions of the midbrain that involve crossed cerebellothalamic fibers result in motor deficits on the side of the body contralateral to the lesion (pp. 447–448).
- General features of a cerebellar lesion include dyssynergia, ataxia, and unsteady gait (p. 448).
- The inability to point quickly and accurately to a moving or stationary target is dysmetria (p. 448).
- When attempting to point to a target, patients with cerebellar lesions may overshoot (hypermetria) or undershoot (hypometria) the target (p. 448).
- An intention tremor (kinetic tremor) is characteristic of a cerebellar lesion (p. 448).
- A resting tremor is characteristic of Parkinson disease (p. 448).
- The inability to perform rapid alternating movements is dysdiadochokinesia (pp. 448–449).
- Impaired check (rebound phenomenon) is the inability of agonist and antagonist muscles to rapidly respond to changes in load (p. 449).
- The dysarthria seen in patients with cerebellar lesions reflects dyssynergia of the vocal muscles (p. 449).
- In addition to somatomotor deficits, medial cerebellar lesions may also result in visceromotor alterations (p. 449).
- Damage to the cerebellum may affect the ability to learn motor tasks (pp. 449–450).

Sources and Additional Reading

Bloedel JR, Dichgans J, Precht W: Cerebellar Functions. New York, Springer-Verlag, 1985.

Brooks VB, Thach WT: Cerebellar control of posture. In Brooks VB (ed): Handbook of Physiology, Section 1: The Nervous System, vol II: Motor Control, Part 2. Bethesda, MD, American Physiological Society, 1981.

Dietrichs E, Haines DE, Roste GK, Roste LS: Hypothalamo-cerebellar and cerebellohypothalamic projections—circuits for regulating nonsomatic cerebellar activity. Histol Histopathol 9:603-614, 1994.

Dino MR, Nunzi MG, Anelli R, Muganini E: Unipolar brush cells of the vestibulocerebellum: Afferents and targets. In Gerrits NM, Ruigrok, de Zeeuw CI (eds): Progress in Brain Research, 124, Cerebellar Modules: Molecules, Morphology and Function. Amsterdam, Elsevier, 2000.

Duvernoy HM: The Human Brain Stem and Cerebellum: Surface, Structure, Vascularization, and Three-Dimensional Sectional Anatomy with MRI. Vienna, Springer-Verlag, 1995.

Gerrits NM, Ruigrok TJH, de Zeeuw CI: Cerebellar modules: Molecules, morphology and function. Prog Brain Res 124:1-330, 2000.

Gilman S, Bloedel JR, Lechtenberg R: Disorders of the Cerebellum. Contemporary Neurology Series, vol 21. Philadelphia, FA Davis, 1981.

Haines DE, Patrick GW, Satrulee P: Organization of cerebellar corticonuclear fiber systems. Exp Brain Res Suppl 6:320-371, 1982.

Haines DE, Dietrichs E, Mihailoff GA, McDonald EF: The cerebellar-hypothalamic axis: Basic circuits and clinical observations. In Schmahmann JD (ed): The Cerebellum and Cognition. Int Rev Neurobiol 41:83-107, 1997.

Hore J, Flament D: Evidence that a disordered servo-like mechanism contributes to tremor in movements during cerebellar dysfunction. J Neurophysiol 56:123-136, 1986.

Ito M: The Cerebellum and Neural Control. New York, Raven Press, 1984.

Larsell O, Jansen J: The Comparative Anatomy and Histology of the Cerebellum: The Human Cerebellum, Cerebellar

Connections, and Cerebellar Cortex. Minneapolis, University of Minnesota Press, 1972.

Mihailoff GA: Identification of pontocerebellar axon collateral synaptic boutons in the rat cerebellar nuclei. Brain Res 648:313-318, 1994.

Nunzi MG, Shigemoto R, Mugnaini E: Differential expression of calretinin and metabotropic glutamate receptor mGluR1(alpha) defines subsets of unipolar brush cells in mouse cerebellum. J Comp Neurol 451:189-199, 2002.

Ojakangas CI, Ebner TJ: Purkinje cell complex and simple spike changes during a voluntary arm movement learning task in the monkey. J Neurophysiol 68:2222-2236, 1992.

Robertson L: Organization of climbing fiber representation in the anterior lobe. In King JS (ed): New Concepts in Cerebellar Neurobiology. New York, Alan R. Liss, 1987, pp 281-320.

Sekerkova G, Ilijic E, Mugnaini E: Time of origin of unipolar brush cells in the rat cerebellum as observed by prenatal bromodeoxyuridine labeling. Neuroscience 127:845-858, 2004.

Thach WT, Goodkin HP, Keating JG: The cerebellum and the adaptive coordination of movement. Annu Rev Neurosci 15:403-442, 1992.

Welker W, Blair C, Shambes GM: Somatosensory projections to cerebellar granule cell layer of giant bushbaby, *Galago crassicaudatus*. Brain Behav Evol 31:150-160, 1988.

Visual Motor Systems

P. J. May and J. J. Corbett

All animals use their sensory organs to scan the environment in search of information. Often these organs are actively oriented toward relevant targets. This *orienting behavior* is exhibited by creatures from honey bees to humans. Movement of the eyes, for example, allows closer inspection of the visual environment. Moreover, human eyes have a fovea, a small portion of the central retina that has exquisite visual sensitivity. Accurately directing the fovea to targets of interest represents a crucial orienting behavior in humans. Extraocular muscles orient our highly mobile eyes. These muscles are supplied by cranial nerves III, IV and VI, and the *oculomotor* (or *ocular motor*) *system* controls these muscles. It is one of several *visual motor* systems that support the function of visual sensation.

Overview

The oculomotor system includes *gaze systems* that redirect the eyes to each new target. There are three basic types of "targeting" movements: (1) *saccades*, rapid movements that direct the eyes to each new target; (2) *smooth pursuit*, slower movements that allow the eyes to follow moving targets; and (3) *vergence movements*, which adjust for target distance by changing the angle between the eyes. Vergence is coupled with changes in the curvature of the *lens* and the size of the *pupil* that focus the target image on the fovea. Saccades and smooth pursuit are *conjugate* movements, in which the eyes move in the same direction, often with accompanying movements of the head and body. Vergence movements are *disconjugate* (Table 28-1).

Visual motor systems also mediate a set of reflex actions. *Compensatory reflexes* keep the eyes on target despite body movements. Sensory inputs from the vestibular and visual systems tell the brain that the body is in motion. During movement, the *vestibulo-ocular reflex* compensates for acceleration, which is sensed by the vestibular labyrinth, whereas the *optokinetic reflex* compensates for velocity, which is indicated by movement of the whole visual field (Table 28-1). Visual motor systems also compensate for the amount of light falling on the retina. The *pupillary light reflex* maintains the level of retinal illumination within the working range of the photopigments in the photoreceptor cells (rods or cones). Finally, rhythmic and reflex *blinks* of the eyelids protect the eye.

Disturbances of the visual motor systems are common and often produce the first symptoms recognized by a patient. Understanding these ocular signs provides for timely and effective diagnosis. For instance, *strabismus* is a defect in which the eyes are misaligned. If this defect is left untreated, the brain reacts to the constant diplopia (double vision) by ignoring the input from one eye and failing to focus it *(amblyopia)* and, eventually, failing even to orient it. However, amblyopia can be avoided through early treatment of strabismus.

Peripheral Structures

Extraocular Muscles

The eye is moved in the orbit by six extraocular muscles (Figs. 28-1 and 28-2). These muscles produce movements in the horizontal plane (left and right) around a vertical axis, movements in the vertical plane (up and down) around a horizontal axis, and torsional movements (clockwise and counterclockwise) around an axis running through the center of the pupil to the fovea. There are two pair of rectus muscles, with the members of each antagonistic pair arranged opposite one another on the globe, and a single pair of oblique muscles, which also act as antagonists (Figs. 28-1 and 28-2). For horizontal eye movements, the *medial rectus muscle* rotates the eye toward the nose *(adduction)* and the *lateral rectus muscle* rotates the eye toward the temple *(abduction)*. For vertical eye movements, the primary action of the *superior rectus* is to rotate the eye upward *(elevation)*, and the primary action of the *inferior rectus* is to rotate the eye downward *(depression)*. The direction of pull of the *superior oblique muscle* (Figs. 28-1 and 28-2A, B) is modified because its tendon passes through a loop of connective tissue, the *trochlea*, on the medial wall of the bony orbit. Its insertion on the globe is caudal to that of the superior rectus. As a consequence, the actions of the superior oblique are *intorsion*, depression, and abduction. Conversely, the *inferior oblique muscle* (Figs. 28-1 and 28-2A, C) actions are *extorsion* and elevation, as well as abduction.

The extraocular muscles are supplied by three cranial nerves. The superior oblique muscle is innervated by the *trochlear nerve*, the lateral rectus muscle by the *abducens nerve*, and the medial, superior and inferior recti and inferior oblique muscles by the

Table 28-1. Summary of Eye Movement Characteristics

Class	Function	Conjugate	Speed	Latency (msec)	Clinical Points
Foveation	Hold fovea on target	NA	None Only very small oscillations	NA	Look for drifts, especially holding eccentric gaze
Saccade	Acquisition of new target	Yes	100-700 degrees/sec Amplitude-dependent	200	Sedative-sensitive Test: Look between points
Smooth pursuit	Follow a moving target	Yes	Variable <100 degrees/sec Target speed dependent	100	Test: Follow a slow moving target
Vergence	Direct fovea at targets of different distances	No	≈15 degrees/sec Disconjugate saccades faster	150	Test: Move target toward and away from nose
Vestibular (VOR)	Compensate for initial head movement	Yes	Variable <500 degrees/sec Head acceleration dependent	<15 Lasts 45 sec	Dizziness and nausea Test: Caloric (irrigate ear)
Optokinetic (OKR)	Compensate for continued head movement	Yes	Variable <100 degrees/sec Retinal slip-dependent	50-100	Test: Steady movement of a striped drum or cloth
Nystagmic fast phase	Recenter eye during continuous VOR or OKR	Yes	500 degrees/sec	NA	Nystagmus: Alternating fast and slow phase movements

OKR, optokinetic reflex; VOR, vestibulo-ocular reflex; NA, not applicable.

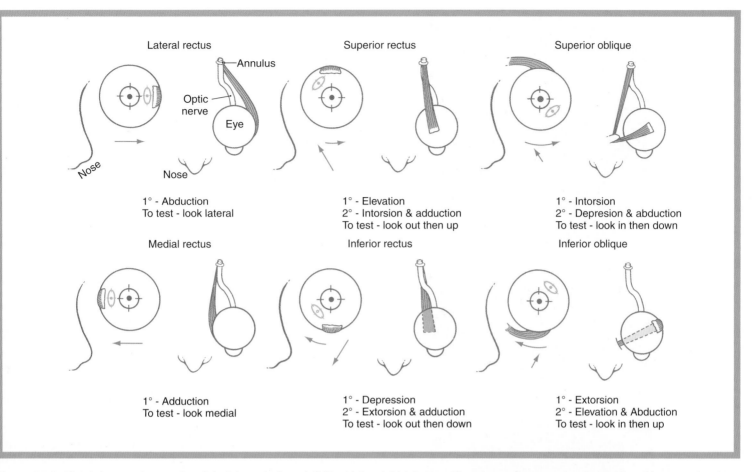

Lateral rectus

Annulus
Optic nerve
Eye
Nose
Nose

1° - Abduction
To test - look lateral

Superior rectus

1° - Elevation
2° - Intorsion & adduction
To test - look out then up

Superior oblique

1° - Intorsion
2° - Depression & abduction
To test - look in then down

Medial rectus

1° - Adduction
To test - look medial

Inferior rectus

1° - Depression
2° - Extorsion & adduction
To test - look out then down

Inferior oblique

1° - Extorsion
2° - Elevation & Abduction
To test - look in then up

Figure 28-1. The six extraocular muscles of the left eye in frontal *(left)* and dorsal *(right)* views. The primary *(long arrow)* and secondary *(short arrow)* actions of each muscle and the position of the pupil after the movement *(red oval)* are indicated on the frontal view. These muscles originate at the common tendon (annulus of Zinn), with the exception of the inferior rectus, which originates from the orbit's nasal wall. Rectus muscles insert in front of the equator of the globe, and the oblique muscles insert behind it. Secondary actions are important for clinical evaluation of muscle function. In these cases, the eye is first rotated to align its axis with that of the muscle; for example, for the inferior oblique, the eye is first adducted and then elevated.

oculomotor nerve. The formula "(SO4 LR6) 3" (superior oblique 4, lateral rectus 6, all others 3) is a convenient memory aid for this pattern. The extraocular muscles are striated and contain fibers adapted to produce extremely high contraction velocities and nearly constant tension. These muscles contain some of the smallest motor units in the body, giving them great precision of movement. The muscles run through connective tissue sheaths that act as pulleys controlling their pulling directions. Each muscle has an inner *global* layer and an outer *orbital* layer. The thick global layer inserts onto the sclera of the eye, whereas the thin orbital layer inserts into the connective tissue sheath to regulate the muscle's pulling direction. Some forms of strabismus may be due to misaligned pulleys. The trigeminal nerve carries sensory information from the extraocular muscles. This proprioceptive signal appears to be critical for normal development of *stereoscopic vision* (perception of three-dimensional space) and may have other roles. Visual feedback is the primary source of information revealing eye movement accuracy.

Intraocular Muscles

The eyes contain three intrinsic smooth muscles (Fig. 28-3). The *ciliary muscle* changes the curvature of the lens to bring visual targets into focus on the retina. The *sphincter* (or *constrictor*) *pupillae muscle* and *dilator pupillae muscle* control the size of the pupils in an antagonistic fashion, to regulate the amount of light entering the eyes and the depth of field.

The ciliary muscle, found in the *ciliary body,* is connected to the lens by the *suspensory ligaments (zonule of Zinn)*. These fine connective tissue threads resemble the spokes of a bicycle wheel. The action of the ciliary muscle changes the shape of the lens

(via the zonule) to adjust its refractive state and focus the image on the retina (Fig. 28-3E, F). These changes are termed *lens accommodation.* Constriction of the ciliary muscle is produced by activation of cholinergic postganglionic parasympathetic fibers from the ciliary ganglion. With age, the lens grows less elastic, so that the actions of the ciliary muscle have less effect on refraction. This loss of accommodation produces a blurring of near vision termed *presbyopia. Myopia,* a loss of distant acuity, generally appears at an early age and may be due to genetic factors or overwork at close focal distances (e.g., reading).

The sphincter pupillae is a ring-shaped muscle that lies along the pupillary margin (Fig. 28-3A, C). It contracts in response to activation of cholinergic parasympathetic fibers from the ciliary ganglion, to constrict the pupil *(miosis).* The dilator muscle is radially arranged, so that its action folds the iris and draws open the pupil *(mydriasis).* The dilator is activated by adrenergic postganglionic sympathetic fibers from the superior cervical ganglion.

Eyelid

The eyelid is controlled by the *levator palpebrae superioris,* the *orbicularis oculi,* and the tarsal or *Müller muscles* (Fig. 28-4). The levator palpebrae is supplied by cranial nerve III. This muscle originates with and travels parallel to the superior rectus but continues forward to insert into the upper lid (Fig. 28-2A, C). The levator holds the eyelid up when the eyes are open, and it functions in concert with the superior rectus, increasing the elevation of the lids when the eyes look up. The orbicularis oculi, supplied by cranial nerve VII, closes the eyes by depressing the upper lid and elevating the lower lid. At the same time, co-

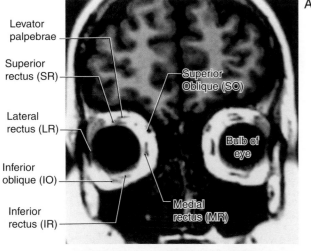

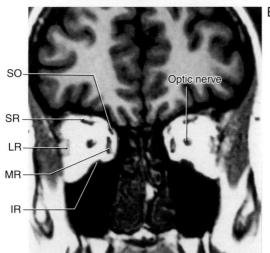

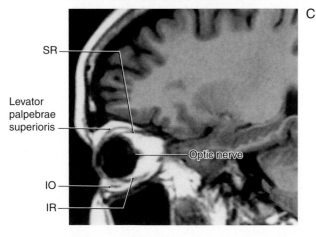

Figure 28-2. Coronal (**A, B**) and sagittal (**C**) T2-weighted MR images showing the relationships of the extraocular muscles within the orbit. The coronal planes are through (**A**) and caudal to (**B**) the bulb of the eye. Compare these images with the drawing in Figure 28-1.

contraction of the rectus muscles retracts the eye. The tarsal muscles are small smooth muscles at the edge of the bony orbit. They are supplied by postganglionic sympathetic fibers and help keep the lids open.

Central Structures

Oculomotor Nucleus

The oculomotor nucleus (Fig. 28-5) lies near the midline in the inferior part of the periaqueductal gray of the rostral midbrain. Beneath it lie the fibers of the *medial longitudinal fasciculus*, many of which synapse within the oculomotor nucleus. Axons

from oculomotor motor neurons generally pass medial to the red nucleus and exit the midbrain just medial to the crus cerebri. These structures are supplied by paramedian branches of the basilar artery and the proximal part of the posterior cerebral artery (P_1 segment). Vascular lesions in this region produce oculomotor deficits in combination with other symptoms (Table 28-2).

The third cranial nerve passes along the wall of the cavernous sinus and enters the ipsilateral orbit by way of the superior orbital fissure. Its three branches supply the superior rectus and levator palpebrae muscles, the inferior rectus and inferior oblique muscles, and the medial rectus muscle. The motor neurons supplying each of these individual muscles form rostrocaudally oriented columns within the nucleus (Fig. 28-6). The motor neurons supplying the levator palpebrae superioris muscle form a separate dorsal midline subnucleus called the *caudal central subdivision*.

Edinger-Westphal Nucleus

The nucleus of *Edinger and Westphal* contains the cholinergic, preganglionic parasympathetic motor neurons that control lens accommodation and pupillary constriction. In humans, the Edinger-Westphal nuclei form a pair of cell columns that lie near the midline, between the superior poles of the oculomotor nuclei (Fig. 28-6). The preganglionic fibers travel with the ipsilateral oculomotor nerve and synapse in the *ciliary ganglion*. Cholinergic, postganglionic motor neurons send their axons to the globe via the *short ciliary nerves*. These motor neurons supply the ciliary muscle and pupillary constrictor, with the great majority supplying the former. Thus, in Weber syndrome (Table 28-2) or other lesions of the oculomotor nerve, loss of the preganglionic fibers may result in ipsilateral *mydriasis* (dilation of the pupil) and paralysis of accommodation.

Trochlear Nucleus

The trochlear nucleus is a small, ovoid group of neurons nestled in the medial longitudinal fasciculus of the caudal midbrain (Fig. 28-7). These motor neurons supply the contralateral superior oblique muscle. The axons forming the trochlear nerve arch dorsally and caudally around the periaqueductal gray, cross the midline in the anterior medullary vellum, and exit the dorsal surface of the brainstem at the base of the inferior colliculus. The nerve courses laterally and then anteriorly, hugging the surface of the midbrain. It passes rostrally along the wall of the cavernous sinus, before entering the orbit via the superior orbital fissure, to innervate the superior oblique muscle.

Abducens Nucleus

The abducens nucleus is a spherical cell group located in the facial colliculus, adjacent to the internal genu of the facial nerve in the caudal pons (Fig. 28-8; also see Figs. 12-10 and 12-12). Abducens fibers pass slightly caudally and then anteriorly (ventrally) to exit near the midline at the pontomedullary junction. En route, they pass adjacent to the medial lemniscus and corticospinal tract. Owing to this relationship, loss of paramedian branches of the basilar artery compromises both the corticospinal tract and the exiting abducens fibers, resulting in a *contralateral hemiplegia* and paralysis of abduction in the *ipsilateral* eye *(Foville syndrome)*. This pairing of motor symptoms is called an *alternating hemiplegia*, or crossed deficit, and it can also occur in association with cranial nerves III and XII. After exiting the brainstem, the abducens nerve (cranial nerve VI) enters the dura and ascends the clivus. It then passes beneath the petroclinoid ligament (the Dorello canal) to enter and pass through the cavernous sinus. Cranial nerves III, IV, and VI and branches of cranial nerve V may be damaged in this sinus, singly or in combination, by pituitary tumors or carotid

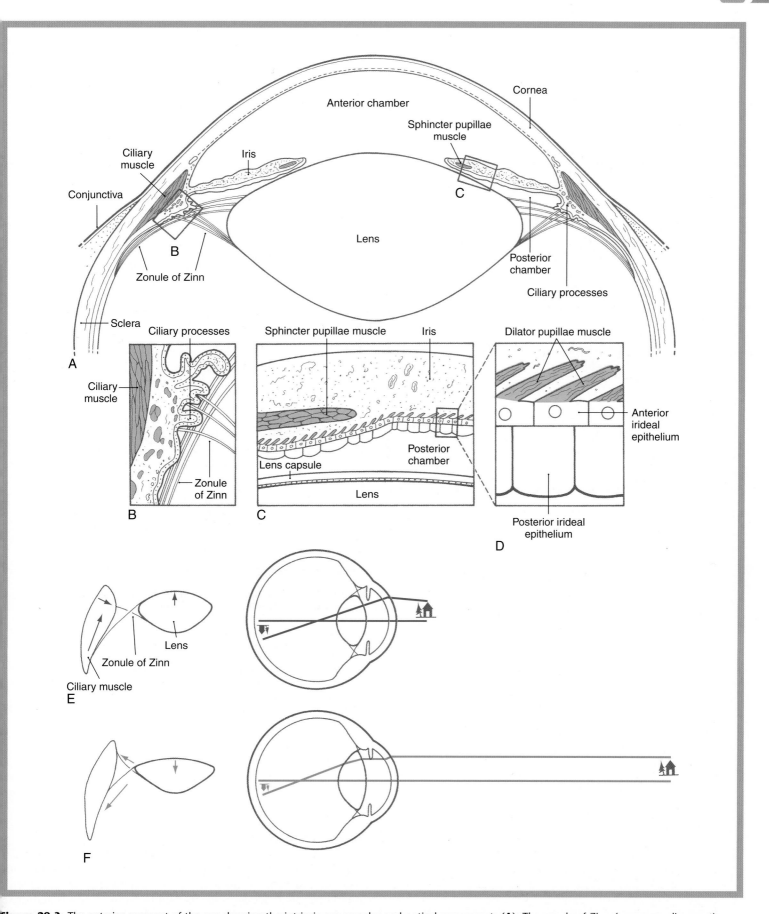

Figure 28-3. The anterior segment of the eye showing the intrinsic eye muscles and optical components (**A**). The zonule of Zinn (suspensory ligament) extends from the lens capsule and inserts into the epithelium covering the ciliary muscle (**B**). The pupillary sphincter and dilator muscles are separate muscles in the iris (**C**). The latter is actually made up of the myoid processes of the anterior iridial epithelium, as shown in **D**. The mechanism (left) and effects (right) of accommodation (**E, F**) are shown. On looking at a nearby target (**E**), the ciliary muscle contracts (arrows), releasing tension in the zonule and allowing the anterior surface of the lens to round up (arrow) owing to its own elasticity. On looking at a distant target (**F**), the ciliary muscle relaxes, and the unopposed tension in the zonule (arrows) flattens the lens (arrow).

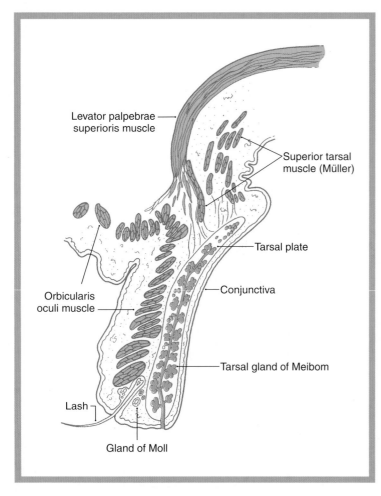

Figure 28-4. The structure of the upper eyelid.

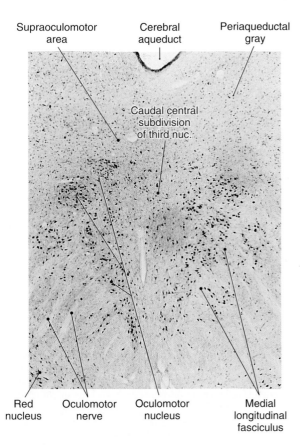

Figure 28-5. The human oculomotor nucleus (nuc.) and adjacent structures in a Nissl-stained cross section showing neuron cell bodies.

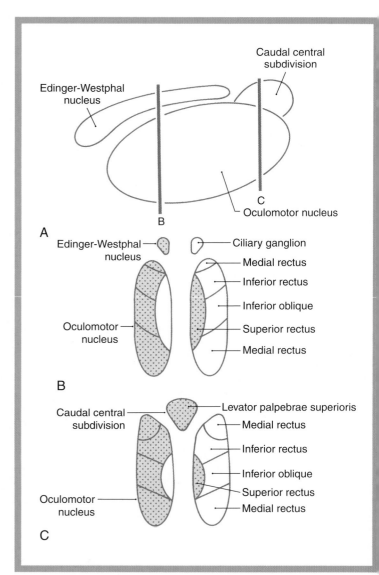

Figure 28-6. Lateral view of the oculomotor and related nuclei (**A**). The motor neuron pools in the nucleus are shown in frontal sections through anterior (**B**) and posterior (**C**) parts of the nucleus. The names of the major nuclei are indicated on the left in **B** and **C**, and the targets of each subdivision are indicated on the right in **B** and **C**. As indicated by the *stippled* and *clear* areas, these motor neurons project ipsilaterally, with the exception of the contralaterally projecting superior rectus motor neurons and the bilaterally distributed levator motor neurons. The axons of contralateral motor neurons cross immediately to join the ipsilateral oculomotor nerve. Thus, the oculomotor nerve projects entirely to ipsilateral muscles.

aneurysms. Cranial nerve VI supplies the lateral rectus muscle, so damage to this nerve in isolation will paralyze abduction ipsilaterally (Fig. 28-9).

Abducens Internuclear Neurons

Conjugate eye movement is achieved in the horizontal plane by a pathway from the abducens nucleus to the contralateral medial rectus subdivision of the oculomotor nucleus (Fig. 28-13, green). Inputs to the abducens nucleus supply motor neurons and drive *abducens internuclear neurons* found in this nucleus. Abducens internuclear neurons transmit signals to medial rectus motor neurons on the contralateral side via the medial longitudinal fasciculus (MLF). In this way, the lateral rectus of one eye works in tandem with the medial rectus of the other eye. Lesions in the MLF *between the abducens and oculomotor nuclei* damage the abducens internuclear neuron axons, producing *internuclear ophthalmoplegia*. In this situation, the lateral rectus contracts appropriately during horizontal eye movements, but the medial

Table 28-2. Summary of Lesions of the Exiting Oculomotor Nerve

Syndromes and Structures Involved	Corresponding Deficits
Weber Syndrome	

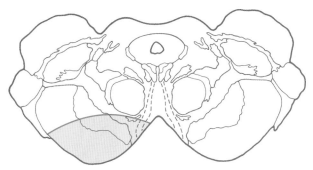

Oculomotor nerve	Ipsilateral oculomotor palsy with muscle atrophy, ptosis, mydriasis.
Corticospinal and corticonuclear fibers in the crus cerebri	Contralateral hemiparesis of upper and lower extremities, contralateral paralysis of lower face and deviation of tongue to contralateral side on protrusion.

Claude Syndrome

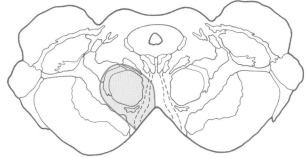

Oculomotor nerve	Oculomotor palsy, muscle atrophy, ptosis, mydriasis.
Red nucleus and cerebellothalamic fibers	Contralateral tremor and ataxia (contralateral loss of position sense, vibratory sense, and discriminative touch if medial lemniscus involved).

Benedikt Syndrome

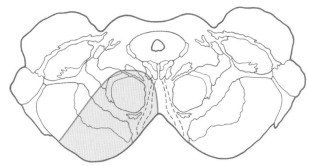

Structures in Weber + Claude Syndromes	The deficits in Benedikt represent a combination of those seen in Weber + Claude syndromes. In addition these patients may have a contralateral rigidity due to damage to the substantia nigra.

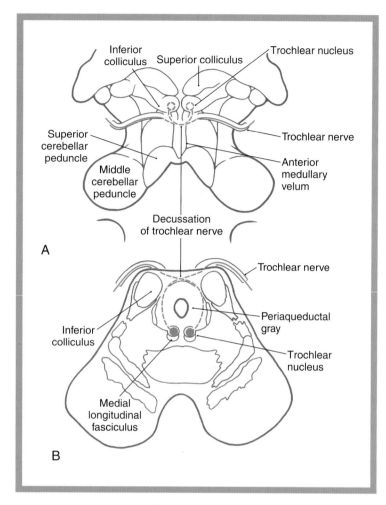

A

B

Figure 28-7. The trochlear nucleus and nerve shown in a dorsal view of the midbrain (**A**) and in a coronal section through the nucleus (**B**).

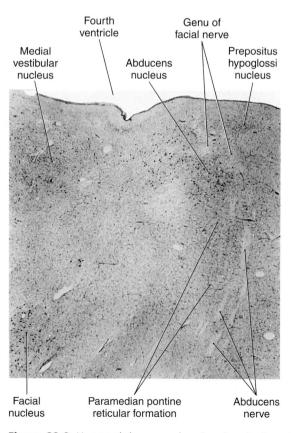

Figure 28-8. Human abducens nucleus (nuc.) and adjacent structures in Nissl-stained cross section showing neuron cell bodies.

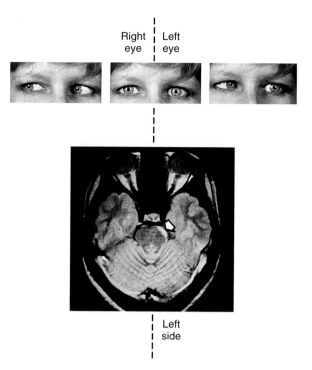

Figure 28-9. Paralysis of abduction in the patient's left eye on looking to the left. The CT scan shows demyelination of the pons at the level of the exiting left abducens nerve *(arrow)*.

rectus for the opposite eye does not. However, because the oculomotor nerve and nucleus are intact, no deficits are present on convergence. The presence of internuclear neurons also explains why the symptoms of abducens nerve lesions differ from those of abducens nucleus lesions. In the latter, the action of the contralateral medial rectus muscle is impaired during conjugate horizontal movements, in addition to the expected paralysis of the ipsilateral lateral rectus muscle. Large abducens nucleus lesions may also include the crossing fibers entering the medial longitudinal fasciculus from the opposite abducens. This produces a *one and a half syndrome* in which the ipsilateral eye does not move in either direction for horizontal gaze and the contralateral eye can only abduct.

Sympathetic Supply to the Orbit

The sympathetic innervation of the orbital contents is from the ipsilateral *superior cervical ganglion* (Fig. 28-10). These adrenergic postganglionic fibers enter the cranium on the internal carotid artery. In the cavernous sinus, they run briefly with cranial nerve VI and then join cranial nerves III and V. Sympathetic fibers traveling with the levator branch of cranial nerve III supply the superior tarsal muscle. Fibers traveling with the trigeminal nasociliary nerve exit as the *long ciliary nerves* to supply the eye, including the dilator pupillae muscle.

The cholinergic preganglionic motor neurons that supply the superior cervical ganglion are located at spinal cord levels T1 to T3. Their axons enter and ascend in the sympathetic trunk, to terminate in the ipsilateral superior cervical ganglion. Damage along this long path produces the *Horner syndrome*. The cardinal symptoms of this loss of sympathetic input to the head are partial *ptosis* (a drooping lid resulting from relaxation of the superior tarsal muscle), *miosis* (constriction of the pupil that occurs because the action of the sphincter is no longer opposed by the action of the dilator), and *anhidrosis* (loss of facial sweating). The Horner syndrome may also result from interruption of pathways linking the hypothalamus and brainstem to preganglionic motor neurons in the thoracic cord.

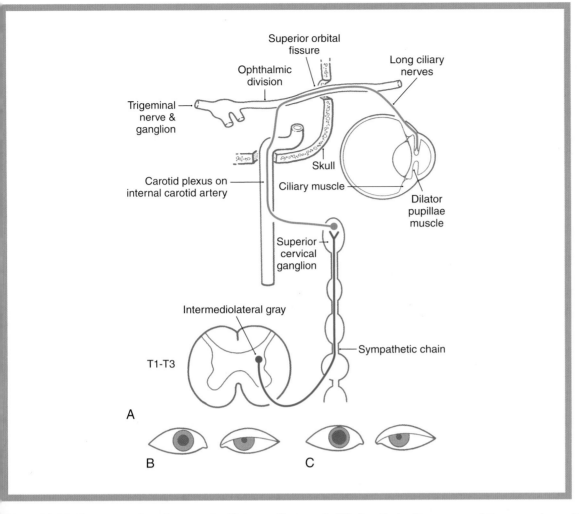

Figure 28-10. The autonomic pathway to the dilator pupillae muscle (**A**). A patient with a presumed Horner syndrome (disruption of this pathway) presents with a partial *ptosis* and *miosis* (**B**). Application of cocaine drops to both eyes establishes that the *anisocoria* is not due to natural or pharmacologic causes (**C**). The normal eye dilates in response to blockade of norepinephrine reuptake, but the deafferented eye shows no change.

Targeting Movements

Saccades

To obtain detailed information about the visual world, the eyes make a series of very rapid movements (200 to 700 degrees/second) from one point to another, stopping briefly at each point to allow detailed foveal inspection. These rapid conjugate eye movements are *saccades,* and the places at which the detailed visual inspection occurs are *fixation points.* During the saccade, the visual system suppresses incoming visual input. Consequently, one is not aware of these movements. Other processes in visual association cortex provide *visual constancy* by weaving together the information obtained at each fixation into a seamless view of the visual world.

Extraocular Muscle Motor Neurons

Extraocular muscle motor neurons have a characteristic *burst-tonic* firing pattern for saccadic eye movements. For example, before a leftward horizontal movement (Fig. 28-11, *points A and B*), left lateral and right medial rectus motor neurons show an initial burst of action potentials, which is then reduced to a sustained tonic level of activity. At the new eye position, the firing rate is slower than during the initial burst but higher than the rate for the previous eye position (Fig. 28-11, *points B and C*).

These two parts of the motor neuron and target muscle response are referred to as a *pulse* and *step* of activity. The pulse, the initial burst of motor neuron activity, directs the phasic

portion of the movement, producing the muscle contraction necessary to overcome the viscosity of the orbit and send the globe toward the target. The step in the activity supports the tonic action of the muscle, which is required to maintain the eye at its new position. The activity of the antagonists is silenced for the saccade and then resumes at a lower rate. However, when the eyes look to the right (Fig. 28-11, *points C and D*), motor neurons for the left medial rectus and right lateral rectus muscles are activated. The brainstem distribution of activated motor neurons defines which muscles are activated and hence the direction of movement. The number of cells activated and their firing rates define the speed and distance (metrics) of the movement.

Horizontal and Vertical Gaze Centers

The brainstem circuitry that controls saccades is subdivided into systems controlling horizontal and vertical eye movement. The pontine reticular formation near the midline, which contains neurons that project to the extraocular motor nuclei, is sometimes called the *paramedian pontine reticular formation* (PPRF) or the *horizontal gaze center* (Figs. 28-12 and 28-13). The PPRF occupies portions of the *oral* and *caudal pontine reticular nuclei.* Cells of this premotor region show activity related to horizontal saccades, and lesions in this region produce *horizontal gaze palsies.* PPRF cells that project to extraocular motor neurons include *excitatory burst neurons* (EBNs), found rostral to the sixth nucleus, and *inhibitory burst neurons* (IBNs), found caudal to the sixth nucleus. Both of these cell types have phasic activity

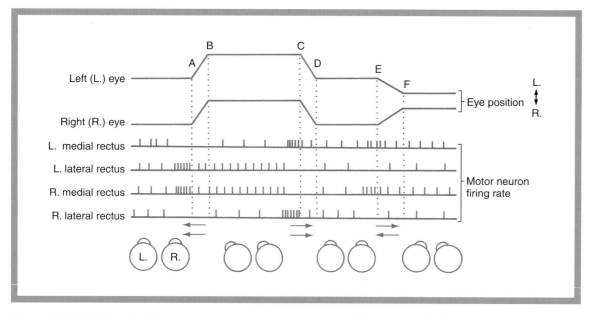

Figure 28-11. Relationship between eye movements and motor neuron firing patterns for horizontal saccades and vergence movements. The top two traces illustrate the changes in eye position. The bottom four traces show idealized firing patterns for motor neurons during horizontal movements. The cartoons at the bottom indicate that the eyes make a saccade to the left (A, B) and then to the right (C, D) and, finally, a convergent movement (E, F).

patterns; that is, they produce a burst of action potentials that slightly precedes the activity of the motor neurons (Fig. 28-13). When gaze shifts to the right, the EBNs activate the abducens nucleus neurons on the right side, as the IBNs suppress the abducens nucleus neurons on the left side. If this inhibition of antagonists does not occur, eye movements are slowed and undershoot.

The pattern of activity in PPRF neurons is a product of the signal (coded in the cell firing pattern) sent from supranuclear structures, including the superior colliculus and the frontal eye field, and processed through interneurons within the PPRF. In addition, the burst of action potentials produced by EBNs and IBNs is gated by inhibition from cells found in the midline of the pontine tegmentum (Figs. 28-12 and 28-13). These inhibitory neurons are called *omnipause cells* because they fire spontaneously during fixation but are silent during a saccadic eye movement in any direction. Thus, the burst of action potentials in PPRF neurons is due, in part, to release from inhibition. PPRF neurons directly contribute to the pulse of motor neuron activity that produces a saccade but not to the step change in activity that maintains eye position. The "where the eye is going" signal produced by the PPRF is transformed (integrated) into a "keep the eye in that position" signal by another brainstem structure. The likely source of this tonic position signal for horizontal saccades is the *nucleus prepositus hypoglossi* (Figs. 28-12 and 28-13).

Vertical gaze palsies are often encountered with lesions of the midbrain-diencephalon junction. The *vertical gaze center* is located in the *rostral interstitial nucleus* of the *medial longitudinal fasciculus* (riMLF), found at the rostral end of the MLF (Fig. 28-12). This region receives supranuclear input from the superior colliculus and frontal eye field, as well as input from omnipause cells. It also contains burst neurons. These neurons provide the phasic signal for the saccade-related pulse of activity present in vertical gaze motor neurons. The tonic signal for the step in vertical gaze motor neuron activity is provided by neurons in the *interstitial nucleus of Cajal* (Fig. 28-12). Because the superior and inferior rectus muscles act in pairs during vertical eye movements, of the riMLF and interstitial nucleus of Cajal on both sides of the brainstem must work in concert. (Unilateral activation produces torsion.) The connections between the two interstitial nuclei of Cajal and the crossed projections to the oculomotor nucleus pass through the posterior commissure.

Consequently, pinealomas pressing on the commissure produce vertical gaze deficits. Oblique saccades are produced by the vertical and horizontal gaze centers working in concert.

Saccadic eye movements are often accompanied by orienting movements of the head. Cells in or near the PPRF, riMLF, and interstitial nucleus of Cajal are responsible for combined head and eye movements. These areas receive collicular and cortical projections, and they project to the extraocular motor neurons and to the cervical spinal cord as *reticulospinal* and *interstitiospinal* fibers. The superior colliculus also projects to the cervical spinal cord, but the tectospinal portion of the tectoreticulospinal system is very small.

Supranuclear Control

For each saccade, the central nervous system must determine the position of the next target of interest and transform this position, which is coded in a sensory map, into the appropriate pattern of motor neuron activity. The areas of the brain that direct saccadic eye movements include the *cortical eye fields* and the *superior colliculus*. In each area, stimulation will initiate contralaterally directed saccades, and single cell recordings reveal neuronal activity before saccades occur. Specifically, stimulation of a location in which cells are active before a 20-degree saccade to the left will produce a 20-degree leftward saccade.

The *frontal eye field* (primarily in area 8 of Brodmann) is located rostral to motor cortex (Figs. 28-14 and 28-15). It is apprised of the location of targets via input from visual association cortex and thalamic relays (paralamellar dorsomedial nucleus) (Fig. 28-15). The frontal eye field influences eye movements through projections to the vertical and horizontal gaze centers and to the superior colliculus. Additional cortical regions influencing saccades include the *supplemental eye field* and the *parietal eye field* in the lateral intraparietal cortex (area 7 of Brodmann) (Fig. 28-14). They have features similar to those of the frontal eye field but are less directly connected to the brainstem saccade circuits. These three cortical eye fields are reciprocally connected, and all three project to the superior colliculus. Perhaps for this reason, loss of any one of these four structures produces few visual motor symptoms.

The *superior colliculus (optic tectum)* is a layered structure found in the roof of the midbrain (Fig. 28-16). This area of the midbrain tectum receives its blood supply from the *quadrigeminal*

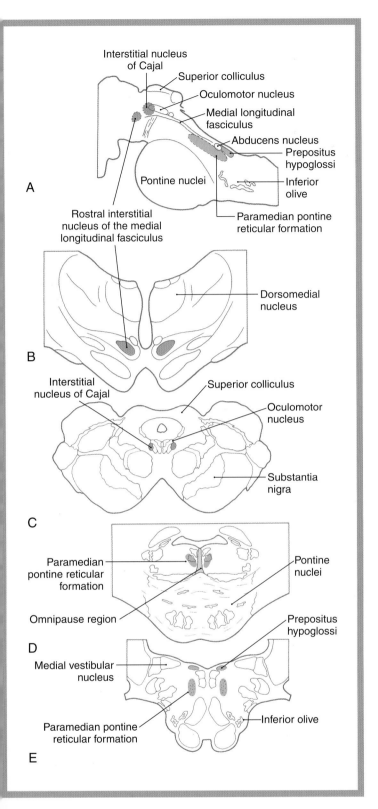

Figure 28-12. The positions of the horizontal and vertical gaze centers in the sagittal (**A**) and frontal (**B-E**) planes.

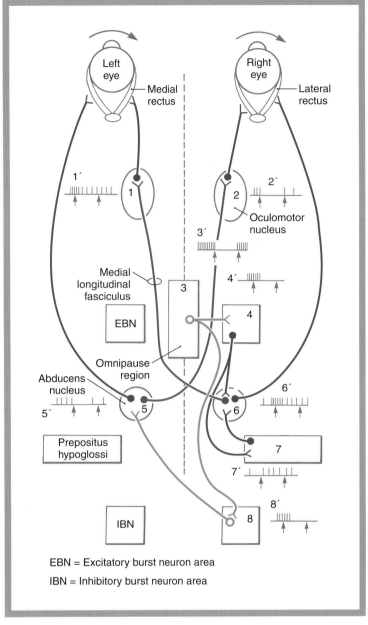

EBN = Excitatory burst neuron area

IBN = Inhibitory burst neuron area

Figure 28-13. Pathway for horizontal saccades. Inhibitory circuits are indicated by *open circles* (red neurons). Idealized firing patterns *(1' etc.)* for a saccade to the right are indicated for each nucleus *(numbers)*. The beginning and the end of the saccade are indicated by *arrows* on the firing patterns. Cells indicated by *green* neurons are abducens internuclear neurons.

artery, a branch of the posterior cerebral artery. The superficial layer of the superior colliculus is visual sensory. It is a target of retinal axons with "Y"- and "W"-type physiologic characteristics and projects to the dorsal lateral geniculate and pulvinar nuclei. In contrast, the intermediate layer is visual motor. It is the source of the *crossed tectoreticulospinal system* that runs ventral to the MLF and terminates in the vertical and horizontal gaze centers (Fig. 28-17).

Major inputs to the intermediate layers of the superior colliculus arise from the parietal association cortex and substantia nigra (Fig. 28-17). GABAergic nigrotectal cells in the substantia

nigra pars lateralis and pars reticulata are spontaneously active but cease firing before saccadic eye movements. Tectal saccade-related activity is partly the result of release from this nigral inhibition. Similar pathways connect the nigra and frontal eye fields. Basal nuclei diseases produce eye movement disorders; for example, patients with Parkinson disease have a dearth of spontaneous eye movements because of unmodulated activity in the nigrotectal pathway.

The superior colliculus and the frontal eye field differ in the types of saccades they control. The frontal eye field is important for *voluntary* and *memory-guided eye movements*, and the superior colliculus directs *reflexive orienting movements*. With loss of either structure, few deficits remain after recovery because the remaining structure compensates for the loss, but loss of both produces profound visuomotor impairment.

Smooth Pursuit

The eyes also make conjugate movements that allow the foveas to follow a moving target (Fig. 28-18). Usually, *smooth pursuit*

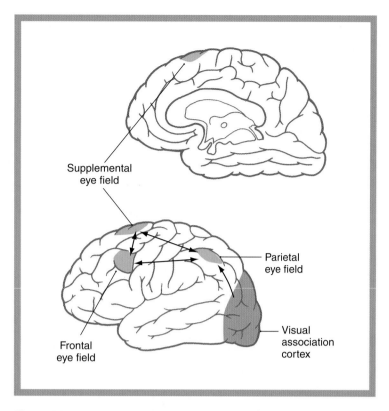

Figure 28-14. Locations and interconnections of the cortical eye fields on medial *(upper)* and lateral *(lower)* views of the cerebral cortex.

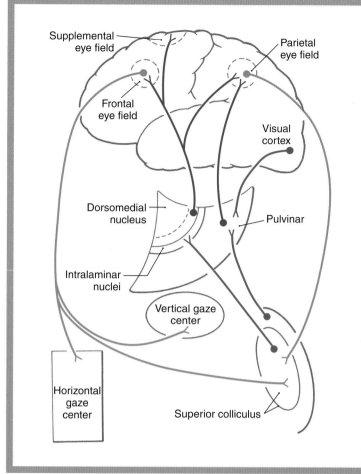

Figure 28-15. Inputs to and outputs of the frontal and parietal eye fields. The *dashed line* in the dorsomedial nucleus indicates the paralamellar subdivision. The pathway to the horizontal gaze center is crossed.

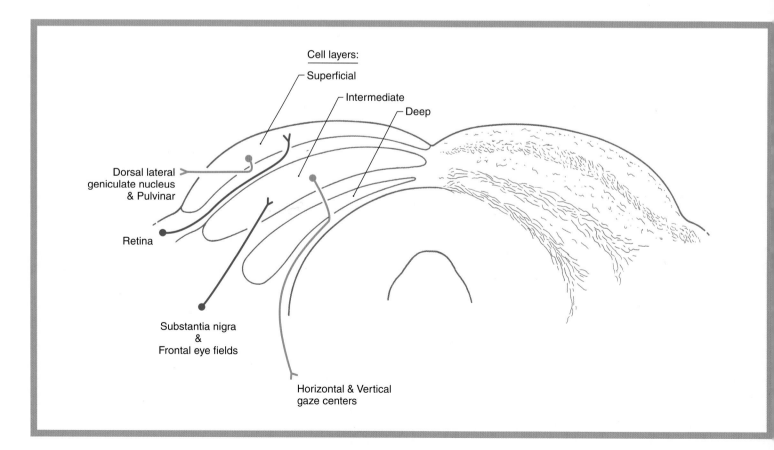

Figure 28-16. The superior colliculus in frontal section. The *right* side shows the layering seen in myelin stains, and the major inputs and outputs are indicated on the *left*.

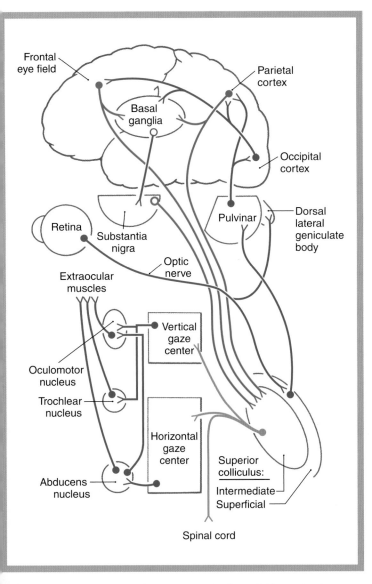

Figure 28-17. Pathways for the superior colliculus. Inhibitory circuits are indicated by *open circles.* The tectoreticulospinal pathway *(red)* to the horizontal gaze center and spinal cord is crossed.

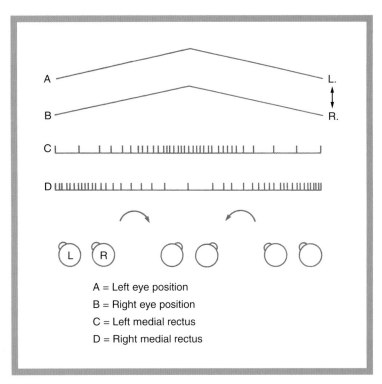

A = Left eye position
B = Right eye position
C = Left medial rectus
D = Right medial rectus

Figure 28-18. The relationship between eye movements and motor neuron firing for smooth pursuit. The eyes change position as they follow a slow-moving target from the left to the right and back to the left (**A, B**). Idealized and graded firing patterns in left (**C**) and right (**B**) medial rectus motor neurons.

eye movements are used to follow slow-moving, predictable targets (30 degrees/second or less). They are, however, capable of following targets at speeds up to 100 degrees/second. The lateral parietal and midtemporal cortices contain neurons that are sensitive to the speed and direction of a target moving across the retina (Fig. 28-19). This input determines the speed and direction of the pursuit eye movements needed to keep the foveas on target. Neurons that display pursuit-related motor activity are found in a portion of the frontal eye field. These three cortical regions project to the *flocculus* and *paraflocculus* of the cerebellum, by way of a synaptic relay in the *posterolateral (dorsolateral) pons.* This portion of the cerebellum, in turn, provides input to the *vestibular nuclei.* Although located in a "sensory" nucleus, vestibular smooth pursuit cells fire with respect to the position and velocity of the eyes, not the visual sensory input. They are, in fact, *premotor neurons,* which project to the third, fourth, and sixth cranial nerve nuclei.

Smooth pursuit premotor neurons fire in a graded manner, depending on the degree and rate of eye excursion. This firing pattern is similar to that displayed by their motor neuron targets during smooth pursuit movements (Fig. 28-18). They do not have the pulse-and-step form seen with saccades. Presumably, the cerebellum plays a role in precisely determining the rate of movement and predicting target trajectory. Floccular lesions do, in fact, produce deficits in smooth pursuit movements.

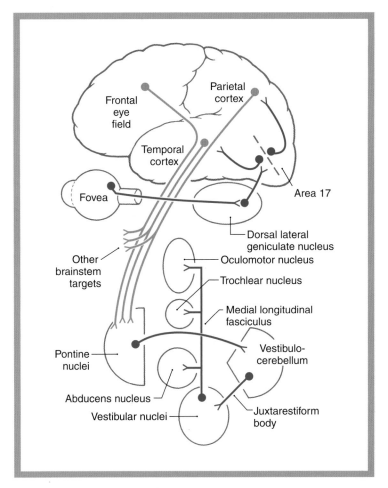

Figure 28-19. Pathways for smooth pursuit eye movements. The retinogeniculostriate pathway is the source of relevant visual sensory input to parietal and temporal association cortices.

Vergence Movements and the Near Triad

Foveation involves directing the eyes toward targets in three-dimensional space. To look from a distant target to a closer one, three changes are made in the eyes. *First*, the eyes converge by the simultaneous activation of both medial rectus muscles to point both foveas at the closer target (Fig. 28-11, *points E and F*). This is a disconjugate movement because the eyes move in opposite directions. *Second*, the curvature of the lens is increased, producing increased refractive power, to focus the closer target on the fovea (Fig. 28-3). *Third*, the pupil is constricted, thereby increasing the depth of field of the eye. The combination of these three actions is termed the *near triad* or *near response*. The opposite effects (*divergence*, flattening of the lens, and pupillary dilation) occur when the gaze is shifted from a closer target to one farther away.

As the term "near triad" suggests, the three actions are generally yoked. Although vergence and accommodation can be dissociated under special conditions (closing one eye and bringing the target straight at the open eye), under normal conditions the vergence angle is used by the brain to adjust the accommodation of the lens. Other cues used to direct the near response include *retinal disparity* and focus, which is indicated by blurring of the image. Cells in visual cortex with binocular visual fields are activated when the retinal images have a specific degree of disparity (the difference in the points on each retina where an image falls). This difference is an appropriate signal for the control of vergence.

Vergence movements are generally slower than saccades, and the initial burst of motor neuron activity is less evident (Fig. 28-11, *points E and F*). Premotor neurons whose activity correlates with the near response are found in a *midbrain near response region* located in the *supraoculomotor area* (SOA) (Fig. 28-20). Cells in the SOA project to the medial and lateral rectus motor neurons and also to the preganglionic motor neurons in the Edinger-Westphal nucleus that control the lens and pupil. The cerebellum influences vergence and accommodation through projections to the SOA, but other near response pathways remain undefined.

Vergence and saccade movements often occur in combination. When combined they have a similar time course, but the saccadic and vergence systems can also act independently. For instance, following a lesion in the paramedian pontine reticular formation, horizontal saccades are disrupted but vergence movements in the horizontal plane are unaltered.

Reflex Movements

The body is equipped with compensatory systems that keep the eyes directed at a target despite external perturbations of the body or head. The vestibular system specializes in sensing the acceleration that usually occurs at the beginning of a movement, and it also senses gravity. Activation of the vestibular labyrinths elicits a series of compensatory eye movements commonly termed the *vestibulo-ocular reflexes* (VOR). The pathways subserving these reflexes are discussed in Chapter 22. In contrast, the *optokinetic system* compensates for continuous-velocity movements. This section covers the optokinetic system, as well as the pupillary and blink reflexes.

Optokinetic Eye Movements

As we move in the world, or move our heads, the entire visual scene moves across the retina. This whole-field movement of the visual scene is called *retinal slip*. Under these conditions, the eyes automatically move in a compensatory fashion to stabilize the image on the retina. For example, if the body is rotating to the left, the visual world will seem to move to the right, and rightward compensatory eye movements match the velocity and direction of this retinal slip (Fig. 28-21). As with smooth pursuit, these *optokinetic eye movements* are produced by graded increases and decreases in the tonic firing rate of the appropriate motor neurons (Fig. 28-21). When the eyes approach the limit of their rotation, a quick saccade brings them back to their primary position and another slow following movement begins. This set of alternating *slow* and *fast* (saccadic) *phases* of movement is called *optokinetic nystagmus* (OKN) (Fig. 28-21). The direction of OKN is specified by the fast phase direction. A series of stripes can be moved in front of a subject to elicit nystagmus and test the *optokinetic reflex*.

The afferent limb of this reflex begins with stimulation of wide-field retinal ganglion cells that are sensitive to slow movements of the whole receptive field (Fig. 28-22). These receptive fields are tuned to directions that are comparable to the orientations

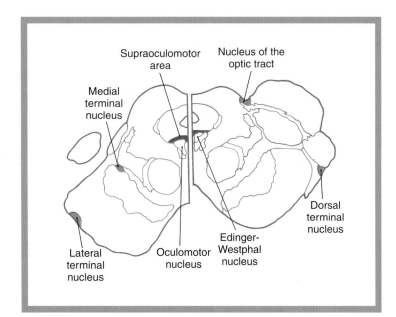

Figure 28-20. Nuclei of the accessory optic system and the supraoculomotor area in caudal (*left*) and rostral (*right*) coronal sections through the rostral midbrain.

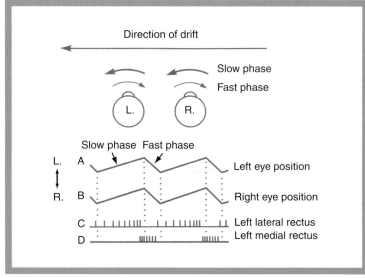

Figure 28-21. The relationship between eye movements and motor neuron firing during optokinetic nystagmus (OKN). The *long arrow* indicates the drift of the visual scene. The *thick arrow* shows the slow optokinetic movement of the eye as it follows the visual scene, and the *thin arrow* indicates the fast saccadic resetting movement. These changes in eye position are illustrated in A and B. Idealized motor neuron firing patterns are shown in C and D. This would be rightward OKN.

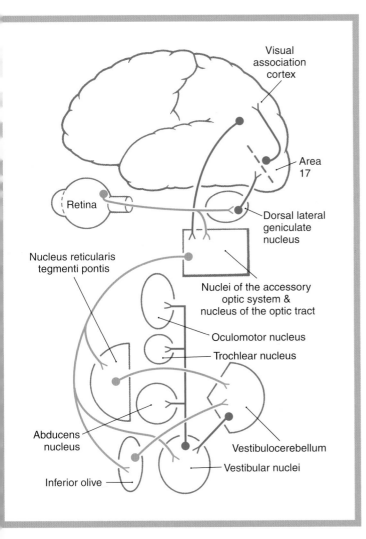

Figure 28-22. Pathway for the optokinetic system.

foveal target movement. Otherwise, the pursuit system overrides the optokinetic system.

The AOS nuclei project to the portions of the *nucleus reticularis tegmenti pontis* and the *inferior olive* that supply the vestibulocerebellum, and to the vestibular nuclei (Fig. 28-22). In addition to vestibulo-ocular premotor neurons, the latter nuclei contain optokinetic neurons that influence extraocular motor neurons. In fact, lesions in the vestibular nuclei produce severe deficits in both reflexes. The pathways through the cerebellum are involved in adapting the gains of the optokinetic and vestibulo-ocular reflexes so that they combine to produce appropriate eye movements.

Pupillary Light Reflex

In addition to the changes in pupillary size that result from the near response, the pupil also responds to the amount of ambient light. The actions of the iris in each eye are yoked, so that light directed into one eye results in pupillary constriction in both the illuminated eye *(direct response)* and the opposite eye *(consensual response)*. The pupil changes diameter to maintain luminance of the retina in the optimal range of the receptor photopigments. Many of the structures involved in the pupillary light reflex pathway are clearly visible in a magnetic resonance image oriented specifically to the long axis of the optic nerve (Fig. 28-23).

The pupillary light reflex is a four-neuron arc (Figs. 28-23 and 28-24). A set of retinal ganglion cells that respond in a linear fashion to luminance levels project via the optic nerve and tract to the midbrain. The decussation of approximately half of these fibers in the chiasm is one of the structural features responsible for the consensual response. The retinal axons terminate in the pretectum within the *olivary pretectal nucleus*, which, in turn, projects bilaterally to the Edinger-Westphal nucleus, with the decussating fibers crossing in the posterior commissure. Parasympathetic, preganglionic fibers from the Edinger-Westphal nucleus exit with the oculomotor nerve and terminate in the ciliary ganglion. The postganglionic fibers reach the iris, where they excite the pupillary constrictor muscle. Damage to these postganglionic fibers produces a *tonic* dilated pupil (the *Adie syndrome*) in which the constrictor muscle is supersensitive to cholinergic drugs.

The pupillary light reflex is a useful diagnostic tool for testing brainstem and cranial nerve function (Figs. 28-23 and 28-24). Lesions may result in loss of the direct or consensual pupillary responses or in uneven pupil size *(anisocoria)*. A dilated, unresponsive (fixed) pupil (or pupils) in the unconscious victim of head trauma is a grave sign. For example, it may indicate that a space-occupying lesion has forced the parahippocampal gyrus or uncus over the edge of the tentorium *(uncal herniation)*, compressing the third cranial nerve. The pupillary fibers are superficially located in the oculomotor nerve and are particularly

of the vestibular semicircular canals. Axons of these retinal ganglion cells terminate in a series of small nuclei along the incoming optic tract, termed the *accessory optic system* (AOS) (Fig. 28-20). These nuclei consist of the *nucleus of the optic tract* and the *accessory optic nuclei*. Each nucleus contains cells that are activated by retinal slip in specific directions. For example, the nucleus of the optic tract is sensitive to temporal-to-nasal retinal slip. So, activation of one nucleus of the optic tract indicates a turn toward the activated side, and bilateral activation indicates backward movement. The AOS nuclei also receive input from visual sensory association cortex, presumably from neurons of the smooth pursuit system (Fig. 28-22). In fact, the human optokinetic reflex comes into play only when the AOS indicates retinal slip and the pursuit system notes equivalent

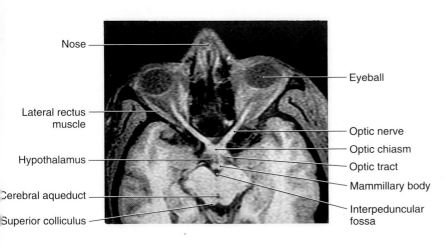

Figure 28-23. T1-weighted MR image of optic structures (nerve, chiasm, and tract) in relation to the hypothalamus and midbrain. Compare with Figure 28-24.

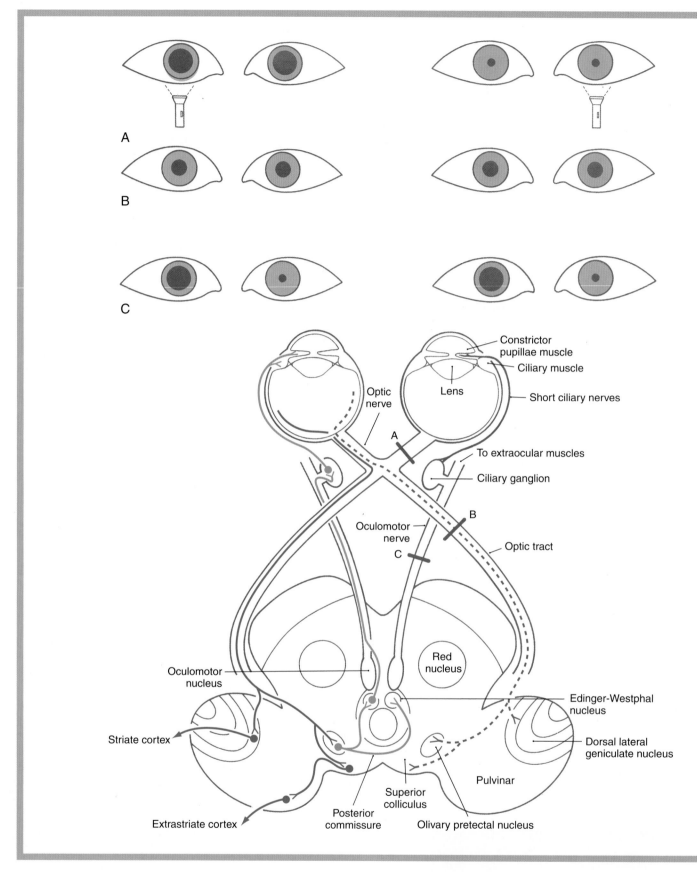

Figure 28-24. Pupillary light reflex pathways. If the optic nerve is partially damaged (**A**), shining a light into that eye will produce a diminished direct and consensual response *(left);* but both will be present when the undamaged side is illuminated *(right).* This is termed a *relative afferent pupillary defect.* A total lesion at **A** would produce a blind eye, which would induce neither a direct nor a consensual response when illuminated. If the lesion occurs in the optic tract (**B**) or pretectum, neither response is lost. Although the reflexes may be weaker, this is *not* easily discerned clinically. However, a large lesion in the posterior (dorsal) midbrain (e.g., pinealoma) would weaken pupillary responses bilaterally. If the lesion occurs in the oculomotor nucleus or nerve (**C**), both direct and consensual responses will be lost in the eye on the lesion side, but they will be present in the other eye.

ensitive to pressure. Their loss may indicate that compression of the brainstem is imminent.

The effects of lesions in the sympathetic pathways (Horner syndrome) have already been discussed. Another syndrome, called *Argyll Robertson pupil*, is found in cases of *tabes dorsalis* (central nervous system syphilis). Affected patients show small pupils with very weak or absent pupillary light reflexes bilaterally, but there is no loss of visual acuity, and the pupils do constrict in the near response. This sparing indicates that the afferent and efferent limbs of the pupillary light reflex must be intact. Consequently, it is assumed that bilateral degeneration in either the olivary pretectal nuclei or the pathways connecting them to the Edinger-Westphal nuclei must be the source of the pupillary dysfunction.

Pupil size also reflects visceromotor tone. Greater levels of excitement, including desire, result in dilation of the pupil via sympathetic activation. This fact was known to Elizabethan women, who used tincture of belladonna to dilate their eyes for cosmetic purposes. Today, cholinergic blockers are used to dilate the pupils for ophthalmologic examination.

Blinking and Other Lid Movements

The delicate structures of the eye are protected by the eyelids. Blinks, some of which occur in response to somatosensory stimulation, ensure protection for the eye. The *corneal blink reflex* is used to assess trigeminal sensory and facial motor nerve function, as well as the integrity of the lid pathways through the lateral pons. Trigeminal nerve fibers with free nerve endings in the cornea and lash follicle receptors have central processes terminating in the spinal portion of the trigeminal sensory nucleus (Fig. 28-25). Second-order trigeminal neurons project directly and indirectly to the facial nucleus to excite orbicularis oculi motor neurons, which produces lid closure. In addition, an inhibitory pathway suppresses the activity of antagonist levator palpebrae motor neurons in the oculomotor nucleus.

Blinks also occur at regular intervals (averaging 12 blinks/minute), as automatically triggered movements that spread the tear film over the cornea. The constant dispersal of the tear film produced by rhythmic blinks prevents corneal lesions and scarring. *Blepharospasm* is a disorder in this rhythmic behavior that results in bouts of high-frequency blinking, whereas parkinsonism produces a decreased blink rate. To keep out of the line of vision, the lids also move with the eyes during vertical eye movements. These movements are produced by actions of the levator palpebrae muscle, which works in concert with the superior rectus. Levator motor neurons receive inputs from cells in and near the vertical gaze centers. The orbicularis oculi muscle is not involved. Consequently, *Bell palsy*, in which the facial nerve is damaged, often due to a herpetic infection of the nerve, results in a loss of the blink reflex on the affected side, but no ptosis or loss of vertical gaze-related lid movements. Lesions of the oculomotor nerve produce just the opposite results.

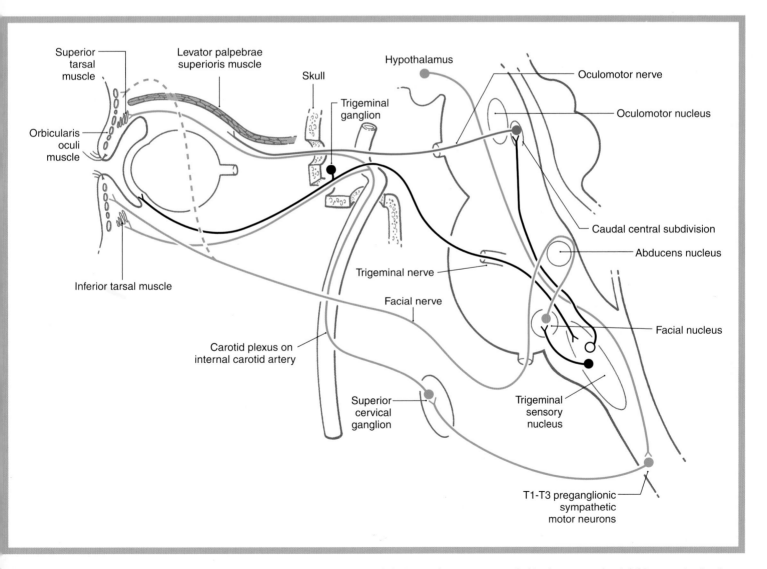

Figure 28-25. Pathways for control of eyelid movements. The motor nerves and their muscle targets are coded in the same color. Inhibitory projection is indicated by the *open circle*.

The tarsal muscles help to keep the lids open, as indicated by the partial ptosis present in the Horner syndrome. Their sympathetic innervation suggests that they regulate lid position with respect to emotional state. For example, high sympathetic tone produces widely opened eyes. Relaxation of the tarsal muscles leads to the feeling of "heavy lids," which signals the general tone of the autonomic system, as the brain prepares to rest.

Synopsis of Clinical Points

- Blinks spread a tear film that protects the cornea (p. 469).
- Strabismus, if left untreated, will usually result in amblyopia (p. 454).
- Proprioceptive feedback from the extraocular muscles may be critical for the development of stereoscopic vision (p. 455).
- The loss of accommodation with age produces presbyopia (p. 455).
- Myopia generally occurs in younger patients (p. 455).
- The sphincter and dilator pupillae muscles are active during reflexive and voluntary ocular activities (p. 455).
- Damage to the parasympathetic fibers from the Edinger-Westphal nucleus results in mydriasis and paralysis of accommodation (p. 456).
- The Foville syndrome is a pontine lesion resulting in an ipsilateral loss of lateral gaze (CN VI) and a contralateral hemiplegia (p. 456).
- Internuclear ophthalmoplegia is seen in patients with lesions of the medial longitudinal fasciculus between the IIIrd and VIth nuclei (p. 458).
- A patient with a one-and-a-half syndrome has lost almost all horizontal gaze in either direction (p. 460).
- The Horner syndrome can be seen following lesions at a variety of locations, one being of the sympathetic postganglionic fibers leaving the superior cervical ganglion (p. 460).
- Patients with the Horner syndrome have ptosis, miosis, and anhidrosis, all on the ipsilateral side (p. 460).
- Lesions of the pons that damage the paramedian pontine reticular formation result in horizontal gaze palsies (p. 462).
- Pinealoma impinging on the rostral midbrain may produce a vertical gaze palsy (p. 462).
- The near response (near triad) includes eye convergence, increased curvature of the lens, and pupil constriction (p. 466).
- Optokinetic eye movements keep the image stabilized on the retina (p. 466).
- Optokinetic nystagmus is the alternating fast and slow phases of saccadic eye movements (p. 466).
- The pupillary light reflex has both direct and consensual responses (p. 467).
- The afferent limb of the pupillary light reflex is via the IInd cranial nerve and the efferent limb via the IIIrd cranial nerve (p. 467).
- In the Adie syndrome the pupil is tonically dilated (p. 467).
- Uncal herniation may result in a dilated and unresponsive pupil, usually on the side of the herniation (p. 467).
- An Argyll Robertson pupil may be seen in tabes dorsalis (p. 469).
- The afferent limb of the corneal reflex is via the Vth cranial nerve and the efferent limb is via the VIIth cranial nerve (p. 469).
- Blepharospasm is a condition in which the patient has periods of high-frequency blinking (p. 469).
- Patients with Parkinson disease have a decreased rate of blinking (p. 469).
- A lesion of the facial nerve will result in weakness of the facial muscles on the side ipsilateral to the lesion (p. 469).

Sources and Additional Reading

Brandt T: Vertigo: Its Multisensory Syndromes, 2nd ed. London, Springer-Verlag, 1999, p 503.

Büttner-Ennever JA (ed): Neuroanatomy of the oculomotor system. Rev Oculomot Res 2:489, 1988.

Clark RA, Miller JM, Demer JL: Three-dimensional location of human rectus pulleys by path inflections in secondary gaze position. Invest Ophthalmol Vis Sci 41:3787-3797, 2000.

Evinger C: A brainstem reflex in the blink of an eye. News Physiolog Sci 10:147-153, 1995.

Gamlin PDR: The functions of the Edinger-Westphal nucleus. In Burnstock G, Sillito. A (eds): Nervous Control of the Eye. Harwood, Academic Publishers, 2000, pp 117-154.

Hikosaka O, Takikawa Y, Kawogoe R: Role of the basal ganglia in the control of purposive saccadic eye movements. Physiol Rev 80: 953-978, 2000.

Huerta MF, Harting JK: The mammalian superior colliculus: Studies of its morphology and connections. In Vanegas H (ed): Comparative Neurology of the Optic Tectum. New York, Plenum Press, 1984, pp 678-773.

Keller EL, Heinen SJ: Generation of smooth-pursuit eye movements: Neuronal mechanism and pathways. Neurosci Res 11:79-107, 1991.

Leigh RJ, Zee DS: The Neurology of Eye Movements. Contemp Neurol 55(entire volume), 1999.

Loewenfeld IE: The Pupil. Anatomy, Physiology and Clinical Applications. Ames, Iowa State University Press, 1993.

Lynch JC, Tian JR: Corticocortical networks and cortico-subcortical loops for the higher control of eye movements. In Buttner-Ennever JA (ed): Neuroanatomy of the Oculomotor System. Amsterdam, Elsevier, 2005, vol 151, pp 467-508.

May PJ: Superior colliculus. In Aminoff M, Daroff R (eds): Encyclopedia of Neurological Sciences. San Diego, Academic Press, 2003, vol 4, pp 443-446.

May PJ: The mammalian superior colliculus. In Buttner-Ennever

JA (ed): Neuroanatomy of the Oculomotor System. Amsterdam, Elsevier, 2005, vol 151, pp 321-379.

Mays LE: Neural control of vergence eye movements: Convergence and divergence neurons in midbrain. J Neurophysiol 51:1091-1108, 1984.

Ong E, Ciuffreda KJ: Nearwork-induced transient myopia. Doc Ophthalmol 91:57-85, 1995.

Schlag J, Schlag-Rey M: Evidence for a supplementary eye field. J Neurophysiol 57:179-200, 1987.

Scudder CA, Fuchs AF, Langer TP: Characteristics and functional identification of inhibitory burst neurons in the trained monkey. J Neurophysiol 59:1430-1454, 1988.

Sparks DL: Functional properties of neurons in the monkey superior colliculus: Coupling of neural activity with saccade onset. Brain Res 156:1-16, 1978.

Tehovnik EJ, Sommer MA, Chou IH, Slocum WM, Schiller PH: Eye fields in the frontal lobes of primates. Brain Res Rev 32:413-448, 2000.

Wurtz RH, Goldberg ME (eds): The neurobiology of saccadic eye movements. Rev Oculomot Res 3:429, 1989.

Chapter 29

Visceral Motor Pathways

J. P. Naftel and S. G. P. Hardy

The primary function of the visceral motor system is the regulation of cardiovascular, respiratory, digestive, urinary, and reproductive organs. These organs are the main effectors of *homeostasis*, the maintenance of a stable internal environment against perturbing influences, both external and internal. In general, visceral motor neurons innervate smooth and cardiac muscles and glandular epithelium, or structures made up of combinations of these tissues.

Overview

The *visceral motor (autonomic) system* ensures that tissues of the body receive appropriate nutrients, electrolytes, and oxygen and that functions such as osmolarity and temperature are properly regulated. The nervous system contributes significantly to the control and coordination of homeostatic mechanisms in response to continually changing requirements. Two overlapping control systems influence visceral effectors. One is *humoral (endocrine)*. Hormonal responses tend to develop slowly, but the effects are prolonged. The other system is *neural (autonomic)*. Visceral motor responses tend to be immediate, but their effects are short term.

The endocrine and autonomic systems are interdependent. They are both under the control of widely distributed central nervous system (CNS) structures, which generate commands after integrating inputs from a wide variety of sources. Thus, visceral motor output is influenced by emotional status, as well as by sensory signals reporting conditions inside and outside the body.

The visceral motor system has two major subdivisions, *sympathetic* and *parasympathetic*. In addition, neurons located in the wall of the alimentary canal form a somewhat autonomous component called the *enteric nervous system*. This is sometimes regarded as a third subdivision of the autonomic system. Within each of these components are populations of chemically coded, target-specific neurons.

Organization of the Visceral Motor System

Targets of Visceral Motor Outflow

The autonomic system provides neural control of *smooth muscle*, *cardiac muscle*, or *glandular secretory cells*, or combinations of these tissues. For example, the gut wall is composed of smooth muscle and glandular epithelium. The *sympathetic* and *parasympathetic divisions* have overlapping and generally antagonistic influences on those viscera located in body cavities and on some structures of the head, such as the iris (Table 29-1). There are also visceral targets in the body wall and limbs. These are found in skeletal muscle (blood vessels) and in the skin (blood vessels, sweat glands, and arrector pili muscles). Visceral structures of the body wall and extremities are generally regulated by the sympathetic division alone. The sympathetic outflow thus has a global distribution in that it innervates visceral structures in all parts of the body, whereas the parasympathetic outflow serves only targets in the head and body cavities (Table 29-1).

General Features of Peripheral Visceral Motor Outflow

There are similarities and differences between the neural control of skeletal muscle and visceral effectors such as smooth muscle (Fig. 29-1). As described in Chapter 24, lower motor neurons (alpha motor neurons) function as the final common pathway linking the CNS to skeletal muscle fibers (Fig. 29-1A). Similarly, sympathetic and parasympathetic outflows serve as the final, but often dual, common neural pathway from the CNS to visceral effectors. However, unlike the somatic motor system,

Table 29-1. Comparisan of Effects of Sympathetic and Parasympathetic Activity on Some Visceral Functions

Physiologic Process	Sympathetic Stimulation	Parasympathetic Stimulation
Eye		
Pupil diameter	+	–
Lens refraction	0	+
Palpebral fissure width	+	0
Tear flow	0	+
Salivary gland flow	–	+
Skin		
Piloerection	+	0
Sweating	+	0
Blood flow	–	0
Skeletal muscle blood flow	±	0
Cardiovascular system		
Cardiac output	+	–
Total peripheral resistance	+	0
Bronchial diameter	+	–
Gut		
Peristalsis	–	+
Secretion	–	+
Sphincter tone	+	–
Blood flow	–	+
Liver glycogenolysis	+	0
Pancreatic insulin secretion	–	+
Pancreatic glycagon secretion	+	+
Urinary bladder detrusor tone	–	+
Urethra sphincter tone	+	±
Penile or clitoral erection	0	+
Ejaculation	+	0

*+, positive effect; –, negative effect; 0, no effect; ±, variable effect.

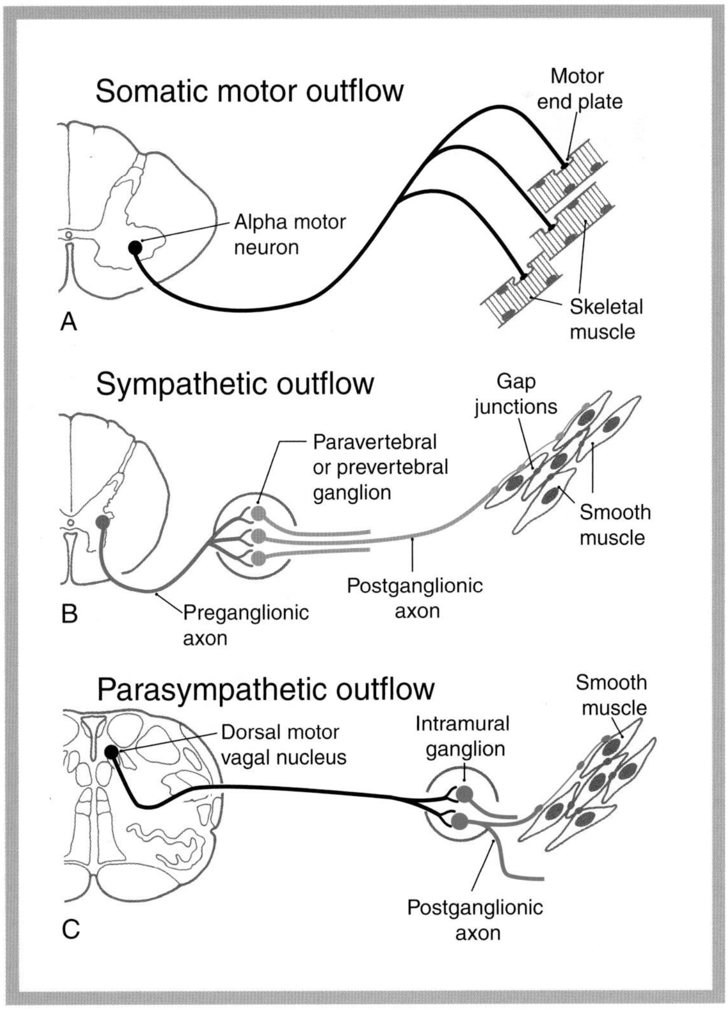

Figure 29-1. Comparison of somatic motor outflow (**A**) with sympathetic (**B**) and parasympathetic (**C**) outflow.

the peripheral visceral motor pathway consists of two neurons (Fig. 29-1B, C). The first, the *preganglionic neuron*, has its cell body in either the brainstem or the spinal cord. Its axon projects as a thinly myelinated *preganglionic fiber* to an autonomic ganglion. The second, the *postganglionic neuron*, has its cell body in the ganglion and sends an unmyelinated axon *(postganglionic fiber)* to visceral effector cells such as smooth muscle. In general, parasympathetic ganglia are close to the effector tissue and sympathetic ganglia are close to the CNS. Consequently, *parasympathetic pathways typically have long preganglionic fibers and short postganglionic fibers whereas sympathetic pathways more often have short preganglionic fibers and long postganglionic fibers.*

Visceral motor neurons and their targets are not organized into discrete motor units like those of the somatic motor system. Recall that an alpha motor neuron makes synaptic contacts with a definite group of skeletal muscle fibers over which it has exclusive control. In contrast, the terminal branches of a postganglionic visceral motor axon typically have a series of swellings containing neurotransmitter vesicles along their length, giving them a beaded (varicose) appearance (Fig. 29-1B, C). The neurotransmitters released from these terminals may act on effector cells at a distance of up to 100 μm. Moreover, unlike skeletal muscle fibers, cardiac muscle fibers and the smooth muscle cells of some organs are electrically coupled by *gap junctions.* Because of this, neurochemical signaling to a few cells is sufficient to regulate a large group of cells that act as a unit. The main features of sympathetic and parasympathetic divisions are summarized in Table 29-2.

Development

Preganglionic Visceral Motor Neurons
Cell bodies of these neurons are located in nuclei or cell columns embryologically derived from the *general visceral efferent* cell column. This column arises from neuroblasts in the basal (motor) plate of the brainstem and spinal cord portions of the neural tube.

Postganglionic Visceral Motor Neurons
Cell bodies of these multipolar neurons are located in autonomic ganglia, which may be either well-defined, encapsulated structures, such as the superior cervical ganglion, or clusters of somata found in nerve plexuses or in the walls and capsules of viscera organs. Like most primary sensory neurons, autonomic ganglion cells are derived from *neural crest cells* that migrate to appropriate locations during development.

One result of this cell migration is the advent, in the adult of the *myenteric (Auerbach)* and the *submucosal (Meissner)* plexuses and the normal muscular and secretory functions of the intestinal wall.

Congenital megacolon, or *Hirschsprung disease*, results from a failure of these enteric neuronal precursor cells to migrate into the wall of the developing lower gut. As a result, the affected segment of the gut (the portion lacking enteric ganglion cells, the aganglionic segment), usually the colon, is paralyzed in a constricted state, with consequent distention of the proximal, and normally innervated (the portion containing enteric ganglion cells, the ganglionic segment), portion of the intestine (Fig. 29-2). This disease is most commonly seen in the very young (newborn to 6 years) but may be seen in adults. Although the presentation of the disease is strikingly characteristic on a radiograph or with magnetic resonance imaging (MRI) (Fig. 29-2), definitive diagnosis relies on a biopsy and histologic confirmation of a lack of enteric ganglion neurons in the affected segment. The treatment of choice is to resect the aganglionic segment and join the remaining normal portions of the gut.

Development of the autonomic nervous system requires an elaborate sequence of intercellular signaling that involves two major families of neurotrophic factors. One is the glial cell

Table 29-2. Comparison of the Sympathetic and Parasympathetic Divisions of Autonomic Outflow

Feature	Sympathetic (Thoracolumbar)	Parasympathetic (Craniosacral)
Location of preganglionic cell bodies	Spinal segments T1 ro T2, mainly intermediolateral cell column	Spinal segments S2 to S4, intermediate gray; general visceral efferent nuclei of cranial nerves III, VII, IX, X
Location of preganglionic fibers	White rami T1 to L2, sympathetic trunks, splanchnic nerves	Pelvic nerves, cranial nerves III, VII, IX, X
Location of postganglionic cell bodies	Paravertebral ganglia, prevertebral ganglia (celiac, aorticorenal, superior mesenteric, inferior mesenteric)	Ganglion cell clusters in walls of viscera, cranial nerve autonomic ganglia (ciliary—III; pterygopalatine and submandibular—VII; otic—IX)
Location of postganglionic nerve fibers	Fibers to structures of body wall and limbs in gray rami and spinal nerves, plexuses associated with arteries supplying visceral structures of the head and body cavities	Within the viscera of body cavities; short nerves or plexuses extending from cranial ganglia to target organs; often accompany trigeminal nerve branches in head
Target effectors	Smooth muscle, cardiac muscle, and secretory cells throughout body	Mostly viscera of the head and the thoracic, abdominal, and pelvic cavities
Primary neurotransmitter of preganglionic neurons	Acetylcholine	Acetylcholine
Primary neurotransmitter of postganglionic neurons	Norepinephrine; cells supplying sweat glands use acetylcholine	Acetylcholine
Neuropeptides of postganglionic neurons	Neuropeptide Y and others	Vasoactive intestinal polypeptide and others
General physiologic effects	Mobilization of resources for intensive activity	Promotion of restorative processes

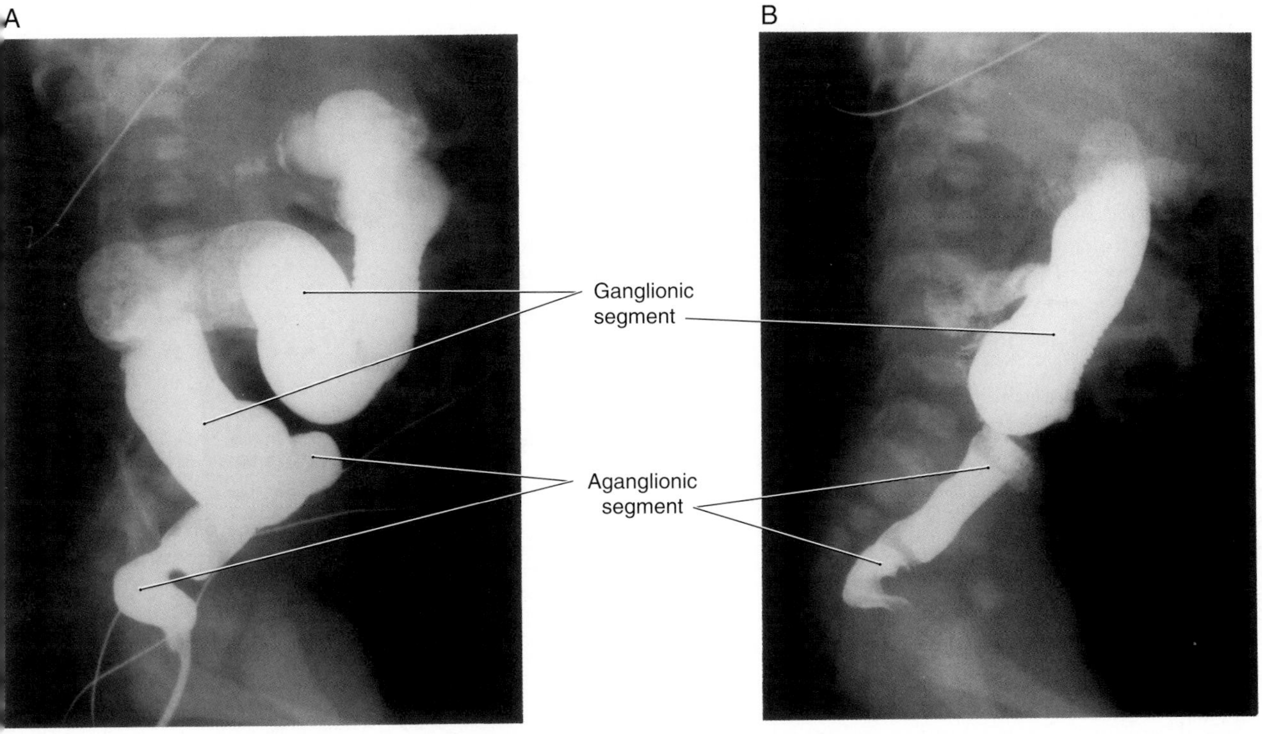
A
B
Ganglionic segment
Aganglionic segment

Figure 29-2. Congenital megacolon in a neonate prior to (**A**) and following (**B**) evacuation. The affected large portion of the large bowel is lacking ganglion cells and is in a chronically constricted state; the dilated portion of the bowel contains ganglion cells (**A**, **B**).

line-derived neurotrophic factor (GDNF) family, which consists of several distinct signaling molecules and their receptors. Mutations of one of these receptors, designated RET, is the underlying cause of some cases of congenital megacolon. The *neurotrophins* are the other large family of neurotrophic factors. As with the GDNF family, each neurotrophin regulates development and function of specific populations of peripheral nervous system (PNS) and CNS neurons via binding to specific receptors. The existence of these neuronal growth factors was first demonstrated when the neurotrophin nerve growth factor (NGF) was discovered as a target-derived messenger molecule that is absolutely essential for survival and development of sympathetic postganglionic neurons (Fig. 29-3) as well as those primary sensory neurons that are involved in pain (Fig. 29-3). The pathologic changes in animals deprived of NGF or its high affinity receptor are similar to those seen in patients with *congenital insensitivity to pain with anhidrosis* (hereditary sensory and autonomic neuropathy type IV), an autosomal recessive disease. Indeed, mutations that impair the function of the NGF receptor have recently been identified in patients with this disease.

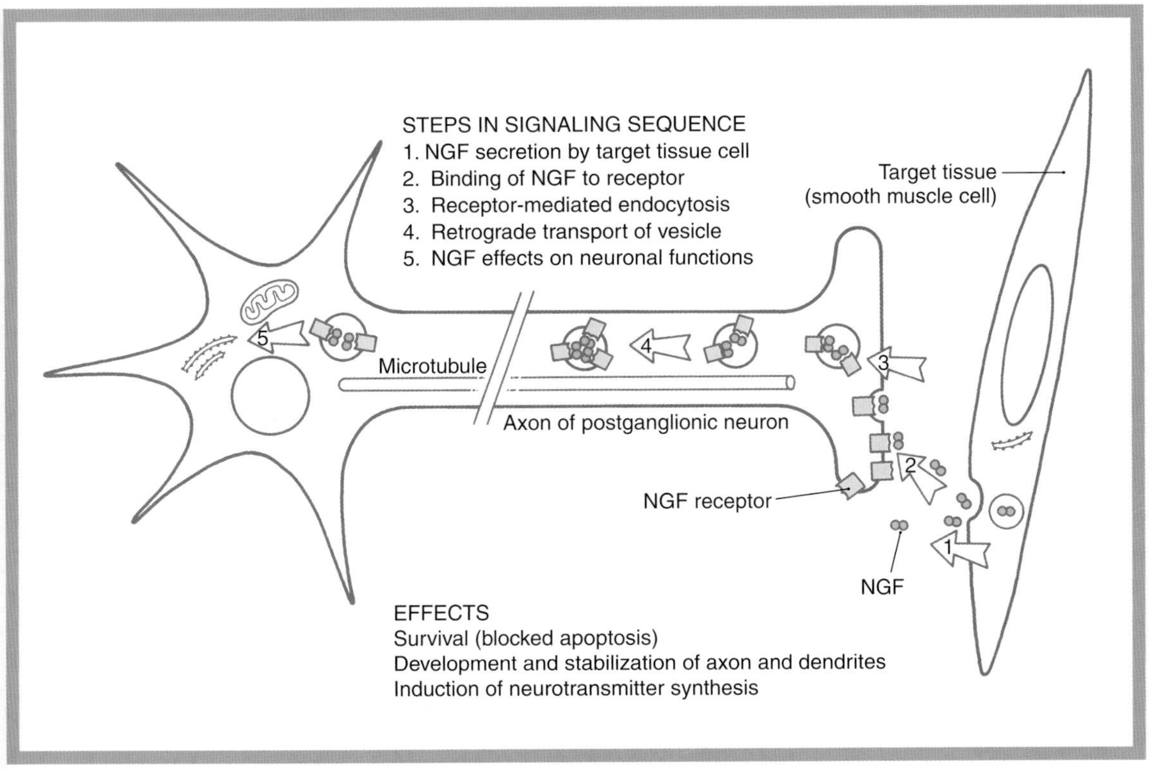
STEPS IN SIGNALING SEQUENCE
1. NGF secretion by target tissue cell
2. Binding of NGF to receptor
3. Receptor-mediated endocytosis
4. Retrograde transport of vesicle
5. NGF effects on neuronal functions
Target tissue
(smooth muscle cell)
Microtubule
Axon of postganglionic neuron
NGF receptor
NGF
1
2
3
4
5
EFFECTS
Survival (blocked apoptosis)
Development and stabilization of axon and dendrites
Induction of neurotransmitter synthesis

Figure 29-3. Mechanism by which the neurotrophin *nerve growth factor* (NGF) regulates the development and function of sympathetic ganglion neurons.

Sympathetic Division

Sympathetic Preganglionic Neurons

Although the sympathetic outflow influences visceral targets throughout the body, sympathetic preganglionic neurons are found only in spinal cord segments T1 through L2 (sometimes in C8 and L3). These cell bodies are located in Rexed lamina VII, primarily in the *intermediolateral nucleus (cell column)* of the lateral horn. The axons of these preganglionic cells exit the spinal cord in the *ventral root* and enter the *sympathetic trunk* via the *white communicating ramus*. Once in the sympathetic chain, a preganglionic fiber may (1) synapse at that level, with postganglionic neurons whose unmyelinated axons join that spinal nerve; (2) ascend or descend in the sympathetic chain to synapse on postganglionic neurons whose axons either join spinal nerves or project to targets in the thoracic cavity or head; or (3) pass through the chain ganglion as a preganglionic fiber to form part of a *splanchnic nerve* (Fig. 29-4).

The sympathetic outflow for the entire body originates from thoracic and upper lumbar spinal cord segments. Although the segmental pattern of innervation is not straightforward, there is a general viscerotopic organization (Figs. 29-5 and 29-6). Neurons of the *superior, middle,* and *inferior cervical ganglia* receive input, via the sympathetic trunk, from preganglionic neurons of the upper thoracic spinal segments. Lower lumbar and sacral ganglia are supplied by neurons of the lower thoracic and upper lumbar spinal segments. The ganglia between these regions are supplied by their corresponding spinal levels. Thus, visceral targets in the head, neck, and upper extremity, as well as the viscera of the thoracic cavity, are served by preganglionic sympathetic neurons in the upper thoracic segments. The main abdominal viscera and other targets in the trunk are served by the central and lower thoracic spinal cord segments, whereas the pelvic viscera, the lower trunk, and the lower extremity are served by the lower thoracic and upper lumbar spinal cord segments.

Preganglionic sympathetic neurons also target the adrenal gland (Fig. 29-6). Chromaffin cells of the adrenal medulla are related to sympathetic ganglion neurons in both derivation (neural crest) and function. These cells secrete catecholamines (mostly epinephrine) into the bloodstream in response to signals from preganglionic neurons. Thus, the sympathetic system, through this endocrine pathway, regulates functions of cells that are not directly contacted by nerve terminals.

Sympathetic Ganglia

Cell bodies of sympathetic postganglionic neurons are generally grouped into discrete ganglia that are located at some distance from the target tissue. Most of them make up the *sympathetic chain (paravertebral) ganglia* and the *prevertebral ganglia* associated with the abdominal aorta or its large branches (the celiac, aorticorenal, superior mesenteric, and inferior mesenteric ganglia; see Fig. 29-6). In addition, small clusters of cell bodies are also scattered among nerve fibers in communicating rami, the sympathetic trunk, and peripheral plexuses.

The *sympathetic chain* extends along the full length of the vertebral column, but the number of ganglia does not exactly match the number of spinal nerves. Generally, there are 3 cervical, 10 to 11 thoracic, 3 to 5 lumbar, and 3 to 5 sacral sympathetic ganglia on each side, and a single *coccygeal ganglion (ganglion impar)* where the two chains meet caudally (Figs. 29-5 and 29-6). Typically, the inferior cervical ganglion and the first thoracic ganglion fuse to form the *stellate ganglion*.

The sympathetic chain ganglia are connected to spinal nerves via *white* and *gray communicating rami*. The former appear white because they contain myelinated *preganglionic fibers*, and

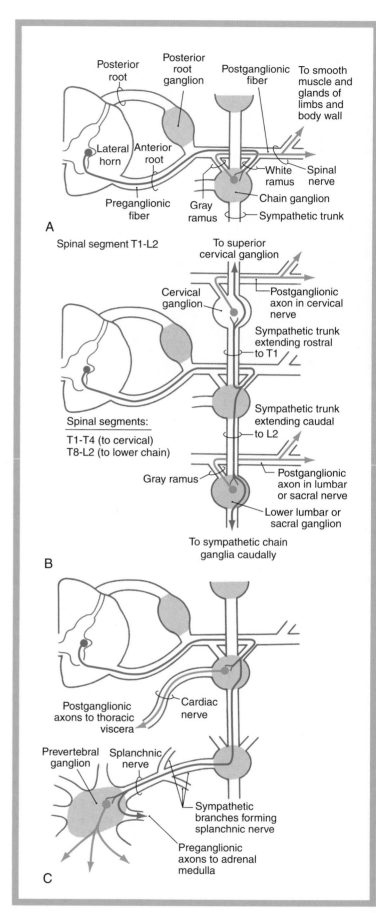

Figure 29-4. The types of routes that can be taken by peripheral sympathetic pathways. A preganglionic fiber may either (**A**) terminate in the chain ganglion at its level of origin, (**B**) ascend or descend in the chain to terminate in different ganglia, or (**C**) traverse the ganglion to enter a splanchnic nerve and terminate in a prevertebral ganglion. Postganglionic neurons that originate in a sympathetic chain ganglion may exit via either the gray ramus and spinal nerve (**A** and **B**) or directly via a nerve such as the cardiac nerve shown in **C**.

Sympathetic postganglionic neurons in paravertebral ganglia send their axons in two general directions. First, some postganglionic fibers join the spinal nerve via a gray ramus. These fibers distribute to blood vessels, sweat glands, and arrector pili muscles in the body wall and extremities (Figs. 29-4A, B and 29-5). These structures receive little or no parasympathetic innervation, so they are exceptions to the dual arrangement of visceral innervation. Second, some of the postganglionic fibers that arise from cervical and upper thoracic sympathetic chain ganglia form *cervical* and *thoracic cardiac nerves* and *pulmonary nerves* that emerge directly from the ganglia (Figs. 29-4C and 29-6). These fibers innervate the vascular smooth muscle of the esophagus, heart, and lung; the glandular epithelium of respiratory structures; the smooth muscles of the esophagus; and cardiac muscle. Axons of these sympathetic neurons mingle with parasympathetic fibers of the vagus nerve to form the autonomic plexuses of the thorax.

The largest of the paravertebral (sympathetic chain) ganglia is the *superior cervical ganglion.* Postganglionic fibers from these cells innervate blood vessels and cutaneous targets of the face and scalp and neck of the territories supplied by the first four cervical nerves (Figs. 29-5 and 29-6). The superior cervical ganglion also innervates the salivary glands, nasal glands, lacrimal gland, and structures of the eye such as the pupillary dilator muscle and the superior and inferior tarsal muscles (Fig. 29-6). Accordingly, a constellation of signs and symptoms results from interruption (central or peripheral) of the sympathetic pathway through the superior cervical ganglion (Fig. 29-7). These include constriction of the pupil *(miosis)* caused by the unopposed action of the parasympathetically innervated pupillary constrictor, drooping of the upper eyelid *(ptosis)* resulting from paralysis of the superior tarsal muscle (of Müller), *flushing of the face* from loss of sympathetically mediated vascular tone, and diminished or absent sweating *(anhidrosis)* on the face. Collectively, these signs and symptoms are known as the *Horner syndrome* (Fig. 29-7).

The *prevertebral sympathetic ganglia* are found in visceral motor plexuses associated with the abdominal aorta and its major branches, and they receive input via the splanchnic nerves (Figs. 29-4C and 29-6). In general, the postganglionic fibers arising from each of these ganglia supply the same visceral targets as the corresponding branch of the aorta. Thus, the *celiac ganglion* is located at the origin of the celiac artery and supplies postganglionic fibers to the spleen and to viscera derived from the embryonic foregut. The *aorticorenal ganglion*, associated with the renal arteries, contains cell bodies of neurons that innervate the blood vessels of the kidneys. The *superior mesenteric ganglion* provides postganglionic fibers that supply the territory of the superior mesenteric artery (derivatives of the midgut). *Inferior mesenteric ganglion* neurons project to hindgut derivatives and to the urinary bladder, urethra, and reproductive organs. All abdominal aortic plexuses contain sympathetic fibers mixed with parasympathetic preganglionic fibers of either vagal or sacral origin.

Internal Organization of Sympathetic Ganglia
Axons of preganglionic sympathetic neurons branch in the periphery and synapse on many postganglionic neurons; the output of the preganglionic neurons is thus widely *divergent* (Figs. 29-1 and 29-8). The number of postganglionic neurons exceeds preganglionic neurons by over 100-fold. Each postganglionic neuron, however, receives synaptic input from a number of preganglionic neurons, so there is also considerable *convergence* within sympathetic ganglia.

Sympathetic ganglia are commonly referred to as "relay ganglia," implying they are sites of simple signal transduction between preganglionic and postganglionic neurons. However, it is clear that more complicated signal processing takes place

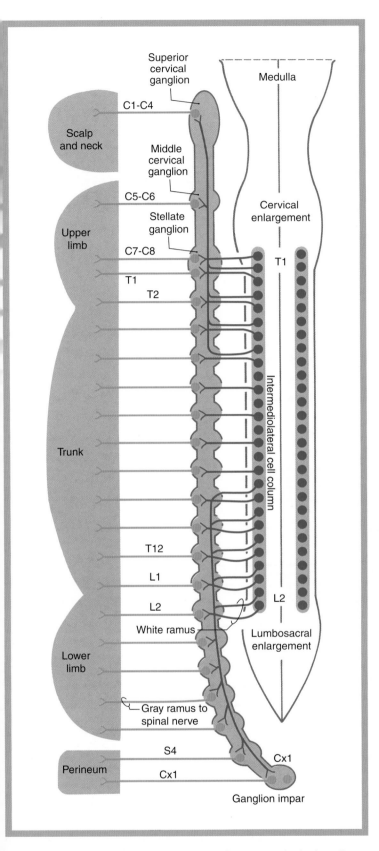

Figure 29-5. Sympathetic pathways to visceral targets in the body wall, limbs, and scalp and neck. Postganglionic sympathetic fibers that distribute to targets of the head are shown in Figure 29-6.

the latter appear gray because they are composed of unmyelinated *postganglionic fibers* that serve the limbs and body wall (Fig. 29-4). Consequently, only spinal nerves T1 to L2 have white rami (and contain preganglionic axons), whereas every spinal nerve is connected to the sympathetic trunk by a gray ramus that conveys postganglionic axons (Fig. 29-5).

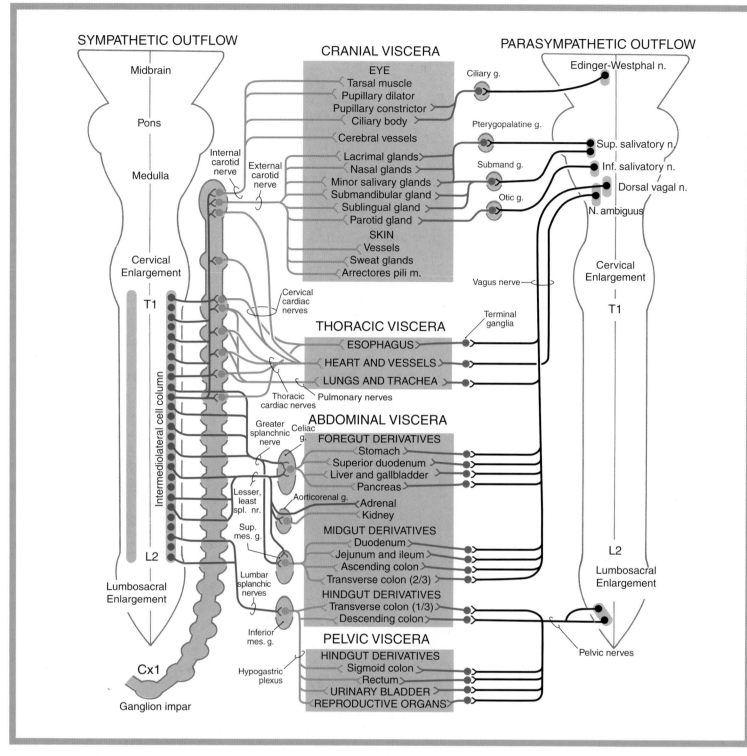

Figure 29-6. Sympathetic and parasympathetic pathways to visceral targets in the head and body cavities. g., ganglion; inf., inferior; m., muscle; mes., mesenteric; n., nucleus; nr., nerve; spl., splanchnic; submand., submandibular; sup., superior.

in prevertebral ganglia. In addition to receiving diverging and converging input from functionally coded preganglionic neurons, postganglionic neurons are influenced by a variety of other sources. These sources include synaptic inputs from collaterals of general visceral afferent fibers and from local neurons (Fig. 29-8). These connections indicate a high degree of integration in prevertebral ganglia.

Functional and Chemical Coding

Conditions of extreme excitement or exertion bring about a comprehensive ("en masse") activation of sympathetic outflow, with widespread effects. These effects include increases in heart rate, blood pressure, blood flow to skeletal muscles, blood glucose level, sweating, and pupil diameter. Concurrently, there

are decreases in gut motility, digestive gland secretion, and blood flow to abdominal viscera and skin (Table 29-1). This constellation of effects has led to the concept that the sympathetic system acts in a global, nonselective manner. However, in less extreme conditions, there is ongoing, selective control of function-specific and target-specific subpopulations of preganglionic and postganglionic neurons. Such selectivity can be found, for example, among cell groups that control vascular tone. For instance, sympathetic pathways to blood vessels in the skin are primarily influenced by temperature, whereas sympathetic outflow to vessels in skeletal muscle responds mainly to changes in blood pressure signaled by baroreceptors. Also, stabilization of blood flow to the head during movement from a reclining to a standing position is a function of the sympathetic division. This

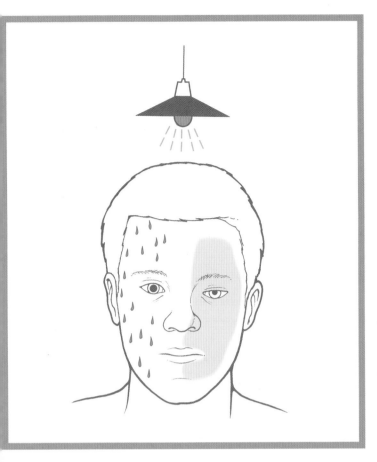

Figure 29-7. Features of the Horner syndrome. Note the lack of sweating on the affected side in response to radiant heat.

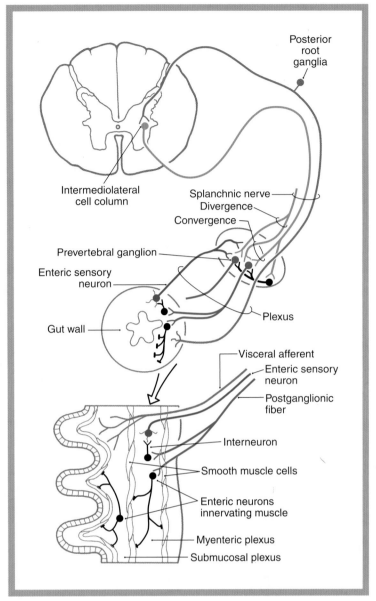

Figure 29-8. Sources of synaptic input to postganglionic neurons in prevertebral ganglia, and the organization of the enteric nervous system. The *lower drawing* is a detail of the gut wall.

adaptation to posture requires rapid changes in vascular tone that must vary according to the region of the body.

Just as components of the sympathetic system can be regulated independently, there is evidence that distinct populations of preganglionic and postganglionic neurons exist. For example, even though preganglionic neurons are all cholinergic, some also express one or more neuropeptides, such as substance P and enkephalins. In addition, distinct populations of preganglionic neurons have been identified on the basis of (1) location of the cell body in the visceral motor cell groups of the spinal cord, (2) morphology of the dendritic tree, and (3) specific target cell type among ganglion cells.

More is known about the functional significance of chemical coding in postganglionic sympathetic neurons. Although most of these cells use *norepinephrine* as a transmitter, some are *cholinergic*. The latter neurons provide secretomotor innervation to most sweat glands and possibly innervation to other targets such as arrector pili muscles and arterioles of skeletal muscle. In addition, postganglionic cells express a variety of neuropeptides, some of which have been linked to specific functional populations of cells (Fig. 29-9 and Table 29-2). Most prevalent among sympathetic peptides is *neuropeptide Y*, which is released along with norepinephrine by vasoconstrictor postganglionic fibers. This peptide has multiple effects at the adrenergic ending. These effects include stimulation of vascular smooth muscle contraction, potentiation of epinephrine effects, and, paradoxically, inhibition of norepinephrine release.

Receptor Types in Sympathetic Targets

The effect of a neurotransmitter on a target cell is determined by the nature of the target cell receptor and the particular signal transduction mechanism to which it is linked. Thus, the effects of norepinephrine, the main neurotransmitter of most postganglionic neurons, and of epinephrine, the main hormone of the

adrenal medulla, vary among different target cells according to the type or types of adrenergic receptor they express (subclasses of α- and β-adrenergic receptors). For example, α_1 receptors on vascular smooth muscle cells mediate vasoconstriction, whereas activation of β_2 receptors results in relaxation. Increases in heart rate and cardiac output are mediated by β_1 receptors on cardiac muscle. Epinephrine is a more potent ligand than norepinephrine at most α- and β-adrenergic receptors. Consequently, epinephrine is administered to counteract symptoms of anaphylactic shock, including bronchospasm, edema, congestion of mucous membranes, and cardiovascular collapse. As mentioned, some tissues receive cholinergic sympathetic innervation (Fig. 29-9). For example, stimulation of sweat gland secretion is mediated by muscarinic acetylcholine receptors.

Causalgia

In special circumstances, sympathetic activation can become linked to pain. Causalgia (complex regional pain syndrome type II) is a syndrome that can result from partial injury to a peripheral nerve, typically a nerve serving an extremity. Signs and symptoms include spontaneous burning pain, hypersensitivity of the skin, pain triggered by loud noises or strong emotions, sweating and reduced temperature of the limb, mottling of the

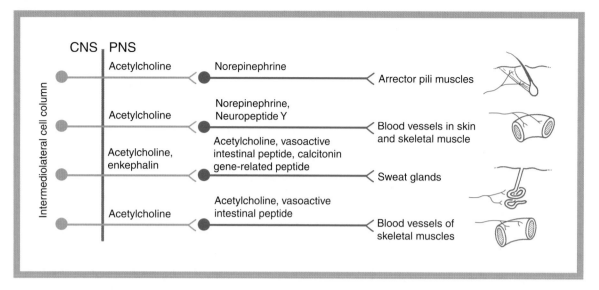

Figure 29-9. Chemical coding of sympathetic preganglionic and postganglionic neurons. Note that some details are based on animal studies and have not been confirmed in humans. CNS, central nervous system; PNS, peripheral nervous system.

skin, and swelling of the extremity. A striking feature of causalgia is that symptoms can often be alleviated by sympathectomy or otherwise blocking sympathetic function. Thus, a prevailing theory of the etiology of the pain associated with the syndrome is that sympathetic postganglionic neurons coursing in the injured nerve develop abnormal connections to nociceptive dorsal root ganglion neurons. This pathologic process could occur either in the tangle of regenerated nerve fibers that form a neuroma or within the sensory ganglion. The nociceptive neurons, in turn, may develop abnormal responsiveness to adrenergic stimulation.

Parasympathetic Division

Preganglionic and Postganglionic Neurons
Compared with the sympathetic division, the parasympathetic division is more restricted in its distribution. The cell bodies of parasympathetic preganglionic neurons are located in either sacral segments S2 to S4 or in the nuclei that provide the *general visceral efferent* (GVE) fibers that travel in cranial nerves III, VII, IX, and X (Table 29-3 and Fig. 29-6). The parasympathetic division of the visceral motor system is accordingly called the *craniosacral* system, as distinct from the sympathetic division, which is *thoracolumbar*.

The cell bodies of postganglionic parasympathetic neurons supplying cranial structures are located in discrete ganglia, and, in general, their axons travel distally with branches of the trigeminal nerve. Cell bodies of parasympathetic postganglionic neurons supplying viscera of the body cavities are not grouped into macroscopic ganglia. Rather, these cells are scattered within nerve plexuses of the target organ or in the wall of the gut *(terminal* or *intramural ganglia)*, where they intermingle with neurons of the *enteric nervous system*.

Parasympathetic Outflow Pathways
The visceral motor component of the oculomotor nerve arises from the *Edinger-Westphal nucleus*. These preganglionic fibers terminate in the ciliary ganglion. Axons of postganglionic cells of the ciliary ganglion innervate the sphincter muscle of the iris (for pupillary constriction) and the ciliary muscle (for near vision accommodation) (Table 29-3 and Fig. 29-6).

The GVE preganglionic parasympathetic fibers of the *facial nerve* originate in the *superior salivatory nucleus*. Some investigators distinguish a separate lacrimal nucleus that targets the lacrimal gland. Preganglionic GVE axons from the superior salivatory nucleus exit the brainstem in the *intermediate nerve*, which is classically considered a part of the facial nerve. Some of these fibers course via the greater petrosal nerve to terminate in the *pterygopalatine ganglion*, which supplies the lacrimal gland and nasal and palatal mucous glands. Other preganglionic fibers travel via the chorda tympani to the *submandibular ganglion*, which innervates the submandibular and sublingual salivary glands (Table 29-3 and Fig. 29-6).

The *glossopharyngeal nerve* contains preganglionic parasympathetic fibers that originate in the *inferior salivatory nucleus*. These fibers take a tortuous course, via the tympanic nerve and plexus, to form the lesser petrosal nerve, which ends in the *otic ganglion*. Postganglionic fibers from the otic ganglion join the auriculotemporal nerve to reach the parotid gland (Table 29-3 and Fig. 29-6).

The visceral motor component of the *vagus nerve* provides parasympathetic innervation to organs of the thoracic and abdominal cavities. Preganglionic GVE fibers of the vagus nerve originate in the *dorsal motor vagal nucleus*. In addition, a part of the *nucleus ambiguus* contains GVE preganglionic cells, whose axons travel with the vagus to innervate the heart. It should be emphasized, however, that the main outflow from the nucleus ambiguus consists of SVE fibers to the glossopharyngeal and vagus nerves. Preganglionic fibers of the vagus terminate on postganglionic neurons located in the walls of viscera of the thorax and abdomen (Table 29-3 and Fig. 29-6). Thus, postganglionic neurons of the vagus nerve are not aggregated into discrete ganglia, as they are for cranial nerves III, VII, and IX.

The *sacral component of the parasympathetic division* innervates the lower digestive tract (beginning at about the left colic flexure) and the urinary bladder, urethra, and reproductive organs. Preganglionic neurons of the *sacral parasympathetic nucleus* occupy a position at sacral levels S2 to S4 comparable to the intermediolateral cell column at thoracic levels (Fig. 29-10). Preganglionic fibers exit the spinal cord via ventral roots and form the *pelvic nerves (nervi erigentes)*. These nerves mingle with sympathetic fibers of the inferior hypogastric plexuses to form the pelvic visceral plexus lateral to the rectum, bladder, and uterus (Table 29-3).

Functional and Chemical Coding
Preganglionic parasympathetic neurons, like preganglionic sympathetic neurons, use *acetylcholine* as their main neurotransmitter. Postganglionic parasympathetic neurons are also cholinergic. Both preganglionic and postganglionic parasympathetic neurons release molecules in addition to the principal transmitter

Table 29-3. Peripheral Pathways of Parasympathetic Outflow

Cranial Nerve	Location of Preganglionic Cell Bodies	Course of Preganglionic Fibers	Location of Postganglionic Cell Bodies	Target Tissue(s)	Effect on Target
Oculomotor	Midbrain: Edinger-Westphal nucleus	With cranial nerve III	Ciliary ganglion	Ciliary bodt, pupillary constrictor	Ciliary muscle contraction; contraction of puplillary sphincter
Facial	Pons: superior salivatory nucleus	Nervus intermedius, greater petrosal nerve to pterygopalatine ganglion or chorda tympani to submandibular ganglion	Pterygopalatine ganglion and submandibular ganglion	Lacrimal gland, nasal glands, submandibular and sublinngual glands	↑ secretion
Glossopharyngeal	Medulla: inferior salivatory nucleus	Tympanic branch of cranial nerve IX, tympanic plexus, lesser petrosal nerve	Otic ganglion	Parotid gland	↑ secretion
Vagus	Medulla: dorsal motor vagal nucleus and nucleus ambiguus*	Various branches of cranial nerve X	Terminal ganglia in or on wall of target organ	Heart and great vessels, respiratory system, esophagus, foregut and midgut derivatives	↓ heart rate; bronchial constriction; ↑ blood flow to gut; ↑ peristalsis and secretion
Sacral splanchnic	S2 to S4 of spinal cord: intermediate gray matter	Pelvic nerve	Terminal ganglia in or on wall of target organ	Hindgut derivatives, reproductive organs, urinary bladder	

*Some general visceral efferent preganglionic parasympathetic cells that innervate the heart are found in this nucleus, although its main function is to provide special visceral efferent fibers that distribute on cranial nerves IX and X.
↑, increase; ↓, decrease.

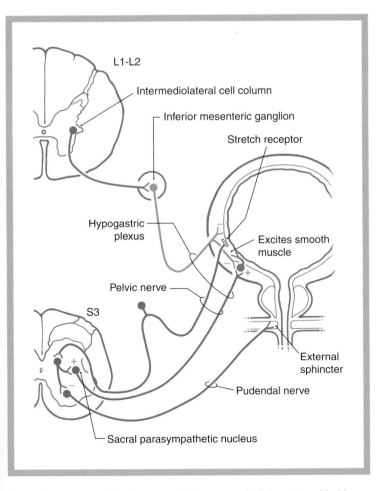

Figure 29-10. Neural pathways mediating control of the urinary bladder.

at their terminals. These include neuropeptides, most prominently vasoactive intestinal peptides, which act as modulators of the postsynaptic response to the main transmitter.

Receptor Types in Parasympathetic Targets

Nicotinic receptors are limited to skeletal muscle and cholinergic synapses in autonomic ganglia and the CNS. Muscarinic cholinergic receptors appear to be the only class involved in the response of smooth muscle, cardiac muscle, and glandular cells to acetylcholine. The nature of the response depends on which type of muscarinic receptor (M_1, M_2, and so on) is expressed. For example, parasympathetic stimulation of gastric acid secretion is mediated by M_1 muscarinic receptors, whereas M_2 receptors mediate parasympathetic depression of heart rate and contraction of cardiac muscle.

The cholinergic receptor blocker atropine has effects that are clinically useful in certain circumstances. These effects include pupillary dilation, relaxation of bronchiolar muscle, and reduction of peristalsis and secretion in the stomach.

Enteric Nervous System

CNS influence over activities of the digestive system is conveyed by sympathetic and parasympathetic pathways. However, the digestive tract is able to perform its basic reflexive functions of secretion, absorption, and mixing and movement of luminal contents with a remarkable degree of independence from regulation by the CNS. This high degree of autonomy of digestive functions is possible because the wall of the gut (from esophagus to anus) is equipped with an elaborate intrinsic network of neurons termed the *enteric nervous system* or *intrinsic nervous system of the gut* (Fig. 29-11). The enteric nervous system is regarded by some authorities as the third division (along with the sympathetic and

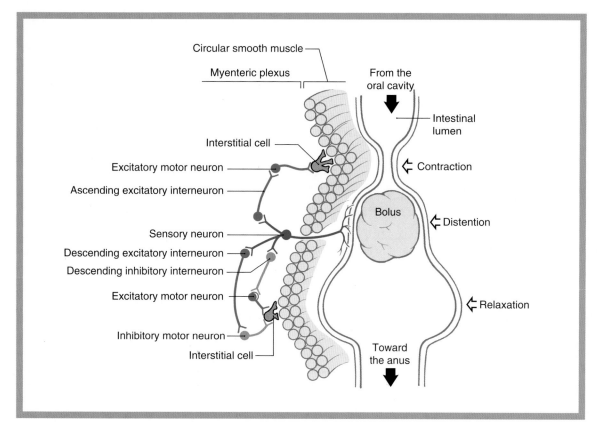

Figure 29-11. Neural pathways mediating the peristaltic reflex. Distention of the intestinal lumen by a bolus of ingested material activates an elaborate intrinsic network that includes sensory neurons, motor neurons, and several types of interneurons. The result is contraction of circular smooth muscle upstream from the bolus and relaxation of circular smooth muscle downstream from the bolus so that it is propelled toward the anus.

parasympathetic divisions) of the autonomic nervous system. It has been estimated to comprise roughly 100 million neurons, approximately the same number found in the spinal cord. The majority of enteric neurons are distributed within the *myenteric* and *submucosal plexuses*, although there are additional *plexuses in the mucosa and serosa* (Fig. 29-11). Over a dozen distinct functional types of intrinsic neurons have been identified, including several kinds of sensory neurons (mechanoreceptors, chemoreceptors, nociceptors), interneurons (excitatory, inhibitory, orally projecting, caudally projecting), and motor neurons (secretomotor, excitatory and inhibitory muscle motor).

In addition to its intrinsic nervous system, the gut wall is endowed with widely distributed smooth muscle–like cells, called interstitial cells of Cajal (ICC), that spontaneously initiate rhythmic electrical activity, much like the pacemaker cells of the heart (Fig. 29-11). These cells have extensive connections both with each other and with conventional smooth muscle cells, which are themselves electrically coupled. Thus, ICC are responsible for generation and propagation of slow waves of depolarization in the smooth muscle layers of the gut wall. Although this ongoing wave pattern of electrical activity of smooth muscle is an intrinsic property of the gut wall, input from the enteric nervous system is necessary to translate the slow waves of depolarization into useful waves of contraction.

A prominent specific function of the enteric nervous system is the peristaltic reflex whereby the presence of ingested material in the intestine evokes waves of contraction and relaxation that slowly propel the material toward the anus (Fig. 29-11). The peristaltic reflex can be initiated either when the presence of a food bolus distends the intestinal wall and activates intrinsic mechanoreceptive sensory neurons or when the enteroendocrine cells in the lining epithelium respond to contents in the lumen by signaling chemoreceptive sensory neurons. In either case, the sensory neurons, in turn, activate populations of excitatory and inhibitory interneurons in the myenteric plexus (Fig. 29-11).

Excitatory interneurons activate excitatory motor neurons upstream from the bolus and inhibitory motor neurons downstream from the bolus. Inhibitory interneurons act on excitatory motor neurons downstream. The result is propulsion of the bolus toward the anus by a combination of constriction of the segment of intestine above the bolus and relaxation (dilation) of the intestinal segment below the bolus.

In addition to intrinsic reflex pathways that generate peristalsis, additional local neural circuits bring about reflexive changes in other activities such as absorption, local blood flow, and secretion. The latter reflex is initiated in the epithelium by enteroendocrine cells that monitor the chemical composition of the luminal contents and activate sensory neurons. The sensory neurons then activate secretomotor pathways that bring about appropriate secretions by glandular cells. It is important to note that although the peristaltic reflex and other basic reflexes can occur independently of external signaling they are normally subject to extrinsic regulation by parasympathetic input (generally enhancement) and sympathetic input (generally inhibitory). Indeed, several more complex reflexes of the digestive tract, such as the defecation and enterogastric reflexes, are generated by parasympathetic and sympathetic circuits.

An extremely diverse array of neurotransmitters and neuromodulators is involved in the functions of the enteric nervous system. These include small molecules (acetylcholine, norepinephrine, adenosine triphosphate, serotonin), a gas (nitric oxide), and numerous polypeptides (substance P, calcitonin gene–related peptide, vasoactive intestinal peptide, cholecystokinin, dynorphin, enkephalins, neuropeptide Y). Some of the chemical messengers, such as serotonin (5-hydroxytryptamine), can be either excitatory or inhibitory, depending on the subtype of receptor expressed by the responding cell. The various molecular signaling systems provide important targets of present and future pharmacologic therapies for disorders of gut motility and secretion. For example, agonists and antagonists that target specific subtypes of neurotransmitter receptors are used to treat irritable bowel syndrome.

Regulation of Visceral Motor Outflow

Sensory input occurs at every level of the visceral motor pathway, including prevertebral postganglionic neurons, preganglionic neurons, and a wide variety of CNS structures that project, either directly or indirectly, to preganglionic neurons. Many different kinds of sensory information are integrated by a series of CNS structures collectively termed the *central autonomic network* (CAN), which generates coordinated signals to the visceral motor, endocrine, and somatic motor outflow pathways. Although visceral motor activities are generally beyond conscious control, emotional status and mental activity clearly influence visceral structures. Accordingly, the CAN integrates input from higher CNS centers involved in cognition and complex behavioral functions.

Major Central Nervous System Components

The preganglionic neurons of the autonomic motor pathways are influenced by cells in various brainstem and forebrain areas. The *hypothalamus* is the highest integrator of autonomic and endocrine functions. It directly regulates the secretory activity of the anterior and posterior pituitary and has reciprocal connections with the solitary nucleus and other components of the CAN in the forebrain and brainstem. Some hypothalamic nuclei project directly to preganglionic visceral motor neurons in the dorsal vagal nucleus, nucleus ambiguus, and intermediolateral cell column. The organization and functions of the hypothalamus are considered in Chapter 30.

Because of its diverse connections, the solitary nucleus is the most important brainstem structure coordinating autonomic functions. It receives general and special visceral sensory input, and it projects to vagal motor neurons, to salivatory and reticular nuclei, and to populations of brainstem neurons, which in turn project to sympathetic preganglionic neurons. The solitary nucleus also has reciprocal connections with other components of the CAN.

Other cell groups that are important in autonomic regulation reside in the reticular formation of the brainstem. These neurons are not always restricted to specific nuclei, and they are therefore sometimes designated by their relative positions. For example, cells in the *rostral ventrolateral medulla* project to the intermediolateral cell column, particularly to preganglionic neurons involved in cardiovascular regulation. This area is called the *vasopressor center* because stimulation results in increased peripheral vascular resistance and increased cardiac output. Areas such as this have been designated *centers*—for example, the respiration center, micturition center, and vomiting center. Although this terminology is convenient, it should be understood that these are not well-defined anatomic entities but are components of widely distributed neural networks.

The importance of the supraspinal control of autonomic function is illustrated by some of the deficits associated with spinal cord injuries at higher levels (T6 or above). Initially, the interruption of descending reticulospinal and hypothalamospinal fibers that regulate sympathetic preganglionic neurons in the intermediolateral cell column is manifested as an overall reduction in sympathetic activity. Thus, clinical signs include lowered blood pressure, orthostatic hypotension, and reduced heart rate (bradycardia). With time, hyperactivity of sympathetic reflexes (termed *autonomic dysreflexia*) develops, probably as a result of denervation hypersensitivity of sympathetic neurons and target tissues. Signs and symptoms include hypertension, urinary retention, piloerection, profuse sweating, and reduction of blood flow to peripheral tissues in response to any of a wide variety of noxious stimuli below the level of the spinal cord injury.

Cardiovascular System

The function of the cardiovascular system is influenced by mental activity, emotional state, posture, muscular exertion, visceral activity, body temperature, and concentrations of blood gases and electrolytes. In addition to mechanisms that regulate blood pressure, there is precise neural control of blood flow to specific organs and regions of the body.

The *baroreceptor reflex* (Fig. 29-12) functions to buffer blood pressure against a sudden change in posture. Failure of this reflex results in *orthostatic hypotension*, a severe drop in blood pressure when the patient assumes an upright position. Primary visceral sensory neurons of the glossopharyngeal and vagus nerves convey signals from mechanoreceptors in the carotid and aortic sinuses centrally, where they terminate in the solitary nucleus (see Fig. 19-8). Projections of solitary neurons influence the tonic activity of parasympathetic (vagal) output to the heart and sympathetic output to the heart and peripheral vessels.

When a reclining individual stands there is a rapid reduction in baroreceptor discharge that results in a *decrease* in signals from the solitary nucleus to two brainstem targets (Fig. 29-12). The first of these targets, the vagal preganglionic parasympathetic neurons that suppress heart rate and cardiac output, receive an excitatory drive from neurons of the solitary nucleus. Thus, a reduction of baroreceptor discharge results in a release of the heart from this inhibitory parasympathetic drive. The second target of solitary cells consists of *vasopressor neurons* in the *rostral ventrolateral medulla*. The neurons in this region have intrinsic pacemaker features and receive inhibitory inputs from the solitary nucleus. When these rostral neurons are released from the inhibitory drive of solitary neurons, the result is

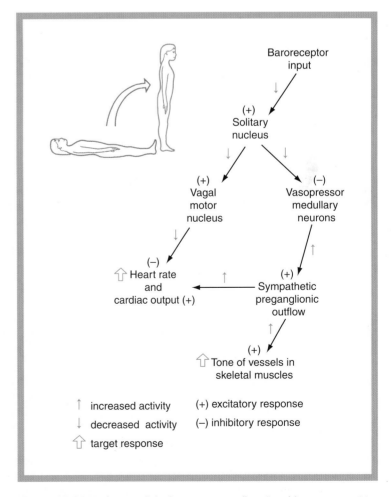

Figure 29-12. Pathways of the baroreceptor reflex. A sudden movement to an upright position results in modification of neuronal activity *(red)* in these pathways to produce the compensatory changes in the cardiovascular system.

increased sympathetic outflow (Fig. 29-12). This input is mediated via a major descending projection from these rostral medullary cells to the sympathetic preganglionic neurons in the intermediolateral cell column. Reduced inhibition of this excitatory projection results in increased cardiac output and increased resistance in vascular beds of skeletal muscle and abdominal visceral organs, but not of the skin, heart, and brain. Some of this solitary input to vasopressor neurons may be relayed through vasodepressor cell groups in the caudal ventrolateral medulla. Thus, when *a person moves from a reclining to standing posture, the resultant pooling of blood in the lower half of the body is quickly countered by increased vascular tone and increased cardiac output.* Without this reflex, movement to a standing position results in dizziness or fainting because of decreased blood flow to the brain. This manifestation of orthostatic hypotension is a serious consequence of many forms of autonomic dysfunction.

The *chemoreceptor reflex* maintains homeostasis of blood gas composition by adjusting respiration, cardiac output, and peripheral blood flow. Decreased PO_2 and increased PCO_2, detected by receptors in the carotid and aortic bodies, are signaled by glossopharyngeal and vagal afferents that terminate in the solitary nucleus. Within the medulla, the reflex pathway for cardiovascular effects parallels that for the baroreceptor reflex. A decrease in blood PO_2 activates this reflex and promotes increased heart rate and vascular tone. These changes result in a decreased blood flow to skeletal muscles and viscera, whereas blood flow to the brain is maintained. Thus, proportionately more oxygenated blood is available to the brain than to skeletal muscle and viscera. The resulting conservation of oxygen preserves vital functioning of the CNS.

The cardiovascular component of the chemoreceptor reflex is closely coordinated with respiration, a somatic motor function coordinated by other neurons of the brainstem reticular formation. For example, if breathing is suspended (as in diving), heart rate is slowed *(bradycardia)* rather than accelerated *(tachycardia)*.

Urinary Bladder and Micturition

Emptying of the urinary bladder, *micturition*, is brought about by contraction of smooth muscle of the bladder wall *(detrusor muscle)* and relaxation of skeletal muscle of the *external urethral sphincter* (Fig. 29-10). Contraction of the detrusor is mediated by parasympathetic outflow. Preganglionic neurons from the sacral cord innervate postganglionic neurons in the bladder wall (Fig. 29-10). The bladder wall also has a sympathetic innervation. Its influence is mainly inhibitory on both the detrusor muscle and the parasympathetic postganglionic neurons in the bladder wall (Fig. 29-10). The external urethral sphincter, which is subject to both reflex and voluntary control, is supplied by alpha motor neurons in segments S3 and S4.

During periods of urine storage, activity of bladder afferent neurons is low. The low activity of the sensory neurons results in (1) low activity of parasympathetic excitatory innervation to the detrusor, (2) tonic activity of sympathetic neurons that inhibit both the parasympathetic ganglion cells in the bladder wall and the detrusor muscle directly, and (3) tonic activity of sacral somatic motor neurons mediating constriction of the external sphincter. As urine accumulates, pressure on the bladder wall activates tension receptors until bladder afferent activity rises to a threshold level. This increased activity of bladder afferents induces micturition by way of both spinal and brainstem reflexes that result in inhibition of sympathetic outflow, activation of parasympathetic outflow, and inhibition of somatic motor neurons supplying external sphincter muscle.

Synopsis of Clinical Points

■ Visceral motor axons innervate smooth muscle, cardiac muscle, or glandular epithelium, or a combination of these (p. 473).
■ The sympathetic division generally serves to function in states of heightened activity (pp. 474, 478).
■ The parasympathetic division generally serves to function in states of quiescence (p. 474).
■ Congenital megacolon results from a failure of migrating neural crest cells to reach the large gut and form the ganglion cells of the intestinal wall (p. 474).
■ Hirschsprung disease (or congenital megacolon) is primarily a disorder of the very young (p. 474).
■ Neurotrophic factors have an important influence on the development of the visceromotor system (pp. 474–475).
■ Congenital insensitivity to pain with anhidrosis may be seen in humans deprived of nerve growth factor or its receptors (p. 475).
■ Horner syndrome may result from a central or peripheral lesion (p. 477).
■ Sympathetic activation increases pupil diameter, cardiac output, and sweating but decreases intestinal motility (p. 473, 478).
■ Causalgia may be the result of sympathetic nerves establishing aberrant reconnections following peripheral nerve injuries (p. 480).
■ The enteric nervous system makes it possible for the gut tube to function somewhat independent of the CNS (p. 481).
■ The enteric nervous system has sensory neurons that respond to changes in the gut wall and interneurons and motor neurons that mediate responses (p. 482).
■ Autonomic dysreflexia is a state of increased sympathetic activity that may result from central lesions (p. 483).
■ Orthostatic hypotension is a severe drop in blood pressure (p. 483).
■ The baroreceptor reflex serves to keep blood pressure within normal ranges in the face of sudden postural changes (p. 483).
■ The vasopressor response increases heart rate and blood pressure (pp. 483–484).
■ The vasodepressor response decreases heart rate and blood pressure (pp. 483–484).
■ Erection is a parasympathetic response whereas ejaculation is a sympathetic response (p. 473).
■ The chemoreceptor reflex is sensitive to oxygen and carbon dioxide in the blood (p. 484).
■ Emptying the bladder is a combination of lower motor neuron and parasympathetic activity (p. 484).
■ Sympathetic activity is highest during urine storage (p. 484).

Sources and Additional Reading

Appenzeller O: The Autonomic Nervous System, 4th ed. Amsterdam, Elsevier, 1990.

Bannister R, Mathias CJ (eds): Autonomic Failure. A Textbook of Clinical Disorders of the Autonomic Nervous System, 3rd ed. Oxford, Oxford University Press, 1992.

Baron R, Levine JD, Fields HL: Causalgia and reflex sympathetic dystrophy: Does the sympathetic nervous system contribute to the generation of pain? Muscle Nerve 22:678-695, 1999.

Benarroch EE: Neuropeptides in the sympathetic system: Presence, plasticity, modulation, and implications. Ann Neurol 36:6-13, 1994.

Brodal P: The Central Nervous System: Structure and Function. Oxford, Oxford University Press, 1998.

Gabella G: Structure of the Autonomic Nervous System. London, Chapman and Hall, 1976.

Hansen MB: The enteric nervous system I: Organisation and classification. Pharmacol Toxicol 92:105-113, 2003.

Hansen MB: The enteric nervous system II: Gastrointestinal functions. Pharmacol Toxicol 92:249-257, 2003.

Hansen MB: The enteric nervous system III: A target for pharmacological treatment. Pharmacol Toxicol 93:1-13, 2003.

Jänig W, Schmidt RF (eds): Reflex Sympathetic Dystrophy. New York, VHC Publishers, 1990.

Jänig W, Stanton-Hicks M (eds): Reflex Sympathetic Dystrophy: A Reappraisal. Seattle, IASP Press, 1996.

Loewy AD, Spyer KM (eds): Central Regulation of Autonomic Functions. New York, Oxford University Press, 1990.

Low PA (ed): Clinical Autonomic Disorders. Evaluation and Management. Boston, Little, Brown, 1992.

Pick J: The Autonomic Nervous System. Morphological, Comparative, Clinical and Surgical Aspects. Philadelphia, JB Lippincott, 1970.

Shephard GM: Neurobiology, 3rd ed. New York, Oxford University Press, 1994.

Teasell RW, Arnold JM, Krassioukov A, Delaney GA: Cardio-vascular consequences of loss of supraspinal control of the sympathetic nervous system after spinal cord injury. Arch Phys Med Rehabil 81:506-516, 2000.

Ward SM, Sanders KM: Physiology and pathophysiology of the interstitial cell of Cajal: From bench to bedside: I. Functional development and plasticity of interstitial cells of Cajal networks. Am J Physiol Gastrointest Liver Physiol 281:G602-G611, 2001.

Chapter 30

The Hypothalamus

S. G. P. Hardy, R. B. Chronister, and A. D. Parent

One of the most rostral cell groups to influence visceral function, and the one that has direct input to all other visceral nuclei in the neuraxis, is the hypothalamus. In addition to its role in regulating visceromotor functions, the hypothalamus also influences neural circuits that modify behavior.

Overview

The hypothalamus is the part of the diencephalon involved in the central control of visceral functions (through the *visceromotor* and *endocrine systems*) and affective or emotional behavior (via the *limbic system*) (Fig. 30-1). Although its primary role is in the maintenance of *homeostasis*, the hypothalamus partially regulates numerous functions, including water and electrolyte balance, food intake, temperature, blood pressure, possibly the sleep-waking mechanism, circadian rhythmicity, and general body metabolism. The hypothalamus (at about 4 g) is dwarfed in size by the rest of the brain (weighing approximately 1400 g). However, it is perhaps the most important 4 g in the entire body. In short, the hypothalamus influences our responses to both the internal and external environments (Fig. 30-1) and is necessary for life.

Boundaries of the Hypothalamus

The rostral boundary of the hypothalamus is the *lamina terminalis*, a thin membrane that extends ventrally from the anterior commissure to the rostral edge of the optic chiasm (Fig. 30-2A). The lamina terminalis separates the hypothalamus from the more rostrally located septal nuclei. Superiorly, the hypothalamus is bounded by the *hypothalamic sulcus*, a shallow groove that separates the hypothalamus from the dorsal thalamus (Fig. 30-2A, C). The lateral boundary of the hypothalamus is formed rostrally by the substantia innominata and caudally by the medial edge of the posterior limb of the *internal capsule* (Fig. 30-2B, C; see also Fig. 15-7). Medially, the hypothalamus is bordered by the inferior portion of the *third ventricle*. Caudally, the hypothalamus is not sharply demarcated, merging instead into the *midbrain tegmentum* and the *periaqueductal gray*. Externally, the boundary between the hypothalamus and the midbrain is represented by the caudal edge of the mammillary body. This is an especially good landmark to use when viewing a sagittal MRI in the diagnosis of hypothalamic lesions.

Hypothalamus and Pituitary

Inferiorly, the hypothalamus is continuous with the pituitary gland (located in the *sella turcica* and covered by the *diaphragma sella*) by way of the *infundibulum* and the *hypophysial stalk* (Fig. 30-3). The *infundibulum* is located immediately caudal to the optic chiasm, is somewhat funnel-shaped (hence its name),

and contains a small portion of the third ventricle, the *infundibular recess*. The infundibulum continues into the pituitary by a stalk of tissue that is sometimes called the *hypophysial stalk*. This stalk passes through an opening in the diaphragma sella.

The pituitary originates from two sources and directions. The *posterior lobe (pars nervosa)* arises as an outpocketing of the inferior surface of the developing diencephalon (Fig. 30-3). The *anterior lobe (adenohypophysis)* arises as an infolding of the ectodermal lining of the roof of the developing oral cavity (the stomodeum) and is commonly referred to as the *Rathke pouch* (Fig. 30-3). The smaller portions of the pituitary, the *tuberal part (pars tuberalis)* and the *intermediate part (pars intermedia)*, also originate in association with the anterior lobe. As development progresses these separate structures join to form the pituitary of the adult (Fig. 30-3).

The pituitary is well protected in the sella turcica. At the same time, it is subject to a variety of potential insults (tumor, vascular, surgical) in this confined location. In addition, the extension of the hypophysial stalk and infundibulum through the diaphragma sella is a vulnerable relationship. For example, trauma to the head may result is a shearing of the stalk and the eventual development of *diabetes insipidus*.

Divisions of the Hypothalamus

The hypothalamus can be divided into the *preoptic area* and the *lateral, medial,* and *periventricular zones* (Fig. 30-4). The preoptic area is a transition region that extends rostrally, by passing laterally to the lamina terminalis, to form a continuation with structures in the basal forebrain. Three zones are located caudal to the preoptic area. The thin periventricular zone is the most medial and is subjacent to the ependymal cells that line the third ventricle. The medial zone is located lateral to the periventricular zone, and a line drawn from the postcommissural fornix to the mammillothalamic tract separates it from the lateral zone (Fig. 30-4).

Preoptic Area
The preoptic area, although functionally a part of the hypothalamus (and diencephalon) is embryologically derived from the telencephalon. This area is composed primarily of the medial and lateral preoptic nuclei (Fig. 30-4). The *medial preoptic nucleus* contains neurons that manufacture gonadotropin-releasing hormone (GnRH). GnRH is transported along the *tuberoinfundibular tract* to capillaries of the hypophysial portal system and thence to the anterior lobe of the pituitary gland (Fig. 30-5; see Table 30-2), where it causes the release of gonadotropins (luteinizing hormone and follicle-stimulating hormone). Because gonadotropin release is continuous in males and cyclical in females, the medial preoptic nucleus of males tends to be more active and consequently larger than that of females. Accordingly, the medial preoptic nucleus is often referred to as the *sexually dimorphic* nucleus of the preoptic area. The medial preoptic nucleus also influences behaviors that are related to eating, reproductive activities, and locomotion. The *lateral preoptic nucleus* is located immediately rostral to the lateral hypothalamic zone (Fig. 30-4). The function of this nucleus is not fully established. However, through its connections with the ventral pallidum, it may function in part in locomotor regulation. Some investigators consider the nuclei of the preoptic area to be part of the supraoptic region of the medial hypothalamic zone.

Lateral Zone
The *lateral zone* (Fig. 30-4) contains a large bundle of axons collectively called the *medial forebrain bundle* (Figs. 30-4 and 30-9). This diffuse bundle of fibers traverses the lateral

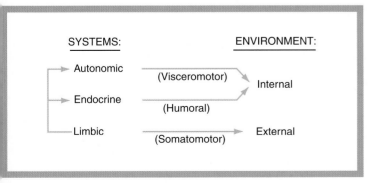

Figure 30-1. The interrelationships among the autonomic, endocrine, and limbic systems. All three systems are under the control of the hypothalamus.

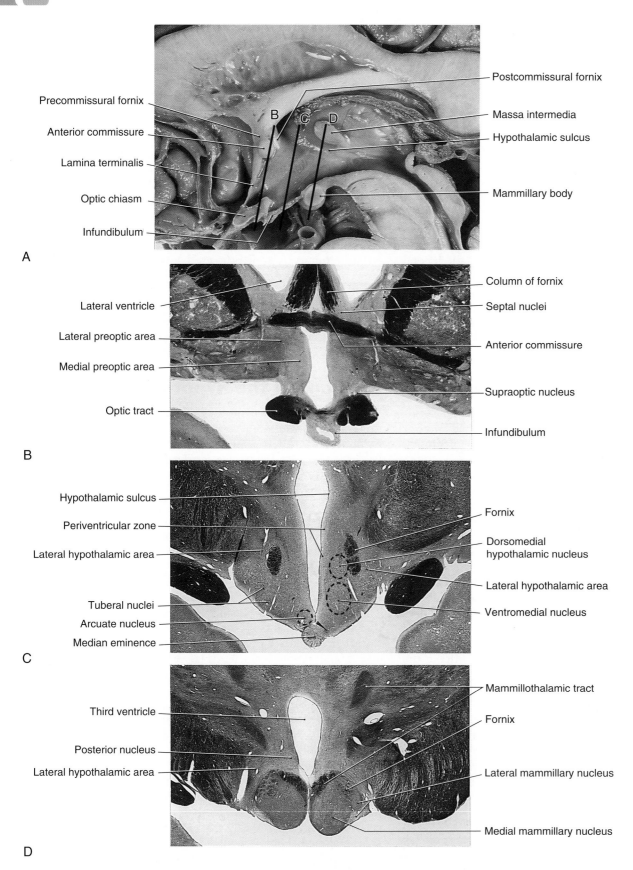

Precommissural fornix
Anterior commissure
Lamina terminalis
Optic chiasm
Infundibulum

Postcommissural fornix
Massa intermedia
Hypothalamic sulcus
Mammillary body

A

Lateral ventricle
Lateral preoptic area
Medial preoptic area
Optic tract

Column of fornix
Septal nuclei
Anterior commissure
Supraoptic nucleus
Infundibulum

B

Hypothalamic sulcus
Periventricular zone
Lateral hypothalamic area
Tuberal nuclei
Arcuate nucleus
Median eminence

Fornix
Dorsomedial hypothalamic nucleus
Lateral hypothalamic area
Ventromedial nucleus

C

Third ventricle
Posterior nucleus
Lateral hypothalamic area

Mammillothalamic tract
Fornix
Lateral mammillary nucleus
Medial mammillary nucleus

D

Figure 30-2. Midsagittal view (**A**) of the brain emphasizing hypothalamic structures. Cross sections of the hypothalamus through preoptic (**B**), tuberal (**C**), and mammillary (**D**) regions. The myelin-stained sections in **B**, **C**, and **D** correspond to the comparably labeled lines in **A**. (B from Haines DE: Neuroanatomy: An Atlas of Structures, Sections, and Systems, 5th ed. Philadelphia, Lippincott Williams & Wilkins, 2000.)

hypothalamic zone and interconnects the hypothalamus with rostral areas such as the septal nuclei and with caudal regions such as the brainstem reticular formation.

The *lateral hypothalamic zone* comprises a large, diffuse population of neurons commonly called the *lateral hypothalamic area* as well as smaller condensations of cells located in its anterior (ventral) portions. The latter cell groups are the *lateral*

hypothalamic nucleus and the *tuberal nuclei*. The *lateral hypothalamic nucleus* is a loose aggregation of relatively large cells that extends throughout the rostrocaudal extent of the lateral hypothalamic zone. This nucleus constitutes a "feeding center." Stimulation of this nucleus in laboratory animals promotes feeding behavior; destruction of it causes feeding behavior to attenuate and the animal loses weight (Table 30-1). The *tuberal*

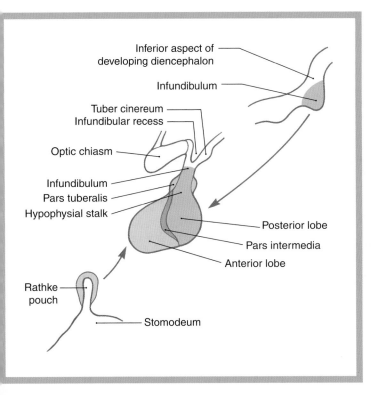

nuclei consist of small clusters of neurons, each containing small, pale, multipolar cells. Some tuberal neurons project into the tuberoinfundibular tract and therefore may convey releasing hormones to the hypophysial portal system. Others send a histaminergic input to the cerebellum that may be involved in the regulation of motor activity.

Medial Zone

The *medial zone* is a cell-rich region composed of many individual nuclei (Figs. 30-4 and 30-5). It is divided into three regions: the *supraoptic (chiasmatic) region*, the *tuberal region*, and the *mammillary region* (Fig. 30-4).

Before considering the major nuclei of the medial zone, it should be stressed that the nuclei comprising each region of this zone are located internal to surface structures that specify the location/position of that specific region (Fig. 30-6). For example, the *supraoptic region* is located internal to the position of the optic chiasm (Figs. 30-5 and 30-6). The *tuberal region* is the widest part of the hypothalamus and, in general, is located internal to the position of the *tuber cinereum* (Figs. 30-5 and 30-6). The *mammillary region* is the most posterior of the three regions of the medial zone and it is located internal to the mammillary bodies (Figs. 30-5 and 30-6).

The *supraoptic region* contains four nuclei: the *supraoptic, paraventricular, suprachiasmatic,* and *anterior nuclei* (Fig. 30-5). Neurons of the *supraoptic* and *paraventricular nuclei* contain oxytocin and antidiuretic hormone (ADH) (i.e., vasopressin) and transmit these substances to the posterior pituitary by way of the *supraopticohypophysial tract* for release into the circulatory system (Fig. 30-5). The functions of these hormones are discussed later in this chapter. The *suprachiasmatic nucleus* receives direct input from the retina and can influence other hypothalamic structures such as the medial preoptic nucleus. It is believed that the suprachiasmatic nucleus may mediate *circadian rhythms*, these being the hormonal fluctuations that are secondary to light-dark cycles. The *anterior nucleus* is located immediately caudal to the preoptic area. Although this nucleus participates in a wide range of visceral and somatic functions, many of its neurons are involved in the maintenance of body temperature.

The *tuberal region* contains three nuclei: the *ventromedial, dorsomedial,* and *arcuate nuclei* (Figs. 30-2C and 30-5). The *ventromedial nucleus,* one of the largest and best-defined of the hypothalamic nuclei, is considered to be a "satiety center." If this nucleus is stimulated in the laboratory, the experimental animal will not engage in feeding behavior. Conversely, a lesion

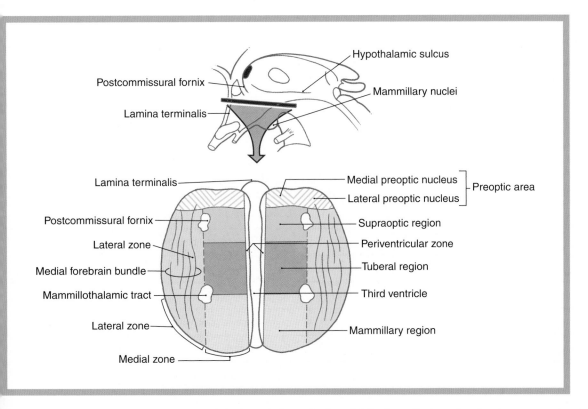

Figure 30-4. Diagrammatic representation of the hypothalamus in the axial (horizontal) plane showing the zones and regions.

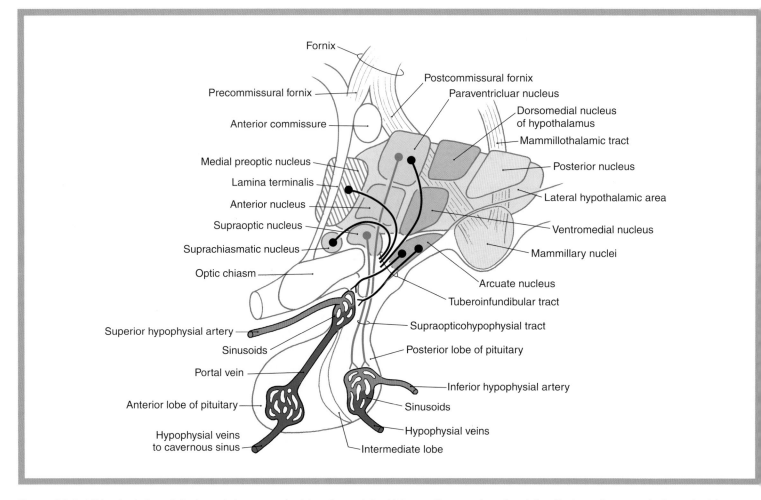

Figure 30-5. Midsagittal view of the hypothalamus emphasizing the nuclei, which contribute to the tuberoinfundibular and supraopticohypophysial tracts, the hypophysial portal system, and the general relations of the fornix and mammillothalamic tract.

to this nucleus causes the animal to eat excessively and gain weight (Table 30-1). The *dorsomedial nucleus*, located immediately posterior (dorsal) to the ventromedial nucleus, subserves a function relating to emotion or, at least, to emotional behavior. In laboratory animals, stimulation of the dorsomedial nucleus results in unusually aggressive behavior, which lasts only so long as the stimulation is present (Table 30-1). This phenomenon, known as *sham rage*, can also be elicited by the stimulation of other hypothalamic and extrahypothalamic sites. The *arcuate nucleus* is the primary location of neurons that contain releasing hormones. These substances are transmitted to the anterior pituitary by way of the tuberoinfundibular tract and hypophysial

portal system, whereupon they influence the release of various pituitary hormones (Fig. 30-5).

The *mammillary region* contains four nuclei: the *medial, intermediate,* and *lateral mammillary* and the *posterior hypothalamic nuclei* (Figs. 30-2A, D and 30-5). The *medial mammillary nucleus* is large and especially well developed in the human. It represents the primary termination point for the axons of the postcommissural fornix, which originate primarily from the subiculum of the hippocampal complex. The medial mammillary nucleus is also the source of axons that are directed to the anterior nucleus of the dorsal thalamus as the *mammillothalamic tract* (Fig. 30-5; see also Fig. 30-8). The latter pathway represents

Table 30-1. The Effect of Stimulation or Lesion of the Principal Hypothalamic Nuclei

Nucleus	Stimulation of	Lesion of
Suprachiasmatic nucleus	Adjusts the circadian clock phase	Abolishes circadian rhythms
Supraoptic or paraventricular nuclei	Increased blood volume, blood pressure, and metabolism	Diabetes insipidus
Lateral hypothalamic nucleus	Increased feeding	Decreased feeding
Ventromedial nucleus	Decreased feeding	Increased feeding
Dorsomedial nucleus	Sham rage	Decreased aggression and decreased feeding
Mammillary body	?	Short-term memory is not processed into long-term memory

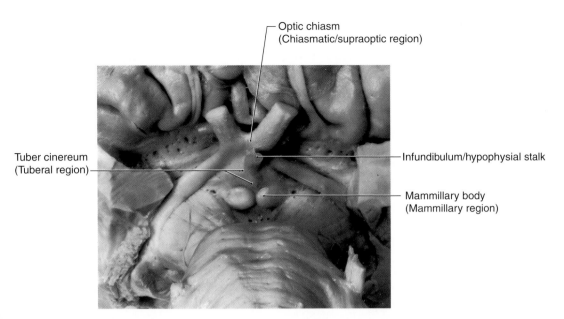

- Optic chiasm
  (Chiasmatic/supraoptic region)

Tuber cinereum
(Tuberal region)

Infundibulum/hypophysial stalk

Mammillary body
(Mammillary region)

Figure 30-6. The inferior aspect of the forebrain showing the external structures that correspond with the locations of the three internal regions that collectively comprise the medial hypothalamic zone; each region has its own respective nuclei (compare with Figures 30-4 and 30-5). The internal region appears in parentheses under the name of the corresponding external structure.

an important part of the limbic system. The much smaller *intermediate* and *lateral mammillary nuclei* are located lateral to the medial mammillary nucleus. The lateral mammillary nucleus receives input from the medial aspects of the midbrain reticular formation by way of the *mammillary peduncle* (see Fig. 30-9).

Insight into the function of the mammillary nuclei comes from experimental and clinical observations. For example, lesions of the mammillary bodies tend to impede the retention of newly acquired memory, so that an immediate memory or a *short-term memory* is not processed into *long-term memory* (Table 30-1). A patient with a mammillary lesion has no difficulty in remembering events occurring months or years prior to the lesion. Memory for events occurring *after* the lesion is, however, limited to the short term (a period of minutes), and long-term memories are not established. As a result of this *anterograde amnesia*, affected patients typically have severe difficulties learning new tasks and transforming these experiences into long-term memory. These specific memory deficits are characteristic of the *Korsakoff syndrome*, a condition that is caused by thiamine deficiency and is typically associated with chronic alcoholism. The memory deficits in this syndrome are caused by progressive degeneration in the mammillary bodies and in functionally related brain structures, such as the hippocampal complex and the dorsomedial thalamic nucleus.

Patients with the Korsakoff syndrome may have difficulty in understanding written material and in conducting meaningful conversations because they tend to forget what was just read or said. An interesting feature of this syndrome is the patient's tendency to *confabulate*, that is, to string together fragmentary memories from various events into a synthesized memory of an "event" that never occurred.

The *posterior hypothalamic nucleus* merges almost imperceptibly with the midbrain periaqueductal gray. Accordingly, this nucleus is associated with the same myriad of emotional, cardiovascular, and analgesic functions that have been attributed to the periaqueductal gray.

Periventricular Zone

The periventricular zone (Fig. 30-4), not to be confused with the paraventricular nucleus, is a very thin region composed of small cell bodies lying medial to the medial zone and immediately subjacent to the ependymal cells of the third ventricle. Many neurons of the periventricular zone synthesize releasing hormones. These neurons project by way of the *tuberoinfundibular tract* to the hypophysial portal system and thus influence the release of various hormones by the anterior pituitary. Consequently, many of the neurons in the periventricular zone serve a function similar to that of neurons located in the arcuate nucleus.

Feeding Motivation

The lateral hypothalamic nucleus, as stated earlier, is commonly referred to as a "feeding center." This is because stimulation of this nucleus will elicit feeding behaviors, whereas a lesion of this nucleus will inhibit the motivation to feed. Stimulation and lesions applied to the ventromedial nucleus have the opposite effects (Table 30-1). Consequently, the ventromedial nucleus is generally thought of as a "satiety center." In recent years, new concepts about feeding motivation have emerged that expand what is known about this topic. These concepts, involving a variety of hormones and peptides, are only briefly explained as follows.

Fat cells secrete a hormone (leptin) that is carried to leptin receptors on various neurons of the arcuate nucleus. Some of these neurons contain the peptides α-melanocyte-stimulating hormone (αMSH) and cocaine- and amphetamine-regulated transcript (CART). Other neurons within the arcuate nucleus contain neuropeptide Y (NPY) and agoutin-related peptide (AgRP).

Neurons containing αMSH and CART project to the lateral hypothalamus, paraventricular nucleus, and lateral horn of the spinal cord. These projections promote an increase of thyroid-stimulating hormone (TSH) and adrenocorticotropic hormone (ACTH). This causes an increase in metabolism, an increase in sympathetic tone, and a *decrease in feeding*.

Neurons containing NPY and AgRP also project to the lateral hypothalamus and paraventricular nucleus. These projections promote the decrease of TSH and ACTH and cause a decrease in metabolism, an increase in parasympathetic tone, and an *increase in feeding*. This increase in feeding is thought to be partly mediated by lateral hypothalamic neurons containing the peptide neurotransmitters melanin-concentrating hormone

(MCH) and orexin. Neurons containing these peptides project to widespread areas of cerebral cortex and are thought to be involved in the promotion of various feeding strategies.

Blood Supply of the Hypothalamus

The hypothalamus and some immediately adjacent structures are served by small perforating arteries that arise from the *circle of Willis* (Fig. 30-7). Those branches from the anterior communicating artery and the A$_1$ segment of the anterior cerebral artery constitute the *anteromedial group* of perforating arteries (also see Fig. 8-16). In general, these vessels serve the nuclei of the preoptic area and supraoptic region, the septal nuclei, and rostral portions of the lateral hypothalamic area. A few perforating arteries may also arise from the bifurcation of the internal carotid artery.

The small perforating arteries that originate from the posterior communicating artery and the P$_1$ segment of the posterior cerebral artery constitute the *posteromedial group* (see Fig. 30-7; also see Fig. 8-16). These vessels serve primarily the nuclei of the tuberal and mammillary regions. Branches arising from the rostral portion of the posterior communicating artery distribute to the former region, whereas the latter region is served by branches of the caudal parts of the posterior communicating artery and of P$_1$. In addition, the posteromedial group also sends branches into the middle and caudal parts of the lateral hypothalamic area. The large *thalamoperforating arteries* usually arise from P$_1$. Although these vessels distribute mainly to rostral areas of the dorsal thalamus, they do give rise to some small branches that enter the posterior hypothalamus.

The *hypophysial arteries* arise from the internal carotid artery. The *inferior branches* (or rami) originate from the cavernous part of this large vessel, whereas the *superior branches* (Fig. 30-5) are from the cerebral (supraclinoid) part of the internal carotid. Although small, these are important vessels.

Hypothalamic Afferent Fibers

The hypothalamus is connected to diverse sites, including the hippocampus, amygdala, brainstem tegmentum, various thalamic nuclei, septal nuclei, and even neocortical areas such as the infralimbic and cingulate cortex. With very few exceptions, these connections are reciprocal. The following are the most important input-output relationships of the hypothalamus.

Fornix

The *fornix* arises from neurons in the *subiculum* and the *hippocampus* (two components of the *hippocampal complex*) and is the largest single input to the hypothalamus (Figs. 30-5 and 30-9). As the fornix approaches the anterior commissure, it divides into a small *precommissural bundle*, derived largely from the hippocampus, and a large *postcommissural bundle*, arising mainly from the subiculum. The former passes to septal and preoptic nuclei and to the anterior hypothalamic region, whereas the latter projects primarily to the medial mammillary nucleus, with lesser inputs to the anterior thalamic nucleus and lateral hypothalamus (Figs. 30-8 and 30-9).

Medial Forebrain Bundle

The *medial forebrain bundle* is a diffuse, composite structure containing mainly fibers that course rostrocaudally through the lateral hypothalamic zone. It contains ascending and descending fibers that interconnect the septal nuclei (including the nucleus accumbens septi), hypothalamus, and midbrain tegmentum (Fig. 30-9).

Amygdalohypothalamic Fibers

Two major afferent fiber systems project to the hypothalamus from the amygdaloid complex: the stria terminalis, which is phylogenetically older, and a newer composite bundle called the ventral amygdalofugal pathway (Fig. 30-9). The *stria terminalis* originates from the corticomedial portion of the amygdala and terminates in the septal nuclei, preoptic area, and medial hypothalamic zone (Fig. 30-9). This bundle, which accompanies the terminal vein at the juncture of the caudate nucleus and the thalamus, follows the arched configuration of the caudate nucleus and thus takes a path quite similar to that of the fornix (Fig. 30-9). The *ventral amygdalofugal pathway* originates from the basolateral portion of the amygdaloid complex and passes rostromedially beneath the lentiform nucleus and through the area of the substantia innominata to enter the hypothalamus (Fig. 30-9). The axons in this pathway terminate primarily in the lateral hypothalamic zone and the septal and preoptic nuclei. This bundle also contains fibers that pass from the hypothalamus to the amygdala.

Other Afferent Fibers

The *mammillary peduncle* is a diffuse bundle of fibers that originates from medial portions of the midbrain reticular formation

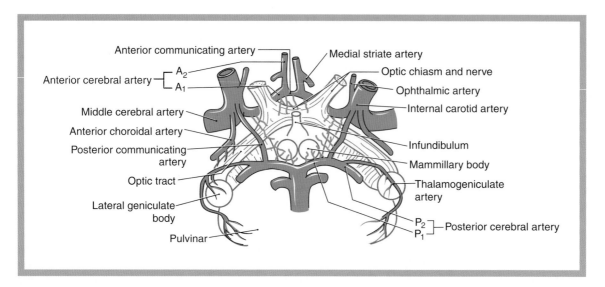

Figure 30-7. The blood supply to the hypothalamus.

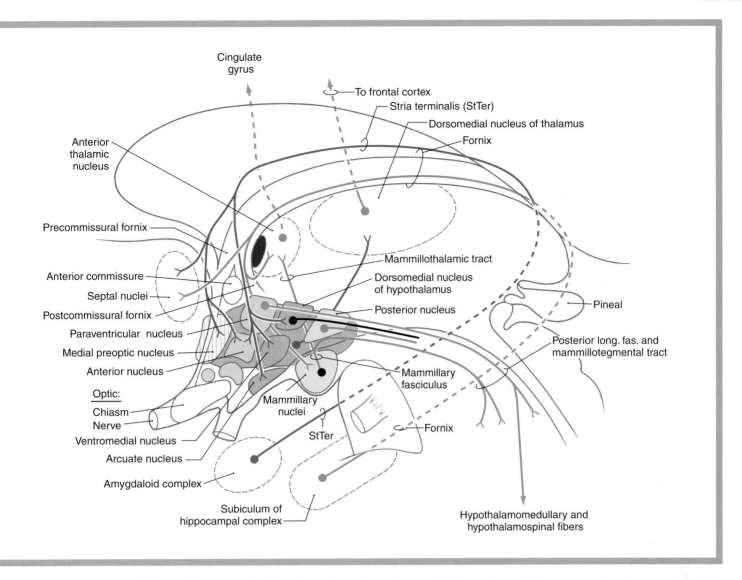

Figure 30-8. Midsagittal view of the hypothalamus emphasizing afferent inputs from the amygdaloid complex and hippocampus. Also shown are the origins of descending fibers to the brainstem and spinal cord. long. fas., longitudinal fasciculus; nuc., nucleus.

and terminates primarily in the lateral mammillary nucleus. Some of these axons enter the medial forebrain bundle and project to the septal nuclei. The dorsomedial nucleus of the thalamus gives rise to *thalamohypothalamic fibers* that course anteriorly (ventrally) to enter the lateral hypothalamus. The only direct neocortical projection to the hypothalamus originates from the prefrontal cortex. This *corticohypothalamic fiber* projection is sparse and terminates primarily in the lateral hypothalamic area. As mentioned earlier, the suprachiasmatic nucleus receives a projection from the retina that is involved in behavioral rhythms and light-dark cycles. These *retinohypothalamic fibers* arise as direct axons from the optic chiasm or as collaterals of retinogeniculate fibers.

Hypothalamic Efferent Fibers

The various subdivisions of the hypothalamus have diffuse projections to numerous sites throughout the neuraxis. Only the major projections are summarized here. A useful generalization is that most structures projecting to the hypothalamus receive a reciprocal input from the hypothalamus. For example, the hypothalamus receives an amygdalohypothalamic projection and gives rise to hypothalamoamygdaloid fibers. For ease of discussion, the efferents are divided into those to forebrain structures (ascending) and those to brainstem and spinal targets (descending).

Ascending Projections

The *mammillary fasciculus* originates as a well-defined bundle from the medial mammillary nucleus (Figs. 30-8 and 30-9). It passes posteriorly (dorsally) for a short distance then bifurcates into the *mammillothalamic tract* and the *mammillotegmental tract* (Fig. 30-8). The former projects to the anterior nucleus of the thalamus and is an important part of the circuit of Papez (see Chapter 31). The latter (discussed further on) turns caudally and distributes to the tegmental nuclei of the midbrain reticular formation, thus reciprocating the mammillary peduncle. *Hypothalamothalamic fibers* arise mainly from the lateral preoptic area and project to the dorsomedial nucleus of the thalamus. The hypothalamus also projects to the amygdaloid nucleus *(hypothalamoamygdaloid fibers)* via the stria terminalis and the ventral amygdalofugal pathway. These fibers originate from various hypothalamic nuclei and project primarily to corticomedial nuclei of the amygdaloid complex.

Descending Projections

There are four main descending projections from the hypothalamus. These are *hypothalamospinal* and *hypothalamomedullary* fibers, the *posterior* (dorsal) *longitudinal fasciculus,* and the *mammillotegmental tract* (Figs. 30-8 and 30-9).

Hypothalamospinal and *hypothalamomedullary fibers* arise mainly from the paraventricular nucleus, although some originate

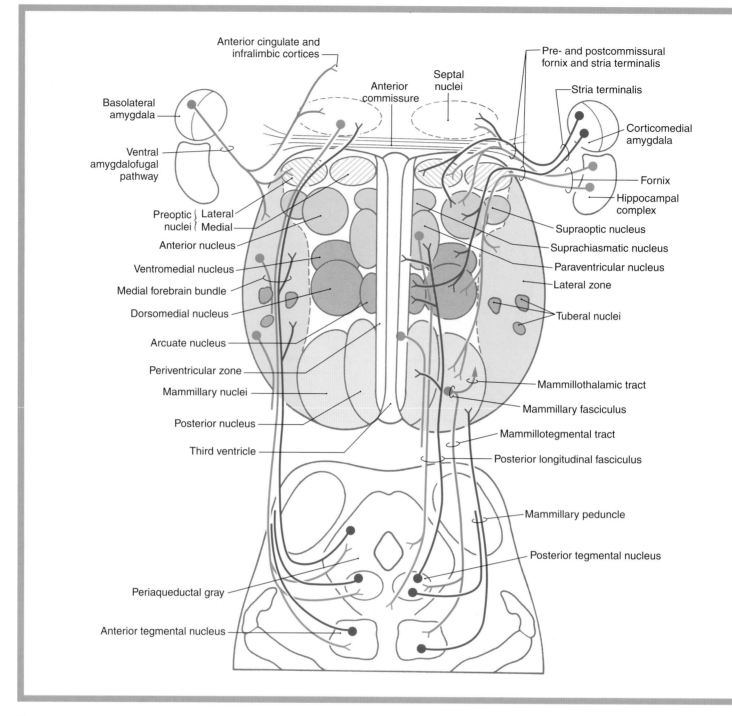

Figure 30-9. Diagrammatic representation of hypothalamic connections as seen in the axial (horizontal) plane. Note the distribution of fibers of the ventral amygdalofugal pathway, the precommissural and postcommissural fornix, and the stria terminalis.

from cells located in the lateral and posterior hypothalamic areas (Fig. 30-8). These fibers descend through the periaqueductal gray and adjacent reticular formation of the midbrain and rostral pons, and then shift to an anterolateral (ventrolateral) position in the medulla. *Hypothalamomedullary fibers* terminate in the solitary nucleus, dorsal vagal motor nucleus, nucleus ambiguus, and other nuclei of the anterolateral medulla. *Hypothalamospinal fibers* traverse the periaqueductal gray and dorsal tegmentum of the midbrain and pons. These fibers then shift laterally, passing through the anterolateral medulla and lateral funiculus of the spinal cord, to terminate on neurons of the intermediolateral cell column (general visceral efferent preganglionic cells). Hypothalamomedullary and hypothalamospinal fibers form an essential and *direct* link between the hypothalamus and autonomic nuclei of the medulla and spinal cord. Lesions in the anterolateral medulla may disrupt these fibers. Although the functional effect

of disrupting hypothalamomedullary fibers is not well understood, injury to hypothalamospinal fibers results in a loss of sympathetic outflow to the ipsilateral face and head (causing a *Horner syndrome*) and to the ipsilateral side of the body.

The *posterior (dorsal) longitudinal fasciculus* originates from nuclei of the medial hypothalamic zone, whereas fibers of the *mammillotegmental tract* arise from the medial mammillary nucleus (Figs. 30-8 and 30-9). Fibers of these pathways descend through, and largely terminate in, the periaqueductal gray. The mammillotegmental tract, being more anteriorly (ventrally) located, also terminates on neurons of the *posterior (dorsal) and anterior (ventral) tegmental nuclei* situated in the periaqueductal gray of the caudal midbrain (Fig. 30-9). Some neurons of the periaqueductal gray function, at least in part, in relaying information to visceral areas of the brainstem, such as the solitary and dorsal motor vagal nuclei. Consequently, the posterior ngitudinal fasciculus and mammillotegmental tract are generally viewed as relatively short tracts that *indirectly* influence the autonomic nuclei of the brainstem.

Intrinsic Hypothalamic Connections

The pathways that interconnect the many nuclei of the hypothalamus are numerous and complex. Only two especially important ones are considered here: the *supraopticohypophysial tract* and the *tuberoinfundibular tract*. Both of these tracts link the hypothalamus to the pituitary (Fig. 30-5).

Supraopticohypophysial Tract

Two hormones are released by the posterior pituitary: *oxytocin* and *antidiuretic hormone* (ADH, vasopressin) (Table 30-2). These hormones are synthesized in large (magnocellular) neurons of the *supraoptic* and *paraventricular nuclei*. They are transported to the posterior pituitary in the axons of these neurons, which form the *supraopticohypophysial tract*. In the posterior pituitary, they are stored in specialized axon terminals, sometimes called *Herring bodies*, which release them in response to the arrival of action potentials from the nerve cell body. The activity of these hypothalamic neurons—and thus the release of the hormones—is regulated in response to appropriate stimuli. Once released, the hormones enter a capillary plexus in the posterior pituitary and are conveyed to the general circulation by hypophysial veins.

Neurons containing oxytocin release this hormone during coitus, nipple suckling, and periods in which there is an increased level of estrogen. The release of oxytocin induces the contraction of smooth muscle in the uterus and of the myoepithelial cells in the mammary gland. The effect of oxytocin on the uterus is critical during and after childbirth. A synthetic form of oxytocin (Pitocin) is often administered to hasten labor and delivery. After the baby is born, oxytocin continues to be important. During nursing, for example, the baby's suckling causes oxytocin to be released from the posterior pituitary, and oxytocin in turn causes the myoepithelial cells of the milk glands to contract, expelling milk. The oxytocin released during nursing also has beneficial effects on the postpartum uterus. Specifically, the contractions of uterine muscles caused by oxytocin help this organ to gradually regain its original form and size.

Neurons containing antidiuretic hormone (ADH, vasopressin) (Table 30-2) are influenced primarily by fluctuations in the osmolarity of the blood. The relative concentration of sodium chloride in blood plasma is normally about 300 milliosmoles. This osmolarity is largely a function of how much water is retained within the body. In the process of maintaining fluid balance homeostasis, small deviations from normal blood osmolarity occur throughout each day. These deviations serve as stimuli that influence the release of ADH from the posterior pituitary. Because these stimuli occur frequently, the neurons containing ADH (unlike those containing oxytocin) are tonically active. Thus, small amounts of ADH are released numerous times each day.

When the blood osmolarity is high, the release of ADH from the posterior pituitary is facilitated. On entering the systemic circulation, ADH has a primary effect on the kidneys. Specifically, ADH causes the collecting tubules to increase their resorption of water from the developing urine, thereby returning water to the circulatory system. The additional water serves to dilute the blood, causing the blood osmolarity to be decreased. Consequently, however, the urine becomes more concentrated. As a result, urine output is diminished and the urine that is produced has a darker color.

When the blood osmolarity is low, the release of ADH from the posterior pituitary is inhibited. Consequently, the amount of ADH in the systemic circulation will be diminished. In response, the collecting tubules of the kidneys decrease their resorption of water from the developing urine. Consequently, water remains in the urine and is not returned to the circulatory system. The effect of this renal conservation of water is an increase in

Table 30-2. Hypothalamic Releasing Hormones and the Pituitary Hormones They Influence

Nucleus	Releasing Hormone	Pituitary Hormone
Medial preoptic nucleus	Gonadotropin-releasing h. Thyrotropin-releasing h. Corticotropin-releasing h. Growth hormone–releasing inhibitor h. (somatostatin)	Gonadotropins Thyrotropin Corticotropin Inhibits release of growth hormone
Anterior nucleus	Growth hormone–releasing inhibitor h. (somatostatin)	Inhibits release of growth hormone
Supraoptic nucleus	 Corticotropin-releasing h.	Oxytocin and antidiuretic h. (vasopressin) Corticotropin
Paraventricular nucleus	 Thyrotropin-releasing h. Corticotropin-releasing h. Growth hormone–releasing h. Growth hormone–releasing inhibitor h. (somatostatin)	Oxytocin and antidiuretic h. (vasopressin) Thyrotropin Corticotropin Growth hormone Inhibits release of growth hormone
Ventromedial nucleus	Growth hormone–releasing h.	Growth hormone
Dorsomedial nucleus	Growth hormone–releasing h. Thyrotropin-releasing h.	Growth hormone Thyrotropin
Arcuate nucleus	Gonadotropin-releasing h. Growth hormone-releasing h. Prolactin-releasing inhibition h. (dopamine)	Gonadotropins Growth hormone Prolactin inhibition
Lateral hypothalamic zone	Thyrotropin-releasing h. Growth hormone–releasing h. Growth hormone–releasing inhibitor h. (somatostatin)	Thyrotropin Growth hormone Inhibits release of growth hormone

the concentration of the blood, causing the blood osmolarity to be increased. Accordingly, there is also an increased output of pale-colored (dilute) urine.

Lesions of the supraoptic or paraventricular nucleus or of the supraopticohypophysial tract produce a syndrome known as *diabetes insipidus*, which is characterized by *polyuria* (increased urination) and *polydipsia* (increased consumption of water) (Table 30-1). This condition is due to a deficit of circulating ADH. It is of interest that ethanol causes a decrease in the release of ADH from the posterior pituitary. This is the reason why consumption of alcoholic beverages tends to cause copious urination and consequent dehydration and thirst.

The main function of ADH (vasopressin) is to assist in the maintenance of normal blood osmolarity and blood pressure. Normally, ADH increases blood pressure by increasing blood volume. However, ADH at high levels will cause contraction of vascular smooth muscle and may also result in increased blood pressure. In this regard, the release of ADH from the posterior pituitary often occurs in those situations in which an increase of blood pressure would be beneficial. For example, the hypotension that occurs in conjunction with *hypovolemia* (decreased blood volume) represents a stimulus that promotes the release of ADH. As a result, arterial constriction takes place and blood pressure is elevated. Accordingly, the hypotensive state is partially alleviated.

Tuberoinfundibular Tract

Most of the input to the pituitary through the tuberoinfundibular tract comes from small (parvicellular) neurons located in the arcuate nucleus and the *periventricular zone*. Neurons of the paraventricular, suprachiasmatic, tuberal, and medial preoptic nuclei also contribute to this tract (Fig. 30-5). These axons convey various *releasing hormones* to the median eminence (the most inferior aspect of the tuberal area) and to the infundibulum of the pituitary gland (Table 30-2). The substances are then released into a *primary plexus* of fenestrated capillaries (sinusoids), from which they are carried by *portal veins* to a *secondary plexus* of fenestrated capillaries in the pituitary (Fig. 30-5). The releasing hormones of the hypothalamus include thyrotropin-releasing hormone, growth hormone-releasing hormone, growth hormone release inhibition hormone (somatostatin), corticotropin-releasing hormone, gonadotropin-releasing hormone, and prolactin-releasing hormone (Table 30-2).

In the anterior lobe, the hypothalamic hormones regulate the functioning of hormone-producing adenohypophysial cells. The hormones of the adenohypophysis include *growth hormone* (primarily affecting the development of the musculoskeletal system), *gonadotropins* (affecting the ovary and testis), *corticotropin* (affecting the cortex of the adrenal gland), *thyrotropin* (affecting the thyroid gland), and *prolactin* (affecting milk production) (Table 30-2). Hormones leave the anterior pituitary via hypophysial veins and are distributed in the systemic circulation.

Pituitary Tumors

The pituitary gland is anatomically and functionally linked to the hypothalamus. Indeed, it is through the pituitary that many hypothalamic functions are expressed. Hormones and releasing hormones manufactured in the hypothalamus are transported via the supraopticohypophysial and tuberoinfundibular tracts and are released into the hypophysial portal system. Small lesions within the hypothalamus can block the manufacture and transportation of these substances, thereby adversely affecting pituitary functions. Similarly, tumors (*adenomas*) occurring within the pituitary can easily encroach on the neighboring hypothalamus and thus jeopardize its functions. It is therefore appropriate to briefly consider pituitary tumors at this point.

Although visual deficits are not a specific topic of this chapter (see Chapter 20), it should be noted that such deficits are frequently experienced by patients with pituitary tumors. These deficits may reflect damage to the optic nerve immediately rostral to the chiasm, to the chiasm itself (uncrossed fibers or decussating fibers), or to the optic tract immediately caudal to the chiasm. For example, a pituitary tumor pressing on the optic chiasm may damage axons originating from the nasal half of each retina. This may result in a loss of vision in the temporal half of the visual field for each eye (a *bitemporal hemianopia*), thereby reducing peripheral vision.

Tumors occurring within the pituitary gland account for 12% of primary brain tumors. In autopsy studies, the overall occurrence of incidental (undiagnosed) pituitary adenomas has been as high as 22.5% and as low as 3.2%, depending on the thickness of sectioned pituitary glands. These tumors, occurring most frequently in young adults, are generally noncancerous. Incidental adenomas occur with increasing frequency in the fifth, sixth, and seventh decades of life.

Pituitary tumors can be classified according to their secretory characteristics, size, or biologic invasiveness. Secreting tumors produce an excess of one or more pituitary hormones; prolactin is the most commonly affected of these hormones. A second classification of these tumors is by size; *microadenomas* are tumors less than 1 cm in greatest dimension, whereas tumors greater than 1 cm across are referred to as *macroadenomas*. A third classification of these tumors is according to invasiveness; invasive tumors may erode and extend into the dura mater and even the sphenoid bone.

Nonsecreting pituitary tumors do not secrete hormones and as a result are often undiagnosed until they grow to a considerable size and exert pressure on nearby structures (e.g., the optic chiasm and hypothalamus). Patients with these large pituitary tumors have symptoms that often include visual disturbances (in 60% to 70% of patients) and headaches.

Secreting Tumors

In the clinical setting, secreting tumors are also commonly referred to as *hormonally active tumors* or *hypersecreting tumors*. The clinical manifestations of a secreting tumor are the effects of the biologic activity of the specific pituitary hormone that is overproduced. In cases of excessive production of *growth hormone*, patients experience uncontrolled growth in height referred to as *gigantism* (Fig. 30-10), if the growth occurs before closure of the epiphyseal plates of the long bones. These patients may have large muscles, but they are actually rather weak because these muscles contain excessive amounts of connective tissue rather than muscle fibers.

On the other hand, the overproduction of growth hormone after the growth plates have closed results in a condition termed *acromegaly*, referring to the enlargement of the digits of the patient (Fig. 30-11A). Patients with acromegaly have typical facial changes (Fig. 30-11B), with elongation of the face, malocclusion of the jaw, and gaps in the lower dentition. Other changes include frontal and mastoid sinus bulges, a bulbous nose, thickened lips, and very large hands and feet (Fig. 30-11). Associated with these external manifestations are excessive cortical thickening of bone, cardiac failure secondary to heart enlargement *(cardiomegaly)*, as well as hypertension, and diabetes mellitus.

A much rarer form of pituitary tumor can result from the overproduction of *thyrotropin hormone*. The result may be either hypothyroidism or hyperthyroidism. Frequently, the patients suffer from abnormal cardiovascular function, as well as tremor. With the progression of these tumors, symptoms such as headaches, visual disturbances, and parasellar cranial nerve (i.e., cranial nerves III, IV, and VI) dysfunction may be recognized.

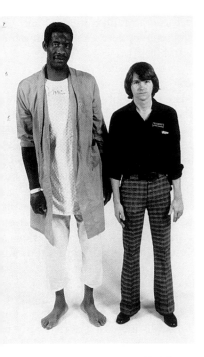

Figure 30-10. Gigantism resulting from overproduction of growth hormone. The normal adult male *(right)* is 6 feet 2.5 inches in height. The patient *(left)* was 7 feet 6 inches in height, wore size 17EEE shoes, and had a 12-inch span from the tip of his little finger to the tip of his thumb when his hand was spread.

The cranial nerve dysfunction generally involves the abducens nerve(s) first, and then the oculomotor and trochlear nerves, as the tumor enlarges in a lateral direction.

Cushing Disease

An overproduction of *corticotropin* leads to a form of hyper-adrenalism known as *Cushing disease* (Fig. 30-12). In this instance, the excessive ACTH from the pituitary gland results in excessive adrenal cortisol secretion with the resultant classic clinical features of Cushing disease. In general, affected patients have central truncal obesity, including moon-like facies, facial hirsutism, and a dorsal cervical hump, commonly called a buffalo hump, which results from enlargement of the fat pad in this area (Fig. 30-12A). The centropedal obesity has a hallmark finding of violaceous striae (stretch marks). These striae are clearly

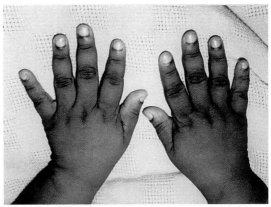

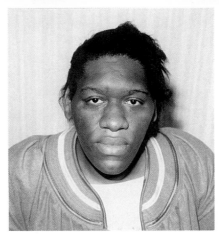

Figure 30-11. A female patient with acromegaly. Note the characteristic appearance of the enlarged hands (**A**) and the facial features (**B**).

different from those seen in pregnancy or in excessive weight gain. Striae in Cushing disease (Fig. 30-12B) are purple to violet, whereas striae in other situations are usually white. These patients also suffer from hyperpigmentation (Fig. 30-12C), easy bruising, hypertension, osteopenia, and emotional lability.

Prolactin-Secreting Tumors

An overproduction of *prolactin* in women results in the syndrome of *galactorrhea (milk production)* (Fig. 30-13) and *amenorrhea (absence of menstrual periods)*. *Hyperprolactinemia* is seen

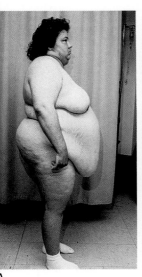

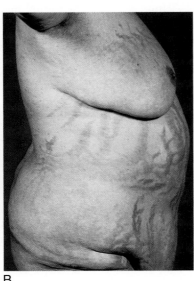

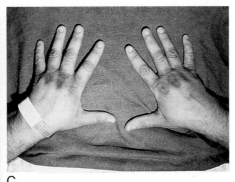

Figure 30-12. Cushing disease resulting from an overproduction of corticotropin. Note the characteristic central (truncal) obesity, the moonlike face, and the cervical hump (**A**). The striae in Cushing disease (**B**) can be very prominent and are purplish. Hyperpigmentation (**C**), here seen as dark oval areas over the knuckles, is also a characteristic feature.

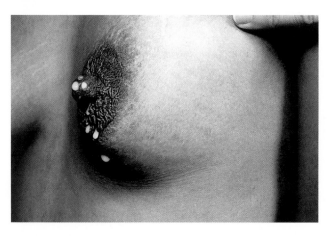

Figure 30-13. Milk production in a nonpregnant woman resulting from a prolactinoma.

physiologically as part of a normal pregnancy. There are, however, other causes of hyperprolactinemia that require differentiation from either tumor or pregnancy (e.g., hypothyroidism, drug use). In men, hyperprolactinemia may be indicated by decreased libido, impotency, or infertility. This type of hypersecretory tumor is the most common pathologic cause of infertility.

Gonadotrope Tumors

These tumors consist of cells that produce either excessive luteinizing hormone (LH) or follicle-stimulating hormone (FSH). Excessive secretion of FSH causes no known symptoms in either men or postmenopausal women. Excessive LH secretion has been reported to cause premature pubertal changes *(precocious puberty)* in males and possibly disruption of the ovarian cyclicity in females. In most instances, however, gonadotrope adenomas come to clinical attention because of their mass effect, with visual impairment, headaches, and occasionally diplopia *(double vision)* caused by optic nerve compression due to lateral extension of the tumor.

Regional Functions of the Hypothalamus

Because of the interrelationships existing among the autonomic, endocrine, and limbic systems (Fig. 30-1), and because of the small size of the hypothalamus, it is difficult to assign a specific function to each of its individual nuclei. Some hypothalamic nuclei participate in functions that are shared with other nuclei within the same vicinity. Consequently, these latter nuclei may participate in functions that are not uniquely their own. Instead, they may act in concert to affect functions that are attributable to hypothalamic *regions*, rather than specific nuclei.

Although the functions of some hypothalamic nuclei are largely known, the functions of others are poorly understood. Because of this and the fact that many hypothalamic nuclei participate in regional functions, some investigators believe that the hypothalamus should not be described as containing functional "centers," such as a "feeding center" or a "satiety center" (Table 30-1). Furthermore, because of the functional interrelationships that exist among certain nuclei within given hypothalamic regions, there is merit in thinking of the hypothalamus in terms of regional functions. Clinical observations are consistent with this view.

On the basis of clinical observations and experimental data, it is appropriate to divide the hypothalamus into two areas that share similar but opposing functions. These regions are the caudolateral and rostromedial areas of the hypothalamus (Fig. 30-4). In general, the *caudolateral area* consists of the lateral hypothalamic zone and the mammillary region, and the *rostromedial area* consists of the supraoptic region and much of the tuberal regions (Figs. 30-8 and 30-9).

Caudolateral Hypothalamus

Activation (stimulation) of the caudolateral hypothalamus produces behavioral manifestations that are generally associated with anxiety. These include (1) increased activity of the *sympathetic* division of the visceromotor system, (2) increased *aggressive* behavior, (3) increased *hunger,* and (4) *increased body temperature* (resulting from cutaneous vasoconstriction and shivering).

A *lesion* in the caudolateral hypothalamus typically results in manifestations opposite to those caused by stimulation. For example, damage in this area results in the inhibition of sympathetic activities and the reduction of body temperature.

Rostromedial Hypothalamus

Activation (stimulation) of the rostromedial hypothalamus produces behavioral manifestations that are generally associated with contentment. These include (1) increased activity of the *parasympathetic* division of the visceromotor system, (2) increased *passive* behavior, (3) increased *satiety,* and (4) *decreased body temperature* (owing to cutaneous vasodilation and sweating).

The phenomenon of sweating is something of an oddity. Even though sweat glands are innervated by sympathetic nerve fibers, sweating is compatible with parasympathetic function in that it helps keep us cool. That the sympathetic terminals innervating most sweat glands are cholinergic, like the parasympathetic terminals innervating viscera, and that sweating can be elicited from the rostromedial hypothalamus support this observation.

Lesions in the rostromedial hypothalamus usually elicit behaviors opposite to those described for stimulation. For example, a lesion in this area results in the inhibition of parasympathetic activities and an increase in body temperature.

Hypothalamic Reflexes

All the vital functions of the hypothalamus, including the maintenance of blood pressure, body temperature, and water balance, are controlled through reflexes and are *typically* not subject to conscious control. However, through meditation or other means, some people can learn to alter certain hypothalamic responses. For example, *biofeedback* training enables some people to alter blood pressure and body temperature, which are generally under hypothalamic control. The neural mechanisms underlying these feats are largely unknown.

The internal environment is controlled partly through hypothalamic reflexes, which are typically mediated by the autonomic or endocrine systems (Fig. 30-1). Three examples are described in the following sections.

Baroreceptor Reflex

The baroreceptor reflex (which is discussed in more detail in Chapter 19 and is illustrated in Figs. 19-8, 19-9) regulates blood pressure in response to input from baroreceptors in the aortic arch and carotid sinus. These receptors are called extrinsic because they are outside the central nervous system. They sense variations in blood pressure and transmit the information to neurons in the solitary nucleus of the medulla. Neurons of the solitary nucleus project to and activate cells in the dorsal vagal nucleus, which in turn project to the terminal ganglia of the heart and influence heart rate. A blood pressure level above normal activates the solitary nucleus, leading to a decrease in heart rate and force of cardiac contraction, and consequently a decrease in blood pressure; a blood pressure level below normal has the opposite effect.

The hypothalamus is capable of influencing the baroreceptor reflex via a somewhat more complex pathway. The solitary nucleus contains cells that transmit baroreceptor information to the paraventricular, dorsomedial, and lateral hypothalamic nuclei. In turn, neurons in these hypothalamic areas project to the dorsal vagal nucleus of the medulla. By this route, the hypothalamus can powerfully modulate the responsiveness of the baroreceptor reflex.

Temperature Regulation Reflex

The reflex that maintains a constant body temperature depends on input from specialized temperature-sensing neurons in the hypothalamus (called *intrinsic receptors* because they are inside the central nervous system). When temperature of the blood reaching the hypothalamus rises above normal, these neurons stimulate regions in the *rostral hypothalamus* that are responsible for activating physiologic mechanisms for *heat dissipation—* sweating and cutaneous vasodilation. These effects are mediated by autonomic pathways. Conversely, when the blood temperature is below normal, the temperature sensors stimulate regions in the *caudal hypothalamus* that activate mechanisms for *heat*

conservation (cutaneous vasoconstriction, mediated by autonomic pathways) and for *heat production* (shivering, mediated by reticulospinal pathways).

Water Balance Reflex

As noted previously, the volume and osmolarity of the blood are kept constant by reflex mechanisms. Unlike the baroreceptor and temperature regulation reflexes, which are entirely neural, the water balance reflex is *neurohumoral*; its efferent limb consists of a hormonal signal carried by ADH. In brief, the reflex works as follows. The osmolarity of the blood is monitored by specialized osmolarity-sensitive neurons located in the anterior hypothalamus near the preoptic and paraventricular nuclei. The output from these receptors influences the release of ADH by ADH-producing neurons in the supraoptic and paraventricular nuclei. When blood osmolarity is too high, more ADH is released and water resorption from the collecting tubules of the kidney is increased. When blood osmolarity is too low, the release of ADH is inhibited and renal water resorption is reduced. Accordingly, water is not resorbed into the blood but stays in the urine.

Synopsis of Clinical Points

- A developmental defect in the formation of the pituitary may be the cause of a Rathke pouch tumor (p. 487).
- Head trauma may result in diabetes insipidus (p. 487).
- A lesion of the feeding center in the lateral hypothalamic zone attenuates feeding and will produce weight loss (p. 491).
- Damage to the ventromedial nucleus, regarded as a satiety center, may result in excessive eating and weight gain (p. 491).
- Lesions of the mammillary region of the hypothalamus produce memory deficits (p. 491).
- The Korsakoff syndrome is seen in chronic alcoholics and may improve with thiamine treatment (p. 491).
- Confabulation is seen in patients with the Korsakoff syndrome (p. 491).
- A lesion that involves descending hypothalamospinal fibers in the brainstem or cervical spinal cord produces an ipsilateral Horner syndrome (p. 494).
- Lesions of the supraoptic and paraventricular nuclei produce diabetes insipidus (p. 496).
- Polyuria (increased urination) and polydipsia (increased water intake) are characteristic of diabetes insipidus (p. 496).
- Pituitary lesions smaller than 1 cm are microadenomas and those larger than 1 cm are macroadenomas (p. 496).
- A hypersecreting pituitary tumor that produces excessive growth hormone may, depending on the patient's age, result in gigantism or acromegaly (p. 496).
- A pituitary tumor producing excessive corticotropin results in the signs and symptoms characteristic of Cushing disease (p. 497).
- Amenorrhea and/or galactorrhea is seen in female patients with a prolactin-secreting tumor (p. 497).
- Lesions of the pituitary, because of its apposition to optic structures, frequently result in visual deficits (p. 496).
- Lesions of the hypothalamus may affect the blood pressure and/or body temperature of the patient (p. 499).

Sources and Additional Reading

Friedman JM, Halaas JL: Leptin and the regulation of body weight in mammals. Nature 395:763-770, 1998.

Haymaker W, Anderson E, Nauta WJH: The Hypothalamus. Springfield, IL, Charles C Thomas, 1969.

Koizumi K, Kollai M, Oomura Y, Yamashita H, Wayner MJ (eds): The hypothalamus: Selected topics. Brain Res Bull 20:651-902, 1988.

Renaud LP: A neurophysiological approach to the identification, connections and pharmacology of the hypothalamic tubero-infundibular system. Neuroendocrinology 33:186-191, 1981.

Saper CB, Lowey AD, Swanson LW, Cowan WM: Direct hypo thalamo-autonomic connections. Brain Res 117:305-312, 1976.

Swanson LW, Sawchenko PE: Hypothalamic integration: Organization of the paraventricular and supraoptic nuclei. Annu Rev Neurosci 6:269-324, 1983.

Ter Horst GJ, de Boer P, Luiten PGM, van Willigen JD: Ascending projections from the solitary tract nucleus to the hypothalamus. A *Phaseolus vulgaris* lectin tracing study in the rat. Neuroscience 31:785-797, 1989.

van der Kooy D, Koda LY, McGinty JF, Gerfin CR, Bloom FE: The organization of projections from the cortex, amygdala, and hypothalamus to the nucleus of the solitary tract in rat. J Comp Neurol 224:1-24, 1984.

The Limbic System

R. B. Chronister and S. G. P. Hardy

Many complex brain systems are organized in a way that allows their function to be readily deduced. For example, even though the connections of the somatosensory pathways with the brainstem, thalamus, and cortex are complex, each component plays a fairly clear-cut role. The processing of somatosensory information is generally well understood. In contrast, some systems are interconnected in such a way that a given function may be carried out by several components acting in cooperation, and a given component may participate in several functions. The *limbic system* is a case in point. This system comprises structures that receive inputs from diverse areas of the neuraxis and participate in complicated and interrelated behaviors such as memory, learning, and social interactions. Thus, lesions involving the limbic system generally result in a wide range of deficits.

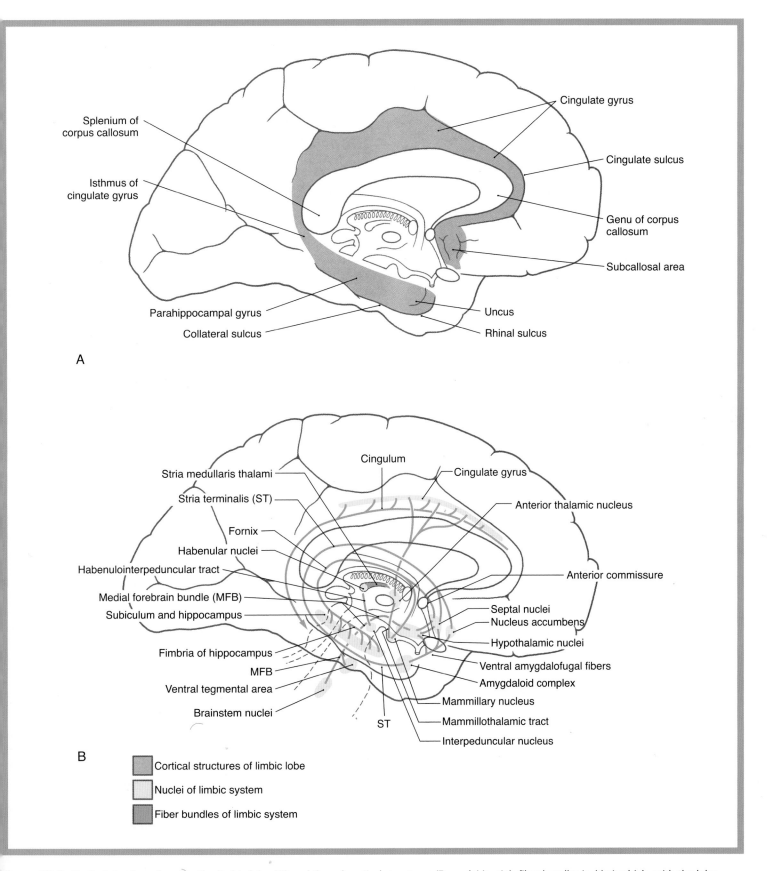

Figure 31-1. Cortical structures forming the limbic lobe (**A**) and the subcortical structures (**B**, nuclei in *pink,* fiber bundles in *blue*) which, with the lobe, represent the main components of the limbic system.

Overview

The concept of a *"limbic system"* actually encompasses two levels of structural and functional organization. The *first level* consists of the cortical structures on the most medial edge (the limbus) of the hemisphere; these collectively form the *limbic lobe* (Fig. 31-1A). Beginning just anterior to the lamina terminalis and proceeding caudally, these are the *subcallosal area*, containing the parolfactory and paraterminal gyri; the *cingulate gyrus;* the *isthmus of the cingulate gyrus;* the *parahippocampal gyrus;* and the *uncus* (Fig. 31-2). The limbic lobe also includes the *hippocampal formation.*

In 1878, Broca noted that the limbic lobe, which is present in all mammals, represents a relatively large part of the cerebral cortex in phylogenetically lower forms, and he postulated that it might be related to olfaction. Because of this latter point, the term *rhinencephalon* ("smell-brain") was later coined, and used interchangeably with *limbic lobe.* However, it is now known that the limbic lobe has little olfactory function in humans. Thus, the term "rhinencephalon" is antiquated and has largely disappeared from use.

The *second level* includes structures of the limbic lobe plus a variety of subcortical nuclei and tracts that collectively form the *limbic system* (Fig. 31-1B). The subcortical nuclei of the limbic system include, among others, the *septal nuclei* and *nucleus accumbens (nucleus accumbens septi);* various nuclei of the hypothalamus, especially those associated with the *mammillary body;* the nuclei of the *amygdaloid complex* and adjacent *substantia innominata;* and parts of the dorsal thalamus, particularly the *anterior* and *dorsomedial nuclei.* Additional structures connected with the limbic system include the *habenular nuclei, ventral tegmental area,* and *periaqueductal gray.* Furthermore, the *prefrontal cortex* is considered by some investigators to be an important component of the limbic system, primarily because of its potential influence on various other cortical and subcortical parts of the limbic system. Cortical targets of the prefrontal cortex include the cingulate gyrus, whereas the hypothalamus, dorsal thalamus, amygdaloid complex, and nuclei of the midbrain represent subcortical targets.

The main efferent fiber bundles of the limbic system are the *fornix* (primarily efferents of the hippocampus and subiculum), the *stria terminalis* and *ventral amygdalofugal pathway* (both are mainly efferents of the amygdaloid complex), and the *mammillothalamic tract* (efferents of the medial mammillary nucleus, Fig. 31-1B). A few additional nuclei and smaller tracts will be introduced as connections and functions of the limbic system.

Cytoarchitectural Definitions of the Limbic Cortex

The human cerebral cortex can be divided into several areas on the basis of the number of cell layers present. Most of the cerebral cortex (more than 90%) has six cell layers and is called the *neocortex* or *neopallium (isocortex).* Examples of neocortex include the primary sensory, motor, and association cortices. The cortical regions that have less than six layers are structurally and functionally associated with the limbic system or with olfaction and are classified as *allocortex.* Those structures that comprise three to five cellular layers are called the *paleocortex (paleopallium* or *periallocortex)* and are represented by the cortex of the parahippocampal gyrus (the *entorhinal cortex*), the uncus (the *piriform cortex*), and the cortex overlying the termination of the lateral olfactory stria (lateral olfactory gyrus) (Fig. 31-2). The lateral olfactory stria is directly rostromedial to the piriform cortex. Structures having only three cellular layers are classified as *archicortex (archipallium* or *allocortex)* and are represented by the dentate gyrus and hippocampus.

The separation between neocortex and allocortex is never sharp but instead consists of transitional areas where one cortical region blends into the next. Such areas are represented by caudal parts of the orbitofrontal cortex, the temporal pole, parts of the insula, and portions of the parahippocampal and cingulate gyri. They are especially important because they funnel input from association areas of the neocortex into the allocortex.

Early Functional Concepts

In the late 1930s, two pivotal observations were made that formed the basis for the concept of a limbic system. First, based largely on the morphology of the brain, a circuit for the elaboration of emotion was proposed. This pathway is now called the *Papez circuit* in recognition of James Papez, who initially described its components. This model, although surprisingly simple, has proved to be quite important in understanding limbic function. The circuit suggested that emotion, mediated through the hypothalamus, is controlled and modulated by fibers from the fornix. Specifically, the cortical control of emotional activity is presumed to originate from cingulate and hippocampal regions. These cortical influences are ultimately conveyed to the mammillary body of the hypothalamus via the fornix. In turn, the medial mammillary nucleus, via the mammillothalamic tract, projects to the anterior nucleus of the thalamus, and this cell group sends axons to the cingulate gyrus. This was the first time a specific anatomic substrate was proposed for a phenomenon as complex as emotion.

The second pivotal observation was that bilateral removal of large parts of the temporal lobe in monkeys resulted in a constellation of dysfunctions that came to be known as the

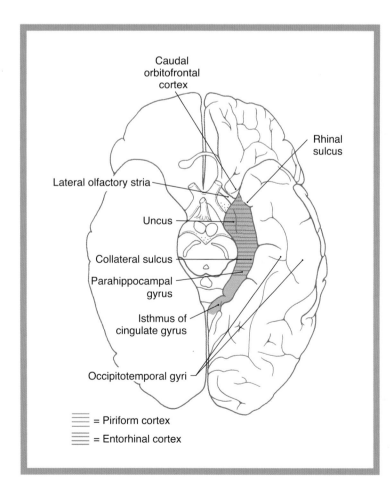

Figure 31-2. Cortical structures of the limbic lobe as seen on an anterior (ventral) view of the hemisphere.

Klüver-Bucy syndrome. This syndrome can also be caused in humans by temporal lobe injuries that involve primarily the amygdaloid complex. Its nature and significance are discussed later in the chapter.

Blood Supply to the Limbic System

The blood supply to the limbic system originates from several sources. The main vessels that serve much of the limbic system are the *anterior* and *posterior cerebral arteries*, the *anterior choroidal artery*, and branches arising from the *circle of Willis.*

The subcallosal area and rostral parts of the cingulate gyrus are supplied by branches of the anterior cerebral artery as it loops around the genu of the corpus callosum (see Fig. 8-6). Most of the cingulate gyrus and its isthmus receives its blood supply via the *pericallosal artery,* a branch of the anterior cerebral artery. *Temporal branches* of the posterior cerebral artery supply the parahippocampal gyrus. Although the uncus may receive some small branches from the posterior cerebral artery, it is served primarily by *uncal arteries,* which are branches of the M_1 segment of the middle cerebral artery (see Fig. 8-5).

The anterior choroidal artery usually originates from the internal carotid artery and follows the general trajectory of the optic tract. En route it sends branches into the choroidal fissure of the temporal horn of the lateral ventricle. This vessel serves the choroid plexus of the temporal horn, the hippocampal formation, parts of the amygdaloid complex, and adjacent structures such as the tail of the caudate nucleus, the stria terminalis, and the sublenticular and retrolenticular limbs of the internal capsule.

Vessels serving hypothalamic nuclei that are functionally associated with the limbic system originate from the circle of Willis. In general, rostral areas of the hypothalamus are served by branches from the anterior communicating artery and anterior cerebral artery, and posterior areas, by branches from the posterior communicating artery and proximal posterior cerebral artery (see Fig. 8-16). The anterior nucleus of the thalamus, an important synaptic station in the limbic system, is supplied by *thalamoperforating arteries* that arise from the P_1 segment of the posterior cerebral artery.

Hippocampal Formation

The *hippocampal formation* is composed of the *subiculum, hippocampus* (also called the hippocampus proper or horn of Ammon), and the *dentate gyrus* (see Fig. 31-4), all of which constitute the allocortex of Brodmann. The subiculum is laterally continuous with the cortex of the parahippocampal gyrus and area of the periallocortex. Medially the edge of the hippocampal formation is formed by the dentate gyrus and the fimbria of the hippocampus.

Developmentally, the hippocampal formation originates dorsally and migrates into its ventral and medial position in the temporal lobe. During this migration, small remnants of the hippocampal formation remain behind to form the *medial* and *lateral longitudinal striae* and their associated gray matter, the *indusium griseum* (Fig. 31-3). These structures are quite small in the human brain and extend rostrally along the dorsal aspect of the corpus callosum into the subcallosal area.

Structure

The *subiculum* of the hippocampal formation is the transitional area between the three-layered hippocampus (archicortex or allocortex) and the five-layered entorhinal cortex (paleocortex or periallocortex) of the parahippocampal gyrus (Fig. 31-4). This transitional zone, although small, can be divided into a prosubiculum, subiculum proper, presubiculum, and parasubiculum.

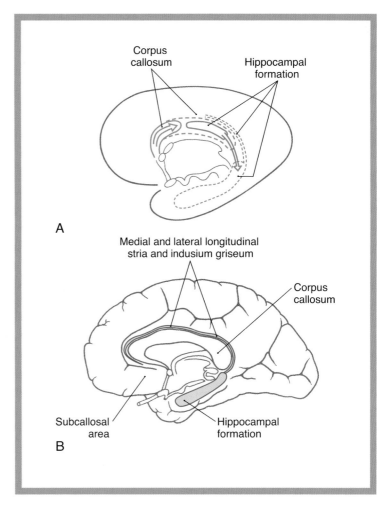

Figure 31-3. Developmental relationships between the corpus callosum (in *red*) and the hippocampal formation (in *green*). As the corpus callosum expands caudally from the general area of the anterior commissure (**A**), the hippocampal primordium migrates into the temporal lobe. In the adult brain, remnants of the hippocampal formation left behind during development are located dorsal to the corpus callosum (**B**).

These areas are essential for the flow of information into the hippocampal formation.

The dentate gyrus and the hippocampus are each composed of three layers, which are characteristic of archicortex (Fig. 31-4). The external layer is called the *molecular layer* and contains afferent axons and dendrites of cells intrinsic to each structure. The middle layer, called the *granule cell layer* in the dentate gyrus and the *pyramidal layer* in the hippocampus, contains the efferent neurons of each structure (Fig. 31-4). These layers are named according to the shape of the cell body of the principal type of neuron found therein. The dendrites of granule and pyramidal cells radiate into the molecular layer. The inner layer, called the *polymorphic layer* (also called the stratum oriens in the hippocampus), contains the axons of pyramidal and granule cells, a few intrinsic neurons, and many glial elements. In addition, the polymorphic layer of the hippocampus contains the elaborate basal dendrites of some larger pyramidal somata that are located in the pyramidal layer. These are called *double pyramid cells* because they have dendrites extending into both molecular and polymorphic layers (Fig. 31-4). The innermost part of the hippocampus borders on the wall of the lateral ventricle and is a layer of myelinated axons arising from cell bodies located in the subiculum and hippocampus. This layer, called the *alveus,* is continuous with the *fimbria of the hippocampus,* which, in turn, becomes the *fornix* (Fig. 31-4).

The hippocampus can be divided into four regions on the basis of a variety of cytoarchitectural criteria (Fig. 31-4). These

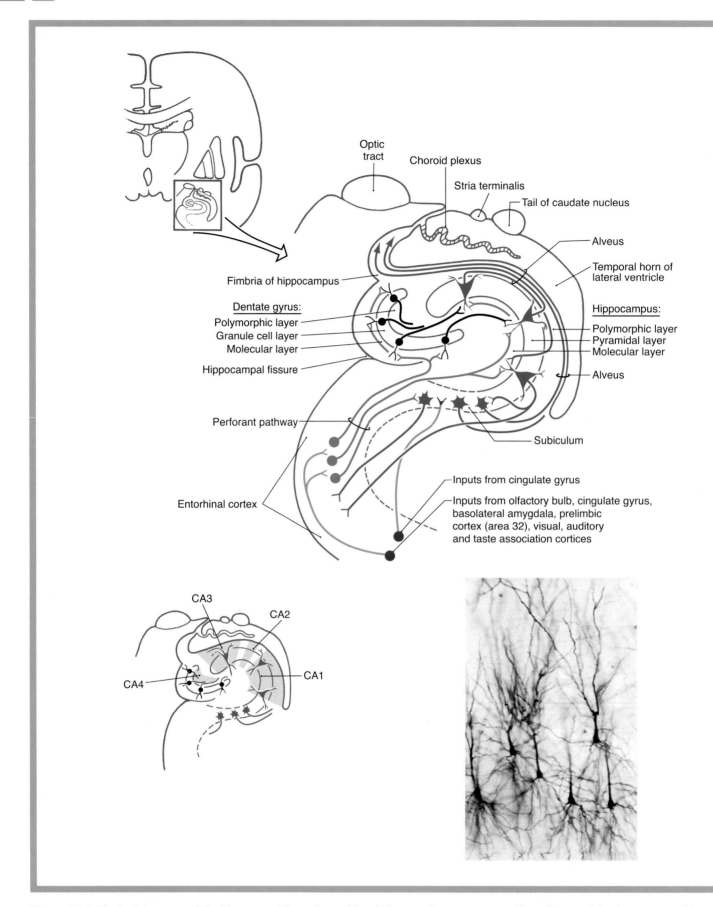

Figure 31-4. The basic structure of the hippocampal formation and its relation to adjacent structures. The cell types of the dentate gyrus, hippocampus, and subiculum are shown diagrammatically. The general locations of fields C1 to C4 are shown on the lower left; a Golgi stain of double pyramid cells is shown at the lower right. (Golgi stain courtesy of Dr. José Rafols, Wayne State University.)

areas are designated CA1 to CA4, where *CA* stands for cornu ammonis (horn of Ammon). Area CA1 (a parvocellular region that can be separated into two cell layers in humans) is located at the subiculum-hippocampal interface. Area CA2 (a mixed zone) and area CA3 (a magnocellular zone) are located within the hippocampus. Area CA4 is located at the junction of the hippocampus with the dentate gyrus, but within the hilus of the dentate gyrus.

Afferent Fibers

The major input to the hippocampal formation is from cells of the entorhinal cortex via a diffuse projection called the *perforant pathway* (Figs. 31-4 and 31-5). Most fibers of the perforant pathway terminate in the molecular layer of the dentate gyrus, although a few terminate in the subiculum and hippocampus. Granule cells in the dentate gyrus project into the molecular layer of the CA3 region of the hippocampus. CA3 neurons project into CA1 of the hippocampus, which, in turn, provides an input to the subiculum. In addition, the subiculum also receives a modest projection from the amygdaloid complex. Although the fornix is mainly an efferent path from the hippocampus, it also conveys cholinergic septohippocampal projections to the hippocampal formation and entorhinal cortex.

Efferent Fibers

The outflow of the hippocampal formation originates primarily from cells of the subiculum and, to a lesser degree, from pyramidal cells of the hippocampus (Figs. 31-4 and 31-5). In both cases, axons of these neurons enter the alveus, coalesce to form the fimbria of the hippocampus, and then continue as the fornix. These glutaminergic fibers traverse the entire extent of the fornix, although some cross the midline in the *hippocampal decussation* just anterior (ventral) to the splenium of the corpus callosum.

At the level of the anterior commissure, the fornix divides into postcommissural and precommissural parts (Fig. 31-5). The fibers originating in the subiculum mainly form the *postcommissural fornix*. Most of these fibers terminate in the *medial mammillary nucleus*, although some enter the ventromedial nucleus of the hypothalamus and the anterior nucleus of the dorsal thalamus (Fig. 31-5). The *precommissural fornix* is composed of fibers arising primarily in the hippocampus. These fibers are somewhat diffusely organized and distribute to the septal nuclei, the medial areas of the frontal cortex, the preoptic and anterior nuclei of the hypothalamus, and the nucleus accumbens (Fig. 31-5).

Complete Circuit of Papez

As noted previously, the initial segment of the *Papez circuit* is a projection primarily from the subiculum, to the medial mammillary nucleus via the postcommissural fornix. The circuit is completed by the following connections (Fig. 31-5): (1) a *mammillothalamic tract* that connects the *medial mammillary nucleus* to the *anterior nucleus* of the thalamus; (2) *thalamocortical fibers* from the anterior nucleus to broad expanses of the cortex of the *cingulate gyrus;* and (3) a projection from the cingulate cortex, via the cingulum, to the entorhinal cortex and also directly to the subiculum and hippocampus. The subiculum returns information to the mammillary body.

Other areas of the cerebral cortex are recruited into the various functions associated with the Papez circuit largely through connections of the cingulate gyrus. For example, the cingulate cortex receives input from premotor and prefrontal areas and from visual, auditory, and somatosensory association cortices. In turn, the cingulate cortex not only is a major source of afferent fibers to the hippocampal formation but also projects to most cortical areas from which it receives input. The cingulate gyrus thus is not only an integral part of the Papez circuit but also an

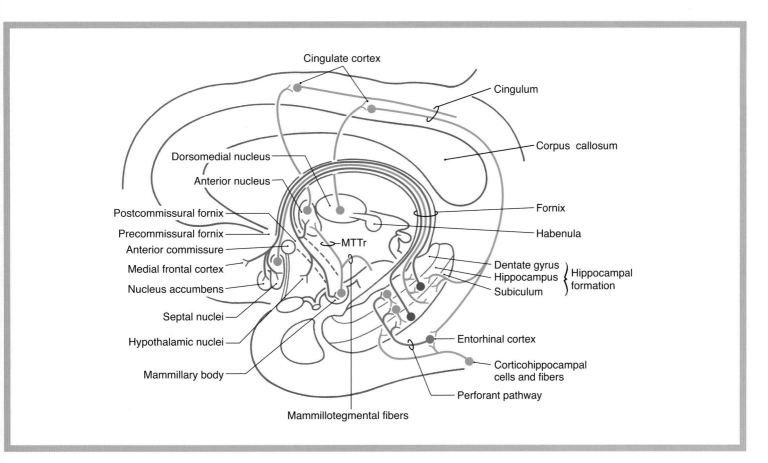

Figure 31-5. Semidiagrammatic representation of afferent and efferent connections of the hippocampal formation. MTTr, mammillothalamic tract.

important conduit through which a wide range of information can reach the limbic system.

Dysfunctions and Korsakoff Syndrome

The basic function of the hippocampal formation appears to be the consolidation of long-term memories from immediate and short-term memories—a point first observed in 1900 by Bechterew but essentially ignored until the 1950s. *Immediate memory* and *short-term memory* refer to types of memory that persist for seconds and minutes, respectively. Normally, these memories can be incorporated into long-term memory, which can be recalled days, months, or years later. However, in persons with hippocampal lesions, this conversion is not accomplished. Although patients may be able to perform a task for seconds or minutes, if distracted from the task they are unable to return to it. In other words, they do not "remember" what they were doing; the short-term experience is not incorporated into long-term memory. The redundancy and feedback in the hippocampus are ideal for this imprinting of memory.

One condition in which loss of memory and cognitive function is particularly obvious is *Alzheimer disease*. This disease is characterized, in part, by the presence of neurofibrillary tangles, neuritic plaques, and neuronal loss in specific brain regions. The subiculum and entorhinal cortices are among the first sites in which these abnormalities appear. As a result, the relay of information through the hippocampal formation is markedly impeded. It is believed that this damage is at least partially responsible for the memory deficits characteristic of Alzheimer disease.

As mentioned previously, the *Korsakoff syndrome* (Korsakoff psychosis) is a condition that is caused by prolonged thiamine deficiency and is typically seen in chronic alcoholics. The thiamine deficiency causes a characteristic pattern of degeneration in the brain. Typically, the mammillary bodies are involved, with some incursion into the dorsomedial nucleus of the thalamus and the columns of the fornix. There is also a loss of neurons in the hippocampal formation. These patients show a defect in short-term memory and consequently also in long-term memory for events occurring since the onset of disease. They may appear demented, and they are prone to *confabulation;* that is, they tend to string together fragments of memory from several different events to form a synthetic "memory" of an event that never occurred. In some chronic alcoholics, the memory loss and general confusion are accompanied by gaze palsies and ataxia, which occur secondary to cerebellar damage. When these deficits accompany profound memory losses and learning difficulties, the condition is called *Wernicke-Korsakoff syndrome*.

Bilateral damage to the hippocampal formation sometimes occurs in victims of heart attack or near-drownings as a result of transient cerebral ischemia. The part of the hippocampal formation most vulnerable to anoxia during an ischemic episode is the CA1 area. The CA1-subiculum interface region is referred to as the *Sommer sector* in pathologic conditions. Affected patients retain their long-term memories from the time before the ischemic event, but they are unable to retain memories for events occurring after the ischemic episode. Consequently, they also have difficulty learning new skills because the new information is not retained (remembered) long enough to become a long-term memory. Damage to the Sommer sector is also related to epilepsy. It is known that malfunction of the hippocampus is indeed related to the genesis of epileptic activity. It is well established that most areas of the hippocampus are involved in the pathogenesis of epilepsy. Surprisingly, area CA2 is the most resistant to sustained seizure activity whereas the Sommer sector and CA4 are the most vulnerable. Understanding the organization of the hippocampal subfields is clinically apparent.

Bilateral lesions of the anterior part of the cingulate gyrus greatly diminish the emotional responses of the patient and may result in *akinetic mutism*. This is a state in which the patient is immobile, mute, and unresponsive but not in a coma. Other patients with cingulate damage may be alert but have no idea of who they are. Patients may also be unable to recall the order in which past events occurred.

Long-Term Potentiation and Memory

The process of *long-term potentiation* at individual synapses is the probable mechanism that underlies the consolidation of short-term into long-term memory. When several synapses are present on a single cell, the input from these synapses is *integrated;* that is, the small potential changes (EPSP and IPSP, see Chapter 3) are added together. In long-term potentiation, one synapse fires in a particular temporal pattern (such as bursts or trains of action potentials). This synaptic activity increases the likelihood that the target cells will be activated by that synapse and other synapses. This increased likelihood may be due to an increased probability that transmitter will be released from the presynaptic cell, or to an increased response in the postsynaptic cell to the same amount of neurotransmitter, or to both. Long-term potentiation has been demonstrated at terminals of the perforant pathway in the dentate gyrus and at the synapses of CA3 pyramidal cells on CA1 cells. These connections use the neurotransmitter glutamate.

According to one current model, the release of glutamate causes a change in the biochemistry of the N-methyl-D-aspartate (NMDA)-type glutamate receptors of the hippocampal cells, allowing an increased number of calcium ions to enter the cell. The calcium influx causes a second postsynaptic biochemical change. The gaseous neuromodulator nitric oxide is released and diffuses back to the presynaptic terminal. It acts on the presynaptic terminal to permanently increase the release of glutamate. At this type of synapse, *a brief, sustained increase in current synaptic activity increases the probability that future synaptic activity will take place.* That is, the more the circuit is activated, the easier it is to activate. This mechanism causes stimuli and responses to be paired in the process we call "memory." The increased probability of activation lasts in isolated preparations for hours; it cannot be measured in human brains but may be permanent.

Amygdaloid Complex

Structure

The amygdaloid complex is an almond-shaped group of cells in the rostromedial part of the temporal lobe internal to the uncus (Fig. 31-1). It is immediately rostral to the hippocampal formation and the anterior end of the temporal horn of the lateral ventricle. The amygdaloid complex is composed of a number of nuclei. For our purposes, these nuclei can be grouped into a larger *basolateral group* and a smaller *corticomedial group* (including the *central nucleus*). The latter group is more closely related to olfaction, whereas the former has extensive interconnections with cortical structures.

Afferent Fibers

The basolateral cell groups of the amygdala receive inputs from the dorsal thalamus, the prefrontal cortex, the cingulate and parahippocampal gyri, the temporal lobe and insular cortex, and the subiculum (Fig. 31-6A). These fibers supply a wide range of somatosensory, visual, and visceral information to the amygdaloid complex.

The corticomedial cell group receives olfactory input, fibers from the hypothalamus (ventromedial nucleus, lateral

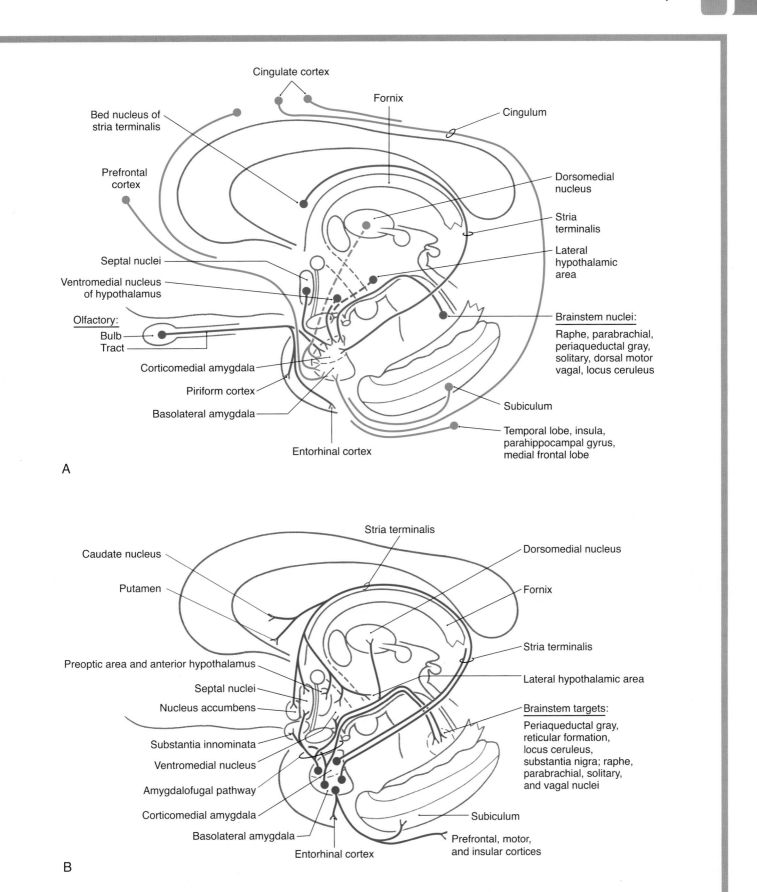

Figure 31-6. Semidiagrammatic representation of the afferent (**A**) and efferent (**B**) connections of the amygdaloid complex.

hypothalamic area), and fibers from the dorsomedial and medial nuclei of the dorsal thalamus (Fig. 31-6A). In addition, this cell group, particularly its central nucleus, receives ascending input from nuclei in the brainstem known to be involved in visceral functions. Among others, these include the parabrachial nuclei, the solitary nucleus, and portions of the periaqueductal gray.

Efferent Fibers

The two major efferent pathways of the amygdaloid complex are the stria terminalis and the ventral amygdalofugal pathway (Figs. 31-1B and 31-6B). The *stria terminalis* is a small fiber bundle that arises primarily from cells of the corticomedial group. Through most of its course, this bundle lies in the groove between the caudate nucleus and the dorsal thalamus, where it is accompanied by the terminal vein. It is associated along its length with discontinuous aggregations of cells, which collectively are called the *bed nucleus of the stria terminalis*. This tract distributes to various nuclei of the *hypothalamus* (the preoptic nuclei, ventromedial nucleus, anterior nucleus, and lateral hypothalamic area), to the *nucleus accumbens* and the *septal nuclei*, and to the rostral areas of the caudate nucleus and putamen (Fig. 31-6B).

The *ventral amygdalofugal pathway* is the major efferent fiber bundle of the amygdaloid complex. These fibers arise from the basolateral cell group and the central nucleus of the corticomedial cell group and follow two general trajectories (Fig. 31-6B). Axons primarily from the basolateral cells pass medially through the substantia innominata (in which some of these fibers terminate) to eventually synapse in the hypothalamus and septal nuclei. The substantia innominata gives rise to a diffuse cholinergic projection to the cerebral cortex. It is probable that these fibers play a role in the activation of the cerebral cortex in response to behaviorally significant stimuli. In addition, cells of the basolateral group also project diffusely to frontal and prefrontal, cingulate, insular, and inferior temporal cortices (Fig. 31-6B). Other fibers, mainly from the central nucleus, turn caudally and descend diffusely in the brainstem to terminate in visceral (dorsal motor vagal) nuclei, raphe nuclei (magnus, obscurus, pallidus), and other areas such as the locus ceruleus, parabrachial nuclei, and periaqueductal gray (Fig. 31-6B). As noted previously, most of those brainstem areas that receive input from the amygdala project back to this structure.

Another route by which hippocampal and amygdaloid efferents influence the brainstem is through the *stria medullaris thalami*. This bundle conveys fibers from the septal nuclei (targets of amygdaloid and hippocampal inputs) to the *habenular nuclei* (Fig. 31-7A). The latter cell groups, in turn, give rise to the *habenulointerpeduncular tract*, which projects to the interpeduncular nucleus and other midbrain sites, including the ventral tegmental area and periaqueductal gray.

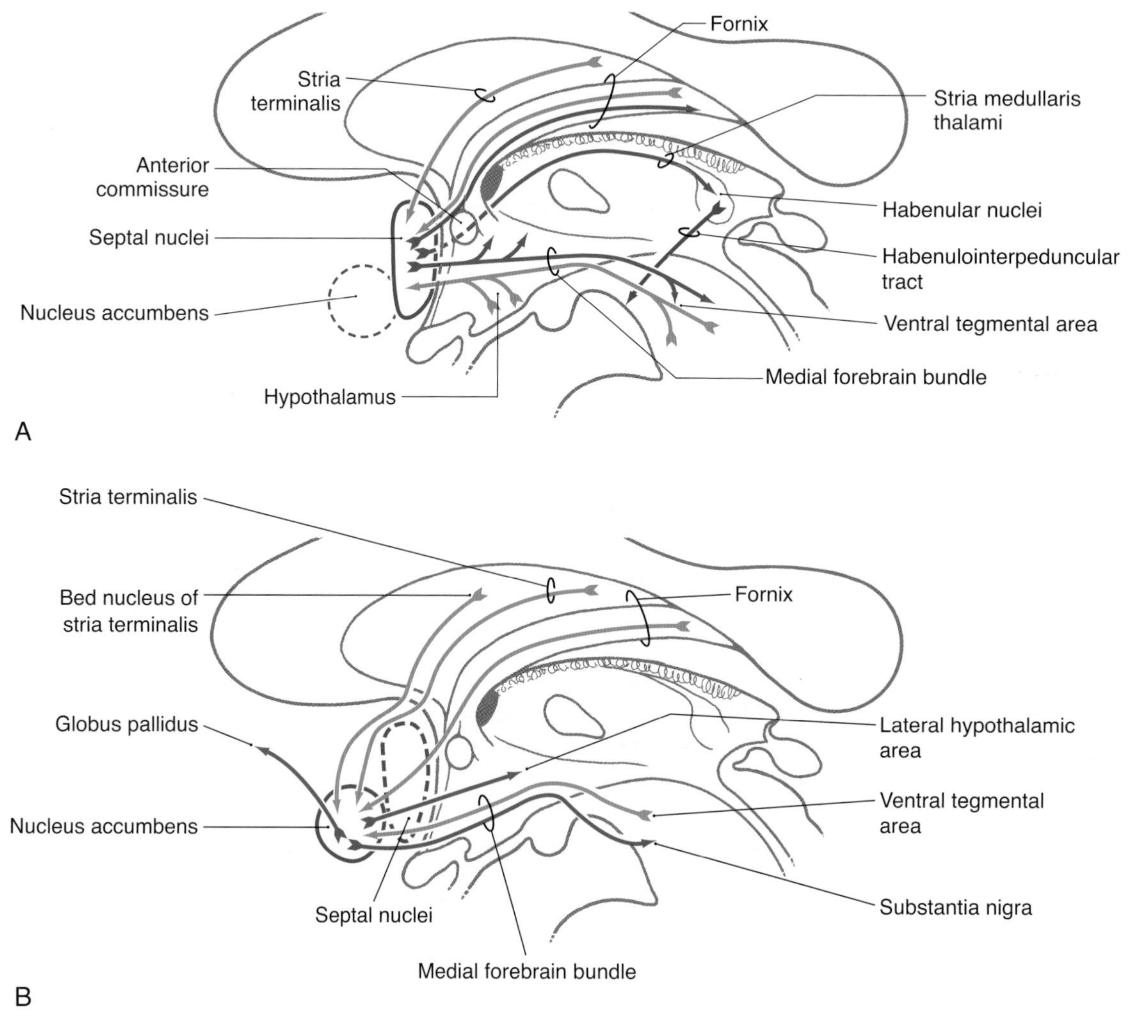

Figure 31-7. Summary of the main afferent *(red arrows)* and efferent *(green arrows)* connections of the septal nuclei (**A**) and of the nucleus accumbens (**B**).

Klüver-Bucy Syndrome

As mentioned previously, bilateral temporal lobe lesions that largely abolish the amygdaloid complex cause a set of behavioral changes called the *Klüver-Bucy syndrome*. These deficits were initially described in a series of animal experiments, but they have also been seen in patients as a result of either trauma to the temporal lobe or temporal lobe surgery for epilepsy. Damage to the amygdaloid complex frequently involves portions of adjacent structures and of the surrounding white matter, and these incursions into other structures may contribute to the clinical picture. Damage to the amygdala and the hippocampus results in a greater memory deficit than the deficit noted with damage to either one alone.

The Klüver-Bucy syndrome is characterized by the following deficits. First, the patient is no longer able to recognize objects by sight (*visual agnosia*) and may also exhibit *tactile* and *auditory agnosia*. Second, there is the tendency to examine objects excessively by mouth (*hyperorality*) or to smell them. Even a harmful object such as a lit match may be examined by being brought to the lips or touched with the tongue. Third, the patient may have a compulsion to intensively explore the immediate environment (*hypermetamorphosis*) and to overreact to visual stimuli. Fourth, *placidity* is characteristically seen. The animal or the patient may no longer show fear or anger, even when such a reaction is appropriate. Fifth, the subject may eat in excessive amounts (*hyperphagia*), even when not hungry, or may eat objects that are not food, or food that is inappropriate to the species. For example, a monkey may eat raw meat or a patient may eat leaves. Sixth, there is a striking augmentation in sexual behavior (*hypersexuality*). In humans, this takes the form of suggestive behavior and talk and vague, ill-conceived attempts at sexual contact. In addition to these predictable deficits, these patients may also experience *amnesia*, *dementia*, or *aphasia*, depending on the extent of the lesion of the temporal lobe.

Temporal Lobe Seizures

Limbic structures are very sensitive to seizure activity. Such seizures have the tendency to spread to adjacent structures of the temporal lobe or to both temporal lobes. In these cases there can be a release of a wide range of physical and emotional behaviors in concert with the predictions of the Kluver-Bucy syndrome. In seizures that start in the area of the uncus there typically is an aura associated with olfactory or gustatory hallucinations. These seizures, commonly referred to as *uncinate fits*, are explainable given the functions of the amygdala and the destinations of the olfactory-gustatory fiber systems. Older literature referred to these seizures as psychomotor seizures referring to the emotional/behavioral behaviors seen. Contemporary literature refers to these seizures as *complex partial seizures*.

Septal Region

The septal region (septal nuclei), excluding the nucleus accumbens, is a small area just rostral to the anterior commissure and in the medial wall of the hemisphere (Figs. 31-1B and 31-7A). These nuclei extend into the base of the septum pellucidum. Despite their relatively small size, the septal nuclei have been implicated in a myriad of functions in animal models on the basis of the patterns of their inputs and outputs. In contrast, there is little clinical information regarding their function in humans. Rage behavior has been seen in a small group of patients with midline infarcts in this area.

The principal afferent pathways to the septal nuclei include fibers from the hippocampus (via the fornix), the amygdaloid complex (via the stria terminalis and ventral amygdalofugal pathways), and the ventral tegmental area of the midbrain

(Fig. 31-7A). Fibers also originate from the preoptic, anterior, and paraventricular hypothalamic nuclei and from the lateral hypothalamic area. Many of the fibers in the stria terminalis and fornix also send branches into the nucleus accumbens.

The main efferent projections from the septal nuclei (Fig. 31-7A) are septohippocampal fibers (in the fornix), projections to the habenular nuclei, the medial thalamic nuclei (via the stria medullaris thalami), and the ventral tegmental area (via the medial forebrain bundle). The preoptic, anterior, and ventromedial nuclei and the lateral hypothalamic areas also receive input from the septal nuclei.

The *medial forebrain bundle* is a diffuse group of fibers that courses rostrocaudally through the lateral hypothalamic area (Fig. 31-7A). This bundle is complex in that it conveys ascending inputs into the hypothalamus and through this area into the septal region. It also is a major conduit through which the septal nuclei and portions of the hypothalamus communicate with the brainstem (Fig. 30-7). The dopamine-containing fibers in this area are thought to be related to perceptions of pleasure or drive reduction.

Nucleus Accumbens

The nucleus accumbens (nucleus accumbens septi) is located in the rostral and ventral forebrain where the head of the caudate nucleus and the putamen are continuous (see Fig. 26-3). These cells receive input from the amygdaloid complex (primarily via the ventral amygdalofugal pathway), from the hippocampal formation (through the precommissural fornix), and from cells of the bed nucleus of the stria terminalis (Fig. 31-7B). The ventral tegmental area also gives rise to ascending fibers that enter the nucleus accumbens via the medial forebrain bundle. In addition, amygdalofugal fibers traversing the stria terminalis also enter the nucleus accumbens.

Cells within the nucleus accumbens have receptors for a variety of neurotransmitters, including endogenous opiates. Studies in animal models indicate that the nucleus accumbens may play an important role in behaviors related to addiction. Recent observations in addicted humans likewise reinforce the concept that nucleus accumbens is a gratification site. These patients show marked binding of substances to cells in nucleus accumbens.

Efferent projections of the nucleus accumbens include fibers to the hypothalamus, nuclei of the brainstem, and the globus pallidus (Fig. 31-7B). Nucleus accumbens fibers to the latter target represent an important route through which the limbic system may access the motor system.

Limbic System and Emotions

In recent years, the term *limbic system* has been used mainly in reference to emotion-related areas of the brain and the pathways that interconnect them. These areas are generally composed of sites that function to alter the emotions. These sites, which are often interspersed in a given region of the brain, are frequently called either *aversion centers* or *gratification centers*. If an aversion center is stimulated, the person will experience fear or sorrow. On the other hand, stimulation of a gratification center will result in pleasure. Functional interconnections between aversion and gratifications centers probably contribute to emotional stability.

Although most limbic structures contain both gratification and aversion centers, in some structures one or the other type of center seems to predominate. For example, the hippocampus and amygdala have an abundance of aversion centers, whereas the nucleus accumbens contains an abundance of gratification centers. Consequently, stimulation of the amygdala may elicit fear, whereas stimulation of the nucleus accumbens results in feelings of joy or pleasure.

The emotion-related deficits resulting from small lesions in the limbic system are difficult to predict. However, the effects of relatively large lesions are more stereotypic. They typically result in the flattening of emotions, as reflected by the fact that emotional extremes (joy and anxiety) are reduced. This phenomenon, presumably resulting from the loss of both aversion and gratification centers, commonly results from large lesions in the amygdala, hippocampus, fornix, or cingulate or prefrontal cortices.

Limbic System and Cognitive Function

There is a trend to look at the limbic system as a set of structures that influence not only emotion per se but also cognitive functions. The area on which there is the most agreement in this regard is memory. Other influences, however, are mediated through the nucleus basalis and are undoubtedly related to the control of cortical excitability. The full contribution of this upstream control is related to the transfer of information from limbic structures to the cerebral cortex. The manner in which limbic structures and the cortex interact is undergoing extensive revision. We know that visual information enters the entorhinal cortex by first synapsing in the perirhinal cortex (area 35) of the proisocortex. Thus, visual place memories are formed in the hippocampus by specific pathways only recently elaborated. Undoubtedly, other sensory modalities enter the hippocampus through similar transitional regions. Such inputs can perhaps account for the cognitive deficits seen following selective limbic system damage.

Synopsis of Clinical Points

- Circuits within the brain presumably associated with emotions and/or emotional behavior were proposed by James Papez (p. 502).
- Regions of the cerebral cortex designated as the limbic cortex, as broadly defined, are characterized as having three (archicortex) or five (paleocortex) cytoarchitectural layers (p. 502).
- The blood supply to the limbic cortex and system originates from a variety of sources (p. 503).
- The hippocampal formation is archicortex; the adjacent entorhinal cortex is paleocortex (p. 503).
- The circuit of Papez interconnects thalamic and cortical structures (p. 505).
- Bilateral damage to the hippocampal formation may profoundly impair the ability of the patient to consolidate immediate- and short-term memory into long-term memory (p. 506).
- A patient with Alzheimer disease may have a progressive loss of memory and cognitive dysfunction (p. 506).
- A patient with the Korsakoff syndrome may appear demented but is actually suffering a memory deficit (p. 506).
- Individuals with a thiamine deficiency, as is characteristic of chronic alcoholics, have memory deficits (p. 506).
- Confabulation is the creation of an artificial memory (p. 506).
- A patient with Wernicke-Korsakoff syndrome has memory losses and learning difficulties accompanied by motor deficits (p. 506).
- Bilateral lesions in the anterior portions of the cingulate gyrus may result in akinetic mutism (p. 506).
- Bilateral damage to the temporal lobes that largely abolish the amygdaloid complex result in the Klüver-Bucy syndrome (p. 509).
- The Klüver-Bucy syndrome is mainly characterized by visual agnosia, hyperorality, hypermetamorphosis, hyperphagia, placidity, and hypersexuality (p. 509).
- A compulsion to examine objects by placing them in the mouth is hyperorality (p. 509).
- A compulsion to examine the details of one's immediate environment is hypermetamorphosis (p. 509).
- A patient with bilateral temporal lobe lesions, in addition to the Klüver-Bucy syndrome, may also experience amnesia, aphasia, and/or dementia depending on the extent of the lesion (p. 509).
- Uncinate fits are seizures that originate in the area of the uncus and have olfactory and gustatory components (p. 509).
- Uncinate fits are also called complex partial seizures (p. 509).

Sources and Additional Reading

Hodges JR, Patterson K: Is semantic memory consistently impaired early in the course of Alzheimer's disease? Neuroanatomical and diagnostic implications. Neuropsychologia 33:441-459, 1995.

Isaacson RL: The Limbic System. New York, Plenum Press, 1974.

Kalivas PW, Barnes CD (eds): Limbic Motor Circuits and Neuropsychiatry. Boca Raton, FL, CRC Press, 1993.

Kötter R, Meyer N: The limbic system: A review of its empirical foundation. Behav Brain Res 52:105-127, 1992.

Masliah E, Mallory M, Hansen L, DeTeresa R, Alford M, Terry R: Synaptic and neuritic alterations during the progression of Alzheimer's disease. Neurosci Lett 174:67-72, 1994.

Nauta WJH: Hippocampal projections and related neural pathways to the midbrain in the cat. Brain 81:319-340, 1958.

Reep R: Relationship between prefrontal and limbic cortex: A comparative anatomical review. Brain Behav Evol 25:5-80, 1984.

Sandner G, Oberling P, Silveira MC, Di Scala G, Rocha B, Bagri A, Depoortere R: What brain structures are active during emotions? Effects of brain stimulation elicited aversion on c-fos immunoreactivity and behavior. Behav Brain Res 58:9-18, 1993.

Squire LR: Memory and Brain. New York, Oxford University Press, 1987.

Zola-Morgan S, Squire LR, Amaral DG: Human amnesia and the medial temporal region: Enduring memory impairment following a bilateral lesion limited to field CA1 of the hippocampus. J Neurosci 6:2950-2967, 1986.

The Cerebral Cortex

J. C. Lynch

The cerebral cortex is the organ of thought. More than any other part of the nervous system, the cerebral cortex is the site of the intellectual functions that make us human and that make each of us a unique individual. These intellectual functions include the ability to use language and logic and to exercise imagination and judgment.

Overview

The cerebral cortex is a dense aggregation of neuron cell bodies that ranges from 2 to 4 mm in thickness and forms the surface of each cerebral hemisphere. The total area of the cerebral cortex is about 2500 cm², a little larger than a single page of a newspaper. Neurons in the cortex receive input from many subcortical structures by way of the thalamus and also from other regions of the cortex via association fibers. Cortical neurons, in turn, project to a wide range of neural structures, including other areas of the cerebral cortex, the thalamus, the basal nuclei, the cerebellum via the pontine nuclei, many of the brainstem nuclei, and the spinal cord.

The cerebral cortex is divided into distinct functional areas, some of which are devoted to the processing of incoming sensory information, others to the organization of motor activity, and still others primarily to what are considered "higher intellectual functions." These functions include memory, judgment, the planning of complex activities, the processing of language, mathematical calculations, and the construction of an internal image of an individual's surroundings. In this chapter the focus is on (1) the basic internal organization of the cerebral cortex at the cellular level, (2) the parceling of the cortex into distinct subregions on the basis of cellular organization and neural connections, and (3) the functional properties of some higher-order association cortical regions.

Histology of the Cerebral Cortex

The gray matter of the cerebral cortex is composed of neuron cell bodies of variable sizes and shapes, intermixed with myelinated and unmyelinated fibers (Figs. 32-1 and 32-2A). These cell bodies may be visualized with stains that bind to the rough endoplasmic reticulum (Nissl substance). Such stains leave the axons and dendrites almost invisible. Substances that bind to the lipoprotein of the myelin sheath surrounding some axons will make the myelinated portion of the fibers visible (Figs. 32-1 and 32-2B). Yet another way of looking at cortical cells is to immerse small blocks of tissue in dilute silver salts, which precipitate on the membranes of the entire neuron. This reaction causes the cell body, its dendrites, and portions of the axon to become visible (Fig. 32-2C); this technique is called the *Golgi method*. The basic connections of a given region of cortex include *projection fibers* to subcortical structures, *callosal fibers* to cortex in the opposite hemisphere, *association fibers* to cortex in the same hemisphere, and *thalamocortical fibers*, which provide virtually all of the neural input to the cortex that originates in noncortical structures (Fig. 32-1).

The pattern of distribution of neuron cell bodies is, in general, called *cytoarchitecture*. Specifically, the cytoarchitecture of the cerebral cortex is characterized by layers. Most of the cerebral cortex has six distinct layers of neurons and is classified as *neocortex*. Two regions of the cerebral cortex have fewer than six layers. The first contains only three layers, is classified as *archicortex*, and includes the hippocampal formation. The second contains from three to five layers, is classified as *paleocortex*, and includes the olfactory sensory area and the nearby entorhinal and periamygdaloid cortices. The following discussion concentrates primarily on the neocortex.

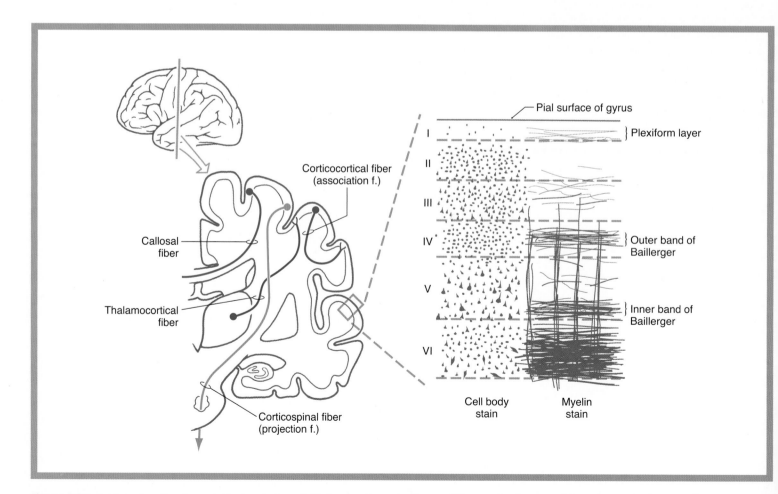

Figure 32-1. A coronal section through the hemisphere *(left)* showing the major types of fibers projecting to and from the cerebral cortex. The representation on the *right* shows layers (I to VI) of the cerebral cortex as they appear after staining for cell bodies of the myelin sheath.

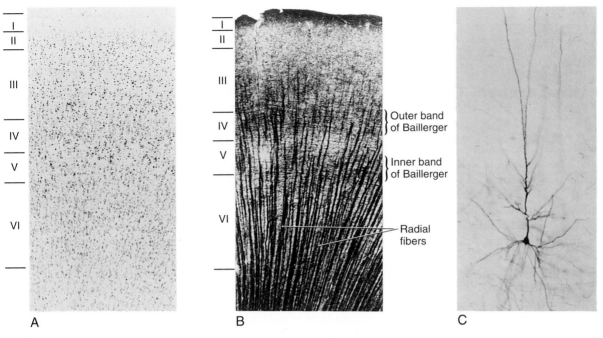

Figure 32-2. Nissl (**A**) and myelin (**B**) stains of adjacent sections of the human cerebral cortex and a Golgi impregnation (**C**) of a pyramidal neuron in the primate neocortex. (**A** and **B** courtesy of Drs. Grayzna Rajkowska and Patricia Goldman-Rakic, University of Mississippi Medical Center and Yale University; **C** courtesy of Dr. José Rafols, Wayne State University.)

Layers of the Cerebral Cortex

The neuronal layers in the neocortex are designated by Roman numerals, beginning at the pial surface (Fig. 32-1). There are six layers in the neocortex, with three of these layers being subdivided based on their architectural features.

Layer I, the *molecular layer*, contains very few neuron cell bodies and consists primarily of axons running parallel (horizontal) to the surface of the cortex. The apical dendrites of cells located in deeper layers also ramify within layer I.

Layer II, the *external granular layer*, is composed of a mixture of small neurons called *granule cells* and slightly larger neurons, which are called *pyramidal cells* based on the shape of their cell body. The apical dendrites of these pyramidal cells extend into layer I and their axons descend into, and through, the deeper cortical layers.

Layer III, the *external pyramidal layer*, contains primarily small- to medium-sized pyramidal cells, along with some neurons of other types. In general the smaller pyramidal cells are sequestered in the outer, or superficial, portion of layer III while the larger pyramidal cells are located in the inner, or deeper, portion of this layer. Their apical dendrites ascend into layer I and their axons descend into, and through, the deeper layers.

Layer IV, the *internal granular layer*, consists almost exclusively of *smooth (aspiny) stellate (star-like) neurons* and *spiny stellate neurons*, both of which have sometimes been categorized as "granule cells." This layer is free of pyramidal-shaped cells. It can be divided into outer (IVa) and inner (IVb) portions in many neocortical areas and into three portions (IVa, IVb, IVc) in the primary visual cortex. Layer IV is the primary target for ascending sensory information from the thalamus.

Layer V, the *internal pyramidal layer*, consists predominantly of medium to large pyramidal cells. Apical dendrites of the medium pyramidal cells may extend upward one or two layers while those of the large pyramidal cells extend outward to layer I. The large pyramidal cells of this layer are a major source of cortical efferent fibers including axons to the basal nuclei, brainstem, and spinal cord. Some corticocortical axons also originate in layer V. These are probably collateral branches of axons that are projecting to some subcortical target.

Layer VI, the *multiform layer*, contains an assortment of neuron types including some with *pyramidal* and *fusiform* cell bodies. The dendrites of the larger cells extend into layer I while those arising from the smaller cells usually extend no farther than layer IV. The axons of the cells of this layer project to subcortical targets, such as the thalamus, and to other cortical regions as corticocortical connections.

Two features of the myelinated fibers in the neocortex are noteworthy. First, there are prominent plexuses of horizontally running myelinated fibers in layers IV and V. These are called the *outer* and *inner bands of Baillerger*, respectively (Fig. 32-1). In the primary visual cortex, bordering on the calcarine sulcus, the outer band of Baillerger is greatly expanded. This band can be seen with the naked eye in fresh and stained sections and is called the *stria (line) of Gennari* (see Fig. 20-17). Second, in most regions of the neocortex, there are many radially oriented bundles of axons passing between the subcortical white matter and various parts of the cortex or between inner and outer cortical layers (Fig. 32-2B).

Neurotransmitters of the Cerebral Cortex

There are a variety of neuroactive substances associated with neurons of the cerebral cortex. Principal among these are *glutamate, aspartate*, and *γ-aminobutyric acid* (GABA). Pyramidal cells are the efferent neurons of the cerebral cortex. They are predominantly *glutaminergic* and are excitatory to their targets. Most interneurons within the cortex are *GABAergic* and are inhibitory. The pyramidal cells of the cortex, and therefore the output of the cortex, are modulated by a variety of cortical afferents. The influence of these afferent fibers is to act on pyramidal cells either directly or via interneurons. A variety of *neuropeptides (monoamines)* are also found in the cerebral cortex; they influence not only populations of neurons but also local metabolic activity and vascular smooth muscle. The most important monoamines in the cortex are (1) *norepinephrine*, which originates from the locus ceruleus of the pons and distributes sparsely to all cortical layers, (2) *dopamine*, which arises from the substantia nigra–pars compacta and the adjacent ventral tegmental area and is found in moderate amounts in layers I and VI and sparsely in II-V, and (3) *serotonin*, which arises from the raphe nuclei and distributes heavily to all cortical layers.

Neuron Types in the Cerebral Cortex

Pyramidal Cells
The most common type of neuron in the cerebral cortex is the pyramidal cell (Figs. 32-2 and 32-3A). Pyramidal cells are found in all layers of the cortex with the exception of the molecular layer (layer I), and they are the predominant cell type in layers II, III, and V (Fig. 32-4). Pyramidal cells are characterized by (1) a roughly triangular cell body; (2) a single large *apical dendrite* that arises from the apex of the cell body and usually extends toward the molecular layer, giving off branches along the way; (3) an array of *basal dendrites* that run in a predominantly horizontal direction; and (4) an axon that originates from the base of the soma, leaves the cortex, and passes through the white matter.

The cell bodies of most pyramidal neurons range in size from 10 to 50 μm in height. The largest, called *giant pyramidal cells of Betz* or *Betz cells*, are found almost exclusively in the primary motor cortex, which is located in the precentral and anterior paracentral gyri. Their somata may reach 100 μm in height. Betz cells are most common in the region of motor cortex that projects to the anterior horn of the lumbar spinal cord and hence are concerned with the control of leg movement. These cells are so large that they can be distinguished with the naked eye in Nissl-stained sections of the human brain.

Both apical and basal dendrites of pyramidal cells are characterized by membrane specializations called *dendritic spines*. These spines are small outgrowths from the dendrite that give

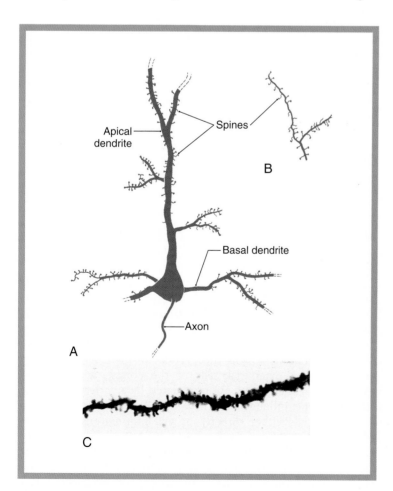

Figure 32-3. Examples of spines on basal and apical dendrites (**A** and **C**) and on the terminal ramifications of apical dendrites (**B**).

the impression of thorns on a rose bush (Fig. 32-3). The vast majority of synaptic contacts received by a pyramidal cell are located on dendritic spines rather than directly on the dendrite shaft or on the cell body.

Pyramidal neurons represent virtually the only output pathway for the cerebral cortex. Almost all other cell types in the cortex are local circuit neurons that exert their influence within their own immediate vicinity. Axons of pyramidal cells may terminate in another region of the cortex in the same hemisphere *(association fibers)*, decussate in the corpus callosum to terminate in the cerebral cortex of the opposite hemisphere *(callosal fibers)*, or course through the white matter to any of the numerous subcortical targets in the forebrain, brainstem, or spinal cord *(projection fibers)*.

Pyramidal cells display a laminar organization, with the cell bodies in a given layer projecting to specific neural targets (Fig. 32-4). In general, pyramidal neurons in layers II and III give rise to association and callosal fibers. Pyramidal cells in layer V project to many subcortical structures, including the spinal cord, as projection fibers. The neurons in layer VI send their axons to a variety of locations, including thalamic nuclei and other regions of cortex. Within the cortex, axons of pyramidal cells send off an extensive and relatively dense array of *axon collaterals*. These collaterals terminate in all cortical layers and extend through a horizontal area covering several millimeters around the cell body (Fig. 32-5).

Local Circuit Neurons
As mentioned previously, all the various nonpyramidal neurons of the cerebral cortex function as cortical *interneurons;* that is, their axons do not leave the immediate region of the cell body. These cells are often referred to as *local circuit neurons* or *intrinsic cortical neurons.*

Santiago Ramón y Cajal, working in the late 1800s and early 1900s, described a rich variety of intrinsic cortical neurons. However, by the 1950s it had become customary to refer to virtually all intrinsic cortical neurons as *stellate cells*, even though many were not actually star shaped. Now the pendulum has swung in the other direction, and a number of distinct morphologic types are recognized. Some of the more important of these are illustrated in Figure 32-4: *spiny* and *aspiny stellate cells*, *basket cells*, and *chandelier cells*.

Three types of intrinsic neurons receive thalamocortical axon terminals in layer IV: the *small spiny cells*, the *aspiny stellate cells*, and dendrites of the *large basket cells*. Of these, the spiny cells are believed to be excitatory, whereas basket cells and aspiny stellate cells use the neurotransmitter GABA and are thus considered to be inhibitory interneurons. Most other intrinsic neurons are presumed to be inhibitory. On the other hand, pyramidal neurons are uniformly associated with excitatory neurotransmitters, *glutamate* and *aspartate* in particular.

Laminar Organization

Intrinsic Circuitry of the Cerebral Cortex
The *basic framework* of the internal circuit diagram of small regions of the cerebral cortex is well understood. In contrast, the *details* of this circuitry are only partially known and are in fact so complex as to defy the construction of a detailed circuit diagram like those used to represent a computer's electronic hardware. For example, a single axon may branch repeatedly and contact hundreds of other neurons. A single neuron may also receive synaptic contacts from thousands of other neurons. Within a small volume of cortex, there may be *millions* of neurons.

The basic framework of cortical circuitry consists of afferent fibers, local circuits for the processing of this afferent information, and efferent fibers that convey the processed information

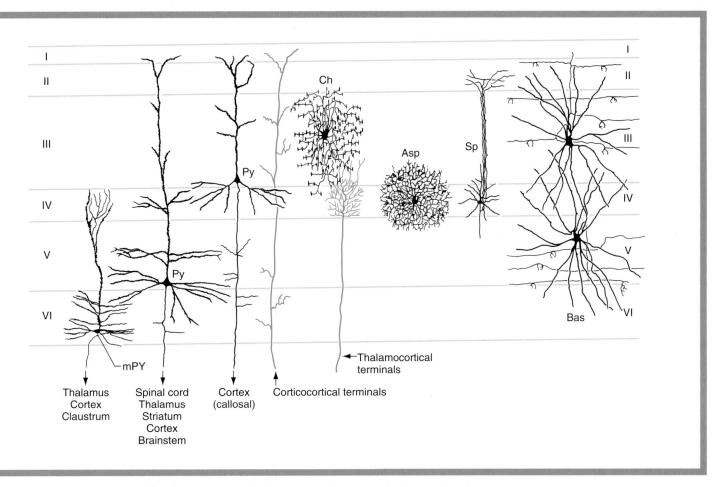

Figure 32-4. Representative cell types in the cerebral cortex and the layers in which their cell bodies and dendrites are found. Dendrites of pyramidal cells (Py) of layers II, III, and V extend into layer I, whereas those of modified pyramidal cells (mPy) in layer VI extend only to about layer IV. Chandelier cells (Ch) are restricted almost entirely to layer III. The somata of aspiny and spiny stellate neurons (Asp, Sp) are in layer IV, although their processes extend into other layers. Basket cells (Bas) have processes that collectively extend into all cortical layers from cell bodies located mainly in layers III and V. (Adapted from Hendry SHC, Jones EG: Sizes and distributions of intrinsic neurons incorporating tritiated GABA in monkey sensory-motor cortex. J Neurosci 1:390-408, 1981 and from Jones EG: Laminar distribution of cortical efferent cells. In Cerebral Cortex, vol 1. New York, Plenum Press, 1984, pp 521-553, with permission.)

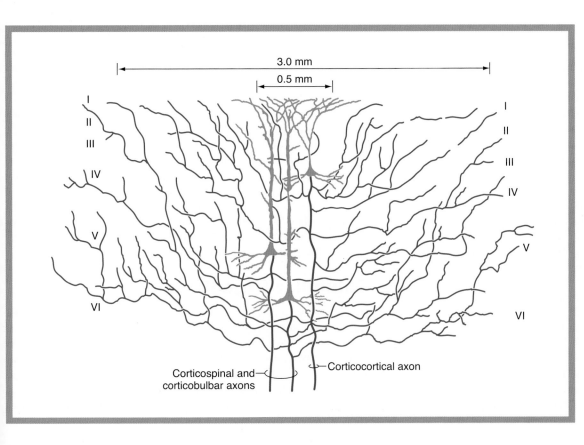

Figure 32-5. The cell bodies and dendrites (in *red*) of three pyramidal cells in the cerebral cortex compared with the intracortical distribution of axons (in *blue*) arising from these cells. Axon collaterals distribute over a much wider area than do the dendrites arising from the same cell. (Adapted from Scheibel ME, Scheibel AB: Elementary processes in selected thalamic and cortical subsystems-the structural substrates. In The Neurosciences, Second Study Programs, vol 2. New York, Rockefeller University Press, 1970, pp 443-457, with permission.)

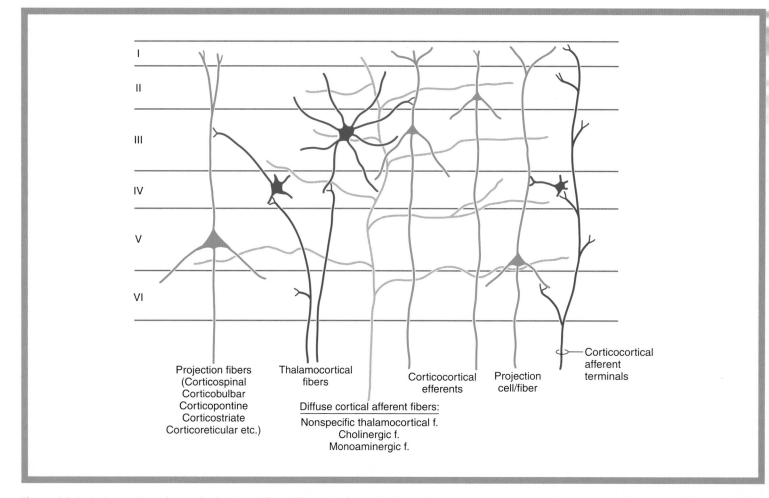

Figure 32-6. Basic circuits in the cerebral cortex. Afferent fibers are shown in *blue* and *gray,* interneurons in *green,* and efferent fibers in *red.* Thalamocortical fibers terminate primarily in layer IV, whereas corticocortical fibers and diffuse cortical afferents synapse in all layers. Pyramidal cells in the outer layers give rise to corticocortical projections, and those in layer V project to a wide range of subcortical targets.

to another site (Fig. 32-6). Thalamocortical axons terminate primarily in layer IV and to a lesser extent in layers III and VI. In layer IV, they terminate on excitatory and inhibitory interneurons as well as on dendrites from neurons in other layers (Fig. 32-4). The axons of interneurons, in turn, may end on dendrites of pyramidal cells or of other interneurons. The local processing of information culminates in connections to pyramidal cells, which carry the information to other cortical or subcortical regions. A copy of the information also goes to neurons in the immediate vicinity via *axon collaterals* (Fig. 32-5).

The general pattern of termination of *corticocortical* axons is quite different from that of thalamocortical axons. Corticocortical axons branch repeatedly and make synaptic contacts on neurons in *all* layers of the cortex (Fig. 32-4).

The cerebral cortex receives a third set of inputs, called *diffuse inputs*, which consists of fibers that branch extensively and end diffusely over a wide area of cortex without respect for cytoarchitectural boundaries (Fig. 32-6). These inputs arise from a variety of sources, including certain *nonspecific nuclei of the thalamus* (for example, the ventral anterior, central lateral, and midline nuclei), the *locus ceruleus,* and the *basal nucleus (of Meynert)*. These structures are generally concerned with regulating overall levels of cortical excitability and the associated phenomena of arousal, sleep, and wakefulness.

Cytoarchitecture

The cytoarchitecture of cortex differs from one area to another in ways that are related to function (Fig. 32-7). In primary sensory cortex, layer IV, the major *input* layer of cortex, is especially thick, whereas layer V, the major *projection layer,* is

narrow and indistinct. Cortex with this pattern is called *heterotypical granular cortex.* In primary motor cortex, the pattern is reversed: layer IV is almost invisible, and layer V is very thick, seeming to merge directly with layer III. Thus, the *projection* layer is prominent and the *input* layer is small. Cortex of this type is called *heterotypical agranular cortex.* In most other areas of the neocortex, including the association cortices, the six layers are all clearly represented and are of roughly equal thickness. This type of cortex is called *homotypical.*

The cerebral cortex has been subdivided on the basis of cytoarchitectural differences by many different investigators. The most famous of these, Korbinian Brodmann, worked in the early part of the 20th century. He identified 47 distinct areas (Fig. 32-8), and his numbering scheme is still in common use today in both research and clinical settings. For example, the primary visual cortex is Brodmann area 17, and the primary motor cortex is area 4. In most instances, Brodmann cytoarchitectural areas are coextensive with cortical regions that have specific functional characteristics.

Columnar Organization

A second, vertical pattern of organization is superimposed on the horizontal layered pattern described earlier. Unlike the cortical layers, this vertical pattern is not immediately obvious in histologic sections stained for neuron cell bodies (Nissl stains). However, when Golgi-stained material is studied, it is clear that neurons are often grouped together so that their cell bodies, axons, and apical dendrites form clusters that are oriented at right angles to the surface of the cortex.

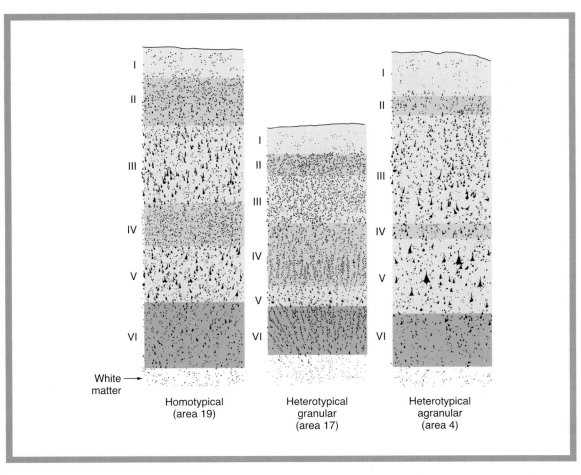

Figure 32-7. Typical cytoarchitectural patterns for homotypical, heterotypical granular, and heterotypical agranular regions. (Adapted from Campbell AW: *Histological Studies on the Localization of Cerebral Function.* Cambridge, Cambridge University Press, 1905.)

Mountcastle was the first to demonstrate physiologically the existence of a vertical ("columnar") organization in the cerebral cortex by recording the activity of hundreds of individual neurons in the primary somatosensory cortex of cats and monkeys. Within an area of cortex a few millimeters in diameter, all neurons had overlapping or adjacent receptive fields. For example, in one cortical region, all neurons might have receptive fields on a finger, whereas in a nearby region, the neurons might have receptive fields on the wrist. Within a cortical region in which all neurons had about the same receptive field, the neurons responded to different *sensory submodalities*. Some neurons were activated by light touch on the skin, others by joint rotation, and still others by strong pressure on deep tissue. However, when a microelectrode was inserted at right angles to the surface of the cortex, all the neurons encountered were activated by only one of these submodalities (Fig. 32-9B). In contrast, when a microelectrode was moved parallel or obliquely relative to the surface of the cortex, it encountered neurons of different submodalities as it moved from one functionally related group of neurons to another (Fig. 32-9A).

The basis of columnar organization in primary sensory cortices is selective input from relay nuclei of the thalamus. Obviously, if all of the cells in one column respond to maintained pressure on the skin while the cells in an adjacent column respond to joint position, the signals from the respective sensory receptors must have been continuously segregated all the way from the periphery through the posterior column nuclei and the ventrobasal complex of the thalamus to terminate in the cortex.

The anatomic basis of the *columnar organization* of the cortex is understood in the greatest detail in the visual cortex. In this region, at least three types of regularly repeating features are superimposed on the laminar patterns of neurons: the stimulus orientation columns, the ocular dominance columns, and the cytochrome oxidase-rich blobs. These features are discussed in detail in Chapter 20.

The ocular dominance columns in the visual cortex provide a clear example of the role of thalamic input in columnar organization. Neurons in the layers of the lateral geniculate nucleus that receive input from the right eye send their axons to layer IV of the right eye–dominant columns (Fig. 32-10). Here, the axons terminate predominantly on spiny and aspiny stellate cells, which, in turn, project to pyramidal cells. Collaterals of pyramidal cell axons provide one pathway by which neural signals can spread from one column to influence activity in adjacent columns (Fig. 32-5). This influence may be either excitatory via direct connections or inhibitory via interneurons. The right eye, therefore, has a direct and strong influence on neurons in right-eye–dominant columns (R_L in Fig. 32-10) and an indirect and weaker influence on neurons in the adjacent left-eye–dominant columns (L_R in Fig. 32-10).

Connections between one region of the cortex and another, through either association fibers or callosal fibers, may also be arranged in a columnar pattern. For example, axons that originate in the inferior parietal lobule terminate in multiple columns in the ipsilateral and contralateral cingulate cortices. Columns of corticocortical axon terminals that originate in different functional regions may either overlap each other or interdigitate with each other.

Synopsis of Thalamocortical Relationships

The details of thalamocortical projections are described in the chapters devoted to specific systems. At this juncture, however, it is appropriate to briefly review what areas of the cortex

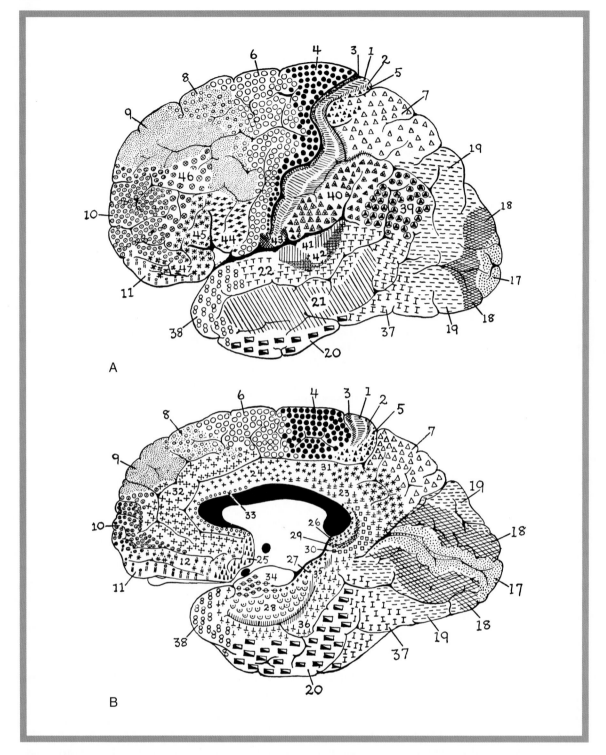

Figure 32-8. Cytoarchitectural map showing Brodmann areas on the lateral (**A**) and medial (**B**) surfaces of the hemisphere. (Modified after Brodmann K, from Carpenter MB, Sutin J: Human Neuroanatomy. Baltimore, Williams & Wilkins, 1983, with permission.)

are functionally related to which of the thalamic nuclei (Fig. 32-11).

The cortex of the frontal lobe encompasses Brodmann areas 4, 6, 8 to 12, 32, and 44 to 47 (Fig. 32-8). The primary somatomotor cortex (area 4) and the premotor and supplementary motor cortices (area 6) receive input mainly from the ventral lateral nucleus of the thalamus and subserve important motor functions. Lateral, medial, and orbital aspects of the frontal lobe receive thalamocortical fibers mainly from the dorsomedial and anterior nuclei of the thalamus (Fig. 32-11). These latter cortical areas, through a variety of direct and indirect connections, relate primarily to functions of the limbic system. Of particular note are the pars orbitalis and pars triangularis of the inferior frontal gyrus, damage to which results in Broca aphasia (discussed below).

Areas 3, 1, 2, 5, 7, 39, 40, and 43 are located in the parietal lobe (Fig. 32-8). The primary somatosensory cortex (areas 3, 1, and 2) receives inputs from the ventral posterolateral and ventral posteromedial nuclei. These thalamic nuclei receive a full range of somatosensory input through synaptic relays in the spinal cord and brainstem and transmit this information to the cerebral cortex. The inferior parietal lobule comprises, in general, areas 39 and 40. Along with area 22, these areas are the cortical regions associated with Wernicke aphasia (discussed below).

The occipital and temporal lobes encompass areas 17 to 22, 36 to 38, and 41 and 42 (Fig. 32-8). These areas of the cortex, plus portions of the parietal lobe, have extensive connections with the pulvinar nucleus of the thalamus and are involved in the processing of visual and auditory information at several different

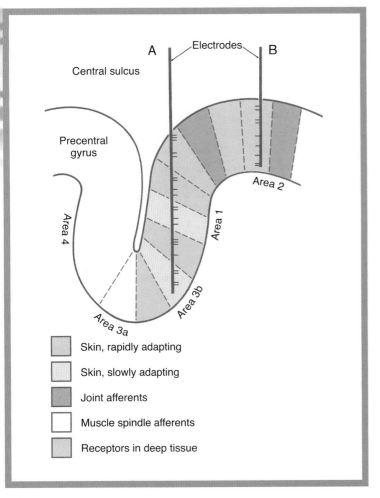

Figure 32-9. Diagrammatic section through the precentral and postcentral gyri showing the organization of columns in the somatosensory cortex. The columns are shown as colored compartments oriented, in general, perpendicular to the surface of the cortex. An electrode (at A) passing parallel to the surface of the cortex will pass through several columns with resultant recordings of the several modalities represented by the types of afferent information arriving at each column. An electrode passing through one column (at B) passing perpendicular to the surface of the cortex penetrates only a single column. Therefore, it records activity related to the single submodality received by that column.

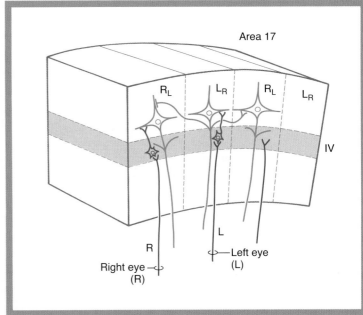

Figure 32-10. Functional columnar organization of sensory cortices, using the visual cortex (ocular dominance columns) as an example. Axons from the layers of the lateral geniculate nucleus related to the right (R) and left (L) eyes terminate in alternating columns. In right eye–dominant columns (R_L), cortical neurons are influenced predominantly by visual stimulation of the right retina, although they are also influenced to a lesser degree by stimulation of the left retina. The reverse is true for left eye–dominant columns (L_R). The neurons in each column influence the adjacent columns (dominant for the other eye) via axon collaterals of pyramidal cells or through the action of cortical interneurons. In general, other sensory cortices are organized similarly in regard to their sensory inputs.

functional levels (Fig. 32-11). Located in this geographic area are the primary sensory cortices for vision and hearing. Area 17, on the banks of the calcarine sulcus, is the primary visual cortex; areas 41 and 42, in the depth of the lateral fissure in the transverse temporal gyri, constitute the primary auditory cortex (Fig. 32-8). These cortical areas receive input from the lateral and medial geniculate nuclei of the thalamus, respectively.

The limbic lobe, which forms the most medial edge of the hemisphere, contains areas 23 to 31 and 33 to 35. The cingulate cortex receives fibers primarily from the anterior nucleus of the thalamus but also from the lateral dorsal nucleus (Fig. 32-11). Other regions of the limbic lobe have some connections with the dorsomedial nucleus. However, many of the subcortical targets of the parahippocampal and uncal cortices are structures such as the hippocampal formation. This area, in turn, projects to a variety of thalamic and basal forebrain targets.

Blood Supply to the Cerebral Cortex

The blood supply to the cerebral cortex and to subcortical structures of the telencephalon, including the internal capsule, is discussed in Chapters 8 and 16. In this section the general nature of these patterns is summarized.

The cerebral cortex is served, in toto, by the *anterior, middle,* and *posterior cerebral arteries.* The anterior and middle cerebral arteries are the terminal branches of the internal carotid artery, and the posterior cerebral artery is formed by the bifurcation of the basilar artery (see Figs. 8-2, 8-6, 8-13).

The anterior cerebral artery is joined to its counterpart just anterior to the optic chiasm by the anterior communicating artery. Proximal to the anterior communicating artery the A_1 segment of the anterior cerebral artery gives rise to small branches that serve rostral portions of the hypothalamus and immediately adjacent optic structures. Segments of the anterior cerebral artery distal to the anterior communicating artery are A_2 (infracallosal), A_3 (precallosal), and $A_4 + A_5$ (supracallosal + postcallosal). Cortical branches of the anterior cerebral artery (A_2 to A_5) distribute to the medial surface of the hemisphere caudally to about the position of the parieto-occipital fissure. The distal portions of these branches arch over the edge of the hemisphere (from its medial to its lateral surface) for a short distance (see Figs. 8-3, 8-7, and 16-11). Located in the domain of the branches of this major vessel (especially segments $A_4 + A_5$) are the foot, lower extremity, and hip areas of the primary somatomotor and primary somatosensory cortices.

The middle cerebral artery passes laterally from its origin and branches, in general, into superior and inferior trunks (these are M_2 branches) over the insular cortex. These proceed as the M_3 segment over the inner surface of the operculum and exit the lateral sulcus to fan out as the cortical branches that collectively comprise the M_4 segment. Terminal branches of the superior and inferior trunks (as the M_4 segment) serve the cortex on the lateral surface of the hemisphere above and below the lateral fissure, respectively (see Figs. 8-9 and 16-11). In addition to lateral portions of the frontal cortex, parietal and temporal association cortices are served by branches of the middle cerebral

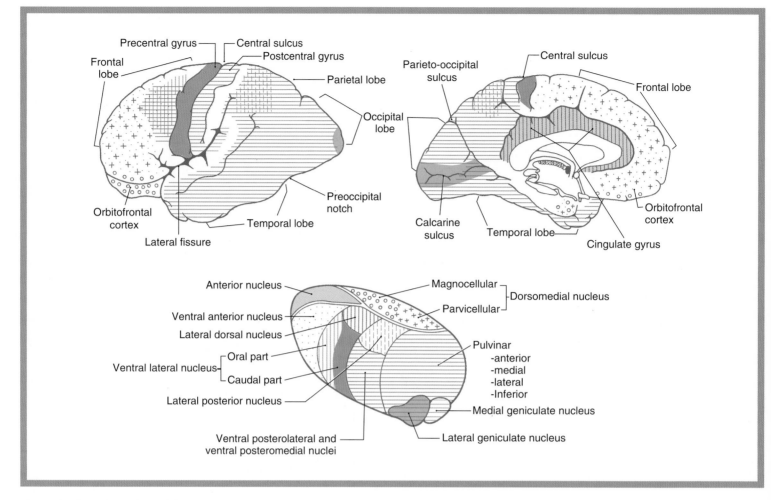

Figure 32-11. Relationships of the thalamic nuclei to the cerebral cortex as revealed by the patterns of thalamocortical connections. Each thalamic nucleus is pattern coded or color coded to match its target area in the cerebral cortex.

artery. Also located in the distribution area of this vessel are the trunk, upper extremity, and head regions of the primary somatomotor and primary somatosensory cortices (via branches of the superior trunk) and the primary auditory cortex (inferior trunk).

The cortex forming the inferior surface of the temporal lobe and the medial aspect of the occipital lobe is served by branches of the posterior cerebral artery (see Figs. 8-5, 8-13, and 16-11). As with the anterior cerebral artery, the terminal rami of the posterior cerebral artery loop over the edge of the inferior and medial surface of the hemisphere to serve small portions of the lateral aspect of the hemisphere. The posterior cerebral artery serves large expanses of visual association cortex and some of the cortical structures associated with the limbic system. In addition, the calcarine artery supplies the primary visual cortex located on and in the banks of the calcarine sulcus.

The wedge-shaped areas of overlap between the distal branches of the anterior and middle cerebral arteries and the posterior and middle cerebral arteries form what are called *border zones* (see Fig. 8-14). These areas are particularly susceptible to hypoperfusion during episodes of systemic hypotension. Such events may result in *watershed infarcts*.

Higher Cortical Functions

The cerebral cortex is generally considered to be the seat of *higher intellectual functions*, those faculties of thought that have reached their most complex levels in humans. Although other brain structures, including the thalamus, corpus striatum, claustrum, and cerebellum, contribute to these functions, the *multimodal association cortex* is closely linked to the most complex intellectual functions, such as logical analysis, judgment, language, and imagination.

The cerebral cortex can be divided into four general functional categories: *sensory, motor, unimodal association cortex*, and *multimodal association cortex* (Fig. 32-12). The primary sensory areas, except that for olfaction, receive thalamocortical fibers from diencephalic relay nuclei that are functionally related to each modality. For example, the ventral posterior complex of the thalamus projects to primary somatosensory cortex (Brodmann areas 3, 1, and 2) in the postcentral gyrus. Similarly, the lateral geniculate nucleus projects to primary visual cortex (area 17) in the banks of the calcarine sulcus, and the medial geniculate nucleus projects to primary auditory cortex in the transverse temporal gyri (areas 41 and 42).

Adjacent to each primary sensory area is a region of cortex that is devoted to a higher level of information processing relevant to that specific sensory modality. These areas are called *unimodal association cortices* (Fig. 32-12). For example, *visual unimodal association cortex* (areas 18, 19, 20, 21, and 37) occupies all of the occipital lobe outside area 17 (the primary visual sensory area), as well as much of the inferior gyrus of the temporal lobe. Within these visual association areas the basic elements of visual sensation are molded into an overall perception of the visual world. Similarly, the *somatosensory association cortex* lies just posterior to the postcentral gyrus in area 5 and the *auditory association cortex* is in the superior temporal gyrus (area 22) next to primary auditory cortex. In all of these examples, the primary sensory cortices (i.e., areas 3, 1, 2; 17; and 41 and 42) receive input from their respective thalamic relay nuclei. In turn,

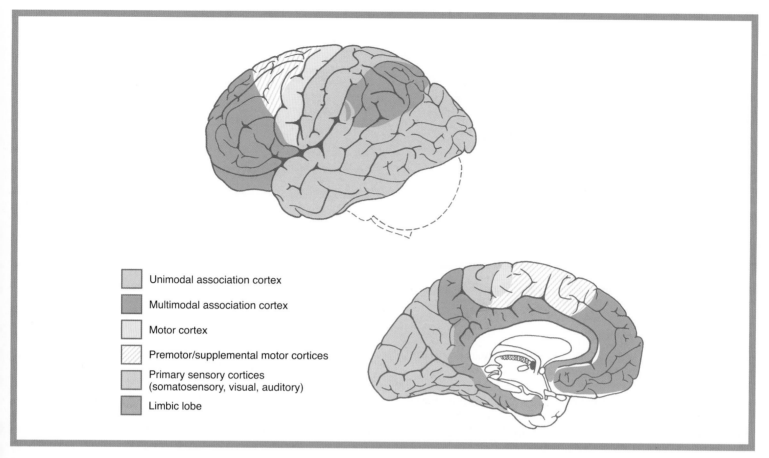

Figure 32-12. Primary motor and sensory *(blue)*, unimodal association *(green)*, and multimodal association *(pink)* areas of the cerebral cortex are shown on lateral *(upper)* and medial *(lower)* surfaces of the hemisphere.

Unimodal association cortex

Multimodal association cortex

Motor cortex

Premotor/supplemental motor cortices

Primary sensory cortices
(somatosensory, visual, auditory)

Limbic lobe

the primary sensory areas project, via corticocortical fibers, to their corresponding association cortices (i.e., areas 3, 1, 2 to area 5; area 17 to areas 18 and 19; and areas 41 and 42 to area 22).

The remaining portions of the cerebral cortex that are not motor in function are classified as *multimodal association cortex* (Fig. 32-12). These areas receive information from several different sensory modalities and create for us a complete experience of our surroundings. Multimodal association areas are critical to our ability to communicate using language, to use reason to extrapolate future events on the basis of present experience, to make complex and long-range plans, and to imagine and create things that have never existed. An example of long-range planning is going to college so you can go to medical school so you can do a residency and become a physician. This section concentrates on the cortical areas responsible for three of these higher functions: language, the appreciation of space, and the planning of behavior.

Dominant Hemisphere and Language
The cerebral hemisphere that controls language is called the *dominant hemisphere*. In the vast majority of people, language functions are processed in the *left hemisphere*. As evidence of this left brain dominance, brain lesions that adversely affect language are found in the left hemisphere in about 95% of cases. Almost all right-handed individuals and about half of left-handed individuals are *left cerebral dominant*. It follows that the right cerebral hemisphere, in most of the general population, is the *nondominant hemisphere*.

Language is the faculty of communication using symbols organized by a system of grammar to describe things and events and to express ideas. In humans, the senses of vision and audition are closely linked to language, but language itself transcends any particular sensory system. Helen Keller was blind and deaf but used language eloquently to communicate very complex

and subtle ideas. Language ability can be impaired selectively, with little or no change in the senses of vision or hearing, by brain damage in either the parietal-temporal junction or the frontal lobe. This impairment, termed *aphasia*, is a *disturbance of the comprehension and formulation of language, not a disorder of hearing, vision, or motor control.*

Wernicke and Broca Aphasia
The two classic types of aphasia are *Broca aphasia* and *Wernicke aphasia*. Broca aphasia, also termed *expressive aphasia* or *nonfluent aphasia*, consists of a loss of the ability to speak fluently. Lesions that produce this deficit are located in the inferior frontal gyrus of the *left hemisphere*, primarily in Brodmann areas 44 and 45 (Fig. 32-13). Wernicke aphasia is primarily a defect of the *comprehension* rather than the *expression* of language. This deficit is seen after injury to the supramarginal and angular gyri (areas 37, 39, and 40) and the posterior part of the superior temporal gyrus (area 22) in the *left hemisphere* (Fig. 32-13).

Patients with the most severe form of *Broca aphasia* are unable to speak *(mutism)*, although they are able to swallow and breathe normally and make guttural sounds. Their problem is not one of paralysis of the vocal apparatus. Rather, it is a difficulty in turning a concept or thought into a sequence of meaningful sounds. In less severe cases, or in patients in the recovery process, limited speech is possible. Short, habitual phrases such as "hi," "fine, thank you," and "yes" and "no" are the first to come back. However, speech is slow and labored, enunciation is poor, and nonessential words are commonly omitted *(telegraphic speech)*. Affected persons typically have as much difficulty with writing *(agraphia)* as with speaking. Although the patient is able to understand spoken or written language and can communicate verbally to some degree, the extremely laborious nature of the process of communication causes considerable frustration. Under

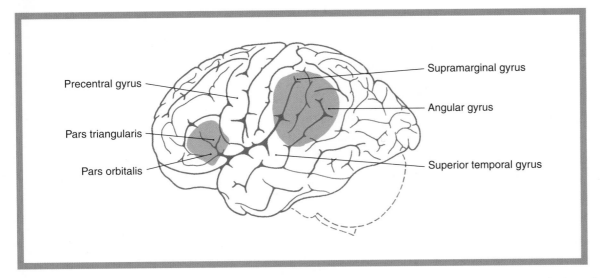

Figure 32-13. Cortical areas that mediate the processing of language. Lesions in the pars orbitalis and pars triangularis of the inferior frontal lobe will result in Broca aphasia, whereas damage in the supramarginal and angular gyri and adjacent superior temporal gyrus will result in Wernicke aphasia.

particular emotional stress, patients may use inappropriate or vulgar words or phrases to express their distress.

The most common causes of Broca aphasia are tumors and occlusions of frontal M_4 branches of the middle cerebral artery. Mild aphasia without other deficits indicates that the damage affects only cortical areas. However, full-blown Broca aphasia indicates that the damage extends beyond the Broca area of the cortex to include insular cortex and subjacent white matter. Patients typically have *contralateral motor signs and symptoms*, such as weakness *(paresis)* of the lower part of the face, lateral deviation of the tongue when protruded, and weakness of the arm. Aphasia plus these motor problems suggests an occlusion of branches from the proximal parts of the middle cerebral artery (M_1), including the lenticulostriate arteries, which serve the internal capsule (see Fig. 16-12).

The second major type of aphasia is *Wernicke aphasia* (also described as *receptive* or *fluent* aphasia). Patients with severe Wernicke aphasia (1) are unable to understand what is said to them; (2) are unable to read *(alexia)*; (3) are unable to write comprehensible language *(agraphia)*; and (4) display *fluent paraphasic speech*. Paraphasic speech refers to the ability of patients to produce clear, fluent, melodic speech at a normal or even faster than normal rate. The content of the speech, however, may be unintelligible because of frequent errors of word choice, inappropriate use of words, or use of made-up nonsense words. An example of this type of speech is "we went to drive in the bridge for red pymarids (sic) were crooking the lawn browsers." Such speech is sometimes called "word salad." In less severe cases, *paraphasias* frequently occur. For example, in trying to say "the cat has claws," the patient may use an incorrect but similar-sounding word ("the cat has clads"—a *literal paraphasia*) or a word that seems appropriate to the patient but is incorrect ("the cat has tires"—a *verbal paraphasia*). A surprising finding is that patients with Wernicke aphasia are much less aware of the extent of their disability than patients with Broca aphasia, and they are usually less frustrated and depressed about it. In contrast, patients with Broca aphasia are completely conscious of their communication problems and are often exceedingly frustrated or despairing.

Wernicke aphasia may result from occlusion of temporal and parietal M_4 branches of the middle cerebral artery. In addition, hemorrhage into the thalamus (or tumors in the thalamus) may produce Wernicke aphasia by extending laterally and caudally to invade the subcortical white matter. If this damage impinges on the Meyer loop and interrupts the optic radiations (see

Chapter 20), a contralateral homonymous hemianopia may accompany the patient's other disabilities.

Conduction and Global Aphasia

The severity and duration of the aphasia depend on the severity of the associated brain damage. In mild cases, only one or two symptoms may be discernible, and those may resolve quickly. A major stroke or severe traumatic injury, however, may produce a full-blown set of signs and symptoms that will never completely disappear.

Other, less common types of aphasia have also been described. These include *conduction aphasia*, which results from interruption of the connections linking the Broca and Wernicke areas. In this disorder, comprehension is normal and expression is fluent but the patient has difficulty translating what someone has said to him or her into an appropriate reply. A more profound disorder is *global aphasia*, which occurs when occlusion of the left internal carotid or the most proximal portion of the middle cerebral artery (M_1 segment) produces damage that encroaches on both the Broca and the Wernicke areas, and the loss of language is virtually complete.

Several additional points should be mentioned. First, damage to the basal nuclei, particularly to the head of the caudate on the *left side*, has been associated with language disorders similar to Wernicke aphasia. Second, although we have referred so far to spoken and written language (i.e., *verbal language*), aphasia can also affect *nonverbal* language. A deaf person who uses American Sign Language can lose the ability to use or understand sign language after focal brain damage in the left hemisphere. Third, although most aspects of language are processed in the left hemisphere, some features are influenced by lesions in the nondominant parietal lobe. In particular, a patient with a right parietal lesion may have difficulty appreciating the *prosody* of speech. This term refers to the variations in vocal inflections, emotional content, and melody that may alter the meaning of a spoken sentence, as in: "George is here." versus "*George* is here!" versus "George is *here*?" versus "George *is* here!"

Parietal Association Cortex: Space and Attention

A completely different set of intellectual functions is mediated in the parietal association cortex of the nondominant hemisphere. Although the segregation of functions between the two parietal lobes is not complete, the parietal association cortex is nevertheless the most highly *lateralized* in the brain, with language functions concentrated in the left hemisphere and spatial relationships and related selective attention concentrated in the right hemisphere.

Much of our knowledge of the functional properties of different regions of the cerebral cortex has been gained from neurologic case studies of patients with cortical damage produced by stroke or head trauma. In this respect, the two great wars of the first half of the 20th century led, inadvertently, to great progress in our understanding of the effects of brain injuries. One of the most striking symptoms of damage to *right parietal association cortex* (nondominant) is a defect of *attention,* in which the patient seems to be completely unaware of objects and events in the left half of his or her surrounding space. This symptom is termed *contralateral neglect* (Fig. 32-14A, B).

Contralateral Neglect and Related Symptoms

In its milder forms, contralateral neglect may simply be a tendency to ignore things on the left side of the patient's surroundings. For example, the patient may be asked to read a short passage and check off each word in the process. As the patient reads, words on the left side of the passage are progressively ignored, and only those on the right part are perceived (Fig. 32-14A). Another way to demonstrate contralateral neglect is to draw a circle and ask the patient to draw in the numbers of a clock face. Typically, the patient with right parietal damage will put all of the numbers (1 to 12) on the right side of the circle (the side ipsilateral to the lesion), completely ignoring the left (contralateral) side of the circle (Fig. 32-14B). A patient with contralateral neglect may not be aware of people standing to the left, may bump into large stationary objects on the left, and may not respond to sounds or words coming from the left. In extreme cases, the patient may not even recognize the left side of his or her own body *(asomatognosia).* For example, the patient may ignore the left side when dressing or grooming *(dressing apraxia)* or, if in a hospital, may even demand that the staff get this "other person" (the left side of his or her own body) out of the bed.

Another characteristic group of symptoms of right parietal lobe lesions concerns the ability to function successfully within the *spatial surroundings.* For example, the affected person may be unable to describe his route between home and work, draw a floor plan of his house (Fig. 32-14C), or find a soft drink machine that is just down the hall. In extreme cases, the patient may not be able to navigate successfully from the bed to a chair that is just across the room and in full view.

Yet another difficulty is an inability to successfully manipulate objects in space. The patient may be unable to duplicate a simple block construction while looking at a model (Fig. 32-14D). This

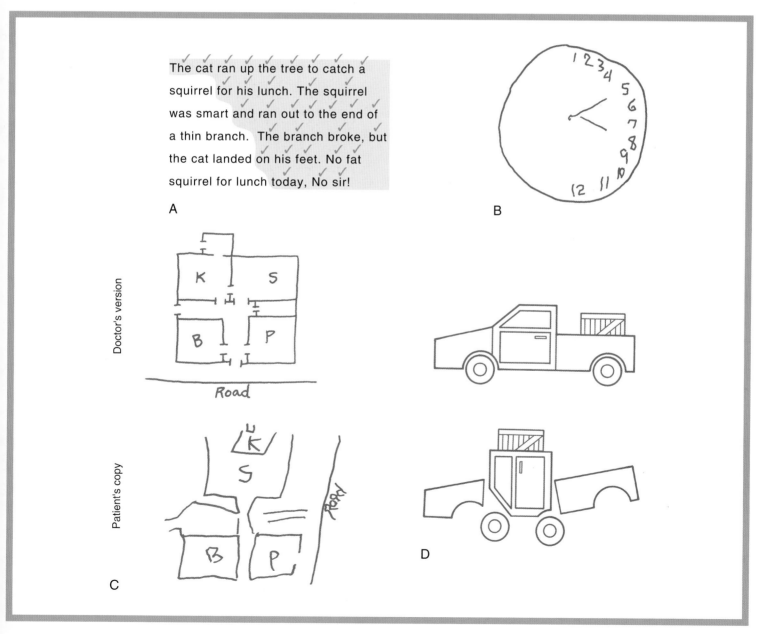

Figure 32-14. Signs (**A-D**) of damage to the nondominant parietal association cortex. See text for details.

difficulty is termed *constructional apraxia;* it is related not to visual acuity or to fine motor control but rather to an inability to internalize and duplicate the spatial relationships of the individual parts of the model. In addition, disorders of *affect* are common, including a reduced ability to understand and appreciate humor, a loss of the ability to appreciate the *prosody* of speech, and often an inappropriate cheerfulness and lack of concern for, or even awareness of, the implications of the illness. This lack of concern may be noted even when the deficit is as serious as total left hemiplegia.

Apraxia and Agnosia

Damage in many areas of association cortex can produce higher-level disorders of behavior. *Apraxia* is a disorder of motor control that may occur after damage in parietal association cortex, premotor cortex, or supplementary motor cortex. In this disorder, there is no paralysis of individual muscles or limbs and muscle strength may be undiminished. Nevertheless, the affected individual is unable to coordinate his or her muscles to execute complex behavior. For example, a patient who can visually recognize a hammer, can name it, can explain what it is used for, and has the strength to pick it up will be unable to demonstrate how it is used to drive a nail into a board. Apraxia may affect the muscles of speech, and thus make speech difficult. Apraxia of speech is a separate disorder from *aphasia* (described earlier), in which the internal processing of the symbols of language is impaired, thus affecting the understanding and production of spoken language, written language, and sign languages.

Agnosia is a general term used to describe a large group of higher-level disorders of sensory perception. The term "agnosia" is derived from two Greek terms that mean a "lack of knowledge." Agnosias are typically confined to a single sensory modality and are characterized by a patient's difficulty in recognizing complex sensory stimuli, for example, faces or letters in the visual modality or tunes or spoken words in the auditory modality. In the clinical setting these deficits are commonly named according to the sensory perception that is disrupted. For example, an inability to recognize a familiar object by sight is *visual agnosia* whereas the inability to recognize noises or sounds is *auditory agnosia.* A somatosensory agnosia might involve a patient's inability to recognize a common object such as a coin, pencil, or key using the sense of touch alone *(tactile agnosia, astereognosis)* or to recognize a letter or number drawn on the palm of the patient's hand while the patient had his or her eyes closed. There are a number of variations on this general theme. This type of deficit also extends to the sense of smell *(olfactory agnosia),* the sense of taste *(gustatory agnosia),* and even the inability to identify colors *(color agnosia).* Agnosias are not a loss of the primary sensation (touch, vision, hearing, etc.) but are a loss of the *ability to interpret the sensation.* They are commonly produced by damage in modality-specific areas of the sensory association cortex.

Prefrontal Cortex and "Plans for Future Operation"

The other major region of multimodal association cortex is the large expanse anterior to the primary motor and premotor cortices, the *prefrontal association cortex.* This region has historically been connected with some of the most distinctly human intellectual traits, such as *judgment, foresight,* a sense of *purpose,* a sense of *responsibility,* and a sense of *social propriety.*

One of the earliest accounts of the effect of brain injury on higher intellectual functions described a series of events that began on September 13, 1848. A crew of railroad construction workers was blasting a right-of-way through the rugged granite mountains of Vermont. The well-liked young foreman of the crew, Phineas Gage, was in charge of placing a black powder

charge in a deep hole drilled in the rock, adding a fuse, covering the powder with sand, and finally tamping the sand and powder down firmly with an iron rod before lighting the fuse and running for cover. On this day, something apparently distracted Gage, and he began to tamp down a charge before the sand had been added. The iron rod struck the granite wall of the hole and a spark ignited the powder. The 3.5-ft-long, 13-lb rod was propelled out of the hole like a giant bullet.

The rod struck Gage just beneath the left eye and exited through the top of his head, destroying most of his prefrontal cortex. Amazingly, Gage was not killed instantly, and even more incredibly, he survived the inevitable serious wound infection that followed. Eventually he recovered his health, or at least the physical portion of it. Mentally, however, he was changed forever. Although he did not suffer paralysis, language disorders, or memory loss, his personality was radically altered. John Harlow, one of the doctors who attended Gage, perceived the importance of this case with respect to the localization of intellectual functions in the brain. In an article describing the injury and Gage's persisting intellectual symptoms, Harlow said:

> His physical health is good, and I am inclined to say that he has recovered....The equilibrium or balance, so to speak, between his intellectual faculties and animal propensities seems to have been destroyed. He is fitful, irreverent, indulging at times in the grossest profanity (which was not previously his custom), manifesting but little deference for his fellows, impatient of restraint or advice when it conflicts with his desires, at times pertinaciously obstinate, yet capricious and vacillating, devising many plans for future operation, which are no sooner arranged than they are abandoned.... In this regard his mind was radically changed, so decidedly that his friends and acquaintances said that he was "no longer Gage."

This passage, written almost 160 years ago, provides an accurate and insightful description of the major symptoms associated with destruction of prefrontal cortex. Patients with significant bilateral damage to the prefrontal cortex have a constellation of deficits that can be summarized as follows. First, they are *highly distractible,* turning from one activity to another according to the novelty of a new stimulus rather than according to a plan. This deficit is sometimes described as a *lack of consistency of purpose.* Second, these persons have a *lack of foresight.* They are not able to anticipate or predict future events on the basis of past events or present conditions. Third, they may be *unusually stubborn* in the face of advice with which they do not agree, and they may also *perseverate* in the performance of a task. Fourth, the patient with prefrontal damage displays a profound *lack of ambition,* a loss of the *sense of responsibility,* and a loss of a *sense of social propriety.* The first and third symptoms *(distractibility versus perseveration)* are obviously in conflict. It is impossible to predict which will dominate at a given moment, but *both* exemplify the affected person's loss of the ability to govern his own actions and life according to a *plan.* The person is instead imprisoned in a chaotic world, with his or her actions governed by randomly changing whims.

It was this set of symptoms that prompted the Portuguese neurosurgeon Egas Moniz to develop the prefrontal lobotomy procedure in the late 1930s to treat a range of severe, intractable mental problems. At that time, mental hospitals ("insane asylums") all over the world contained many patients who were so immobilized by anxiety that they could not even take care of their own bodily needs. They were warehoused under reprehensible conditions. The discovery that a neurosurgical procedure could alleviate the anxiety to the extent that the patients could lead a somewhat more normal existence (albeit still within the confines of a mental institution) was hailed as a great breakthrough. In these desperate patients, the symptoms as described above seemed a justifiable price to pay for freedom from the crushing anxiety that had immobilized them. Unfortunately, by the late 1940s and early 1950s, the procedure had acquired a popularity out of all proportion to its actual benefits, and it was widely misapplied (as in the movie "One Flew Over the Cuckoo's Nest"). The discovery of tranquilizers in the late 1950s provided a more effective method of treatment, having fewer undesirable side effects, and prefrontal lobotomy was rapidly abandoned as a method of treatment.

Synopsis of Clinical Points

- The vast majority of cerebral cortical efferent fibers to subcortical structures arise from large pyramidal cells of layer V and are excitatory to their forebrain, brainstem, and spinal cord targets (p. 513).
- Layer IV is the primary cortical layer for the receipt of sensory input (p. 513).
- Cortical arousal and wakefulness is partially regulated by inputs from the thalamus, locus ceruleus, and basal nuclei (p. 513).
- Many functional regions of the cerebral cortex correlate with the numbering schema of Brodmann (p. 516).
- Lesions located on Brodmann areas 39, 40, and extending into 22 produce a Wernicke aphasia (pp. 521–522).
- Lesions involving Brodmann areas 44 and 45 produce a Broca aphasia (pp. 521–522).
- Damage to Brodmann area 17 results in visual deficits (p. 520).
- The vast majority of patients have a left cerebral dominance (p. 521).
- A lesion in the dominant hemisphere may, depending on its location, result in some type of aphasia (p. 521).
- Aphasia is a disturbance of the comprehension and formulation of language (p. 521).
- A lesion involving primarily the dominant inferior parietal lobule will result in a Wernicke aphasia (p. 521).
- Wernicke aphasia is also called a receptive or fluent aphasia (p. 522).
- A lesion centered in the dominant inferior frontal gyrus, especially its pars opercularis and pars triangularis portions, results in a Broca aphasia (pp. 521–522).
- Broca aphasia is also known as an expressive or nonfluent aphasia (p. 521).
- A patient with a Broca aphasia has great difficulty speaking although the muscles of speech are not paralyzed (p. 521).
- A patient who can speak but whose speech makes no sense has a Wernicke aphasia (p. 522).
- Patients with severe Wernicke aphasia may have alexia, agraphia, or paraphasic speech (p. 522).
- A large hemisphere lesion following the occlusion of the M1 segment may result in a global aphasia (p. 522).
- A patient with a nondominant parietal lobe lesion may demonstrate a loss of appreciation for the prosody of speech (p. 522).
- Lesions in the parietal area of the nondominant hemisphere result in hemineglect or contralateral neglect (pp. 522–523).
- Hemineglect may cause the ambulatory patient considerable difficulties in daily life (pp. 523–524).
- Apraxia is a disorder of motor control even though strength may not be diminished (p. 524).
- Agnosia is a disorder of sensory perception (p. 524).
- An inability to recognize an object in spite of the fact that the patient can see the object is visual agnosia (p. 524).
- The inability to recognize the significance of sounds is auditory agnosia (p. 524).
- The patient who can feel the object in his or her hand but is not able to recognize the object has tactile agnosia (p. 524).
- Forebrain lesions may cause a variety of sensory agnosias (p. 524).
- Agnosia is not a loss of sensation but a loss of the ability to interpret the sensation (p. 524).
- The interesting case of Phineas Gage (p. 524).
- Although once thought to be a potentially revolutionary medical treatment, prefrontal lobotomy is no longer considered acceptable medical care (pp. 524–525).

Sources and Additional Reading

Blakemore C: Mechanics of the Mind. Cambridge, Cambridge University Press, 1977.

Casanova, Manuel F (ed): Neocortical Modularity and the Cell Minicolumn. New York, Nova Science Publishers, 2005.

Damasio AR: Aphasia. N Engl J Med 326:531-538, 1992.

Damasio H, Grabowski T, Frank R, Galaburda AM, Damasio AR: The return of Phineas Gage: Clues about the brain from the skull of a famous patient. Science 264:1102-1105, 1994.

Harlow JM: Recovery from the passage of an iron bar through the head. Pub Mass Med Soc 2:327-347, 1868.

Hendry SHC, Jones EG: Sizes and distributions of intrinsic neurons incorporating tritiated GABA in monkey sensory-motor cortex. J Neurosci 1:390-408, 1981.

Hubel DH, Wiesel TN: Functional architecture of macaque monkey visual cortex. Proc R Soc Lond B Biol Sci 198:1-59, 1977.

Jones EG: Varieties and distribution of non-pyramidal cells in the somatic sensory cortex of the squirrel monkey. J Comp Neurol 160:205-268, 1975.

Jones EG: Laminar distribution of cortical efferent cells. In Cerebral Cortex, vol 1. New York, Plenum Press, 1984, pp 521-553.

Lynch JC: Parietal association cortex. In Encyclopedia of Neuroscience, vol 2. Boston, Birkhauser, 1987, pp 925-926.

Lynch JC: Columnar organization of the cerebral cortex (cortical columns). In Neuroscience Year (Supplement to Encyclopedia of Neuroscience). Boston, Birkhauser, 1989, pp 37-40.

Lynch JC, Tian JR: Corticocortical networks and cortico-subcortical loops for the higher control of eye movement. In Buttner-Ennever JA (ed): Neuroanatomy of the Oculomotor System. Amsterdam, Elsevier, 2005, vol 151, pp 467-508.

Mountcastle VB: The cortical organization of the neocortex. Brain 120:701-722, 1997.

Mountcastle VB: Modality and topographic properties of single neurons of cat's somatic sensory cortex. J Neurophysiol 20:408-434, 1957.

Peters A, Jones EG: Cerebral Cortex. New York, Plenum Press, 1984-1999, vols 1-14.

Rowland LP: Merritt's Neurology, 10th ed. Baltimore, Lippincott Williams & Wilkins, 2000.

Scheibel ME, Scheibel AB: Elementary processes in selected thalamic and cortical subsystems-the structural substrates. In The Neurosciences, Second Study Programs, vol 2. New York, Rockefeller University Press, 1970, pp 443-457.

Valenstein ES: Great and Desperate Cures. New York, Basic Books, 1986.

Victor M, Ropper AH: Adams and Victor's Principles of Neurology, 7th ed. New 1York, McGraw-Hill, 2001.

Chapter 33

The Neurologic Examination

M. E. Santiago and J. J. Corbett

In many respects this chapter is a prologue to the experience of working directly with the patient. Now that many aspects of functional systems neurobiology have been mastered, the opportunity to apply this knowledge is at hand. Performing the neurologic examination is an excellent example of how basic neuroscience can apply directly to events (both normal and abnormal) encountered in the clinical setting. After all, the neurologically compromised patient is simply a normal person whose nervous system is not functioning properly.

Overview

No other branch of medicine lends itself so well to the correlation of the signs and symptoms of disease with structure and function as does neurology. The neurologic diagnosis of the impaired patient is a deductive process and is reached by a synthesis of all of the details from the history, the examination, and laboratory studies. The neurologic examination is divided into four main segments: mental status, cranial nerves, motor and cerebellar, and sensory.

Figure 33-1 shows a sample set of tools necessary to perform a routine neurologic examination: visual acuity card and eye occluder, ophthalmoscope, dilating eye drops, a flashlight, test tube with coffee to assess smell, disposable tongue blade, safety pin, tissue paper, and cotton-tipped applicator. Tuning forks, measuring tape, and a reflex hammer should also be included, as well as a quarter or a wooden cube for sensation testing.

Evaluation versus Examination

The *evaluation* and the *examination* of a patient are different but intimately integrated aspects of the patient-physician encounter. In general, the examination is a small umbrella under the larger umbrella of evaluation (Fig. 33-2).

Evaluation covers all the aspects related to a specific medical event (Fig. 33-2). It includes the *current complaint*, which is the main reason why the patient seeks medical attention at that time, and the *history of present illness*, which focuses on the details and circumstances surrounding the main complaint, such as time course (abrupt onset as opposed to slowly progressive), associated symptoms (pain, blurred vision, headache, inability to talk, and so on), and predisposing or concurrent factors (with exercise or physical activity, warm weather or exposure to drugs).

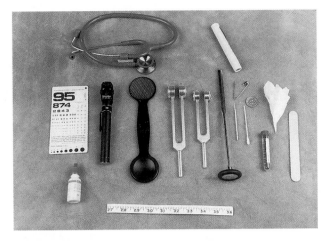

Figure 33-1. Instruments used to conduct a general neurologic examination.

Remember that getting information from an observer, such as a family member or friend, is essential to characterize many neurologic conditions such as seizures, dementia or loss of consciousness when the patient may not be aware of the events. The *past medical and surgical histories* focus on learning facts about past illnesses; concurrent medical problems such as arterial hypertension, diabetes mellitus, or history of cancer may be pertinent to the new medical complaint. Surgical procedures that the patient may have had in the past are also important clues in the medical history. *Family history* is an essential part of the medical history and may explain the present medical issue. For example, some forms of hand tremors or strokes at an early age may be genetically determined. *Social history* inquiries about the patient's habits like smoking, alcohol or illicit drug abuse, life style, and occupation. *Medications* that the patient is taking are also detailed in the history. *Review of systems* is a systematic general review of all systems including cardiovascular, respiratory, genitourinary, and gastrointestinal.

Physical examination, or simply *examination*, is an important part of the more extensive evaluation of the patient (Fig. 33-2). In general, it includes the patient's vital signs and a general examination by systems with a more focused examination of the

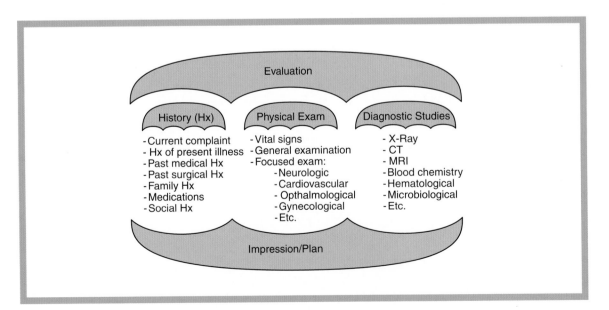

Figure 33-2. Diagrammatic representation of the relationship between the overall evaluation, and its specific components, and the examination when evaluating the neurologically compromised patient.

ystem involved in the current medical problem. For example, f the patient presents with complains of acute onset of chest ain and shortness of breath a detailed *cardiovascular examination* is in order with a general examination of the abdomen and brief neurologic examination. On the other hand, if a patient resents with sudden onset of weakness of the right side of the ody and difficulty speaking, a detailed *neurologic examination* is alled for.

Diagnostic studies (Fig. 33-2) may be ordered as a result of the verall evaluation of the patient in order to confirm a possible iagnostic hypothesis. For example, cerebrospinal fluid (CSF) hemical, cytologic, and bacteriologic examination can be done o confirm suspected meningitis, or computed tomography (CT) r magnetic resonance imaging (MRI) of the brain can be ordered o confirm the localization of a stroke and determine if it is schemic or hemorrhagic.

Finally, the *impression* (Fig. 33-2) of the evaluating physician n what and where the problem might be and *recommendations* n management and therapy indicated simply puts together he overall evaluation by the examiner and sets the immediate ourse of treatment and future health care plans for the patient.

The Mental Status Examination

The mental status examination starts first with an assessment f the level of consciousness of the patient. Orientation to time, lace, and person should also be documented. Memory of past vents and short-term memory, as well as the ability to calculate, re also evaluated at this time. This basic examination is known s the Folstein Mini-Mental Status test (Fig. 33-3). Special tests f parietal lobe function include drawing a clock face (Fig. 33-4), isecting a line, and copying a picture of a daisy or drawing a set f intersecting pentagons.

Speech disorders such as *dysarthria* are detectable in ordinary onversation and result from defects of articulation of the words econdary to tongue (cranial nerve XII), palate (cranial nerves IX nd X), lips (cranial nerve VII), or pharyngeal muscle weakness r incoordination. Evidence of a speech disorder is usually ursued by asking the patient to repeat a difficult phrase like Methodist Episcopal" or to repeat the sounds "puh-tuh-kuh" apidly.

Language is the ability to use and understand written and poken speech and is a function of the cortical, thalamic, and asal nuclei language circuits located in the dominant cerebral emisphere. Language is assessed by asking the patient to epeat words or phrases ("no, ifs, ands, or buts"), to name simple bjects (watch, finger, pen), to follow commands (touch your eft shoulder, close your eyes, point to the ceiling), and to write a sentence and read it aloud.

Language abnormalities are called aphasias. There are two najor types: *nonfluent aphasia* and *fluent aphasia*. In nonfluent phasia the patient has difficulty with verbal self-expression, roducing the words only with great effort, but is able to understand and follow commands appropriately. Nonfluent aphasia s also called an *expressive*, or Broca, aphasia; a lesion resulting n this type of deficit is found in the inferior frontal gyrus sometimes called the Broca convolution) specifically involving he *pars opercularis* and the *pars triangularis*. In fluent aphasia he patient has normal or even increased production of words, ometimes in long sentences with normal prosody (rhythm of peech); well-articulated but frequent neologisms (a series of neaningless words) give these sentences no content or meaning. n fluent aphasia, also called a *receptive*, or Wernicke, aphasia, neither the patient nor the examiner is able to understand the neaning of the patient's speech. A lesion of the lateral aspect f the dominant hemisphere in the area of the *supramarginal*

and *angular gyri* (and sometimes adjacent portions of the superior temporal lobe) may result in fluent aphasia.

Cranial Nerve Function Testing

Cranial Nerve I

The *olfactory nerve (cranial nerve I)* is rarely tested, because of the deleterious effects of smoking and sinus disease on the sense of smell in the general population. The nerve can be unilaterally damaged by trauma or a tumor of the skull base in the olfactory groove such as an olfactory groove meningioma (see Fig. 7-10). Total loss of the ability to smell *(anosmia)* is always associated with the inability to taste food *(ageusia)* as well—a familiar example being the unappealing taste of food associated with the nasal congestion of a head cold. *Dysageusia* is an unappealing or altered sense of taste, and *parosmia* is an altered or perverted perception of odors.

Olfactory stimuli should be nontrigeminal, that is, it should not tickle or irritate the inside of the nose (as does ammonia, for example), which is innervated by the trigeminal nerve. Commonly used substances are vanilla, coffee, and perfumed soap. With the patient's eyes closed, occlude one nostril and bring a vial of the substance near the open nostril (Fig. 33-5). Ask the patient whether he or she smells something or not. The sensing of odor is more important than its identification. The process is then repeated for the other nostril.

Cranial Nerve II

The *optic nerve (cranial nerve II)* is tested by measuring visual acuity (a measurement of the ability to detect fine detail and contrast in an image) and assessing the extent of peripheral vision by examining visual fields and by inspecting the retina and the optic nerve head using the ophthalmoscope. Visual acuity (also called visual resolution) is tested separately for each eye and should be recorded using the patient's best spectacle correction and a handheld visual acuity chart or a Snellen chart at 20 feet (Fig. 33-6). The number beside each line of letters indicates the number of feet at which the letters can be read by a person who has normal vision; thus, normally, the letters in the line designated 20 can be read at 20 feet, and the visual acuity is recorded as 20/20.

Examination of the visual fields is an important part of the ophthalmologic and neurologic examination. This procedure provides information about the entire visual pathway from the optic nerve to the occipital cortex. Because lesions interrupting various parts of the pathway cause specific types of defects in the visual field, it is frequently possible to determine the location of the lesion (see Chapter 20 for examples). There are several different methods for evaluation of the visual field. The most common method used by most neurologists at the bedside is the *confrontation visual field examination*. The examiner faces the patient being examined. The patient should cover one eye with the palm of the hand, or with an eye occluder, and fixate the gaze of the eye to be examined on the examiner's nose. Then the examiner presents a stimulus in each of the four quadrants—upper and lower nasal and upper and lower temporal—of the visual field; finger movement, rapid finger counting, or hand comparison may be used for this purpose (Fig. 33-7).

Lesions of the various structures collectively making up the visual pathway give rise to deficits that are characteristic of the specific portion of the pathway compromised. These lesions and corresponding deficits are considered in detail in Chapter 20 and are only summarized here (Fig. 33-8). A *scotoma* (Greek for "spot") is a defect of the visual field surrounded by normal vision. A scotoma is most frequently the result of a lesion within the retina or the optic nerve but may also be seen in cases of

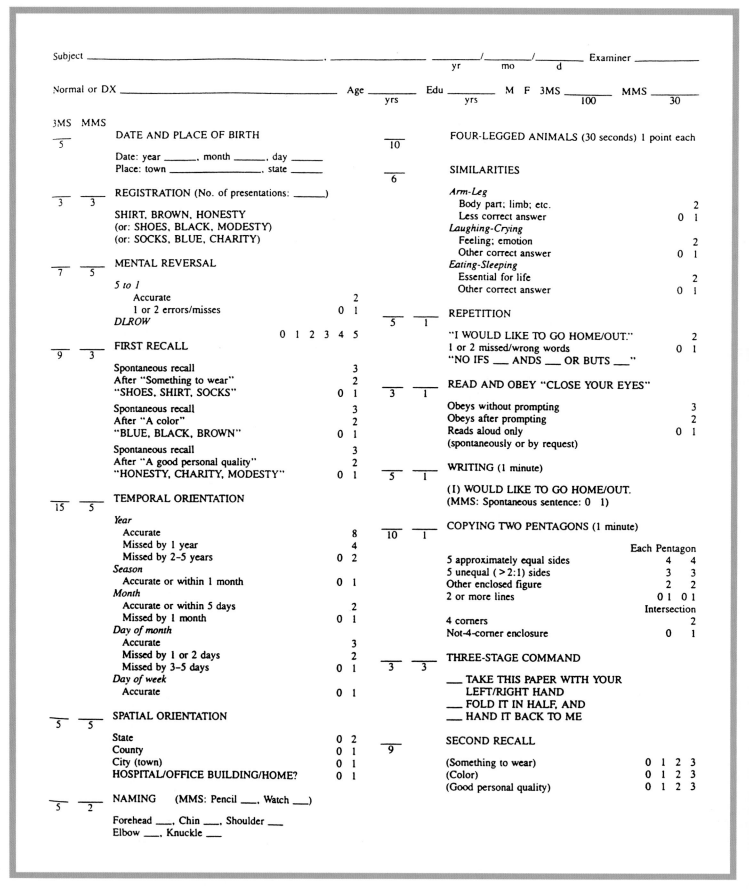

Subject _____, _____ _____/_____/_____ Examiner _____
                                                                    yr   mo   d

Normal or DX _____ Age _____ Edu _____ M F 3MS _____ MMS _____
                                                            yrs   yrs   100   30

3MS	MMS				
__5__		**DATE AND PLACE OF BIRTH**		__10__	**FOUR-LEGGED ANIMALS** (30 seconds) 1 point each

Date: year _____, month _____, day _____
Place: town _____, state _____

__3__ __3__ **REGISTRATION** (No. of presentations: _____)

SHIRT, BROWN, HONESTY
(or: SHOES, BLACK, MODESTY)
(or: SOCKS, BLUE, CHARITY)

__7__ __5__ **MENTAL REVERSAL**

5 to 1
    Accurate   2
    1 or 2 errors/misses   0 1
DLROW
    0 1 2 3 4 5

__9__ __3__ **FIRST RECALL**

Spontaneous recall   3
After "Something to wear"   2
"SHOES, SHIRT, SOCKS"   0 1

Spontaneous recall   3
After "A color"   2
"BLUE, BLACK, BROWN"   0 1

Spontaneous recall   3
After "A good personal quality"   2
"HONESTY, CHARITY, MODESTY"   0 1

__15__ __5__ **TEMPORAL ORIENTATION**

Year
    Accurate   8
    Missed by 1 year   4
    Missed by 2–5 years   0 2
Season
    Accurate or within 1 month   0 1
Month
    Accurate or within 5 days   2
    Missed by 1 month   0 1
Day of month
    Accurate   3
    Missed by 1 or 2 days   2
    Missed by 3–5 days   0 1
Day of week
    Accurate   0 1

__5__ __5__ **SPATIAL ORIENTATION**

State   0 2
County   0 1
City (town)   0 1
HOSPITAL/OFFICE BUILDING/HOME?   0 1

__5__ __2__ **NAMING** (MMS: Pencil ___, Watch ___)

Forehead ___, Chin ___, Shoulder ___
Elbow ___, Knuckle ___

__6__ **SIMILARITIES**

Arm-Leg
    Body part; limb; etc.   2
    Less correct answer   0 1
Laughing-Crying
    Feeling; emotion   2
    Other correct answer   0 1
Eating-Sleeping
    Essential for life   2
    Other correct answer   0 1

__5__ __1__ **REPETITION**

"I WOULD LIKE TO GO HOME/OUT."   2
1 or 2 missed/wrong words   0 1
"NO IFS ___ ANDS ___ OR BUTS ___"

__3__ __1__ **READ AND OBEY "CLOSE YOUR EYES"**

Obeys without prompting   3
Obeys after prompting   2
Reads aloud only   0 1
(spontaneously or by request)

__5__ __1__ **WRITING** (1 minute)

(I) WOULD LIKE TO GO HOME/OUT.
(MMS: Spontaneous sentence: 0 1)

__10__ __1__ **COPYING TWO PENTAGONS** (1 minute)

	Each Pentagon	
5 approximately equal sides	4	4
5 unequal (>2:1) sides	3	3
Other enclosed figure	2	2
2 or more lines	0 1	0 1
	Intersection	
4 corners		2
Not-4-corner enclosure	0	1

__3__ __3__ **THREE-STAGE COMMAND**

___ TAKE THIS PAPER WITH YOUR
    LEFT/RIGHT HAND
___ FOLD IT IN HALF, AND
___ HAND IT BACK TO ME

__9__ **SECOND RECALL**

(Something to wear)   0 1 2 3
(Color)   0 1 2 3
(Good personal quality)   0 1 2 3

Figure 33-3. The Folstein Mini-Mental examination.

stroke or tumor along the course of the visual pathway. It is perceived as an area within the field of vision where the patient cannot see. The *blind spot* is a physiologic scotoma that represents the position of the optic disc within the visual field (the optic disc has no rods, cones, or ganglion cells; see Chapter 20).

Lesions of the visual pathway result in characteristic visual deficits. There are many variations to this theme, and only a few examples are illustrated in Figure 33-8 (for more detail on the visual system consult Chapter 20). For example, loss of vision in one half of the field in one eye is called *hemianopsia*, and loss

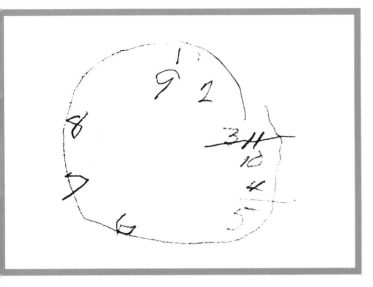

Figure 33-4. A clock face drawn by a patient with a parietal lobe lesion.

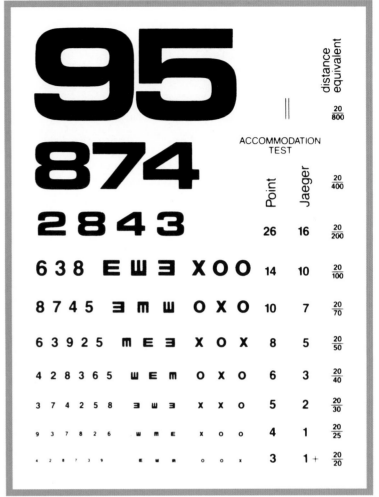

	Point	Jaeger	distance equivalent
95			20/800
874			20/400
2843	26	16	20/200
638 EШƎ XOO	14	10	20/100
8745 ƎMШ OXO	10	7	20/70
63925 MEƎ XOX	8	5	20/50
428365 ШEM OXO	6	3	20/40
374258 ƎШƎ XXO	5	2	20/30
937826 ШME XOO	4	1	20/25
	3	1+	20/20

ACCOMMODATION TEST

Figure 33-6. The handheld visual acuity chart.

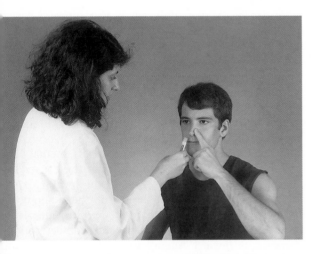

Figure 33-5. Testing the sense of smell (olfaction). The patient presses one nostril closed, and the open nostril is exposed to an aromatic substance.

of vision in corresponding halves of the visual fields of both eyes is called *right* or *left homonymous hemianopsia* depending on which visual fields are lost. Loss of vision in the temporal halves of the visual fields of both eyes is called *bitemporal hemianopia*. The loss of a quadrant of the visual field, a *quadrantanopia*, is most commonly seen in lesions involving the white matter between the lateral geniculate body and the visual cortex. The retinotopic organization is well preserved throughout the visual pathway and a careful examination of visual field deficits may be instrumental in precisely localizing these lesions (Fig. 33-8).

The appearance of the optic nerve head or the optic disc is examined with an ophthalmoscope (Fig. 33-9) while the patient looks at a distant object. To examine the patient's right eye, the examiner holds the ophthalmoscope with the right hand

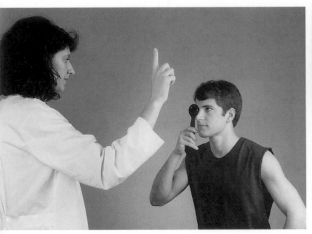 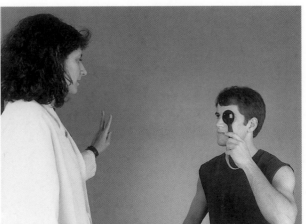

A   B

Figure 33-7. Visual field examination by confrontation. One eye is covered (**A**), and all visual quadrants are tested for that eye. The procedure is repeated for the other eye (**B**).

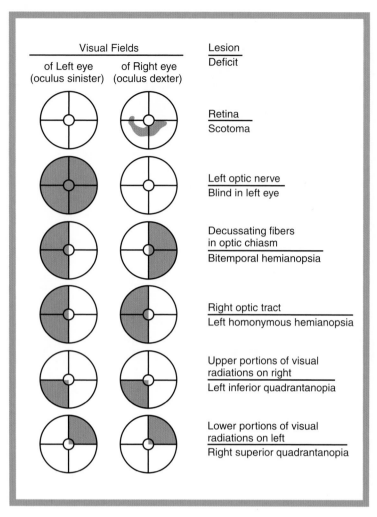

Visual Fields

of Left eye (oculus sinister)   of Right eye (oculus dexter)

Lesion
Deficit

Retina
Scotoma

Left optic nerve
Blind in left eye

Decussating fibers in optic chiasm
Bitemporal hemianopsia

Right optic tract
Left homonymous hemianopsia

Upper portions of visual radiations on right
Left inferior quadrantanopia

Lower portions of visual radiations on left
Right superior quadrantanopia

Figure 33-8. Representative visual field deficits as correlated with the name of the deficit and the location of the lesion. Also consult Chapter 20 for more information on the visual system.

and uses his or her own right eye; this technique is reversed for examination of the patient's left eye. With the ophthalmoscope dial set on zero, the pupillary red reflex (the point at which the retinal reflex is seen "glowing" in the pupil) is located from a distance of 2 or 3 feet (Fig. 33-9A). The examiner slowly approaches the patient's eye as if viewing the eye through a keyhole. At the same time, plus or minus lenses, as needed, are dialed on the ophthalmoscope to focus on the patient's retina. The *optic disc* is located by directing the ophthalmoscope slightly

toward the nasal side of the patient's retina (Fig. 33-9B). The appearance of the optic disc is important. Normally it is round or slightly oval and of a yellowish-red color, with clearly defined margins (Fig. 33-10A). Veins are darker in color and slightly larger in diameter than arterioles. The presence of the *central cup*, or excavation, and its size should be documented (Fig. 33-10B).

Papilledema, or swelling of the optic disc, is usually due to increased intracranial pressure, regardless of the cause of the pressure increase. Early signs of papilledema include disappearance of the normal cup, blurring of the disc margins, and arching and elevation of the vessels as they pass over the margin of the disc. As papilledema progresses, exudates and hemorrhages appear, as well as tortuosity of the vessels (Fig. 33-11).

Optic atrophy may be primary or secondary. Primary optic atrophy results from different processes involving the optic nerve such as retrobulbar optic nerve injury, compression by a tumor or demyelination. Secondary optic atrophy is a consequence of chronic increased intracranial pressure, infarctions, or diseases such as syphilis (Fig. 33-12).

Cranial Nerves III, IV, and VI

The *oculomotor, trochlear, and abducens nerves (cranial nerves III, IV, and VI)* are usually examined as a group because they act together in controlling ocular muscles to ensure that the eyes remain parallel throughout their range of motion. A lesion affecting one or more of these nerves results in weakness of the corresponding muscles, manifested by *diplopia* or *double vision*. Ocular motility is tested by having the patient follow the examiner's finger in upgaze and downgaze and from side to side (Fig. 33-13A, C).

The oculomotor nerve innervates the superior, medial, and inferior rectus muscles; the inferior oblique; and the constrictor of the pupil and the ciliary body as well as the levator of the eyelid (see Fig. 28-1). A complete lesion of the oculomotor nerve results in paralysis of the ipsilateral muscles innervated by the nerve and ptosis, pupillary dilation, and inability to look upward, downward, or inward. Aneurysms of the internal carotid artery or posterior communicating artery and pressure from herniation of the uncinate gyrus (uncus) in expanding lesions of the cerebral hemisphere are common causes of a peripheral complete third nerve palsy with pupillary involvement.

The trochlear nerve innervates the superior oblique muscle (see Fig. 28-1). When the fourth nerve is damaged, the affected ipsilateral eye is higher than the normal opposite eye and it cannot be turned downward when the eye is rotated inward (adducted). The position of the globe (eyeball) is higher relative to the position of the other globe because the superior oblique

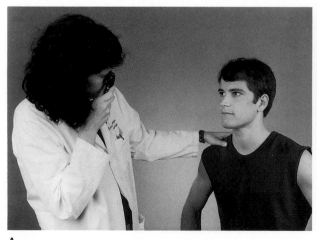

A

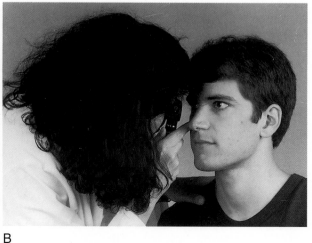

B

Figure 33-9. Ophthalmoscopic examination. The examiner locates the red reflex (**A**) and then focuses on the details of the optic nerve (**B**) through the pupil.

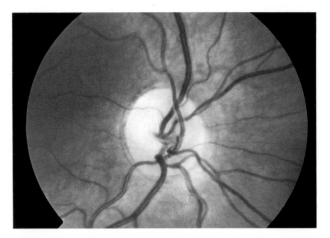

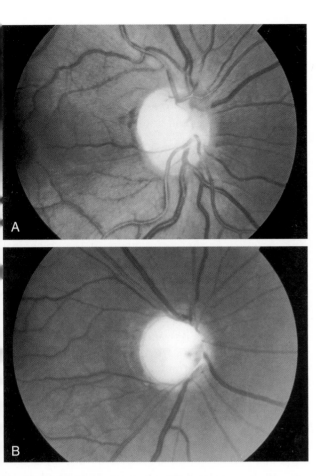

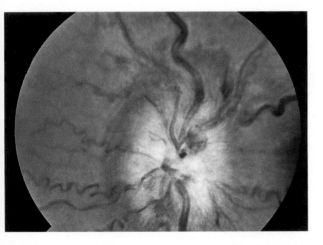

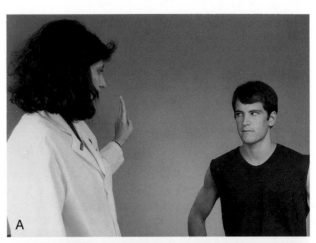

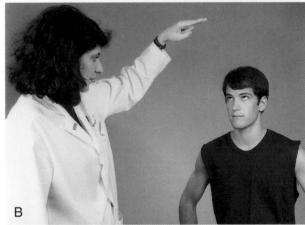

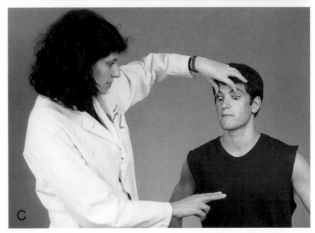

Figure 33-12. Optic atrophy. Note the pale appearance of the optic disc.

Figure 33-10. Normal optic disc (**A**) and an example of an abnormally enlarged central cup (**B**) in a patient with glaucoma.

Figure 33-11. Papilledema with hemorrhages. Observe the tortuosity of vessels.

muscle normally depresses the eyeball. When this muscle is weak or paralyzed, the eyeball will not depress normally relative to the other eye. Thus, it is "higher" than the normal eye.

The abducens nerve controls the ipsilateral lateral rectus muscle, which makes the eye look outward (laterally). Defects in abduction (from a lesion of the sixth cranial nerve, for example) give the patient a "cross-eyed" appearance, because the normal eye is oriented straight ahead and the affected eye is rotated slightly inward (medially), owing to the unopposed action of the medial rectus muscle on that side.

Cranial Nerve V

The *trigeminal nerve (cranial nerve V)* is both motor and sensory. In sensory testing, its innervation includes the face up to the vertex of the scalp but spares the angle of the mandible (which

Figure 33-13. Test of ocular motility to evaluate the function of the extraocular muscles. The patient holds the head still and follows the examiner's fingers with the eyes. Examples here show the patient looking to his right (**A**), upward (**B**), and downward (**C**).

is innervated by C3). The sensation from the oral and nasal cavities is transmitted through the trigeminal nerve, although these areas are not usually included in the routine neurologic examination (see Chapter 18).

Pain and temperature should be tested in the three divisions of the fifth cranial nerve: the ophthalmic, the maxillary, and the mandibular (Fig. 33-14A, B; also see Figs. 18-4, 18-14, and 18-15). The ophthalmic division innervates the scalp as far back as the vertex of the skull, forehead, cornea, conjunctiva, and skin of the side and tip of the nose. Corneal sensation is tested by gently touching the cornea with a cotton-tipped applicator or tissue paper while the patient looks in the other direction (Fig. 33-14C). *This maneuver constitutes the afferent limb of the corneal reflex.* The normal response is a rapid, partial or complete blinking movement of the eyelid elicited by the efferent limb of the corneal reflex via the facial nerve. The second trigeminal division, the maxillary nerve, conducts stimuli from the skin of the cheek, far lateral aspect of the nose, upper teeth, and jaw. The third division, the mandibular nerve, carries sensory and motor impulses. The sensory distribution is skin of the lower jaw, pinna of the ear, and lower teeth and gums as well as the side of the tongue.

The motor fibers supply the muscles of mastication: the temporal, masseter, and pterygoid muscles. The temporal and masseter muscles are examined by having the patient close the jaws together while the examiner palpates these muscles (Fig. 33-15A). The pterygoid muscles are responsible for side-to-side movements of the jaw, as well as aiding closure of the jaw (Fig. 33-15B). A lesion of the motor fibers of the trigeminal nerve results in weakness of the masticatory muscles on that side and a slight deviation of the jaw toward the weak side, on jaw closing, owing to the unopposed action of the healthy contralateral pterygoid muscles. The *jaw jerk reflex* is elicited by a gentle tap on the chin, with resultant closure of the jaw by the masticatory muscles. The afferent limb of this reflex is via receptors in the muscles of mastication that enter the brainstem on fibers of the mesencephalic tract, and the efferent limb is in response to collaterals of these fibers that bilaterally innervate the motor trigeminal muscles (also see Fig. 14-18).

Cranial Nerve VII

The *facial nerve (cranial nerve VII)* is a complex nerve with motor, sensory, and parasympathetic (visceromotor) fibers. The motor portion of the nerve innervates the muscles of facial expression and is tested by instructing the patient to wrinkle

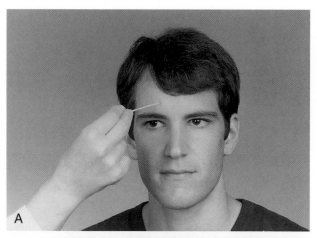

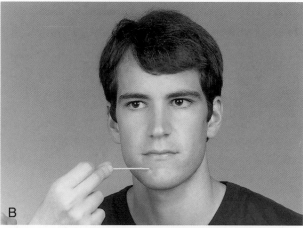

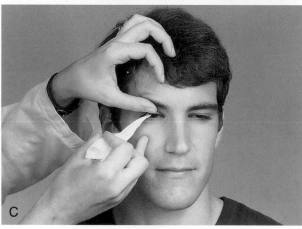

Figure 33-14. Testing sensory portions of the trigeminal nerve. Examples show a probe touching the ophthalmic (**A**) and mandibular (**B**) territories of the trigeminal nerve; the maxillary division is tested by touching the cheek below the eye. A wisp of tissue touched to the cornea (**C**) activates the afferent limb of the corneal reflex and results in closing of the eyes; the efferent limb is mediated by the facial nerve.

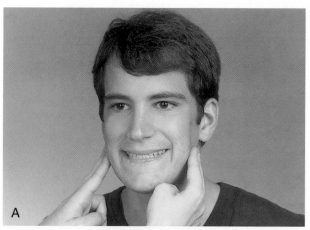

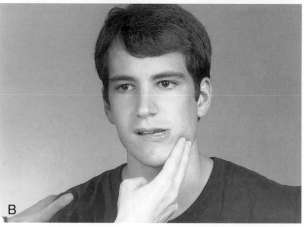

Figure 33-15. Testing the muscles of mastication. The patient clenches the masticatory muscles while they are palpated by the examiner (**A**) and deviates the jaw against resistance (**B**); this maneuver tests the pterygoid muscles.

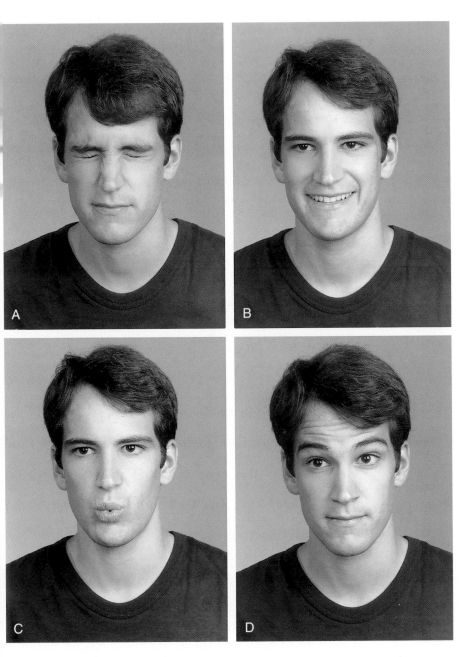

Figure 33-16. Testing the muscles of facial expression. The patient is asked to tightly close the eyes (**A**), smile (**B**), purse the lips (**C**), and wrinkle the forehead (**D**). In each case, the examiner carefully assesses the symmetry of the face.

the forehead, to close the eyelids tightly, to smile or grimace showing the teeth, and to whistle (Fig. 33-16). There are two types of facial motor weakness, one with involvement of the upper motor neuron or corticonuclear (corticobulbar) pathways, and the other with involvement of the lower motor neuron, or "peripheral" seventh nerve palsy. The "central" or upper motor neuron facial palsy is characterized by inability to retract the corner of the mouth, while forehead function and eyelid closure remain for the most part unaffected. Lesions in the facial nucleus or the nerve proper will cause paralysis of half of the entire face, with inability to wrinkle the forehead or to close the eyelids and lips on the affected side (Fig. 33-17; also see Fig. 25-14).

The sensory portions of the seventh nerve originate from the taste buds in the anterior two thirds of the tongue and from the posterior wall of the external ear canal. Taste is examined using sugar, salt, or quinine solutions. The patient is instructed to protrude the tongue; then the test substance is applied with a cotton-tipped applicator on one side of the tongue. The patient must identify the test substance before drawing the tongue back into the mouth, where function of the posterior portion of the tongue or the contralateral side masks the result of the test. The facial nerve also carries parasympathetic fibers to the maxillary and lacrimal glands (see Chapter 14).

Cranial Nerve VIII

The *eighth cranial nerve* is made up of two divisions: cochlear, subserving the sense of hearing, and vestibular, subserving the sense of balance—hence its common name, the *vestibulocochlear nerve.*

The cochlear division is usually tested using a tuning fork with a frequency of 256 vibrations per second to compare bone and air conduction (Fig. 33-18). This examination is known as the *Rinne test.* In the normal ear, air conduction is greater than bone conduction. The vibrating tuning fork is placed against the mastoid bone (Fig. 33-18C), and the patient is instructed to indicate when he or she no longer senses the vibration. Then the tuning fork is placed near the external auditory canal (Fig. 33-18D), and the time for air conduction is estimated. With a normal test result, the time for air conduction is about twice that for bone conduction. Bone conduction will be louder in conductive hearing loss; both air and bone conduction are abnormal in neurogenic hearing loss. The *Weber test* is performed by placing the tuning fork on the vertex of the skull (Fig. 33-18B); normally, the vibration is perceived equally in both ears. If there is disease of the middle ear or the external ear is blocked (conductive hearing loss), the vibration is lateralized to the affected side. If the cochlear nerve is involved on one side (neurogenic

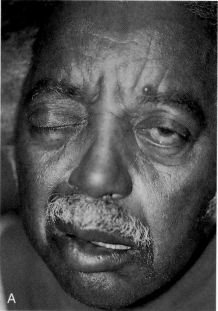

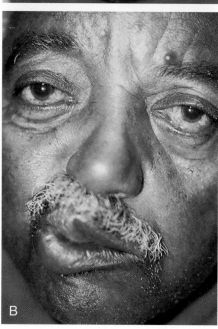

Figure 33-17. A patient with a lesion of the facial nerve. The patient has difficulty in closing his left eye and the left corner of his mouth droops (**A**; compare with Fig. 33-13A, B). The latter defect is especially evident when the patient attempts to purse his lips (**B**; compare with Fig. 33-13C).

opposite/warm—same) refers to the direction of the fast phase of the nystagmus.

Cranial Nerves IX and X

The *glossopharyngeal and vagus nerves (cranial nerves IX and X)* are usually examined at the same time. Touching the posterior wall of the pharynx with a tongue depressor tests the general sensory fibers of the ninth nerve. The normal response is the prompt contraction of the pharyngeal muscles, including the stylopharyngeus muscle. Afferent information conducted on the ninth nerve and the resultant contraction of the stylopharyngeus muscle constitute the *circuit of the gag reflex.*

Vagus nerve dysfunction will result in ipsilateral paralysis of the palatal, pharyngeal, and laryngeal muscles. In such cases, the voice is hoarse *(dysarthria)* as a result of weakness of the vocal cord (and vocalis muscle) and speech has a nasal sound. In addition, the patient may experience difficulty swallowing, or *dysphagia.* The soft palate should be observed while the patient says "Ah." Normally, the uvula remains in the midline, but in cases of weakness of the palate on one side, it is pulled toward the contralateral side because of the unopposed action of muscles on the healthy side (also see Fig. 25-15).

Cranial Nerve XI

The *spinal accessory nerve (cranial nerve XI)* innervates the ipsilateral sternocleidomastoid and trapezius muscles. It is examined by having the patient turn the head forcibly against the examiner's hand away from the muscle being tested while the muscle is palpated (Fig. 33-19). In this respect it is important to remember that contraction of the sternocleidomastoid muscle turns the head to the opposite side. Damage to this nerve causes inability to shrug (elevate) the shoulder against resistance (weakness of the trapezius muscle) and winging of the scapula on the side of the lesion.

Cranial Nerve XII

The *hypoglossal nerve (cranial nerve XII)* supplies the extrinsic and intrinsic muscles of the tongue. To test the integrity of the hypoglossal nerve, the patient is asked to protrude the tongue in the midline and move it from side to side (Fig. 33-20). In the presence of a lesion of the hypoglossal nerve, the tongue is seen to deviate toward the side of the lesion, toward the weak half, on attempted protrusion (Fig. 33-21). This deficit is due to a paralysis of the genioglossus muscle.

The Motor Examination

The motor examination includes a consideration of muscle tone and strength. Tone examination requires that the patient be as relaxed as possible. The patient may respond to suggestions such as "Go loose" or "Let me do all the work and go floppy," thereby permitting the examiner to move the patient's limbs freely. Normally, a mild resistance to movement is noted during the whole range of motion. In *hypertonicity,* increased resistance is present in extensor and flexor muscles. Flexor resistance can range between very mild to so severe as to prevent passive movement. This increased tone is called *lead pipe rigidity* and is a feature of Parkinson disease (see Chapter 26).

Spasticity is a phasic change in muscle tone brought out by a rapid snap of the limb in extension or flexion. The spastic "catch" is an abrupt increase in the tone followed by a slow release, much as in the operation of the hydraulic hinge on the rear door of a hatchback automobile. Spasticity is seen with corticospinal tract lesions. *Hypotonia* is characterized by increased ease of passive movements, as exemplified by the pendular swing of a leg extended and released in the sitting position.

hearing loss), the sound is heard better on the opposite or the normal side.

The vestibular division of the acoustic nerve is assessed using rotational and caloric stimuli to produce changes in the endolymph current in the semicircular canals (see Chapter 22). Typically, patients with vestibular dysfunction complain of vertigo, nausea and vomiting, and difficulty with balance, especially with movement of the head. Vertigo may be perceived by the patient as movement of the environment around him or her, or the patient perceives that he or she is moving and the environment remains still. Vertigo may be induced by visual input or by changes of the body space. The *water caloric test,* or *Barány test,* is done by irrigating the external auditory canal with 10 mL of cold water while holding the patient's head at 30 degrees above the horizontal. The patient is then examined for horizontal nystagmus with the slow component toward the side of the stimulus past the midline and the fast corrective phase of the nystagmus to the opposite side. The mnemonic COWS (cold—

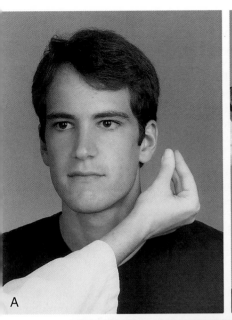

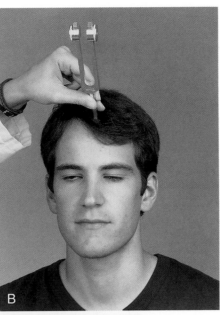

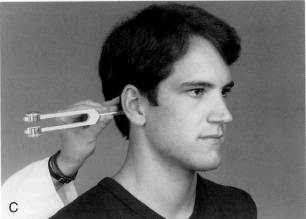

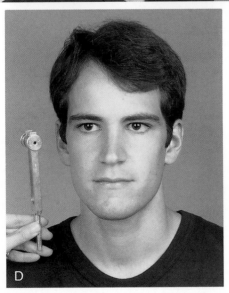

Figure 33-18. Test of auditory function (hearing). If the patient is unable to identify a sound made with the fingers (**A**), the examination then proceeds to a test of bone conduction for both ears together (**B**) and for each ear separately (**C**), and of air conduction for each ear (**D**).

Muscle strength testing (Fig. 33-22) requires the patient's cooperation. Results are usually graded as follows:

+0 = paralysis
+1 = minimal muscle contraction
+2 = muscle contracts but the patient is unable to lift the limb
+3 = able to hold the limb against gravity
+4 = able to hold against resistance but the examiner is able to overcome
+5 = not able to overcome resistance

The different muscle groups are examined in an organized fashion, proximal to distal in the upper and lower extremities, documenting the degree and pattern of strength or weakness observed (Fig. 33-22). A lesion in the cerebral hemisphere produces hemiparesis with weakness involving the face and upper and lower extremities on the contralateral side (see Chapter 25). A midthoracic (or slightly lower) lesion in the spinal cord may produce weakness in both lower extremities *(paraplegia)*, with an associated *sensory deficit* and abnormal sphincter control. Weakness involving only one limb is called *monoparesis;* it is

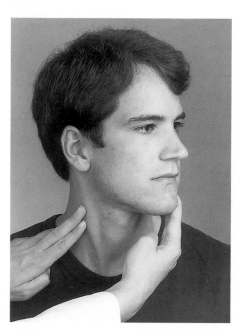

Figure 33-19. Testing the strength of the sternocleidomastoid muscle by rotating the head against resistance. A test of the integrity of the accessory nerve also includes asking the patient to shrug the shoulders (trapezius muscle).

commonly, but not invariably, localized to a plexus or a peripheral nerve. A midcervical lesion of the spinal cord may result in *quadriplegia* (bilateral paralysis of both upper and lower extremities) with a corresponding sensory loss; if the lesion is at the C1 or C2 level, the patient may also experience difficulty breathing without assistance. A lesion of one side of the spinal cord at midcervical levels may result in paralysis of the upper and lower extremities on that side; this deficit is a *hemiplegia* and is usually accompanied by characteristic sensory deficits (Brown-Séquard syndrome) (also see Fig. 25-12).

Muscle Stretch Reflexes

The muscle stretch reflexes (also called "deep tendon" reflexes—a misnomer) are obtained by percussing the tendons of major muscles (Fig. 33-23). The muscles are innervated by nerves from specific spinal cord levels. The afferent impulses are conducted to the spinal cord, or the brainstem, by the sensory fibers in the peripheral nerve and the corresponding posterior root or cranial nerve. The impulse then acts on the anterior horn cells of the cord (or motor cells of cranial nerves), and the action potential travels through the motor roots and peripheral nerve back to the muscle (see also Chapter 9). Normal reflexes indicate that the sensory-motor loop to and from the spinal cord (or brainstem) is intact.

Reflexes are modulated by down-coming inhibitory and excitatory influences from the cortical, vestibular, and reticular regions of the cerebral hemispheres and brainstem (see Chapter 24). When the inhibitory influences are damaged, the resulting reflex elicited by tapping a tendon may be very brisk or hyperactive, called *hyperreflexia*. If the nerve leading to or from the muscle is injured, reflexes may be hypoactive *(hyporeflexia)* or absent *(areflexia)*.

In the upper extremity, four reflexes are usually tested: *the biceps reflex* (Fig. 33-23A), mediated by C5-C6 through the musculocutaneous nerve; the *triceps reflex* (Fig. 33-23B), mediated by C7-C8 through the radial nerve; the *brachioradialis reflex*, mediated by C5-C6 radial nerve; and the *finger flexor reflex*, mediated by C7-C8 through the ulnar and median nerves. In the lower extremity, two reflexes are commonly tested: the *quadriceps reflex*, commonly called the *patellar* or *knee-jerk reflex*, elicited by tapping the patellar tendon (Fig. 33-23C) and mediated by L2-L4 through the femoral nerve, and the *"Achilles reflex"* or *ankle jerk reflex*, mediated by S1 through the sciatic (tibial) nerve and elicited by tapping the tendon of the gastrocnemius muscle (Fig. 33-23D).

An example of a pathologic reflex is the *Babinski sign*, seen on stroking the lateral border of the sole of the foot from the heel to the base of the great toe (Fig. 33-24). This reflex consists of dorsiflexion of the great toe, sometimes with fanning of the other toes (Fig. 33-24B). The normal response is flexion of all of the toes (Fig. 33-24A). In an adult, the Babinski sign indicates some type of abnormal process, whereas this sign may be present in a normal infant. The incomplete myelination seen in newborns or infants is the likely explanation of this latter observation.

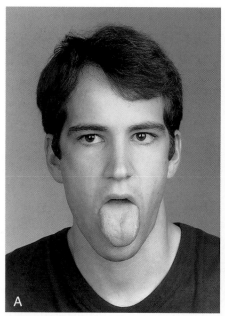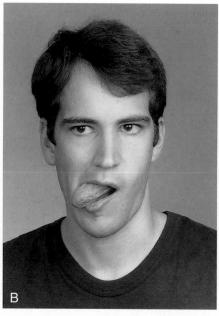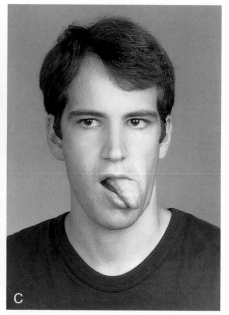

Figure 33-20. Testing the hypoglossal nerve. The patient is asked to protrude the tongue straight out (**A**), to the right (**B**), and to the left (**C**). The examiner looks for asymmetry in these movements or for an inability to perform these movements.

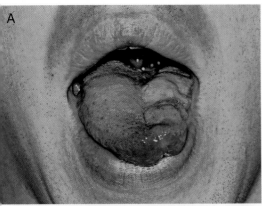

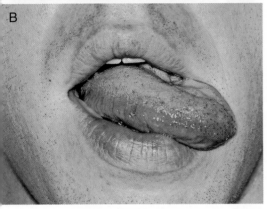

Figure 33-21. Lesion of the hypoglossal nerve results in deficits characteristic of a lower motor neuron lesion. The surface of the tongue on the lesion side appears rough and the muscles atrophic, and there may be fasciculations (**A**). On attempted protrusion (**B**) the tongue deviates toward the side of the lesion.

Cerebellar Testing

Cerebellar testing can be thought of as a mix of motor and sensory testing that assesses the accuracy of movement. In addition to normal cerebellar function, the patient must have normal strength, tone, and sensory input to carry out coordinated movements. It is important to compare coordination of one side of the body with the other. The cerebellum is usually tested by having the patient perform a *finger-to-nose-to-finger maneuver* (in which the patient touches alternately the examiner's finger and then his or her own nose rapidly) (Fig. 33-25A, B); the *heel-knee-shin maneuver* (in which the patient puts the heel on the opposite knee and runs it down the shin) is performed to test the accuracy of appendicular movement (Fig. 33-25C, D). The inability to perform this maneuver is also called *limb ataxia*. These types of dysfunctions, largely relegated to the more distal parts of the body—the extremities—are indicative of damage to more lateral portions (the hemispheres) of the cerebellum (also see Figs. 27-20 and 27-21).

Truncal ataxia (titubation, from the Greek word meaning "to stagger or lurch") is present when the patient exhibits unsteadiness while sitting, standing, or walking in tandem. This finding, in which primarily axial parts of the body are affected, is evidence of midline cerebellar dysfunction.

The Sensory Examination

Sensory testing is purely subjective; results obtained depend heavily on the patient's accuracy and cooperation. The sensory examination is most conveniently divided into *anterolateral system testing of pain and temperature sense* and *posterior column testing of vibration and position sense*.

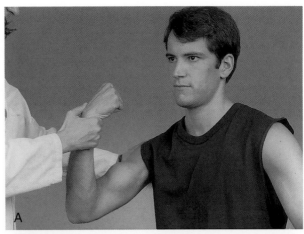

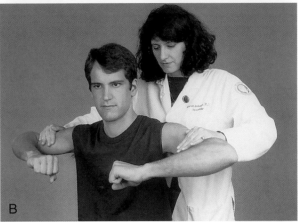

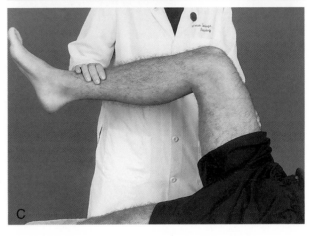

Figure 33-22. Test of muscle strength. Many muscles can be used. The examples shown here are the biceps (**A**), deltoid (**B**), and quadriceps femoris (**C**) muscles.

The standard method of evaluating pain perception is to stimulate the skin with a pin and ask the patient if the stimulus is perceived as sharp. Because the entire body surface cannot be evaluated, the examination must be guided by the nature and location of signs and symptoms, such as numbness or tingling in a specific distribution. Temperature sensation may also be tested using a cold metallic object or a small tube of warm water.

To test *position sense*, the patient is instructed to relax and, with the eyes closed, to indicate whether he or she feels the finger (or toe) moving up or down (Fig. 33-26). The *Romberg test* evaluates the sense of position of the legs and trunk when the visual information is blocked. While the patient stands with feet together and the eyes closed, the examiner looks for the presence of any sway or imbalance. These patients may be relatively steady during testing with eyes open but rapidly lose

Figure 33-23. Examination for muscle stretch reflexes (tendon reflexes) of the biceps (**A**), triceps (**B**), the quadriceps femoris (**C**, patellar tendon), and gastrocnemius (**D**, Achilles tendon) muscles.

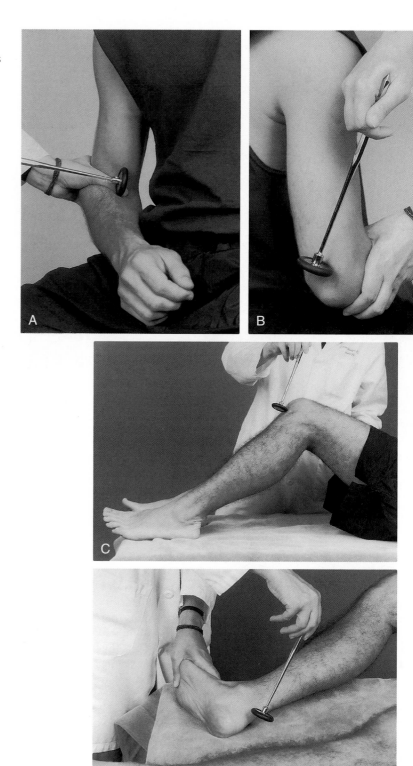

balance and sway or fall in any direction when visual compensation is eliminated by eye closure. Remember that ability to stand and maintain balance is the result of vestibular, cerebellar, and peripheral nerve information and patients with dysfunction of any of these systems may be unable to stand for Romberg testing. *Vibration sense* is tested with a 128-Hz tuning fork usually applied to the bony prominences of the terminal phalanges of the thumbs and great toes (Fig. 33-27). The patient is instructed to close the eyes and indicate whether a "buzzing" sensation is experienced. Vibration changes may be seen in peripheral nerve disease and spinal cord problems. Selective loss of proprioception and vibration sense may localize the dysfunction to the posterior columns, as seen in patients with vitamin B$_{12}$ deficiency or early *tabes dorsalis.*

Cortical sensory function is evaluated only if there is no loss of primary sensation. Testing is done using familiar objects such as a quarter, a wooden cube, or a plastic pen placed in the patient's hand while the patient's eyes are closed (Fig. 33-28). The patient is then asked to identify the object(s). *Stereognosis* is the perception of the form and nature of an object. Two-point discrimination testing is also valuable. Using two pointed objects, the stimuli are applied at the same time, and the patient is asked whether one or two points are detected. *Agnosia* is a "percept stripped of its meaning." *Stereoagnosia* is an inability to identify objects by touch *(tactile agnosia)* or by sight *(visual agnosia),* sounds or words *(auditory agnosia),* colors *(color agnosia),* or the location or position of an extremity *(position agnosia).* This type of deficit results from lesions in the cerebral hemisphere.

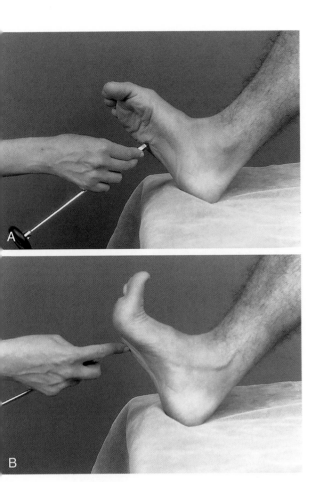

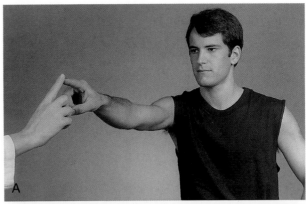

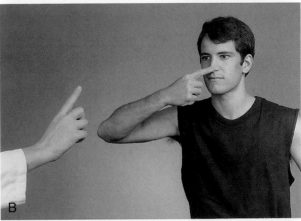

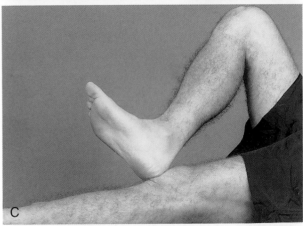

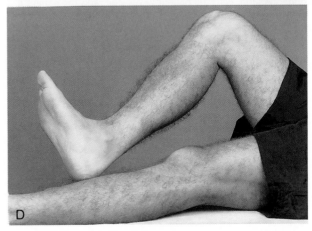

Figure 33-24. The Babinski sign. Rubbing a probe on the plantar aspect of the foot in a normal person results in a plantar flexion of the toes (**A**). Dorsiflexion of the toes (**B**)—the Babinski sign—elicited by briskly rubbing the plantar surface of the foot is indicative of a lesion involving descending fibers from the cortex and brainstem that influence spinal motor neurons.

Figure 33-25. Testing of cerebellar function. The normal patient can touch the physician's finger and then his own nose and repeat the movement rapidly and without difficulty (**A, B**). For the heel-to-shin test, the patient slides the heel of one foot down the shin of the other leg (**C, D**).

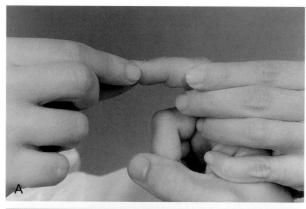

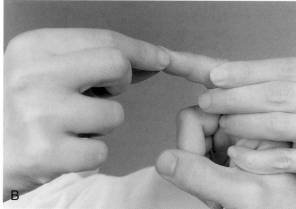

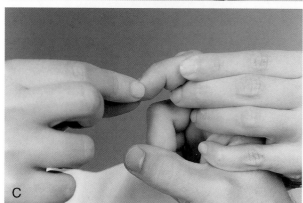

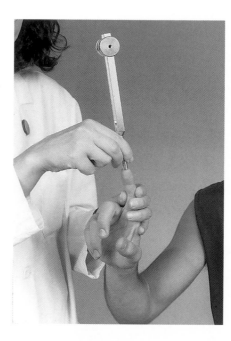

Figure 33-27. Test of vibratory sense. The tuning fork may be placed on the fingertip, tips of the toes, or bony prominences.

Figure 33-26. Test of proprioception/position sense. The physician holds the patient's finger (**A**) and, with the patient's eyes shut, asks the patient if the finger is being moved up (**B**) or down (**C**). The same test can be conducted using, for example, the toe, hand, or foot.

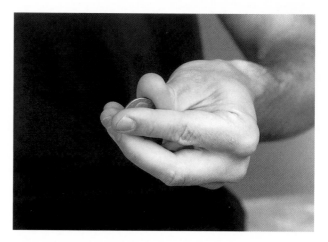

Figure 33-28. Test for shape and texture of an object (stereognosis). This portion of the neurologic examination evaluates cortical function.

Synopsis of Clinical Points

- The physical examination is a part of the larger evaluation (p. 528).
- Diagnostic studies, such as MRI, may be ordered as part of the evaluation (p. 529).
- The mental status examination provides information on the level of relative alertness and orientation to time, place, and other persons (p. 529).
- Speech disorders may be evident during the examination; these may or may not signal an organic problem (p. 529).
- Nonfluent, or expressive, aphasia is seen in a patient with a lesion in the pars opercularis and pars triangularis (p. 529).
- Fluent, or receptive, aphasia is seen in a patient with a lesion in the general area of the inferior parietal lobule (p. 529).
- Broca aphasia results from a lesion in the dominant inferior frontal gyrus (p. 529).
- Wernicke aphasia results from a lesion located mainly in the area of the dominant inferior parietal lobule (p. 529).
- Visual acuity is the ability to detect fine detail and contrast (p. 529).
- A scotoma is a defect in the visual field surrounded by normal vision (p. 529).
- Lesions at various points in the visual system result in characteristic visual deficits (p. 530).
- A hemianopia is loss of vision in one half of a visual field (p. 530).
- A quadrantanopia is the loss of a quadrant of the visual field and is more frequently seen in lesions between the lateral geniculate body and the visual cortex (p. 531).
- Papilledema may result from increased intracranial pressure (p. 532).
- Diplopia is commonly seen in patients with damage to cranial nerves III, IV, or VI (p. 532).
- A lesion of one abducens nerve may give the patient a cross-eyed appearance (p. 533).
- Destruction of the root of the oculomotor nerve results in paralysis of most eye movement; the eye is oriented down and out (p. 532).
- The ophthalmic division of the trigeminal nerve contains the afferent limb of the corneal reflex (p. 534).
- A lesion of the sensory root of the trigeminal nerve will result in an ipsilateral loss of sensation over the forehead to the vertex of the skull, the face and cheek, the jaw, and much of the oral cavity including the teeth (p. 534).
- Both afferent and efferent limbs of the jaw jerk reflex are carried on the trigeminal nerve (p. 534).
- Damage to the root of the facial nerve will result in a paralysis of the ipsilateral muscles of facial expression and a loss of taste on the anterior two thirds of the tongue (p. 535).
- The Rinne and Weber tests are used to evaluate the cochlear division of the eighth nerve (p. 535).
- Lesion of the cochlear division of the eighth nerve will result in deafness in that ear (p. 535).
- Damage to the vestibular division of the eighth nerve will result in vertigo, nausea and vomiting, and balance problems (p. 536).
- The afferent and efferent limbs of the gag reflex are transmitted via the glossopharyngeal nerve (p. 536).
- Dysarthria may result from a lesion of the vagus nerve (p. 536).
- Dysphagia is difficulty in swallowing (p. 536).
- A lesion of the spinal accessory nerve results in an inability to shrug the ipsilateral shoulder and to turn the head to the contralateral side, both against resistance (p. 536).
- Damage to the hypoglossal nerve results in deviation of the tongue to the ipsilateral side on attempted protrusion (p. 536).
- Paralysis of the genioglossus muscle results in an ipsilateral deviation of the tongue (p. 536).
- Hypertonia is an increase in muscle tone (p. 536).
- A decrease in muscle tone is hypotonia (p. 536).
- Paralysis of one extremity, monoparesis, is usually the result of a peripheral nerve lesion (p. 537).
- Paraplegia is the paralysis of both lower extremities (p. 537).
- A lesion at high cervical levels results in quadriplegia, a paralysis of all four extremities (p. 538).
- A hemisection of the spinal cord at high cervical levels results in a hemiparesis, a paralysis of the upper and lower extremities on the side of the lesion (p. 538).
- Muscle stretch reflexes may be very brisk (hyperreflexia), very slow (hyporeflexia), or absent (p. 538).
- There are a number of muscle stretch reflexes used to test the integrity of the extremities (p. 538).
- The Babinski sign is indicative of a neuropathologic process in adults but is commonly seen in normal newborns and infants (p. 538).
- Cerebellar function may be tested by the finger-to-nose and heel-knee-shin maneuvers (p. 539).
- Various types of ataxia are seen in patients with lesions of the cerebellum (p. 539).
- Testing for pain perception can be done with a pin; it is important to compare sides of the body and face (p. 539).
- Position sense may be evaluated using the Romberg test (p. 539).
- A 128-Hz tuning fork is used to test vibratory sense, a function of the posterior columns (p. 540).
- Agnosia is the inability to recognize an object by touch (tactile agnosia), sight (visual agnosia), sound (auditory agnosia), color (color agnosia), or location (position agnosia) (p. 540).

Sources and Additional Reading

Adams AC: Neurology in Primary Care. Philadelphia, FA Davis, 2000.

Aminoff MJ, Greenberg DA, Simon RP: Clinical Neurology, 3rd ed. Stamford, CT, Appleton & Lange, 1996.

Brazis PW, Masdeu JC, Biller J: Localization in Clinical Neurology, 4th ed. Philadelphia, Lippincott Williams & Wilkins, 2001.

Caplan LR: Caplan's Stroke: A Clinical Approach, 3rd ed. Boston, Butterworth Heinemann, 2000.

Donaghy M: Neurology. New York, Oxford University Press, 1997.

Duus P: Topical Diagnosis in Neurology: Anatomy, Physiology, Signs, Symptoms, 2nd rev. ed. Stuttgart, Thieme, 1989.

Haerer AF: DeJong's The Neurologic Examination, 5th ed. Philadelphia, JB Lippincott, 1992.

Hankey GJ, Wardlaw JM: Clinical Neurology. New York, Demos Medical Publishing, 2002.

Martin TJ, Corbett JJ: Neuro-Ophthalmology: The Requisites in Ophthalmology. St. Louis, Mosby, 2000.

Pryse-Phillips W: Companion to Clinical Neurology, 2nd ed. New York, Oxford University Press, 2003.

Rowland LP: Merrits Neurology, 10th ed. Philadelphia, Lippincott Williams & Wilkins, 2000.

Victor M, Ropper AH: Adams and Victor's Principles of Neurology, 7th ed. New York, McGraw-Hill, 2001.

Figure Acknowledgments

The editor acknowledges the following publishers for permission to use borrowed, and modified, illustrations.

From Haines DE: On the question of a subdural space. Anat Rec 230:3-21, 1991.
In *Fundamental Neuroscience for Basic and Clinical Applications*, 3rd ed., Figure 7-3 (adapted from original).

From Haines DE: *Neuroanatomy: An Atlas of Structures, Sections, and Systems*, 6th ed. Lippincott, Williams & Wilkins, Batimore, 2004.
In *Fundamental Neuroscience for Basic and Clinical Applications*, 3rd ed., Figure 16-12B and 16-14 (MRI only).
Figures 7-2, 8-12, 8-13, 8-20 (adapted from originals).
Figures 13-4, 13-15, 15-6, 15-15, 16-17E and F, 16-19A and B, 26-3A and B, 30-2B (modified from originals).

Atlas Figure	Fundamental Neuroscience for Basic and Clinical Applications, 3rd ed.
2-54A	6-11A
2-54D	6-11C
2-48B	7-15B
8-10A	8-15
2-37	10-4
2-29	12-6, 12-20, 27-7
2-45B	14-5
2-44D	14-9
2-41C	14-20A
2-40B	14-20B
2-23	15-5
4-2	15-8A
4-3	15-8B
4-5	15-8C
4-7	15-8D
4-12	15-9
2-9	16-5A
2-28	16-5B
2-39B	20-13
5-29	20-17A
6-7	20-17B
2-31B	27-4B
2-31C	27-4C
2-32A	27-4D
2-31E	27-4F
2-31F	27-4G
2-32C	27-4J

From Haines DE, Frederickson RG: The meninges. In Al-Mefty O (ed.): *Meningiomas*. Raven Press, New York, 1991.
In *Fundamental Neuroscience for Basic and Clinical Applications*, 3rd ed., Figures 7-3, 7-4, and 7-17 (adapted from original).

Modified from Parent A: *Carpenter's Human Neuroanatomy*, 9th ed., Lippincott, Williams & Wilkins, 1995.
In *Fundamental Neuroscience for Basic and Clinical Applications*, 3rd ed., Figure 14-1.

Adapted from Penfield W, Rasmussen T: *The Cerebral Cortex of Man: A Clinical Study of Localization of Function*. Hafner Publishing, New York, 1968 (facsimile of 1950 ed.).
In *Fundamental Neuroscience for Basic and Clinical Applications*, 3rd ed., Figures 16-8A and 17-12.

Adapted from Mistretta CM: Anatomy and neurophysiology of the taste system in aged animals. In Murphy C, Cain WS, Hegsted DM (eds): *Nutrition and the Chemical Senses in Aging: Recurrent Advances and Current Research Needs*. Ann NY Acad Sci 561:277-290, 1989.
In *Fundamental Neuroscience for Basic and Clinical Applications*, 3rd ed., Figure 23-9.

Adapted from Kinnamon SC: Taster transduction: A diversity of mechanisms. Trends Neurosci 11:491-496, 1988
In *Fundamental Neuroscience for Basic and Clinical Applications*, 3rd ed., Figure 23-12

Adapted from Nieuwenhuys R: *The Human Central Nervous System*, 3rd ed. Springer-Verlag, Berlin, 1988.
In *Fundamental Neuroscience for Basic and Clinical Applications*, 3rd ed., Figure 16-8.

Adapted from Welker W, Blair C, Shambes GM: Somatosensory projections to cerebellar granule cell layer of giant bushbaby, *Galago crassicaudatus*. Brain Behav Evol 31:150-160, 1988.
In *Fundamental Neuroscience for Basic and Clinical Applications*, 3rd ed., Figure 27-12B.

Additional borrowed illustrations in *Fundamental Neuroscience for Basic and Clinical Applications*, 3rd ed., are acknowledged in their figure captions.

Index

Page numbers followed by the letter f refer to figures; those followed by the letter t refer to tables.